BASIC HANDBOOK

OF

Child Psychiatry

VOLUME FIVE

BASIC HANDBOOK

OF

Child Psychiatry

Joseph D. Noshpitz / *Editor-in-Chief*

VOLUME FIVE

Advances and New Directions

JUSTIN D. CALL, RICHARD L. COHEN,
SAUL I. HARRISON, IRVING N. BERLIN,
LAWRENCE A. STONE

EDITORS

Basic Books, Inc., Publishers / New York

To all those

who strive to ease the pain

and better the lives of troubled children

these books are dedicated

Library of Congress Cataloging-in-Publication Data
(Revised for vol. 5)

Basic handbook of child psychiatry.

Includes bibliographies and indexes.
Contents: v. 1. Development—v. 2. Disturbances
in development.—[etc.]—v. 5. Advances and new
directions.
1. Child psychiatry. I. Noshpitz, Joseph D.
[DNLM: 1. Child psychiatry—Handbooks. WS350 B311]
RJ499.B33 618.92'89 78-7082
ISBN 0–465–00602–7

CONTENTS

SECTION ONE / Development

SECTION TWO / Varieties of Development

Contents

SECTION THREE   /   Assessment

SECTION FOUR   /   Deviations of Development: Etiology, Nosology, and Syndromes

PART A   ETIOLOGY

Contents

SECTION FIVE / Therapeutics

Contents

SECTION SIX / Prevention

Contents

CONTRIBUTORS

JULES R. BEMPORAD, M.D.
  Associate Professor of Psychiatry, Harvard Medical School; Director of Training and Education, Massachusetts Mental Health Center, Boston, Massachusetts.

ELLEN G. BENSWANGER, PH.D.
  Assistant Professor of Psychiatry, Regional Activities on Children and Youth, Office of Education and Regional Programming, University of Pittsburgh, School of Medicine, Western Psychiatric Institute and Clinic, Pittsburgh, Pennsylvania.

KAREN BERGER, M.S.W.
  Research Social Worker, Health in Adolescence Research Project, Children's Hospital National Medical Center, Washington, D.C.

IRVING N. BERLIN, M.D.
  Professor of Psychiatry and Pediatrics and Director, Division of Child and Adolescent Psychiatry, University of New Mexico School of Medicine; and Director, Children's Psychiatric Hospital, University of New Mexico, Albuquerque, New Mexico.

EFRAIN BLEIBERG, M.D.
  Associate Dean, Division of Psychiatric Training Programs, Karl Menninger School of Psychiatry and Mental Health Sciences; Director, General Psychiatry and Child Psychiatry Training, The Menninger Foundation, Topeka, Kansas.

LINDA CANFIELD BLICK, L.C.S.W.
  Executive Director, Chesapeake Institute, Inc., Kensington, Maryland.

RICHARD W. BRUNSTETTER, M.D.
  Director, Division of Adolescent and Child Psychia-try, The Institute of Pennsylvania Hospital, Philadelphia, Pennsylvania.

NANCY U. CAIRNS, PH.D.
  Clinical Supervisor, Children and Family Services, Northland Mental Health Center, Grand Rapids, Minnesota.

JUSTIN D. CALL, M.D.
  Professor and Chief of Child and Adolescent Psychiatry and Professor of Pediatrics, California College of Medicine, University of California, Irvine; and Training and Supervising Analyst, Los Angeles Psychoanalytic Society and Institute, Los Angeles, California.

MAGDA CAMPBELL, M.D.
  Professor of Psychiatry and Director, Children's Psychopharmacology Unit, New York University School of Medicine, New York, New York.

IRENE CHATOOR, M.D.
  Director of Psychiatric Consultation and Liaison, Children's Hospital National Medical Center; and Associate Professor of Psychiatry and Behavioral Sciences and of Child Health and Development, George Washington University School of Medicine, Washington, D.C.

WILLIAM B. CLOTWORTHY, JR., M.D.
  Associate Clinical Professor of Psychiatry, Georgetown University; and Faculty, Washington School of Psychiatry, Washington, D.C.

R. DEAN CODDINGTON, M.D.
  Professor Emeritus, Department of Psychiatry, Louisiana State University School of Medicine, New Orleans, Louisiana.

Contributors

DONALD J. COHEN, M.D.
Professor of Pediatrics, Psychiatry, and Psychology, Yale Child Study Center; and Chief, Department of Child Psychiatry, Yale-New Haven Hospital, New Haven, Connecticut.

RICHARD L. COHEN, M.D.
Vice Chairman and Professor of Child Psychiatry, Department of Psychiatry, University of Pittsburgh School of Medicine, Western Psychiatric Institute and Clinic, Pittsburgh, Pennsylvania.

CYNTHIA D. CONRAD, M.D., PH.D.
Assistant Professor of Psychiatry, Department of Psychiatry, Yale University School of Medicine; and Unit Chief, Adolescent Treatment, Yale Psychiatric Institute, New Haven, Connecticut.

ANTHONY J. COSTELLO, M.D., B.CH., M.R.C. PSYCH., D.P.M.
Associate Professor of Child Psychiatry, University of Pittsburgh, Pittsburgh, Pennsylvania.

JOSEPH T. COYLE, M.D.
Distinguished Service Professor of Child Psychiatry and Director, Division of Child Psychiatry, The Johns Hopkins University School of Medicine, Baltimore, Maryland.

LEON CYTRYN, M.D.
Senior Investigator, Intramural Research Program, National Institute of Mental Health, Bethesda, Maryland; Clinical Professor of Psychiatry and Clinical Professor of Psychiatry and Behavioral Sciences, and of Child Health and Development, George Washington University, School of Medicine, Washington, D.C.

SHERRY E. DAVIS, PH.D.
Assistant Professor of Research, Department of Psychiatry, Health in Adolescence Research Project, Children's Hospital, National Medical Center, Washington, D.C.

MARIAN K. DEMYER, M.D.
Professor of Psychiatry, Institute of Psychiatric Research, Indiana University School of Medicine, Indianapolis, Indiana.

MAUREEN DENNIS, PH.D.
Associate Professor, Research Institute, The Hospital for Sick Children; and Associate Professor, Department of Behavioural Science, University of Toronto, Toronto, Ontario, Canada.

ANDRE P. DERDEYN, M.D.
Professor of Psychiatry and Director, Child and Family Psychiatry, University of Virginia School of Medicine, Charlottesville, Virginia.

MARIAN CLEEVES DIAMOND, PH.D.
Professor of Anatomy, University of California, Berkeley; Former Associate Dean, College of Letters and Science, University of California, Berkeley, California.

CRAIG EDELBROCK, PH.D.
Associate Professor of Psychiatry and Director, Child and Adolescent Research, Department of Psychiatry, University of Massachusetts Medical School, Worcester, Massachusetts.

JAMES EGAN, M.D.
Chairman, Department of Psychiatry, Children's Hospital National Medical Center; and Professor of Psychiatry and the Behavioral Sciences and of Child Health and Development, George Washington University School of Medicine, Washington, D.C.

CARL FEINSTEIN, M.D.
Director, Program in Autism and Developmental Disabilities, Emma Pendleton Bradley Hospital, East Providence, Rhode Island; and Assistant Professor, Division of Psychiatry, Department of Psychiatry and Human Behavior, Brown University, Providence, Rhode Island.

RICHARD FERBER, M.D.
Director, Center for Pediatric Sleep Disorders and the Sleep Laboratory, Children's Hospital, Harvard Medical School, Boston, Massachusetts.

H. BRUCE FERGUSON, PH.D.
Professor, Department of Psychology, Carleton University; and Adjunct Professor, Department of Psychiatry, University of Ottawa School of Medicine, Ottawa, Canada.

Contributors

M. JEROME FIALKOV, M.D.

Medical Director, Children's Psychiatric Treatment Center, Mayview State Hospital, Bridgeville, Pennsylvania; and Assistant Professor of Child Psychiatry, University of Pittsburgh School of Medicine, Pittsburgh, Pennsylvania.

JOSEPH FISCHHOFF, M.D.

Hamburger Professor and Director, Child and Adolescent Psychiatry, Wayne State University School of Medicine; and Director of Psychiatric Services, Children's Hospital of Michigan, Detroit, Michigan.

MICHAEL E. FISHMAN, M.D.

Associate Director for Children and Youth, Office of Policy Analysis and Coordination, National Institute of Mental Health, Rockville, Maryland.

RICHARD GALDSTON, M.D.

Principal Investigator, The Parents' Centre Project for the Study in Prevention of Child Abuse; and Private Practice in Psychoanalysis, Boston, Massachusetts

ELEANOR GALENSON, M.D.

Clinical Professor of Psychiatry, Mount Sinai School of Medicine; and Vice President, New York Psychoanalytic Society, New York, New York.

RICHARD A. GARDNER, M.D.

Clinical Professor of Child Psychiatry, Columbia University College of Physicians and Surgeons; and Attending Psychiatrist, Presbyterian Hospital and New York Psychiatric Institute, New York, New York.

MARGARET P. GEAN, M.D.

Director, Infant-Toddler Program, New England Medical Center; and Assistant Professor of Psychiatry, Tufts University School of Medicine, Boston, Massachusetts.

JEAN GOODWIN, M.D., M.P.H.

Professor of Psychiatry, Medical College of Wisconsin, and Director of Joint Educational Programs, Milwaukee County Mental Health Complex, Milwaukee, Wisconsin.

MADELYN S. GOULD, PH.D., M.P.H.

Assistant Professor of Clinical Social Sciences in Psychiatry and Public Health (Epidemiology), Columbia University College of Physicians and Surgeons; and Research Scientist, New York State Psychiatric Institute, New York, New York.

WAYNE H. GREEN, M.D.

Associate Professor of Clinical Psychiatry, New York University Medical Center; and Director, Child and Adolescent Outpatient Services, New York University-Bellevue Medical Center, New York, New York.

STANLEY I. GREENSPAN, M.D.

Chief, Infant/Child Clinical Development Services Program, Division of Maternal and Child Health, Health Resources and Services Administration, Department of Health and Human Services, Rockville, Maryland; and Clinical Professor of Psychiatry and Behavioral Science and Child Health and Development, George Washington University Medical School, Washington, D.C.

LEE H. HALLER, M.D.

Assistant Clinical Professor of Psychiatry, George Washington University and Georgetown University, Washington, D.C.; and Member of the American Bar Association Project on Child Kidnapping.

EDWARD HALLOWELL, M.D.

Instructor in Psychiatry, Harvard Medical School at Massachusetts Mental Health Center, Boston, Massachusetts.

JEAN A. HAMILTON, M.D.

Private Practice and Scientific Director, Institute for Research on Women's Health, Washington, D.C.; formerly Clinical Research Fellow in Adolescence, Michael Reese Medical Center and University of Chicago, Chicago, Illinois, and Head, Biology of Depression Research Unit, National Institute of Mental Health, Rockville, Maryland.

GRAEME HANSON, M.D.

Director, Pediatric Mental Health Services, San Francisco General Hospital; and Assistant Clinical Professor of Pediatrics and Psychiatry, University of California, San Francisco, California.

JAMES C. HARRIS, M.D.

Associate Professor of Psychiatry and Pediatrics, The

Contributors

Johns Hopkins University School of Medicine, Baltimore, Maryland.

SAUL I. HARRISON, M.D.
Professor and Director of Child and Adolescent Psychiatry, Harbor-UCLA Medical Center, Torrance, California; and Professor Emeritus, University of Michigan, Ann Arbor, Michigan.

KENNETH I. HOWARD, PH.D.
Professor of Psychology, Northwestern University, Evanston, Illinois; and Senior Research Consultant, Department of Psychiatry, Michael Reese Hospital and Medical Center, Chicago, Illinois.

L. K. GEORGE HSU, M.D.
Director, Eating Disorders Clinic, Western Psychiatric Institute and Clinic, Pittsburgh, Pennsylvania.

ROBERT D. HUNT, M.D.
Director of Research and Training, Director of Neuropsychiatric Unit, and Associate Professor of Psychiatry and Pharmacology, Division of Child and Adolescent Psychiatry, Vanderbilt Medical School, Nashville, Tennessee.

DOROTHY STEVENSON JENKINS, A.C.S.W.
Associate Member of Graduate Faculty, School of Social Work, Wayne State University; and School Social Worker, Detroit Board of Education, Detroit, Michigan.

JEROME KAGAN, PH.D.
Professor of Psychology, Harvard University, Cambridge, Massachusetts.

ALAN E. KAZDIN, PH.D.
Professor of Child Psychiatry and Psychology, University of Pittsburgh School of Medicine; and Research Director, Child Psychiatric Treatment Service, Western Psychiatric Institute and Clinic, Pittsburgh, Pennsylvania.

CHARLES R. KEITH, M.D.
Associate Professor of Psychiatry, Division of Child and Adolescent Psychiatry, Duke University Medical Center; and Training/Supervising Analyst and Child Supervisor, UNC-Duke Psychoanalytic Training Program, Durham, North Carolina.

KEITH G. KRAMLINGER, M.D.
Senior Resident in Psychiatry, Mayo Graduate School of Medicine, Rochester, Minnesota.

SHIRLEY B. LANSKY, M.D.
Professor of Psychiatry and Pediatrics, University of Illinois; and Director, Illinois Cancer Council, Chicago, Illinois.

JAMES F. LECKMAN, M.D.
Associate Professor of Psychiatry and Pediatrics, Yale Child Study Center; and Co-Director, Children's Clinical Research Center, Yale-New Haven Hospital, New Haven, Connecticut.

NADINE A. LEVINSON, D.D.S.
Assistant Clinical Professor, Department of Psychiatry and Human Behavior, Division of Child and Adolescent Psychiatry, School of Medicine, University of California at Irvine; and Clinical Associate, San Diego Psychoanalytic Institute, San Diego, California.

DOROTHY OTNOW LEWIS, M.D., F.A.C.P.
Professor of Psychiatry, New York University School of Medicine, New York, New York; and Clinical Professor of Psychiatry, Yale Child Study Center, New Haven, Connecticut.

IRA S. LOURIE, M.D.
Director, Child and Adolescent Service System Program, National Institute of Mental Health, Rockville, Maryland; and Assistant Clinical Professor of Child Psychiatry, Georgetown University School of Medicine, Washington, D.C.

ALEXANDER R. LUCAS, M.D.
Consultant, Section of Child and Adolescent Psychiatry, Mayo Clinic and Mayo Foundation; and Professor in Psychiatry, Mayo Medical School, Rochester, Minnesota.

JOHN B. McDEVITT, M.D.
Research Director, The Margaret S. Mahler Psychiatric Research Foundation; and Instructor, New York Psychiatric Institute, New York, New York.

JOHN E. MACK, M.D.
Professor of Psychiatry, Harvard Medical School,

Contributors

The Cambridge Hospital, Cambridge, Massachusetts.

DONALD H. MCKNEW, JR., M.D.

Research Psychiatrist, Laboratory of Developmental Psychology, National Institute of Mental Health, Bethesda, Maryland; and Clinical Professor of Child Health and Development and of Psychiatry and Behavioral Sciences, George Washington University School of Medicine, Washington, D.C.

J. GARY MAY, M.D.

Assistant Clinical Professor, University of Colorado Medical Center, Denver, Colorado.

JOHN E. MEEKS, M.D.

Medical Director and Chief Executive Officer, Psychiatric Institute of Montgomery County, Rockville, Maryland; and Associate Clinical Professor, Department of Psychiatry, George Washington University Medical School, Washington, D.C.

H. DAVID MOSIER, JR., M.D.

Professor of Pediatrics and Head, Division of Pediatric Endocrinology, University of California, Irvine, California.

CAROL C. NADELSON, M.D.

Professor and Vice Chairman of Academic Affairs, Department of Psychiatry, Tufts University School of Medicine, and Director of Training and Education, Department of Psychiatry, New England Medical Center Hospitals, Boston, Massachusetts.

JOSEPH D. NOSHPITZ, M.D.

Professor of Psychiatry and Behavioral Sciences, George Washington University; and Senior Attending Staff Psychiatrist, Children's Hospital National Medical Center, Washington, D.C.

MALKAH T. NOTMAN, M.D.

Clinical Professor of Psychiatry, Tufts Medical School and New England Medical Center; and Director, Women's Resource Center, New England Medical Center, Boston, Massachusetts.

DANIEL OFFER, M.D.

Chairman, Department of Psychiatry, Michael Reese Hospital and Medical Center; and Professor of Psychiatry, University of Chicago, Chicago, Illinois.

ERIC OSTROV, J.D., PH.D.

Director of Forensic Psychology, Department of Psychiatry, Michael Reese Hospital and Medical Center, Chicago, Illinois.

THEODORE A. PETTI, M.D., M.P.H.

Associate Professor of Child Psychiatry and Director, Regional Activities on Children and Youth, Office of Education and Regional Programming, Western Psychiatric Institute and Clinic, Pittsburgh, Pennsylvania.

JOAQUIM PUIG-ANTICH, M.D.

Chief of Child and Adolescent Psychiatry, Western Psychiatric Institute and Clinic, University of Pittsburgh School of Medicine, Pittsburgh, Pennsylvania.

MARK A. RIDDLE, M.D.

Assistant Professor of Pediatrics and Psychiatry, Yale Child Study Center; and Associate Medical Director of Children's Psychiatric Inpatient Service, Yale-New Haven Hospital, New Haven, Connecticut.

MARIA SAUZIER, M.D.

Staff, Child Psychiatry Department, Cambridge Hospital, Cambridge, Massachusetts; and Clinical Instructor in Psychiatry, Harvard Medical School, Boston, Massachusetts.

ELIZABETH S. SCOTT, J.D.

Director, Center for the Study of Children and the Law, University of Virginia School of Law, Charlottesville, Virginia.

DAVID SHAFFER, M.R.C.P., F.R.C. PSYCH.

Director, Division of Child Psychiatry, New York State Psychiatric Institute; and Professor of Clinical Psychiatry and Pediatrics, Columbia University College of Physicians and Surgeons, New York, New York.

MILTON F. SHORE, PH.D.

Formerly Psychologist, National Institute of Mental Health, Rockville, Maryland; Adjunct Professor of Psychology, Catholic University of America, Washington, D.C.; and Adjunct Professor of Psychology, The American University, Washington, D.C.

LARRY B. SILVER, M.D.

Director, National Institute of Dyslexia;

Contributors

and Clinical Professor of Psychiatry, Georgetown University School of Medicine, Washington, D.C.

JOVAN G. SIMEON, M.D.
Professor of Psychiatry, Department of Psychiatry, University of Ottawa School of Medicine; and Director, Child Psychiatry Research, Royal Ottawa Hospital, Ottawa, Ontario, Canada.

HENRY F. SMITH, M.D.
Clinical Instructor in Psychiatry, Harvard Medical School at the Massachusetts Mental Health Center, Boston, Massachusetts.

FREDERICK J. STODDARD, M.D.
Chief of Psychiatry, Shriners Burns Institute; and Assistant Clinical Professor of Psychiatry, Harvard Medical School, Boston, Massachusetts.

LAWRENCE A. STONE, M.D.
Associate Clinical Professor of Child Psychiatry, University of Texas Health Science Center, San Antonio, Texas.

PETER E. TANGUAY, M.D.
Professor and Associate Director of Child Psychiatry, and Director, Child Psychiatry Clinical Research Center, UCLA Department of Psychiatry, Los Angeles, California.

LENORE CAGEN TERR, M.D.
Clinical Professor of Psychiatry, University of California, San Francisco School of Medicine, San Francisco, California.

DANIEL WEINBERGER, M.D.
Chief, Section on Clinical Neuropsychiatry, Neuropsychiatry Branch, Division of Intramural Research, National Institute of Mental Health, Washington, D.C.

KARL R. WHITE, PH.D.
Associate Professor of Special Education and Psychology, Early Intervention Research Institute, Utah State University, Logan, Utah.

CHARLES D. YINGLING, PH.D.
Associate Professor of Medical Psychology, Department of Psychiatry and Neurological Surgery, University of California, San Francisco, California.

PREFACE

This fifth volume of the *Basic Handbook of Child Psychiatry* is compiled some eleven years after the work was originally conceived and seven years after the first four volumes were published. Thus, for over a decade, the editors have been observing our profession evolve and have been seeking to find ways to encode it and to communicate its contents in a definitive manner. This fifth volume is integral to the series and makes no attempt to stand alone. Instead it seeks to fulfill the promise of the original work and to maintain the *Handbook* as a current and functional part of the equipment of the mental health professional in general and of the child psychiatrist in particular.

Among other things, Volume V is designed as an update, a collection of materials that attends especially to information which has emerged during the past seven years and which thus keeps the reader abreast of current developments. To be sure, for the researcher there is no substitute for the original sources, whether in journals or in the many personal exchanges with colleagues working in parallel areas, to challenge new conceptions and enrich methods. But for the practitioner, or for the researcher who wishes to get some background in a less familiar realm, the availability of dependable compendia gives ready access to a rich trove of information about particular areas, and thus plays a vital role in professional adaptation. This, then, is one of the primary missions of the fifth volume, to facilitate the readiness with which the working professional can seek out data about current cases and to encourage him or her to sharpen knowledge about the recent advances in our field. The work is intended to educate, to enrich, and to widen the perspective of practitioners, to make them aware of the newest clinical data, and to alert them to the frontiers where novel developments are most likely to arise.

The volume has an additional mission that merits address. A part of the task that dogs the editor always is to seek in some measure to undo or to redo the past. Inevitably, it is inherent in the nature of a handbook that it tries to be encyclopedic in scope. As a result, it immediately becomes vulnerable to two classic critiques: On the one hand, it will always face the charge that it is not complete, that it omitted something important—and indeed, so vast is the field that child psychiatry now subtends that there is no escaping this criticism; one can hope only to minimize it. And on the other hand, in regard to the material that *is* included, there will always be the critic who feels that the treatment accorded a particular topic was insufficient, excessive, or in any case could have been better done. The way the encyclopedist addresses these difficulties is to work in a group with a number of thoughtful and well-informed colleagues joining forces to consider both what should and should not go into the work, and to allow this group mind (as it were) to review and evaluate the quality of what is planned for inclusion. In the present instance, the same group of editors who produced the first four volumes of the *Handbook* participated in its update; indeed, the very form of the new publication reflects in microcosm the outline and structure of the original work.

In the years that have elapsed since the publication of the first four volumes, we have had time in which to discover something of what was left out and in which to review the substance of what was included and to ponder what changes could be made. Along with its update function, then, this volume permits for certain additions and for some measure of revision, limited in extent to be sure, yet helpful all the same in the endless struggle to convey more perfectly the sense of the field.

The passage of years allows for a number of additional changes as well—in knowledge, in perspective, and in the milieu within which the field itself lives and grows. There are new technologies to be described, new details to be added to the maps of experience already depicted, and new economic forces with which the child psychiatrist must reckon to be accounted for. All these impinge on practitioners and shape and influence what they do and what they think. And all must be presented and illustrated if the *Handbook* is to do its work.

Since the goal of the present effort is to enrich and expand the existing four volumes, it seemed best to the editors to hew to the general outline of the original work and use the same section titles that were used in the earlier volumes. Hence Volume V opens with several chapters on development, proceeds to a section on varieties of development, continues with an extension of the studies on assessment, moves then to etiology, nosology, and syndromes, which in turn logically builds toward therapeutics, and finally addresses prevention and current trends. The authors were requested to provide an update of the field in respect to their particular realm of expertise; except for the chapters dealing with material that was altogether new, the authors were urged to emphasize references from the writings of the last five years. In general, the work displays the influence of this editorial approach.

In this sense, the current effort sits as a sort of capstone on the original volumes; it can certainly be read as an independent work, and as such it has much to say about current trends and recent developments in child mental health. But it comes into its own most fully if each section is viewed as an extension of the studies already assembled within the structure of the *Handbook*.

Before addressing the contents of this volume, it seems appropriate to observe some of the general directions of the field. A great drift is clearly in evidence in child psychiatry, and it flows with almost a visible direction as the studies continue to pour out and the professionals' grasp on the field widens and deepens. To best perceive the nature of this current, it may be wise to study it first from the vantage point of the past. For many years the classical position for the American child psychiatrist had been to favor clear and precise clinical description and a crisp and incisive statement of the dynamics of a case. In a sense, it was a tighter and more focused version of child psychoanalytic work. Indeed, from the point of view of publication, in the immediate post–World War II era, the individual case report was one of the mainstays of the field. In effect, one watched the expert perform; the case report gave the reader a picture of good clinicians at work, and it allowed a glimpse as well of their thinking about their work. It seems safe to say that most of the earlier generation of child psychiatrists were schooled in this way.

In recent years, however, this approach has undergone a radical transformation. The great weakness of the individual case study is that it suggests generalizations which cannot be substantiated by means of one case; the only way to know whether the conclusions reached are valid is for the study to be controlled and extended to many cases, or at least to look for the longitudinal outcome of what took place in the given instance. As a result, the gradual accumulation of experience and the refinement of methods gave rise to a new generation of researchers and practitioners and a new sense of the kind of knowledge to seek.

Much of this change was heralded by the English school led by Michael Rutter, which made a fine art of demographic studies and began to base clinical reports on the survey findings arising from subtle and complex comparisons made among the data from multiple cases. In the United States, comparable work by the Offers was revising the standard picture of adolescent development. But ideas were pouring in from everywhere. Another great revolution arose out of the change in our understanding of brain physiology that followed in the wake of the discovery of the neurotransmitters. This led to generative new conceptualizations of mental illness, and these formulations extended to work with children no less than to our grasp on the psychophysiology of adults. As a result, the psychopharmacology of childhood is one of the great new frontiers.

In another realm, behavioral methods, operant conditioning, and social learning theory were providing new approaches with which to redefine many forms of disturbance and new treatment tactics with which to engage them. Zealous workers applied these measures to a wide array of childhood disorders and began to sift out the methods that helped from those that merely glittered.

In yet another domain, those concerned with diagnosis and the establishment of the categories and subcategories of mental illness had long been at work in a patient effort to refine the concepts and the means for designating the many varieties of psychopathology. This undertaking had been going on for years and was spurred on by the demands of researchers that some standardization be introduced into diagnosis so that findings in different centers should be comparable. Ultimately, in the late 1970s, all this bore fruit: In a novel approach to assessment, the idea arose that a case must meet specific descriptive criteria in order to be given a particular label. DSM-III appeared and the art of diagnosis took a new, albeit hotly debated, turn.

For child psychiatrists in particular, a major catalyst in effecting a change in their views was the ever-increasing interest in that complex form of disturbance (with its associated hyperactivity and learning difficulties) now designated as attention deficit disorder. This had a peculiarly alerting impact on the field. Here was a condition that was primarily an illness of childhood, that in fact affected a great many children, that had a significant biological component, that did not lend itself to dynamic etiologic explication (or to exclusive dynamically based intervention), that involved primarily cognitive instead of the familiar defensive/emotional components of the ego, and that often—although not altogether predictably—seemed to respond to specific medication. It opened up whole new vistas of study, understanding, and conceptualization and did much to foster an expanded way of looking at children.

This then is some of the context within which child psychiatric practice is evolving. The former emphasis on the clinical, the dynamic, the intuitive, and the experiential is still very much there. When decisions must be made, clinicians often call on their dynamic thinking in order to determine how best to respond to a clinical situation and how then to proceed with the care of the patient. But a new quality has been added. There is an additional increment of rigor in the way that the child psychiatrist thinks, a sense that one can know more about a case than dynamic thinking can offer. Now it is taken for granted that there is a biological dimension to explore, a behavioral aspect to consider, a cultural component to weigh. More than that, there is a hunger among the many practitioners for ever greater precision, a yearning for things that can be concretely specified, measured, and compared. Child psychiatrists have an ever-widening array of therapies to offer; they want to know which is the correct approach for which condition. They are using powerful psychoactive agents; they want to know which cases merit which treatments, and what dosage is the optimal one. They are concerned about therapeutic efficiency, and they want to know whether they are getting placebo effects from their interventions or whether what they are doing is making a real difference. There is a new diagnostic framework to which to adapt; they want to be certain that they know how to arrive at the correct formulation. Hence many practitioners are interested in the latest wrinkle in semistructured interviews or abbreviated forms of some extensive and recondite research questionnaire, something the office assistant can administer, something that comes up with a value, that gives a quantitative answer. The former emphasis on clear clinical description with its strong humane and subjective flavor is now rubbing shoulders with this hunger for the precise. Inevitably, in some instances, this has led to a polarization of views, with particular groups of colleagues moving radically and totally toward the one extreme or clinging steadfastly to the other. But overall, child psychiatry is a field with roots deep in both the dynamic process of the interpersonal and the scientific and methodological substrate of medicine. Hence despite the fascination with the new emergents and advances, the sense of the immediacy and relevance of the descriptive experiential is still looked for and needed; nor will it be quickly abandoned, no matter how precise the tools the field develops. For just as the great weakness of the dynamic is the tendency to overgeneralize from too few cases, the parallel problem of the precise and the scientific is the risk of losing sight of the subjective and the humane. And child psychiatry is above all things a field of compassionate endeavor, sensitively attuned to the nuances of the deepest human emotions; ultimately, every act of the serious professional bears the stamp of this commitment. Perhaps it is the fate of practitioners to be eternally torn between the subjective and the objective as we go through our daily routine.

It seems fair to say that today, the optimal approach is one that gives full and heartfelt attention to the inner world of the troubled child and family, empathizes with their sense of panic or dismay, and shares in some measure the turmoil and pain of their subjective experience. Then, having done all that, the work proceeds toward a considered recounting in column form of how many of what kinds and what severity of symptoms are here displayed, plus the scores recorded by the child and family on a variety of instruments. And these data too become factored into the equation and lend to the understanding, the formulation, and the character of the chosen intervention.

In this connection, a second trend that bears remark is the continued emphasis on development as the basic science of child psychiatry. This powerful conception has been the backbone of the field for years, and it is evident that the developmental history will continue to be a mainstay of our understanding. Ultimately, all the objective data and the behavioral items will be considered within the framework of the child's personality unfolding, and the modes of intervention selected will be subserving the long-range goal of developmental repair.

Let us now consider the sections of the book and review some of the contents. In the Development section (edited by Justin D. Call), the opening chapters deal with the relationship of brain development to environment. Marion C. Diamond makes the point by showing how relatively simple additions to the richness of environmental experience for newborn rats can thicken the cortex of their developing brains (as compared to the brains of controls). In a different kind of report, Joseph T. Coyle and James C. Harris demonstrate that neurotransmitter systems, too, have a timetable and a sequencing of development that make for a newly understandable coherence in the way many functions appear. More new ground is broken as H. David Mosier, Jr., demonstrates the vital role of endocrine metabolism in fetal development. Then, on a more macroscopic level, Jerome Kagan asserts that the emergence of new function is not merely an example of continuity, an elaboration of existing potentials; it is a product of discontinuity, a new encounter with the environment and a new adaptive position.

As the child grows through the first year of life, the issues of separation-individuation come to the fore and the account of the rapproachement crisis given by John

B. McDevitt, one of early workers in that field, becomes a central presence in the explication of much later psychopathology. Parallel with this process is the elaboration of the beginnings of speech and language, a sequence described by Nadine A. Levinson and Call.

Presently the issues of gender identity assume special salience, and the recent important work in this realm is summed up and annotated by Eleanor Galenson; the earliest descriptions of the sense of gender and their implications for future development are at last receiving the thorough documentation they have so long needed.

As we proceed up the ladder of development, we find that various psychopharmacological agents become ever more commonly employed. But are the reactions of children and adolescents the same as those of adults? Will the immature psychoendocrine and neurological structures respond in quite the same fashion as do the later forms of these systems in adulthood? Jean A. Hamilton and Cynthia Conrad explore this for us in an unusual chapter.

And finally, the ever-sharpening focus on the adolescent gives rise to a remarkable study by Daniel Offer, Eric Ostrov, and Kenneth I. Howard that yields a highly precise epidemiologic measure of the presence of psychopathology among a large population of high-school students.

In the next section, which deals with varieties of development (edited by Joseph D. Noshpitz), the work is devoted to presenting cross sections of childhood where youngsters have grown up under special cultural or physical conditions. To begin with, siblings, who have so long been neglected both in theory and in practice, begin now to come in for a share of the attention they have so richly merited. Carl Feinstein and Sherry Davis take a look at the siblings of chronically ill or disabled children and what it means to grow up in a home with a needy, suffering, and dependent family member. From here the material moves ahead in the form of a thoughtful look by Joseph Fischhoff and Dorothy Jenkins at the meaning of sickle cell anemia in the life of a child. The family theme recurs with a study by Jean Goodwin on the developmental impact of incest on children. Charles R. Keith sums up another major area in his concise and comprehensive account of the enormous increase of our knowledge about youth and violence. Finally there is an exploration by Feinstein and Karen Berger into the ever-increasing research realm of the child with developmental disabilities.

Of all the fields of endeavor treated in this volume, perhaps none reflects as much novelty and change as does the work on assessment (edited by Richard L. Cohen). This dimension of child psychiatry has taken off in a manner that is at once enormously intriguing and thoroughly baffling. There has been a sharpening of the instruments of observation with both the emergence of new techniques and the refinement of older methods. Brand-new modalities of observation are appearing now, with preliminary papers coming out almost monthly, and the field stands by a bit breathlessly waiting for what will happen next. Hence the section on assessment is perforce filled with new research, novel methods, and much reference to opening horizons.

The section is led off by a thoughtful review and critique by David Shaffer and Madelyn S. Gould of that newest and sharpest of instruments to be currently applied to children and youth, the third edition of the *Diagnostic and Statistical Manual of Mental Disorders* by the American Psychiatric Association. This work has shaken the field out of any former state of self-satisfied comfort; it has invigorated some and provoked others, but it has aroused everyone. The authors review both its strengths and its problems.

Among the characteristic devices that are finding their way ever more frequently from the workbenches of the researchers into the offices of the practitioners are the various rating scales and (more or less) structured interviews. Some have become almost standard diagnostic equipment, and others are still being developed. This turbulent and exciting area is reviewed in two chapters, one by Anthony J. Costello and one by Craig Edelbrock. The techniques elaborated are in the process of changing a great many diagnostic procedures. Rich resources being mined in other realms as well. One of the most rewarding is the more regular recourse to neuropsychological testing, an idea whose time has come. Maureen Dennis updates this approach.

Perhaps an even more novel and exciting new area, so new that some of its subrealms have barely reached the stage of clinical utility, is the host of brain imaging techniques that are emerging. New worlds of acronyms are coming into play, with the several combinations being thrown about like the first names of movie stars among fan club members. PET scans, NMR, and several other new devices are becoming available in some areas, and indeed the promise of their help in the future is one of the truly exciting aspects of current professional development. Feinstein and Daniel Weinberger offer at least a basic explanation of the way these several new methods function and something about their strengths and limitations.

A somewhat less well established but still novel and promising area is the use of biological tests for the diagnosis of affective disorders. Joaquim Puig-Antich considers these instruments. Sleep research, no longer so exotic as once it seemed, continues to deepen our understanding of brain function and is becoming more and more readily translated into clinical practice. Richard Ferber discusses some of the current findings and their clinical applications. Charles D. Yingling reviews the status of the much-debated automated EEG techniques as screening devices in the evluation of children. And the section closes with a most intriguing addition to the way that the individual practitioner could work, the possibility and the method for conducting meaningful research by the artful management of a single case. Alan E. Kazdin has been teaching such methodology for many years and shares his knowledge with us here.

Section 4 (edited by Joseph D. Noshpitz and Saul I. Harrison) is entitled "Deviations of Development: Etiology, Nosology, and Syndromes." The etiology material is composed of two chapters, both dealing with seminal aspects of the field and both covering topics not dealt with in detail in the first four volumes of the *Handbook*. The first, by R. Dean Coddington, looks at the current status of stress research and its relationship to clinical child psychiatry. The other, by Peter E. Tanguay, addresses the often overlooked relationship between cognition and psychopathology. The work with stress is becoming one of the great organizing concepts in psychiatric thinking, and our attention to cognition has moved out of the merely intellectual and into the therapeutic. Indeed, both areas will command ever more attention in the future.

Nosology is discussed in a chapter wherein J. Gary May continues his initial work on diagnostic categories, this time by a study of the DSM-III system. This in turn leads into the Syndromes section in which some fifteen conditions of primary interest to child psychiatrists are updated. Call addresses that newest of the emerging offshoots of traditional child psychiatry, the syndromes and diagnostic categories of infancy. A realm of study that is likely to become a major focus of theory in American psychiatry within the next decade is explored with unusual richness by Lenore Cagen Terr in her presentation on children caught up in catastrophes, where the unexpected, profound, and far-reaching reverberations of severe traumatic experiences are given a definitive description. Another of the pressing problems of our time is the proliferation of that group of disturbances known as the eating disorders, and Irene Chatoor and James Egan look at the earlier forms of these conditions in their chapter on failure to thrive and growth disorders.

Among the many new emphases in the past few years, the area of child sexual abuse has become a central cultural as well as psychiatric concern. Ira S. Lourie and Linda C. Blick review this field. Parallel with this is the newly emerging awareness of the prevalence of childhood depression. Leon Cytryn and Donald H. McKnew address some of the puzzling and still unresolved issues presented by the childhood forms of the depressive syndromes. In a similar vein, Efrain

Bleiberg has submitted the first chapter in the *Handbook* to deal with the critical area of the narcissistic disorders of childhood. In the associated realm of the borderline child, the diagnosis is often made but very few careful objective surveys of children bearing this diagnosis have ever been made; Jules R. Bemporad, Henry F. Smith, and Graeme Hanson have conducted what is almost a unique project of this kind and tell about it in their chapter.

With the advent of DSM-III, the classical term neurosis was called into question and the concept of anxiety-related disorders was substituted; Alexander R. Lucas and Keith G. Kramlinger write on this topic, giving due heed to the many fascinating biological data that have recently emerged in this connection. In a similar vein, Donald J. Cohen, Mark A. Riddle, and James F. Leckman reconsider from a psychobiological perspective the intriguing and ever more beckoning area for exploration, Tourette syndrome and the movement disorders of childhood. Jovan G. Simeon brings the reader up to date with the current findings concerning sleep disorders. Robert D. Hunt, Richard W. Brunstetter, and Larry B. Silver throw a noose about what is easily the most richly explored condition in the field and write on ADD. Silver and Brunstetter round out this topic with a chapter on the associated turbulent realm of learning disabilities.

A number of topics in the field have long been under study yet remain baffling and elusive. Next to ADD and perhaps childhood depression, perhaps no realm of clinical research is currently more active than that concerned with the psychoses of childhood. Marian K. DeMyer brings us up to date with the new knowledge about these conditions. With this we move into adolescence, and we encounter the issues of abuse in their more mature forms. First there is that great realm of abuse, the self-abuse that accompanies so many of the food-related syndromes and that is becoming so widespread and so prominent a concern in the everyday practice of child psychiatry: L. K. George Hsu reviews this in a study of the eating disorders. And finally, John E. Meeks looks back on several decades of various attempts to deal with the abuse of an ever-increasing number of psychoactive substances and describes what we have learned and how very much remains to be done.

Overall it is safe to say that all the authors of these chapters were at some pains to concentrate on material that has emerged within the last five years in order to make their presentation as topical as possible.

Section 5, which deals with therapeutics (and is edited by Saul I. Harrison), parallels the Syndrome material in many ways but diverges in a few significant instances. There are nineteen chapters in this section, launched by two overview chapters, each of which updates an important sector of the field. In particular, Wayne H. Green and Magda Campbell continue and extend Campbell's previous study of the psychopharmacology of childhood, and Kazdin gives the reader an account of advances in child behavior therapy. Both chapters are immediate and cogent accounts of major movements within the domain of child psychiatric therapeutics.

They are then followed by sixteen chapters in which the authors of fourteen of the Syndrome chapters write about the therapeutics of each of the several conditions they had described earlier. In addition, woven in among these there is an updating of two conditions not specifically included within the Syndrome section, with Richard Galdston addressing the management of child abuse and Bemporad and Edward Hallowell reviewing the most recent developments in the treatment of disorders of elimination.

Finally, Milton F. Shore closes the section with an account of the role of alternative mental health services (such as the self-help groups), a tactic of support that is gaining momentum on the national scene. This is becoming an important interventional mode, one with which child psychiatrists should be more familiar and within which they should be ever more active.

Section 6 (edited by Irving N. Berlin) is devoted to current trends in prevention. The material is led off by a chapter on a particularly significant topic, the epidemiology of child mental health disorders. This is a rich wellspring of knowledge that has been a driving force in bringing about much of the change in child psychiatric thinking in the post–World War II years and is now coming into its own as a basis for preventive and interventional strategies. Brunstetter reviews the recent studies and their implications for prevention. There follow a series of chapters on the impact of some of the newer interventional efforts on a number of different populations. In two intriguing chapters, Karl R. White and Stanley I. Greenspan describe the status of work with infants, how early intervention affects their development, and how such interventional programs can be studied. This is followed by two chapters that explore the sometimes excruciating problems of preventive work with the sick child. Irving N. Berlin deals with the parents of children with chronic disease, and, in a separate study, Shirley B. Lansky and Nancy U. Cairns consider the needs of those children afflicted with cancer, who are surviving these days in ever greater numbers. Next come two chapters that focus on the problems of teenagers. Dorothy Otnow Lewis considers approaches to a more rational and comprehensive address to juvenile delinquents, and Malkah Notman, Carol Nadelson, Maria Sauzier, and Margaret Gean look at programs targeted toward the ever-increasing crisis

posed by the growing number of pregnant adolescents. Finally Berlin closes the section with the socially induced psychiatric problems of American Indian children. All in all, preventive measures are beginning to shake free of their long dormancy and are proposing strategies that seem to offer both method and hope.

The volume closes with a section entitled "Impact of Current Events" (edited by Lawrence A. Stone) on the development and mental health of children. This topic involves us with the world of technology and its impact on the way children grow and adapt. Fredrick J. Stoddard and John E. Mack collaborate to talk of that most distressing of all technological advances, children and the threat of nuclear war. On a more optimistic note, a topic that will fill the journals of the future is adumbrated by Richard A. Gardner's provocative chapter on video games, computer-assisted instruction and their implications for mental health. A second area of major interest in terms of current events is the new developments in law as these address the problems of children. Gardner tells of the stresses of new child custody arrangements on the lives of children; Lee H. Haller discusses the kidnapping of children by disaffected parents who steal them from one another; and Elizabeth S. Scott and Andre P. Derdeyn continue the theme with a chapter on the work of the child psychiatrist as court consultant. Theodore A. Petti, Ellen G. Benswanger, and M. Jerome Fialkov offer a description of that relative rarity in the United States, the rural child, and his or her needs for child psychiatric services. From the overall legislative point of view, Michael E. Fishman and Silver consider the multifarious ways in which the federal government offers programs for children, and, by way of contrast, William B. Clotworthy considers the classic antithesis to federal programs, the private practice of child psychiatry.

Putting this volume together has been a considerable effort and a work accomplished under intense time pressure. One of the goals of the undertaking has been to create a book that is topical and includes some of the more recent efforts in study and research. This meant demanding deadlines and rapid editing efforts. Another goal was to maintain the basic position of the *Handbook* as an authoritative and thorough source book in child psychiatry. This in turn meant meticulous care, both by authors and editors, in their address to the data that were included. All in all, the editors sought to attain a combination of the novel and the comprehensive; time and their readers will tell them how close they have come to their goal, and how far they still must go.

Joseph D. Noshpitz
Washington, D.C.

SECTION I

Development

Justin D. Call / Editor

Introduction

Justin D. Call

The interplay between normality and psychopathology continues to pose intriguing new questions to all the basic sciences and clinical sciences of human development, including child psychiatry. The old adage from physiology and pathology that pathology is an exaggeration of normal processes still seems true, but not true enough to define adequately either normality or pathology. Normality in child development is infinitely more difficult to define than is psychopathology because of the adaptive nature of much early unusual, or "deviant," development. Some distortions in development may reflect individual differences and lead to specialized adaptive capacities. Sociobiologists have suggested that the *less* robust members of a species are more likely to initiate and/or make use of unusual adaptations. Such adaptations allow survival of the species under unusual environmental circumstances. The optimally functioning, robust organism has, on the other hand, already committed many functional capacities to usual environmental situations. All of this suggests that what is normal for the individual may not be what is optimal for species survival over time.

Nevertheless, we proceed bravely on with the assumption that we can say what is normal in developing children. (For a more systematic review of this issue, see Chapter 1 in Volume I of this *Handbook* series.) Chapters on normal development were chosen for this volume on the basis of which new findings in current research were most important and relevant to the task of the clinician in dealing with a definition of psychopathology, in preventing psychopathology, and in treating psychopathology.

In chapter 1, Marian C. Diamond discusses environmental influences on the developing brain. How does nutritional sensory stimulation and patterning of sensory stimulation influence brain mass, the number of developing neurons and the development of dendritic processes in nerve cells which go on to form neuronal networks? *Answer:* By increasing each of these. Is there any evidence that a variety of playful experiences with peers and with adult members of the species has any effect upon brain development? *Answer:* Yes. Is there any evidence to suggest that infants with brain injury or those who have suffered sensory or nutritional deprivation during early brain development have any capacity whatsoever to recover? *Answer:* Yes. More detailed answers to these questions and others can be found in the beautiful experiments described in this chapter, although Diamond's findings will not be convincing to anyone who continues to believe that the human mammal comes from entirely different stuff and does not share a common biological heritage with the lowly rat.

Where can the clinician find a concise description of current knowledge of the various neurotransmitter systems, their anatomic location, and how they effect brain function? Whence do the cell bodies of a fully functioning brain come? Do developing neurons produce the same brain neurotransmitters they are destined to produce when mature? Do the connections between neurons effect neurotransmitter production during development of the neuron? Is it possible in considering the embryological physiology of neurotransmitter production to correlate findings with landmarks of normal development and with the occurrence of specific psychiatric syndromes of infancy and childhood? Can the anatomic location of the neurotransmitter lesion which could account for characteristic symptoms, neurotransmitter deficiencies and response of the child to psychopharmacologic agents be postulated? The reader does not have to be a neurophysiologist or a researcher to find the answers to these important questions in the chapter provided by Dr. Joseph Coyle.

What hormone systems influence prenatal and postnatal growth of the brain and the body? Does birth in the human infant suddenly increase the production of thyroid releasing hormone (TRH) and the subsequent production of thyroid stimulating hormone (TSH), thyroxine-3, and thyroxine-4? Is fetal production of meletonin effected by light transmitted through the cranium during gestation? Does the fetal pituitary respond to stress in connection to the birth process? What underlying hormonal difficulties account for ambiguous sex development? What kinds of hormones are produced by the placenta? Is hormone production by the placenta effected by the physiology of the fetus? Answering these questions, the chapter, "Endocrine Factors and Fetal Development," by David Mosier is a most impressive synthesis of what is presently known about how hormones influence growth. Many other fundamental issues in understanding the nature of fetal growth and the evolution of central nervous system functioning are also addressed.

SECTION I / Development

The idea that development is continuous, that earlier events profoundly determine the nature of subsequent events seems deeply embedded in our thinking about normal development and psychopathological development. Yet there is much evidence to suggest that this is not quite true. The problems posed and the underlying assumptions of these two viewpoints are elegantly presented by Jerome Kagan in his chapter. What is a mental schema? What is a category of information? How are categories of information influenced by language function? How do schemas, categories, actions, states of consciousness, and finally persons influence ongoing development? Have longitudinal studies supported the continuity of individual differences over time? "No," says Kagan, and he offers considerable evidence to suggest that as far as intellectual and cognitive functioning is concerned, the individual is in the process of constant change, redefining his or her approach to life. In fact, continuity of earlier trends is difficult to substantiate. Kagan summarizes the Kauai study by Werner and Smith of 600 children studied from birth to eighteen years of age. The study showed that among the sixty-nine infants born with mild to moderate perinatal stress, the appearance of various syndromes such as mental retardation, psychosis, neurosis, or delinquency was no greater than among infants born without risk, and further, that a supportive home environment can ameliorate the vulnerabilities imposed by earlier problems vulnerability.

In their chapter, Levinson and Call point out the philosophical and practical difficulties in actually coming to a definition of language, propose a method of operationally defining language for the purpose of study, and summarize what is presently known in their own and others' work about how the infant and very young child actually acquire the capacity for that form of communication conventionally known as language. Studies of language acquisition and disturbances of language function cut across many fields and have often been central to an understanding of other important phenomena in normal and psychopathological development. For example, such studies interdigitate with almost all forms of psychopathology in infancy which affect and are affected by speech and language development, brain development, psychodynamic mechanisms underlying psychopathology in infancy and later life, individual differences in style of language acquisition in infants as a reflection of inherent constitutional differences in children, and the differences between cultures as reflected by the difficulties children experience in learning the language of each culture. Some sample questions and answers will illustrate more specifically the richness of this chapter.

In what ways can language be operationally defined? *Answer:* By phonological, syntactic, semantic, and pragmatic functions of language. What is the difference between language disorder and speech disorder? *Answer:* A language disorder is a reflection of distortions in the basic functions of language (i.e., syntax pragmatics, phonological, semantic, and symbolic functions), whereas a speech disorder is a problem in articulation or other peculiarity of speech production. Language disorder is more profound and serious. Disorders of speech are less pervasive and do not necessarily reflect a profound disturbance in the functioning of the central nervous system or of developmental arrests and distortions of development itself. Is there any evidence at birth to suggest anatomic differences between the right and left temporal lobes? *Answer:* Yes, and this recent work suggests some anatomical confirmation of Chomsky's postulation of a language acquisition device (LAD). Of what significance is pragmatics in explaining language acquisition? *Answer:* The search for an understanding of how the child acquires language has shifted among linguists from a concern of vocabulary and syntax to pragmatics—the study of how the child makes use of language in negotiating transactions with others. Both sides of this transaction are studied, and many recent discoveries are based upon this exploration.

The basic challenge of identifying exactly how the child progresses from prelinguistic forms of communication in infancy to the formal use of language as the main communication after the age of two to two and one-half remains as a heuristically valuable no-man's-land, or more properly, every-man's-land.

Eleanor Galenson explores the origins of gender identity, which she defines as "the kind of man or woman the individual is, particularly in the sexual area." Her chapter presents a summary of findings from direct observation of infants, including her own work with Roiphe, is presented in well-organized stages following the infant's development from birth through early childhood. At what age do boys and girls discover the genitals? *Answer:* Boys discover the penis at six to eight months, about two or three months before girls are aware of their genitals. Of what significance is urination and anal phase masturbation in the evolution of gender identity in boys and in girls? *Answer:* The visible urinary stream is a source of great excitement and interest for both boys and girls and, as a clear marker for the anatomical distinctions between the sexes, is linked with interest in how the mother and father urinate. The anxiety associated with this observation leads to intense investigative activities concerning urination on the part of both boys and girls during the late part of the second year of life and has an early influence on the child's growing awareness of his own anatomical sex. This is carried further by the child's anal phase masturbation at the same developmental phase and leads to the emer-

4

gence of genital awareness. Why are little boys more inclined to use the toilet without engaging the mother, while little girls readily engage the mother in toileting? *Answer:* Dr. Galenson states, "It is likely that the boy's emerging awareness of the genital anatomical differences promotes the development of a defensive denial in relation to the mother's perineum." What is the special role of the father in aiding the girl in developing an untroubled sense of herself as a girl early in the course of development of gender identity and prior to the time that she can fully comprehend her potentiality for producing a baby and nourishing an infant? *Answer:* The father can provide his daughter a much needed assurance of her sense of gender identity by providing opportunities and encouragement of a close psychological relationship when genital differences are first discovered. The father's increased availability, nurturance, and support for her development at this time seem to be especially important for the girl's future unconflicted functioning.

Dr. Galenson goes on to describe differences in castration anxiety between boys and girls and the later impact of oedipal events upon the growing sense of gender identity. This is a fundamentally important chapter for anyone who wishes to understand the current state of our knowledge about how boys and girls each come to terms with their own anatomy and sexual functioning.

Perhaps nowhere in the extensive literature on infant and child development does one find a more helpful, well-written, and comprehensive summary of the important works of Mahler and her coworkers in describing the phases of development from early infancy through the stages of separation-individualtion, an epic of research which has had, and continues to have, a profound effect upon our thinking about these continuing life-long processes. What is the significance of the symbiotic phase? *Answer:* It is during this phase that the infant (1) anticipates and initiates the pleasure provided by interaction with the caregiver; (2) develops a sense of confidence and basic trust in the caregiver and in his own initiative; and (3) responds to the caregiver with a non-specific social smile and with eye-to-eye contact. As Galenson notes, "Mutual cueing is at its peak indicating the symbiotic phase is well under way."

What is the difference between Piaget's concept of object permanence and libidinal object constancy? *Answer:* Piaget's studies concern the infant's cognitive development within a well-defined experimental setting with conflictual variables minimized. The concept of libidinal object constancy refers to the capacity of the infant to maintain a stable representation of the love object (i.e., the mother), even in the presence of powerful affects, libidinal strivings and frustrations. What is meant by hatching? *Answer:* Hatching refers

to the emergence of the child from the symbiotic envelope with the mother. Usually occurring in the last half of the first year of life, it marks the child's emergence from psychobiological unity with the mother to the beginning phases of awareness of separateness from her. Children's capacity to bring themselves to the sitting position and move their torso in various directions gives them a whole new sense of awareness about the world and themselves. This achievement, reached at eight months, is the midwife to what is described as hatching, the time at which children begin to establish a clear awareness of themselves as entities, correlating with separation anxiety and with Piaget's fourth stage of sensorimotor development. In his chapter, John McDevitt observes that, "When the symbiotic phase is satisfactory, it serves as a prerequisite for the infant's successful disengagement from the mother during the subsequent separation-individuation phase and furthers both self-object differentiation and the emergence of the sense of self." How does the infant normally cope with separation distress? *Answer:* By forming a more stable representation of the mother and by active mastery. Why is the rapprochement subphase of development also described as a rapprochement crisis? *Answer:* Because the establishment of libidinal object constancy is subject to many vicissitudes and irregularities and leaves the child exposed to anxiety, which in turn may lead to regression and the expression of violent angry feelings related to the internal struggle the child experiences with the shifting nature of libidinal object representation. It is during this period, late in the second year of life, that splitting and projective mechanisms play such an important role in the child's defenses, and it is here that a link with later pathology is so clearly shown. At approximately what age does the child respond to his own image in the mirror with an apparent recognition of himself? *Answer:* At nine to twelve months. McDevitt summarizes his extensive observations of the infant's response to a mirrored image beginning from the early months and proceeding well into the second year, supporting other observations made during the symbiotic and separation-individuation phases. On completion of the rapprochement subphase late in the second year a strong sense of self should emerge.

These brief comments do not do justice to the way in which McDevitt summarizes and assembles the observations of infancy into a coherently organized theory of how the infant's sense of self actually emerges. His theory does vary considerably from the propositions set forth by Kohut and by Kernberg and will provide the reader a better grasp of this important question now occupying center stage among psychoanalysts concerned with issues of normality and psychopathology.

Chapter 8, by Jean Hamilton and Cynthia Conrad, deals with developmental psychopharmacology, particularly during adolescence, and provides an early glimpse into a field that is likely to become of central importance in understanding both the normal development of biological predispositions as they unfold in relationship to age and sex, and the response of a specific individual to the use of psychopharmacological agents in treating major psychopathology during childhood and adolescence. This chapter is an original contribution which presents for the first time a coherently organized summary of our knowledge in this arena and from which more studies will undoubtedly proceed.

A review of normal adolescence, which only infrequently is associated with family crisis, together with an epidemiologic study of mental health and mental illness among adolescents is presented by Offer, Ostrov, and

Howard. This well designed epidemiologic study of mental illness during adolescence sheds considerable light upon psychopathological as well as normal processes of development and correlates with earlier studies showing that not every adolescent—in fact, only 20 percent in a random sample—is disturbed. Mentally ill girls are more likely to be quiet in their disturbance than are boys. Boys who are "quietly" disturbed tend to have relatively good impulse control in family relationships, but do show evidence of affective, body image and social relationship disturbances. Quietly disturbed girls had healthier body images than boys.

The chapters contained in this section are of interest to a variety of readers. Reporting on a range of child development issues, the authors present exciting new findings that reflect the most current research in this field relevant to clinical practice.

1 / Environmental Influences on the Young Brain

Marian Cleeves Diamond

Introduction

One December morning my husband, Arnold Scheibel, a psychiatrist-anatomist and I, discussed possible types of enriched environments for a child. Arnold began to describe the environmental enrichment provided to him by his father. Between the years of five to eight, Arnold received some magnificently illustrated stories from the Bible. These were followed by *The Child's History of the World,* and *The Child's Geography of the World* by Henrik W. van Loon. The *Compton Encyclopedia* became another source of solid information. Then there were the short biographies of world leaders and men who became President. What a vast, varied amount of information to offer stimulation and somehow storage in the growing brain of a very young boy!

This is but one example of enriching the input into a human brain. Youngsters in the foothills of the Himalayas may gather stones and sticks of various sizes to construct a game as complicated as chess. The point of this discussion is that wherever we are in the world, new and stimulating input is essential to challenge nerve cells in the developing brain.

As the individual experiences a constant flow of new stimuli, what kind of changes are actually occurring in

the brain cells within the skull? At birth the brains of most mammals are structurally and functionally underdeveloped. During the early neonatal period, rapid development occurs before brain growth tapers off in early life. Ideally, with controlled environmental input, detailed stages of development in the mammalian brain could be identified in order to study the so-called normal stages of growth and maturation. Unfortunately, until recently, environments have not been controlled. It is now essential, therefore, to examine the growth curve of the mammalian brain under a given set of circumstances and then to consider how changes in the environment can alter this basic pattern. Since it is the cerebral cortex that appears most responsive to changes in the external environment, this chapter will focus on this region of the brain.

Obviously the knowledge we seek could best be attained if we were to examine the brains of human beings. However, because of both ethical and practical considerations, we cannot control the environmental input into human brains. Nor is it possible to make precise measurements over time of identical areas on fixed human cortices. Even with computed tomography and positron emission tomography scanning techniques, the resolution is not sensitive enough to allow us to measure living human brains; in particular, we are unable to differentiate the boundaries of the gray matter constituting the cerebral cortex from the underlying white matter. While we cannot at this time follow the growth of cortical thickness with these techniques, newly developed magnetic resonance technology may allow us to do so in the future. In the meantime, we must turn to animal models where we can control the environment and make precise measurements of cortical dimensions on preserved tissue. In this chapter, much of the work will deal with the rat brain, a circumstance that evokes the usual cautions about extrapolating from rats to man. And indeed differences do exist on many levels. In the cerebral cortex of the rat, neuronal cell division is complete at birth at which time dendritic branching begins to develop profusely. This period of rapid cortical development in the rat occurs during the first thirty days postnatally. In contrast to this, cell division in human brains continues for about five months postnatally.[38] In humans, rapid dendritic growth takes place during the first three to four postnatal years. On the other hand, according to Dobbing and Sands,[15] at least five-sixths of human brain growth is postnatal and in this respect humans resemble rats more closely than formerly thought. In any case, to promote optimum human or rat brain growth it is important to establish appropriate environmental conditions during these early years. The fact that the plasticity of the cerebral cortex has been demonstrated throughout the rat's lifetime offers an optimistic view of the brain's adaptability to its environment at any age.[15]

Until the early 1960s, the fact that the brain could structurally change with experience was not generally accepted. In 1911 Ramon y Cajal, the great neurohistologist, stated that cerebral exercise must undoubtedly affect neuronal structure.[27] Nevertheless, scientists believed that after the initial development the brain became structurally stable. With aging it might decrease in size, but that it could grow with use and shrink with disuse was not a widely held notion. Now that plasticity of the morphology of the cerebral cortex has been clearly demonstrated by several laboratories, there has been a turnabout toward acceptance. Nonetheless, there are still many variables to be considered in learning about plasticity: age, duration of stimulation, sex, nutrition, brain regions involved, chemical supplements, sleep, and so forth.

Normal Cortical Development

In order to understand the brain's structural and chemical responses to alterations in the environment, it is essential first to examine the normal curve of development. In 1975 such a curve was published, present-

ing the cerebral cortical thickness of the male rat.[12] In general, the whole cortex, whether frontal, parietal, occipital, medial, or lateral, grows very rapidly for the first ten days postnatally and then continues to grow more slowly until somewhere between twenty-six and forty-one days of age. At this time a gradual decrease in cortical thickness begins and continues until death. These slopes were found in the brains of male rats that lived in cages (32 by 20 by 20 cm) with their mothers prior to weaning and in rats that were weaned at twenty-three to twenty-five days of age before living three per cage. (This study is part of a larger ongoing histological exploration; it includes male rats from the following age groups, with fifteen to twenty-five rats per age group: 6, 10, 14, 20, 26, 41, 55, 77, 90, 108, 185, 300, 400, 650, and 904 days of age.)

Figure 1–1 presents a representative sample of a rat brain. This transverse section illustrates the method of measuring cortical thickness in the occipital cortex. Figure 1–2 presents the developing cortical curves for each of the areas measured from birth to fifty-five days of age (frontal cortex, somatosensory $[B, C, D]$, and occipital $[B, C, D]$). The areas are shown separately to indicate that, in general, the total mantle increases in a similar fashion, that certain areas do have different developmental patterns. For example, the frontal cortex develops similarly to the rest of the cortex until age fourteen days; at that point its growth curve maintains a plateau until twenty days of age, when once again the slope follows the pattern of the other cortical areas.

Because of the possible use of these brain developmental data as guidelines in the modern human educational system for how the brain grows, the whole and the parts are presented separately. There are no comparable data available on human brains. It has been proposed that "the brain grows in spurts" and that intellectual inputs are most effective during the growth spurts.[16] Rat data from our laboratory do not support this hypothesis of cycles of growth advances. Measuring skull dimensions alone is evidently not adequate to determine the dimensions of intracranial structures. By means of measuring roentgenograms of the skulls of enriched and impoverished rats, we have found that the intracranial size was not significantly different between the two groups of animals, although the external cranial dimensions were.[10] The isolated rats with greater body weights had larger external skull dimensions.

Our data suggest that for the first month postnatally the male rat cerebral cortex increases its dimensions rapidly and then decreases slowly thereafter. The next important questions are: Can one accelerate maturation during the increasing slope of the curve or alter the curve during its decline?

All of the preceding discussion has dealt with the male rat's cortex. The developmental curve of the cor-

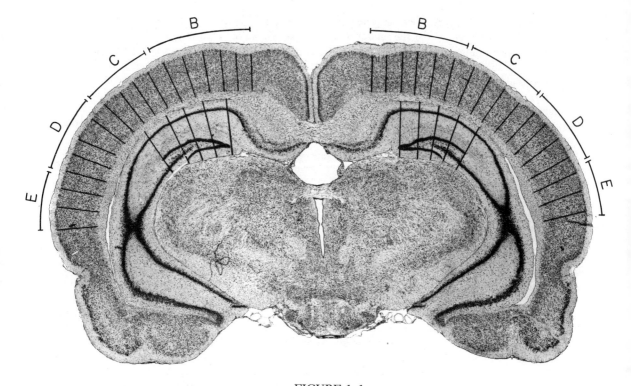

FIGURE 1–1

A Transverse Section of the Rat Brain Indicating the Method by Which Cortical Thickness Was Measured

NOTE: The letters B, C, D, and E were used to illustrate the general divisions of cortical measurements. The divisions vary numerically depending upon the section. For the somatosensory cortex: B = area 4; C = area 3; D = area 2; for the occipital cortex: B = area 18; C = area 17; D = area 18a and E = area 39.

SOURCE: reprinted from a chapter by Marian C. Diamond in *Knowing, Thinking and Believing,* Eds., J. McGaugh and L. Petrinovich (New York: Plenum Press, 1976), 218.

tical thickness for the female rat is still being determined. Nonetheless, it is of interest to point out one obvious difference in the developmental pattern of the female compared to the male. Between seven and fourteen days of age, area 39 (as identified by Krieg[22]) grows at a much more rapid rate than do the other regions of the cortex. In fact, in the second week this area increases by 40 percent. What determines the rapidity of this growth, so out of proportion to the rest of the cortex at this time, is not clear. Area 39 is reportedly a region where extensive sensory integration takes place. Is it possible that the eventual demands of child bearing and rearing require early development of this region, which is considered to be the integrative area of integrated areas.

Investigators have reported that histological changes occur in the cortex during maturation and the accompanying behavioral patterns. Before ten days of age, when cortical neuronal cell bodies are expanding but not sending out branches in any number, reflex actions are well developed. After ten days of age, as the dendrites and axons increase richly and synaptogenesis

proceeds rapidly, the infant rats begin to crawl over their littermates and show signs of more mature behavior. By thirty days of age, the animals have attained adult behavior and the cortex has reached its maximum thickness. These observations were made while the animals were living in the uneventful laboratory environment.

Enriched Environments During the Preweaning Period

CEREBRAL CORTICAL THICKNESS

Let us now explore how the external environment can modify the developmental curve of the thickness of the male rat cerebral cortex. The only available work on the preweaned cortex is that of Malkasian and Diamond.[23] The aims of these experiments were to deter-

8

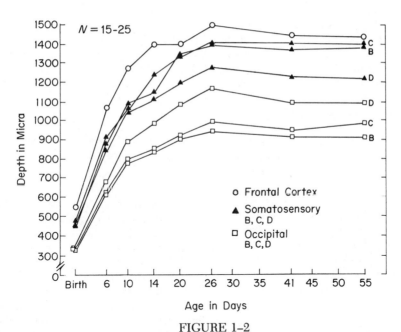

FIGURE 1–2

Cortical Thickness Growth Curves in Male Long-Evans Rats from Birth to Fifty-Five Days of Age

mine the effects on cortical neurogenesis of an enriched condition plus a multifamily environment compared to a nonenriched unifamily condition. An additional experiment was conducted in order to examine the effect of a tranquilizer on the morphological cortical response in the enriched multifamily environment. The response of the preweaned rats' cortex to the environmental conditions were also compared with that of the adult animals.

At birth all litters for these preweaned enriched and nonenriched environments were reduced to three pups per mother. At six days of age, three conditions were established: one mother and her three pups remained in the standard colony cage (32 by 20 by 20 cm) (unifamily environment); three mothers with three pups each were placed in a single large cage (70 by 70 by 46 cm) (multifamily environment); and three mothers, each with three pups, were placed in a single large cage that contained objects to explore, climb, and sniff (multifamily environment, enriched condition).

None of the pups was weaned at the usual time (between twenty-one to twenty-three days of age). Instead they lived continuously with the mothers. I know of no data available about the direct effect of weaning on cerebral cortical development.

Since the major thrust of the experiment was to determine whether stimulating living conditions could enhance brain development, more animals were studied in the experiment between the nonenriched (small cage) and enriched (large cage) environments than between the nonenriched (small cage) and the nonenriched (large cage) animals. In the first type of experiment, three different age groups were studied: fourteen, nineteen, and twenty-eight days of age respectively. In the second type of experiment only one age group was examined, twenty-eight days of age.

The results from these experiments indicated that when comparing the brains of the animals from the multifamily enriched conditions with those of the nonenriched group in small cages, the changes in cortical thickness were striking. As early as fourteen days of age—that is, eight days after being placed in the enriched environment—the somatosensory cortex showed increases of 7 to 11 percent ($p < 0.001$) compared to the unifamily littermate controls. In particular, on the lateral aspect of the occipital cortical section, area 39 increased as much as 16 percent ($p < 0.001$). It is noteworthy that during this early period, the primary visual cortex did not change, undoubtedly because the eyes had not yet opened.

By nineteen days of age in response to the enriched conditions, all cortical areas measured showed significant increases in thickness, with differences ranging from 6 to 14 percent. At twenty-eight days of age, after twenty-two days of enrichment, the same order of magnitude of differences was found. These differences ranged from 7 to 12 percent, and statistically all were highly significant.

However, there were no significant differences in cortical thickness between the multifamily nonenriched condition and the unifamily nonenriched condition. Thus it is the presence of the objects or toys, rather than grouped living in a large cage, that is essential to bring about the cortical changes. At the same time, it is not clear what aspect of the interaction with the toys is necessary—that is, whether the increase is due primarily to touch, pressure, temperature, vision, or other factors.

These results clearly indicate that it is possible to accelerate the maturation of the developing cerebral cortex by exposing an animal to reasonably stimulating environments. Many additional experiments need to be carried out to answer the numerous questions arising from these studies. For example, how much stimulation is optimal, and at which point does it become excessive? Is there a ceiling effect that the cortex will reach with increased activity during this early developing period? Can normal neuronal cell loss be prevented by providing an enriched environment during this early period? Needless to say, endless experiments could be done to attempt to learn the optimum conditions for the growing cortex. Priority is the key word. What are the most important questions to ask? What environmental input should be given and when? Many parents have succeeded in stimulating their children positively with their own versions of enriched conditions, and many have brought about negative effects.

My associates and I are interested primarily in how the cortex develops and ages without the use of severe artificial conditions; as a rule, our laboratory does not study the effects of drugs on the brain. However, in the case of these enriched preweaned rats, one group was given 0.1 mg reserpine injected subcutaneously each day from day 6 to 28. This tranquilizer is a catecholamine-depleting agent and was chosen for its possible effect on the increased cortical dimensions brought about by the enrichment. In spite of the known tranquilizing effect of this drug, the medial somatosensory cortex increased by as much as 7 percent ($p < 0.001$). Without the drug, this medial cortical area increased by 8 percent ($p < 0.002$). However, in the more lateral portions of the somatosensory cortex (areas 3 and 2 of Krieg[22]), reserpine damped the enrichment effects. Without the drug, these areas increased by 7 and 9 percent, but with the drug, the changes were only 5 and −1.5 percent. Evidently different areas of the cortex respond individually to such a systemically introduced tranquilizer.

the mean neuronal nuclear and perikaryon areas indicated increases by as much as 19 and 15 percent in layers II and III, respectively. In the occipital cortex (area 18), the neuronal nuclear area of the enriched animals exceeded that of the nonenriched by as much as 25 percent!

LATERAL GENICULATE NEURONAL AREA

The lateral geniculate nucleus is a thalamic station for visual impulses; in the course of our study, it too was examined for possible plasticity of response to an enriched environment. No significant differences were discovered between the enriched and nonenriched animals in the neuronal nuclear *area*, but the proportion of neuronal constituents was 20 percent ($p < 0.01$) less in the enriched than in the nonenriched rats. This means that when the lateral geniculate nucleus from the enriched animals was compared to that of the nonenriched ones, significantly more neuropil was present. Such results demonstrate one pathway that is involved in creating the enriched cortical differences, namely, the visual path. These conclusions were not anticipated, for Krech, Rosenzweig, and Bennett[21] had shown that blind enriched rats or rats raised in darkness during the experimental period developed an increase in occipital cortical weight.

BEHAVIOR

Some behavioral observations were made on these pups, but no specific maze tests were used, as was done with the older animals. At the time of feeding and cleaning, no striking differences were noted between the enriched and nonenriched pups in respect to gregariousness or behavior. However, since the enriched animals did have more room to explore, they were observed to interact actively with their toys during the twelve-hour dark period. Thus the interaction with the toys was evidently an important factor in creating the brain changes.

Enriched Environments During the Postweaning Period

CEREBRAL CORTICAL NEURONAL AREA

One can ask at this time what intracortical structures are changing dimensions in order to create the differences in cortical thickness. When the somatosensory cortex of the enriched pups was compared to that of the nonenriched pups, planimetric measurements of

CEREBRAL CORTICAL THICKNESS

As mentioned earlier, in the young rat there are two slopes to the cortical thickness curve, one increasing and the other decreasing. Now that I have shown that the developing curve can be further accelerated, the next question is whether it is possible to counteract the decrease in slope by placing animals in enriched environments. For this group of experiments it was no longer essential for the animals to live with their mothers. Three other basic conditions were used:[29] enriched, standard colony, and impoverished. The enriched environment consisted of twelve rats living in the large cage with the stimulus objects (in order to maintain the increased cortical dimensions, it is essential that the objects be changed frequently). The standard-colony environment included three rats per small cage, and the impoverished one rat per small cage. Food and water were available equally to all animals.

These experiments provided much new information. They proved that an enriched environment increased cortical thickness at any age, from the very young to the extremely elderly rat. Significant changes were noted as early as four days. As mentioned earlier, it was found that continued substitution of the toys was essential. With constant exposure to the same objects, the rats' cortices decreased in size; the animals apparently became bored with the unchanging living conditions, much as people do.

If the rats were separated immediately after weaning into enriched and impoverished conditions, the effects of the latter were stronger than those of the former. In other words, isolation immediately after weaning was detrimental to cortical development. If the rats were first placed into standard-colony conditions for a month and then transferred into the enriched or impoverished conditions for a month, the grouping of the animals was more effective than if done immediately after weaning. Indeed this timing sequence established the largest overall cortical thickness encountered in these experiments. Also, isolation was not as detrimental to the cortex if the movement of the animals into a single small cage took place gradually, from weaning to standard colony and then finally to isolation.

NEURONAL SIZE AND GLIAL MEASURES

Once cortical structure had been shown to change with response to a positive environmental condition, many investigators, utilizing various techniques and measurements, found ways to support the basic findings.*

These enriched and nonenriched experiments have distinctly demonstrated that at any age, the cerebral cortex can, in response to the environmental input, change its structure either positively or negatively.[14] Cummins and Livesey[7] suggest that the primary cause

---

*(For dimensions of the cerebral cortex, see Altman et al.[2] and Walsh et al.[36] For dendritic branching, see Connor, Wang, and Diamond[6]; Greenough, Volkmar, and Jaraska[18]; and Holloway.[19] For synaptic length, see Diamond et al.[12]; Mollgaard et al.[25]; Walsh and Cummins[35]; and West and Greenough.[37] For the hippocampus, see Altschuler.[3] For glial cells, see Altman and Das[1]; and Diamond et al.[11]

of differential development could be traced to retarded neurological growth in the isolated animals. Jorgenson and Bock[20] too interpret their results as delayed development in the isolated rats. However, this theory has been refuted; results of experiments by Uylings and associates[34] showed that growth of dendrites had taken place in the adult enriched rats, rather than retardation alone in the isolated animals.

CHEMICAL CHANGES DUE TO ENVIRONMENTAL ALTERATIONS

Most of the studies on chemical changes in the brain in response to the environment have been carried out on postweaned rats. Brenner and associates[5] experimented with pups placed into enriched environments at one, three, five, and seven days of age postnatally. If the pups received saline until twenty-five days of age, the cortical weight increased. If, however, they received 6-hydroxydopamine (60HDA), cortical weight was lowered. The investigators concluded that norepinephrine influenced early cortical development. A very thorough review of the literature on chemical alteration with environment has been presented by Rosenzweig and Bennett.[28]

Findings Due to Modifications of the Original Enriched Environmental Paradigm

NEGATIVE AIR IONS

Experiments indicated that if the level of small negative air ions was raised (10^5) while the preweaned animals lived in enriched versus nonenriched conditions, the cerebral cortex increased in wet weight and the amounts of endogenous serotonin and cyclic adenosine monophosphate decreased. It is of particular interest that the cortical changes with ions were more marked if the rats lived in enriched rather than in nonenriched conditions. This experiment shows the unusual sensitivity of the cerebral cortex to external environmental conditions.[13]

SLEEPING PATTERNS AND THE ENVIRONMENT

According to Mirmiran, Uylings, and Corner,[24] if clonidine hydrochloride was given to rats from eight to twenty-one days after birth, the amount of rapid-eye-movement sleep was diminished. When this suppressing agent was employed, it prevented the usual enriched-versus standard-colony cortical weight increases. These authors reported that under enriched conditions, active sleep and noradrenaline play a role in the growth of the cortex.

Tagney[33] found that environmental conditions altered the sleeping patterns of postweaned rats. In the impoverished condition the rats spent only 45 percent of their time sleeping, whereas in the enriched condition, they spent 56 percent of the time asleep. However, if the animals were transferred from the impoverished to the enriched condition, their sleeping patterns followed those of the enriched rats.

LEARNING ABILITY AFTER ENRICHMENT

At every age at which the animals have been tested, the enriched rats ran a maze better than the nonenriched animals. Forgays and Reed[17] found improvement in learning at 123 days of age if the animals had begun an enriched condition at birth, 22, 44, or 66 days of age. Nyman[26] found that from thirty to forty, fifty to sixty, and seventy to eighty days, the rats benefitted from only eight hours per day of environmental enrichment and proved better at spatial learning than did the nonenriched rats. An enriched environment after weaning improved problem-solving ability. Of course, it can always be questioned whether the laboratory enriched environment is comparable to that of the wild rat's. The answer is simply and clearly no. The natural environment is more challenging because life is threatened every moment. However, laboratory conditions do provide graded degrees of stimulation whose effectiveness can be estimated from the results obtained from the reported cortical measurements.

NUTRITION AND ENRICHED CONDITIONS

Bhide and Bedi[4] concluded that eighty days of enriched environments could bring about changes in both undernourished and well-fed pups. The pups were nutritionally deprived from the sixteenth day of gestation until the twenty-fifth postnatal day. They were then divided into isolated or enriched conditions until eighty days later. These data are presented with some reservations because the usual cortical thickness changes with healthy rats in enriched and impoverished conditions were not obtained.

In another group of nutritionally deprived and normally fed animals followed by enriched conditions, the cerebrum showed deficits due to the undernutrition in weight and size but not in cortical thickness.[8] Changes in cerebral weight and size also occurred as a result of differential housing; relative to their impoverished littermates, the enriched rats showed increased values.

SEXUAL MATURATION AND ENRICHED ENVIRONMENTS

Swanson and Van de Poll[32] handled rats from birth to thirty days of age before placing them in enriched or standard-colony or isolated environments. Isolation advanced vaginal opening in both handled and nonhandled rats. Isolation also improved sexual performance more than either the standard or the enriched condition.

Conclusion

The plasticity of the cerebral cortex is evident in both preweaned and postweaned rats. Whether they are from rats or humans, nerve cells are designed to receive stimuli, somehow store information, and transmit impulses. The results obtained from animal studies can be used as guidelines to help understand the human brain. Such questions as how much stimulation is beneficial or detrimental, when is stimulation optimal, and whether there is a ceiling to cortical growth are yet to be answered.

REFERENCES

1. ALTMAN, J., and DAS, G. D. "Autoradiographic Examination of the Effects of Enriched Environment on the Rate of Glial Multiplication in the Adult Rat Brain," *Nature,* 204 (1964):1161–1163.

2. ALTMAN, J., et al. "Behaviorally Induced Changes in Length of Cerebrum in Rats," *Developmental Psychobiology,* 1 (1968):112–117.

3. ALTSCHULER, R. "Changes in Hippocampal Synaptic Density with Increased Learning Experiences in the Rat," *Neuroscience Abstracts,* 2 (1976):438.

4. BHIDE, P. G., and BEDI, K. S. "The Effects of Environmental Diversity on Well Fed and Previously Undernourished Rats: Neuronal and Glial Cell measurements in the Visual Cortex (Area 17)," *Journal of Anatomy,* 138 (1984):-447–461.

5. BRENNER, E., et al. "Impaired Growth of the Cerebral Cortex of Rats Treated Neonatally with 6-hydroxydopamine Under Different Environmental Conditions," *Neuroscience Letters,* 42 (1983):13–17.

6. CONNOR, J. R., WANG, E. C., and DIAMOND, M. C. "Increased Length of Terminal Dendritic Segments in Old Rats' Somatosensory Cortex: An Environmentally Induced Response," *Experimental Neurology,* 78 (1982):466–470.

7. CUMMINS, R. A., and LIVESEY, P. J. "Enrichment-

Isolation, Cortex Length and Rank Order Effect," *Brain Research*, 178 (1979):89–98.

8. DAVIES, C. A., and KATZ, H. B. "The Comparative Effects of Early-life Under-nutrition and Subsequent Differential Environments on the Dendritic Branching of Pyramidal Cells in Rat Visual Cortex," *Journal of Comparative Neurology*, 218 (1983):345–350.

9. DIAMOND, M. C., JOHNSON, R. E., and INGHAM, C. A. "Morphological Changes in the Young, Adult and Aging Rat Cerebral Cortex, Hippocampus and Diencephalon," *Behavioral Biology*, 14 (1975):163–174.

10. DIAMOND, M. D., ROSENZWEIG, M. R., and KRECH, D. "Relationships Between Body Weight and Skull Development in Rats Raised in Enriched and Impoverished Conditions," *Journal of Experimental Zoology*, 160 (1965):29–36.

11. DIAMOND, M. C., et al. "Increases in Cortical Depth and Glia Numbers in Rats Subjected to Enriched Environment," *Journal of Comparative Neurology*, 128 (1966):117–126.

12. DIAMOND, M. C., et al. "Differences in Occipital Cortical Synapses from Environmentally Enriched, Impoverished, and Standard Colony Rats," *Journal of Neuroscience Research*, 1 (1975):109–119.

13. DIAMOND, M. C., et al. "Environmental Influences on Serotonin and Cyclic Nucleotides in Rat Cerebral Cortex," *Science*, 210 (1980):652–654.

14. DIAMOND, M. C., et al. "Plasticity in the 904-day-old Male Rat Cerebral Cortex," *Experimental Neurology*, 87 (1985):309–317.

15. DOBBING, J., and SANDS, J. "Quantitative Growth and Development of the Human Brain," *Archives of Diseases in Childhood*, 48 (1973):757–767.

16. EPSTEIN, H. T. "Growth Spurts During Brain Development: Implications for Educational Policy and Practice," in J. S. Chall and A. F. Mirsky, eds., *Education and the Brain*. Chicago: University of Chicago Press, 1978.

17. FORGAYS, D. G., and READ, J. M. "Crucial Periods for Free-Environmental Experience in the Rat," *Journal of Comparative and Physiological Psychology*, 55 (1962):816–818.

18. GREENOUGH, W. T., VOLKMAR, F. R., and JURASKA, J. M. "Effects of Rearing Complexity on Dendritic Branching in Frontolateral and Temporal Cortex of the Rat," *Experimental Neurology*, 41 (1973):371–378.

19. HOLLOWAY, R. R. L. "Dendritic Branching in Rat Visual Cortex. Effects of Extra Environmental Complexity and Training," *Brain Research*, 2 (1966):393.

20. JORGENSON, O. S., and BOCK, E. "Brain Specific Proteins in the Occipital Cortex of Rats Housed in Enriched and Impoverished Environments," *Neurochemistry Research*, 4 (1979):175–187.

21. KRECH, D., ROSENZWEIG, M. R., and BENNETT, E. L. "Effects of Complex Environment and Blindness on the Rat Brain," *Archives of Neurology*, 8 (1963):403–412.

22. KRIEG, W. "Connections of the Cerebral Cortex. I. The Albino Rat. B. Structure of the Cortical Areas," *Journal of Comparative Neurology*, 84 (1946):278–323.

23. MALKASIAN, D. R., and DIAMOND, M. C. "The Effects of Environmental Manipulation on the Morphology of the Neonate Rat Brain," *International Journal of Neuroscience*, 2 (1971):161–170.

24. MIRMIRAN, M., UYLINGS, H. B., and CORNER, M. A. "Pharmacological Suppression of REM Sleep Prior to Weaning Counteracts the Effectiveness of Subsequent Environmental Enrichment on Cortical Growth in Rats," *Brain Research*, 283 (1983):102–105.

25. MOLLGAARD, K., et al. "Quantitative Synaptic Changes with Differential Experience in Rat Brain," *International Journal of Neuroscience*, 2 (1971):113–128.

26. NYMAN, A. J. "Problem Solving in Rats as a Function of Experience at Different Ages," *Journal of Genetic Psychology*, 110 (1967):31–39.

27. RAMON Y CAJAL, S, *Histologie du Systeme Nerveux de l'Homme et des Vertébrés*. Madrid: Consojo Superior de Investigaciones Cientificas, 1911 (reprint).

28. ROSENZWEIG, M. R., and BENNETT, E. L. "Experiential Influences on Brain Anatomy and Brain Chemistry in Rodents," in G. Gottlich, ed., *Studies of the Development of Behavior and the Nervous System*. New York: Academic Press, 1978, pp. 289–327.

29. ROSENZWEIG, M. R., BENNETT, E. L., and DIAMOND, M. C. "Chemical and Anatomical Plasticity of Brain: Replication and Extensions, 1970," in J. Gaito, ed., *Macromolecules and Behavior*, 2nd ed. New York: Appleton-Century-Crofts, 1972, pp. 205–277.

30. SHAPIRO, S. "Hormonal and Environmental Influences on Rat Brain Development and Behavior," in M. B. Sterman, D. J. McGinty, and A. M. Adinolfi, eds., *Brain Development and Behavior*. New York: Academic Press, 1971, pp. 307–334.

31. SHAPIRO, S., and VUKOVICH, K. R. "Early Experience Effects Upon Cortical Dendrites: A Proposed Model for Development," *Science*, 167 (1970):292–294.

32. SWANSON, H. H., and VAN DE POLL, N. E. "Effects of an Isolated or Enriched Environment After Handling on Sexual Maturation and Behavior in Male and Female Rats," *Journal of Reproduction and Fertility*, 69 (1983):165–171.

33. TAGNEY, J. "Sleep Patterns Related to Rearing Rats in Enriched and Impoverished Environments," *Brain Research*, 53 (1973):353–361.

34. UYLINGS, H. B. M., et al. "Dendritic Outgrowth in the Visual Cortex of Adult Rats Under Different Environmental Conditions," *Experimental Neurology*, 62 (1979):658–677.

35. WALSH, R. N., and CUMMINS, R. A. "Effects of Differential Sensory Environments on the Electron Microscopy of the Rat Occipital Cortex," *Proceedings of the Society of Neuroscience Annual Meeting*, 2 (1976):839.

36. WALSH, R. N., et al. "Environmentally Induced Changes in the Dimensions of the Rat Cerebrum," *Developmental Psychobiology*, 4 (1971):115–122.

37. WEST, R. W., and GREENOUGH, W. T. "Effect of Environmental Complexity on Cortical Synapses of Rats: Preliminary Results," *Behavioral Biology*, 7 (1972):279–284.

38. WINICK, M. *Malnutrition and Brain Development*. New York: Oxford University Press, 1976.

2 / The Development of Neurotransmitters and Neuropeptides

Joseph T. Coyle and James C. Harris

Introduction

Development has been emphasized as the organizing focus for basic and clinical science in child psychiatry. Psychosocial,* family developmental,[7] and neuromaturational[22] phases or stages have been described as having etiological significance in the genesis of psychiatric disorders in children. Similarly, from a biomedical perspective, in assessing potential vulnerability to neuropsychiatric disorders, specific attention has been paid to ontogenetic events and the impact of brain dysfunction and damage occurring during development.[50] There is increasing evidence of an important interaction among psychodynamic, psychological, and neurobiological factors in the etiology of psychiatric disorders. This interaction has been elaborated in the integrated biopsychosocial approach to psychiatry.[15]

During the last decade, due to a growing appreciation of the role of chemical neurotransmitters, in the pathophysiology of certain psychiatric disorders and as the mediators of the effects of virtually all psychotropic medications, there has been increasing focus on child disorders. These issues have been extensively reviewed recently.[9,10] Since the processes involved in chemical synaptic neurotransmission play a critical role in normal as well as pathological brain function, the ontogeny of these processes may be linked to the emergence of behaviors, to developmental stages, and to the age-related appearance of certain psychiatric disorders, such as infantile autism, attention deficit disorder, Tourette syndrome, schizophrenia, anorexia nervosa, and the affective disorders. This chapter represents an attempt to relate our current understanding of the development of brain neurotransmitter systems to the onset of psychiatric disorders during the developmental periods.

*See references 17, 18, 19, 20, 23, 44, and 60.

General Principles of Brain Development

Brain development can be likened to a symphony; there is an overall theme, which is punctuated by brief, percussive events that provide the critical rhythm.[30] Brain development at the cellular level can be divided into four primary events: neuroblast cell division, neuronal migration, transmitter specific differentiation, and synaptogenesis. Nests of epidermal germinal cells are the source of immature neurons that ultimately form the component regions of the brain; these cells typically lie within the center of the primordial brain. These dividing neuroblasts generate the immature, postmitotic neurons that make up the nervous system. Neuroblast cell division is not a continuous process but rather involves locally discrete and synchronized periods of cell multiplication. There is a precisely timed gradient of regional formation of the brain; the most primitive and caudal aspects are laid down before the more recently evolved structures, such as the cerebral cortex.

The postmitotic immature neuron typically migrates from the germinal zone to its final resting place within the brain. In the brain stem, populations of neurons grouped together in "nuclei" are generated during a brief period of mitotic activity and migrate together to coalesce into functionally discrete neuronal cell groupings, such as the noradrenergic locus coeruleus, the serotonergic raphe nuclei, or the dopaminergic substantia nigra. In cortical structures, which have a laminar organization, the early-formed neurons migrate to the surface and the subsequently formed neurons are layered upon them, so that cortical development occurs by an "inside-out" sequence. The mechanisms that organize the migration of these immature neurons remain poorly understood, although certain types of glial cells may serve as the scaffolding and neuron-neuron interactions appear to provide the cues. [47]

The migration of the immature neurons to their ultimate resting place also appears to be involved in the biochemical differentiation into the type of neurotransmitter that they will utilize. The appearance of the specialized biochemical mechanisms responsible for neurotransmitter synthesis generally takes place after the immature neuron has reached its final destination. Recent studies have provided evidence that immature neurons may transiently manifest the biochemical characteristics typical for one neurotransmitter before assuming those neurotransmitter characteristics that they will retain throughout their mature life. [33] The factors that control the phenotypic expression of neurotransmitter characteristics have yet to be precisely identified. Working with less complex peripheral systems, neuroscientists have demonstrated that local interactions with neighboring neurons and neurotrophic cues, such as the hormone nerve growth factor (NGF), play important roles in the epigenetic decision of neurotransmitter specification. [6,43]

The final process of brain development involves the elaboration of the receptive portion of neurons—the dendrite—and the communicational portion of the neurons—the axons—which ultimately meet to form the synaptic contacts. While most of this process occurs during the early stages of brain development—before two years of age in humans—it is becoming increasingly apparent that the elaboration and modification of axonal-dendritic synaptic contacts continues to occur, although to a much more limited degree, throughout maturation. In fact, a critical characteristic of senescence may be the loss of the ability to develop new synaptic contacts. The length of axonal projections may range from a few millimeters or less, as in local circuit GABAergic neurons in the cerebral cortex, to a meter, as in noradrenergic and serotonergic pathways innervating the spinal cord.

The factors that control the arborization of the axonal processes are the subject of intense investigation; and experiments have revealed a remarkable cellular precision in the formation of axonal contacts. For example, studies in the frog indicate that transsection of the optic nerve and rotation of the eye after a critical period of development will result in regrowth of axons to the appropriate neurons in the geniculate[30]; and studies in the rodent indicate that disruption of the normal laminar distribution of cortical neurons will not prevent the ultimate development of appropriate synaptic connections between the thalamus and the maldistributed cortical pyramidal cells. [8] Nevertheless, serotonergic and noradrenergic components of the reticular core of the brain appear to be relatively insensitive to the integrity of their postsynaptic neurons

within the cerebral cortex and will develop a quantitatively normal terminal arbor even in the absence of a full complement of cortical neurons. [31]

In summary, evidence obtained thus far in fundamental developmental neurobiological studies indicates that the maturation of the nervous system is a remarkably complicated process, which involves an interplay between precisely timed developmental events orchestrated by genetically determined programs. Because of the limited information contained in the cellular DNA, all developmental events are not directly controlled by the genes but rather are also determined by cell-cell interactions. There is growing evidence that neurotransmitters themselves may be intimately involved in the intercellular communication that regulates the development of neuronal systems. [6] Genetic defects or environmental insults that occur during the period of neurogenesis, which takes place in man during the first trimester, are associated with gross teratogenic or structural defects in brain development. Later-appearing genetically expressed disturbances or environmental insults are more likely to affect the emerging neuronal connectivity in the brain.

Synaptic Neurotransmission

Before we discuss the development of specific neurotransmitters, we shall review the concepts involved in synaptic chemical neurotransmission. The intraneuronal transmission of information from the receptive area of neurones, the dendritic extensions from their cell bodies, down the axon to the nerve terminals, occurs by a means of electical chemical wave of depolarization (see figure 2–1). However, the communication between neurones occurs by chemical messengers, known as neurotransmitters, that are released by the nerve terminals when a wave of depolarization reaches them.

Neurotransmitters can be divided into different classes based on their mode of synthesis and their neurophysiological effects. With regard to mode of synthesis, neuropeptides represent the most rapidly expanding class of neurotransmitters, whose synthesis occurs by a messenger RNA–dependent process within the neuronal cell body; the neuropeptide is then transported down the axon to the nerve terminal, where the active neuropeptide is released on demand. [10] A second class, the nonpeptide neurotransmitters, includes biogenic amines, amino acids, and certain other substances, whose synthesis occurs within the nerve terminal and is regulated by enzymes contained within it. Neurotransmitter synthesis in these nonpeptide neuro-

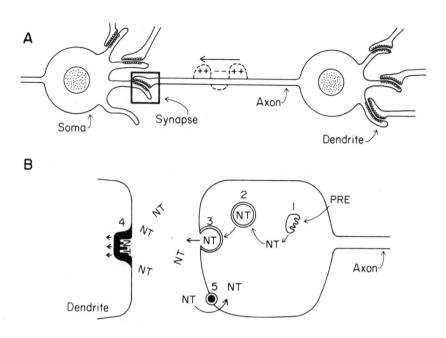

FIGURE 2–1

Schematic Representation of Synaptic Transmission

LEGEND: Part A. The structural components of the neuron include the soma (cell body), the receptive extension known as dendrites, the axon, and the specialized contact between the axon terminal and dendrite known as the synapse. Part B. The processes involved in chemical synaptic transmission at the synapse are illustrated. Precursors (PRE) for the neurotransmitter (NT) are taken up into the terminal and converted by enzymes to the neurotransmitter (1). The neurotransmitter is stored in vesicles (2) for release (3) into the synaptic cleft, where it interacts with receptors (4) on the dendrite. In many cases the neurotransmitter is inactivated by reuptake (5) into the nerve terminal.

transmitters is not closely tied to translational events within the neuronal cell body but rather is controlled at the level of the nerve terminal and therefore is much better able to respond to rapid changes in neurotransmitter demand.

Postsynaptic responses to neurotransmitters can be divided into three broad categories: excitatory, inhibitory, and modulatory. This simple, three-way division, however, does not do justice to the important and subtle relations between the neurotransmitter receptors and the various ion channels and enzymatic processes that mediate the neuronal effects of the neurotransmitters. Excitatory or inhibitory response represents the "hard" information communicated in the brain—for example, the decision whether a receptive neuron fires or not. In contrast, neuromodulators such as the biogenic amines appear to alter neuronal responsiveness to excitatory or inhibitory inputs. The neurotransmitter receptors, which are located on the postsynaptic neurones, translate the message encoded in the neurotransmitter; this highly specific interaction has been likened to the relationship between a key (the neurotransmitter) and a lock (receptor-transducer).

The neurotransmitter released by a given neuron is used throughout all its axonal extensions and nerve terminal ramifications, thus conferring upon it a biochemical identity. The neuron contains the biochemical processes necessary for synthesis, storage, release, and inactivation of the neurotransmitter. Conversely, the neuron does not possess the biochemical processes required for the disposition of other neurotransmitters. However, in a growing number of neuronal systems, there is evidence of colocalization of more than one neurotransmitter in the same nerve terminal field.[27] Colocalization generally involves a neuropeptide and a nonpeptide neurotransmitter such as a biogenic amine. Neurons that use specific neurotransmitters tend to be grouped together in clumps of cell bodies known as nuclei or to have specific laminar distributions, for example, in cortical structures.

Currently the number of substances in the brain thought to serve as neurotransmitters is approaching fifty and is increasing rapidly. The number implicated in the pathophysiology of psychiatric disorders or in the mechanism of action of psychotropic medications, however, is far more restricted. This fact reflects our current state of ignorance about the roles most neurotransmitters play in normal and abnormal behavior. The following discussion focuses on a review of the former neurotransmitters.

Development of Brain Neurotransmitters

The most detailed studies on development of specific neurotransmitter systems in the brain have been carried out in subprimate species, particularly the laboratory rat. However, limited information available thus far from studies on the developing human and subhuman primate brain suggest that the general principles defined in the rat are applicable to man.[24] The reticular core neurons—the noradrenergic, dopaminergic, serotonergic, and cholinergic neuronal systems—are located in the brain stem and therefore are among the neuronal systems that are formed particularly early in development. In contrast, the GABAergic intraneurons within the cortex are formed much later in brain development, during the genesis of the cerebral cortex.

RETICULAR CORE

An important group of neurons involved in the mechanism of action of several classes of psychotropic drugs is located in the reticular core of the brain. The cell bodies of the reticular core neurons are distributed in the midbrain and brain stem and have highly diffuse and arborized axonal projections that innervate large areas of the nervous system, particularly the forebrain. The localization of the cell bodies in the reticular core ensures that they receive diverse inputs from neuronal systems coming from the periphery and from neuronal systems projecting from the forebrain to lower brain regions. This organization suggests that the reticular core plays an integrative role in broadly regulating the activity of neurons located in the cerebral cortex, the corpus striatum, and the limbic system. Consistent with this anatomic organization, neurophysiological studies suggest that the reticular core neuronal systems act to "modulate" neuronal activity in the cortex and related structures rather than to convey excitatory or inhibitory information to discrete neurons within these regions.

Noradrenergic Neurons. The primary source of noradrenergic innervation for the cerebral cortex, limbic system, midbrain, and cerebellum is the locus coeruleus, a small group of pigmented neurons situated bilaterally on the floor of the fourth ventricle under the cerebellum (see figure 2–2). These neurons utilize norepinephrine (NE) as their neurotransmitter, synthesizing it within their nerve terminals from the amino acid tyrosine. The postsynaptic effects of NE are mediated by alpha- and beta-adrenergic receptors. The noradrenergic neuronal cell bodies send axons that inner-

vate virtually all neurons in the cerebral cortex and limbic system; accordingly, an individual noradrenergic neuron may contact more than ten[6] other neurons.

The noradrenergic neurons in the locus coeruleus are among the most caudal aspects of the reticular core and accordingly are formed remarkably early in brain development. This NE nucleus issues from a brief period of intense cell division, which in the rodent lasts approximately thirty-six hours.[37] The nucleus is established in the rodent when the brain represents less than 1 percent of the adult weight, which would be equivalent to the middle of the first trimester of pregnancy in man. As this nucleus coalesces, the neurons express in a coordinate fashion all the biochemical processes required for the synthesis, storage, and release of its neurotransmitter, NE.[12] It is remarkable to note that the nascent axons that grow from the newly formed noradrenergic neurons contain NE. The noradrenergic axons are among the very earliest to appear in the primordial cerebral cortex during its formation. Although noradrenergic terminals contribute to a very small percentage of the total number of synaptic contacts in the adult cerebral cortex, at this early stage of development up to 30 percent of the synapses in the immature cortex may be noradrenergic.[12]

This early and transient developmental predominance of noradrenergic terminals in the cortex suggests that the pioneering noradrenergic innervation may play a critical role in cortical development. Indeed, lesions of the noradrenergic system early in development affect cortical synaptic plasticity, which is the process whereby cortical synaptic contacts are altered on the basis of sensory input.[32] The noradrenergic innervation of the primordial cortex is subsequently diluted by the development of other cortical inputs, such as the thalamo-cortical pathways, as well as the elaboration of the rich synaptic arbors of neurons intrinsic to the cortex. It is important to make a distinction between the relative contribution of noradrenergic input at early developmental stages and the total elaboration of noradrenergic processes throughout the brain with maturation. Although the noradrenergic input to the cortex is relatively large early in development, the volume of the cortex is quite small at this time; with the progressive increase in cortical volume during maturation, the noradrenergic terminal arbor is diluted by the appearance of many other types of synaptic input. Thus the small group of noradrenergic neuronal cell bodies in the locus coeruleus elaborate a remarkably arborized group of axons and terminals that develop in lockstep fashion with the brain regions that they innervate. These noradrenergic neurons have been implicated in the modulation of arousal, anxiety, and affective state.

Serotonergic Neurons. The serotonergic neurons

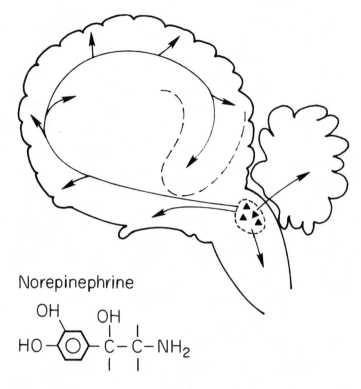

Norepinephrine

FIGURE 2–2
Noradrenergic Neuronal Pathways

utilize the indolamine serotonin (5HT) as their neurotransmitter. It is synthesized from the essential acid tryptophan by enzymes contained in the nerve terminal. Like the noradrenergic neurons, the serotonergic neurons provide an extremely diffuse innervation to the cerebral cortex, corpus striatum, and limbic system. Recent evidence indicates that the dual input by noradrenergic and serotonergic neurons may interact in modulating neuronal activity in the brain regions.[40] The serotonergic neurons have been implicated in mood, aggression, and rapid-eye-movement sleep.[57]

The serotonergic neurons (see figure 2–3) located in the raphe nuclei in the midbrain, anterior to the locus coeruleus, are formed somewhat later in brain development than the noradrenergic system. The serotonergic neurons send axons to virtually all areas of the fetal nervous system, as do the noradrenergic neurons. The early innervation of the primordial cortex by serotonergic neurons appears to play a role in modulating neuronal development, since disruption of the serotonergic neuronal system alters the rate of cell division in the fetal cerebral cortex.[38] In contrast to the noradrenergic input, the serotonergic input to the cerebral cortex develops more gradually in spite of its early appearance in the cortex.[39]

Dopaminergic Neurons. The dopaminergic neurons utilize dopamine (DA) as their neurotransmitter (see figure 2–4). DA is synthesized by enzymes contained within their nerve terminals from the amino acid tyrosine. The dopaminergic neurons in the substantia nigra proper provide a very diffuse and massive innervation to the corpus striatum (i.e., the caudate and putamen). It is estimated that 15 percent of the nerve terminal synapses in the corpus striatum are dopaminergic. This system plays a critical role in modulating motor activity, as evidenced by the the symptoms of Parkinson's disease, a disorder resulting from a selective degeneration of dopaminergic neurons and involving the nigrostriatal DA system.[28] The more medially located DA neurons in the ventral tegmentrum innervate the limbic system and the frontal cortex, providing the origins of the mesolimbic and mesocortical DA systems. There is indirect evidence supporting the notion that these DA neurons play a role in reward systems, attentional mechanisms, and cognitive integration.[41,61]

The nigral dopaminergic neurons, which lie even more anteriorly in the midbrain, are formed in man during a brief period of cell division in the late first trimester. The dopaminergic neurons send axons to the primordial striatum (caudate-putamen) soon after their formation. Although the striatal innervation by

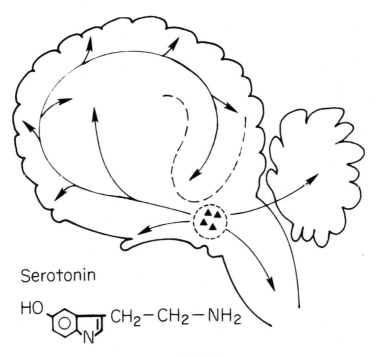

FIGURE 2–3
Serotonergic Neuronal Pathways

dopaminergic afferents is particularly dense in adulthood and virtually confluent when viewed by histofluorescent techniques that reveal the neurotransmitter itself, the initial input to the striatum involves localized islands of dopaminergic innervation.[25] These islands appear to be important developmental organizational points for the striatum since their distribution correlates with the ingrowth of other inputs to the striatum as well as cell divisional activity of striatal intrinsic neurons. With maturation, these initial outposts of striatal dopaminergic innervation soon spread to achieve the confluent pattern observed in the adult striatum. Quantitative neurochemical studies indicate that striatal dopaminergic innervation develops very gradually and reaches its apex around puberty in rats as well as man. Information about the development of the more medially located dopaminergic neurons, whose axons innervate the limbic system as well as the frontal and cingulate cortex, is quite limited; but this system also appears to exhibit a fairly gradual development that continues on past late childhood.

Cholinergic Neurons. Cholinergic cell bodies are scattered from the base of the midbrain overlying the hypothalamus anteriorly to the medial septum. The cholinergic neurons utilize acetylcholine as their neurotransmitter; it is synthesized within the nerve terminals from choline. These neurons provide a diffuse innervation to all areas of the cerebral cortex, hippocampus, and limbic system. Studies with Alzheimer's disease, a disorder involving a striking degeneration of cholinergic neurons, indicate that this cholinergic pathway plays an important role in memory and perhaps in other higher cognitive functions.[14]

The most anterior components of the reticular core are the cholinergic neurons of the basal forebrain complex (see figure 2–5). Because of the size and anterior-posterior extent of this complex, the neurons that form it undergo division over a longer period of time and later in development than the more caudally located components of the reticular core. Nevertheless, the cholinergic basal forebrain complex is formed well in advance of the development of its target areas of innervation in the cortex, hippocampus, and limbic system. In contrast to the early appearance of noradrenergic and serotonergic fibers in the primordial cortex, invasion by cholinergic axons occurs quite late. In the rodent, cholinergic innervation to the cortex does not occur until a full week after birth; the limited information from studies with primate cortex suggests that the peak of development of cholinergic innervation to the cortex occurs during the first year after birth.[13] As the cortical cholinergic projections appear to be the last developing component of the reticular core, it may be speculated that they may play a role in finalizing or cementing synaptogenesis in the cortex.

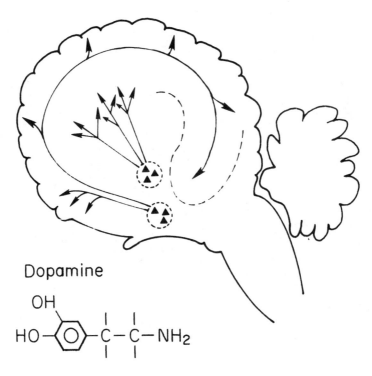

Dopamine

FIGURE 2–4
Dopamine Neuronal Pathways

GABAERGIC NEURONS

The GABAergic neurons are local circuit neurons in the cerebral cortex, cerebellum, and spinal cord, and projecting neurons from the striatum; thus they are not components of the reticular core. In the cerebral cortex, they play a critical role in local processing of information. A major class of local circuit neurons, they utilize gamma-aminobutyric acid (GABA) synthesized from the amino acid l-glutamic acid as their neurotransmitter. GABA is the primary inhibitory neurotransmitter that may be used by up to 30 percent of brain synapses.[16] The GABAergic neurons intrinsic to the cortex are scattered throughout all cortical layers and provide important inhibitory input to the pyramidal cells, which form the primary output system from the cortex. The GABA receptors mediating the effect of this neurotransmitter are also linked to receptor sites for the benzodiazepines. Several anticonvulsants interact directly with the GABA receptor; in addition, the anxiolytic benzodiazepines indirectly enhance the sensitivity of the GABA receptors to its neurotransmitter.[14] Thus pharmacological evidence indicates that GABAergic neurons are involved in seizure susceptibility, sedation, and anxiety.

In contrast to the systems already described, which are components of the reticular core, the cortical GABAergic neurons are local circuit neurons. Their progenitors reside in the subcortical ventricular germinal zone, which generates immature GABAergic neurons throughout the period of cortical formation (consistent with the fact that the GABAergic neurons are located in virtually all cortical layers).[48] Thus the appearance of GABAergic neurons occurs much later in brain development than do the reticular core neurons; and GABAergic neuronal maturation coincides with the progressive differentiation of neurons within the cerebral cortex. Synaptic neurochemical studies, however, indicate that the biochemical components involved in the synthesis, release, and inactivation of GABA do not develop in a coordinate fashion as do the noradrenergic, serotonergic, and dopaminergic systems.[11] Curiously, the levels of GABA in the immature brain are disproportionately high in comparison to the relative activity of its synthetic enzyme, glutamic acid decarboxylase; and at early stages of development, the high-affinity uptake-inactivation process for GABA surpasses the activity in adulthood. In contrast, the postsynaptic GABA receptors and their modulatory benzodiazepine receptors exhibit a much more gradual developmental increase in the cerebral cortex. The physiological implications of the developmental disparities in the pre- and postsynaptic components of the GABAergic system remain unclear at present.

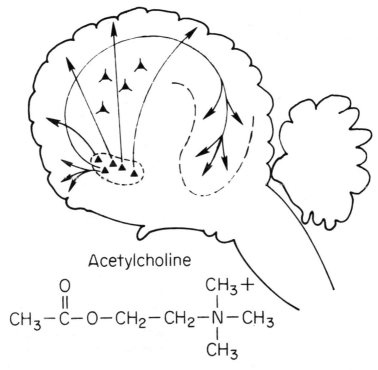

Acetylcholine

$$CH_3-\overset{\overset{\textstyle O}{\|}}{C}-O-CH_2-CH_2-\overset{\overset{\textstyle CH_3}{|}}{\underset{\underset{\textstyle CH_3}{|}}{N}}+CH_3$$

FIGURE 2–5
Cholinergic Neuronal Pathways

ENDOGENOUS OPIOID PEPTIDES

From recombinant DNA techniques, multiple endogenous opioid systems belonging to three genetically distinct families have been identified.[1,34,35] These are the (1) opiocortin (beta-endorphin, adrenocorticotrophic hormone [ACTH]), (2) enkephalin, and (3) dynorphin groups. Just as differences in function have been demonstrated between the monoamines previously discussed (the catecholaminergic and serotonergic systems), differences in opioid systems cannot be ignored. Less clear at this time is the issue of multiple opioid receptors. It remains to be established whether each family has its own receptor or whether a family can interact with more than one subtype and each subtype with more than one family.[1] An understanding of psychological effects will depend on· further clarification of the roles of the separate opioid families and receptor subtypes.

OPIOCORTIN SYSTEM

Derived from a larger peptide precursor, pro-opiomelanocortin, or POMC, contains one opioid peptide (beta-endorphin), ACTH, and potentially three melanocyte-stimulating hormone (MSH)–like peptides. These peptides are generated by the enzymatic cleavage of the larger precursor. In subprimate species, peptides from POMC have been found in several major brain sites. The primary site is the corticotrophes of the anterior lobe of the pituitary and all the cells of the pars intermedia. Within the brain, the main cell group is located in the region of the arcuate nucleus of the medial basal hypothalamus; its fibers project widely to areas of the limbic system and brain stem. Another group of brain POMC is found in the nucleus of the solitary tract and in the nucleus commissuralis. There is colocalization with NE and corticotropin-releasing factor (CRF) in brain stem nerve terminal areas. The endorphin systems appear to develop contemporaneously in the rat brain.[5] However, no correlation was found in regional distribution of developing endorphin and enkephalin systems. A developmental study of this system in the rat brain stem[2] indicates a twentyfold increase in total content of endorphin in the medulla, with minimal alterations in the concentration of beta-endorphin.

Enkephalins. Unlike POMC, the enkephalin precursor, pro-enkephalin, produces only active opioid peptides, seven copies of which are contained in its core. It is very widespread, with both endocrine and brain distribution. In the brain, these peptides are located in neuronal systems throughout the neuraxis, including cells of the cerebral cortex down to the spinal cord. Fiber tracts are being mapped and include local circuit and long-tract systems associated with pain, respiration, endocrine actions, motor activity, and limbic system functions. In the periphery, an apparently similar precursor is found in the adrenal medulla (with catecholamines) and in the gastrointestinal tract. Bayon and associates[5] indicate that developmentally local enkephalin interneurons frequently migrate and differentiate later than larger enkephalin neurons, which form neural pathways projecting over long distances.

Dynorphin/Neo-endorphin. Prodynorphin, the dynorphin/neo-endorphin precursor, produces three opioid peptides. They have been found in the brain, posterior pituitary, gastrointestinal tracts, and in several hypothalamic cell groups, and are widely scattered in the brain stem. Pathways identified to date include those from the supraoptic nucleus to the posterior pituitary.

Developing Neurotransmitter Systems and Human Psychopathology

The integration of our current knowledge on the development of brain neurotransmitter systems into concepts about the pathophysiology of major mental disorders must remain highly speculative at present, since conclusive evidence of the involvement of these specific neurotransmitter systems in any major mental disorder has yet to be established. Nevertheless, because of the clear role played by neurotransmitters in the mechanism of action of psychotropic drugs in several neuropsychiatric disorders, there would appear to be adequate justification for inferring neurotransmitter dysfunction in these disorders.

It seems appropriate that the noradrenergic neuronal system, which mediates arousal and anxiety, two primitive defenses necessary for survival, would appear at the earliest stages of brain development. Indeed, the noradrenergic system is represented in the brains of the lowest vertebrates on the phylogenetic tree. And it is clear that in the first year of development, arousal, fear of strangers, and separation anxiety emerge early in the infant's behavioral repertoire. The role of cortical noradrenergic input in modulating synaptic plasticity and modifiability early in development[32] provides a basis for a hypothesized relationship between affect-laden experiences in infancy and the establishment of the synaptic organization of the cerebral cortex.

Through the action of antidepressant drugs, the noradrenergic system has also been implicated in the pathophysiology of mood disorders. The last decade has witnessed mounting evidence of the occurrence of major depressive disorder not only in adolescents but also in prepubertal children.[36,46] These depressive episodes have the same cognitive and physiological features as those in adults, including anhedonia, suicidal preoccupation, and a high incidence of abnormal dexamethasone suppression tests.[46] Furthermore, mood disorders in children respond to antidepressant treatment in a manner similar to those in adults. Notably, the capability of developing severe mood disturbances may be present even in infancy, as evidenced by marasmus and anaclytic depression.

The serotonergic system, aside from its potential role in the mood disorders,[42] has long been implicated in the pathophysiology of infantile autism. Consistent with the early innervation of cortical and limbic structures by the serotonergic system, the symptoms of infantile autism appear within the first eighteen months of life. Over the last decade, there have been several reports of elevated levels of 5HT in whole blood in a significant number of individuals suffering from infantile autism.[63] Recently, Geller and his colleagues[21] have reported that fenfluramine hydrochloride, a drug that enhances central serotonergic neurotransmission, caused both behavioral as well as cognitive improvement in two children with infantile autism; however, this has not been confirmed by other investigators.[4] Whether or not this treatment proves useful, recent findings by Todd and Ciaranello[56] provide additional support for a role of central serotonergic dysfunction in some infantile autism patients. These investigators have demonstrated the presence of antibodies against brain 5HT receptor both in serum and in the cerebrospinal fluid (CSF). Seven of thirteen of the autistic individuals studied exhibited this receptor antibody, which was not found in a matched group of controls.

The dopaminergic system has long been considered to be involved in the pathophysiology of attention deficit disorder with hyperactivity.[58] Stimulants, such as d-amphetamine and methylphenidate hydrochloride, which reputedly enhance central dopaminergic neurotransmission, reduce activity and increase attention span in affected children. Paradoxically, neuroleptics that block the DA receptor can also reduce the hyperactivity, although their effects on cognition may be less salutory.[59] Shaywitz and his colleagues[52] have demonstrated in experimental animals that neonatal destruction of the dopaminergic neurons innervating the forebrain results in a marked enhancement of the normally increased motoric activity of prepubescent rat pups and that this hyperactivity can be reduced by administration of stimulants. However, Hunt, Minderaa, and

Cohen[29] have reported improvements in behavior with clonidine hydrochloride, an alpha$_2$adrenergic receptor agonist, suggesting that the role of DA systems may not be as specific as previously suggested.

The gradual development of striatal-limbic dopaminergic pathways may account for the age-related emergence of two disorders thought to involve enhanced dopaminergic neurotransmission: Tourette syndrome and schizophrenia. In the case of Tourette syndrome, symptoms typically emerge between five and twelve years of age with the appearance of hyperactivity, motor tics, and vocal tics that evolve over time. Since the symptoms of the disorder are exacerbated by stimulants that enhance dopaminergic neurotransmission and are attenuated by neuroleptics that block DA receptors, symptoms would likely emerge from the development of altered dopaminergic neurotransmission.[54] In light of evidence of decreased levels of the DA metabolite homovanillic acid (HVA) in the CSF of Tourette patients, there is reason to believe that the syndrome involves an increased post-synaptic response to DA, possibly due to a supersensitivity of the DA receptors.[54] With the recent, more restrictive definition of schizophrenia in childhood, it is apparent that this disorder represents an earlier age of onset of a disorder that is phenomenologically identical to that which typically has its onset in mid- to late adolescence. Thus the appearance of positive symptoms of schizophrenia, the symptoms most responsive to neuroleptic medications, occurs on an age-related continuum, beginning in childhood but peaking in late adolescence when DA levels in the forebrain have reached their apex.

Studies on the levels of biogenic amine metabolites in CSF provide an indirect assessment of neurotransmitter disposition in developing neurons. CSF levels of monoamine metabolites change with age from infancy throughout childhood until adulthood. Interestingly, levels are highest in infants[3] and decline with age.[51,53] As this pattern conflicts with the developmental profile for the endogenous amines in the brain, these changes provide indirect evidence of a reduction in neurotransmitter turnover with age but may also suggest reduced clearance of the metabolites from the toddlers' brain. Shaywitz and associates[53] noted a difference in ratio of 5HT to DA metabolites (5-hydroxyindoleacetic acid [5-HIAA]/HVA ratio) between a group of boys and girls with neurological disorders. Compared with boys, girls had a lower accumulation of the DA metabolite and a higher accumulation of the 5HT metabolite. The authors question whether these differences may relate to the increased prevalence of neuropsychiatric disorders such as Tourette syndrome, attention deficit disorder, and autism in boys during middle childhood compared to girls. Based on positron emission tomography (PET) scan studies, it has been determined that DA receptors reach their peak density by age eighteen in males.[62]

Clinical psychopharmacological and lesion studies in experimental animals have implicated the forebrain cholinergic projections in higher cognitive functions, especially memory. This finding has been strengthened by the demonstration of rather selective and striking impairments in cortical and hippocampal cholinergic integrity in Alzheimer's dementia.[14] Thus it appears more than coincidental that the postnatal development of cholinergic innervation to the cerebral cortex and hippocampal formation corresponds with the emergence, at the end of the first year of life, of complex cognitive functions such as speech and memory in the infant. Although there is little direct evidence at present to support the hypothesis, one must wonder whether dysfunction of selective aspects of cortical cholinergic projections might not contribute to hereditary and acquired learning disorders. In this regard, evidence has accumulated of rather selective cortical cholinergic deficits in middle-aged individuals with Down's syndrome who exhibit the neuropathology of Alzheimer's disease.[45] While the functional integrity of these cholinergic pathways in younger Down's individuals whose brains do not exhibit the pathology of Alzheimer's disease remains to be determined, there is pharmacological evidence of a compromised cholinergic system even in young Down's syndrome patients.[26] Furthermore, studies on the fetal brain of a mouse that suffers from trisomy of the genes coded on chromosome 21 in man indicate a developmental failure of the cholinergic neurons.[55]

As the potential role of brain endogenous opioid systems in human psychopathology remains highly speculative at present and the development of these systems has not yet been adequately characterized, it is not possible to link them to the emergence of psychiatric symptoms except in one area. Self-injurious behavior is a frequent complication of severe and profound mental retardation. Because of the critical role of the endogenous opioid systems in pain perception and stress-induced analgesia, several authors[49] have proposed that secondary abnormalities in the endogenous opioid systems might be responsible for the maintenance of certain forms of self-injurious behavior.

Conclusion

Over the last decade, considerable advances have been made in our understanding of the neuroanatomic and neurochemical process of brain development. These advances have occurred in the context of a rapid expansion in the identification and characterization of the substances involved in chemical synaptic neurotransmission. While information is regrettably scanty with regard to the development of neurotransmitter systems in the human and subhuman primate brain, neuroanatomic studies suggest a general validity for extrapolation from observations in the rodent. Current findings point to intriguing relationships between the development of components of the reticular core neuronal systems and the emergence of age-related behavioral and psychiatric disorders. These relationships provide heuristically valuable leads that may assist us in better understanding the pathophysi-

ology of psychiatric disorders. In addition, they suggest ways in which early developmental experiences may affect cortical maturation and provide an experimental context to integrate the biopsychosocial approach to psychiatry.

ACKNOWLEDGMENTS

Joseph T. Coyle, M.D., receives support from the Surdna Foundation, the McKnight Foundation, and a National Institute of Mental Health Research Career Development Award (MH-00125). The excellent secretarial assistance of Deborah Culp is gratefully acknowledged.

REFERENCES

1. AKIL, H., et al. "Endogenous Opioids: Biology and Function," *Annual Review of Neuroscience,* 7 (1984):223–255.

2. ALESSI, N. E., and KHACHATURIAN, H. "Postnatal Development of Beta-Endorphin Immunoreactivity in the Medulla Oblongata of Rat," *Neuropeptides,* 5 (1985):473–476.

3. ANDERSON, G. M., et al. "Neurotransmitter Precursors and Metabolites in CSF of Human Neonates," *Developmental Medicine and Child Neurology,* 27 (1985):207–214.

4. AUGUST, G., et al. "Fenfluramine Treatment in Infantile Autism. Neurochemical, Electrophysiological and Behavioral Effects," *Journal of Nervous and Mental Disease,* 172 (1984): 604–612.

5. BAYON, A. "Perinatal Development of the Endorphin and Enkephalin Containing System in the Rat Brain," *Brain Research,* 179 (1979):93–101.

6. BLACK, I. B. "Stages of Neurotransmitter Development in Autonomic Neurons," *Science,* 215 (1982):1198–1204.

7. BROWN, S. L. "The Developmental Cycle of Families: Clinical Implications," *Psychiatric Clinics of North America,* 3 (1980):369–381.

8. CAVINESS V. S., and RAKIC P. "Mechanisms of Cortical Development: A View from Mutations in Mice," *Annual Review Neuroscience,* 1 (1978):297–326.

9. COOPER, J., BLOOM, F. E., and ROTH, R. *The Biochemical Basis of Neuropharmacology.* New York: Oxford University Press, 1983.

10. COYLE, J. T. "Introduction to the World of Neurotransmitters and Neuroreceptors," in R. F. Hales and A. J. Frances, eds., *Annual Review,* vol 4. Washington, D.C.: American Psychiatric Press, 1985, pp. 3–97.

11. COYLE, J. T., and ENNA, S. J. "Neurochemical Aspects of the Ontogenesis of GABAergic Neurons in the Rat Brain," *Brain Research,* 111 (1976):119–133.

12. COYLE, J. T., and MOLLIVER, M. E. "Major Innervation of Newborn Rat Cortex by Monoaminergic Neurons," *Science,* 196 (1977):444–447.

13. COYLE, J. T., and YAMAMURA, H. "Neurochemical Aspects of the Ontongenesis of Cholinergic Neurons in the Rat Brain," *Brain Research,* 118 (1976):429–440.

14. COYLE, J. T., PRICE, D., and DELONG, M. R. "Alzheimer's Disease: A Disorder of Cortical Cholinergic Innervation," *Science,* 219 (1983):1184–1190.

15. ENGEL, G. "The Need for a New Medical Model: A Challenge for Biomedicine," *Science,* 196 (1977):129–136.

16. ENNA, S. J., and GALLAGHER, J. P. "Biochemical and Electrophysiologic Characteristics of Mammalian GABA Receptors," *International Review of Neurobiology,* 24 (1983): 181–212.

17. ERIKSON, E. H. *Childhood and Society.* New York: W. W. Norton, 1950.

18. FREUD, A. "The Concept of Developmental Lines," *Psychoanalytical Study of the Child,* 18 (1963):245–266.

19. ———. *Normality and Pathology in Childhood.* London: Hogarth Press, 1966.

20. FREUD, S. "Analysis of a Phobia in a Five Year Old Boy," in J. Strachey, ed., *The Standard Edition of the Complete Psychological Works of Sigmund Freud,* vol. 10. London: Hogarth Press, 1958, pp. 3–153. (Originally published 1909.)

21. GELLER, E., et. al. "Preliminary Observations on the Effect of Fenfluramine on Blood Serotonin and Symptoms in Three Autistic Boys," *New England Journal of Medicine,* 307 (1983):165–168.

22. GESELL., A., and AMATRUDA, C. S. *Developmental Diagnosis.* New York: Paul B. Hoeber, 1947.

23. GINSBERG, H., and OPPER, S. *Piaget's Theory of Intellectual Development: An Introduction.* Englewood Cliffs, N.J.: Prentice-Hall, 1969.

24. GOLDMAN-RAKICK, P. S., and BROWN, R. M. "Postnatal Development of Monoamine Content and Activity in the Cerebral Cortex of Rhesus Monkeys," *Developmental Brain Research,* 4 (1982):339–349.

25. GRAYBIEL, A. M., et al. "Direct Demonstration of a Correspondence Between Dopamine Islands and Acetylcholinesterase Patches in the Developing Striatum," *Proceedings of the National Academy of Science* (USA), 78 (1981): 5871–5875. 1981.

26. HARRIS, W. S., and GOODMAN, R. M. "Hyper-reactivity to Atropine in Down's Syndrome," *New England Journal of Medicine,* 279 (1968):407–410.

27. HOKFELT, T., et. al. "Peptidergic Neurons," *Nature* (London), 284 (1980):515–521.

28. HORNJIKIEWICZ, O. "Dopamine and Brain Function," *Pharmacologic Reviews,* 18 (1966):925–964.

29. HUNT, R. D., MINDERAA, R., and COHEN, D. J.

"Clonidine Benefits Children with Attention Deficit Disorder," *Journal of the American Academy of Child Psychiatry*, 24 (1985):617–629.

30. JACOBSON, M. *Developmental Neurobiology*. New York: Plenum Press, 1978.

31. JOHNSTON, M. V., GRZANNA, R., and COYLE, J. T. "Abnormally Dense Noradrenergic Innervation of Rat Neocortex Follows Fetal Treatment with Methyazoxymethanol," *Science*, 203 (1979):435–469.

32. KASAMATSU, T., and PETTIGREW, J. D. "Depletion of Brain Catecholamines: Failure of Ocular Dominance Shift After Monoculary Occlusion in Kittens," *Science*, 194 (1976): 206–209.

33. KATZ, D. M., et al. "Expression of Catecholaminergic Characteristics by Primary Sensory Neurons In the Normal Adult Rat *in vivo*," *Proceedings of the National Academy of Science* (USA), 80 (1983):3526–3530.

34. KHACHATURIAN, H., et al. "Anatomy of the CNS Opioid Systmes," *Trends in Neuroscience*, March (1985): 111–119.

35. KNIGGE, K. M., and JOSEPH, S. A. Anatomy of the Opioid-Systems of the Brain. *Canadian Journal of Neurological Sciences*, 11 (1984):14–23.

36. KOVACS, M., et al. "Depressive Disorders in Childhood: A Longitudinal Study of the Risk for a Subsequent Major Depression," *Archives of General Psychiatry*, 41 (1984):643–649.

37. LAUDER, J. M., and BLOOM, F. E. "Ontogeny of Monoamine Neurons in the Locus Coeruleus, Raphe Nuclei and Substantia Nigra of the Rat," *Journal of Comparative Neurology*, 155 (1974):469–482.

38. LAUDER, J. M., and KREBS, H. "Effects of p-chlorophenylalamine on Time of Neuronal Origin During Embryogenesis in the Rat," *Brain Research*, 107 (1976):638–644.

39. LIDOV, H., and MOLLIVER, M. E. "An Immunocytochemical Study of the Development of Serotonergic Neurons in the Rat CNS," *Brain Research Bulletin*, 8 (1982):389–430.

40. MOLLIVER, M. E., et al. "Monoamine Systems in Cerebral Cortex," in S. Palay and V. Chan-Palay, eds., *Cytochemical Methods in Neuroanatomy*. New York: Alan R. Liss, 1982, pp. 255–277.

41. MORAL-MAROGER, A. "Effects of Levodopa on Frontal Signs in Parkinsonism," *British Medical Journal*, 2 (1977):1543.

42. MURPHY, D. L., CAMPBELL, I., and COSTA, J. L. "Current Status of the Indolamine Hypothesis of Affective Disorders," in M. A. Lipton, A. DiMascio, and K. F. Killam, eds., *Psychopharmacology: A Generation of Progress*. New York: Raven Press, 1978, pp. 1235–1248.

43. PATTERSON, P. H. "Environmental Determination of Autonomic Neurotransmitter Functions," *Annual Review of Neuroscience*, 1 (1978):1–17.

44. PIAGET, J. "The Stages of Intellectual Development of the Child," *Bulletin of the Menninger Clinic*, 26 (1962):120–128.

45. PRICE, D. L., et al. "Alzheimer's Disease and Down's Syndrome," *Annals of the New York Academy of Science*, 396 (1982):145–164.

46. PUIG-ANTICH, J., and WESTON, B. "The Diagnosis and Treatment of Major Depressive Disorder in Childhood," *Annual Review of Medicine*, 34 (1983):231–245.

47. RAKIC, P. "Neuronal Migration and Contact Guidance in Primate Telencephalon," *Postgraduate Medical Journal*, 54 (1978):25–40.

48. RIBAK, C. "Aspinous and Sparsely-spinous Stellate Neurons in the Visual Cortex of Rats Contain Glutamic Acidic Decarboxylase," *Neurocytology*, 7 (1978):461–478.

49. RICHARDSON, J. S., and ZALESKI, W. A. "Naloxone and Self-Mutilation," *Biological Psychiatry*, 18 (1983):99–101.

50. RUTTER, M. "Psychological Sequelae of Brain Damage in Children," *American Journal of Psychiatry*, 138 (1981):-1533–1544

51. SEIFERT, W. E., FOX, J. L., and BUTLER, I. J. "Age Effects on Dopamine and Serotonin Metabolite Levels in Cerebrospinal Fluid," *Annals of Neurology*, 8 (1980):38–42.

52. SHAYWITZ, B. A., et al. "Paradoxical Response to Amphetamine in Developing Rats Treated with 6-hydroxydopamine," *Nature*, 261 (1976):153–155.

53. SHAYWITZ, B. A., et al. "Ontogeny of Dopamine and Serotonin Metabolites in the Cerebrospinal Fluid of Children with Neurological Disorders," *Developmental Medicine and Child Neurology*, 22 (1980):748–754.

54. SINGER, H. S., et al. "Dopamine Dysfunction in Tourette Syndrome," *Annals of Neurology*, 12 (1982):361–366.

55. SINGER, H. S., et al. "Morphologic and Neurochemical Studies of Embryonic Brain Development in Murine Trisomy 16," *Developmental Brain Research*, 15 (1984):155–166.

56. TODD, R. D., and CIARANELLO, R. D. "Demonstration of Inter- and Intraspecies Differences in Serotonin Binding Sites by Antibodies from an Autistic Child," *Proceedings of the National Academy of Science* (USA), 82 (1985):612–616.

57. VANPRAAG, H. M. "Depression, Suicide and the Metabolism of Serotonin in the Brain," *Journal of Affective Disorders*, 4 (1982):275–290.

58. WENDER, P. "Hypothesis for a Possible Biochemical Basis of Minimal Brain Dysfunction," in R. M. Knights and D. J. Baker, eds., *Neuropsychology of Learning Disorders*. Baltimore: University Park Press, 1976, pp. 126–142.

59. WERRY, J. S., and AMAN, M. G. "Methylphenidate and Haloperidol in Children: Effects on Attention, Memory and Activity," *Archives of General Psychiatry*, 32 (1975):-790–796.

60. WHITE, R. "Competence and the Psychosexual Stages of Development," in *Nebraska Symposium on Motivation*. Lincoln: University of Nebraska Press, 1960, pp. 97–141.

61. WISE, R. A. "Neuroleptics and Operant Behavior: The Anhedonia Hypothesis," *Behavioral & Brain Sciences*, 5 (1982):39–87.

62. WONG, D. F., et al. "Effects of Age on Dopamine and Serotonin Receptors Measured by Positron Tomography in the Living Human Brain," *Science*, 226 (1984):1393–1396.

63. YOUNG, J. G., et al. "Clinical Neurochemistry of Autism and Associated Disorders," *Journal of Autism and Developmental Disorders*, 12 (1982):147–156.

3 / Endocrine Factors in Fetal Development

H. David Mosier, Jr.

Neuroendocrine–Adenohypophysical System

In the human fetus the definitive anatomic structures of the hypothamo-hypophyseal system are well established by midgestation.[38] Secretory function closely follows the morphological development of the system. Thyrotropin-releasing hormone (TRH), gonadotropin-releasing hormone (GnRH), and growth hormone release-inhibiting hormone (SRIH) can be identified in the hypothalamus as early as eight to ten weeks of gestation.[38] Secretory granules are present in pituitary cells by ten to twelve weeks. By this time the presence of growth hormone (GH), follicle-stimulating hormone (FSH), luteinizing hormone (LH), thyrotropin (TSH), adrenocorticotropin (ACTH), prolactin (PRL), oxytocin, vasotocin, and vasopressin have been demonstrated in the pituitary.[21] Recent observations indicate that early in fetal development blood levels of GH, LH, FSH, TSH, and ACTH are relatively high; this demonstrates that maturation of the normal central nervous system inhibition of anterior pituitary secretion occurs later in fetal life or after birth.[38]

Control of Fetal Growth

In addition to GH, insulin and a number of recently discovered peptides are known to influence postnatal growth; however, the role of these substances in fetal life is still unclear. Results of fetal decapitation experiments in animals indicate that during gestation, pituitary GH is not required for growth[9,30,34,68]; indeed, in the human, pituitary aplasia and hypoplasia have been associated with normal fetal growth.[4,45] Humans with anencephaly approach normal size at birth.[49] This is frequently cited as the human counterpart of the decapitation experiments, but the presence of pituitary tissue in the majority of anencephalics[2] leaves open the

possibility that even under such circumstances, the pituitary may continue to function to some extent (see the next section).

Circumstantial evidence supports a significant role for insulin in fetal growth. This is based on observations of fetal overgrowth in hyperinsulinemia, a well-known example of which is the infant of the diabetic mother. Other fetal hyperinsulinemic states are also associated with overgrowth.[27,58] The converse, decreased fetal growth, has occurred in hypoinsulinemia[27] and in insulin-resistant states.[18,59] The growth-promoting actions of insulin—for example, increased protein synthesis—are well established, but the role of insulin in fetal growth is not clear. Somatomedin-C (IGF-I, insulinlike growth factor-I), a peptide capable of stimulating cartilage growth functions *in vivo*, has been shown to be GH-dependent postnatally. (For a review, see Daughaday.[13]) Various fetal tissues have been shown to produce somatomedin-C in organ culture in the rodent.[17] In various mammalian species, other growth factors such as insulinlike growth factor-II (IGF-II), epithelial growth factor (EGF), platelet-derived growth factor (PDGF), multiplication stimulating activity (MSA, equivalent to rat IGF-II), fibroblast growth factor (FGF), and nerve growth factor (NGF) have growth-stimulating effects. This is only a partial list of known factors; it is likely that others will be discovered. A full discussion of the status of this field is beyond the scope of this chapter. At present, the role of the peptide growth factors and their mechanisms of action in fetal development in animals and humans are not well understood. (For a review, see Underwood and D'Ercole[69])

Thyrotropin–Releasing Hormone and Thyrotropin

Fetal TSH has been reported low in cord serum of anencephalic infants,[1,38] suggesting that the pituitary is dependent on an intact hypothalamus.[21] However, in three recently studied anencephalic infants, TSH levels in cord blood were normal at birth, indicating that pituitary TSH secreting cells were present and were receiving TRH stimulation. Injection of TRH into the cysts of the amorphous cerebral tissue of the anencephalic infants was shown to evoke TSH release, indicating that extrahypothalamic transport to the hypophysial vessels may occur in this malformation.[55]

Although TRH was first identified as a factor causing TSH release, in some pathological states it has been shown to promote GH release. (For a review, see Mosier.[46]) Intravenous administration of TRH to term pregnant women resulted first in a progressive rise and then in a fall of cord blood GH levels. This suggests that TRH that crosses the placenta[60] is capable of stimulating GH release by the fetus.[61]

The ability to degrade TRH is undetectable in cord blood at term. After three days of life, however, it appears, and by five days of age it reaches adult levels. The role of this phenomenon is unknown.[3] It is well known that within thirty minutes after birth TSH is abruptly released and rapidly peaks, and that plasma levels of triiodothyronine (T_3) and thyroxine (T_4) continue to increase, with peaks occurring twenty-four to forty-eight hours after birth.

Oxytocin and Vasopressin

Vasopressin, oxytocin, and their related neurophysins (specific binding proteins) have been demonstrated in the hypothalamus and pituitary gland of midtrimester human fetuses. Vasopressin is present in the tissues of both organs approximately three to four weeks before oxytocin. In the pituitary gland, the levels of the hormones increase greatly over the next three to four months. Vasopressin and oxytocin neurophysins appear in the pituitary gland at about the same gestational age.[6] The concentrations of the nonapeptides, oxytocin and vasopressin, in fetal blood appear to increase with increasing gestational age.[21] At the time of delivery measurements of antidiuretic hormone (ADH) in cord arterial blood by radioimmunoassay showed concentrations fifty times the basal adult level. Plasma ADH decreased rapidly within an hour after birth; indeed, during the first day of life, its concentration usually fell to adult basal levels.

In a recent study, plasma oxytocin levels in the umbilical artery exceeded umbilical venous levels in newborns born of cesarean section ($p < 0.05$) and after labor, although the results after labor were not statistically significant.[42] Following delivery of a paraplegic woman, plasma oxytocin values were found to be much

higher in the infant than in the mother. It was thought that fetal oxytocins may have contributed to maternal uterine contractions.[14]

In stressed babies and babies subjected to difficult deliveries, ADH levels in plasma are reported to be increased.[43] Animal experiments indicate that plasma vasopressin concentration correlates inversely with fetal oxygenation.[62]

Thyroid Gland

In the human the formation of follicles by the fetal thyroid gland begins at about eight weeks of gestation. The ratio of thyroid weight to body weight attains the mature level at about ten weeks of gestation. After seventy-four days of gestation, upon administration of radioiodine, a full spectrum of organically bound iodinated products is observable in the human fetal thyroid. Fetal thyrotrophs appears as early as thirteen weeks of gestation, at about the time the thyroid gland begins to trap iodine. The typical polyhedral thyrotroph does not appear until about twenty-eight weeks. During very early stages of thyroid development, the gland appears to be self-differentiating and not under the influence of the pituitary. Maturation of the pituitary thyroid system occurs about midgestation. (For a review, see Mosier.[46])

Late in pregnancy the placenta has been observed to be nearly impermeable to the passage of thyroid hormone.[21] This has led to a widely held view that the fetus depends on its own thyroid gland for its main supply of hormone. There are few data bearing on placental crossover of thyroid hormone during early pregnancy. However, the sensitivity of embryonic tissues to the growth-stimulating effects of T_4 has been well established, as has the capability of thyroid hormone to stimulate the metabolic and differentiating functions of cells and organs in culture. That fetal tissues are highly susceptible to the influence of thyroid hormone suggests the possibility that small amounts, even traces, of thyroid hormone crossing the placenta during early fetal life may play a role in fetal growth. (For a review, see Mosier.[46])

Reverse triiodothyronine (rT_3) levels are increased in fetal serum relative to the adult. A significant negative correlation exists between rT_3 and gestational age.[29] In a recent study, the concentration of rT_3 in cord blood was found to have no correlation with concentrations of T_3, T_4, and TSH.[7] Moreover, when the cord blood rT_3 values of hypothyroid and normal newborns were measured, the overlap was so great that it eliminated any advantage of this test over screening of T_4 in the detection of neonatal hypothyroidism.[39] There is a significant decrease in rT_3 concentration from eight to fifty days of age.[50]

Parathyroid Gland, Calcitonin, Calcium, Phosphorus, and Vitamin D

The parathyroid glands differentiate between five and fourteen weeks of gestation; this suggests that fetal calcium metabolism is under hormonal influence.[20] Parathyroid hormone (PTH) appears to be present by twelve to thirteen weeks.[64] In the neonate the thyroid gland contains prominent C-cells containing calcitonin in tissue concentrations greater than the adult level.[71] Fetal accretion rates of calcium and phosphorus are approximately 150 mg and 96 mg per kg, respectively.[72]

After parturition, the main function of vitamin D is to enhance intestinal absorption of calcium and phosphorus. (For reviews, see DeLuca[16] and Fraser.[22]) In the fetus, the principal supply of vitamin D appears to be from the mother. The active form of the vitamin is $1,25\text{-}(OH)_2D$, which is formed by 25-hydroxylation in the liver and 1-hydroxylation in the kidneys. The circulating concentration of $1,25\text{-}(OH)_2D$ is regulated according to the body's needs for calcium and phosphorus. Another chemical variant, $24,25\text{-}(OH)_2D$, is also found in the circulation; its function remains to be established.[16,22] The fetus has a high potential for synthesis of $1,25\text{-}(OH)_2D$ as evidenced by a rapid increase of this substance to high levels in the blood of premature infants placed on a low-calcium, low-phosphorus intake.[44]

It has been shown that exposure to light decreases pineal melatonin synthesis; presumably this comes about through stimulation of photoreceptors of the pineal by light transmitted through the cranium.[15] Recent work has shown that melatonin administration in newborn rats prevents the hypocalcemic response to light. This finding supports the hypothesis that hypocalcemia during phototherapy in the human neonate results from transcranial photic inhibition of melatonin synthesis.[26]

Adrenal Cortex

The human adrenal cortex begins to differentiate about the fourth week of gestation. At that time it is composed predominantly of acidophilic cells. In the fifth week, a smaller basophilic cell appears, spreads over the acidophilic cells, and forms the definitive cortex. The initial layer becomes the fetal zone. In fetuses between six and seventeen weeks of gestation, ultrastructural studies indicate that the definitive cortex is inactive but that the fetal zone appears to be active. The relative prominance of the fetal zone increases throughout pregnancy; during the last trimester it comprises approximately 80 percent of the cortex. However, there is an almost complete involution of the fetal zone during the first month of postnatal life. (For a review, see Orti.[51])

Between twelve and twenty-two weeks, the fetal adrenal cortex is capable of full synthesis of cortisol from acetate.[5] However, the function of the fetal adrenal cortex is not well understood; it has been shown in fetal animals that the adrenal cortex influences the size of thymus and the deposition of glycogen in the liver and myocardium. (For reviews, see Jost.[35,36]) However, experiments in rabbits and rats have established that in those species the adrenal cortex is not required for fetal growth.[37]

Both the fetal adrenal cortex and the placenta are actively steroidogenic. However, the steroid spectrum secreted by the fetal adrenal differs from that of the adult gland. The principal differences result from a deficiency of 3-beta-hydroxysteroid dehydrogenase (3-B-HSD) and from the capability of the fetal adrenal for 16-hydroxylation. The placenta produces pregnenolone and progesterone from circulating cholesterol which are then utilized by the fetal adrenal as precursors for corticosteroid synthesis. The placenta also carries out important steroid transformations, one example of which is conversion of 16-alpha-hydroxydehydroandrosterone sulfate to estriol sulfate, the principal estrogen of the fetal circulation. Based on the predictable surge at around thirty-six weeks of gestation, plasma estriol has been used to time gestational age. However, a recent study showed only 66 percent accuracy in this prediction.[32] The placenta transfers corticosteroids as well as estrogens from mother to fetus, and possibly androgens from fetus to mother. The fetus conjugates most steroids in its circulation as sulfates; the placenta splits the sulfates and transfers the steroids to the maternal circulation. (For a review, see Orti.[51])

In late pregnancy, whether or not labor takes place, there appears to be a rise in the fetal level of cortisol with gestational age. This rise is steepest immediately before the normal time of onset of labor and cannot be attributed to the stress associated with labor.[47]

Desoxycorticosterone sulfate and desoxycorticosterone are synthesized in the human fetal kidney in high concentration. These steroids are found in the fetal blood; the kidney may be an important site for their formation.[8]

In prenatal and early postnatal life, total cortisol and cortisol binding globulin are low; indeed, except for elevated values immediately after birth, free cortisol values are not significantly different from those of normal adults.[66] Dehydroepiandrosterone sulfate concentration in fetal plasma increases coincidentally with fetal adrenal growth. The rapid increase in maternal estrogen levels near term can be explained by an increased availability of the fetal precursor dehydroepiandrosterone sulfate.[52] Controversy exists as to whether cortisol acts physiologically to accelerate human fetal lung maturation, but recent evidence indicates that there is a link between fetal lung maturation and fetal steroid production.[48]

In a recent study, full-term newborns had higher cord artery blood ACTH concentration after vaginal delivery than after cesarean section; this indicates that the fetal anterior pituitary is capable of responding to partial stress.[57] The fetal pituitary also appears to be responsible for the maintenance of the fetal zone. (For a review, see Lanman.[41]) In addition, other factors may play a role in the growth of the fetal adrenal. Proliferation of human fetal adrenal cells *in vitro* has been shown to be responsive to either fibroblast growth factor or epidermal growth factor.[12]

Adrenal Medulla and Autonomic Nervous System

During the fifth week of gestation, neural crest cells migrate toward the region behind the dorsal aorta and form the segmentally arranged sympathetic ganglia. Cells originating in the sympathetic system invade the developing adrenal cortex and arrange themselves in the cords and clusters that give rise to the adrenal medulla.[40] These specialized cells stain brownish with chromic acid salts, hence the term chromaffin cells. Clusters of chromaffin cells also locate in close proximity to each of the chain ganglia, where they are known as paraganglionic chromaffin bodies, or paraganglia. At birth the paraganglia are approximately a millimeter in diameter; thereafter, they tend to become smaller. Several small masses of chromaffin cells aggregate in the region of the abdominal sympathetic plexus near the root of the mesenteric artery. One of the larger and more caudally located of these masses is the so-called aortic chromaffin body (organ of Zuckerkandl).

The largest and most constant masses of chromaffin tissue are those that form the adrenal medulla.[53] By ten to twelve weeks the paired adrenal medullary masses are well developed.[24] Coincident with the chromaffin reaction, catecholamines can be measured in the extraadrenal tissues of the human fetus.[11] Extramedullary chromaffin tissue contains only norepinephrine, while epinephrine is found in the adrenal medulla as early as the 130 mm stage (approximately sixteen weeks gestation).[25]

There is little information on how control of catecholamine secretion develops in the human. By term, the human fetus is capable of responding to hypoglycemia and to cold exposure with increased epinephrine secretion.[58] However, catecholamine responses figure prominently in the adaptation of the neonate to the extrauterine environment. (For reviews, see Hill[27] and Phillippe.[56]) Epinephrine secretion in the adrenal seems to be dependent on the development of adrenal splanchnic innervation; norepinephrine secretion presumably occurs through direct stimulation of norepinephrine cells—for example, by hypoxia.[10,33]

Pancreas, Insulin, and Glucagon

The pancreas differentiates at about the fourth week of gestation. The specific secretory products of the primordial tissue include hydrolytic enzymes and insulin; these can be recognized before differentiation of exocrine or islet beta-cells is evident. By the time the islet can be distinguished, well-differentiated alpha-cells containing glucagon granules are present. The alpha-cells predominate early in gestation, but by the time of birth the alpha-to-beta cell ratio is approximately 1. (For a review, see Sperling.[65]) Insulin concentration in the fetal pancreas is higher than in the adult. In spite of this, fetal insulin response to glucose is relatively blunted[28]; however, it shows an increase with increasing fetal age. Insulin responses of infants of gestationally diabetic mothers are enhanced, suggesting that hyperglycemia may accelerate the maturation of the insulin secretory mechanism. With respect to insulin biosynthesis and release, the pancreatic islet cells isolated from fetuses of diabetic mothers are glucose sensitive whereas the islets of fetuses of nondiabetic women are not.[31] It is well known that there is a marked increase in fetal growth and fat deposition in the infants of diabetic mothers; these data are highly suggestive of a role that insulin plays in fetal metabolism. (For a review, see Sperling.[65]) Specific functions ascribed to insulin have been shown in fetal tissues in *in vitro* studies, but *in vivo* functions are not well delineated.

As fetal age advances, the human fetal pancreas contains glucagon in increasing quantities. The metabolic functions of glucagon in the fetus are not known. *In vitro* studies indicate that glucagon may influence organogenesis by increasing cyclic adenosine monophosphate (AMP) in tissues. (For a review, see Sperling.[65]) Gastrin and gastric inhibitory polypeptide (GIP) have been demonstrated in the human pancreas at fetal ages of twelve to forty-one weeks. GIP immunoreactive cells were observed in fetuses of gestational ages of eighteen to twenty weeks. No gastrin-immunoreactive cells were observed.[19]

Gonads and Sex Differentiation

The gonads are derived from primordial germ cells, the coelomic epithelium and the mesonephric mesenchyme. Differentiation of the primordial gonad can follow either of two routes; its conversion into testis depends on the presence of a gene probably located in the Y chromosome. In the absence of a Y chromosome, for a time the gonad remains undifferentiated; it then proceeds to differentiate into an ovary. Where testicular differentiation does take place, Leydig cells appear early and produce androgen; this in turn induces male differentiation of the mesonephric duct, the accessory sex glands, the external genitalia, and the neuroendocrine system. Synthesis and secretion of androgens by the testis are evident by eight weeks, and the testes descend at six months of fetal age. By way of contrast, the female genital system differentiates without known hormonal control by the ovary. Around seven weeks, medullary cords appear in the fetal ovary, and one week later, estrogen synthesis by the ovary is evident. Oogonal meiosis begins about the twelfth week. (For reviews, see Pelliniemi and Dym[54]; Schlegel[63]; and Stempfel.[67])

In the fetus, it is convenient to stage the progression of sex differentiation as (1) genetic sex, (2) gonadal sex, and (3) genital sex. Organization of testicular cords begins around six weeks of fetal age. Genetic sex is determined most commonly by chromosomal karyotyping. Recent work has shown that several genes located on the X and Y chromosomes are involved in sex differentiation of the gonad. The X chromosome contains genes for ovarian differentiation. (For a review, see Pelliniemi and Dym.[54]) The short arm of the Y chromosome appears to contain the testis-organizing gene, the H-Y (histocompatibility-Y) antigen. Differentiation of the external genitalia is determined principally by the presence or absence of testosterone. Normal male differentiation also requires secretion of the nonsteroidal müllerian-inhibitory factor by the fetal testis.[70] Under the influence of testosterone, fusion of the urogenital folds and enlargement of the genital tubercle begin during the third fetal month. Male external genitalia are completely differentiated late in the fourth fetal month.

Ambiguous Sex Development

In the female, or in fetuses lacking testes, the urogenital folds remain unfused and the genital tubercle fails to enlarge. Fetal testicular insufficiency or excessive androgen stimulation in the female will result in partial masculinization of the internal and external genitalia. The timing of the disturbance is obviously an important factor in determining the anatomical pattern of ambiguous development of the genital ducts and external genitalia. (For reviews, see Patten[53]; Schlegel[63]; and Stempfel.[67])

Placenta

Most of the information available on the endocrine aspects of placental function results from animal studies. These indicate impermeability to passage of GH, ACTH, LH, and TSH. Minimal transfer of vasopressin, insulin, glucagon, parathyroid hormone, and calcitonin may occur. The placenta appears to be permeable to most adrenal corticosteroids, aldosterone, progesterone, androgens, and estrogens. Passage of thyroid hormones is minimal (see the section entitled "Thyroid Gland"). (For a review, see Fisher.[21])

Hormone production in the human feto-placental unit has been extensively investigated. The placenta synthesizes peptides that are structurally homologous to pituitary hormones or hypothalamic-releasing factors. The list includes placental lactogen, chorionic gonadotropin, prolactin, and LH-releasing factor. The placenta also participates in steroidogenesis and synthesizes nerve growth factor. (For a review, see Underwood and D'Ercole.[69]) Regulation of placental hormone production is poorly understood. In placental tissue culture, various adrenal metabolites have inhibited progesterone production, whereas LH-releasing hormone has inhibited both estrogen and progesterone biosynthesis. Thus placental steroidogenesis can be influenced by both fetal and placental factors.[23]

ACKNOWLEDGMENT

Work on this chapter was supported in part by grant HD 07074 from the National Institutes of Health.

REFERENCES

1. ALLEN, J. P., et al. "Endocrine Function in an Anencephalic Infant," *Journal of Clinical Endocrinology and Metabolism,* 38 (1974):94–98.

2. ANGEVINE, D. M. "Pathologic Anatomy of Hypophysis and Adrenals in Anencephaly," *Archives of Pathology,* 26 (1938):507–518.

3. ARATAN-SPIRE, S., and CZERNICHOW, P. "Thyrotropin-releasing Hormone-degrading Activity of Neonatal Human Plasma," *Journal of Clinical Endocrinology and Metabolism,* 50 (1980):88–92.

4. BLIZZARD, R M., and ALBERTS, M. "Hypopituitarism, Hypoadrenalism, and Hypogonadism in the Newborn Infant," *Journal of Pediatrics,* 48 (1956):782–792.

5. BLOCK, E., and BENERSCHKE, K. "Synthesis *in vitro* of Steroids by Human Fetal Adrenal Gland Slices," *Journal of Biological Chemistry,* 234 (1959):1085–1089.

6. BURFORD, G. D., and ROBINSON, I. C. "Oxytocin, Vasopressin and Neurophysins in the Hypothalamo-neurohypophysial System of the Human Fetus," *Journal of Endocrinology,* 95 (1982):403–408.

7. BYFIELD, P. G., et al. "Reverse Triiodothyronine, Thyroid Hormone, and Thyrotrophin Concentrations in Placental Cord Blood," *Archives of Disease in Childhood,* 53 (1978): 620–624.

8. CASEY, M. L., et al. "Deoxycorticosterone Sulfate Biosynthesis in Human Fetal Kidney," *Journal of Clinical Endocrinology and Metabolism,* 53 (1981):990–996.

9. CHEZ, R. A., et al. "Some Effects of Fetal and Maternal Hypophysectomy in Pregnancy," *American Journal of Obstetrics and Gynecology,* 108 (1970):643–650.

10. COMLINE, R. S., and SILVER, M. "Development of Activity in the Adrenal Medulla of the Foetus and New-born Animal," *British Medical Bulletin,* 22 (1966):16–20.

11. COUPLAND, R. E. *The Natural History of the Chromaffin Cell.* London: Longmans, Green, 1965.

12. CRICKARE, K., ILL, C. R., and JAFFE, R. B. "Control and Proliferation of Human Fetal Adrenal Cells *in vitro,*" *Journal of Clinical Endocrinology and Metabolism,* 53 (1981):790–796.

13. DAUGHADAY, W. H. "Growth Hormone and the Somatomedins," in W. H. Daughaday, ed., *Endocrine Control of Growth.* New York: Elsevier, 1981, pp. 1–24.

14. DAWOOD, M. Y., and FUCHS, F. "Maternal and Fetal Oxytocin Levels at Parturation in a Paraplegic Woman," *European Journal of Obstetrics, Gynecology, and Reproductive Biology,* 12 (1981):1–6.

15. DEGUCHI, T., and AXELROD, J. "Control of Circadian Change of Serotonin N-acetyltransferase Activity in the Pineal Organ by the B-adrenergic Receptor," *Proceedings of the National Academy of Science,* 69 (1972):2547–2550.

16. DELUCA, H. F. *Vitamin D, Metabolism and Function,* Monographs on Endocrinology. New York: Springer-Verlag, 1979.

17. D'ERCOLE, A. J., APPLEWHITE, G. T., and UNDERWOOD, L. E. "Evidence That Somatomedin Is Synthesized by Multiple Tissues in the Fetus," *Developmental Biology,* 75 (1980):315–328.

18. D'ERCOLE, A. J., et al. "Leprechaunism: Studies of the Relationship Among Hyperinsulinism, Insulin Resistance, and Growth Retardation," *Journal of Clinical Endocrinology and Metabolism,* 48 (1979):495–502.

19. EL-SALHY, M., WILANDER, E., and GRIMELIUS, L. "Immunocytochemical Localization of Gastric Inhibitory Peptide (GIP) in the Human Foetal Pancreas," *Uppsala Journal of Medical Sciences,* 87 (1982):81–85.

20. FISHER, D. A. "Endocrine Physiology I and II," in C. A. Smith and N. M. Nelson, eds., *The Physiology of the Newborn Infant,* 4th ed. Springfield, Ill.: Charles C Thomas, 1976, p. 554.

21. ———. "Fetal Endocrinology: Endocrine Disease and Pregnancy," in L. J. DeGroot, et al., eds. *Endocrinology,* vol. 3. New York: Grune & Stratton, 1979, pp. 1649–1663.

22. FRASER, D. R. "Regulation of the Metabolism of Vitamin D," *Physiological Reviews,* 60 (1980):551–613.

23. GOODYER, C G , and BRANCHAUD, C. L. "Regulation of Hormone Production in the Human Feto-placental Unit," *Ciba Foundation Symposia,* 86 (1981):89–123.

24. GREENBERG, R. E. "The Physiology and Metabolism of Catecholamines," in L. I. Gardner, ed., *Endocrine and Genetic Diseases of Childhood and Adolescence,* 2nd ed. Philadelphia: W. B. Saunders, 1969, pp. 886–898.

25. GREENBERG, R. E., and LIND, J. "Catecholamines in Tissues of the Human Fetus," *Pediatrics,* 27 (1961):904–911.

26. HAKANSON, D. O., PENNY, R., and BERGSTROM, W. H. "Calcemic Responses to Photic and Pharmacologic Manipulation of Serum Melatonin," *Pediatric Research,* 18 (1984):168A.

27. HILL, D. E. "Effect of Insulin on Fetal Growth," *Seminars in Perinatology,* 2 (1978):319–328.

28. HOFFMAN, L., et al. "Insulin Secretion by Fetal Human Pancreas in Organ Culture," *Diabetologia,* 23 (1982):426–430.

29. ISAAC, R. M., et al. "Reverse Tri-iodothyronine to Tri-iodothyronine Ratio and Gestational Age," *Journal of Pediatrics,* 94 (1979):477–479.

30. JACK, P.M.B., and MILNER, R.D.G. "Effect of Decapitation and ACTH on Somatic Development of the Rabbit Fetus," *Biology of the Neonate,* 26 (1975):195–204.

31. JAHR, H., et al. "Secretion and Biosynthesis of (Pro)insulin by Pancreatic Islets Isolated from Fetuses of Normal and Diabetic Women," *Diabetes and Metabolism,* 7 (1981): 71–75.

32. JOHNSON, T. R., Jr., et al. "Plasma Estriol in the Evaluation of Third-trimester Gestational Age," *Obstetrics and Gynecology,* 55 (1980):621–624.

33. JONES, C. T., and ROBINSON, R. O. "Plasma Catecholamines in Foetal and Adult Sheep," *Journal of Physiology,* 248 (1975):15–33.

34. JOST, A. "Expériences de Décapitation de l'embryon de Lapin," *Academy of Sciences* (Paris), 225 (1947):322–324.

35. ———. "Problems of Fetal Endocrinology: The Adrenal Glands," *Recent Progress in Hormone Research,* 22 (1966):541–574.

36. ———. "The Function of the Fetal Adrenal Cortex," in G. E. W. Wolstonholm and R. Porter, eds., *The Human Adrenal Cortex: Its Function Throughout Life,* Ciba Foundation Study Group No. 27. Boston: Little, Brown, 1967, pp. 11–28.

37. JOST, A., JACQUOT, R., and COHEN, A. "The Pituitary Control of the Fetal Adrenal Cortex," in A. R. Currie et al., eds., *The Human Adrenal Cortex.* Baltimore: Williams & Wilkins, 1962, pp. 569–579.

38. KAPLAN, S. L., GRUMBACH, M. M., and AUBERT M. L. "The Ontogenesis of Pituitary Hormones and Hypothalamic Factors in the Human Fetus: Maturation of Central Nervous System Regulation of Anterior Pituitary Function," *Recent Progress in Hormone Research,* 32 (1976):161–243.

39. KLEIN, A. H., et al. "Cord Blood Reverse T3 in Congenital Hypothyroidism," *Journal of Clinical Endocrinology and Metabolism,* 46 (1978):336–368.

40. LANGMAN, J. *Medical Embryology.* Baltimore: Williams & Williams, 1963.

41. LANMAN, J. T. "The Adrenal Gland in the Human Fetus: An Interpretation of Its Physiology and Unusual Developmental Patterns," *Pediatrics,* 27 (1961):140–158.

42. LEAKE, R. D., WEITZMAN, R. S., and FISHER, D. A. "Oxytocin Concentrations During the Neonatal Period," *Biology of the Neonate,* 39 (1981):127–131.

43. LEUNG, A. K., et al. "Circulating Antidiuretic Hormone During Labour and in the Newborn," *Acta Paediatrica Scandinavica,* 69 (1980):505–510.

44. MARKESTAD, T., et al. "Plasma Concentrations of Vitamin D Metabolites in Premature Infants," *Pediatric Research,* 18 (1984):269–272.

45. MOSIER, H. D., Jr. "Hypoplasia of the Pituitary and Adrenal Cortex," *Journal of Pediatrics,* 48 (1956):633–639.

46. ———. "Thyroid Hormone," in W. H. Daughaday, ed., *Endocrine Control of Growth.* New York: Elsevier, 1981, pp. 25–66.

47. MURPHY, B. E. "Human Fetal Serum Cortisol Levels Related to Gestational Age: Evidence of a Midgestational Fall and a Steep Late Gestational Rise, Independent of Sex or Mode of Delivery," *American Journal of Obstetrics and Gynecology,* 144 (1982):276–282.

48. MURPHY, B. E., and SILVERMAN, A. Y. "Comparison of Glucocorticoid Conjugates with Other Indexes of Fetal Maturation," *Obstetrics and Gynecology,* 54 (1979):35–38.

49. NANAGAS, J. C. "A Comparison of the Body Dimensions of Anencephalic Human Fetuses with Normal Fetal Growth as Determined by Graphic Analysis and Empirical Formulas," *American Journal of Anatomy,* 35 (1925):455–494.

50. ODDIE, T. H., et al. "Comparison of T4, T3, rT3 and TSH Concentrations in Cord Blood and Serum of Infants Up to 3 Months of Age," *Early Human Development,* 3 (1979): 239–244.

51. ORTI, E. "Steroid Hormone Formation and Metabolism," in U. Stave, ed., *Perinatal Physiology.* New York: Plenum Press, 1979, pp. 775–792.

52. PARKER, C. R., Jr., et al. "Umbilical Cord Plasma Levels of Dehydroepiandrosterone Sulfate During Human Gestation," *Journal of Clinical Endocrinology and Metabolism,* 54 (1982):1216–1220.

53. PATTEN, B. M. *Human Embryology.* Philadelphia: Blakiston, 1946.

54. PELLINIEMI, L. J., and DYM, M. "The Fetal Gonad and Sexual Differentiation," in D. Tulchinsky and K. J. Ryan, eds., *Maternal and Fetal Endocrinology.* Philadelphia: W. B. Saunders, 1980, pp. 252–280.

55. PEZZINO, V., et al. "Possible Role of Extrahypothalamic TRH in the Development of Pituitary-thyroid Axis in Anencephalic Infants," in G. Chiunello and M. Sperling, eds., *Research Progress in Pediatric Endocrinology.* New York: Raven Press, 1983, pp. 345–350.

56. PHILLIPPE, M. "Fetal Catecholamines," *American Journal of Obstetrics and Gynecology,* 146 (1983):840–855.

57. PUOLAKKA, J., et al. "Fetal Adrenocorticotropic Hormone and Prolactin at Delivery," *Obstetrics and Gynecology,* 60 (1982):71–73.

58. ROE, T. F., et al. "Beckwith's Syndrome with Extreme Organ Hyperplasia," *Pediatrics,* 52 (1973):372–381.

59. ROSENBERG, A. M., et al. "A case of Leprechaunism with Severe Hyperinsulinemia," *American Journal of Diseases of Children,* 134 (1980):170–175.

60. ROTI, E. et al. "Human Cord Blood Concentrations of Thyrotropin, Thyroglobulin, and Iodothyronines After Maternal Administration of Thyrotropin-releasing Hormone," *Journal of Clinical Endocrinology and Metabolism,* 53 (1981):813–817.

61. ROTI, E., et al. "Response of Growth Hormone to Thyrotropin-releasing Hormone During Fetal Life," *Journal of Clinical Endocrinology and Metabolism,* 54 (1982):1255–1257.

62. RURAK, D. W. "Plasma Vasopressin Levels During Hypoxaemia and the Cardiovascular Effects of Exogenous Vasopressin in Foetal and Adult Sheep," *Journal of Physiology* (London), 277 (1978):341–357.

63. SCHLEGEL, R. J. "Ostogenesis of the Gonads," in L. I. Gardner, ed., *Endocrine and Genetic Diseases of Childhood.* Philadelphia: W. B. Saunders, 1969, pp. 469–499.

64. SCOTHORNE, R. J. "Functional Capacity of the Fetal Parathyroid Glands with Reference to Their Clinical Use as Homografts," *Annals of the New York Academy of Sciences,* 120 (1964):669–676.

65. SPERLING, M. A. "Insulin and Glucagon," in U. Stave, ed., *Perinatal Physiology.* New York: Plenum Press, 1979, pp. 813–829.

66. STAHL, F., AMENDT, P., and DORNER, G. "Total and Free Cortisol Plasma Levels in Pre- and Postnatal Life," *Endokrinologie,* 74 (1979):243–246.

67. STEMPFEL, R. S., Jr. "Abnormalities of Sexual Differentiation," in L. I. Gardner, ed., *Endocrine and Genetic Diseases of Childhood.* Philadelphia: W. B. Saunders, 1969, pp. 500–521.

68. STRYKER, J. L., and DZIUK, P. J. "Effects of Fetal Decapitation on Fetal Development, Parturition and Lactation in Pigs," *Journal of Animal Science,* 40 (1980):282–287.

69. UNDERWOOD, L. E., and D'ERCOLE, A. J. "Growth Factors in Fetal Growth," in W. H. Daughaday, ed., *Tissue Growth Factors, Clinics in Endocrinology and Metabolism,* vol. 13, no. 1. Philadelphia: W. B. Saunders, 1984, pp. 69–89.

70. WINTER, J. S., FAIMAN, C., and REYES, F. I. "Sex Steroid Production by the Human Fetus: Its Role in Morphogenesis and Control by Gonadotropins," *Birth Defects Original Article Series,* 13 (1977):41–58.

71. WOLFE, H. J., et al. "Distribution of Calcitonin-containing Cells in the Normal Neonatal Human Thyroid Gland: A Correlation of Morphology and Peptide Content," *Journal of Clinical Endocrinology and Metabolism,* 41 (1975):1076–1081.

72. ZIEGLER, E. E., et al. "Body Composition of the Reference Fetus," *Growth,* 40 (1976):329–341.

4 / Continuity and Discontinuity in Development

Jerome Kagan

Continuities and discontinuities in development are themes with two different meanings in the growth of children. One concerns the connectedness between the structures that define the successive stages of development. Scholars who follow Freud[6] maintain that all children carry forward into successive psychodynamic stages some remnants of the experiences of infancy. Clinicians and scientists who follow Bowlby[2] and Erikson[5] believe that the attachment to and trust in adults established during infancy are a necessary foundation for the next phase of development when autonomy is required. Students of Piaget[14] claim that the psychological achievements of the sensorimotor stage are necessary precursors for the stage of concrete operations. Although these ideas are so popular some investigators regard them as proven facts, it is possible to maintain that even though all children pass through the same sequence of milestones—an attachment to the mother followed by autonomous behavior—there is not a necessarily dependent relation between the successive competences. Almost all children crawl before they stand, but a child prevented from crawling will stand at one year.

Discontinuity in Development

Although most psychiatrists and psychologists favor a connected view of the milestones that define the successive stages of ontogeny, a skepticism has arisen which claims that some of the psychological milestones are adaptive only for a specific developmental period. Like the notochord and the trellis cells of the embryo, these patterns disappear when their mission is accomplished, leaving few heirs. Each life phase makes special demands, and each phase is accompanied by a special set of qualities. Succeeding phases have a different set of demands; hence some of the past is discarded or inhibited. Separation distress occurs toward the end of the first year because children are able to locomote away from the mother and so need a way to recall the care-taker when they confront a dangerous situation. The older child is more self-reliant; hence there is no need to cry if the caretaker is not present. Separation anxiety might even be omitted from the first year with no untoward consequences. Separation anxiety, therefore, is a temporarily adaptive response, similar to the actions of birds that are about to hatch, for the special behaviors accompanying hatching are used once and once only and have no future function. These actions are like the stepping reflex of the fetus, whose presumed function is to ensure normal positioning of the head for delivery. The animal literature is supportive of this claim, for infant rats that are prevented from suckling their mother will ultimately show adult feeding patterns that are not different from those of normally reared rats.[7] Further, in some species of young squirrel monkeys, infantile play behavior is not necessary for the later appearance of normal social behavior.

The Attraction to Continuity

There are several reasons why many scholars prefer the philosophy of connectedness to one of discontinuity. First, such a doctrine makes original forms useful. If the characteristics of adulthood originate during later childhood or adolescence, the first few years of life would seem to have no special purpose. By contrast, if the adolescent's qualities are determined by early experience, the future is to some degree knowable through careful attention to each day. Second, connectedness has the illusion of being mechanistic. If each new property is preceded by a different one that makes a substantial contribution to it, the scientist feels it is easier to state a cause-effect sequence. The connectedness doctrine seems to be in greater accord with egalitarian principles than is a belief in discontinuity. Discontinuities in early development are likely to be due to maturational changes in the central nervous system, and such an emphasis on the role of biological changes in the brain implies that an individual's inheritance has formative force. This conclusion is regarded by some theorists as inconsistent with egalitarian premises, although it need not be. Legitimizing discontinuities in development due to biological maturation, genetic variation, or revolutionary social arrangements implies that the benevolent products of early experience might be abrogated by new social encounters, quality of schools, social unrest, or changes in physiology. Awarding power to these forces is regarded by some—incorrectly, I add—as inconsistent with egalitarian suppositions, for it seems to make it more difficult to arrange similar benevolent experiences for all young children. Finally, the belief in connectedness gains persuasive force because of the manner in which schoolchildren are ranked in modern societies. The parents of preschool children are aware of the fact that at the end of the first grade their child will be ranked with respect to academic ability and that such evaluations will influence the quality of education the child will receive from that time forward. As a result, parents assume that the half-dozen years prior to school determine the initial evaluation, and they interpret the kindergarten profile as a complex derivative of all that has occurred before.

Preservation of Differences in Qualities

A second, quite different meaning of continuity-discontinuity refers to the preservation of individual differences in psychological qualities from infancy and early childhood to adolescence and adulthood. This meaning of continuity is of great interest to parents and psychiatrists who wish to know whether a child's unique personality provides a preview of adult character. But before we can decide on what psychological qualities are preserved, we need agreement as to which individual qualities are likely to enjoy the privilege of continuity. I suggest that there are five hypothetical qualities or processes that might be preserved over time. They are: schemata, categories, actions, states of consciousness, and, finally, classes of persons.

A schema is the infant's way to represent an event, whether it be the father's face, the feeling of hunger, or the anticipation of the mother's arrival. Schemata allow older children and adults to recognize that a voice, a room, a melody, or a fragrance that is now in the perceptual field has been encountered previously. But schemata do not lend themselves very well either to linguistic description or to logical reasoning; hence

a more discrete unit that can be communicated easily and is amenable to manipulation and thought is required.

A category, defined as a symbolic representation of the quality shared by a set of events, fills that function. Linguistic categories are the essential components of beliefs, for a belief is a relation between categories. The belief "boys are tough" represents the relation between the categories *boy* and *tough*. Linguistic philosophers and psychologists treat beliefs as part of a larger class of units called propositions. Because many beliefs are preserved, some for long periods of time, it would seem wise to make propositions basic units. Such a decision would not be an error. However, we can avoid positing the extra unit by suggesting that a belief like "boys are tough" can also be regarded as meaning that the category *boy* has toughness as one of its salient qualities. And most propositions can be treated as statements about one or more salient attributes of a concept. When a person's belief changes, the salient attributes of the underlying categories change too. A girl whose attitude of hostility toward her mother is transformed to one of respect alters a salient attribute of the category *mother*. There are few propositions that cannot be transformed in this way. For this reason, we treat category as the basic entity and proposition as a derivative.

Schemata, categories, and propositions are mental units; the person also possesses entities that will allow him or her to stay alive and out of danger. Thus the third primary unit is an action that produces some change in the environment. Behaviors that produce a change in the environment provide the person with information that can be used to perfect the actions that at the behavioral surface can move toward adaptation.

Each person, however, possesses many actions, schemata, and categories, and we need a unit that selects the relevant few from the larger array. The nineteenth century nominated will to serve this function. But will was purely cognitive in its connotations, and chronic emotional states or moods, which control the selection of behavior, can be preserved for a long time. Thus a state of consciousness, which includes perceived feeling tone and the intentions that dominate awareness at a particular moment, is a fourth unit. Although the specific contents of states of consciousness are more transient than the reservoir of schemata, categories, or actions, a state of consciousness is the executor of a large but limited proportion of an individual's behaviors, desires, and emotions.

Finally, psychologists find it useful to invent categories for coherences of schemata, categories, acts, and states of consciousness. These four elementary units form clusters that are treated as classes of persons, a fifth entity. Adolescents who feel anxious in test situations, believe they are incompetent, and behaviorally avoid situations that contain intellectual challenge are classified by the scientist as "ones who are afraid of failure." Because investigators who study preservation of human qualities theorize about such coherences, we need to posit *a class of person* as a fundamental theoretical unit.

A number of empirical investigations have been concerned with the continuity of human qualities from childhood forward. Unfortunately, almost all of these studies have focused on actions and classes of persons, in part because of the lack of sensitive methods to evaluate schemata, categories, and states of consciousness. When actions and classes of persons are the primary units, long-term continuity is minimal for most qualities until late in childhood. However, it is possible that when scientists are able to evaluate schemata, categories, and states of consciousness with greater precision, they might find support for the folk belief that some early memories or intense states of anxiety are preserved from infancy to adolescence.

Before considering the evidence regarding continuity, we have to decide on how to measure preservation. All statements about the degree of preservation of an action, a category, or a mood must be relative. Suppose we have filmed a woman's behavior in her home for the first hour after she awakens for one hundred successive mornings and wish to know if her actions during this hour are preserved across one hundred days. We cannot know whether her behavior is preserved to a significant degree unless we have some point of comparison. The comparison could be her behavior during another part of the day, her behavior at another place, or the early-morning behavior of another person. Most research shows that the most frequently used comparison is the behavior of another person or persons. But the selection of the other person is extremely important. The comparison of the morning routine of our woman with that of her neighbor will probably reveal small differences in behavior, while the comparison with an Eskimo woman living at Hudson Bay will surely reveal dramatic differences.

The vast majority of investigations of the continuity of human qualities over time rely on differences among persons with respect to a single attribute or set of related attributes.

adolescence.[9,13] Over fourteen different longitudinal studies from both American and European laboratories reveal continuity of aggressive behavior, especially among boys, over periods of two to three years. As the age interval increases, there is a gradual drop in the degree of preservation of individual differences in aggression. However, even for intervals as long as twenty years the differences in aggressive behavior are preserved.[13] Hence for some actions and classes of persons, individual differences are preserved from childhood to adulthood.

However, the existing data, albeit vulnerable to criticism, are much less supportive of the proposition that the characteristics displayed during the first two years of life, with the exception of the temperamental qualities of inhibition and lack of inhibition to the unfamiliar, provide a sensitive preview of the future.[12] These findings are reviewed in Kagan,[8] Kagan, Kearsley, and Zelazo,[10] and Brim and Kagan.[3] Oddly enough, studies of laboratory-reared animals from infancy to reproductive maturity also reveal minimal preservation of individual differences in qualities like aggressiveness, activity, or excitability.[4]

In contrast to the difficulty of using a one- or two-year-old's qualities to predict his or her future, the family's social class is an excellent predictor of many aspects of the child's behavior at adolescence. Thus discovery of a relation between variation in a quality during infancy and one seen in a ten-year-old need not mean that some aspect of the original quality has been preserved. Rather it could indicate that the same forces that produced the behavior in the one-year-old continued to operate for the next decade (see Kagan, Lapidus, and Moore,[11]). In general, about 10 to 15 percent of adolescents in a typical modern community fail to adjust to the demands of the school or to other local norms for socialized behavior. The best predictor of these apparent failures in adaptation is continued rearing in a family that is under economic stress and believes itself powerless to change its status. The child's social class represents a continuing set of influences on his or her development, and it is this constancy in the envelope of daily events that determines the degree of continuity of a psychological quality.

The Evidence for Continuity

Examination of the available evidence suggests that the differences among children in specific actions—such as aggression, dominance, dependence, or sociability—are preserved from about age five or six years through

The Preservation of Inhibition to the Unfamiliar

Of the many temperamental qualities that have been studied—activity, irritability, and fearfulness are the most popular—an initial display of inhibition to the unfamiliar—what parents call shyness, caution, or timidity—and its opposite—what they call sociability, boldness, or fearlessness—are two qualities that seem to persist from the first birthday to late childhood. Inhibition to the unfamiliar can be seen in the eight-month-old, but it is displayed most clearly after the first birthday. Most two-year-olds will stop playing and become quiet in the face of events that are surprising or puzzling. But children differ in how readily they exhibit these reactions and how regularly they display inhibition or lack of inhibition across different situations. I have suggested that about 10 percent of American two-year-olds consistently show an extreme degree of inhibition or lack of inhibition to nonthreatening but unfamiliar events, such as an unfamiliar woman talking to them.[8] The inhibited children stop playing, become quiet, and assume a wary facial expression. The uninhibited infants smile, talk to the adult stranger, and allow her to play with them. The inhibited child may recover after ten to twenty minutes and play with considerable zeal; nonetheless, despite its temporary quality the inhibition is a reliable reaction during the preschool years. A larger proportion of the consistently inhibited four-year-olds, compared with their uninhibited peers, have frequent nightmares and unusual fears. Moreover, because they are sensitive to parental reprimand, they are generally obedient to parental requests. When tested by an unfamiliar woman, the inhibited children rarely make interrupting comments. They tend to look at the examiner frequently and speak in soft, hesitant voices. The uninhibited children interrupt the examiner, laugh frequently, and speak with confident, vital voices. In searching for the best adjectives to capture the differences between the two classes of children, recognizing that any word distorts what is observed, the terms restrained, watchful, and gentle come close to capturing the essence of the inhibited child, while free, energetic, and spontaneous depict the profile of the uninhibited youngster.

The inhibited children show physiological reactions to unfamiliar or mildly challenging situations that imply they are easily aroused by mild stress. Nearly 50 percent of the inhibited children, but only 10 percent of the uninhibited ones, show higher and more stable heart rates when they are looking at pictures or listening to sounds or stories that are difficult to understand. When a child or adult is psychologically involved in a mental task, the accompanying physiological arousal can inhibit vagal control of the heart. As a result, the heart rate rises slightly and becomes much less variable. The fact that the inhibited children usually have higher and more stable heart rates while processing information that is difficult to understand suggests they are physiologically more aroused.

This behavioral quality might be stable for many years. One group of eighty-nine children from the Fels Research Institute's longitudinal population was studied from birth to age fourteen and again during young adulthood. Seven boys in this group were extremely inhibited during the first three years of life. Throughout childhood, adolescence, and early adulthood, these boys remained different from the extremely uninhibited boys. The inhibited males avoided traditional masculine sexual activities, chose less masculine vocations, and, as adults, were introverted and very anxious in new social situations.[9] Throughout his first ten years, one of the boys was described as shy, timid, and anxious. Observers used phrases like insecure, gentle, delicate, meek, vulnerable, and a shrinking violet. When this young man was interviewed at age twenty, he complained of his extreme anxiety in social situations: "I'd like to go up and be able to talk to people that I don't know but I can't."

However, the behavioral surface of the inhibited child can be changed if parents gently encourage a less fearful approach to unfamiliar situations. Because most American parents prefer a bold child to a timid one, they self-consciously try to make their inhibited three-year-old less cautious. And they are often successful. But if the basic temperamental quality is preserved, such children might reveal it in subtle ways under special circumstances and perhaps show signs of conflict.

It is likely that genetic influences can create conditions that make some children vulnerable to becoming inhibited or uninhibited. Identical one-year-old twins are much more similar in their tendency to be inhibited or uninhibited than are nonidentical twins.[15] Further, the adult tendency to be shy and introverted always shows strong evidence for the operation of heredity.[16] Finally, longitudinal observations on groups of laboratory-reared macaque monkeys reveal that the only one of three qualities that persisted over several years was absence of fearfulness to novel situations.[17] However, if the home environment is unusually benevolent, the biological vulnerability to inhibition may not be actualized. This will occur if, for example, the child has unusually sensitive parents and is protected from bullying by an older sibling.

Summary

The existing corpus of data is not firm enough to permit the conclusion that early experiences or the qualities of infants are of no consequence for later childhood. The evidence only implies that if the profiles created by early encounters are not supported by current and future environments, change is likely. There is probably a broad range of early environments that have similar effects on infants. As long as caretakers provide children with food, warmth, protection from pain, and playful interaction on a regular schedule, the small differences among two-year-olds raised on such regimens will have little predictive consequence for individual differences ten years hence. But, of course, infants who experience prolonged periods of distress frequently will be more fearful, irritable, perhaps more aggressive, and less cognitively competent than children treated in a benevolent fashion. But infants whose experiences have created such pathology will continue to grow anomalously only if they remain in the same environment. Two- and three-year-olds do change, often dramatically, if their neglecting environments become benevolent and conducive to desirable growth.

A long-term study was conducted on over six-hundred children growing up on the Hawaiian island of Kauai.[18] The youngsters were followed from birth to eighteen years of age. The data revealed that only a small group of fourteen infants were born with serious perinatal stress. Of this group four were mentally retarded at age ten, two had health problems, and three were delinquent. Thus perinatal stress did place the infant at risk. But of the sixty-nine infants born with mild perinatal stress, the occurrence of mental retardation, psychosis, neurosis, or delinquency was not greater than it was for infants born without risk, because a supportive home environment can ameliorate the vulnerabilities imposed by the earlier mild stress. The authors wrote, "As we watched these children grow from babyhood to adulthood, we could not help but respect the self-righting tendencies within them

that produced normal development under all but the most persistently adverse circumstances"[18] (p. 159).

The evolutionary tree may be a good metaphor for psychological development. Biologists do not explain the appearance of man in phylogeny by pointing to the prior existence of protozoa, even though the fact that protozoa existed in the remote past made the evolution of humans a little more likely. Similarly, one cannot explain the ten-year-old's phobia of horses by listing all the experiences of infancy. Each person can be understood only as a coherence of many, many past events. The older the child, the less satisfying are explanations that rely too heavily on early experience. The embryological development of the neural crest cells provides the most informative analogy for an individual life. The final fate of the cells is determined by other cells they will encounter in their journey and is not completely inherent in their intrinsic structure before their migration begins. I suspect this principle applies to psychological development, for once the child begins to interpret experience as having implications for his or her talent, gender, virtue, and acceptability to others, dispositions become a little more resistant to change. It appears that a major enhancement in the components of a sense of self emerge late in the second year. This fact suggests that the events that occur prior to this milestone may be less well preserved than those that follow the emergence of this organizing structure.

ACKNOWLEDGMENT

Preparation of this chapter was supported in part by a grant from the John D. and Catherine T. MacArthur Foundation.

REFERENCES

1. BALDWIN, J. D., and BALDWIN, J. I. "The Role of Play in Social Organization," *Primates,* 14 (1973):369–381.

2. BOWLBY, J. *Attachment and Loss,* vol. 1, *Attachment.* New York: Basic Books, 1969.

3. BRIM, O. G., and KAGAN, J., eds. *Constancy and Change in Human Development.* Cambridge, Mass.: Harvard University Press, 1980.

4. CAIRNS, R. B., and HOOD, K. E. "Continuity in Social Development," in P. Baltes and O. G. Brim, eds., *Life Span Development,* vol. 5. New York: Academic Press, 1983, pp. 301–358.

5. ERIKSON, E. H. *Childhood and Society.* New York: W. W. Norton, 1963.

6. FREUD, S. "An Outline of Psychoanalysis," in J. Strachey, ed., *The Standard Edition of the Complete Psychological Works of Sigmund Freud,* vol. 23. London: Hogarth Press, 1964, pp. 141–207.

7. HALL, W. G. "Weaning and Growth of Artificially Reared Rats," *Science,* 190 (1975):1313–1315.

8. KAGAN, J. *The Nature of the Child.* New York: Basic Books, 1984.

9. KAGAN, J., and MOSS, H. A. *Birth to Maturity.* New York: John Wiley & Sons, 1962; rev. ed., New Haven: Yale University Press, 1983.

10. KAGAN, J., KEARSLEY, R. B., and ZELAZO, P. R. *Infancy: Its Place in Human Development.* Cambridge, Mass.: Harvard University Press, 1978.

11. KAGAN, J., LAPIDUS, D., and MOORE, M. "Infant Antecedents of Cognitive Functioning," *Child Development,* 49 (1978):1005–1023.

12. MOSS, H. A., and SUSMAN, E. J. "Longitudinal Study of Personality Development," in O. G. Brim and J. Kagan, eds., *Constancy and Change in Human Development.* Cambridge, Mass.: Harvard University Press, 1980, pp. 530–595.

13. OLWEUS, D. "Stability in Aggressive, Inhibited, and Withdrawn Behavior Patterns. Paper presented at the meeting of the Society for Research in Child Development, Boston, April 1981.

14. PIAGET, J. *Play, Dreams, and Imitation in Childhood*, trans. C. Gattegno and F. M. Hodgson. London: Routledge and Kegan Paul, 1951.

15. PLOMIN, R., and ROWE, D. C. "Genetic and Environmental Etiology of Social Behavior in Infancy," *Developmental Psychology*, 15 (1979):62–72.

16. SCARR, S. "Social Introversion-extroversion as a Heritable Response," *Child Development*, 40 (1969):823–832.

17. STEVENSON-HINDE, J., STILLWELL-BARNES, R., and ZUNZ, M. "Individual Differences in Young Rhesus Monkeys," *Primates*, 21 (1980):498–509.

18. WERNER, E. E., and SMITH, R. S. *Vulnerable but Invincible*. New York: McGraw-Hill, 1982.

5 / Separation-Individuation and the Beginning Emergence of the Sense of Self

John B. McDevitt

Introduction

Margaret Mahler's concept of the separation-individuation process addresses a number of crucial developmental issues. It is a framework for ordering and organizing complex observational data and for making inferences about intrapsychic development in the first three years of life. It also sets forth a theory about the symbiotic origin of the human condition and the subsequent psychological birth of the human infant. Finally, it provides a sound basis for the prevention of developmental disturbances when these might occur, and offers a model for early intervention when they do occur.

In 1955 Mahler introduced into psychoanalytic theory the hypothesis of an obligatory separation-individuation process. [44] In order to validate and elaborate on this hypothesis, she undertook observational research studies of average mothers with their normal infants during the first three years of life. Later she developed a framework for inference consisting of four subphases of the separation-individuation process. This offered a more detailed means by which to order and organize observational data, both of the behavior of infants and of their interactions with the caregiver.

The findings and the theory of the separation-individuation process apply both to data from experimental research study of infants and to those that derive from the psychoanalysis of young children. In turn, the material from these realms contributes to a better understanding of the separation-individuation process.

The research strategy and yield of this naturalistic observational study is represented by Mahler's published work—her *Selected Papers* [40] and *The Psychological Birth of the Human Infant* (with Pine and Bergman) [48]—and by her two narrated films, *The Basic Films of the Separation-Individuation Process"* and *The Emergence of the Sense of Self.* *

The "psychological birth" of the individual takes place during the separation-individuation process as it proceeds from about the fifth to the thirty-sixth month of age. In contrast to the dramatic, clearly observable and well-defined biological birth of human infants, their psychological birth is a slowly unfolding intrapsychic process. The fundamental task of children during this process is to establish a measure of object- and self-constancy, the beginnings of stable object relations, and enduring individuality. Subphase development based on Mahler's work will be presented from this point of view.

The Forerunners of the Separation–Individuation Phase

Newborns have the task of adjusting to extrauterine existence, that is, to finding their own niche in the extramural world. They have to achieve adequate inner regulation in synchrony with the outside world by means of their own innate, phylogenetically programmed equipment.

In the first few weeks, infants achieve physiological homeostasis (the normal autistic phase). At the same

*These films were produced by The Margaret S. Mahler Psychiatric Research Foundation. They are available from The Mahler Research Film Library, P.O. Box 315, Franklin Lake, New Jersey, 07417.

time, during limited periods of alert inactivity, they are biologically predesigned to respond to certain complex species-specific stimuli, particularly the details and features of the human face. From the first day on, infants attune themselves to the mother's vocal and gestural rhythms (see Brazelton[6]; Emde, Gaensbaur, and Harmon[11]; Stern[70]). In other words, each neonate elicits his or her particular mother's caregiving in a unique way, and the competent mother responds with intuitive coenesthetic empathy to her particular infant.

In the second month of life, there is a shift to an increased attentiveness to regularly repeated caretaking stimuli. As a result, infants begin gradually and vaguely to sense that relief from tension and hunger must come from an outside source and begin to initiate interaction with the caregiver in order to attain relief from distress as well as gratification and pleasure. In particular, it would appear that infants do not experience the caregiver or themselves as separate entities. This is the beginning of the symbiotic phase.

Through repeated experiences of relief, memory traces of the sense of caregiving are established. By two to three months, infants (1) both anticipate and initiate the pleasure provided by interaction with the caregiver, (2) develop a sense of confidence and basic trust in the caregiver and in their own initiative, and (3) respond to the caregiver with a nonspecific social smile and with eye-to-eye contact. At this point, mutual cueing is at its peak, indicating that the symbiotic phase is well on its way.

As the mother ministers to her infant, she begins to interpret his or her varying signs of distress and contentment as communications. The quality of the exchange depends on how clearly baby signals needs and on how well mother is attuned to the cues. Infants give many cues; mothers pick up some of them. In time, infants adapt and continue to employ primarily those cues to which mother responds. This results in selective mutual cueing. The ensuing attunement between mother and infant influences the development of the self within the framework of the mother-child dual unit. Playfulness between mother and infant promotes and enriches the important—primarily affective—symbiotic attachment and mutual interaction between baby and mother.[71] Mutual gaze and gaze aversion contribute to the baby's sense of self as an active agent initiating interactions with the mother.

The term symbiosis has several implications. It speaks for the infant's almost exclusive attachment to, mutual interaction with, and dependence on the mother along with the latter's complementary involvement with the infant. It refers as well to a state in which infants gradually begin to sense some degree of differentiation between themselves and the source of caregiving. Although their initiative and their response are to some extent experienced as "their own," they seem

to be embedded primarily within the matrix of their interactions with their mother.[8,71] The primary focus seems to be on the synchrony of the mother-infant interplay.

The infant's specific smiling response, which appears at six to eight weeks, achieves a certain specificity in respect to the mother. This peaks during the symbiotic phase at around five months and indicates that the child is responding to the symbiotic partner in a unique manner. The infant has achieved a specific symbiotic relationship with the mother. In order to arrive at this level of attachment, an additional step must occur.

The normal symbiotic phase thus reveals the all-important phylogenetic capacity of the human infant to form an emotional tie to the mother. It is this synchronous mutual attachment that furnishes the soil out of which grow all subsequent human relationships.

The Beginning Attainment of Object Constancy

It has been widely believed that "libidinal" object constancy[18] is attained between six and eighteen months of age.* Those who place it earlier within this age range use as their criterion the infant's libidinal attachment to the love object; those who place it later add the establishment of some form of mental representation of the love object (in line with Piaget's criteria[52] for the emergence of the mental representation of inanimate objects at about eighteen months of age).

In Mahler's view, however, such "libidinal" object constancy begins to be attained only in the third year of life.† In terms of precursors, it is based on the child's libidinal attachment to the mother and on the cognitive achievement of person permanence and representational intelligence.[5,23,52] Its eventual establishment, however, depends on the gradual internalization of a constant, positively cathected, functionally available representation of the mother. The availability of such an inner presence permits the child to tolerate brief separations from her. These representations become functional following the resolution of ambivalence typical of the rapprochement crisis, a phenomenon that occurs between eighteen and twenty-four months (or later). This crisis achieves resolution primarily by means of internalization. The presence of the actual mother is no longer necessary; during her physical absence she can now be substituted for, at least in part, by the presence of an internal image that remains relatively stable. Provided the absence is not prolonged,

*See references 7, 9, 14, 16, 21, 22, 49, 64, and 65.
†See references 28, 34, 35, 36, 37, and 48.

she will not be rejected (hated) or exchanged for another. This will be true even when she no longer provides satisfaction or when she is absent.

These changes allow senior toddlers to tolerate their mother's absences for ever longer periods of time, provided they are placed in familiar surroundings. In fact, in the nurserylike research setting, the senior toddlers often preferred to play in the toddler playroom, leaving their mothers behind in the infant room. If toddlers busily engaged in play are asked where their mother is or whether they miss her, they usually provide a simple answer without needing to seek her out. During the practicing subphase the actual mother served as a secure base from which to explore; now, however, she is represented increasingly by a stable mental image. Toddlers are thus able to engage in a variety of activities independent of her physical presence.[28]

Object Constancy

The establishment of object constancy is a slow, complex process that involves all aspects of the personality. The emergence spans several different subphases, and it is best regarded as a continuing process rather than simply as a specific stage—a process that has its beginning in infancy, continues throughout childhood and adolescence, and probably is never fully completed.

By the fifth month, as a rule, infants have developed a specific libidinal attachment to and recognition memory of the mother. Soon afterward they begin to react to others either with interest, tactually and visually exploring and comparing their faces with their mother's face as well as with the "inner image" they have of her (a behavior pattern that has been called customs inspection and comparative scanning). Or they may display apprehension (stranger anxiety). When apprehensive, infants begin to "check back" to the mother's face for reassurance.

By seven to eight months, infants begin to show characteristic responses to brief separations from the mother. They miss her, long for her, and may become quite distressed. They now start to perceive her to a greater extent as separate from themselves. Furthermore, when the mother leaves the room temporarily, infants look repeatedly, in apparent distress at the door through which she has gone. This suggests that even at this age infants have a rudimentary ability to remember the absent love object as well as a primitive notion of "person permanence."

This would be in agreement with Piaget's findings with regard to the inanimate object.* Not until stage

*See references 9, 13, 50, 51, and 52.

IV (eight to twelve months) in sensorimotor development will infants search for an inanimate object that before their eyes has been hidden behind a screen. They will remove that screen in order to recover the object. They evidently remember the object and can now attribute some "objectivity" to things hidden from their perception. There is thus a beginning practical sense of "object permanence."

The degree of children's distress and their repeated looking at the door through which the mother left suggest that children's attachment to the love object persists for a much longer time than their interest in the inanimate object.

According to Fraiberg,[14] the ability to remember the absent mother at this age (seven to eight months) is dependent on the stimulus of the infant's "need states," just as "recognition memory" is dependent on the stimulus of external perception. Such "need states," however, refer not only to the intermittent physiological needs, which had been characteristic of the earlier need-satisfying relationship; now they refer also to the more continuous and enduring object cathexis of the mother. In her absence infants seem to miss her; they may look sad, cry, and protest helplessly. This memory is not yet able to help them tolerate their mother's absence. In a similar manner, the memory of the mother's face is still too unstable to prevent the occurrence of "stranger anxiety" when infants are confronted with a face that is similar to, although different from, the mother's face.[63]

Passive Separation Experiences

From about eight to fourteen months infants seem to have only two ways of coping with marked separation distress: One is to accept the comforting of a mother substitute; the other is to withdraw regressively into the self.[46] As they withdraw, they appear to lose all interest in their surroundings; instead they seem to become preoccupied with an inner feeling of the previous state of sensorimotor and affective closeness or "oneness" with the mother. Apparently, during her absence there is an attempt to undo their painful sense of separation and to maintain their equilibrium. They shut out affective and perceptual claims emanating from other sources and endeavor to maintain their emotional balance by diminution of activity, reduction of perceptual intake, underresponsiveness, and regression in their ability to relate—a regressive defense I have called "low-keyedness" (see also Engel and Reichman[12]; Kaufman and Rosenblum[24]; Rubinfine[56]; Tennes and Lampl[73]). Their memory or image of their mother, as it becomes more discrete, probably exists in the form of its previous sensorimotor and sensoriaffective context, such as "being-cuddled-by-mother," rather than retaining its form as an exclusively visual image.

In the early part of the differentiation subphase (from five to seven months), the specific libidinal attachment to the mother has already been established, and "recognition memory" exists. Presumably it is evoked only when infants are actually perceiving either the mother herself or something that represents her. Toward the end of this subphase (from seven to nine months), there are indications of a beginning capacity to retain a rudimentary memory of the absent mother. This can be evoked at times of need, but it is apparently too unstable to sustain infants during the mother's absence. Even though children's bodily needs may be gratified while the mother is absent, they still miss her and are distressed. The object is no longer interchangeable; mother has become *the* love object. [62] The object cathexis tends to persist irrespective of frustration of satisfaction or the mother's temporary absence.* At this age, however, the object cathexis is too fragile to endure prolonged absence. [15] The infants' sense of well-being is now dependent on the presence of the mother or of a mother substitute to whom they have also become attached.

As infants progress from the differentiation to the practicing subphase (from ten to sixteen months), [35,42] they become more consciously aware of the relation between their mother's absence and their own distress. As early as nine months they begin to anticipate the possibility of her leaving (signal anxiety); if they sense she is about to depart, they will try to keep her from doing so by protesting in advance. When the mother does leave the room, infants are likely to creep or toddle to the door in an attempt to follow her; while she is absent, they may repeatedly go to the door, and, at around one year of age or a little later, they may even say "mama" over and over again. These behaviors suggest that by the end of the first year infants have developed a more differentiated image of their mother, a picture that comes to mind whenever they are reminded of her or need her. Later in the practicing period (fourteen to sixteen months) the infants' sense of well-being is no longer so completely dependent on their mother's presence. They are now better able to cope with separation distress by means of a more stable mental representation of the mother and by active mastery, as opposed to their previous passive helplessness.

The more stable the representation of the mother, based on former experiences of trust and confidence, the better able are the children to tolerate her brief absences from the room and the more cheerfully they greet her on her return. This is in contrast to other

children who, for example, would typically fret, cry, or avoid their mother on her return. [2]

Toward the end of the first year, "recognition memory" becomes sufficiently stable so that stranger anxiety diminishes markedly. A few months later, the memory of the absent mother, activated by the stimulus of inner need, becomes sufficiently stable to sustain children briefly during her absence. They are now able to obtain some degree of well-being by turning to a supportive maternal representation rather than by seeking the physical presence of the mother. This representation has by now gained some degree of autonomy from the demands of immediate need-satisfaction. It permits children to use advances to ego development to make the need for the mother less urgent, just as the mother's actual presence formerly enabled them to start to move away from her to explore and play. The children's pleasure in practicing their recently acquired motor skills and exploring their expanding environment, as well as their pleasure in experiencing new capacities, resources, and interests, enable them to resort to play and to make use of substitute adults in the service of tolerating and coping actively with separation distress. Other advances in ego development—for example, the taming of affect and the increased tolerance of frustration—also contribute to a greater ability to "handle" mother's absence.

Toward the end of the practicing subphase we see the beginnings of deferred imitation and symbolic play as well as the verbal evocation of the mother in her absence. [50,51,52] During the mother's absence or in anticipation of it, children may go to the door and say "bye-bye" or "mama." The junior toddler—especially the little girl—may mother her doll in symbolic play, using this play to comfort herself while her mother is away. She may be heard to say "mama" and "baba" while cradling and rocking her doll.

These behaviors are significant for several reasons. First, they indicate that the junior toddler is now able to construct mental representations of behavior patterns, thereby implying the evocation of the mother at a time when she is neither present nor perceived. In these behaviors, action becomes detached from its previous motoric context and rests instead on representation in thought. Second, this is the beginning of identifications that are patterned on a representational model. By re-creating in play an actual experience with the mother, the junior toddler is able to function better during her absence. Third, symbolic play based on identification serves as an intermediate step between the actual mother-child relationship and the transfer of that relationship to the child's inner world. It is striking how often such play appears to be an exact replication of the actual mother-child relation and its significant qualities. This transfer of the mother-child relation to the child's inner world permits a continuing

*See references 1, 3, 15, 16, 60, and 61.

relationship with the love object during the latter's absence. [53,59]

At first, deferred imitation, symbolic play, and verbal evocation of the absent mother are enacted as the result of an inner need for the mother. As a further step in cognitive development, at around sixteen to eighteen months of age, behaviors (primarily verbal) occur that indicate a beginning capacity to evoke a more complex and differentiated mental image of the mother, one that has an even greater autonomy from outer and inner stimuli. With the acquisition of this capacity, children are on the verge of representational thought. [50,51,52] These achievements would not be possible, of course, without advances in other areas of ego development—for example, in the capacity for delay, neutralization, reality testing—that are dependent on satisfactory object relations. At the same time, these exert an influence on both object relations and drive development.

Active Separation Experiences

So far, I have been describing behavioral phenomena that reflect passive separation experiences. The focus will now be shifted to active separation experiences, to the infant's active approach and distancing behaviors.

Beginning in the differentiation subphase and continuing into the practicing subphase, infants approach the mother actively with expressions of affection. They enjoy communicating with her and begin to comply with her requests and prohibitions. Paradoxically, it is during this time, when children's libidinal attachment to the mother is growing stronger, that the nature of their development is requiring them gradually to detach themselves from her. [66]

During the differentiation subphase, infants at first like to play near their mother's feet; later they play at a somewhat greater distance, all the while, however, maintaining full visual contact with her and showing constant concern for her presence. [45] When they enter the practicing subphase, once their stranger anxiety has diminished and their locomotor skills permit, they move farther and farther away from the mother, both physically and emotionally, seeking pleasure in exploring their newfound world. [35] This is when children may even leave their mother in the "infant room" and creep or toddle to the adjoining "toddler room."

Those children who have had the most gratifying relationship with their mother show the greatest curiosity about their surroundings; they move away from her more freely and do their exploring at greater distances from her, seemingly unconcerned with her whereabouts. In the practicing subphase, whenever

they choose to move away from her, infants seem to maintain an "illusion" that the mother is with them or is nearby. They probably need to do so because at this point, self-object differentiation is still far from complete. Toward the end of the first year and the beginning of the second, however, children will move away from the mother cheerfully, often with a mood elation. Albeit seemingly unconcerned with the mother's whereabouts, at the same time they appear to be secure in their awareness that she is somewhere at hand and available. Mother seems to be taken for granted; she has become a secure base, not to be thought about except when the need arises. When such a need does arise, infants periodically return to her for brief physical and emotional closeness ("refueling"). Like those patterns that enable infants to cope with passive separation experiences better late in the practicing subphase, these behaviors also suggest the gradual development of a more stable and secure mental representation of the mother, as well as a practical, sensorimotor knowledge of the mother's whereabouts and how to reach her.

During the course of the rapprochement subphase, which lasts from about the sixteenth to the twenty-fourth month and beyond, considerable change occurs in children's behavior. The relative obliviousness to the mother's presence, the tolerance of her absence, and the overall "good mood" that were characteristic of the practicing subphase more or less give way to feelings of separateness, loneliness, and helplessness. There is a constant concern with the mother's presence, increased separation distress, and a tendency toward a depressive mood. [33,35,36]

This rapprochement subphase is a critical period, during which profound changes occur in children's mental and emotional development. These include more advanced independent walking, the capacity for evocative memory, the beginnings of representational thought, a more precise demarcation of the self and object representations, and a shift to the anal-sadistic and early genital phases of psychosexual development. [55] Children's capacity for mental representations of the mother, the self, body parts, prohibitions, feelings and wishes, and so forth, as well as for the complex relations among these, is advancing rapidly. Thoughts and feelings now persist routinely beyond the situation in which they had their origin. Conflicts with the mother no longer simply flare up and disappear; they appear to continue in children's minds for ever longer periods of time. There is an increased sensitivity to the mother's approval or disapproval; ambivalence is clearly evident; and the beginning internalization of prohibitions and regulations becomes apparent.

There is a resurgence of stranger and separation anxiety. Presumably, as a consequence of their greater awareness of separateness, children are confronted by a renewed fear of object loss. In the earlier differentiation subphase, fear of object loss was related to the distinguishing of mother from nonmother (stranger anxiety) as well as to the beginning differentiation of self and mother (grief reactions to mother's absence). Now, in the rapprochement subphase, once again these fears surge up. This time they are determined by two factors: the complex intrapsychic differentiation of the self-representation and the maternal representation and the projection of aggression, which contributes both to a renewed distrust of strangers as well as to the fears that are typical of this subphase.

Junior toddlers not only recognize that they and their mother are separate human beings, they are also beginning to recognize another very frightening state of affairs, namely that there are causes of events that exist outside themselves that are quite independent of their needs and their wishes. It is difficult for them to accept the fact that they are not omnipotent. There is often a conflict between their wish to get their own way and their need to please the mother; their wish to assert their independence and their autonomy by moving away from her and their need to remain near her. Often they cling to her and literally "shadow" her. Furthermore, their former relative obliviousness to the mother's presence is now replaced by active approach behavior—a wish to share their new skills and experiences with her—a need for her love and a constant concern with her whereabouts. Their previous elated preoccupation with locomotion and exploration wanes; they are no longer as impervious as they were to knocks and falls, and they can become upset merely by a sudden realization of their separateness. Their greatest source of pleasure now shifts to social interaction. They employ all kinds of mechanisms to ward off and to undo their painful sense of separateness from the mother, while at the same time they experience a great desire to expand their newly developing autonomy. They are torn between the wish to stay near the mother and the compulsion to move away from her.

These changes place a considerable strain on junior toddlers. Everything is happening to them at once. At the very time that they are becoming painfully aware of their physical and emotional separateness, their limitations and their helplessness, the junior toddlers' anger at the mother is mounting in the face of the inevitable frustrations, jealousies, envy, and possessiveness they are experiencing toward her. This brings about a crisis in their relationship. This is especially stressful since they still consider the mother omnipotent and since they have not yet achieved a satisfactory and consistent integration of the "good" and "bad" object. Anger at the mother may be compounded fur-

ther by the castration reactions that occur at this age (albeit predominantly in little girls).[55]

These "rapprochement crises" are frequently precipitated by traumatic events. The intensity and duration of the crises seem to depend largely on the nature of the past or present mother-child relationship. Generally speaking, there seems to be an inverse relationship between children's ability to assert themselves pleasurably in independent play and hostile aggression against the mother when it is expressed in a need to cling anxiously to her. The three basic fears in early development—the fear of the loss of the object, of the loss of the object's love, and of punishment and castration anxiety—come together during this subphase.

Most children experience such a "rapprochement crisis." To be sure, at times some degree of "libidinal" object constancy is present during this subphase. Nevertheless, it is still too infrequent, too inconsistent, and too subject to momentary moods and regression to permit us to say that children have attained a significant degree of object constancy. During times of crisis, the mental representation of the mother is buffeted by violent and angry feelings; as a result, the stability of this maternal image—at least from the affective as distinguished from the cognitive side—is disrupted. At such times, children experience severe separation anxiety. To cope with this, the children will then attempt to maintain a "good" object image during the mother's absence. To do this, they will not infrequently displace their anger onto the caregiver who, as a consequence, becomes the "bad" object. This mechanism thus entails a "splitting" of the object representation. In this way, the longed-for image of the love object is separated from the hated component.[37,48]

When the aggressive forces outweigh the libidinal ones, the junior toddlers' representation of the mother becomes unstable. Such an image cannot sustain them during her absence; in order to maintain it they must seek repeated contacts with her. Even these contacts (often physical in nature) do not provide sufficient relief. Neither the actual presence of the mother nor her representation in their mind enables the children to use already acquired resources or other adults as a way of tolerating brief separations. In addition, the children's intense ambivalence and their need to cling to mother combine to disrupt their identification with her. Once identification again becomes possible, however, it plays a significant role in resolving the crises of the rapprochement subphase. A similar interference with identification is seen in young children separated from their parents for longer periods of time.[19]

The mother is often perplexed by her child's eagerness, on the one hand, to become more independent while, on the other, insisting that she share every aspect of his or her life. It is particularly important at this time that the mother not withdraw or react harshly to her toddler's ambivalence, that she continue to be emotionally available and behaviorally predictable, and that she provide a general push in the direction of the child's independence. Only in this way can toddlers' previous love of self and their unrealistic belief in their magical powers be replaced by a realistic recognition of and belief in their newly developed individual autonomy.

The fourth subphase of the separation-individuation process spans the interval from twenty-four to thirty-six months of age. It is only gradually during the course of this epoch that senior toddlers become able to tolerate their mother's absence for longer periods of time (and only if they are in familiar surroundings). In fact, they often were seen to prefer to play in the nearby research observational toddler room, leaving their mother in the research observational infant room. This ability to play comfortably and even to function better in the adjacent room without the mother is one indication that children have begun to attain a greater degree of object constancy.[35] Senior toddlers also become more consistently loving, friendly, and cooperative. They are better able to withstand frustration, delay gratification, and accept substitute satisfactions. The children experience the unfolding of such complex cognitive functions as verbal communication and reality testing, along with pleasure in their own autonomous attainments. Together these contribute to the development of a beginning measure of self-constancy as well as a unified self-image.

When such children choose to play at some distance from the mother, they do not show the same lack of concern for the mother's whereabouts that had been characteristic of the practicing subphase. Instead, they are now very much more aware of where their mother is and may even have some idea of what she is doing; yet this awareness does not give rise to the sort of concern that was present during the differentiation and rapprochement subphases. Similarly, when the mother chooses to leave them, they are better able to tolerate her absence. Their sense of comfort seems to rest on the existence of a relatively secure and stable mental representation of the mother. For example, if children who are busily engaged in play are asked where their mother is or whether they miss her, they will provide a simple answer, without needing to seek her out. The mother whose actual presence served as a secure base from which to explore in the practicing subphase now begins to take the form of a secure and stable mental representation, thereby enabling toddlers to engage in a variety of activities separately and independently of her.

The specific libidinal attachment to the mother, along with progress in the invariant, largely autono-

mous sequences in cognitive development, are necessary conditions for the gradual attainment of object constancy. However, this ability to tolerate separation from the mother during the third year of life indicates that they are not sufficient conditions. The essential determinants are the nature of the cathexis of the mental representation of the mother and what might be called the "quality" of this representation.

The ambivalence that is characteristic of the rapprochement subphase does not begin to be resolved until well into, or even toward the end of, the third year of life. Only then does there exist a stable mental representation of the mother, an image invested predominantly with libidinal as opposed to aggressive cathexis, and one capable of persisting in the same form regardless of frustration, instinctual need, or the temporary absence of the mother. This object representation is no longer readily subject to regression or to the mechanism of splitting.[43] Libido outweighs and counteracts aggression; the "good" and "bad" aspects of the mother are solidly united into a single representation. Disappointment and rage become tempered and are better tolerated, since they are now counteracted to a greater degree by memories of the loving as well as the frustrating behavior of the mother.[53]

Identification plays an important role in bringing about these changes. The "quality" of the representation of the mother produces a sense of security and comfort in the child, just as the actual mother had. As Mahler[43] so aptly put it, "By object constancy we mean that the maternal image has become intrapsychically available to the child in the same way as the actual mother had been libidinally available—for sustenance, comfort, and love" (p. 222).

Even in the third year, however, children's tolerance of separation fluctuates just as it had during the previous subphase; a tolerance that had already been achieved can break down again under such stresses as toilet training and castration reactions. Even so, when they are upset, children may cling to the mother only part of the time; the rest of the time they are free to play independently. As a consequence of difficulties in previous subphases, there are some children, however, who do not attain sufficient object constancy in the fourth subphase. These "problem children" continue to show the danger signals typical of the rapprochement subphase. They are vulnerable to the development of an infantile neurosis and to a variety of disturbances in later life.[26,27]

We have now reached the end of the third year of life, at which time a degree of object constancy has ordinarily been attained. As a result, children can tolerate separation sufficiently well to be ready to enter nursery school and can even benefit by doing so.[16]

The Beginning Emergence of the Sense of Self

It is much more difficult to find behavioral referents or to make inferences about the emerging sense of self than to find referents to the developing sense of the object. For example, one can readily see evidence for and make inferences about infants' feelings about the mother and their recognition memory of her. Comparable data regarding feelings about, or recognition and awareness of, the emerging self is either nonexistent in early infancy or highly elusive. We can only assume that infants who are to become a self must experience from the first a variety of bodily sensations and feeling states along the pleasure-unpleasure continuum within the framework of the mother-infant dual unit.[31] These sensations are at first largely proprioceptive; later, sensory stimuli coming from the outside predominate. These, along with a sense of caregiving by the libidinal object, form the primitive core of infants' emerging sense of self, particularly their bodily self or body ego.

Because the sense of self emerges in the context of the interaction with the mother during early development, it will bear the imprint of her caregiving. During symbiosis and the differentiation subphase, for example, the caregiver's "mirroring" is a vital ingredient in the development of the sense of self, as are games between mother and baby, which help to delineate the infant's own body image from that of the mother. In fact, it is not possible to speak of self-development separately from the development of object relations or to attempt to separate out the perceptive and cognitive from the affective elements responsible for the demarcation of the body self from the object world.[47] Infants begin to distinguish not only mother from stranger but similarly mother from self. The ability to remember and recall the absent mother by six to eight months as well as the capacity to experience and defend against the painful sadness brought on by her absence also makes infants more exquisitely aware of their separateness.

The emergence of the sense of self is more gradual than Stern[72] believes, even if many more elements necessary for its development are inborn than we previously thought. Emde[10] has written convincingly that the continuity of experience is guaranteed by the "affective core" of the self in the first fifteen months of life. Probably the most sophisticated approach to the beginning development of the self is that of Stechler and Kaplan,[69] who emphasize complex self-regulatory, self-initiatory, and self-inhibitory behaviors as well as the ability to carry out plans, to hold intentions in abeyance, and to resolve interpersonal conflicts as criteria for self-awareness and the emergence of the self. In this chapter further aspects of development necessary for the emergent sense of self are presented. Particular emphasis is placed on certain nodal points in which motor, affective drive, and cognitive development in interaction with object relations come together in a manner that produces qualitative shifts, as opposed to quantitative changes, in the emerging sense of self.

Among the infant's experiences, activity is a most important trigger for the development of the sense of self. An important crossroads occurs at the beginning of the differentiation subphase. Infants become visibly interested in looking and listening beyond the symbiotic orbit. By age four to five months they take in much more of the outside world by way of distance perceptual modalities. As a result they acquire the important abilities of checking back to mother, of scanning the environment, of picking out the toys and objects that interest them. They become more goal-directed and show more intentionality.

When the mother is available, infants take pleasure in tentative experiments in actively moving away from her, of being on their own. This can be seen in such behaviors as pushing away from the mother or sliding down from her lap in order to play on the floor at her feet. In contrast to the previous almost total bodily dependence on the mother and passive molding in her arms, infants now begin to take active pleasure in the use of their own bodies as well as to turn more actively to the outside world for pleasure and stimulation. They now begin to take a first step toward the possession of their own bodies and their functions.

Being able to achieve a sitting position without help is a major attainment at around eight months of age. Being able to freely move the torso in whatever direction at will is the midwife to the most significant achievement in the development of the sense of self during the first fifteen months of life. This achievement Mahler[34] calls "hatching." It coincides with Piaget's stage IV of sensorimotor development[52] and brings together, in a much more integrated form, all previous perceptual, cognitive, motor, and affective developments. A shift in the sensorium results in a more permanently outward directed alert state. Alert children, able to sit securely and to use their hands freely to handle whatever they want to reach out for, can pivot the upper body, have a wider scope for scanning and reaching, and can easily select a preferred toy. They can also examine the mother's features, especially her face as well as her jewelry, eyeglasses, and so forth, seemingly contrasting these inanimate objects with the feel of the mother's skin. At the same time, they move, touch, and examine visually their fingers and other parts of their own bodies. Hoffer[20] has drawn attention to the fact that this "double touch" (touching the self and the other) becomes a lesson in self-discovery.

The hatched child as a matter of course has the need to rapidly crawl in all directions, toward and away from the mother. These behaviors mark the beginning of the early practicing subphase at around nine months of age. Children can now use their bodies in many ways —coasting, playing while standing up, and climbing. Being capable of these new activities and of exploring carries a mood of elation, which lends a new expansiveness to the child's developing sense of self. The sense of self now begins to include the body in motion— powered by the child's intentionality.

As infants explore the inanimate and the animate world with all their sensory modalities, they learn more and more about themselves and their relation to the outside world. During the early practicing period, they learn that they can propel themselves into space by flexing and extending arms and legs. Encounters with the inanimate objects in the environment help to firm up and delineate body-self boundaries. Infants experience pleasure or pain in coming into contact with and exploring or passively enduring the outer world's hard, unyielding, and, at times, hurtful surface.

After the early practicing period, children take the greatest step in human individuation, walking with free, upright locomotion. With this beginning of the practicing period proper, the child's narcissism and pleasure in functioning is at its peak. Love for the mother is shared with love for the self as well as for external objects and objectives. The urge for new sensory experience is like an insatiable hunger, incessantly driving the child on.

The constructive use of forceful activity, often accompanied by anger, provides an essential impetus to the developmentally essential shift from passivity to activity. It promotes appropriate distancing from the mother and, as a consequence, self-object differentiation, which enables infants to begin to experience themselves as separate and distinct from the mother, as autonomous and independent individuals.[41] Early in life this essential adaptive shift from passive to active is enhanced by primitive motor and gestural imitations, later by selective ego identifications.

How infants feel about themselves during the practicing subphase depends both on subphase adequate mothering and fathering and on their own autonomous achievements. If adequate, these experiences create sound secondary narcissism: self-love, self-esteem, and omnipotence. Self-love is enhanced by the child's as well as by the mother's and father's satisfaction in the child's growing competence and is reinforced by the mother's and other adults' admiration.

During these subphases, as well as later, the specific conscious and unconscious needs of the mother activate out of each infant's infinite inborn potentialities those particular patterns of personality organization that create for each mother "the child" who reflects her own unique needs. The "birth" of the child as an individual begins when the infant gradually begins to alter behavior as the result of the mother's selective response to his or her cueing.[37] These personality patterns as well as the child's vulnerabilities seem to remain significant in later phases and beyond.

In addition to active behavior, passive experiences suggest inferences about the developing sense of self. Soon after the specific attachment to the mother occurs, infants show characteristic responses to brief separations from her. By six to eight months their tears and distress indicate that they miss her, long for her, and remember her. As early as nine months of age infants recollect the pain brought on by the mother's previous absences from the room and begin to anticipate that she might leave again. They begin to anticipate the recognized and remembered danger situation of object loss and the consequent feeling of helplessness. They watch the mother closely in order to try to stop her from leaving. Clearly the sense of self is now influenced by past experiences and anticipated outcomes.[68] This is the same critical age period during which infants "hatch." They acquire a beginning object permanence, anticipation, intentionality, and means-ends relations. They also acquire the capacity to experience the emotions of fear and anger[11] as well as a more complex network of interrelated memory systems including beginning recall memory, for example, of the absent mother. Infants also become anxious that the mother might be critical of angry behaviors. As a consequence, between nine and ten months they may cling to her for a few weeks.[30] They anticipate that the mother might leave the room based both on perceptual cues (e.g., the mother's movements) and affective cues (e.g., anger), and both can motivate them, for example, to try to prevent mother from doing so. It seems reasonable to assume that there has been a qualitative jump, alongside the expected quantitative progression, in the development of self-awareness, in the ability to organize and respond selectively to a variety of external (perceptual) and internal (affective and cognitive) stimuli, and in the capacity to initiate adaptive behaviors.

Mahler and I have also followed the infant's developing sense of self by observing behavior in front of the mirror.[47] General impressions stemming from the observations of the reactions of nine infants as they observe themselves in the mirror during the differentiation and practicing subphases form the basis for the inferences that follow. In this study the infants are free to observe and learn about their mirror images from an early age both in the setting of the study and at home. It is probably for this reason that the findings regarding the nine- to twelve-month period are slightly different from those of Lewis and Brooks-Gunn[25] and Amsterdam and Levitt,[4] although they are not altogether different from those of Gesell and Ames.[17]

At the same time that infants develop a nonspecific attachment to and a recognition memory of the human face by two to three months, they also show considerable interest in moving, staring at, examining, playing with, and mouthing fingers and hands, and slightly later, toes and feet. By the time they develop a specific attachment to and a recognition memory of the mother at four to five months, infants' behaviors suggest that they have also developed a specific, though different, attachment to and recognition memory of their own body: They show an increased interest in body parts and a certain familiarity with them.

Infants at four to five months study with interest the same features of their own faces in the mirror as those of the mother—particularly the eyes, the mouth, and the smile. We infer that the perception of themselves in the mirror has two points of reference: an inner, probably mainly kinesthetic and vestibular root and an outer layer consisting of visual-perceptual engrams.

From five to six months on, they begin to pay attention to the movement of fingers, hands, and arms as these are reflected in the mirror. In addition, they shift their gaze back and forth between the mirror reflection of their own faces and the face of the mother or other observer in the mirror and, shortly thereafter, also to the actual mother or observer. The infant's behavior in front of the mirror is similar to, although more complex than, comparative scanning (looking from one object to another at a distance), checking back (looking back to the mother's face as a point of reference after looking at the "other-than-mother-world"), and customs inspection (detailed visual and tactile examination of the mother's and "other's" faces).

Beginning by six months of age, the feedback through the mirror reflection also elicits considerable excitement. This excitement is more marked when the infants look at their own faces and movements, perhaps because they are more novel and more predictably elicted than when they look at the mother's mirror image.

By eight months the novelty of examining their body parts by touching and handling them wears off. By contrast, the infants become even more interested in and more excited than before by their own mirror images. As tactile and visual direct handling of their own body parts diminishes, they show increased interest in initiating and observing the reflection of coordinated movements and facial expressions. The babies wave their arms, move their bodies, rock, and kick their feet; they smile broadly while looking at their mirror images. The excited movements and smiles seen in the mirror are reflected back to themselves, probably acting as a continuous feedback, a reliable source of stimulation. Microanalysis of mirror reactions during these months indicates that each infant has a unique pattern of responding to the mirror.

We inferred from the infants' total behavior further progress, by nine to twelve months, in the integration of the body image. Whereas they still sometimes show excited enjoyment while looking at the mirror, more often than before they soberly look from the image and the movements of limbs to the by-then more familiar image of the face as a point of reference. Although earlier the babies had a recognition memory of their own mirror images as other, albeit familiar infants, they now seem to begin to sense that their self-initiated movements are in some way related to themselves. This vague awareness that the mirror image reflects the baby's own self seems to be disturbing at times, for during these same several months the infants sometimes become fussy and look away from or lose interest in the mirror. They seem disturbed, confused, and perplexed by the uncertain and fluctuating recognition that the familiar "other infant" observed in the mirror begins now to be dimly recognized as a reflection of themselves. This phenomena is reminiscent of the perplexity and distress infants experience when recognizing that another person is similar to but yet somewhat different from the mother or when the mother does not look quite like herself.

As we have seen, it is during the age span of eight to twelve months that infants hatch, acquire the emotions of fear and anger, begin to attain object and possibly some degree of self-permanence, and develop the capacity for intentionality and anticipation. The mother is not only recalled with distress when absent; her absence is anticipated on the basis of both perceptual and affective cues, and infants initiate behaviors in order to prevent her from leaving. It seems likely that infants now begin to link these experiences with a more differentiated and integrated sense of the bodily self and its boundaries. Whereas the "double touch" mentioned earlier is the young infant's first lesson in bodily tactile self-discovery, the fact that the one-year-old can now readily, predictably, and consistently bring about intended behaviors and expressions in a mirror reflection seems to point to the probability that the visual and kinesthetic self-schemata are now of a perceptually and cognitively higher order, which further augments self-awareness. The baby seen in the mirror begins to be the same baby who has sensations and feelings, intentions and anticipations that differ from others. From twelve to eighteen months infants slowly become aware that the body parts seen in the mirror are their own and, by eighteen months, that the child seen is indeed herself or himself.

From nine to fourteen months there are many behaviors indicative of identification that significantly shape the emerging sense of self. Particularly vivid are instances of identification with mother's prohibitions. Donna illustrates this well.[29]

During her eighth month, Donna grabbed a toy from another child without hesitation. During her ninth month, however—the same month she began to anticipate her mother's leaving the room—Donna looked at her mother quickly and searchingly after grabbing a toy from Peter. Instead of enjoying playing with the toy, she seemed bewildered, as if she did not know what to do with it. It was between nine and ten months that Donna developed a crisis in which she feared she would lose her mother completely, a crisis seemingly related to her angry behavior and her fear of mother's response. In her thirteenth month, after hitting Susan on the head with a hammer, Donna seemed confused when Susan cried. She backed away and mouthed her fingers. Soon after this, when Susan reached for Donna's toy, Donna said, "bye-bye" and walked away, seemingly relieved. Donna first obeyed mother's prohibition, then identified with it. She became inhibited, and her sense of self changed. Her inhibitions, strengthened during the rapprochement crisis, were still present at age four.

By fourteen to sixteen months children begin to show deferred imitation, symbolic play, and the verbal evocation of the mother in her absence.[52] Their behavior indicates not only the beginning of identifications that are patterned on a representational model; they also indicate the beginning of the capacity for self-reflection and are another qualitative shift in the emergence of self-awareness.

Up to the age of sixteen to eighteen months, we can speak only of a sense of self and of self-feelings, which are limited by the infants' sensorimotor and sensori-affective level of cognitive development. In the next subphase, which need be mentioned only briefly, we see cognitive and other developments—for example, representational thought—that in time will permit toddlers to begin to have a more crystallized self-awareness, a more fluid ability for self-reflection, as well as beginning fantasies about the self. In all probability the nature of the sense of self that has been built up during the first sixteen to eighteen months will play a role in determining the shape of these fantasies.

During the rapprochement subphase, from fifteen to twenty-four months, a noticeable shift in the sense of self occurs. Toddlers, as they develop a mental awareness of themselves as distinctly separate from their mother, become increasingly aware of their relative smallness and vulnerability. The feeling of omnipotence begins to wane. The mental sense of self is often characterized by envy and ambivalence, by moodiness, and by depressive feelings of sadness, longing, and anger.

It is particularly during intense conflict with the mother over autonomy and closeness and conflict over anger and the need to please (rapprochement crisis) that toddlers are most unhappy with themselves and tend to regress to a clinging, ambivalent relationship with their mothers.[38,39] This developmental conflict may become an intrapsychic conflict that has lasting consequences for the sense of self.

Conclusion

In this chapter inferences have been made about some of the developmental steps that contribute to the gradual attainment of object and self-constancy during the subphases of the separation-individuation process. These steps have been viewed in terms of both the cognitive development of stable object and self-representations and the stability of the cathexis and the "quality" of these representations. These advances are brought about by a number of factors. This includes the changing nature of the libidinal and aggressive cathexis of the love object and the self, the progressively more complex levels of memory organization and mental representation, and the emergence of numerous ego functions, particularly internalization. The attainment of object and self-constancy is a continuing developmental process; yet the emergence of each aspect of this developmental sequence is phase-specific.

When conditions are not favorable, there may be a failure in the development of object relations and the sense of self; the conflicts of the rapprochement crisis are also vulnerable and may not be resolved satisfactorily. Any of these may become points of fixation, with the persistence of excessive ambivalence, "splitting," and intrapsychic conflict. As a result, the attainment of object and self-constancy and the development of psychic structure are impaired, the resolution of oedipal conflicts is made more difficult, and either neurotic symptoms of the narcissistic variety[26,27] or borderline symptoms may occur in latency and adolescence.[48]

Under favorable conditions, a firm libidinal cathexis of object and self-representation will be established by the fourth subphase, the ego will exert substantial control over the aggressive drive, and the "good" and "bad" aspects of the love object as well as the "good" and "bad" aspects of the self will become united in one concept. Major steps along the line of self-object objectivization, differentiation, and integration will take place. Both the love object and the self are presently perceived and represented in closer accordance with reality.

During the fourth subphase there is an integration of self and object on a higher psychobiological and social level of development, far removed from the earlier symbiosis of self and object. The mental self is experienced as an integral part of a larger whole—the family and society. This higher level of integration plus the beginning development of object and self-constancy relieve toddlers of the threats of helplessness and loneliness characteristic of the rapprochement crisis. As a rule they no longer have to struggle against the danger of regressive symbiotic reengulfment. They have achieved internally and externally a close relationship with their love objects; at the same time they have achieved a certain degree of object constancy, autonomy, individuation, and self-constancy.

ACKNOWLEDGMENTS

This chapter is based in part on research supported by NIMH Grant MH-08238, United States Public Health Service, Bethesda, Maryland, and FFRP Grant 069-458 Foundation Fund for Research in Psychiatry, New Haven, Connecticut, Margaret S. Mahler, Principal Investigator, John B. McDevitt, Co-Principal Investigator.

REFERENCES

1. AINSWORTH, M.D.S. *Infancy in Uganda: Infant Care and the Growth of Love.* Baltimore: Johns Hopkins Press, 1967.

2. AINSWORTH, M.D.S., and BELL, S. M. "Attachment, Exploration, and Separation: Illustrated by the Behavior of One-year-olds in a Strange Situation," *Child Development,* 41 (1970):49–67.

3. AINSWORTH, M.D.S., and WITTIG, B. A. "Attachment and Exploratory Behavior of One-year-olds in a Strange Situation," in B. M. Foss, ed., *Determinants of Infant Behavior,* vol. 4. New York: Barnes & Noble, 1969, pp. 111–137.

4. AMSTERDAM, B. K., and LEVITT, M. "Consciousness of Self and Painful Self-consciousness," *Psychoanalytic Study of the Child,* 35 (1980):67–83.

5. BELL, S. M. "The Development of a Concept of Object as Related to Infant-mother Attachment," *Child Development,* 41 (1970):291–311.

6. BRAZELTON, B. "Neonatal Assessment," in S. I. Greenspan and G. H. Pollock, eds., *The Course of Life, vol. 1, Infancy and Early Childhood.* Washington, D.C.: U.S. Government Printing Office, 1981, pp. 203–234.

7. COBLINER, W. G. "Psychoanalysis and the Geneva School of Genetic Psychology: Parallels and Counterparts," *International Journal of Psychiatry,* 3 (1967):82–116.

8. CONDON, W., and SANDER, L. "Neonate Movement Is Synchronized with Adult Speech," *Science,* 183 (1972):99–101.

9. DECARIE, T. G. *Intelligence and Affectivity in Early Childhood.* New York: International Universities Press, 1965.

10. EMDE, R. N. "The Prerepresentational Self and Its Affective Core," *Psychoanalytic Study of the Child,* 38 (1983):165–192.

11. EMDE, R. N., GAENSBAUR, T., and HARMON, R. *Emotional Expression in Infancy: A Biobehavioral Study. Psychological Issues, Monograph 37.* New York: International Universities Press, 1976.

12. ENGEL, G. L., and REICHSMAN, F. "Depression in an Infant with a Gastric Fistula," *Journal of the American Psychoanalytic Association,* 4 (1956):428–452.

13. FLAVELL, J. H. *The Developmental Psychology of Jean Piaget.* New York: D. Van Nostrand, 1963.

14. FRAIBURG, S. "Libidinal Object Constancy and Mental Representation," *Psychoanalytic Study of the Child,* 24 (1969):9–47.

15. FREUD, A. "The Mutual Influences in the Development of Ego and Id, in *The Writings of Anna Freud,* vol. 4. New York: International Universities Press, 1968, pp. 230–244. (Originally published 1952.)

16. ———. *Normality and Pathology in Childhood: Assessments of Development.* New York: International Universities Press, 1965.

17. GESELL, A., and AMES, L. B. "The Infant's Reaction to His Mirror Image," *Journal of Genetic Psychology,* 70 (1947):141–154.

18. HARTMANN, H. "The Mutual Influences in the Development of Ego and Id," in *Essays on Ego Psychology,* New York: International Universities Press, 1952, pp. 155–181.

19. HEINICKE, C. M., and WESTHEIMER, I. J. *Brief Separations.* New York: International Universities Press, 1965.

20. HOFFER, W. "Mouth, Hand, and Ego-Integration," *Psychoanalytic Study of the Child,* 3/4 (1949):49–56.

21. ———. "The Mutual Influences in the Development of Ego and Id: Earliest Stages," *Psychoanalytic Study of the Child,* 7 (1952):31–41.

22. ———. *Psychoanalysis: Practical and Research Aspects. The Flexner Lectures, Series 12.* Baltimore: Vanderbilt University, 1955.

23. KAPLAN, L. "Object Constancy in the Light of Piaget's Vertical Decalage," *Bulletin of the Menninger Clinic,* 36 (1972):322–334.

24. KAUFMAN, I. C., and ROSENBLUM, L. A. "The Reaction to Separation in Infant Monkeys: Anaclitic Depression and Conservation Withdrawal," *Psychosomatic Medicine,* 29 (1967):648–675.

25. LEWIS, M., and BROOKS-GUNN, J. *Social Cognition and the Acquisition of Self.* New York: Plenum Press, 1979.

26. McDEVITT, J. B. "A Separation problem in a Three-year-old Girl," in E. R. Geleerd, ed., *The Child Analyst at Work.* New York: International Universities Press, 1967, pp. 24–58.

27. ———. "Preoedipal Determinants of an Infantile Neurosis," in J. B. McDevitt and C. F. Settlage, eds., *Separation-*

Individuation: Essays in Honor of Margaret S. Mahler. New York: International Universities Press, 1971, pp. 201–226.

28. ———. "Separation-individuation and Object Constancy," *Journal of the American Psychoanalytic Association,* 23 (1975):713–742.

29. ———. "The Role of Internalization in the Development of Object Relations During the Separation-individuation Phase," *Journal of the American Psychoanalytic Association,* 27 (1979):327–343.

30. ———. "The Emergence of Hostile Aggression and Its Defensive and Adaptive Modifications During the Separation-individuation Process," *Journal of the American Psychoanalytic Association,* 31 (Supplement) (1983):273–300.

31. McDEVITT, J. B., and MAHLER, M. S. "Object Constancy, Individuality and Internalization," in S. I. Greenspan and G. H. Pollock, eds., *The Course of Life,* vol. 1. Bethesda, Md.: National Institute of Mental Health, 1980, pp. 407–423.

32. MAHLER, M. S. "On Child Psychosis and Schizophrenia: Autistic and Symbiotic Infantile Psychoses," in *The Selected Papers of Margaret S. Mahler,* vol. 1. New York: Jason Aronson, 1979, pp. 131–154. (Originally published 1952.)

33. ———. "On Sadness and Grief in Infancy and Childhood: Loss and Restoration of the Symbiotic Love Object," in *The Selected Papers of Margaret S. Mahler,* vol. 1. New York: Jason Aronson, 1979, pp. 261–279. (Originally published 1961.)

34. ———. "Thoughts About Development and Individuation," *Psychoanalytic Study of the Child,* 18 (1963): 307–342.

35. ———. "On the Significance of the Normal Separation-individuation Phase with Reference to Research in Symbiotic Child Psychosis," in *The Selected Papers of Margaret S. Mahler,* vol. 2. New York: Jason Aronson, 1979, pp. 49–58. (Originally published 1965.)

36. ———. "Notes on the Development of Basic Moods: The Depressive Affect," in *The Selected Papers of Margaret S. Mahler,* vol. 2. New York: Jason Aronson, 1979, pp. 59–76. (Originally published 1966.)

37. ———. *On Human Symbiosis and the Vicissitudes of Individuation,* vol. 1, *Infantile Psychosis.* New York: International Universities Press, 1968.

38. ———. "Rapprochement Subphase of the Separation-individuation Process," in *The Selected Papers of Margaret S. Mahler,* vol. 2. New York: Jason Aronson, 1979, pp. 131–148. (Originally published 1972.)

39. ———. "Symbiosis and Individuation: The Psychological Birth of the Human Infant," in *The Selected Papers of Margaret S. Mahler,* vol. 2. New York: Jason Aronson, 1979, pp. 149–165. (Originally published 1974.)

40. ———. *Selected Papers,* vol. 1 and 2. New York: Jason Aronson, 1979.

41. ———. "Aggression in the Service of Separation-individuation: Case Study of a Mother-Daughter Relationship," *Psychoanalytic Quarterly,* 50 (1981):625–638.

42. MAHLER, M. S., and FURER, M. Certain aspects of the separation-individuation phase. In *The Selected Papers of Margaret S. Mahler,* vol. 2. New York: Jason Aronson, 1979, pp. 21–34. (Originally published 1963.)

43. ———. *On Human Symbiosis and the Vicissitudes of Individuation.* New York: International Universities Press, 1968.

44. MAHLER, M. S., and GOSLINER, B. J. "On Symbiotic Child Psychosis: Genetic, Dynamic, and Restitutive Aspects," in *The Selected Papers of Margaret S. Mahler,* vol. 1. New York: Jason Aronson, 1979, pp. 109–130. (Originally published 1955.)

45. MAHLER, M. S., and LA PERRIERE, K. "Mother-Child Interaction During Separation-individuation," in *The Selected Papers of Margaret S. Mahler,* vol. 2. New York: Jason Aronson, 1979, pp. 35–38. (Originally published 1965.)

46. MAHLER, M. S., and McDEVITT, J. B. "Observations on Adaptation and Defense *in statu nascendi,*" in *The Selected Papers of Margaret S. Mahler,* vol. 2. New York: Jason Aronson, 1979, pp. 99–118. (Originally published 1968.)

47. ———. "Thoughts on the Emergence of the Sense of Self, with Particular Emphasis on the Body Self," *Journal of the American Psychoanalytic Association,* 30 (1982):827–848.

48. MAHLER, M. S., PINE, F., and BERGMAN, A. *The Psychological Birth of the Human Infant: Symbiosis and Individuation.* New York: Basic Books, 1975.

49. NAGERA, H. "Sleep and Its Disturbances Approached Developmentally," *Psychoanalytic Study of the Child,* 21 (1966):393–447.

50. PIAGET, J. *Play, Dreams and Imitation in Childhood.* New York: W. W. Norton, 1951.

51. ———. *The Construction of Reality in the Child.* New York: Basic Books, 1954.

52. PIAGET, J., and INHELDER, B. *The Psychology of the Child.* New York: Basic Books, 1969.

53. PINE, F. "Libidinal Object Constancy: A Theoretical Note," in L. Goldberger, ed., *Psychoanalysis and Contemporary Science,* vol. 3. New York: International Universities Press, 1975, pp. 307–313.

54. RAPAPORT, D. "The Structure of Psychoanalytic Theory," *Psychological Issues Monograph 6.* New York: International Universities Press, 1960.

55. ROIPHE, H., and GALENSON, E. *Infantile Origins of Sexual Identity.* New York: International Universities Press, 1981.

56. RUBINFINE, D. L. "Perception, Reality Testing, and Symbolism," *Psychoanalytic Study of the Child,* 16 (1961): 73–89.

57. SANDLER, J. "The Background of Safety," *International Journal of Psycho-Analysis,* 41 (1960):352–356.

58. SANDLER, J., and JOFFE, W. G. "On Skill and Sublimation," *Journal of American Psychoanalytic Association,* 14 (1966):335–355.

59. SCHAFER, R. *Aspects of Internalization.* New York: International Universities Press, 1968.

60. SCHAFFER, H. R. "Objective Observations of Personality Development in Early Infancy," *British Journal of Medical Psychology,* 31 (1958):174–183.

61. SCHAFFER, H. R., and CALLENDER, W. M. "Psychobiological Effects of Hospitalization in Infancy," *Pediatrics,* 24 (1959):528–539.

62. SPITZ, R. A. "Relevancy of Direct Infant Observation," *Psychoanalytic Study of the Child,* 5 (1950):66–73.

63. ———. *No and Yes: On the Genesis of Human Communication.* New York: International Universities Press, 1957.

64. ———. (In collaboration with W. G. Cobliner.) *The First Year of Life.* New York: International Universities Press, 1965.

65. ———. "Metapsychology and Direct Infant Observation," in R. M. Loewenstein, et al., eds., *Psychoanalysis—A General Psychology.* New York: International Universities Press, 1966, pp. 123–151.

66. SPOCK, B. "The Striving for Autonomy and Regressive Object Relationships," *Psychoanalytic Study of the Child,* 28 (1963):365–366.

67. SPRUIELL, V. "Three Strands of Narcissism," *Psychoanalytic Quarterly,* 44 (1975):577–595.

68. SROUFE, A. L. "Socioemotional Development," in J. D. Osofsky, ed., *Handbook of Infant Development.* New York: John Wiley & Sons, 1979, pp. 462–516.

69. STECHLER, G., and KAPLAN, S. "The Development of the Self: A Psychoanalytic Perspective," *Psychoanalytic Study of the Child,* 35 (1980):85–105.

70. STERN, D. N. "A Microanalysis of Mother-infant Interaction: Behavior Regulating Social Contact Between a Mother and her 3½ Month Old Twins," in E. Rexford, L. Sander, and T. Shapiro, eds., *Infant Psychiatry.* New Haven: Yale University Press, 1976, pp. 113–126.

71. ———. *The First Relationship.* Cambridge, Mass.: Harvard University Press, 1977.

72. ———. "The Early Development of Schemas of Self, of Other, and of Various Experiences of 'Self with Other,'" in J. D. Lichtenberg and S. Kaplan, eds., *Reflections on Self*

Psychology. New York: International Universities Press, 1982, pp. 49–84.

73. TENNES, K. H., and LAMPL, E. E. "Defensive Reactions to Infantile Separation Anxiety," *Journal of the American Psychoanalytic Association,* 17 (1969):1142–1162.

74. WINNICOTT, D. W. "Mirror-role of Mother and Family in Child Development," in D. W. Winnicott, *Playing and Reality.* New York: Basic Books, 1967, pp. 111–118.

75. YARROW, L. J. "Attachment and Dependency: A Developmental Perspective," in M. L. Hoffman and L. W. Hoffman, eds., *Attachment and Dependency.* Washington, D.C.: Winston, 1972, pp. 81–96.

6 / New Developments in Early Language Acquisition

Nadine A. Levinson and Justin D. Call

. . . for I was no longer a speechless infant; but a speaking boy. This I remember; and have since observed how I learned to speak. It was not that my elders taught me words . . . in any set method; but I . . . did myself . . . practice the sounds in my memory. . . . And thus by constantly hearing words, as they occurred in various sentences . . . I thereby gave utterance to my will.

—St. Augustine[66]

How infants learn to speak has been the focus of extensive discussion for centuries. As we see from his account, St. Augustine[66] believed he knew how he had taught himself to speak. He thus anticipated a trend of language acquisition research of the 1980s. This approach emphasizes the active role of the child in determining his or her own unique style and the possibility that several different roads to language acquisition might be traveled. Each of these depends on the inherent predispositions in the child and the nature of the individual parent-child interaction.

What Is Language?

It is impressive that children by the age of two can master the basic rules of syntax and by four or five years, with little instruction and with limited and imperfect language exposure, can master the intricate and complex rules of a formal language system. More than that, they use this modality to convey, often quite elo-

quently, their inner thoughts and feelings to others.[15] What mental structures or levels of organization do children acquire that enables such achievement? How do children acquire knowledge of how language works? This chapter will attempt an updating of knowledge, even if not a complete answer to these questions, by reviewing and discussing some of the recent findings from biology, neurosciences, developmental psycholinguistics, psychoanalysis, and child psychiatry that contribute to a model of language acquisition.

But first we must attempt an answer to a question that has plagued philosophers and linguists alike: If speech cannot be equated to language, then, what is language?

To define language is as elusive as attempting to define energy. No single viewpoint is sufficient. An operational definition specifies language as a rule-governed, species-specific, creative, symbolic, and displaceable (having the capacity to refer to a distant source) means of communication. A language has systematic rules for pronunciation, word formation, and grammatical construction that determine its usage for communication. Four essential subsystems of linguistic structure systematically studied by linguists include phonology, syntactics, semantics, and pragmatics.

Phonology describes the rules governing the sound system of spoken language. A nondistinctive unit of sound is called a phone while a distinctive unit of sound is called a phoneme. Phonemes alone or in relation to other phonemes form words. "Pat" becomes "bat" by changing the phoneme "p" to "b." A child may know the rules of sound but may be unable to use the rules in forming words correctly.[8] This can be illustrated from an example from our longitudinal study:

Observer: Fish?
Child: Yes, Fis!
Observer: Fis?
Child: NO!!! Fis!!!!
Observer: Fish?
Child: Yes! Fis! That's right.

In the early stages of sound making, infants, ages six to twelve months, can babble and discriminate distinctive sound features. The pitch contours and intonations of these rhythmically organized utterances (identifiable as early as three months) reflect the children's internal state, state gradience, and categories of emotion or affect. Such states are communicated to the mother and understood by her.[77] In the late babbling stage, ages twelve to eighteen months, children can string sounds together randomly so that the sound sequences resemble words and even sentences but contain no conventional words or decipherable meaning. In effect, the children have the music but not the lyrics.

Contrary to earlier research, which suggested that infants learn the phonemes of their native language by six months,[40] recent studies suggest that the learning of phonological rules that determine how words are formed from phonemes is dependent on the nature and context of the first words.[55] Thus rates of phoneme production and articulation are a function of the complexity of the sound system of a given language. Children learning the same language also show considerable variation in the age, rate, and style in which they acquire the basic phonemes of language.

The *semantics* of language is the study of how meaning is embedded in words and sentences (as distinguished from general semantics, which deals with all sources of meaning). The minimal unit of meaning in language is the morpheme, which consists of one or more phonemes. At the one-word stage, age twelve months to fifteen months, children recognize general perceptual or functional features such as shape, size, movement, or texture of objects and then generalize the use of the word for that object to represent other objects. For example, "dog" may mean cat, horse, rabbit, or any four-legged animal.[16,60] These overgeneralizations resemble primary process thinking as shown in dream work and symptom formation.[51]

Syntax describes the rules by which words are meaningfully combined to express thoughts in the form of phrases and sentences. Children who have not yet acquired the complete set of adult rules for organizing word strings generate their own rules for sentence formation.

Motherese and the special language of twins are examples of how children and their parents can create idiosyncratic sound, meaning, and syntax by arbitrarily assigning meaning to phonemes and morphemes. When the mother ascribes meaning to the infantile utterance, she is participating in the formation of infantese, the infant's first sound system of communication. As the mother modifies the complexity of her language to the infant and the infant reciprocates with her, a second system of communication, motherese, is superimposed on the first system.

Pragmatics describes how children participate with others in a conversation using gestures, affects, words, and sentences to negotiate problem solving and mastery of the human environment. Language with mother is a shared event consisting of communicating and being understood. Consider Vana, seventeen months, one of the children in our ongoing longitudinal study. She points at an object while she says:

A ma be pa
A ma be pa
M. You need the paper? (Hands her the paper.)
V. Dank you.

The integration of these four subsystems of linguistic structure comprise language competence as distinguished from communication and speech. *Communication* describes all of the ways in which information, including feelings, thoughts, and bodily states, can be transmitted from one person to another. In contrast to this, *speech* refers to the act or behavior of verbalizing. Speech is only one expression of linguistic competence. Deaf children, utilizing sign language, sign writing, and lip reading, for example, may demonstrate highly skilled linguistic competence in communicating their feelings and thoughts to others while remaining inarticulate using the spoken word.

With ongoing maturation and development, these subsystems of linguistic structure and function are influenced by and influence cognitive, social, affective and neurological maturation.[56] Noam Chomsky[15] has stated that language approaches "the human essence," and Henry Edelheit[61] has described language as the least deceptive mirror of the mind.

Language Acquisition Theories

Systematic child language research can be traced back to the work of Tiedemann,[80] Darwin,[21] and Preyer.[63] Writing in the eighteenth and nineteenth centuries, they established the tradition of observational studies of infants, carried out by parent-scientists, recording language development, affective communication, and gestures of their own children, a type of study that continues to this day. The commonsense notion that children learn language from their parents through imitation, rewards, and punishments was emphasized by Skinner.[73] This conceptual framework was successfully challenged by Chomsky,[14] who noted that, by five years of age, children show the capacity to employ billions of combinations of word strings in forming phrases and sentences. As well, rather than replicating the often imperfect adult language environment to which they are exposed, children generate creative rules of their own for producing word strings. Chomsky's theory of generative transformational grammar[13] postulated a set of biologically derived internal rules for forming sentences, referred to as the language acquisition device (LAD). Linguistic research of the 1960s followed Chomsky's lead and centered almost exclusively on children's acquisition of these internal linguistic structures. Little attention was paid to a system of meaning that regulates the exchanges between people. Although children may indeed be innately predisposed for language development, Chomsky's linguistic theories are not sufficient to explain the processes involved in language acquisition.

A semantic approach to language acquisition was initiated by Bloom[4] and Schlesinger.[69] Their approach considered meaning and the communicative intent of utterances to be as important as linguistic structure. Universal semantic content was viewed as evidence that cognitive, rather than linguistic, achievements formed the primary bases of child utterances.[57,74]

The semantic/cognitive approach specifies that language acquisition is dependent on mastery of sensorimotor intelligence[19] and certain cognitive principles such as means-end behavior. The capacity for object permanence, while important in its own right, was found to be a cognitive achievement that was not necessary for language acquisition.[1] Children are active participants in the process of language learning,[76] and before two years of age they can "map" their knowledge of the world with their utterances.[6]

The study of Genie[31] and her encounter with language provides some interesting data about the acquisition of syntax in relationship to cognitive development. Genie is a young girl with extreme language deprivation who was raised in isolation from twenty months to almost fourteen years. When tested in her late adolescence, Genie was found to show very primitive syntactic utterances and demonstrated greater cognitive sophistication by her expression and comprehension of meanings of words and word combinations. Curtiss[20] suggests that syntax need not develop from a cognitive-

semantic base, but, as was the case with Genie, both capacities may develop independently.

During the 1980s more interest has been devoted to children's ability to exchange in conversations and to respond to communication from others. Linguistic competence, or knowing the rules that govern word and sentence formation, is only one aspect of communicative competence.[2] From a secure base with mother, children learn more about the world around them. Utilizing communicative, affective, and cognitive skills, they can share such knowledge with their mother through conversation.[79] Early prelinguistic, reciprocal interactions such as turn-taking, shared attention, play, and games underlie communicative competence.*

Even though intuition and circumstantial evidence indicate that the social milieu and the developmental history of the child function as influences on language development, Bates[2] concludes that in the normal range of social interaction, the evolutionary "fit" of mother to child has become so good that language development is "buffered" against variability. The concept of "buffering" is similar to the proposition that language is an autonomous ego function[39] that develops in an average expectable environment.[64]

Language Acquisition in Infancy

What differentiates language proper from earlier prelinguistic behavior patterns? Prelinguistic behavior *reflects* bodily and internal states rather than being a conventional system of signs to *represent* symbolically the inner states and affects.[84] However, from the earliest period of infancy, language precursors for content, form, and use are already evident. Children gradually acquire concepts about regularities in the world with regard to objects and the relations among those objects. These concepts serve as a precursor for language content. Later, speaking children not only know empirically about events in the world but know how to represent that knowledge in a conventional language system.

Fetus and infant speech perception studies[3,26,43,59] have demonstrated that babies can perceive and discriminate among phonetic features that are a part of adult language. In carefully controlled studies, fetuses who had prenatal auditory stimulation showed postnatal auditory preferences.[43] This implies both an inherent basis for at least one aspect of linguistic form and the capacity for fetal learning (habituation). There is

*See references 9, 10, 41, 45, and 78.

an early readiness for communication in babies, as shown by their synchronous movements in rhythm with the human voice at birth.[17] However, how children's later language functions develop and relate to these early perceptual and cognitive abilities is still being actively investigated.

When and how does the sound making of the child gain meaning? Many investigators agree that sound making between infant and mother gains meaning in the context of their reciprocal interactions. The infant's internal state finds a subtle outward expression; whether intentional or not, this is perceived by the mother "as if" the infant intended to communicate with her. The smallest movement or sound provided by the infant is endowed by the mother with highly personal meaning, and such meaning, in turn, is often influenced by the mother's state.[25] For example, the "mmm" sound of the five- to six-month-old nursing infant eventually becomes in the nine-month-old an intentional and conventional signal for the wish to nurse. The meaning of "mmm" is enhanced by the way the infant glances at the mother and persists with the "mmm" and glance until the request is arranged. The sounds, looks, and movements become part of the mutually recognized signal system of infantese. Call[10] suggests that affective signals are biologically based in infants. Such signals are internalized in the mother through her narcissistic identification with the infant. They are further modified internally by the mother and then reflected back to the infant so that both infant and mother come to know the subjective feeling states of the other.[62] The process is one of merging affect and sound into a basic matrix for communication and language; Trevarthan[81] has referred to this sequence as intersubjectivity. Emde[27] emphasized this process as a pathway to the affective self.

A useful way to understand language acquisition is in the context of separation-individuation.[51,54] In the symbiotic phase, back-and-forth activities such as mutual gaze,[78] burst pause[41] raspberry game,[10] joint attention,[9] talking, cooing, and touching establish a basis for later back-and-forth listening and speaking. As the mother becomes a separate and important libidinal object, the child becomes increasingly aware of the value of language for obtaining wished-for gratification.

Between seven and twelve months, corresponding with the later part of the differentiating subphase, there is increasing use of gesture for spontaneous and intentional communication. As the child moves away or "hatches" from mother physically, the vocal and visual systems are used to maintain contact. Mahler has called this "the checking-back pattern." The child points, reaches, and rejects with the intention of demanding, requesting, stating, and questioning.[1,38]

Sounds become more phonetically consistent and can accompany or replace gesture.[50]

Most children go through a single-word stage for about six months, using one word at a time for labeling and naming. First words represent conceptual categories of existence, nonexistence, and recurrence.[5] "Hi" and "bye" are among children's first words and are used frequently in separation situations, facilitating the mastery of "object loss." The child uses gestures, affective expressions, and action or play to express affect-laden thoughts until words denoting affects—such as "mad," "bad," "good," "nice," and so forth—can be codified and used in the appropriate context. "Acting-out" in the adult, rather than using language or thought, indicates a regression to this preverbal mode of expression.[36]

The twelve- to eighteen-month period is an exciting time for language acquisition. During the practicing subphase, children practice using multiple utterances that are strung together in a linear fashion, such as; "Here pretty," "truck, truck go." Words that are so strung together are difficult for anyone but the primary care giver to understand. Telegraphic language, a derivative of primary process thinking, is used by many children at fifteen to eighteen months; it is similar to Western Union messages where nonfunctional words, such as articles, prepositions, plurals, adjectives, and adverbs, are deleted.

Vana, at eighteen months, said, "me push button."

As the child passes from single-word to multiword speech, significant individual differences in style, rate, content, and form of communicative competence emerge. Those same differences in style are simultaneously represented in the play situation. In microcosmic play, which takes place from eighteen to twenty-one months, children sequence and use small objects to replicate and master an increasingly complex social and psychological world. Parallel with this, children also begin to organize words into meaningful sequences —phrases and sentences. Like microcosmic play, language can be intrapersonal or interpersonal. At eighteen months, Vana's play patterns were accompanied by a back-and-forth dialogue with mother. When Vana holds up objects and asks, "What's this?" Mother responds, "It's a . . ." illustrating the interpersonal aspect of language. At twenty-five months, Vana plays at a distance from mother while speaking aloud to herself. She verbally references and monitors her own solitary play activities that arise from her inner mentation, illustrating the intrapersonal aspect of language.

At two years of age, in the rapprochement subphase, most children have a vocabulary of two hundred words.[6] They demonstrate many new language functions that reveal the emergence of symbolic thought and other developing ego functions. In addition to serving pragmatic ends, represented by simple phrases such as as "I want" or "give me," children use language to assist learning as shown by asking "What's this?" In addition, other important language functions such as the informative function, commonly demonstrated by children stating "me say," and the imaginative function, shown by children pretending "me mommy, you baby," can be routinely observed.[38] Reference to oneself in language can be observed as early as eighteen months. Language assists children in self-definition as they name parts of the body and begin to use pronouns "I" and "you." David provides an example of how language facilitates a toddler's separation from mother. At twelve months, when mother left the room, David would break down and cry. At fourteen months he was able to use the hand-waving "bye-bye" gesture when mother left, but was still quite visibly upset. At two years of age, he still used the "bye-bye" gesture but was also able to comfort himself by saying, "Mommy bye-bye, be right back," while still continuing to play with his blocks.

In considering the leap from early forms of communication to language proper, Call[11] suggests a developmental sequence for the evolution of syntax, beginning with the use of the pointing gesture as a protosyntactic device followed by the use of idiosyncratic utterances and action sequences as transitional phenomena. He provides examples of how the sequential organization of experience from fifteen months to age two develops into a grammar of experience that in turn sets the stage for the sequencing of words utilizing syntactic rules.

Freud[29] pointed out that language is important in establishing superego precursors. Jordan, eighteen months, wanted to touch the fire and was able to control the wish to touch by speaking out loud to himself, "No, hot! No, hot! No, touch!" The "voice of conscience" can be observed in many children before eighteen months of age. At two years children demonstrate a creative and nonimitative rule system for organizing phrases and questions.

M. "What this is?"
V. "Dog goed."

Corrections of such "improper grammar" by parents are usually based on content rather than form. Exchanges in which parents try to correct for form are futile and can lead to control struggles as shown by this language sample from Fromkin and Rodman[30] (p. 333).

Child: Nobody don't like me.
Mother: No, say "Nobody likes me."
Child: Nobody don't like me.
 [dialogue repeated eight times]
Mother: Now, listen carefully, say "Nobody likes me."
Child: Oh, nobody don't likes me.

Cerebral Lateralization and Early Language Acquisition

The discovery by Broca[7] that the human brain has the capacity for lateralization of language functions may be one of the most important observations of the nineteenth century. Current technological advances in the neurosciences have moved us closer to unlocking some of the mysteries of the maturation of the brain and its structural strategies for language acquisition. The literature on language function in infants and young children and its relationship to the normal anatomy, physiology, and pathology of the brain has led to a variety of hypotheses about the maturation and development of lateralization of language function. How and when does cerebral lateralization take place? Is right-hemispheric language capacity possible, or is all language solely organized by the left hemisphere? Does experience influence the development of cerebral dominance for language, or is dominance determined exclusively by genetic programming? Current studies of cerebral lateralization and hemispheric specialization of language functions and their implications for language acquisition will be reviewed and discussed in the next sections.

CEREBRAL ASYMMETRY IN INFANCY

There is conclusive evidence that gross and subtle cortical asymmetries in language-mediating areas such as the inferior frontal gyrus occur in the fetus[12,88] and in the infant,[83,87] just as with adults.[34] Noninvasive computerized tomographic radiologic techniques have shown bilateral asymmetries in the Sylvian fissures of children and of nonhuman primates.[47,48]

Asymmetry of cytoarchitectonics (the morphology, layered arrangement, and physiology of nerve cells) has also been demonstrated in fetuses and infants.[32] Unlike gross anatomical landmarks, cytoarchitectonics correspond more closely to regions in the brain with distinct neuronal organizations that reflect different language functions.[32] For example, maps of the brain[24] show that in infants, the primary area of the planum temporale is larger on the right side, while the left side has larger association areas. Such findings cast serious doubt on Lenneberg's hypothesis[49] of equipotentiality of both brain hemispheres for language function at birth and supports the concept of anatomical, left-hemisphere specialization for some aspects of language function.[42] Psychophysiological studies have furthered our understanding of the functional asymmetries present in young children. In infants one week to ten months old, Molfese[58] found evoked potential responses to speech sounds greater in the left hemisphere than in the right. At three months of age, dichotic listening studies have shown a right-ear advantage, implying a left-hemisphere dominance for speech sounds in such infants.[28] An attempt to replicate this study was unsuccessful,[82] although similar results were obtained using heart rate instead of sucking as a criteria for right-ear advantage in three-month-old infants.[35]

In six-month-old infants, electroencephalographic recordings[33] comparing perception of music and speech have shown interhemispheric differences. Such infants recognize correspondences in acoustic and optic properties when attending to these acoustic stimuli entering the right ear. This suggests that the capacity to begin prelinguistic babbling may "rest on a predisposition of the left hemisphere to recognize sensorimotor connections between the auditory structure of speech and its articulatory source"[52] (p. 1348).

Adult women exhibit a lesser degree of cerebral lateralization than do men.[53] However, little evidence of lateralization based on sex differences has been found in children.[86] This data is in striking contrast to the empirical observation that up until puberty, girls are more mature linguistically and show a higher mean sentence length (MSL), word usage, level of articulation, and grammatical competence than do boys. Future research will be required to increase our understanding of the role of cultural experience, hormonal effects, and other neuropsychological variables that might account for sex differences in lateralized linguistic functioning.

DEVELOPMENTAL ASPECTS OF RECOVERY FROM BRAIN INJURY AS SHOWN BY CEREBRAL LATERALIZATION OF LANGUAGE FUNCTIONING

Even though the fetal, neonatal, and juvenile brains demonstrate early lateralization of structure and function, the young brain has a remarkable ability to recover from and compensate for serious lesions. (It has been presumed that similar damage would produce language deficits in the adult.) From birth until age five, children have shown the capacity to recover linguistic functioning after serious injury to the left side of the brain.[44] However, recovery from brain damage beyond adolescence has also been observed.[31] The considerable variations in the data concerning the range of recovery in relation to age are due largely to methodological problems. When rigorous criteria for recovery are applied to earlier recovery reports in the literature and when inadequacy of sampling and of failure to control for lateralization, handedness, site of lesion, nature of persisting lesions, and other developmental

concerns are taken into account, age differences and recovery of language functions following severe brain injury are less than convincing.[42]

A systematic study of three infants who had surgical hemidecortication for epilepsy before five months of age was undertaken by Dennis and Whitaker.[23] One of the infants had the cortex of the right hemisphere removed, while the other two infants had the cortex of the left hemisphere removed. Each of the children were assessed at nine and ten years of age, at which time all three were found to have normal IQs in verbal and performance areas. They were functioning adequately in school and had no difficulty with the semantic or conceptual aspects of language. However, subsequent follow-up of the two children with left decortication showed subtly defective language recovery, casting some doubt on the equal potentiality for language of the two hemispheres during infancy.

A comprehensive reinterpretation of the hemispherectomy data by St. James-Roberts[67] suggests that recovery from hemispherectomy is related to the surgical techniques used, duration and extent of epilepsy prior to surgery, the presence of complications, the use of medication, and many other confounding variables. There is some general agreement, however, that the right hemisphere can assume left-hemispheric language functions. However, the exact role of the right hemisphere in language acquisition for normal children is still not thoroughly understood. The processing of nonverbal expression, as in sign language, and of affective signals, as shown in affective, facial expression, vocal intonation, gestural communication, is the dominant mode of communication in the first 18 months of life. The associated functions are organized by the right hemisphere.[22] Just how the right hemisphere may assume left-hemispheric language function when Broca's area of the left cortex is injured or removed is still unclear.

Corballis[18] hypothesizes that right-hemispheric plasticity for language acquisition is based on a left to right maturational gradient. He suggests that both hemispheres are intrinsically similar for language function, but that the left cerebral hemisphere develops earlier than the right and at a time when language acquisition is taking place. The right hemisphere can take over for the left hemisphere as long as it has not gone beyond a critical phase of development. Just when the critical phase occurs is not certain from presently available data.

Another interesting and relevant maturational variable has been introduced by Scheibel, et al.[68] who have demonstrated increased branchiness of layer III pyramidal cell dendrites in the left triangularis-opercularis cortical area (the association area for speech) as contrasted with greater length of first order dendrite branches in the same area on the right cortex. He states,

If the adult dendritic arbor is conceived of as a 'fossilized' record of this dendritic development, we suggest that right-left differences in branching patterns represent differential sequences of growth peculiar to the two hemispheres and to the areas involved. Thus the greater dendritic length of lower-order branches suggests that portions of the right cortex may 'lead' the left during the first year of life, when the infant depends extensively on sensory impressions of a highly concrete nature and is limited to relatively large-scale and undifferentiated motor acts (sensory-motor period of Piaget). Somewhat later, with continuous maturation of the cortical systems, symbolic operations such as language and other 'left-hemisphere tasks' emerge, and motor actions become more discrete. During this period the higher-order dendritic branches develop, and the LOP becomes anatomically more complex, coincident with its emerging functional dominance. (p. 72)

The intact functional corpus collosum is responsible for transfer of information between the two hemispheres. Myelinization of the corpus collosum does not begin until one year of age, is far advanced by age four, and is complete by age ten.[46] The functional immaturity of the corpus collosum in infancy might explain the regular occurrence of play and verbal self-communication in two- and three-year-olds who accompany solitary play with verbal monitoring, as shown, for example, by putting the doll into bed and saying to oneself, "Dolly go sleep." Actions organized by the right hemisphere are presented via the corpus collosum to the left hemisphere, which has the capacity to linguistically code nonverbal communications to verbal statements. Interhemispheric transfer of information from the right hemisphere to the left hemisphere via the corpus collosum may well facilitate tension reduction, mastery of affects, dramatic affect-laden visual memories and fantasy originating in the right hemisphere. Indeed, it may be that by passing such information to the left hemisphere, it can then be verbally encoded and sequenced (i.e., readied for verbal expression rather than acted out). It is reasonable to conclude from present knowledge that both hemispheres mediate language, but that they do so in different ways and according to different rates of growth for each hemisphere and for the connections between them. A preliminary study of children of schizophrenic parents revealed possible defects of interhemispheric integration, suggesting developmental precursors involving the corpus collosum for schizophrenia.[37]

In summary, the evidence seems overwhelmingly in favor of functional and anatomical asymmetry of the two hemispheres at birth, long before children learn language. These studies suggest an innate mechanism for speech perception and support Chomsky's hypothesis about an innate basis for language acquisition.[13]

Developing lateralization is a multidimensional process involving localization of language functioning in the two hemispheres, different dendritic arbolization in the right and left speech association areas and varying rates of maturation of myelinization in the corpus collosum association tracts, and experiential factors.[81,85,86] New noninvasive brain imaging techniques such as nuclear magnetic resonance (NMR) combined with positron emission transmission (PET), more detailed developmental studies of gross and microscopic brain anatomy, and clinically applicable neurophysiologic tools will prove useful in the longitudinal study of language-disordered infants and young children. It is likely that these will advance our knowledge about the maturation and functioning of the hemispheres and the corpus collosum for the development of language. In addition, we will learn more about the degree of hemispheric specialization, the limits of neural plasticity in childhood, and genetic and environmental influences. In light of current data, the concept of left-hemispheric dominance for language function may be relative rather than absolute and, at best, seems oversimplified.

Styles in Language Acquisition

Since the 1960s several conceptual shifts in the study of language acquisition have occurred. Currently, from the very beginning of the process by which children achieve linguistic and communicative competence, children are regarded as active and creative participants in their own development. In the early stages of language acquisition, prior to one year of age, children can be seen to initiate communication in feeding, games, play, gesture, and many other activities, including psychophysiological ones. These individual patterns of communication provide the basis for different styles of language learning in each child. Some children rely on imitation, while others seem to intuit language usage and are capable of astounding their parents with spontaneous and idiosyncratic utterances. In their first fifty words, firstborn children tend to use words that refer to objects while later-born children use words that include social expressions and gestures.[60] In effect, children form their own rules for early expression, which are not copies of adult rules. The child's capacity to utilize parental language input is constrained by the youngster's actual abilities, strategies, and productions.[64,75] In the course of assessing developmental disturbances, a knowledge and appreciation of individual variations of child-originated strategies can be of importance to the child psychotherapist and to the speech pathologist.

For example, consider a male infant who has a quiet, slow, and easygoing temperament, born to a family with two active and energetic older sisters age three and five. The boy fails to talk at three years of age and the parents, who are pediatricians, become concerned about his delay in language acquisition. His sisters talked clearly at two years. He has no organic deficits and he appears to understand various statements, commands, and requests. His motor and gestural responses are variable while his verbal responses consist of grunts. He can say "mama." The little boy has been overgratified and overprotected by his family, who seldom require him to speak in order to express his needs. This has been partially motivated by their own guilt and separation anxiety from an unresolved parenting/working conflict. Does the child have a linguistic disorder? Probably not. His failure to speak is related to his constitutional nature, object relations, variation in his rate and style of language acquisition, and to the way his family bind their own anxiety and guilt.

All children go through stages of developmental transformation and discontinuity, followed by periods of reorganization. Spurts in language acquisition can be observed as the child begins to use word strings followed within weeks by syntactical sentences. Consolidation exists at each new level of development; new language capacity and form may appear different in structure yet it always integrates with the advancements of the preceding stage.

Like other developmental phenomena, whenever there is a deficit, the human organism has a tendency to adapt by self-correction or compensation for the abnormality. Brian, age two and one-half, who we saw for several years in longitudinal study, was born with a severe hearing deficit. He was a bright-eyed, charming, friendly, and intelligent child with warm and engaging parents. They provided him with an enriched homelife and special language classes. Although without the capacity for oral-aural speech, he was able to develop creative and and abstract language and he was able to achieve total communication through the use of sign, lip reading, and limited speech. Brian's case highlights the fact that language capacity involves many sensory modalities. Most importantly, compensation for deficit is facilitated by an optimal language environment and a context of good object relations.

The mutual influences of early parent/child interaction comprise a phenomenon that extends beyond the direct interaction of the two individuals. The behavior of each dyad is not typified by stimulus and response, but by a reciprocal exchange that leads to modification of behavior for each participant. Longitudinal, micro- and macroanalytic studies are needed in order to understand which combination of factors, such as the child's sex, genetic, and constitutional sensory and brain deficits, auditory or visual supersensitivity, plus the parent's personality and language patterns, socioeconomic status, and psychopathology or other family circumstances, might affect the individual styles of language acquisition.

Conclusions

Current research about early language acquisition seeks to understand how the acquisition of syntax is influenced by the unfolding of innate grammatical capacities and how semantic, cognitive, and social abilities influence communicative competence. Social-affective communicative competence has begun to replace the limited concept of linguistic competence. In the 1980s we see more active research into the role of brain structure and function on language acquisition with particular emphasis on the effects of early experience. The scientific community has finally begun to appreciate children as organismic wholes, active participants, even architects of their own development, with individual differences in rate and style. We see a shift in focus to an interactive model of child development with a meshing of linguistic, cognitive, neurolinguistic, and social-affective theories for language acquisition. Separate theoretical models that stress only one component are reductionistic and cannot account for the complexity of language development.

A human mind, like a computer, is not easily programmed to understand language without emotions. ". . . to truly understand what is said or written by humans about humans one must feel human emotion . . . man's most important sentences, human-interest sentences, are rich in metaphor drawn from decades of hoping and fearing, loving and hating, laughing and crying"[72] (p. 1158). The study of language provides an opportunity to postulate and consider theories about mental structure and to account for overt behavior.[71] However, "there is no royal road to language. To learn about language we must be ready to follow the child as he is lolloping on his often circuitous way toward [conflict reduction and] mastery"[70] (p. xvii).

REFERENCES

1. BATES, E., et al. "From Gesture to the First Word: On Cognitive and Social Prerequisites," in M. Lewis and L. Rosenblum, eds., *Interaction, Conservation and the Development of Language*. New York: John Wiley & Sons, 1977, pp. 247–307.

2. BATES, E., et. al. "Social Bases of Language Development: A Reassessment," *Advances in Child Development and Behavior,* 17 (1982):7–75.

3. BIRNHOLZ, J., and BENACERRAF, B. "Development of Human Fetal Hearing," *Science,* 222 (1983):516–518.

4. BLOOM, L. *Language Development: Form and Function in Emerging Grammars.* Cambridge, Mass.: MIT Press, 1970.

5. ———. *One Word at a Time.* The Hague: Mouton, 1973.

6. BLOOM, L., and LAHEY, M. *Language Development and Language Disorders.* New York: John Wiley & Sons, 1978.

7. BROCA, P. "Remarques sur le Siege de la Faculte du Language de la Parole," *Bulletins de la Societe Anatomique,* 6 (1861):330–357.

8. BROWN, R. *A First Language: The Early Stages.* Cambridge, Mass.: Harvard University Press, 1973.

9. BRUNER, J. "From Communication to Language: A Psychological Perspective," *Cognition,* 3 (1974/75):255–287.

10. CALL, J. D. "Some Prelinguistic Aspects of Language Development," *Journal of the American Psychoanalytic Association,* 28 (1980):259–289.

11. ———. "From Early Patterns of Communication to the Grammar of Experience and Syntax in Infancy," in J. D. Call, R. L. Tyson, and E. Galenson, eds., *Frontiers of Infant Psychiatry,* vol. 2. New York: Basic Books, 1984, pp. 15–29.

12. CHI, J. E., DOOLING, E. C., and GILES, F. H. "Left-right Asymmetries of the Temporal Speech Areas of the Human Fetus," *Archives of Neurology,* 34 (1977):346–348.

13. CHOMSKY, N. *Syntactic Structures.* The Hague: Mouton, 1957.

14. ———. "A Review of Skinner's Verbal Behavior," *Language,* 35 (1959):26–58.

15. ———. *Language and Mind.* New York: Harcourt Brace Jovanovich, 1972.

16. CLARK, E. "What's in a Word?" in T. Moore ed., *Cognitive Development and the Acquisition of Language.* New York: Academic Press, 1973, pp. 65–100.

17. CONDON, W., and SANDER, L. "Neonate Movement Is Synchronized with Adult Speech: Interactional Participation and Language Acquisition," *Science,* 183 (1974):99–101.

18. CORBALLIS, M. C. *Human Laterality.* New York: Academic Press, 1983.

19. CROMER, R. F. "Developmental Language Disorders: Cognitive Processes, Semantics, Pragmatics, Phonology and Syntax," *Journal of Autism and Developmental Disorders,* 11 (1981):57–74.

20. CURTISS, S. "Dissociations Between Languages and Cognition: Cases and Implications," *Journal of Autism and Developmental Disorders,* 11 (1981):15–30.

21. DARWIN, C. *The Expression of Emotions in Man and Animals.* London: Murray, 1872.

22. DAVIDSON, R., and FOX, N. "Asymmetrical Brain Activity Discriminates Between Positive and Negative Affective Stimuli in Human Infants," *Science,* 218 (1982):1235–1236.

23. DENNIS, M., and WHITAKER, H. "Language Acquisition Following Hemidecortication: Linguistic Superiority of the Left Over the Right Hemisphere," *Brain and Language,* 3 (1976):404.

24. ECONOMO, C.v., and HORN, L. A. "Uber Windungsrelief Masse und Rindenarchitektonik der Supratemporalflache, ihre Individuellen und ihre Seintenunterschiede," *Zentralblatt Neurologie, Psychiatrie,* 130 (1930):678.

25. EDGCUMBE, R. M. "Toward a Developmental Line for Acquisition of Language," *Psychoanalytic Study of the Child,* 36 (1981):71–103.

26. EIMAS, P. D. "Linguistic Processing of Speech by Young Infants," in R. Schiefelbusch and L. Lloyd, eds., *Language Perspectives: Acquisition, Retardation and Intervention.* Baltimore: University Park Press, 1974, pp. 55–74.

27. EMDE, R. "The Affective Self: Continuities and Transformations from Infancy," in J. D. Call, R. L. Tyson, and E. Galenson, eds., *Frontiers of Infant Psychiatry,* vol. 2, New York: Basic Books, 1984, pp. 38–54.

28. ENTUS, A. K. "Hemispheric Asymmetry in Processing Dichotically Presented Speech and Nonspeech Stimuli by Infants," in S. J. Segalowitz and F. Gruber, eds., *Language Development and Neurological Theory.* New York: Academic Press, 1977, pp. 63–73.

29. FREUD, S., "The Ego and the Id," in J. Strachey, ed., *The Standard Edition of the Complete Psychological Works of Sigmund Freud,* vol. 19. London: Hogarth Press, 1961, pp. 1–66.

30. FROMKIN, V., and RODMAN, R. *An Introduction to Language.* New York: Holt, Rinehart and Winston, 1983.

31. FROMKIN, V., et al. "The Development of Language in Genie: A Case of Language Acquisition Beyond the Critical Period," *Brain and Language,* 1 (1974):81–107.

32. GALABURDA, A. M., and GESCHWIND, N. "Anatomical Asymmetries in the Adult and Developing Brain and Their Implications for Function," *Advances in Pediatrics,* 28 (1981):271–292.

33. GARDNER, M. F., and WALTER, D. O. "Evidence of Hemispheric Specialization from Infant EEG," in S. Harnad, et. al., eds., *Lateralization in the Nervous System.* New York: Academic Press, 1977, pp. 481–516.

34. GESCHWIND, N., and LEVITSKY, W. "Human Brain Left-right Asymmetries in Temporal Speech Region," *Science,* 161 (1968):186–187.

35. GLANVILLE, B., BEST, C., and LEVENSON, R., "A Cardiac Measure of Cerebral Asymmetries in Infant Auditory Perception," *Developmental Psychology,* 13 (1977):54–59.

36. GREENACRE, P. "Problems of Acting Out in the Transference Relationship," in E. Rexford, ed., *The Developmental Approach to Problems of Acting Out, A Symposium,* Monograph 1. New York: International Universities Press, 1966, pp. 144–160.

37. HALLETT, S., and GREEN, P. "Possible Defects of Interhemispheric Integration in Children of Schizophrenics," *Journal of Nervous and Mental Disease,* 171 (1983):421–425.

38. HALLIDAY, M.A.K. *Learning How to Mean: Explorations in the Development of Language.* London: Edward Arnold, 1975.

39. HARTMANN, H. *Ego Psychology and the Problem of Adaptation.* New York: International Universities Press, 1958. (Originally published 1939.)

40. JAKOBSON, R., and HALLE, M. *Fundamentals of Language (Janua Linguanum, 1).* The Hague: Mouton, 1956.

41. KAYE, K. "Toward the Origin of Dialogue," in H.

Schaffer, ed., *Studies in Mother-infant Interaction.* New York: Academic Press, 1977, pp. 89–117.

42. KINSBOURNE, M., and HISCOCK, M. "Does Cerebral Dominance Develop?" in S. Segalowitz and F. Gruber, eds., *Language Development and Neurologic Theory.* New York: Academic Press, 1977, pp. 172–188.

43. KOLATA, G. "Studying Learning in the Womb," *Science,* 225 (1984):302–303.

44. KRASHEN, S. "The Critical Period for Language Acquisition and Its Possible Causes," *Annals of the New York Academy of Sciences,* 263 (1975):211–224.

45. KUSCAJ, S. "Language Play and Language Acquisition," *Advances in Child Development and Behavior,* 17 (1982):197–232.

46. LECOURS, A. R. "Mylegenetic Correlates of the Development of Speech and Language," in E. H. Lenneberg and E. Lenneberg, eds., *Foundations of Language Development.* New York: Academic Press, 1975, pp. 121–135.

47. LeMAY, M. "Morphological Cerebral Asymmetries of Modern Man, Fossil Man and Nonhuman Primate," *Annals of the New York Academy of Science,* 280 (1976):349–366.

48. LeMAY, M., and CULEBRAS, A. "Human Brain-Morphological Differences in the Hemispheres Demonstrable by Carotid Arteriography," *New England Journal of Medicine,* 287 (1972):168–170.

49. LENNEBERG, E. *Biological Foundations in Language.* New York: John Wiley & Sons, 1967.

50. LEVINSON, N. A. "Ontogenesis of the Pointing Gesture," unpublished manuscript, 1978.

51. ———. "Psycholinguistic and Child Psychiatry: A Developmental Perspective," *Psychiatric Clinics of North America,* 3 (1980):563–577.

52. MACKAIN, K. "Infant Intermodal Speech Perception Is a Left-Hemisphere Function," *Science,* 219 (1983):1347–1349.

53. McGLONE, J. "Sex Differences in Human Brain Asymmetry: A Critical Survey," *Behavioral and Brain Sciences,* 3 (1980):215–263.

54. MAHLER, M., PINE, F., and BERGMAN, A. *The Psychological Birth of the Human Infant.* New York: Basic Books, 1975.

55. MENYUK, P., and MENN, L. "Early Strategies for the Perception and Production of Words and Sounds," in P. Fletcher and M. Garman, eds., *Language Acquisition.* Cambridge: Cambridge University Press, 1979, pp. 49–70.

56. MENYUK, P., and WILBUR, R. "Preface to Special Issue on Language Disorders," *Journal of Autism and Developmental Disorders,* 11 (1981):1–13.

57. MOERK, E. L., and WONG, E. "Meaningful and Structured Behavioral Antecedents of Semantics and Syntax in Language," *International Journal of Psycholinguistics,* 5 (1976):23–37.

58. MOLFESE, D. "Cerebral Assymetry in Infants, Children, and Adults: Auditory Evoked Responses to Speech and Noise Stimuli" (Ph.D. diss., Pennsylvania State University, 1972).

59. MORSE, P. "Infant Speech Perception: A Preliminary Model and Review of the Literature," in R. Schiefelbusch and L. Lloyd, eds., *Language Perspectives: Acquisition, Retardation and Intervention.* Baltimore: University Park Press, 1974, pp. 19–54.

60. NELSON, K. *Structure and Strategy in Learning to Talk.* Monograph of the Society for Research in Child Development, vol. 38, nos. 1&2, serial no. 149, 1973.

61. PANEL. "Language and Psychoanalysis," S. Leavy, reporter. *Journal of the American Psychoanalytic Association,* 26 (1978):633–639.

62. PAPOUSEK, H., and PAPOUSEK, M. "Interactional Failures: Their Origins and Significance in Child Psychiatry," in J. Call, E. Galenson, and R. L. Tyson, eds., *Frontiers of Infant Psychiatry,* New York: Basic Books, 1983, pp. 30–37.

63. PREYER, W. *The Mind of the Child,* Part II, "The Development of Intellect," New York: Appleton, 1893.

64. RAPAPORT, D., (1960), "On the Psychoanalytic Theory of Motivation," in M. Gill, ed., *The Collected Papers of David Rapaport,* New York: Basic Books, 1967 (paper originally published in 1960), pp. 853–915.

65. RONDAL, J. A. "On the Nature of Linguistic Input to Language-learning Children," *International Journal of Psycholinguistics,* 8 (1981):75–107.

66. ST. AUGUSTINE. "The Confessions of the City of God on Christian Doctrine," in M. Hutchins, ed., *Great Books of the Western World.* Chicago: William Benton, 1952, p. 4.

67. ST. JAMES-ROBERTS, I. "A Reinterpretation of Hemispherectomy Data Without Functional Plasticity of the Brain," *Brain and Language,* 13 (1981):31–53.

68. SCHEIBEL, A. B., et al. "Differentiating Characteristics of the Human Speech Cortex: A Quantitative Golgi Study," in D. F. Benson and E. Zaidel, eds., *The Dual Brain: Hemispheric Specialization in Humans,* New York, London: Guilford Press, 1985, pp. 65–74.

69. SCHLESINGER, I. M. "Production of Utterances and Language Acquisition," in D. Slobin, ed., *The Ontogenesis of Grammar.* New York: Academic Press, 1971, pp. 63–101.

70. ———. *Steps to Language.* Hillsdale, N.J.: Lawrence Erlbaum Associates, 1982.

71. SHAPIRO, T. *Clinical Psycholinguistics,* New York: Plenum Press, 1979.

72. SHURCLIFF, W. A. "Computers, Intelligence, and Emotion," *Science,* 224 (1984):1158.

73. SKINNER, B. F. *Verbal Behavior.* New York: Appleton-Century-Crofts, 1957.

74. SLOBIN, D. "Cognitive Prerequisites for the Development of Grammar," in C. A. Ferguson and D. Slobin eds., *Studies of Child Language Development.* New York: Holt, Rinehart and Winston, 1973, pp. 175–225.

75. SNOW, C. "Mother's Speech to Children Learning Language," *Child Development,* 43 (1972):549–565.

76. SNYDER, L. K., and McLEAN, J. E. "Deficient Acquisition Strategies: A Proposed Conceptual Framework for Analyzing Severe Language Deficiency," *American Journal of Mental Deficiency,* 81 (1976):338–349.

77. STERN, D., BARNETT, R., and SPIEKER, S. "Transmission of Affect: Some Research Issues," in J. D. Call, E. Galenson, and R. L. Tyson, eds., *Frontiers of Infant Psychiatry.* New York: Basic Books, 1983, pp. 38–52.

78. STERN, D., et al. "Vocalizing in Unison and in Alternation: Two Modes of Communication Within the Mother-Infant Dyad," in D. Aaronson and R. Rieber, eds., *Developmental Psycholinguistics and Communication Disorders. Annals of the New York Academy of Science,* 263 (1975): 89–100.

79. THOMAN, E. B. "Affective Communication as the Prelude and Context for Language Learning," in R. L. Schiefelbusch et al., eds., *Early Language Acquisition and Intervention.* Baltimore: University Park Press, 1981, pp. 181–200.

80. TIEDEMANN, D. *Beobachtungen Uber Die Entwicklung Der Seelenfähigkeiten bei Kindern,* W. Rein, ed. Setenburg: Bonde, 1897 (originally published in 1787).

81. TREVARTHAN, C. "Foundations of Intersubjectivity: Development of Interpersonal and Cooperative Understanding in Infants," in D. R. Olson, ed., *Social Foundations of Language and Thought, Essays in Honor of Jerome S. Bruner,* New York: W.W. Norton, 1977, pp. 316–342.

82. VARGHA-KHADEM, F., and CORBALLIS, M. "Cerebral Assymetry in Infants," *Brain and Language,* 8 (1979): 1–9.

83. WADA, J., CLARKE, R., and HAMM, A. "Cerebral Hemispheric Asymmetry in Humans," *Archives of Neurology,* 32 (1975):239–246.

84. WERNER, H., and KAPLAN, B. *Symbol Formation.* New York: John Wiley & Sons, 1963.

85. WHITAKER, H. A., BUB, D., and LEVENTER, S. "Neurolinguistic Aspects of Language Acquisition and Bilingualism," *Annals of the New York Academy of Sciences,* 379 (1981):59–74.

86. WITELSON, S. "Early Hemispheric Specialization and Interhemispheric Plasticity: An Empirical and Theoretical Review," in S. Segalowitz, and F. Gruber, eds., *Language and Neurologic Theory.* New York: Academic Press, 1977, pp. 213–275.

87. WITELSON, S., and PALIE, W. "Left Hemisphere Specialization for Language in the Newborn: Neuroanatomical Evidence of Asymmetry," *Brain,* 96 (1973):641–646.

88. YAKOVLEV, P., and RAKIC, P. "Patterns of Decussation of Bulbar Pyramids and Distribution of Pyramidal Tracts of Two Sides of the Spinal Cord," *Transactions of the American Neurological Association,* 91 (1966):366–367.

7 / Gender Identity

Eleanor Galenson

Introduction

Gender identity is a special aspect of the development of the sense of self; it has been defined by Moore and Fine[16] as usually representing a predominant identification with the parent of the same sex. In regard to infant sexuality, Freud[3] remarked that the masturbation of early infancy seems to disappear after a short time, although it may persist without interruption until puberty; and Spitz and Wolf[22] described that infants of mothers confined to institutions developed autoerotic behavior during their first year only if they had been able to establish a tie to the mother of good-enough quality. This finding was corroborated by Provence and Lipton.[17]

During the past fifteen years the progressive steps necessary for the acquisition of gender identity have been the subject of a good deal of infant observational research. Kleeman[11,12,13] described the genital development of five infant girls and one infant boy. This began with random fingering of the genitals during the first year and proceeded to genital self-stimulation of a different quality toward the end of the second year. This behavior coincided with the emergence of genital pride and exhibitionism as well as castration anxiety.

In a series of publications Roiphe,[18,19] Galenson and Roiphe,[6,7,8,9] Roiphe and Galenson,[20,21] Galenson and Miller,[5] and Galenson and associates[10] verified Kleeman's initial findings and expanded the available information about the development of gender identity, based on data from their study of seventy normal boys and girls.

Boys discover the penis at about six to eight months of age; this is some two to three months before girls discover the clitoris. The difference probably arises because of the mechanical stimulation of the more directly exposed male genitals. Until the end of the first year, this early casual and intermittent genital touching subserves general bodily exploration. Then, with the emergence of intentionality and upright locomotion, boys and girls are observed to reach for their genitals intentionally and with some degree of pleasure.

Beginning at twelve to fourteen months, as the process of separation-individuation advances, various indications of anal-phase organization and urinary awareness appear. In the boy, excitement and exhibitionistic pride in urination are now coupled with scoptophilic interest, while both sexes become intensely curious about their own urinary function. An intimate interrelationship ensues between the developing psychosexual organization and object relations. In most infants at this time, this is reflected in the appearance of acute separation anxiety as well as in reflections of anal-phase organization, as they are correlated with variations in the progress of the separation-individuation process.

Some time between their twelfth and fourteenth month, both boys and girls begin to show increased negativism and ambivalence. This appears along with direct anal-zone awareness and anal-derivative play. The richness and complexity of the emerging anal-phase behavior indicates that a new level of psychological organization has been attained. Anal-derivative behavior appears only after anal-zone awareness is already present. It is only subsequently that fears of anal loss emerge, with these fears usually reaching their peak intensity near the middle of the second year.

At the anal zone itself, anal-phase emergence is marked by variations in bowel patterning—diarrhea or constipation. Such behaviors as squatting, flushing, and straining and grunting accompany defecation or directly precede it. There is definite interest in the stool itself and in exploring the anal area, and the child begins to employ the gestures and words supplied by the parent for the act of defecation and its product.

There are further phase-related changes, such as ambivalence and bouts of directed aggression. Ego reflections of this new level of organization include anal curiosity, and the children proceed to investigate the anal areas of people, toy animals, and dolls. Moreover, these young toddlers invent many play sequences in which the form, structure, or other attributes (such as an olfactory interest) of the play items resemble those of the anal area itself or of the stool. This is when symbolic play first appears, and there is an enormous variety of play, which is part of the early symbolic function and in which the anal-derivative influence is unmistakable. Some of the activities include collecting and piling games and in-and-out games.

Urinary Awareness

The richness of this aspect of Roiphe's and my research data is particularly striking. In most of the children studied, urinary-zone awareness emerged some time between the twelfth and fourteenth month. Usually, although not always, this was after anal awareness was present (it was independent of attempts at toilet training). Urinary-derivative behavior followed soon afterward. Direct zonal manifestations included changes in urinary diurnal patterning, and the infants now paid selective attention to wet diapers. The boys in the study experimented with interrupting and then resuming urination; in the course of this they would handle the penis itself as well as the urinary stream. Moreover, they now liked to play in the puddles of urine they produced. Curiosity mounted about the urinary function in others—adults and peers and animals—and their play was rich with sequences involving pouring and squirting liquids with faucets, hoses, watering cans, or the mouth. The

structural similarity of this play to the urinary act itself was unmistakable.

Despite parental modesty in several of the families at this period, most of the subjects succeeded in being admitted to the parents' toileting. Particularly in the boys, the new excitement and exhibitionistic pride in urination was coupled with scoptophilia, which then became enmeshed in genital curiosity. Both boys and girls tried to grasp and sometimes to mouth the father's urinary stream. This behavior was not connected with an undue degree of parental exposure but simply expressed the intense curiosity and interest evoked by this newly discovered phenomenon.

The boys and girls differed regarding their response to the mother's urination. The girls clamored consistently to be with the mother during her toileting, but intermittently, many of the boys seemed to avoid this exposure. It is likely that the boy's emerging awareness of the genital anatomical difference promotes the development of a defensive denial in relation to the mother's perineum.

The degree of the father's emotional availability to his son appeared to play an important role in connection with the boy's exhibitionistic pride and his choice of urinary posture. Where the father was more available, this interest in the boy's urinary progress and technique became an important aspect of their mutual involvement. Indeed, these children tended to adopt the upright urinary posture some months earlier than boys whose fathers were less emotionally available to them. During the second part of the second year of life, paternal support for the boy's growing sense of male identity is a crucial factor in providing the boy with confirmation of his own phallic body image. Eventually it is this that allows him to acknowledge the absence of a penis in his mother—a process that extends well into the third year of life.

Young children will thus manifest their urinary curiosity by exploring the spectacle of the male urinary stream by means of both oral and tactile measures. In the face of this, the reactions of even the most psychologically sophisticated fathers are often intense ones involving a high level of anxiety. Some fathers continue to allow occasional touching, while others instantly banish their *daughter* from the bathroom while they urinate, although she is permitted to reenter during the father's bathing, showering, and shaving. As would be expected, in most families the boy is allowed to remain and encouraged to imitate the father. Parents are usually driven to repress the erotic feelings aroused by the primitive urinary and sexual curiosity of the young child; within a week or two many parents will have repressed their own reactions as well as the memory of the child's sexual behavior and curiosity.

The Emergence of Genital Awareness

Sometime between sixteen and nineteen months of age, both boys and girls begin to experience a heightening of their genital sensitivity. This serves as a source of focused pleasure, which is sensuously far more intense than the earlier forms of genital stimulation. Repetitive patterns of intense genital self-stimulation appear, enacted by either manual means or indirect tactics such as straddling objects, rocking, and thigh pressure. The children accompany these activities by visual exploration of their own genitals. Facial expressions of excitement and pleasure, flushing, and rapid respiration all speak for the erotic arousal that occurs in conjunction with the genital self-stimulation. In boys, erections occur frequently with or without masturbation, as they have occurred since the first weeks of life. The testicles are often included in the self-stimulation. In girls, the new type of genital self-stimulation consists of manual, repetitive rubbing, squeezing, and pinching of the labia in the region of the mons and clitoris, and several children have been reported to have introduced a finger into the vaginal opening, although this was not the main site of stimulation.

In both sexes, at the outset, open affectionate behavior to the mother accompanies this self-stimulation; however, within a few weeks this disappears to be replaced by the familiar inward gaze and self-absorbed facial expression. At this point many toddlers begin to use various inanimate objects for masturbation, such as nursing bottles, "transitional object" blankets, stuffed animals, and dolls. Together, the earlier affectionate gestures, the later self-absorption, and the use of the "mother-me" objects indicate that a fantasy feeling state has become a concomitant of the new quality of genitality. This fantasy includes a partial sensory memory of earlier maternal contact during various caretaking activities.

Along with the new quality of genital self-stimulation, genital derivative behavior emerges. In girls, doll play advances in quantity and diversity. The dolls are continually undressed, the crotch area is examined, phallic-shaped objects are placed either at the doll's or the child's own pubic area, and the dolls are often used for direct manual masturbation or placed beneath the girls' genitals at bedtime. At this point, many girls adopt a particular doll as an obligatory companion. In boys, genital derivative play takes the form of greatly increased involvement with phallic-type toys such as cars, trucks, and airplanes.

Simultaneously, the strutting, exhibitionistic body posture and pride of boys offers a decided contrast to the flirtatiousness of girls, who often lift their skirts provocatively or expose their genitals in other ways.

The Emergence of Curiosity About Sexual Differences

As evidence of endogenous genital responsiveness mounts, both girls and boys become curious about genital differences and begin to make visual comparisons. Boys compare the father's penis to their own, and both boys and girls want to view and touch their mother's genitals and breasts. They explore dolls and animals as well in regard to their genitals.

These sexual comparisons are followed, in both sexes, by reactions that appear to constitute attempts to understand and deal with the genital differences— that is, temporary ubiquitous denial of these differences and displacement of interest to the mother's breasts, umbilicus, and buttocks.

Virtually all girls then go on to develop some degree of "preoedipal castration reaction," as Roiphe and I[6] have characterized it. These reactions include a revival of recently allayed fears of object loss—evidenced as increased separation anxiety—and fear of bodily disintegration (fear of loss of the stool, anxiety about small cuts and bruises, etc.). Other regressive behavior may be present as well, depending on the severity of the reaction. Most girls also show developmental advances; fantasy play becomes far more imaginative and elaborate, and early attempts at graphic representation appear. These ego advances reflect defensive efforts to cope with the anxiety provoked in relation to the recognition of genital differences.

In almost every one of the girls we studied, the reaction to the genital difference also affected the child's relationship to her mother, heightening the anal-phase ambivalence. However, in most instances there is a new erotic and flirtatious component in the girl's relationship to her father. This enlarges and intensifies their former attachment to one another. However, the girl's relationship to both parents remains dyadic in nature in that the child wants the exclusive attention of each parent for herself.

Some girls develop a more severe preoedipal reaction, as Roiphe[18] has postulated, if they have experienced either an important threat to their developing body image during their first year of life (such as serious physical illnesses, operations, or restrictive orthopedic devices) or difficult relationships with the mother (due to such factors as maternal depression or prolonged periods of separation). Roiphe has predicted that the impact of such experiences during the first year of life would make the infant more vulnerable to becoming disturbed when awareness of genital differences emerges.

It appears that, as a group, girls are more vulnerable than are boys to the effect of observing the differences in genital anatomy. These preoedipal castration reactions involve almost every area. At the genital zone itself, some girls abandon masturbation entirely, while for others manual masturbation is frequently replaced by other, indirect means of genital stimulation. Still others continue to masturbate, but without pleasure. In the more severe castration responses, fantasy life becomes more constricted, imaginative play becomes sparse and stereotyped, and general intellectual curiosity becomes inhibited.

Concurrently with the preoedipal castration reactions, many girls develop changes in mood with a loss of zest and enthusiasm and the onset of sadness. Mahler[14] described this sadness and loss of zest in many girls during the second part of the second year, mood changes that she ascribed to a more severe rapprochement crisis in girls than in boys. It is likely that these affective shifts reflect developments in both the psychosexual sphere (the preoedipal castration reactions) and the area of object relations.

The castration responses described here appear to influence the girl's development from this time onward, both to enhance and to inhibit. In regard to object relations, both girls and boys develop a special tie to the father before the end of the first year. In girls, however, this tie begins to take on an erotic quality (while they maintain the more ambivalent tie to the mother), thus preparing the way for the girl's oedipal attachment to the father in the third year. A number of factors may influence the progress of this unfolding. Thus, where the girl's earlier relationship with the mother has been of poor quality, where the girl suffered important bodily trauma during the first year of her life, or where she experienced the birth of a sibling during the second half of the second year, then the discovery of the sexual anatomical difference will aggravate hostile dependence on the mother enormously. Under such circumstances, the erotic shift to the father does not occur.

In regard to ego development, part of the impact of the preoedipal castration reactions in girls has already been mentioned—that is, the advance in the complexity and the symbolic function as seen in their play and in their attempts at graphic representation. However, in contrast to the usual sequence, those girls with an overly intense castration reaction suffer a constriction in their symbolic function. Their imaginative play becomes sparse and stereotyped, and the inhibition extends to their general intellectual curiosity as well. As a result, during the critical transitional era of the emerging verbal capacity, their exploration of the world about them narrows in scope.

Reaction of Boys to the Discovery of the Genital Difference

Boys show fewer overt reactions to the discovery of the anatomical difference. A brief upsurge of masturbation somewhere between sixteen and nineteen months of age is then followed by a decline in direct manual masturbation, but there is a definite increase in the level of their general motor activity. This probably reflects some degree of anxiety in relation to the recognition of the genital difference. There is an implied threat of castration, and there is also the danger of regression to the more passive and symbiotic type of attachment to the mother. It appears that the boy attempts to deny the sexual difference by avoiding confrontation with his mother's genitals as well as with those of female peers. He begins to turn more toward his father, seeking identification with him in support of his own phallic identity.

From time to time, the boy's denial of the genital difference appears to break down, and behavioral evidence of anal-genital confusion emerges; at such times attempts at toilet training are apt to be met with strong negativism. There is also periodic regression to an increased demand for bottle feeding, heightened attachment to transitional objects, and an intensification of separation anxiety.

Between sixteen and nineteen months, along with the emergence of genital awareness, most boys display an upsurge in phallic type of play with cars and trucks. There is in addition an increase in rough-and-tumble play with the father as the boy's identification with him increases over the succeeding months. In regard to other types of play, the semisymbolic fantasy elaboration of play that characterizes the reaction of girls as they cope with their discovery of the genital difference does not appear in boys. Nor do boys attempt graphic representation until several months after the girls.

In regard to preoedipal castration reactions in boys, Roiphe[18] has postulated that these would occur, as in girls, if during the first year the child had experienced untoward bodily traumata or a poor relationship with the mother. In contrast to girls, however, only a small number of boys—five in the research sample of thirty-five boys—showed evidence of preoedipal castration reactions; it turned out that all five boys had indeed suffered the predicted untoward experiences during their first year, although several other boys in our sample also had such first-year traumata but did not develop such reactions. During the course of the next year or so these reactions tended to emerge, disappear, and reemerge. The boys' attachment to the mother became increasingly intense but also increasingly ambivalent. They tended to identify with her in their interest in both her clothes, hair, cosmetics, and jewelry and her activities such as housework and handicraft; all in all, they showed confusion in their sense of gender identity. Their semisymbolic play involved dolls and other types of activities usually carried out by girls of this age, but their play was rigid, repetitive, and compulsive in quality—very much like the play of those girls who had suffered the more severe degrees of castration reaction. Thus these boys reflect an underlying maternal identification, forecasting the future formation of a negative oedipal constellation.

In some boys, the onset of genital awareness and curiosity about the genital difference does not occur until the beginning of their third year. These boys tend to have suffered some distortion in their object relations. Some remain locked in an overly close and erotic relationship with their mothers for a longer period, and they display transient confusion in gender identity. Others, such as two sets of twins in our study who were delayed in the progression of their separation-individuation, showed a later onset in the emergence of their genital awareness and in their reactions to it.

The Pathway to the Oedipal Phase

Mahler[15] has emphasized that the period of the rapprochement crisis is more troubled for girls than for boys. It is likely that the recognition of the sexual difference accounts in part for these differences. In girls, there is a heightening of the aggressive aspect of the ambivalence to the mother as a result of the recognition of the genital anatomical difference; this leads to a loosening of the tie to the mother and an increasingly erotic turn to the father. This provides a developmental precondition for the future positive oedipal constellation. In girls with severe castration reactions, the hostile ambivalence to the mother becomes very intense,

the maternal attachment is heightened, and the turn to the father does not occur.

Overtly boys are far less disturbed by the discovery of the genital difference. In fact, however, they defend themselves against castration anxiety by more profound denial and displacement—both of which may affect development in other areas as well. The father's availability at this time plays a crucial role in supporting the boys' gradual distancing from their mother and the increasingly stable sense of their phallic identity.

Recently Edgcumbe and Burgner[2] have offered additional material related to the process of acquiring a sense of sexual identity. They view this as beginning during the second year, continuing during the anal phase, and reaching its peak within the phallic phase. During this "phallic-narcissistic" phase exhibitionism and scoptophilia are the most pronounced components in both sexes, with a gradual divergence between girls and boys becoming evident in regard to drive derivative fantasies, sexual identification, and object relations.

Edgcumbe and Burgner stress that sexual wishes and fantasies are still in a one-to-one relationship. They describe castration anxiety in the preoedipal boy that differs from oedipal castration anxiety. For such a child, the penis becomes a highly valued body part and his main source of narcissistic gratification. He may fear its loss at the hands of envious females, or as talion punishment by his father, or even fear that damage may come to him through masturbation, but he does not anticipate its loss as punishment for his wishes to banish or castrate his father. In the girl, the wish for a penis may build on earlier wishes she has had for other objects she did not possess; these yearnings are intensified by the discovery of the genital difference. Phallic-narcissistic feelings of penis envy with lowering of her self-esteem may interfere with the development of her feminine sexual identification. Exhibitionism may appear as a defense against this sense of devaluation.

The complexities and vicissitudes of feminine preoedipal development have been further amplified by Dahl's detailed material[1] from the analysis of a four-and-one-half-year-old girl. The material provides clinical confirmation of the earlier conclusions about gender identity formation that were based on direct infant observational research.

REFERENCES

1. DAHL, E. K. "First Class or Nothing at All: Aspects of Early Feminine Development," *Psychoanalytic Study of the Child,* 38 (1983):405–429.

2. EDGCUMBE, R., and BURGNER, M. "The Phallic-Narcissistic Phase," *Psychoanalytic Study of the Child,* 30 (1975): 160–180.

3. FREUD, S. "Three Essays on the Theory of Sexuality," in J. Strachey, ed., *The Standard Edition of the Complete Psychological Works of Sigmund Freud* (hereafter *The Standard Edition*), vol. 7. London: Hogarth Press, 1953, pp. 125–143.

4. ———. "The Dissolution of the Oedipus Complex," *The*

Standard Edition, vol. 19. London: Hogarth Press, 1953, pp. 173–179.

5. GALENSON, E., and MILLER, R. "The Choice of Symbols," *Journal of the American Academy of Child Psychiatry,* 15 (1976):83–96.

6. GALENSON, E., and ROIPHE, H. "The Impact of Sexual Discovery on Mood, Defensive Organization and Symbolization," *Psychoanalytic Study of the Child,* 26 (1976):195–216.

7. ———. "Some Suggested Revisions Concerning Early Female Development," *Journal of the American Psychoanalytic Association,* 28 (1976):805–827.

8. ———. "Development of Sexual Identity: Discoveries and Implications," in T. B. Karasu and C. W. Socarides, eds., *On Sexuality.* New York: International Universities Press, 1979, pp. 1–17.

9. ———. "The Pre-Oedipal Development of the Boy," *Journal of the American Psychoanalytic Association,* 28 (1980):805–829.

10. GALENSON, E., et al. "Disturbance in Sexual Identity Beginning at 18 Months of Age," *International Review of Psycho-Analysis,* 2 (1975):389–397.

11. KLEEMAN, J. A. "A Boy Discovers His Penis," *Psychoanalytic Study of the Child,* 20 (1965):239–266.

12. ———. "Genital Discovery During a Boy's Second Year: A Follow-up," *Psychoanalytic Study of the Child,* 21 (1966):358–392.

13. ———. "The Establishment of Core Gender Identity in Normal Girls," *Archives of Sexual Behavior,* 1 (1971): 117–129.

14. MAHLER, M. S. "Notes on the Development of Basic Moods: The Depressive Affect," in R. M. Loewenstein et al., eds., *Psychoanalysis—A General Psychology.* New York: International Universities Press, 1966, pp. 156–168.

15. MAHLER, M. S., PINE, F., and BERGMAN, A. *The Psychological Birth of the Human Infant.* New York: Basic Books, 1975.

16. MOORE, B. E., and FINE, B. D., eds. *A Glossary of Psychoanalytic Terms and Concepts,* 2nd ed. New York. American Psychoanalytic Association, 1968.

17. PROVENCE, S., and LIPTON R. *"Point of View,"* *Infants in Institutions.* New York: International Universities Press, 1962.

18. ROIPHE, H. "On an Early Genital Phase: With an Addendum on Genesis," *Psychoanalytic Study of the Child,* 23 (1968):348–365.

19. ———. "Some Thoughts on Childhood Psychosis," *Psychoanalytic Study of the Child,* 28 (1973):136–145.

20. ROIPHE, H., and GALENSON, E. "Object Loss and Early Sexual Development," *Psychoanalytic Quarterly,* 42 (1973):73–90.

21. ———. *The Infantile Origins of Sexual Identity.* New York: International Universities Press, 1983.

22. SPITZ, R. A., and WOLF, M. "Autoerotism: Some Empirical Findings and Hypothesis on Three of Its Manifestations in the First Year of Life," *Psychoanalytic Study of the Child,* 3/4 (1949):85–120.

8 / Toward a Developmental Psychopharmacology: The Physiological Basis of Age, Gender, and Hormonal Effects on Drug Responsivity

Jean A. Hamilton and Cynthia D. Conrad

Introduction

Pediatrics has long recognized age-linked effects on the drug dosages appropriate for infants[5] and children. More recently, age has been recognized as a crucial variable in geriatric pharmacology. Yet a developmental approach to psychopharmacology that would span the intervening years of the human life cycle has been neglected. New evidence is now available about the effects of drug-hormone interactions. We suggest that this evidence provides the basis for an integrative, conceptual framework that may be useful in advancing the study of both age- and gender-related drug responsivity. Although these effects extend across the life cycle, they are particularly notable around the time of puberty. In this chapter we focus primarily but not exclusively on the pharmacological treatment of affect-related disorders from childhood through adolescence.

We reexamine the magnitude, extent, and time course of pubertal physiological changes known to affect pharmacokinetics. In addition, we summarize new basic science data demonstrating hormonal effects on the neurochemical substrate of drug responsivity. Taken together, we believe that these considerations provide a strong rationale for further clarification of possible age and gender-linked effects. In view of the methodological limitations that characterize existing studies, clinical parallels to animal data are critically assessed.

We then consider clinically relevant subgroups that are defined by age, gender, and both maturational and hormonal status. Finally, we clarify essential methodological issues for future psychopharmacological comparisons across such groupings. Because the documentation of drug effects on treatment outcome depends on adequate diagnoses and methods of follow-up assessment, we examine these issues in detail with respect to studies of children and adolescents. In this age group there is obviously a special need to differentiate pharmacological effects from maturational ones. In recognition of this, we introduce a developmental timeline approach to cognitive, behavioral, and clinical assessments.

Reexamination of Physiological Changes Affecting Pharmacokinetics

PHYSICAL GROWTH AND DEVELOPMENT

Weight, body composition, and proportion of fat to total body water differ by age and gender; these factors are also known to affect the absorption, distribution, biotransformation, and excretion of drugs. The greatest change in body composition occurs during the adolescent growth spurt. For girls, there is an average 120 percent increase in body fat, compared to a 44 percent increase in lean body weight. Further comparison [29] of the body composition of a girl (age eighteen) with a boy (age fifteen) of the same height and weight indicates that the ratio of fat/body weight is 2.3 times greater in females (28 vs. 12 percent). Particularly for girls, the percentage of body water decreases as the percentage of body fat increases so markedly.

Variability in steady-state drug levels is determined largely by genetic differences in drug elimination rates. Studies in adults indicate that in different patients receiving the same dose of the same drug, up to a fortyfold difference exists in the steady-state plasma drug concentrations. [86] Other factors also contribute to variability in steady-state drug levels, including: (1) demographic variables such as race; (2) disease states such as malabsorption, impaired renal function, and liver disease; and (3) drug-drug interactions. Additionally, we know that gender-linked behaviors such as cigarette smoking [103] and alcohol use can significantly affect neuroendocrine indices of drug responsivity.

It has been empirically demonstrated that adult data are not adequate for establishing the drug plasma concentrations that will be optimally therapeutic for children. Among other well-known differences, children differ from adults in protein-binding characteristics and liver-mass to body-mass ratio. [123] They also differ in the content and activity, of hepatic p450 cytochrome oxidase, an important enzyme that helps to metabolize drugs and steroids. [63] Due to their more active enzyme systems, children may in some cases produce and accumulate more metabolites of the parent compound than will adults. This difference might be revealed by lower plasma concentrations of the drug, but if some of the metabolites are biologically active there may be a greater risk for certain side effects. [86] Possible pubertal effects on drug metabolism have not been well described.

AGE-RELATED CHANGES IN NEUROREGULATORS

In animal studies, there is evidence documenting postnatal maturational changes in the central nervous system; these occur both before and after the onset of reproductive maturity. [25] These studies have included the assessment of endogenous levels of putative neuroregulators such as tryptophan, serotonin (5HT), and the main 5HT metabolite, 5-hydroxyindoleacetic acid, [6,20] as well as other monoamines. [94] For example, prior to puberty, a steady rise has been reported in brain catecholamine content. [52] It appears likely, however, that there are marked differences in the onset of functioning and rate of change of the various neurotransmitter systems. [88] These changes may be relevant to age-linked individual differences in drug responsivity.

Alterations in these chemical communicators may in turn be related both to other maturational changes in neuronal development [25,64] and, possibly, to alterations in receptor location, number, or affinity. Receptor function is thought to be a crucial physiological substrate of drug responsivity. Hence, apart from the pharmacokinetic effects that were discussed earlier, there may be a fundamental relationship between age and drug efficacy.

New Basic Science Data: Hormonal Hypotheses of Gender and Age Effects on Drug Responsivity

DRUG–HORMONE INTERACTIONS

As reviewed elsewhere, for at least the past ten years, pharmacologists have been aware of significant gender differences in drug metabolism. [44,48,57] It is known that oral contraceptives, exogenous steroid hormones, affect benzodiazepine metabolism and elimination.[1] More recently, even the relatively subtle endogenous steroid hormone fluctuations of the menstrual cycle have been shown to affect drug metabolism,[74] plasma concentrations, and responsivity.[104]

Perhaps of more fundamental scientific interest than metabolic effects, however, are the effects of steriod hormones on both putative neuroregulators and the physiological mechanisms of drug action in the brain. These hormonal influences on pharmacodynamics may in part account for gender- and age-related effects in the response to psychoactive drugs.[27]

While we argue for exploring possible clinical parallels, the data from studies in nonhuman animals must be viewed with caution. For example, there are species-related variations in reproductive endocrinology, and certain animals provide better models for human functioning than do others. Moreover, there are undoubtedly limitations in extrapolating from drug-hormone interactions in rodents to those in humans. For these and other reasons, the data in animals must be used cautiously, as clues or as guides for further research in humans.

In the following discussion, we specify the different types and sources of data in order to help the reader to remain sensitive to these issues. Particularly with regard to the clinical data, we have tried to identify gaps in knowledge as well as to highlight aspects of our thinking that remain speculative. Because of these gaps in knowledge and the methodological limitations in existing studies, we have also been careful to specify when studies of adult populations are used as guides to possible gender- or hormonally linked processes in adolescents.

Gonadal steroids affect neuronal growth, morphology, and electrical activity. Ongoing effects on monoamine turnover, enzyme regulation, and neurosecretion have also been demonstrated, although this is most clear in animal models. The mechanisms of steroid action on nerve cells are therefore varied and are known to include both rapid, direct actions on pre- and postsynaptic membranes (nongenomic) and indirect actions such as alterations in protein synthesis (genomic) that are mediated by intracellular receptors.[67]

It is difficult to isolate the effects of the different gonadal steroids (estrogens, progestins, and androgens) by sex. In humans both males and females synthesize these hormones by converting progesterone to estradiol or testosterone, and testosterone to estradiol. Hormone levels in any individual fluctuate daily. Concentrations for the sexes overlap depending on physiological conditions. For example, in humans between the ages of ten and fifteen years, plasma estradiol concentrations in females and males overlap. Even for adult women, follicular and luteal phase estradiol concentrations are somewhat overlapping with the levels found in adult males.[7]

Across various species certain hormones found predominantly in one sex have similar effects in both sexes. Others have unique effects in certain brain regions. Thus males and females may show different patterns of responsivity to the same hormone. This depends, in part, on the functional repertoire of the neuronal substrate on which the hormone acts. Initially this substrate specificity may be genetically determined, but it undergoes further differentiation during the course of prenatal and early postnatal development.[66]

As a very brief overview of certain animal models and possible human correlates, we summarize some of the effects of gonadal steroids, primarily estrogen, on several neuroregulatory systems that are especially pertinent to affective disorders research. The presence or absence of beta-endorphin in hypophyseal portal blood in monkeys depends on adequate circulating levels of gonadal steroids. The highest levels occur premenstrually, falling to undetectable levels with the onset of menses. Possible pubertal changes in humans have not been clarified. However, a report by Hamilton and colleagues[47] summarizes the available literature. In addition, it describes a clinical study in which beta-endorphin levels in peripheral blood were measured across the human menstrual cycle and correlated with symptom presentation. Quigley and Yen[93] report that luteinizing hormone (LH) secretion in response to naloxone hydrochloride, an opiate antagonist, varies with the phase of the menstrual cycle.

Estrogen has also been shown to affect central monoaminergic systems.[27] A 30 to 50 percent variation in certain cortical 5HT receptors occurs over the course of the rodent estrous cycle.[8] There are antidepressant-induced changes in 5HT receptor binding, which are thought to be linked to the therapeutic efficacy of this class of drug. These changes are dependent on the presence of adequate gonadal steroids in both sexes.[56] Differences between prepubertal as compared to postpubertal individuals are unknown and require further investigation.

The concentration of dopamine (DA) in hypophyseal portal blood varies by as much as 50 percent across the rodent estrous cycle. Pharmacological doses of estrogen stimulate at least a 20 percent increase in striatal DA receptors, an alteration that may partly account for subsequent hypersensitivity to drugs known to affect dopaminergic neurons.[43,44,50] Estrogen effects are complex, however, because the direction and magnitude of receptor alterations vary with the dosage and the duration of steroid administration. Simpkins [107] has shown that testosterone also has variable effects on brain DA.

THE EXTENT AND TIME COURSE OF HORMONAL CHANGES AT PUBERTY

Puberty is initiated and characterized by a broad spectrum of endocrine changes that are thought to be related to the progressive maturation of the hypothalamo-pituitary-gonadal axis. The magnitude of these changes is striking. For example, once testosterone levels begin to rise in boys, the change occurs relatively rapidly. As shown in table 8–1, as puberty advances, boys have a ten- to twentyfold increase in serum testosterone levels. The male adolescent growth spurt occurs around fourteen years of age. During this time, serum testosterone nearly doubles. On the other hand, in twelve-year-old females, at the time of their growth spurt, serum testosterone changes relatively little and indeed varies only 1.7-fold throughout the pubertal period.[7,59,125] Reciprocally, in girls during puberty, there is a twelve- to fourteenfold increase in estradiol,[125,7] whereas only a 1.8-fold increase is seen in boys. In girls, the increase in circulating estradiol and the related hormonal shifts culminate in menar-che. However, menarche itself is clearly not the end point of the girl's development. Over the five-year period subsequent to the onset of menses, there continues to be a progressive increase in the number of ovulatory cycles.[62]

Perhaps more important than absolute hormone concentration is the fraction of total hormone that is not bound to protein, for it is this unbound (free) fraction that is available for receptor binding on the target cell. Despite conflicting findings, it appears that the binding capacity of plasma sex hormone binding globulin (SHBG) varies with respect to gender and phase of puberty.[30] For both sexes, SHBG binding capacity for dihydrotestosterone and testosterone is highest in prepubertal subjects, intermediate in pubertal subjects, and lowest in adults. It has been observed that gonadal hormone entry into the cerebrospinal fluid (CSF) shows a positive correlation with the free hormone level in plasma.[128] As a result, the dramatic rise in plasma hormone concentration during puberty, which is not accompanied by a compensatory increase in protein binding, is likely to result in an increase in transfer of hormone into the CSF. There may be important gonadal hormone effects on psychoactive drug responsivity, and for that reason, the possibility of increased

TABLE 8–1

Absolute Levels of and Percent Change in Gonadal Hormones

Absolute Hormone Levels in Puberty

Mean Levels	Stage I		Stage V	
	Male	Female	Male	Female
Estradiol (pg/ml)	7.5	8.2	20.7	121
Testosterone (ng/ml)	25	21	500	57

Percent Change in Gonadal Hormone Levels in Puberty (compared to prepubertal baseline)[a]

Mean Levels	Throughout Puberty		Associated with the Adolescent Growth Spurt	
	Male	Female	Male	Female
Estradiol	180	1,200–1,400	39	85
Testosterone	1,000–2,000	170	150–180	6–12

SOURCE: F. Bidlingmaier, et al., "Plasma Estrogens in Childhood and Puberty Under Physiologic and Pathologic Conditions," *Pediatric Research*, 7 (1973): 901–907; H. Kulin and R. Santen, "Normal and Aberrant Pubertal Development in Man," in J. Vaitukaitis, ed., *Clinical Reproductive Neuroendrocrinology* (New York: Elsevier Biomedical, 1982), pp. 19–68; J. Winter and C. Faiman, "Pituitary-Gonadal Relations in Female Children and Adolescents," *Pediatric Research*, 7 (1973): 948–953.
[a]Calculated from figures just cited.

hormone transfer into the CSF and related functional consequences warrant investigation in adolescent age groups.

In addition to gonadal maturation, there are changes in adrenal functioning at or before adolescence. The onset of "adrenarche" (maturation and augmentation of adrenal cortex functioning) is revealed by an increase in 17-ketosteroids. There are also age-related effects on cortisol secretion; in particular with increasing age there ensues an increasing likelihood of cortisol hypersecretion.[4]

Moreover, puberty is marked not only by alterations in circulating levels of steroid hormones but by maturational changes in the temporal patterning of hormonal secretions. For example, episodic secretion of LH during sleep has been reported to be present in pubertal but not in prepubertal children.[125]

Possible Clinical Parallels: Hormonal Changes and the Life-cycle Approach

PHARMACOKINETICS AND ADVERSE DRUG REACTIONS

Several lines of evidence demonstrate the need for a life-cycle approach to gender-related psychopharmacology.[57] The potential clinical importance of the rapid physical growth and development at puberty is illustrated by a report that shows that at a fixed dose of chlorpromazine hydrochloride, plasma levels are significantly higher in adult females than they are in males. The report goes on to demonstrate that this difference can be accounted for simply by differences in body weight.[70] Greater symptomatic improvement at lower dosage regimens in women as compared to men[70,102] may reflect the fact that women achieve higher plasma levels at lower oral doses. The use of lower-dose neuroleptic regimens in women may in turn decrease the risk for later development of tardive dyskinesia (TD).

As recently reviewed by Hamilton,[43] TD, a side effect of drugs that act on dopaminergic neurons, is more common in females. This can be viewed as a gender-linked difference in drug responsivity. In both males and females,[116,117] estrogens appear to have a moderating effect on neuroleptic-induced dyskinesias. Children may be at greater risk for drug-induced TD because they lack high circulating levels of gonadal steroids. One report suggests that adolescents have a greater risk for drug-induced extrapyramidal symptoms,[16] but the data are conflicting.[40] Simple hormonal hypotheses of risk and causality are probably inadequate.

In the case of water-soluble drugs like alcohol, the effective dose depends on the concentration of the drug relative to body water. The gender- and age-linked effects on total body water are accordingly thought to be important in understanding the pharmacokinetics of such agents. In one well-controlled study, compared to men, women subjects showed a 21 percent higher peak blood-alcohol concentration based on a 9 percent lower ratio of body water to kilogram body weight.[113] Additionally, the percentage of heavy drinkers is 60 to 74 percent lower in women than it is in men across comparable age groups.[3] Despite this, there is a higher alcohol mortality ratio documented for women of reproductive ages as could be grouped in this study from fifteen to forty-four years.[2] One can speculate that the higher blood-alcohol levels obtained by women on fixed oral regimens might be related to this outcome, although the age-linked finding would require further clarification.

There is a dramatic decrease in total body water in association with the 120 percent increase in body fat in girls during adolescence. Given that, postpubertal girls may display a heightened variability of drug responses for both water-soluble and fat-soluble drugs.

Preliminary data show that the overall incidence of adverse drug reactions (ADR) is greater for women than for men.[11,22] Although women continue to be prescribed more drugs than men,[17] Domecq and coworkers[22] have shown that possible risk factors such as age, number of drugs administered, and duration of hospitalization do not account for the greater proportions of ADR in women. For both men and women, most adverse reactions were assessed to be dose-related.

In order further to clarify possible gender-related differences, it would be necessary to examine data on the incidence and severity of ADR, drug intake and plasma concentrations, body composition, and the hormonal status of female patients. Unfortunately, to our knowledge this type of data analysis is not generally available. It is a fact that fatal drug reactions are two times greater in women than men. What is of interest, however, is the finding that this is true only during the reproductive years, denoted in this study by ages fifteen to forty-five.[11] While it may be that during their reproductive years women are prescribed more drugs than either before or after as well as that women are prescribed medication more frequently than men, it is possible that the incidence of adverse effects may be affected by stage-related hormonal conditions, with the greatest vulnerability to ADR occurring after puberty and before menopause.

INDICES OF DRUG RESPONSIVITY: CLINICAL NEUROENDOCRINE CORRELATES

Gender differences have been reported for neuroendocrine indices of drug responsivity. In response to chlorpromazine[70] and to environmental stressors, adult women show greater prolactin elevations than do men.[76] In the former study, the higher drug-induced prolactin levels were independent of weight-related differences in serum levels. It has been suggested that prolactin secretion is an indicator of sensitivity to drugs that affect dopaminergic neurons. In some women a correlation has been reported between serum prolactin levels and the presence of TD.[34] It is not clear whether the gender difference in prolactin response is related to differences in the pool of prolactin available for release or to other hormonal factors.

There is a great deal of variability in studies evaluating provocative tests of growth hormone (GH) secretion in major depression. The stimulating effect of estrogen on GH levels may explain some of this inconsistency. The augmentation of GH secretion is under investigation both as a state marker for endogenous depression and as a trait marker for predisposition to the disorder. In ovulating (menstruating) women, the rise in GH levels parallels the cyclic fluctuation of estrogen secretion. Moreover,[28,71] women have mean GH levels many times higher than those of men. As a result, the onset of puberty notably increases the biological heterogeneity between the sexes. On the other hand, the onset of menopause tends to reestablish a degree of hormonal similarity. Thus it is interesting that postmenopausal depressed women show a markedly diminished GH response to hypoglycemic stimulation,[39] not unlike the response documented in prepubertal depressed children.[91] It is not surprising that the results of a study using similar provocative neuroendocrine challenges in a patient population homogeneous for the diagnosis of depression but heterogeneous for sex, age, and estrogen status yielded more variable results.[38]

CLINICAL PARALLELS IN RESEARCH ON AFFECTIVE DISORDERS

Raskin[95] reviewed the age-sex differences in the response of adults to antidepressant drugs. He concluded that although "twice as many women as men are treated for depression, the depression literature suggests that it is the men rather than the women who benefit most from the antidepressant drugs" (p. 120). Using a variety of assessments, Greenblatt, Grossner, and Wechsler[37] suggested a gender-age effect on treatment outcome with certain antidepressants across various diagnostic categories. The Medical Research Council[69] conducted a four-week therapeutic trial of phenelzine sulfate, a nonspecific monoamine oxidase (MAO)–inhibiting antidepressant. They reported that, as assessed by a symptom severity rating scale, a greater percentage of men than women with "primary" depressions improved. Bielski and Friedel[10] reviewed a number of studies that suggested that hysteria, a gender-linked trait, predicted a poor tricyclic antidepressant response. In contrast, Gerner[34] has reviewed studies on the efficacy of amphetamine in the treatment of depression. He found that women and the elderly responded more favorably than did men or younger patients.

In the light of new basic science data that also support gender-related differences, Hamilton and colleagues[48] recently updated Raskin's review. For example, a sex-related difference in the behavioral effects of an MAO-inhibiting drug has been reported in animals.[9] In both male and female rats, gonadal steroids have been shown to affect antidepressant-induced changes in brain receptors.[56] Wirz-Justice and Chappius-Arndt[126] reported that in response to chlorimipramine hydrochloride, a tricyclic antidepressant, they found sex-specific differences in the inhibition of 5HT uptake in human platelets.

Very little research in psychopharmacology has been specifically directed toward the adolescent.[108] This has made the search for clinical parallels relevant to the peripubertal period all the more difficult. In studies designed to assess drug responsivity, postpubertal adolescents are rarely compared to prepubertal children. When children are included in pharmacological research, early adolescents (ages thirteen to fifteen years) are often excluded from consideration. Moreover, psychopharmacological studies in adults have rarely been aimed at clarifying the possible effects of age, gender, and hormonal status (premenopausal versus postmenopausal).[57] It is therefore not surprising that possible age- and gender-linked effects around puberty have also been neglected. Patient samples in "adult" studies may actually include late adolescents (ages sixteen to eighteen years).

Despite these problems, we will focus on two clinical situations that address age- and gender-related effects on the psychopharmacological treatment of affective disorders in children and adolescents. The first example concerns the role of thyroid hormone in depression, while the second highlights the use of lithium carbonate in the treatment of postpubertal bipolar disorder across the menstrual cycle.

PUBERTY AND THYROID FUNCTION

In view of the rapid changes in body composition and metabolic needs during puberty, alterations in thyroid function are not unexpected. In adults, thyroid function is known to be related both to depressive symptomatology and to antidepressant responsivity. It is therefore possible that in the treatment of depression in adolescents, age or gender differences may be pertinent pyschopharmacological considerations. Clinical examples from the adult literature include the attempt to advance the onset of symptomatic improvement in women with major depression by the use of thyroid hormone in conjunction with antidepressant medication.[85] Certain treatment-resistant depressions appear to respond to the addition of low doses of thyroid hormone,[34] and this occurs despite the fact that thyroid function tests are normal. Currently we do not know whether or not adjunctive thyroid would prove useful in the treatment of severe depression in children or adolescents of either sex. In any case, the assessment of this possibility would require knowledge of baseline thyroid function in these age groups.

Unfortunately, the studies in this area have utilized differing methodologies; any conclusions based on overall findings are therefore problematic. Earlier studies more often paid attention to carefully assessing data by sex and pubertal stage; later studies presented data more with reference to chronological age, which is less developmentally appropriate, instead offering updated endocrine assays.

In one of the older studies[60] in which the endocrine assays appear acceptable, skeletal age was assessed across chronological age and by sex. The maturation process in girls was shown to involve an increase in total thyroxine (T_4) and in free T_4 levels. Thyroxine binding globulin (TBG) remained virtually unchanged, but pre-albumin levels increased. A more recent investigation[81] confirmed the increase in T_4 levels in girls older than 13.9 years, but found that TBG also increased in girls older than 15.9 years. This increase in T_4 in adolescent girls contrasts with a decrease in T_4 and TBG in adolescent boys spanning Tanner's pubertal stages.[100]

There is disagreement as to whether the changes in T_4 levels are correlated with parallel changes in thyroid-stimulating hormone (TSH) levels and thyrotropin (TRH) levels. The Lamberg group[61] reported a gradual decrease in TSH for adolescent girls but relatively stable values for boys. In girls, levels declined prior to menarche (by 46 percent), then rose at menarche to previous levels followed by a gradual decline approximating levels seen in mature women. For boys, however, the peripubertal values did not change and indeed were substantially lower, on the average, than those measured in girls at comparable stages of development. If this fluctuation reported for adolescent girls is confirmed, it would suggest that documentation of thyroid dysfunction as a correlate of clinical depression

by absolute measures of TRH, TSH, or T_4 could prove misleading in this age group.

When TSH levels were measured in boys and girls six to seventeen years of age,[26] no differences in TSH values could be demonstrated. Unfortunately, however, the data were analyzed with chronological age rather than pubertal stage as the dependent variable, and the maturational distinctions were therefore obscured. Similarly, studies[82] that combine girls and boys rather than looking at each sex separately can only demonstrate an overall decrease in TSH with increasing age. Although Reichlin[97] concluded that there are no age- or sex-related differences in TSH secretion past neonatal life, the Lamberg data remain of interest because of the care with which pubertal stages were defined and used in the demonstration of a maturational effect on TSH secretion in adolescent girls.

In summary, it appears that there are gender-related shifts in thyroid hormone secretion around puberty. Lamberg's early work on pubertal changes in TSH secretion deserves replication. In order to decrease the confounding variability that arises from the inclusion of patients of mixed maturational levels in the same age range groups, careful definition of pubertal stages is required. Given the data supporting an estrogen effect on the neuroendocrine responsivity to TRH, gender- and age-related differences in thyroid function would not be surprising.[78,127] If confirmed, these sex-based physiological differences might be related to the well-known preponderance of thyroid dysfunction in women as compared to men. For example, hyperthyroidism is largely a disease of adult women, with a female-to-male sex ratio of approximately five to one. The sex ratio for multinodular goiter is even higher, at between ten to twenty to one.[21] In addition to the possible role of subtle thyroid dysregulation in affective disorder, the roles that thyroid[115] and other hormones play in the developmental and evolutionary aspects of drug metabolism have been discussed by Jondorf.[51] As cases in point, Saenger[101] and Vesell[115] have shown that in children and in adults, respectively, with thyroid disturbance, drug kinetics are substantially altered.

LITHIUM CARBONATE AND THE MENSTRUAL CYCLE

We have worked with an adolescent patient with bipolar disorder who was treated with lithium carbonate across the menstrual cycle,* an obvious marker of

*C. D. Conrad and J. A. Hamilton, "Recurrent Premenstrual Decline in Serum Lithium Concentration—Clinical Correlates and Treatment Implications," *Journal of the American Academy of Child Psychiatry,* in press.

gender differences. Our experience suggests a hormonally linked alteration in drug responsivity. Following the onset of menses at age fourteen years, this sixteen-year-old adolescent female experienced a general deterioration in functioning. Within four months of menarche she became suspicious and inattentive. She was easily distracted by racing thoughts, and she experienced auditory hallucinations of accusatory voices telling her she was sinful and worthless. She sometimes believed people could read her mind. Unprovoked outbursts of rage and agitation alternated with periods of mutism. She became hypersexual, especially during the premenstrual and early menstrual phases of her regular monthly cycles. Self-care and personal hygiene were disrupted at these times—the patient would often smear menstrual blood on herself and her surroundings. She would also have thoughts of killing herself and would scratch herself or bang her head. Psychiatric hospitalization was recommended.

The initial clinical impression was that of an atypical psychosis with prominent depressive features intermixed with periodic hyperactivity and hyperarousal. Pharmacotherapy with antipsychotic agents alone (halperidol and perphenazine) resulted in only minimal symptom diminution. Despite the regular antipsychotic regimen, affective and psychotic symptoms continued and flared during the premenstrual and menstrual phases. Increased doses led to oversedation or pronounced tremor and rigidity.

Lithium was added to a low-dose perphenazine regimen. The oral dose was adjusted as needed to maintain a serum lithium concentration between 0.9 and 1.1 mEq/l. With this, attentiveness improved, paranoia diminished, and the accusatory hallucinations and denigrating delusions subsided. The periods of behavioral dyscontrol decreased in frequency and intensity, and the patient reported an enhanced capacity to regulate her aggressive and sexual impulses.

Nevertheless, a progressive exacerbation of symptoms was noted whenever the patient entered the premenstrual phase of her menstrual cycle. Despite a constant oral dose and documentable compliance, this exacerbation in her affective psychosis coincided with a fall in serum lithium concentration. The typical pattern observed on a 1,200 mg oral regimen was a fall in serum lithium from the 0.9 to 1.1 mEq/l maintenance range to 0.6 to 0.8 mEq/l. Symptoms would begin to spontaneously remit by day 2 of menses.

This cyclic premenstrual psychosis could be effectively aborted by means of precisely timed increases in the patient's oral lithium regimen. A daily lithium regimen of between 2,100 and 2,700 mg initiated eight days prior to expected onset of menses and then tapered to maintenance doses of between 1,500 and 1,800 mg at the cessation of menses consistently blunted symptoms

of hyperactivity, aggressivity, hypersexuality, paranoia, and self-denigrating ideation. This oral regimen resulted in serum lithium concentration between 1.3 and 1.6 mEq/l, without demonstrable signs or subjective complaints indicative of toxicity. This phenomenon is similar to that observed in the treatment of acute mania, in which higher serum lithium concentrations are required to block symptoms and are tolerated by the patient.

The onset of this young woman's severe recurrent affective psychosis began within months of menarche. Cyclic exacerbation of a predictable nature, both in terms of symptomatology and duration, occurred premenstrually. The patient's hospitalization provided an opportunity to observe the phenomenon over a two-year period. During this time a pharmacological strategy was developed that involved the regulation of the patient's serum lithium concentration in phase with her menstrual cycle. This effectively blunted the intensity of the syndrome.

The pathophysiological processes responsible for the premenstrual drop in effective lithium concentration remain to be elucidated, and could simply be a dilutional effect. Of note, Ostrow and coworkers[79] have observed a similar phenomenon in female patients with menstrual cycle–related mood disorders. In these cases the red blood cell lithium concentration rose and fell in phase with the premenstrual exacerbation of tension and depressive symptoms. This cyclic variation in the red cell:plasma distribution of lithium is not typical; it is generally not encountered in the majority of individuals with affective disorders. Thus the process peculiar to these cases appears to override a predominantly stable, steady-state pattern of lithium distribution determined at the level of the cellular membrane.

Methodological Issues: Suggestions for Developmental and Gender-related Psychopharmacological Research

CHILDHOOD AND ADOLESCENT MAJOR DEPRESSION

The documentation of drug efficacy and specificity in the treatment of particular psychiatric disorders depends on adequate diagnosis and reliable methods for the assessment of clinical change. There have now been many convincing case reports of persistent and recurrent depressive episodes in children and adolescents.[19,31,65,114] These in turn have led to comprehensive assessments of clinic and hospital populations in which notable percentages of the sampled patients met specified symptomatic criteria for depression.[13,14,119] Continued refinements in technique have resulted in the delineation of groups of children and adolescents who present a clinical picture identical to that described in adults.*[15]

Thus a consensus is developing in the child psychiatric literature to confirm the existence of a clinical syndrome (depressive disorder) characterized by dysphoric mood and a predictable pattern of specific signs and symptoms. Additional external validation has come from studies on children that corroborate findings in the adult literature concerning the effectiveness of tricyclic antidepressants in achieving symptom remission.[87,90,123] In addition, there are studies that document abnormal secretion of cortisol and GH in a subset of child and adolescent depressed patients.[24,84,91,98]

AGE AND GENDER DIFFERENCES IN THE PRESENTATION OF MAJOR DEPRESSION

The clinical syndrome of major depression can be used as a model for discussing the possible physiological bases of differential age and gender effects. This disorder has now been studied in patient populations that span the life cycle—children, adolescents, adults. Several studies have referred to age distinctions in the onset and presentation of major depression. Kashani and colleagues[55] estimate a point prevalence of 1.8 percent in a sample of nine-year-old children compared to a 4.3 percent prevalence for major depression in adults.[122] In a longitudinal study of eight- to thirteen-year-old outpatients, Kovacs and her coworkers[58] note an earlier age of onset for dysthymia, a less intensive and often more chronic disorder, than for major depression. They additionally observe that when either syndrome emerges, the younger the child the more lengthy the natural history (fifteen to eighteen months for major depression and three and one-half years for dysthymia).

These data suggest that depression may be less clearly defined and run a more insidious course in the younger child population. Then as puberty nears, it may become more differentiated and specific. As a result of the increasing clarity and sophistication of these studies, intriguing questions arise related to symptomatology and psychopharmacology. For example, to what extent may age and degree of maturation, genetic sex, and hormonal status influence symptom expression or depressive subtype, onset, and the temporal

*See references 15, 55, 58, 89, 98, and 111.

course (treatment response or natural history) of a psychiatric disorder?

Sex differences in prevalence rates for depression have been documented, but these differences in rate are far from understood. In their 1977 article on the epidemiology of depression, Weissman and Klerman[121] review the evidence for the high rates of depression in females. For adults, a two-to-one sex ratio of women to men is a relatively consistent, though not universal, finding; this holds true both for community surveys and studies of patients coming for treatment. Similar studies of major depression in adolescents reveal that postpubertal girls make up 70 to 78 percent of the samples meeting operationalized criteria for the diagnosis (see table 8–2).

In contrast, a survey of ten studies of childhood (prepubertal) depression fails to demonstrate a notable female preponderance (see table 8–2). Most of the studies, in fact, report depression more frequently among boys than girls. Since similar operationally defined criteria were used, this shift in percent diagnosed according to gender is intriguing and cannot be easily explained by variability in diagnosis. Although the difference may reflect larger numbers of prepubertal boys as compared to adolescent boys or men being seen in the mental health system, data from recent studies speak against this explanation. If one compares the percentage of boys included in each of the samples to the percentage of boys diagnosed as depressed, these frequencies shift substantially (see table 8–3). Thus male patients appear to make up the larger component of prepubertal depressed children.

According to data presented by Kandel and Davies,[53] the adult pattern gender difference in depression first appears in early adolescence. That is, the onset of puberty appears to mark a crucial transition at which female sex begins to predict increased risk for depression. To what extent do the complex endocrine changes occurring at puberty account for the altered sex ratio? This question becomes all the more challenging when one considers the variable results of provocative endocrine tests in the assessment of clinical state (endogenous versus nonendogenous), of hereditary predisposition (trait markers), and of the response to treatment.

Data supporting an association between neuroendocrine dysfunction and the diagnosis of major depression, particularly the endogenous subtype, have been more convincingly documented in prepubertal children[84,91,92] than in adolescents.[41] It may be that the prepubertal hormonal status confers greater baseline biological homogeneity across a studied population. This would enhance the likelihood of uncovering physiological distinctions among different diagnostic groups or diagnostic subtypes. As discussed earlier, for

TABLE 8–2

Sex Differences in Diagnosis of Major Depression

Study	Date	Criteria	Patient Status	Age	Ratio of Males/Females
I. Childhood[a] (prepubertal)					
Weinberg et al.[119]	1973	analogous DSM-III	outpatient	6–12	30/12
Puig-Antich et al.[90]	1979	RDC	inpatient & outpatient	6–12	9/4
Carlson and Cantwell[13]	1979	RDC & DSM-III	inpatient & outpatient	≤12	9/2
Kashani et al.[54]	1982	DSM III	inpatient	9–12	11/2
Preskorn, Weller, and Weller[87]	1982	DSM-III	inpatient	7–12	16/4
Kashani et al.[55]	1983	RDC & DSM-III	general population	9	18/22[b]
Weller et al.[124]	1983	DSM-III	inpatient	7–12	16/4
Geller et al.[33]	1983	RDC & DSM-III	unstated	5–11	8/4
Kovacs et al.[58]	1984	DSM-III	outpatient	8–13	32/33
Puig-Antich et al.[91]		RDC	inpatient	6–12	20/10
II. Adolescence[a] (postpubertal)					
Mezzich and Mezzich[73]	1979	FVDSA[c] from MMPI	inpatient	12–18	10/36
Carlson and Cantwell[13]	1979	RDC & DSM-III	inpatient & outpatient	13+	5/12
Strober, Green, and Carlson[111]	1981	DSM-III	inpatient	12–17	12/28
Strober and Carlson[110]	1982	RDC	inpatient	13–16	13/47

[a]Representative studies of depressive syndrome, diagnostic criteria for which were operationally defined by the authors.
[b]Major depression not distinguished from minor depression (RDC) when sex differences were analyzed; current and past episodes included.
[c]Face Valid Depression Scale for Adolescents.

example, prepubertal children, like postmenopausal women, have consistently low basal estrogen levels.

Research endeavors in biological psychiatry have sought to clarify what might account for the observed physiological differences in patients who present with similar symptom configurations. The assumption is that more definitive pharmacological treatment interventions can be developed if the pathophysiological processes inherent in a given disorder are understood. Attempts to elucidate these processes will be improved if individuals with known variations in hormonal status, metabolic status, or central nervous system maturation are studied independently.

A DEVELOPMENTAL APPROACH TO DRUG
TREATMENT OUTCOME MEASURES
MATURATIONAL EFFECTS

In periods of rapid change such as puberty, it is particularly important to avoid confounding maturational or developmental changes with drug effects. The timing of changes from childhood into adolescence has been assessed by measures including chronological age (in years), skeletal age, height and weight, gynecological age in females (years from menarche), as well as by the direct assessment of secondary sexual characteristics[68] such as facial and pubic hair, breast development

TABLE 8–3

Number of Prepubertal Boys and Girls in General Psychiatric Versus Depressive Populations

Study	Date	Total Sample		Depressed Group	
		Male	Female	Male	Female
Carlson and Cantwell[13]	1979	62 (61%)	40 (39%)	9 (82%)	2 (18%)
Kashani et al.[54]	1982	75 (75%)	25 (25%)	11 (85%)	2 (15%)

in females, and by the measurement of circulating levels of hormones. Because clinical and behavioral norms may vary critically in a matter of months, there is a need to apply not only age but also maturational norms to the criteria used for follow-up assessments. But throughout adolescence, the various indices of change are not necessarily synchronized. Instead, some variables may show a smooth, relatively uniform rate of change, whereas others may show discontinuities, such as the abrupt acceleration in height in adolescent males.

While interrelated, these and other changes usually occur over an interval of about two to three years.[68] Moreover, there are gender differences in the timing of pubertal changes (e.g., the growth spurt around age twelve years in females and around age fourteen years in males). Variables such as age, hormonal status, and body composition may significantly affect drug metabolism and responsivity. To the extent that they do, we suggest that pharmacological studies utilize a variety of these measures in order to standardize, or at least better describe, subgroups; this would also serve to decrease uncontrolled sources of variance. Particularly around the time of puberty, we believe that pharmacological effects must be assessed against a moving baseline of functioning, in which different aspects of maturation may be changing at different times.

THE TIME LINE OF COGNITIVE CHANGES

Our suggestion for studies with early adolescents is for a time-line approach to treatment outcome measures. This idea comes in part from the work of Meyersburg and Post,[72] who originally attempted to integrate findings in neurobiology with psychodynamic theory. We will focus on cognitive measures as one example, not only because learning is a primary developmental task in this age group but also because cognition has recently been demonstrated to be pertinent to outcome assessment in affective disorders research.[46,106] In addition, Piaget's work has provided a major theoretical impetus for examining differences in attention and information processing between childhood and adolescence. In particular, Piaget described the acquisition of formal operational thinking in early adolescence (although by no means will all adolescents in our society acquire this capacity).[83]

As summarized in table 8–4, Hamilton[42] reviewed studies showing that biological, behavioral, and cognitive indices of information processing performance continue to change from childhood through adolescence. The patterning of these changes needs to be appreciated when measuring the cognitive changes related to drug treatment and assessing pharmacological side effects. For example, one study[109] of antidepressant response in adolescents involved measures of cognitive change over a three-to-six-month period. For this age group, apart from normalization due to drug treatment, the passage of six months could be associated with improvement on some cognitive measures due to maturational effects. Furthermore, cognitive dysfunction may well be related to the illness process, and comparisons with nonpsychiatric controls may therefore not be entirely adequate. We suggest that the subjects also be compared to patients receiving other treatments or placebo. Such comparisons may be

TABLE 8–4

Time of Maximum Performance (+) or Time of Greatest Change or Improvement (*)

			Age Group					
	7–8	9–10	11–12	13–14	15–16	17–18	19–20	21–22
Biological								
EEG amplitude of adulthood			⊢—⊣					
Increase in "reducing" of sensory inputs				⊢————————⊣				
Behavioral								
Self-paced tapping	[.....*.....]							
Speed of reaction time					[.....+.....]			
Zuckerman sensation-seeking score						[...+...]		
Cognitive								
Susceptibility to hypnosis			[..........+..........]					
Incidental learning			⊢————⊣					
Selective learning			[......+......]					
Selectivity in retrieval				[.............*.............]				
Field independence						[...*...]		
Typical time of onset of "formal operations"*			⊢————⊣					

SOURCE: J. A. Hamilton, "Development of Interest and Enjoyment in Adolescence, Parts I and II," *Journal of Youth and Adolescence*, 12 (1983): 355–372.

especially needed in order to provide additional controls for possible differential baseline changes, changes that may arise from illness-related alterations in maturational processes.

Times of rapid change may also constitute a critical period of vulnerability to drug-induced side effects. Neff[75] has explored how drug side effects such as somnolence and inhibition of motor activity can block two of the most important characteristic defensive and adaptive responses of adolescents, intellectualization and motor activity. He argues, but does not prove, for example, that drug-related side effects may have residual, long-lasting effects on adolescent ego development.

Alterations in cognition and memory are clinical features of major depression.[120] Gender differences have been reported both in symptom presentation[105] and in pharmacological effects on cognition.[48] Both drugs and hormones have state-dependent effects on learning and memory, and preliminary evidence suggests that the phase of the menstrual cycle may define a relatively specific state for processing information about oneself and the environment.[46] For these reasons, we suggest that during adolescence, clinical investigators should be sensitive to the state-dependent learning that may occur in association with states defined by either drug use or hormonal changes.

Gender Differences in Psychological Response Pattern, Neuroendocrine Measures, and Depressive Symptomatology

In a careful study of hormonal and psychological shifts during early adolescence,[112] a complicated pattern of correlations between gonadal and adrenal changes and mood variables was found for males but not for females. Several positive correlations were noted between hormonal changes and the emergence of behavior problems. The same investigators[77] examined the relationships during early adolescence among pubertal stage, gonadotropin secretion, and gonadal and adrenal hormone secretion on the one hand and changes in self-perception of cognitive, social, and physical competence on the other. Again, there were gender differences in the patterning of the correlations. In males, shifts in adrenal androgen levels paralleled changes in all three measures of competence. In females, shifts in gonadotropin and sex steroid levels paralleled changes in the measures of competence.

Certain situations can also elicit differential responses in males and females. This has been most clearly demonstrated under conditions of stress,[96] where adrenaline excretion in males correlated positively with investment in achievement and negatively with measures of anxiety. In females, however, adrenaline excretion was inversely related to measures of self-esteem and self-fulfilling social expectations. Although both sexes performed equally well in the stressful situation (an examination), the authors noted that feelings of success and confidence were more common among the males. The females more frequently reported discomfort and a sense of failure.

Such differences may play a role in shaping gender-specific depressive symptoms. This is true not only in response to stress but also with respect to self-perception. For example, in a college population, depressed men are more likely to express social withdrawal, cognitive and motivational deficits, and somatic concerns, while depressed women are more likely to report a lack of confidence, a lack of concern about their future, and sensitivity to criticism.[80]

We do not know if similar differences in reported symptoms might be found in samples of children or adolescents. However, Dweck and Reppucci[23] documented sex differences in learned helplessness in children, with girls attributing deficits to a lack of ability, something not in their control, rather than to a lack of effort.

Taken together, we believe these differences in psychological response patterns and the neuroendocrine measures with which they correlate suggest the need to investigate gender differences in children and adolescents in a more comprehensive manner. We have indicated that despite meeting identical diagnostic criteria, the configuration of the symptoms of prepubertal children may differ from that of adolescents. Thus it should also be recognized that clinical presentation may differ by age as well as by sex.

Conclusion

In this chapter we have reexamined the magnitude and time course of physiological changes in puberty that are known to affect pharmacokinetics. New neuroendocrine data demonstrating hormonal effects on the physiological mechanisms of drug responsivity were also summarized. We believe that these considerations, along with preliminary clinical parallels to basic science data, provide a strong rationale for further investigation of developmental and gender-related drug effects.

Clinically relevant questions include the following: In what manner might maturational state, hormonal status, or cognitive development modify the characteristic presentation of a clinical syndrome? Are there dysfunctional behaviors that might be developmentally determined? Would treatment strategies be similarly affected?

In view of the methodological problems that characterize existing studies, we made several suggestions for future clinical research protocols. In particular, in order to generate a reasonable sample size, it is not unusual for individuals spanning several developmental epochs to be studied together. Unfortunately, potential maturational effects may thus be overlooked. For these reasons, we urge clinicians to consider the possible effects that pubertal changes may exert on drug responsivity.

REFERENCES

1. ABERNETHY, D. R., et al. "Impairment of Diazepam Metabolism by Low-Dose Estrogen-Containing Oral-Contraceptive Steriods," New England Journal of Medicine, 306 (1982):791–192.

2. "Alcohol and Health: Second Special Report to the U.S. Congress." Washington, D.C.: Superintendent of Documents, U.S. Government Printing Office, 1974, chap. 4, p. 82.

3. "Alcohol and Health: Fourth Special Report to the U.S. Congress." Washington D.C.: Superintendent of Documents, U.S. Government Printing Office, 1981, chap. 1, p. 21.

4. ASNIS, G., et al. "Cortisol Secretion in Relation to Age in Major Depression," Psychosomatic Medicine, 43 (1981): 235–242.

5. ASSAEL, B. M. "Pharmacokinetics and Drug Distribution During Postnatal Development," Pharmacologic Therapeutics, 8 (1982):159–197.

6. BAKER, P. and GOODRICH, C. "The Effects of the Specific Uptake Inhibitor Citalopram upon Brain Indoleamine Stores in the Maturing Mouse," General Pharmacology, 13 (1982):59–61.

7. BIDLINGMAIER, F. et al. "Plasma Estrogens in Childhood and Puberty Under Physiologic and Pathologic Conditions," Pediatric Research, 7 (1973):901–907.

8. BIEGON, A. H., BERCOVITZ, H., and SAMUEL, D., "Serotonin Receptor Concentration During the Estrous Cycle of the Rat," Brain Research, 187 (1980):221–225.

9. BIEGON, A., SEGAL, M., and SAMUEL, D., "Sex Differences in Behavioral and Thermal Responses to Pargyline and Tryptophan," Psychopharmacologia, 61 (1979):77–80.

10. BIELSKI, R. J., and FRIEDEL, R. O. "Prediction of Tricyclic Antidepressant Response," Archives of General Psychiatry, 33 (1976):1479–1489.

11. BOTTIGER, L. E., FURHOFF, A. K., and HOLMBERG, L. "Fatal Reactions to Drugs," ACTA Medica Scandinavica, 102 (1979):451–456.

12. CAMPBELL, M., and SMALL, A. M. "Chemotherapy," in B. B. Wolman, ed., Handbook of Treatment of Mental Disorders in Childhood and Adolescence. Englewood Cliffs, N.J.: Prentice-Hall, 1978, pp. 9–27.

13. CARLSON, G. A., and CANTWELL, D. P. "A Survey of Depressive Symptoms in a Child and Adolescent Psychiatric Population," Journal of the American Academy of Child Psychiatry, 18 (1979):587–599.

14. ———. "Unmasking Masked Depression in Children and Adolescents," American Journal of Psychiatry, 137 (1980):455–449.

15. ———. "Diagnosis of Childhood Depression: A Comparison of the Weinberg and DSM-III Criteria," Journal of the American Academy of Child Psychiatry, 129 (1982):247–250.

16. CHILES, J. "Extrapyramidal Reactions in Adolescents Treated with High-Potency Antipsychotics," American Journal of Psychiatry, 135 (1978):239–240.

17. CLARK, A. F., et al. "Plasma Testosterone Free Index: A Better Indicator of Plasma Androgen Activity," Fertility and Sterility, 26 (1975):1001–1005.

18. COTTLER, L. B., and ROBINS, L. N. "The Prevalence and Characteristics of Psychoactive Medication Use in a General Population Study," Psychopharmacology Bulletin, 19 (1983):746–751.

19. CYTRYN, L., and McKNEW, D. H. "Proposed Classification of Childhood Depression," American Journal of Psychiatry, 129 (1972):149–155.

20. DASZUTA, A., et. al. "Endogenous Levels of Tryptophan, Serotonin, and 5-Hydroxyindole Acetic Acid in the Developing Brain of the Cat," Neuroscience Letters, 11 (1979):187–192.

21. DEGROOT, L. J. "Thyroid," in P. B. Beeson and W. McDermott, eds., Textbook of Medicine. Philadelphia: W. B. Saunders, 1975, pp. 1703–1733.

22. DOMECQ, C., et al. "Sex-Related Variations in the Frequency and Characteristics of Adverse Drug Reactions," International Journal of Clinical Pharmacology, 18 (1980):326–366.

23. DWECK, C. S., and REPPUCCI, N. D. "Learned Helplessness and Reinforcement in Children," Journal of Personality and Social Psychology, 25 (1973):109–116.

24. EXTEIN, I., et al. "The Dexamethasone Supression Test in Depressed Adolescents," American Journal of Psychiatry, 139 (1982):1617–1619.

25. FINCH, C. "Neuroendocrine and Autonomic Aspects of Aging," in C. Finch and L. Hayflick, eds., Handbook of the Biology of Aging. New York: Van Nostrand Reinhold, 1977, pp. 262–280.

26. FISHER, D. A., et al. "Serum T4, TBG, T3 Uptake, T3, Reverse T3, and TSH Concentrations in Children 1 to 15 Years of Age," Journal of Clinical Endocrinology and Metabolism, 45 (1977):191–198.

27. FLUDDER, M. J., and TONGE, S. R. "Variations in the Concentrations of Monoamines in Eight Regions of Rat Brain During the Aestrous Cycle: A Basis for Interactions Between Hormones and Psychotropic Drugs," Journal of Pharmacology and Pharmacotherapeutics, 27 (Supplement) (1975):39.

28. FRANTZ, A. G., and RABKIN, M. T. "Effects of Estrogen and Sex Difference on Secretion of Human Growth Hormone," Journal of Clinical Endocrinology and Metabolism, 25 (1965):1470–1480.

29. FRISCH, R. "Fatness, Puberty, Menstrual Periodicity and Fertility," in J. Vaitukaitis, ed., Clinical Reproductive Neuroendocrinology. New York: Elsevier Biomedical, 1982, pp. 105–135.

78

30. GAIDANO, G., et al. "Dynamics of the Binding Capacity of Plasma Sex Hormone Binding Globulin (SHBG) for Testosterone and Dihydrotestosterone During Puberty," *Clinica Chimica Acta,* 100 (1980):91–97.

31. GALLEMORE, J. L., and WILSON, W. P. "Adolescent Maladjustment or Affective Disorder?" *American Journal of Psychiatry,* 129 (1972):608–612.

32. GAVALER, J. "Sex-Related Differences in Ethanol-Induced Liver Disease: Artifactual or Real?" *Alcoholism: Clinical and Experimental Research,* 6 (1982):186–196.

33. GELLER, B., et al. "Nortriptyline in Major Depressive Disorder in Children: Responses, Steady-State Plasma Levels, Predictive Kinetics, and Pharmacokinetics," *Psychopharmacology Bulletin,* 19 (1983):62–65.

34. GERNER, R. H. "Systematic Treatment Approach to Depression and Treatment-Resistant Depression," *Psychiatric Annals,* 13 (1983):37–49.

35. GLAZER, W. M., et al. "Serum Prolactin and Tardive Dyskinesia," *American Journal of Psychiatry,* 138 (1981): 1493–1496.

36. GOLDMAN-RAHIC, P., and BROWN, R. "Postnatal Development of Monoamine Content and Synthesis in the Cerebral Cortex of Rhesus Monkeys," *Brain Research,* 256 (1982):339–349.

37. GREENBLATT, M., GROSSNER, G. H., and WECHSLER, H. "Differential Response of Hospitalized Depressed Patients to Somatic Therapy," *American Journal of Psychiatry,* 120 (1964):935–943.

38. GREGOIRE, G., et al. "Hormone Release in Depressed Patients Before and After Recovery," *Psychoneuroendocrinology,* 2 (1977):303–312.

39. GRUEN, P. H., et al. "Growth Hormone Responses to Hypoglycemia in Postmenopausal Depressed Women," *Archives of General Psychiatry,* 32 (1975):31–33.

40. GUALTIERI, C. T., et al. "Tardive Dyskinesia and Other Clinical Consequences of Neuroleptic Treatment in Children and Adolescents," *American Journal of Psychiatry,* 141 (1984):20–23.

41. HA, H., KAPLAN, S., and FOLEY, C. "The Dexamethasone Supression Test in Adolescent Psychiatric Patients," *American Journal of Psychiatry,* 144 (1984):421–423.

42. HAMILTON, J. A. "Development of Interest and Enjoyment in Adolescence, Parts I and II," *Journal of Youth and Adolescence,* 12 (1983):355–372.

43. ———. "An Overview of the Clinical Rationale for Advancing Gender-related Psychopharmacology and Drug Abuse Research," in *Women and Drugs* (monograph). Washington, D.C.: National Institute on Drug Abuse, Government Printing Office, forthcoming.

44. HAMILTON, J. A., and PARRY, B. "Sex-Related Differences in Clinical Drug Response: Implications for Women's Health," *Journal of the American Medical Women's Association,* 38 (1983):126–132.

45. HAMILTON, J. A., ALAGNA, S., and PINKEL, S. "Gender Differences in Antidepressant and Activating Drug Effects on Self-Perceptions," *Journal of Affective Disorders,* 7 (1984):235–243.

46. HAMILTON, J. A., ALAGNA, S. W., and SHARPE, K. "Cognitive Approaches to Understanding and Treating Premenstrual Depressions," in H. J. Osofsky, and S. J. Blumenthal eds., *Premenstrual Syndromes.* Washington, D.C.: American Psychiatric Press, 1985, pp. 69–84.

47. HAMILTON, J. A., et al. "Human Plasma Beta-Endorphin Through the Menstrual Cycle," *Psychopharmacology Bulletin,* 19 (1983):586–587.

48. HAMILTON, J. A., et al. "Gender, Depressive Subtypes, and Gender by Age Effects on Antidepressant Response," *Psychopharmacology Bulletin,* 20 (1984):475–480.

49. HENDNER, T., and LUNDBERG, P. "Neurochemical Characteristics of Cerebral Catecholamine Neurons During Post-Natal Development in the Rat," *Medical Biology,* 59 (1981):212–223.

50. HRUSKA, R., and SILBERGELD, E. "Increased Dopamine Receptor Sensitivity After Estrogen Treatment Using the Rat Rotation Model," *Science,* 289 (1980):1466–1468.

51. JONDORF, W. R. "Developmental Aspects of the Metabolism and Toxicity of Drugs," in J. W. Garrod, ed., *Drug Toxicity.* London: Taylor and Francis, 1979, pp. 25–50.

52. JONES, G., and WENTZ, A. "Adolescence, Menstruation, and the Climacteric," in D. Danforth, ed., *Obsterics and Gynecology.* New York: Harper and Row, 1977, pp. 163–169.

53. KANDEL, D., and DAVIES, M. "Epidemiology of Depressive Mood in Adolescents," *Archives of General Psychiatry,* 39 (1982):1205–1212.

54. KASHANI, J. H., et al. "Major Depressive Disorder in Children Admitted to an Inpatient Community Mental Health Center," *American Journal of Psychiatry,* 139 (1982): 671–672.

55. KASHANI, J. H., et al. "Depression in a Sample of 9-Year-Old Children," *Archives of General Psychiatry,* 40 (1983):1217–1223.

56. KENDALL, D., STANCEL, G., and ENNA, S. "The Influence of Sex Hormones on Antidepressant-Induced Alterations in Neurotransmitter Receptor Binding," *Journal of Neuroscience,* 2 (1982):354–360.

57. KINNEY, E. L. et al. "Underrepresentation of Women in New Drug Trials," *Annals of Internal Medicine,* 95 (1981): 495–499.

58. KOVACS, M., et al. "Depressive Disorders in Childhood. I. Longitudinal Prospective Study of Characteristics and Recovery," *Archives of General Psychiatry,* 41 (1984): 229–237.

59. KULIN, H., and SANTEN, R. "Normal and Aberrant Pubertal Development in Man," in J. Vaitukaitis, ed. *Clinical Reproductive Neuroendocrinology,* New York: Elsevier Biomedical, 1982, pp. 19–68.

60. LAMBERG, B. et al. "Endocrine Changes Before and After the Menarche: III. Total Thyroxine and Free Thyroxine Index, and the Binding Capacity of Thyroxine Binding Proteins in Female Adolescents," *Acta Endocrinologica,* 74 (1973):685–694.

61. LAMBERG, B. A., et al. "Endocrine Changes Before and After the Menarche: IV. Serum Thyrotropin in Female Adolescents," *Acta Endocrinologica,* 74 (1973):695–702.

62. LEMARCHAND-BERAUD, T., et al. "Maturation of the Hypothalamo-Pituitary-Ovarian Axis in Adolescent Girls," *Journal of Clinical Endocrinology and Metabolism,* 54 (1982):241–246.

63. LEVIN, W., and RYAN, D. "Age and Sex Differences in the Turnover of Rat Liver Cytochrome P-450: The Role of Neonatal Imprinting," in P. L. Marselli, S. Garattini, and F. Sereni, eds., *Basic and Therapeutic Aspects of Perinatal Pharmacology.* New York: Raven Press, 1975, pp. 265–275.

64. LIDOR, H., and MOLLIVER, M. "An Immunohistochemical Study of Serotonin Neuron Development in the Rat: Ascending Pathways and Terminal Fields," *Brain Research Bulletin,* 8 (1982):89–430.

65. LING, W., OFFEDAL, G., and WEINBERG, W. "Depressive Illness in Children Presenting as Severe Headache," *American Journal of Diseases of Children,* 120 (1970):122–124.

66. McEwen, B. S. "Neural Gonadal Steroid Actions," *Science,* 211 (1981):1303–1310.

67. McEwen, B. S., and Parsons, B. "Gonadal Steroid Action on the Brain: Neurochemistry and Neuropharmacology," *Annual Review of Pharmacology and Toxicology,* 22 (1982):555–597.

68. Marshall, W. and Tanner, J. "Variations in the Pattern of Pubertal Changes in Girls," *Archives of Disease in Childhood,* 44 (1969):291–303.

69. Medical Research Council. "Clinical Trial of the Treatment of Depressive Illness," *British Medical Journal,* 1 (1965):881–885.

70. Meltzer, H., Busch, D., and Fang, V. "Serum Neuroleptic and Prolactin Levels in Schizophrenic Patients and Clinical Response," *Psychiatry Research,* 9 (1983):271–283.

71. Merimee, T. J., and Fineberg, S. E. "Studies of the Sex-Based Variation of Human Growth Hormone Secretion," *Journal of Clinical Endocrinology and Metabolism,* 33 (1971):896–902.

72. Meyersburg, H., Post, R. "An Holistic Developmental View of Neural and Psychological Process: A Neurobiologic-Psychoanalytic Integration," *British Journal of Psychiatry,* 135 (1979):139–155.

73. Mezzich, A. C., and Mezzich, J. E. "Symptomatology of Depression in Adolescence," *Journal of Personality Assessment,* 43 (1979):267–275.

74. Miskiewicz, S. L., Shively, C. A., and Vesell, E. S. "Sex Differences in Absorption Kinetics of Sodium Salicylate," *Clinical Pharmacology and Therapeutics,* 31 (1982):30–37.

75. Neff, L. "Untoward Responses to Medication in Adolescents," in L. Miller ed., *Fourth International Congress of Social Psychiatry: Abstract of Papers.* Jerusalem: Ahva Cooperative, 1972, p. 171.

76. Noel, G., et al. "Human Prolactin and Growth Hormone Release During Surgery and Other Conditions of Stress," *Journal of Clinical Endocrinology and Metabolism,* 35 (1972):840–851.

77. Nottelmann, E. D. et al. "Gonadal and Adrenal Hormone Correlates of Self-Concept in Early Adolescence," paper presented at the meeting of the Society for Pediatric Research, San Francisco, May 1984.

78. Ojeda, S. R., Castro-Vazques, A., and Jameson, H. E. "Prolactin Release in Response to Blockade of Dopaminergic Receptors and to TRH Injection in Developing and Adult Rats: Role of Estrogen in Determining Sex Differences," *Endocrinology,* 100 (1977):427–439.

79. Ostrow, D. G. et al. "Sodium Dependent Membrane Processes in Major Affective Disorders," in E. Usdin and I. Handin, eds., *Biological Markers in Psychiatry and Neurology.* New York: Pergamon Press, 1982, pp. 153–167.

80. Padesky, C. A., and Hammen, C. L. "Sex Differences in Depressive Symptom Expression and Help-Seeking Among College Students," *Sex Roles,* 7 (1981):309–320.

81. Parra, A., et al. "Thyroid Gland Function During Childhood and Adolescence. Changes in Serum TSH, T_4, T_3, Thyroxine Binding Globulin, Reverse T3 and Free T_4 and T_3 Concentrations," *Acta Endocrinologica,* 93 (1980):306–314.

82. Penny, R. et al. "Thyroid-Stimulating Hormone and Thyroglobulin Levels Decrease with Chronological Age in Children and Adolescents," *Journal of Clinical Endocrinology and Metabolism,* 56 (1983):177–180.

83. Petersen, A., and Offer, D. "Adolescent Development: Sixteen to Nineteen Years," in J. Call et al., eds., *Basic Handbook of Child Psychiatry,* vol. 1. New York: Basic Books, 1979, pp. 213–233.

84. Poznanski, E. O., et al. "The Dexamethasone Suppression Test in Prepubertal Depressed Children," *American Journal of Psychiatry,* 139 (1982):321–324.

85. Prange, A., et al. "Clinical and Theoretical Implications of the Enhancement of Imipramine by Tri-Iodothyronine in the Full Spectrum of Depressive Illness: A Possible Role of Central Aminergic Receptors," in T. Williams, M. Katz, and J. A. Shield, Jr., eds., *Recent Advances in the Psychobiology of the Depressive Illness,* Washington, D.C.: Superintendent of Documents, U.S. Government Printing Office, 1972, pp. 249–255.

86. Preskorn, S. "Clinical Usefulness of Monitoring Imipramine Plasma Levels in Depressed Children," in E. Weller and R. Weller, eds., *Current Perspectives on Major Depressive Disorders in Children.* Washington, D.C.: American Psychiatric Press, 1984, pp. 66–75.

87. Preskorn, S. H., Weller, E. B., and Weller, R. A. "Depression in Children: Relationship Between Plasma Imipramine Levels and Response," *Journal of Clinical Psychiatry,* 43 (1982):450–453.

88. Puig-Antich, J. "Psychobiology of Prepubertal Major Depression," in E. Weller and R. Weller, eds., *Current Perspectives on Major Depressive Disorders in Children.* Washington, D.C.: American Psychiatric Press, 1984, pp. 77–90.

89. Puig-Antich, J., et al. "Prepubertal Major Depressive Disorder," *Journal of the American Academy of Child Psychiatry,* 17 (1978):695–707.

90. Puig-Antich, J., et al. "Plasma Levels of Imipramine (IMI) and Desmethylimipramine (DMI) and Clinical Response in Prepubertal Major Depressive Disorder," *Journal of the American Academy of Child Psychiatry,* 18 (1979):616–627.

91. Puig-Antich, J. et al. "Growth Hormone Secretion in Prepubertal Children with Major Depression, I. Final Report on Responses to Insulin-Induced Hypoglycemia During a Depressive Episode," *Archives of General Psychiatry,* 41 (1984):455–460.

92. Puig-Antich, J. et al. "Growth Hormone Secretion in Prepubertal Children with Major Depression, III. Response to Insulin-Induced Hypoglycemia After Recovery From a Depressive Episode and in a Drug-Free State," *Archives of General Psychiatry,* 41 (1984):471–475.

93. Quigley, M. E., and Yen, S.S.C. "The Role of Endogenous Opiate on LH Secretion During the Menstrual Cycle," *Journal of Clinical Endocrinology and Metabolism,* 51 (1980):179–181.

94. Ramsay, P. Urigmar, M., and Morell, P. "Developmental Studies of the Uptake of Choline, GABA and Dopamine by Crude Synaptosomal Preparations After In Vivo or In Vitro Lead Treatment," *Brain Research,* 187 (1980):383–402.

95. Raskin, A. "Age-Sex Differences in Response to Antidepressant Drugs," *Journal of Nervous and Mental Diseases,* 159 (1974):120–130.

96. Rauste-von Wright, M., von Wright, J., and Frankenhaeuser, M. "Relationships Between Sex-Related Psychological Characteristics During Adolescence and Catecholamine Excretion During Achievement Stress," *Psychophysiology,* 18 (1981):362–370.

97. Reichlin, S. "The Control of Anterior Pituitary Secretion," in P. B. Beeson and W. McDermott, eds., *Textbook of Medicine.* Philadelphia: W. B. Saunders, 1975, pp. 1671–1677.

98. Robbins, D. R. et al. "The Use of the Research Diagnostic Criteria (RDC) for Depression in Adolescent Psychiatric Inpatients," *Journal of the American Academy of Child Psychiatry,* 21 (1982):251–255.

99. Robbins, D. R., et al. "Preliminary Report on the

Dexamethasone Supression Test in Adolescents," *American Journal of Psychiatry,* 139 (1982):942–943.

100. SACK, J., et al. "Serum T_4, T_3 and TBG Concentrations During Puberty in Males," *European Journal of Pediatrics,* 138 (1982):136–137.

101. SAENGER, P., RIFKIND, A. B., and NEW, M. I. "Changes in Drug Metabolism in Children with Thyroid Disorders," *Journal of Clinical Endocrinology and Metabolism,* 42 (1976):155–159.

102. SEEMAN, M. V. "Interaction of Sex, Age, and Neuroleptic Dose," *Comprehensive Psychiatry,* 24 (1983):125–128.

103. SEPKOVIC, D. W., HALEY, N. J., and WYNDER, E. L. "Thyroid Activity in Cigarette Smokers," *Archives of Internal Medicine,* 144 (1984):501–503.

104. SHADER, R. I., and HARMATZ, J. S. "Premenstrual Tension in Biochemical and Psychotropic Drug Assessment," *Psychopharmacology Bulletin,* 18 (1982):113–123.

105. SILBERMAN, E., et al. "Altered Lateralization of Cognitive Processes in Depressed Women," *American Journal of Psychiatry,* 140 (1983):1340–1344.

106. SIMONS, A., GARFIELD, S., and MURPHY, G. "The Process of Change in Cognitive Therapy and Pharmacotherapy," *Archives of General Psychiatry,* 41 (1984):45–54.

107. SIMPKINS, J., KALRA, S. P., and KALRA, P. S. "Variable Effects of Testosterone on Dopamine Activity in Several Microdisected Regions in the Preoptic Area and Medial Basal Hypothalamus," *Endocrinology,* 112 (1983):665–669.

108. SOLOW, R. A. "Psychopharmacology with Adolescents: A Current Review," in S. C. Feinstein, and P. L. Giovacchini, eds., *Adolescent Psychiatry,* vol. 6, *Developmental and Clinical Studies.* Chicago: University of Chicago Press, 1978, pp. 480–494.

109. STANTON, R., WILSON, H., and BRUMBACK, R. "Cognitive Improvement Associated with Tricyclic Antidepressant Treatment of Childhood Major Depressive Illness," *Perceptual and Motor Skills,* 53 (1981):219–234.

110. STROBER, M., and CARLSON, G. "Bipolar Illness in Adolescents with Major Depression," *Archives of General Psychiatry,* 39 (1982):549–555.

111. STROBER, M., GREEN, J., and CARLSON, G. "Phenomenology and Subtypes of Major Depressive Disorder in Adolescence," *Journal of Affective Disorders,* 3 (1981):281–290.

112. SUSMAN, E. J., et al. "Hormones and Mood Variability and Behavior Problems During Early Adolescence," Paper presented at the Seventh International Congress of Endocrinology, Quebec, July 1984.

113. SUTKER, P., et al. "Acute Alcohol Intoxication, Mood States and Alcohol Metabolism in Women and Men," *Pharmacology, Biochemistry and Behavior,* 19 (Supplement 1) (1983):349–354.

114. TOOLAN, J. M. "Depression in Children and Adolescents," *Journal of Orthopsychiatry,* 32 (1962):404–414.

115. VESELL, E. S., et al. "Altered Plasma Half Life of Antipyrine, Propylthiouracil, and Methimazole in Thyroid Dysfunction," *Clinical Pharmacology and Therapeutics,* 17 (1975):48–56.

116. VILLENEUVE, A., CAZEJUST, T., and COTE, M. "Estrogens in Tardive Dyskinesia in Male Psychiatric Patients," *Neuropsychobiology,* 6 (1980):145–151.

117. VILLENEUVE, A., LANGLELIER, P., and BEDARD, P. "Estrogens, Dopamine, and Dyskinesias," *Canadian Psychiatry Association Journal,* 23 (1978):68–70.

118. WEHR, T., and GOODWIN, F. "Rapid Changes in Manic-Depressives Induced by Tricyclic Antidepressants," *Archives of General Psychiatry,* 36 (1979):555–559.

119. WEINBERG, W. A., et al. "Depression in Children Referred to an Educational Diagnostic Center: Diagnosis and Treatment," *Journal of Pediatrics,* 83 (1973):1065–1072.

120. WEINGARTNER, H., et al. "Cognitive Processes in Depression," *Archives of General Psychiatry,* 38 (1981):42–47.

121. WEISSMAN, M. M., and KLERMAN, G. L. "Sex Differences and the Epidemiology of Depression," *Archives of General Psychiatry,* 34 (1977):98–111.

122. WEISSMAN, M. M., and MYERS, J. K. "Affective Disorders in a U.S. Urban Community: The Use of Research Diagnostic Criteria in an Epidemiologic Survey," *Archives of General Psychiatry,* 35 (1979):1304–1311.

123. WELLER, E., WELLER, R., and PRESKORN, S., "Steady-State Plasma Imipramine Levels in Prepubertal Depressed Children," *American Journal of Psychiatry,* 139 (1982):506–508.

124. WELLER, E. B., et al. "Childhood Depression: Imipramine Levels and Response," *Psychopharmacology Bulletin,* 19 (1983):59–62.

125. WINTER, J., and FAIMAN, C. "Pituitary-Gonadal Relations in Female Children and Adolescents," *Pediatric Research,* 7 (1973):948–953.

126. WIRZ-JUSTICE, A., and CHAPPIUS-ARNDT, E. "Sex-Specific Differences in Chlorimpramine Inhibition of Serotonin Uptake in Human Platelets," *European Journal of Pharmacology,* 40 (1976):21–25.

127. WOLLENSEN, F., KNIGGE, U., and LARSEN, K. "Effect of the Plasma Estrone/17 B-Estradiol Ratio on the Prolactin and TSH Responses to TRH," *Neuroendocrinology,* 35 (1982):200–204.

128. WOODS, J. H. "Neuroendocrinology of Cerebrospinal Fluid: Peptides, Steroids, and Other Hormones," *Neurosurgery,* 11 (1982):293–305.

9 / Epidemiology of Mental Health and Mental Illness Among Adolescents

Daniel Offer, Eric Ostrov, and Kenneth I. Howard

Introduction

Many adults, including a surprisingly large number of mental health professionals, believe that adolescence must be a tumultuous developmental period.* These individuals have written that if adolescents do not go through a serious and prolonged identity crisis, they will ultimately become very disturbed persons.

In writing this chapter, we have made several assumptions. First, we have assumed that a theoretical understanding of the psychological phases of development is of critical importance. Such a theoretical formulation is vital for a better grasp on the nature and structure of the life span and its several substages. However, theories formulated without an adequate data base are likely to be greatly misleading. In sum, empirical data are necessary for the formulation of any adequate theory of development. Second, we have assumed that it is possible that there is a high incidence and prevalence of psychopathology among adolescents. To deny serious problems out of a theoretical bias is no more scientific than to assume that universal psychopathology is a necessary characteristic of this age group. Third, we have assumed that the resolution of theoretical conflicts will be extremely complicated and difficult. Descriptions of persons who have pursued a relatively benign course during their adolescence will be questioned by many who will claim that the identity crisis in these teenagers is either submerged (and hence even more insidious) or that the smooth sailing represents a case of "arrested development." Conversely, disturbance among adolescents could be dismissed as representing only the troubled group brought to clinical attention or as a trivial sample reflecting transient, age-typical turmoil. And fourth, we have assumed that the approach to learning more about adolescents must be broad-based in order to gain further insight into the bio-psychosocial aspects of this time of life.

*See references 3, 6, 7, 8, and 23.

Review of Literature

Recently we[19] have shown that mental health professionals who work with adolescents tend to think that normal teenagers are as disturbed and as unhappy as are those teenagers who are hospitalized and psychiatrically ill. To quote Oldham,[21] "The clinician who views adolescence as a period of inevitable turbulence and disruption will approach the problem differently from colleagues who regard normal adolescence as characterized by stability" (p. 267). Among clinicians who believe adolescent turmoil or unhappiness is normative, only the extremely disturbing or the clearly disturbed adolescent may generate concern and intervention.

When studies were performed on large groups of adolescents in the community or in their families, it was uniformly found that the vast majority of adolescents were not in great turmoil. They were not in a state of rebellion in their relationships with other family members, and they underwent relatively smooth transitions from childhood to adulthood.* As we[18] put it:

The results reveal that normal adolescents are not in the throes of turmoil. . . . The vast majority function well, enjoy good relationships with their families and friends, and accept the values of the larger society. In addition, most report having adapted without undue conflict to the bodily changes and emerging sexuality brought on by puberty. (P. 116)

Relevant to the issue of the prevalence of psychiatric disturbance among adolescents, the empirical literature indicates that at any one point in time, approximately 20 percent of adolescents attest to being psychiatrically ill to a clinically significant degree. This rate is virtually identical with that found in epidemiological studies of adults.[27] There is almost no literature bearing on the specific kinds of psychiatric illnesses found among those teenagers in the community who

*See references 4, 5, 17, 18, and 28.

are disturbed. Similarly, almost no literature exists that depicts the prevalence of teenage difficulties or characteristics of disturbed adolescents who do not receive treatment or who are not the subject of intervention efforts.

However, there is evidence that a large proportion of disturbed adolescents do not come to the attention of adults as needing or requiring help. An early epidemiological study was conducted by Krupinski and associates[13] in 1967 in the small Australian town of Heyfield. Based on this research, it was concluded that 16 percent of the male adolescents and 19 percent of the female adolescents in the town had psychiatrically diagnosable conditions. A Scandinavian study[2] of the thirteen- to fourteen-year-old adolescents in an industrial town reported a prevalence rate of moderate or severe disorder of 21 percent for boys and 14 percent for girls.

A key series of studies by Rutter and coworkers[9,24] were conducted on the Isle of Wight, an island off the coast of England. Information was based both on individual interviews of the youngsters by psychiatrists and on interviews with parents and teachers of the youths studied. According to the authors,[9] "More than a fifth of the boys and girls reported that they felt miserable or depressed, and the same proportion reported great difficulty in sleeping and waking unnecessarily early in the morning" (p. 42). Using parents' interviews as the source of information about adolescents, the prevalence of psychiatric disorder among fourteen-year-olds was found to be 13 percent. Based on interviews with the adolescents themselves, it was concluded that 16 percent could be diagnosed as having psychiatric disorders. After compiling the figures from multiple data sources, it was concluded that "the corrected prevalence rate for psychiatric disorder in 14- to 15-year-old children is 21.0%"[9] (p. 1227).

In the United States relatively few studies have attempted to ascertain the prevalence of emotional disturbance among adolescents and, secondarily, to determine the kinds of disturbance shown by those adolescents who are disturbed. While Locksley and Douvan[16] emphasized this fact in 1979, writing: "Although national surveys of the incidence of psychopathology among adolescents have not been conducted as yet, this may be a direction for research ultimately as profitable as those directions heretofore pursued" (p. 73), since then, very few relevant studies have been undertaken.

Langner, Gersten, and Eisenberg[14] conducted one of the few studies of this kind among U.S. adolescents. The methodology involved a questionnaire administered to mothers regarding their children's behavior. The sample population consisted of 1,034 children ages six to eighteen who were randomly selected from a cross-section of Manhattan in New York. The questionnaire results were then rated by a psychiatrist for degree of impairment. The findings indicated that 17 to 20 percent of the black and Spanish children displayed extreme rates of impairment, whereas only 8 to 9 percent of the white children were so characterized. Unfortunately, the data for adolescents were not reported separately from the findings for children in other age groups. In the Locksley and Douvan study cited earlier, sophomores, juniors, and seniors attending a midwestern urban, lower-middle-class high school were evaluated on the basis of a self-report questionnaire. Longitudinal data were obtained by readministering the questionnaire to a subsample of the sophomores during their senior year. Locksley and Douvan[16] observed that males reported aggression and feelings of resentment significantly more frequently than did females, while, on the average, females reported significantly more frequent feelings of tension and psychosomatic symptoms. The sexes did not differ on their accounts of feelings of depression. Unfortunately, Locksley and Douvan's observations do not include an estimate of the prevalence of psychiatric disorder among the adolescents studied.

Other studies have focused on the incidence of depressive symptoms among adolescents and not the incidence of psychiatric illness generally. Schoenbach and associates[25] administered a self-report depressive symptom checklist to 384 junior-high-school students. Elevated symptom scores among blacks and low-socioeconomic-status whites were cited in this study. Prevalence rates of depression were not reported, but the authors do note that compared to adults who were studied by means of the same instruments, the adolescents showed similar symptom "persistence," that is, they reported that they felt symptoms of depression most or all of the time during the preceding week at the same rate as did the adults. Studying small samples of seventh and eight graders from one parochial school in suburban Philadelphia, and using the Beck Depression Inventory as a source of data, Albert and Beck[1] concluded that 33.3 percent of their early-adolescent sample fell into the range of moderate to severe depressive symptomatology, while only 2.2 percent fell into the severe range.

Kandel and Davies[10] studied the epidemiology of depression among adolescents. The subjects were a sample of adolescents, fourteen to eighteen years of age, who were representative of public high school students in New York state in 1971 through 1972. They found that adolescents from families with very low incomes were more depressed than were those from any other social-economic status group. Girls were more depressed than were boys. The one prevalence rate cited in this study indicated that 20 percent of the adolescents reported feeling sad or depressed during the previous year.

Regarding the question of what proportion of psychiatrically ill teenagers seek or obtain professional help, only two studies of help-seeking behavior among adolescents were found. One study[15] was conducted in Britain; it concluded that "the parents of 24 out of the 67 children with psychiatric disorder (or 36%) had not sought advice at any time; some did not perceive abnormality, but others did not know of anyone who would help with such problems" (p. 118). The other study by Kellam and coworkers[11] presents even more dramatic results. According to these authors, an adolescent's acceptance of an offer of help through counseling was associated not with how disturbed the adolescent was but with the characteristics of the persons offering the help. The implication seems to be that many adolescents in need of help probably do not receive it, particularly when it is left up to them to initiate and carry through on the help-seeking behavior.

The 1983 Epidemiological Study

We carried out a study in the Chicago area to learn more about emotional disturbance and mental health resource utilization among adolescents.[22] In general, it turned out that about 20 percent of the adolescents studied were psychologically disturbed. Many of these troubled youngsters had never been seen by a mental health professional, had never come to the attention of the authorities, and had never been perceived by other adults as needing help.

SUBJECTS

As a first step in our study, the authorization of the trustees of a Chicago suburban township was obtained to collect data from adolescents who attended the township high schools. We randomly selected every fourteenth student in the entire high school. Since there were 4,530 students, a list of 324 students was obtained. These 324 students were divided into four groups—the smallest of these groups comprised 65 students. Sixty-five students were then randomly drawn from each of the other three groups, yielding a total of 260 students to be studied.

Questionnaires were mailed to the homes of these teenagers with a request that the youth fill them out and return them to the investigators. As an incentive for the subjects to do so, those who cooperated were promised (and given) a five-dollar gift certificate to a local record store. Adolescents not responding to the mailed questionnaires were telephoned by the investigators as a way of furthering participation, and a hired research assistant went to the teenagers' home to

encourage them to fill out the questionnaires. As a result of these efforts, 87 percent of the students sampled from this suburban high school (who were still in the area when the research was being conducted) completed questionnaires.

The responses obtained from these students comprise the core of the research data. To make the data base demographically more diverse, questionnaires were also collected from two Roman Catholic high schools located in Chicago. One of these high schools is all male, all black, and is located in a lower- to lower-middle-class neighborhood; the other parochial high school is almost entirely white, enrolls only girls, and is located in a lower-middle to upper-middle-class neighborhood. In contrast, the students from the suburban high school are almost all white, attend a coeducational school, and come from an upper-middle to lower-upper-class neighborhood. Limited resources did not allow extensive data collection in the parochial high schools, so only juniors were studied. This age group was chosen because after a year, follow-up would be easier to obtain than it would be with seniors; conversely, it was thought that their self-image would be more stable than that of freshmen or sophomores. Data were obtained from all those present in the school on the day of the testing.

INSTRUMENTS

The instruments given to the suburban adolescents included the Offer Self-Image Questionnaire (OSIQ),[18] the Delinquency CheckList (DCL),[26] a survey of mental health services utilized, and unstructured questions calling for written answers regarding problems and need for mental health services not received. A fact sheet requesting demographic data including parents' marital status was also included. The Catholic school students were just given the OSIQ, the DCL, and the fact sheet to fill out. Questionnaires were given anonymously, but the adolescents surveyed could write their names, addresses, and telephone numbers in a space provided for that purpose if they were willing to participate in future research.

The OSIQ contains 130 items covering adjustment in eleven areas important to the psychological life of adolescents. Adjustment in each area is measured by a scale score; the eleven scale scores, in turn, are clustered into five psychological selves. (See table 9–1.) Scores for each scale are expressed as standard scores. In this metric a score of 50 represents functioning in a given area equal to the mean of a like-age, same-sex, nationwide normative group. The standard scores are adjusted so that the standard deviation of the norming group is 15. In this metric, too, a higher score represents better adjustment in a particular area. OSIQ scale scores are internally consistent and moderately stable.[18]

TABLE 9–1

Offer Self-Image Questionnaire Scales and Self Clusters

Psychological Selves	Scales
Psychological self	Impulse control
Psychological self	Mood
Psychological self	Body image
Social self	Social relations
Social self	Morals
Social self	Vocational and educational goals
Sexual self	Sexual attitudes and behavior
Familial self	Family relations
Coping self	Mastery of the external world
Coping self	Psychopathology
Coping self	Superior adjustment (coping)

The value of the OSIQ as a measure of adolescents' self-image and adjustment has been demonstrated in many studies.[17,18,20] The DCL is a self-report inventory of the extent to which the youth has engaged in delinquent behaviors.

DATA ANALYSIS

As a first step, OSIQ data were scored using the standard score format. As a result, OSIQ standard scores describing functioning in eleven areas relevant to adolescents were obtained for teenagers from each community. These scores were then used as a criterion of disturbance: If a student scored one standard deviation or more below the mean (a score of 35 or less in standard score terms) on three or more OSIQ scales, that student was considered disturbed. In addition, those disturbed students who were "quiet"—that is, by self-report had not received professional help more than once, had not been stopped or apprehended by the police, and had never committed any repetitive serious delinquent acts—were identified. Analyses were performed showing mean OSIQ scale scores for all male and female students, for male and female disturbed students, and for male and female quietly disturbed students.

RESULTS

OSIQ scale score means for boys and girls from the three communities studied are well within the range of the normal. These results imply that the teenagers tested in this study and those tested as part of the national norming group[18] were, on the average, very similar in self-image.

Results show that, combining the three communities studied, 17 percent of the boys and 22 percent of the girls are disturbed. Of the disturbed male adolescents, 35 percent are quietly disturbed; of the disturbed female adolescents, 62 percent are quietly disturbed. In comparing quietly and actively disturbed adolescents' OSIQ means, because the numbers in each group are so small, results are reported if they are significant at the 0.10 level by a two-tailed t-test. Table 9–2 shows quietly disturbed male adolescents reported significantly better impulse control, family relationships, and sense of competency than did disturbed adolescents who acted out and/or have received help. The quietly disturbed adolescents also showed significantly more conservative sexual attitudes than did the actively disturbed adolescents. With respect to emotional tone, body image, social relationships, morals, mastery of external world, and vocational and educational goals, the quietly disturbed males reported self-image within 5 standard score points of that reported by the actively disturbed male adolescents.

Among girls (see table 9–3), results indicate that the quietly disturbed adolescents reported markedly better family relationships and better body image than did actively disturbed adolescents. In all other scales but emotional tone, the quietly disturbed females scored

TABLE 9–2

OSIQ Standard Scores[a] for Quietly Disturbed and Actively Disturbed Male Adolescents in Three Chicago Community High Schools

OSIQ Scale	Quietly Disturbed Males ($N = 10$)	Actively Disturbed Males ($N = 17$)
Impulse control	46[b]	31[b]
Emotional tone	37	34
Body and self-image	32	37
Social relationships	41	37
Morals	43	40
Sexual attitudes	37[b]	49[b]
Family relationships	46[b]	34[b]
Mastery of external world	33	36
Vocational educational goals	44	39
Psychopathology	41	33
Superior adjustment	46[b]	35[b]

[a] A standard score of 50 is equal to the norming group mean for that scale. The standard deviation for the norming group's scores on each scale is 15. A score higher than 50 represents better adjustment in the area measured than that attested to by the norming group on the average.
[b] Difference significant at the 0.10 level or lower by two-tailed t-test.

TABLE 9–3

OSIQ Standard Scores[a] for Quietly Disturbed and Actively Disturbed Female Adolescents in Three Chicago Community High Schools

OSIQ Scale	Quietly Disturbed Females (N = 23)	Actively Disturbed Females (N = 14)
Impulse control	37	36
Emotional tone	33	27
Body and self-image	36[b]	25[b]
Social relationships	37	37
Morals	44	46
Sexual attitudes	43	43
Family relationships	43[b]	24[b]
Mastery of external world	32	30
Vocational-educational goals	45	42
Psychopathology	36	31
Superior adjustment	41	36

[a] A standard score of 50 is equal to the norming group mean for that scale. The standard deviation for the norming group's scores on each scale is 15. A score higher than 50 represents better adjustment in the area measured than that attested to by the norming group on the average.
[b] Difference significant at the 0.10 level of lower by two-tailed t-test.

within 5 standard score points of the average scale scores obtained by the actively disturbed females.

In the suburban high-school sample specific data exist concerning the adolescents' mental health care utilization. (See tables 9–4 and 9–5.) These data show that although more delinquents and disturbed youngsters than normal teenagers used mental health care, a significant number of disturbed adolescents did not ever consult a mental health professional.

DISCUSSION

As has been true whenever research has been conducted with representative groups of adolescents, our results demonstrate that the vast majority of adolescents in this study are happy and well adjusted. Consistent with previous epidemiological studies, the data gathered here indicate that about 20 percent of the adolescents studied are emotionally disturbed to a meaningful degree. Until now, a factor that has been

TABLE 9–4

Midwest Suburban High School Nondelinquent vs. Delinquent Adolescents Using Mental Health Professionals

	Nondelinquent (N = 160)	Delinquent (N = 59)
Consulted mental health professionals more than once	13%	27%
Consulted mental health professionals excluding school counselor one time	22%	20%
Never consulted a mental health professional	65%	53%

largely unknown is the percentage of disturbed adolescents who do not manifest their difficulties through antisocial behavior sufficient to warrant either their being apprehended by the police more than once or their being seen by a mental health professional more than once. The data suggest that about one-third of the boys and two-thirds of those girls who are disturbed have neither received help nor come to the attention of the authorities. In the suburban high schools, more than half of the disturbed or delinquent adolescents had never seen any mental health professional. It is of interest that if the OSIQ scores of the teenagers in these samples identified as disturbed are compared with the OSIQ scores of youths who are hospitalized for psychiatric illness (see Koenig et al.[12]), the profiles are very similar. This suggests that the teenagers identified as disturbed in these samples are notably ill, even though almost none has been treated on an inpatient basis and

TABLE 9–5

Midwest Suburban High School Nondisturbed vs. Disturbed Adolescents Using Mental Health Professionals

	Nondisturbed (N = 167)	Disturbed (N = 32)
Consulted mental health professionals more than once	12%	25%
Consulted mental health professionals excluding school counselor one time	25%	22%
Never consulted a mental health professional	63%	53%

many (in the case of girls, most) have not received any sustained professional help.

Among the boys identified as disturbed in this sample, those who are quietly disturbed have relatively good impulse control and family relationships. But quietly disturbed boys achieved scores in respect to affect, body image, and social relationships that were as low or lower than those recorded by the actively disturbed group. Quietly disturbed girls reported healthier body images than did their actively disturbed counterparts, but the primary difference between the two groups were in the area of family relationships. In most realms, the quietly disturbed girls were as poorly adjusted as were the actively disturbed girls. For both boys and girls, a key difference between the quietly disturbed and the actively disturbed was the better family relationships of the quietly disturbed group.

When comparing boys and girls, it is troublesome to note that proportionately many more girls than boys seem to be quietly disturbed. This may explain why in adolescence, unlike other age groups, more boys than girls receive mental health care or are in treatment. Taking all the adolescents together, a majority of those who reported themselves to be disturbed attested to being quietly disturbed—that is, they had not seen any professional more than once, they had not engaged in serious delinquency, and they had not been stopped or apprehended by the police.

Conclusions

Our study indicates that only a minority of adolescents are disturbed (in terms of feeling bad about themselves in a number of areas). Viewed nationally, however, that minority represents a very large number of teenagers. At this time, there are approximately 18 million adolescents in high school in the United States. If 20 percent of those adolescents are disturbed, the implication is that nearly 3.6 million may require some kind of help or intervention. Our results suggest that of those 3.6 million, approximately 50 percent, or 1.8 million, have not received any mental health care or have not acted out enough to attract attention. Thus 1.8 million adolescents are quietly disturbed and stand in need of mental health care but do not receive it. Future research should determine what developmental course quietly disturbed adolescents follow and what kind of interventions can best help them.

ACKNOWLEDGMENTS

This work was supported, in part, by the Adolescent Research Fund: In Memory of Judith Offer, and by Grant #82085500 from the Grant Foundation, New York City.

REFERENCES

1. ALBERT, N., and BECK, A. T. "Incidence of Depression in Early Adolescence: A Preliminary Study," *Journal of Youth and Adolescence*, 4 (1975):301–107.

2. BJORNSSON, S. "Epidemiological Investigation of Mental Disorders of Children in Reykjavik, Iceland," *Scandinavian Journal of Psychology*, 15 (1974):244–254.

3. BLOS, P. *On Adolescence*. New York: Free Press of Glencoe, 1962.

4. CSIKSZENTMIHALYI, M., and LARSON, R. *Being Adolescent*. New York: Basic Books, 1984.

5. DOUVAN, E., and ADELSON, J. *The Adolescent Experience*. New York: John Wiley & Sons, 1966.

6. ERIKSON, E. H. "Identity and the Life Cycle," *Psychological Issues*, 1 (1959):1–171.

7. FREUD, A. *The Ego and the Mechanism of Defense*. New York: International Universities Press, 1946.

8. ———. "Adolescence," *Psychoanalytic Study of the Child*, 16 (1958):225–278.

9. GRAHAM, P., and RUTTER, M. "Psychiatric Disorder in the Young Adolescent: A Follow-up Study," *Proceedings of the Royal Society of Medicine*, 66 (1973):58–61.

10. KANDEL, D. B., and DAVIES, M. "Epidemiology of Depressive Mood in Adolescents," *Archives of General Psychiatry*, 39 (1982):1205–1212.

11. KELLAM, S. G., et al. "Why Teenagers Come for Treatment: A Ten-Year Prospective Epidemiological Study in Woodlawn," *Journal of the American Academy of Child Psychiatry*, 20 (1981):477–495.

12. KOENIG, L. et al. "Psychopathology and Adolescent Self-Image," in D. Offer, E. Ostrov, and K. I. Howard, eds., *Patterns of Adolescent Self-Image*. New Directions for Mental Health Services Series. San Francisco: Jossey-Bass, 1984, pp. 57–72.

13. KRUPINSKI, J., et al. "A Community Health Survey of Heyfield, Victoria," *Medical Journal of Australia*, 54 (1967): 1204–1211.

14. LANGNER, T. S., GERSTEN, J. C., and EISENBERG, J. G. "Approaches to Measurement and Definition in Epidemiology of Behavior Disorders: Ethnic Background and Child Behavior," *International Journal of Health Services*, 4 (1974):483–501.

15. LESLIE, S. A. 1974. "Psychiatric Disorder in the Young Adolescents of an Industrial Town," *British Journal of Psychiatry*, 125 (1974):113–124.

16. LOCKSLEY, A. and DOUVAN, E. "Problem Behavior in Adolescents," in E. Gombera and V. Frank, eds., *Gender and Disordered Behavior.* New York: Brunner/Mazel, 1979, pp. 71–100.

17. OFFER, D., and OFFER, J. B. *From Teenage to Young Manhood: A Psychological Study.* New York: Basic Books, 1975.

18. OFFER, D., OSTROV, E., and HOWARD, K. I. *The Adolescent: A Psychological Self-Portrait.* New York: Basic Books, 1981.

19. ———. "The Mental Health Professional's Concept of the Normal Adolescent," *Archives of General Psychiatry,* 38 (1981):149–152.

20. OFFER, D., OSTROV, E., and HOWARD, K. I., eds. *Patterns of Adolescent Self-Image.* New Directions for Mental Health Services Series. San Francisco: Jossey-Bass, 1984.

21. OLDHAM, D. G. "Adolescent Turmoil: A Myth Revisited," *Adolescent Psychiatry,* 6 (1978):267–282.

22. OSTROV, E., OFFER, D., and HARTTAGE, S. "The Quietly Disturbed Adolescent," in D. Offer, E. Ostrov, and K. I.

Howard, eds., *Patterns of Adolescent Self-Image.* New Directions for Mental Health Services. San Francisco: Jossey-Bass, 1984, pp. 73–82.

23. RABICHOW, H. G., and SKLANSKY, M. A. *Effective Counseling of Adolescents.* Chicago: Follett, 1980.

24. RUTTER, M., et al. "Adolescent Turmoil: Fact or Fiction," *Journal of Child Psychology and Psychiatry,* 17 (1976): 35–56.

25. SCHOENBACH, V. J., et al. "Depressive Symptoms in Young Adolescents," *Society for Epidemiologic Research Abstracts,* 112 (1980):440.

26. SHORT, J. F., JR., and NYE, F. I. "Reported Behavior as a Criterion of Deviant Behavior," *Social Problems,* 5 (1957):207–213.

27. UHLENHUTH, E. H., et al. "Symptom Checklist Syndromes in the General Population: Correlations with Psychotherapeutic Drug Use," *Archives of General Psychiatry,* 40 (1983):1167–1173.

28. WESTLEY, W. A., and EPSTEIN, N. B. *The Silent Majority.* San Francisco: Jossey-Bass, 1969.

SECTION II

Varieties of Development

Joseph D. Noshpitz / Editor

Introduction

Joseph D. Noshpitz

When the *Basic Handbook of Child Psychiatry* was originally compiled, the concept of personality development was regarded as the central organizing principle that would bind together and give form to the structure of the entire work. Accordingly, the opening section of the Handbook was devoted to development, one of the editors took this on as his sole area of effort, and the resulting array of material in the several chapters extended from the molecular biology of genes to the vicissitudes of late adolescence.

At the same time, however, there was a sense that much more needed to be said. It was all well and good to recount the studies and theories about normal development; that was a kind of laboratory model, an *in vitro* approach, which provided the reader with essential information. But children do not grow in a laboratory and their development is by no means necessarily normal. They grow in a wide variety of environments, and they pursue their individual courses under circumstances that not only vary from the norm but that often enough are extraordinary in terms of the variety of vectors and constellations which shape the form of their emergence. In a volume devoted to studying the mental health and psychological growth of children, how then to represent this complexity?

It was in answer to this question that the second section of this *Handbook,* Varieties of Development, was created. Here we attempt to delineate some of the differing circumstances, normal and pathological, that surround and affect the growth of children and to list some of the types of childhood adaptation that then ensue. This has led to the assemblage of a somewhat unusual array of articles; our aim is to offer the reader a sense of the variety of the ecological niches that children come to occupy and a picture of the life-styles that presently emerge from the shaping forces at work in these several settings.

Not the least important among these are pictures of children affected by illness and surgery and some of the consequences of our attempts to heal the many life-threatening conditions that affect the early years.

In this update volume, the editors seek to continue the earlier undertaking and to add a number of additional categories to the array. Some of these reflect the effects of new investigations, some the uncovering of new realms for description. In any case, it is part of our effort to catch and to present an ever more accurate and more valid description of the children of our times and the way they grow and live.

10 / The Sibling of the Chronically Ill or Disabled Child

Carl Feinstein and Sherry E. Davis

Introduction

Clinicians working with chronically ill or handicapped children and their families have long suspected that the siblings of these children are at risk for the development of emotional problems.[41] However, attempts to explore systematically the emotional well-being of the siblings of handicapped children have taken place only in the last two decades. Although many of the earlier studies reported that siblings of handicapped children are more emotionally vulnerable,[9, 13] the results of these studies must be interpreted with caution because of methodological problems (e.g., use of retrospective data, absence of control groups, etc.). Recent studies that employ more sophisticated research methodology do suggest that siblings of handicapped children may be more psychologically vulnerable, with many studies citing[2, 7, 32, 48] higher levels of anxiety, negative self-esteem, behavioral problems, and somatic complaints among these siblings when compared to control groups. Although a myriad of hypotheses have been generated to explain this phenomenon, the most frequently cited explanation is that the increased demands on the parents detract from the attention they can provide their able-bodied offspring.[4, 16, 46]

Gaps in developmental theories pertaining to sibling effects also have greatly impeded an understanding of this issue. Recently, however, there has been a flurry of valuable books and literature reviews reassessing sibling relationships.* These works have begun to shed light on many aspects of the sibling relationship that had previously been obscured by an overreliance on general status indicators, such as birth order and ordinal position.[30] The old preoccupation with ordinal position, in which generalizations were sought regarding "the first child," "the middle child," and "the youngest child," did not provide clinicians with a sufficiently specific methodology for clinically evaluating the effect of chronically ill or handicapped children on their healthy siblings.

Contemporary researchers have turned increasingly toward the study of a wider range of processes whereby sibling effects are mediated. This chapter categorizes these mediating processes through which the sibling relationship is influenced. The focus is on how well siblings are affected by having a handicapped child in the family; however, it may be readily seen that this same approach can be applied clinically to any situation where there is a need to understand sibling relationships.

The large number of variables that affect the well sibling–handicapped sibling relationship may be organized into four general categories or types of influences: (1) direct parental influences, (2) family influences, (3) sibling relationship influences, and (4) sibling attitude toward disability. Each of these general categories may then be further subdivided into a large number of more specific considerations, any or all of which may play a role in the complex field of family interactions.

Direct Parental Influences

Kris and Ritvo[29] have recently reviewed the ways in which parents may influence the relationships among their children. They found that the role of the parents

in this relationship is "critically important." In general, parents harbor an idealized image of their children's relationships with each other, which includes an elaborate value system regarding such issues as fraternal closeness, rivalry, loyalty, and mutual assistance. These ideas exert a strong effect on both their children's interactions and their inner attitudes. Conscious and unconscious paradigms of the sibling relationships derive from parental experiences with their own siblings and influence the way parents respond to the developing sibling relationships of their offspring. In any clinical evaluation these must be made explicit.

In addition, parents serve as models for identification to their children. Thus well siblings will be strongly influenced by the way their parents respond to the handicapped child.[24, 26, 43, 44] If parents are generally accepting of the condition and the child, siblings often follow their example. However, if parents react with shame, negativism, or anxiety,[43] these parents are not prepared to influence positively their well children. The attitude of the well child toward the handicapped sibling is also greatly influenced by the knowledge the parents possess about the nature of the condition and by the way parents communicate this information to the other children. Lack of communication within the family over the child's disabling condition may contribute to a sense of loneliness and isolation among the well children. Commonly, parents fear that healthy children will undermine their wish to feel "normal" by revealing too much to neighbors, relatives, teachers, and peers.[5, 51] The need to protect the family's image may partially explain the observations that children seem to be poorly informed about their siblings' illnesses.[8, 46]

Differential parental expectations for the well and handicapped children also play an important role in the emotional development of both the handicapped child and the well sibling. Parental demands of the well sib may revolve around household chores and caregiving responsibilities for the handicapped child, resulting in feelings of resentment and jealousy from the well sibling.[20, 28, 44, 49] Trevino[49] notes that healthy siblings may be deprived of their childhood because they have to assume the role of substitute parents. Often parents expect the well sibling to be very tolerant of the handicapped child but are themselves less tolerant of negative behaviors (e.g., hostility, resentment, jealousy)* that are expressed toward the handicapped child. Siblings may also assume responsibility for the inferred psychological needs of parents by feeling that they must overachieve or overcompensate for the limitations of the handicapped child.[44, 49]

Parental attitudes toward sex roles contribute significantly to the response of the well child toward the

*See references 2, 12, 14, 29, 30, 40, 42, and 45.

*See references 3, 38, 43, 44, and 49.

handicapped sibling. In general, many investigators have found that female siblings of handicapped children are at higher risk for emotional problems, although this effect appears to be mediated by birth order. Breslau, Weitzman, and Messenger,[6] Gath,[22] and Trevino[49] have all found that older female siblings experience greater psychological distress than older male siblings and postulate that the older female child is faced with more parental pressure to care for her handicapped sibling than is the older male sibling. However, Lavigne and Ryan[32] found that while females in general had more psychological problems than their well male counterparts, well adolescent female siblings had fewer emotional problems than adolescent males; Tew and Laurence[48] found no sex, age, or birth-order effects in their sample of siblings of handicapped children.

The quality of the marital relationship sets the background for all relationships within the family. Yet this relationship itself is greatly stressed by the fact of having a handicapped child.[17] Severe marital problems, including estrangement and divorce, could then be the source of the well child's difficulties, an indirect effect of the presence of a disabled sibling in the family. The way this stress is manifested will also exert a powerful effect on the way the well sibling views the source of this stress—that is, the handicapped sibling.[17, 21, 50]

The possible effect of decreased parental attention to the well child because of the demands of caring for a handicapped child has also been well documented[4, 35] and may create conflicts between the well child and the parents or between the siblings themselves. The effects of decreased parental attention on the well sibling must be understood in light of the child's developmental level. Lack of parental attention would differentially affect the well infant, the toddler, the oedipal child, the latency child, and the adolescent. For example, a mother's preoccupation with an older handicapped child may interfere with attachment or nurturance issues for a very young child; for the older child or adolescent, the decreased involvement of the mother may intensify feelings of rivalry or envy or may result in impairments with the establishment of autonomous functioning and the acquisition of certain social skills.

Family Influences

A diverse range of experiences deriving from characteristics of the family of the disabled child will influence the well sibling's development. These influences may be socioeconomic, cultural, or related to family composition and dynamics.

The socioeconomic status of the family greatly affects the way it responds to the stress of a disabled child. This in turn will affect the parenting and the general milieu in which the well child develops. Families from middle and upper socioeconomic status backgrounds are more likely to have the financial resources to obtain additional child care and household help[18] to relieve the burden of special caregiving responsibilities. They may also be able to mobilize and have greater access to more effective and specialized support services from the school system and voluntary agencies. Farber[18] characterized the response of wealthier families to the presence of a handicapped child in the family as a "tragic crisis," noting that these parents may become demoralized or resentful when they realize that their disabled child will be unable to obtain postsecondary school education or skills. In contrast, Farber[18] noted that in lower socioeconomic status families, the child's disability was perceived as a burden superimposed on already heavy family demands; he characterized this response as an "organizational crisis." As such, the lower-class family's financial resources may be further restricted because the demands of caring for a handicapped child may prevent a parent (generally the mother) from working. In poorer families, the well siblings, especially older girls, are often obliged to contribute to child care, even when this compromises educational, peer, and/or recreational opportunities.[18, 21] This may in turn breed resentment or depression in the affected able-bodied child.

Family composition is a critical variable in assessing the impact that a disabled child has on a well sibling. Of great importance is whether the family is a single-parent or two-parent nuclear family. Kellam, Ensminger, and Turner[27] have documented the increased vulnerability of children from single-parent households. The added stress of a handicapped child could be expected to drain even further the limited resources a single parent would have for the care of her healthy child. (Note: The vast majority of single parents with handicapped children are female.) If the single-parent family came about as the result of estrangement related to the stress of raising a chronically ill child, then the well sibling also suffers from the loss of a parent.

Family size and the birth order of siblings will also exert an influence on the entire family. In general, siblings from large families are better adapted than siblings from small families.[5, 22, 47] This is probably due to the fact that in large families, the responsibility for care is dispersed among a larger number of people. Also, parents with a large number of children may be less disturbed by the birth of a handicapped child because their aspirations for their offspring can be fulfilled by their other children.

The data on the effect of ordinal position is equivocal, with some studies citing that older siblings are at greater risk [11,21] and others citing that younger siblings are at greater risk. [24,31] Some investigators agree that older siblings, especially female siblings, are at greater risk because they are more likely to assume child care responsibilities, whereas Farber and Rychman [20] argue that the younger sibling is at greater risk because the handicapped child usurps the position of the sibling who is actually the youngest in the family. Thus the younger sibling may be required to grow up faster and perform tasks that he or she would not otherwise perform. The effects of birth order are confounded by several factors, including the sex of the well sibling and the age of the handicapped child. Breslau, Weitzman, and Messenger [6] found that the older female sibling and the younger male sibling were at greater risk. Both Miller [36] and Farber [19] note that handicapped individuals increasingly disrupt family life as they get older. Thus, assessing the effects of an older, as opposed to younger, handicapped child or sibling may reveal more negative attitudes regardless of the sibling ordinal position. [44]

The presence or absence of supportive extended family members in the home or nearby is also an important influence. Such relatives may increase the amount of available parenting or provide a well sib with direct emotional support. Another factor, perhaps less tangible, relates to the stance of the family in the community. A family actively engaged in neighborhood or community affairs not only receives support from this type of "belonging" but increases the likelihood that the well sibling will find supplementary helpful relationships with adults outside the family in situations where the parents are overly burdened by the disabled sibling.

Family system dynamics profoundly affect the emotional status and development of the well child in a home with a chronically ill sibling. As previously discussed, the most critical issue in such a family is the quality and degree of support the marital partners find in each other. In addition, however, to marital estrangement, it is not uncommon for the mother and the ill child to form a tight alliance from which the father and the well siblings are excluded. [41] Such situations may range from those in which the well child receives support and attention from the mother, albeit less intense involvement than the disabled sib, to those where the well child feels excluded and seeks maternal attention by problem behavior.

The manner in which families respond to health crises in the chronically ill child has been shown by Minuchin and colleagues [39] to influence the course of illness. It would seem no less likely that maladaptive patterns here could also adversely affect the well sibling.

Sibling Relationship Influences

The direct effect of the relationship between disabled and well siblings has not yet been subject to systematic research. As Solnit [45] stated in a recent review, there have been no systematic clinical studies of sibling experience that have focused on healthy or progressive development; rather, sibling rivalry and the reaction of the first child to the birth of a sibling have been the main emphasis. This lack in both knowledge and theory only increases the need for the clinician to pay attention to sibling relationships in the families of handicapped children.

Many authors recently have stressed the importance of the sibling relationship. Kris and Ritvo [29] point out the often neglected fact that for one another, siblings become libidinal and aggressive objects. According to Edington and Wilson, [15] a child's first experience of competition, cooperation, mutual dependence, and mutual defiance of authority is with siblings. Lamb and Sutton-Smith [30] remind us that often siblings are the only regular playmates available to each other. Solnit [45] describes the "community of interest and experience shared by siblings." Because of their developmental closeness, Solnit feels siblings can play, fight, love, and compete in a way that is usually protective because their various strengths and weaknesses—physical, emotional, and intellectual—are more proportionately matched than those of children and their parents. In the course of their lifetime, siblings form, in the words of Bank and Kahn, [2] "a semi-autonomous group" who have feelings about each other and affect one another separate from the influence of parents.

Kris and Ritvo [29] describe the sibling relationship as a "second triangular relationship," in which the child experiences and develops ways of coping with conflicts over jealousy, envy, love and hate, but without some of the characteristics found in the child's oedipal complex with the parents. In middle childhood the siblings are often closest playmates and primary confidants. Bank and Kahn [2] describe how important aspects of a child's identity are influenced by sibling comparison and feelings of common background.

The influence of one sibling's chronic illness on the development of another sibling as mediated directly through the relationship is influenced by many factors. Certainly among the most important of these are the characteristics of the illness or disabilities, as they directly influence the types of interactions that siblings could have. The small amount of research in this area has demonstrated that the well sibling plays differently with the disabled child [38]: Helping is emphasized more and the expression of emotion is emphasized less. This same study found that parents were more intolerant of well children's anger and hostility toward the disabled child than when they were directed toward a nonimpaired sibling. Although this research was done with a mentally retardated population, it seems likely that a similar phenomena would occur with certain other types of chronic conditions. A few studies exist regarding the sibling of the deaf child and the blind child; however, the unique problems of these two disabilities may limit the generalization of these findings. Recently Miller and Cantwell[37] and Weinrott[52] reported on the beneficial effect for the disabled child of using a healthy sibling as a "tutor." The value of such studies would be enhanced if information was also obtained about the effects of such interactions on the unimpaired child.

Sibling Attitude Toward Disability

The well child's response to the specific handicap of the disabled sibling may exert an important effect in its own right. Characteristics of the disability itself, such as its chronicity, visibility, severity, and whether or not it was congenital or acquired, all present the well child with different emotional and conceptual problems.[24,34,43] The well child's ability to conceptualize the nature and ramifications of a chronic illness or disability are related both to his or her level of development and the quality and sensitivity with which parents have presented information about the disability or illness to the well child.[10] "Invisible" disabilities in which there are no obvious external stigmata may be misunderstood by the younger well child as volitional behavior. The attention of the parents to the ill child may then be responded to with exaggerated jealousy or self-esteem problems.[33,43]

Fantasies about the meaning and origin of the disability and illness affect the well child's response to his or her disabled sibling and may also stir up fears of body damage to the self.[44] An additional effect on the sibling may be related to his or her acceptance of the disability. The child whose sibling's impairment is obvious must constantly answer peer questions and is influenced by the anxiety and rejecting attitudes of those peers.[25,49] In this regard, parental attitudes toward the disability will exert an important influence. If the illness is a source of shame or discomfort to the parent, it is likely to be so also to the well child. This in turn may affect the well child's self-esteem.

Conclusion

Thus far we have reviewed the many ways in which the presence of a chronic illness or disability in a sibling may influence the emotional status of the well sibling. The discussion has emphasized primarily immediate effects of such conditions. It must be remembered, however, that the sibling relationship is a lifelong one. The effects of this relationship are profoundly formative during adult life in ways that cannot always be predicted. It should also be stressed that the presence of a disabled child in the home, while it may be a source of anguish and even a burden to the family of the well child, is not necessarily harmful. Research to date has failed to document that the sibling of a handicapped child is, in general, more vulnerable; however, certain types of sibling relationships may be exceptions.[6,23] The potential for developing greater emotional depths and empathic capacity as an outgrowth of living in a family that copes well with this adversity has probably been underestimated and warrants further study.

REFERENCES

1. BANK, S., and KAHN, M. "Sisterhood-brotherhood Is Powerful: Sibling Subsystems in Family Therapy," *Family Process,* 14 (1975):311–339.

2. ———. *The Sibling Bond.* New York: Basic Books, 1982.

3. BARDACH, J. L. "Psychological Adjustment of Handicapped Children and Their Families," *White House Conference on Handicapped Individuals.*

4. BERGGREEN, S. "A Study of the Mental Health of Near Relatives of 20 Multihandicapped Children," *Acta Paediatrica Scandinavica,* Supplement 215 (1971).

5. BIRENBAUM, A. "On Managing a Courtesy Stigma," *Journal of Health and Social Behavior,* 2 (1970):196–206.

6. BRESLAU, N., WEITZMAN, M., and MESSENGER, K. "Psychologic Functioning of Siblings of Disabled Children," *Pediatrics,* 67 (1981):344–353.

7. BROWNMILLER, N., and CANTWELL, D. "Siblings as Therapists: A Behavioral Approach," *American Journal of Psychiatry,* 133 (1976):447–450.

8. BURTON, L. *The Family Life of Sick Children.* London: Routledge & Kegan Paul, 1975.

9. CAIN, A. C., and CAIN, G. S. "On Replacing a Child," *Journal of the American Academy of Child Psychiatry,* 3 (1964):443.

10. CARANDANG, M.L.A., et al. "The Role of Cognitive Level and Sibling Illness in Children's Conceptualizations

of Illness," *American Journal of Orthopsychiatry,* 49 (1979):474–481.

11. CLEVELAND, D., and MILLER, N. "Attitudes and Life Commitments of Older Siblings of Mentally Retarded Adults: An Exploratory Study," *Mental Retardation,* (1977):38–41.

12. COLONNA, A. B., and NEWMAN, L. M. "The Psychoanalytic Literature on Siblings," *Psychoanalytic Study of the Child,* 38 (1983):285–309.

13. CRAIN, A.. SUSSMAN, M., and WEIL, W. "Family Interaction, Diabetes and Sibling Relationships," *International Journal of Social Psychiatry,* 12 (1966):35–43.

14. DUNN, J., and KENDRICK, C. *Siblings: Love, Envy and Understanding.* Cambridge, Mass.: Harvard University Press, 1982.

15. EDINGTON, G., and WILSON, B. "Children of Different Ordinal Position," in J. D. Noshpitz, ed., *Basic Handbook of Child Psychiatry,* vol. 1. New York: Basic Books, 1979, pp. 397–406.

16. FALKMAN, C. "Cystic Fibrosis: A Psychological Study of 52 Children and Their Families," *Acta Paediatrica Scandinavia,* Supplement 269 (1977).

17. FARBER, B. "Effects of a Severely Mentally Retarded Child on Family Integration," *Monograph of Social Research on Child Development,* 24 (1959):1.

18. ———. "Family Organization and Crisis: Maintenance of Integration in Families with a Severely Retarded Child," *Monographs of Social Research on Child Development,* 25 (1960):71.

19. ———. *Family: Organization and Interaction.* San Francisco: Chandler, 1964.

20. FARBER, B., and RYCKMAN, J. "Effects of Severely Mentally Retarded Children on Family Relationships," *Mental Retardation Abstracts,* 2 (1965):1–17.

21. GATH, A. "The Mental Health of Siblings of Congenitally Abnormal Children," *Journal of Child Psychology and Psychiatry and Allied Disciplines,* 13 (1972):211–218.

22. ———. "Sibling Reactions to Mental Handicap: A Comparison of the Brothers and Sisters of Mongol Children," *Journal of Child Psychology and Psychiatry and Allied Disciplines,* 15 (1974):187–198.

23. GAYTON, W. F., et al. "Children with Cystic Fibrosis: I. Psychological Test Findings of Patients, Siblings and Parents," *Pediatrics,* 59 (1977):888–894.

24. GROSSMAN, F. K. *Brothers and Sisters of Retarded Children.* Syracuse, N.Y.: Syracuse University Press, 1972.

25. HAYDEN, V. "Reactions of Siblings to a Child's Disability: The Other Children," *Exceptional Parent,* 4 (1974): 26–29.

26. HOLT, K. "The Home Care of Severely Retarded Children," *Pediatrics,* 22 (1958):744–755.

27. KELLAM, S. G., ENSMINGER, M. E., and TURNER, R. J. "Family Structure and the Mental Health of Children: Concurrent and Longitudinal Community-wide Studies," *Archives of General Psychiatry,* 34 (1977):1012–1022.

28. KLEIN, S. "Measuring the Outcome of the Impact of Chronic Childhood Illness on the Family," in G. Grave and I. Pless, eds., *Chronic Childhood Illness: Assessment of Outcome.* Washington, D.C.: U.S. Department of Health, Education and Welfare, No. 76–877, 1976.

29. KRIS, M., and RITVO, S. "Parents and Siblings: Their Mutual Influences," *Psychoanalytic Study of the Child,* 38 (1983):311–324.

30. LAMB, M. E., and SUTTON-SMITH, B., eds. *Sibling Relationships.* Hillsdale, N.J.: Laurence Erlbaum Associates, 1982.

31. LAUTERBACH, C. G. *Socio-behavioral Adaptation of Siblings of the Mentally Handicapped Child.* Scranton, Pa.: Print-shop, 1974.

32. LAVIGNE, J. V., and RYAN, M. "Psychologic Adjustment of Siblings of Children with Chronic Illness," *Pediatrics,* 63 (1979):616–627.

33. LOBATO, P. "Siblings of Handicapped Children: A Review," *Journal of Autism and Developmental Disorders,* 13 (1983):347–364.

34. LUTERMAN, D. *Counseling Parents of Hearing-impaired Children.* Boston: Little, Brown, 1979.

35. MCKEEVER, P. "Siblings of Chronically Ill Children: A Literature Review with Implications for Research and Practice," *American Journal of Orthopsychiatry,* 53 (1983): 209–218.

36. MILLER, L. G. "The Seven Stages in the Life Cycle of a Family with a Mentally Retarded Child," *Washington Institutions Department Proceedings of the 9th Annual Research Meeting,* 2 (1969):78–81.

37. MILLER, N. B., and CANTWELL, D. P. "Siblings as Therapists: A Behavioral Approach," *American Journal of Psychiatry,* 133 (1976):447–450.

38. MILLER, S. G. "An Exploratory Study of Sibling Relationships in Families with Retarded Children," *Dissertation Abstracts International,* 35 (1974):2994B–2995B.

39. MINUCHIN, S., et al. "A Conceptual Model of Psychosomatic Illness in Children," *Archives of General Psychiatry,* 32 (1975):1031–1038.

40. NEUBAUER, P. B. "The Importance of the Sibling Experience," *Psychoanalytic Study of the Child,* 38 (1983):325–336.

41. POZNANSKI, E. "Psychiatric Difficulties in Siblings of Handicapped Children," *Clinical Pediatrics,* 8 (1969):232–234.

42. PROVENCE, S., and SOLNIT, A. J. "Development-promoting Aspects of the Sibling Experience," *Psychoanalytic Study of the Child,* 38 (1983):337–351.

43. SELIGMAN, M. "Sources of Psychological Disturbance Among Siblings of Handicapped Children," *Personnel and Guidance Journal,* 61 (1983):529–531.

44. SIMEONSSON, R. J., and MCHALE, S. M. "Review: Research on Handicapped Children: Sibling Relationships," *Child: Care, Health and Development,* 7 (1981):153–171.

45. SOLNIT, A. J. "The Sibling Experience," *Psychoanalytic Study of the Child,* 38 (1983):281–284.

46. SPINETTA, J., and DEASY-SPINETTA, P., *Living with Childhood Cancer.* St. Louis: C. V. Mosby, 1981.

47. TAYLOR, L. S. "Communication Between Mothers and Normal Siblings of Retarded Children: Nature and Modification" diss.: University of North Carolina, (Ph.D 1974).

48. TEW, B., and LAURENCE, K. M. "Mothers, Brothers and Sisters of Patients with Spina Bifida," *Developmental Medicine and Child Neurology,* 15 (Supplement 29) (1972): 69–76.

49. TREVINO, F. "Siblings of Handicapped Children: Identifying Those at Risk," *Social Casework,* 60 (1979):488–493.

50. VADASY, P. F., et al. "Siblings of Handicapped Children: A Developmental Perspective on Family Interactions," *Family Relations,* 33 (1984):155–167.

51. VOYSEY, M. "Impression Management by Parents of Disabled Children," *Journal of Health and Social Behavior,* 13 (1972):180–189.

52. WEINROTT, M. R. "A Training Program in Behavior Modification for Siblings of the Retarded," *American Journal of Orthopsychiatry,* 44 (1974):362–375.

11 / Sickle Cell Anemia

Joseph Fischhoff and Dorothy Stevenson Jenkins

Introduction

Sickle cell anemia is a hereditary blood disease caused by a basic defect in a mutant, autosomal gene. It predominantly affects the black population in the United States and parts of Africa. Ethnic groups from the Mediterranean and Middle and Near Eastern areas are also affected. Heterozygous occurrence of the sickle gene, which is called sickle cell trait, usually is benign. Rarely, entering into a state of shock or flying at high altitudes in unpressurized aircraft may result in hypoxia and produce vaso-occlusive phenomena in a carrier. Other than that, the heterozygous individual does not develop signs and symptoms. By way of contrast, children who are homozygous for this gene suffer from sickle cell disease, a severe, chronic hemolytic anemia. Deoxygenation results in a change that facilitates stacking of deoxygenated sickle hemoglobin molecules into monofilaments; these aggregate into elongated crystals, distorting the red cell membrane and forming the sickle cell.[2] Such a cell is viable for only fifteen to twenty-five days.

Two major consequences follow when the sickle cells are rapidly destroyed or when conditions allow the occurrence of sickling. First, the body recognizes that the sickle cells present abnormal shapes and rapidly removes them. This rapid destruction causes jaundice. The body strives to compensate by producing new red blood cells as quickly as possible; the rate of regeneration is limited, however, and patients with sickle cell disease will have only one-half to one-third as many red cells as a normal individual. Second, the elongated cells are very rigid and cannot easily pass through small blood vessels. As a result they form logjams that often deprive vital organs, tissues, and muscles of blood and oxygen. This kind of vaso-occlusive phenomenon is traditionally called a crisis and is marked by a considerable degree of pain. Such vaso-occlusion can occur in any organ of the body.

Signs and Symptoms of the Disease

Like other patients who have anemia, children with sickle cell anemia often suffer from chronic fatigue. Jaundice and swollen, painful extremities are not uncommonly present. The "hand-foot syndrome," or sickle cell dactylitis, may be the initial manifestation of sickle cell anemia in infancy but can occur at any age. This is characterized by swollen, warm, and painful extremities. Other symptoms that characteristically afflict younger children are irritability, fussiness, distention of the abdomen, repeated fever, poor appetite, vomiting, siow weight gain, and jaundice. Vaso-occlusion of the spleen is also a noticeable problem at this developmental level, with infarction resulting in severe abdominal pain; other abdominal structures may be similarly involved.

Young children with sickle cell anemia are quite susceptible to infections and, in general, are felt to be at much greater risk than are their nondiseased contemporaries. Repeated vaso-occlusion involving the head of the femur may result in aseptic necrosis, with accompanying symptoms of persistent pain and a limp. Progressive impairment of liver function occurs from infancy on due to vaso-occlusion, and gallstones have occurred in children as young as three years old. Vascular blockage may also result in a stroke or in pulmonary and renal infarctions.[2]

Patients with sickle cell disease may also experience an aplastic crisis, which can last for ten to twenty days, thus placing the afflicted person in a life-threatening position. The symptoms include lethargy, weakness, and fainting. The hyperhemolytic crisis in which the already-rapid destruction of red blood cells is further accelerated causes pallor, jaundice, faintness, and lethargy. In childhood, most children with sickle cell anemia are underweight and smaller in stature than are their peers; as they come into adolescence, puberty frequently is delayed.[2]

Literature Review

In 1974 one of these authors could write that "there are apparently no published studies" on the psychosocial effects of sickle cell anemia.[11] Federal funding then became available for treatment, education, and research into sickle cell anemia, and psychosocial studies have gradually evolved, with findings reported in the literature or at the annual conference on Sickle Cell Disease.* Early reports revealed that parents of children with sickle cell anemia often knew little about the disease or had erroneous information—for example, 50 percent felt that the child needed "special" food and 80 percent did not know why the anemia occurred. Several years later a survey revealed that parents in 50 percent of the families saw the disease as a problem only from time to time and that 25 percent of the children were concerned about their small stature and were the objects of teasing. Almost 25 percent used the disease to avoid chores, 40 percent were concerned about delayed sexual maturation, and 60 percent were behind in school. They had frequent extended absences from school because of illnesses, and they experienced limitations in physical ability due to fatigue.

Some studies have pointed to a greater tendency to withdrawal from relationships; lower self-esteem; an increase in dependency, fear of illness, depression and anxiety; and, sometimes, a preoccupation with death.[3,7] Conversely, other studies have reported that though children with sickle cell anemia may have a greater tendency to withdraw because of frequent episodes of illness, when compared to children with other chronic diseases they did not differ in their global, personal, and social adjustment.[1] Intelligence was not affected by the disease except in those instances where a stroke occurred that damaged a specific area of the brain; however, academic problems due to frequent illnesses and absences were of real concern. Clinical accounts of adolescents report greater than normal difficulty with separation and achieving independence and intensified concerns with body image and sexual identity.[4] Some investigators report depression to be more frequent.[3] Presentations about treatment have focused on family stress and pathology; individual, group, and family therapy; parent education; and special academic supports including home teaching programs, vocational training and rehabilitation, camping programs, and community education programs.[9,10,11]

*See references 1, 3, 4, 5, 6, 7, 8, 9, and 10.

Psychosocial Effects of the Disease

The child or adolescent with sickle cell anemia has to cope with and adapt to a number of manifestations of the disease: pain, fatigue, jaundice with "yellow eyes," the possibility of a cerebrovascular accident, enuresis, thin and small stature, delayed puberty with concern over sexuality, frequent school absences and "running to catch up," unpredictable periods of hospitalization, and repeated transfusions (which may in turn demand treatment for excess iron storage).

The way an individual adapts to a chronic illness involves a number of factors: the individual's existing personality structure with its strengths, ego functions, and defenses; the family's attitudes and behavior; and the community's responses and resources. At any given time, one factor may play a greater role than the others, but overall, it is the character of the interactions among the individual, family, and community that is critical. The following discussion seeks first to identify these aspects of sickle cell anemia that can be stressful, then to clarify the multiple influences and the interrelations that determine the eventual level of adjustment, and finally to recommend mechanisms designed to prevent maladjustment. A developmental or maturational approach to personality development and coping techniques is utilized.

EFFECTS ON THE CHILD

As is true of any illness, the symptoms of sickle cell anemia arouse feelings of helplessness and fear of abandonment in the affected children. This does not mean abandonment in the literal sense; rather, it is a fear that the youngsters will not be taken care of but left to experience the illness without appropriate help, intervention, or psychological support. These feelings have to be met with reassurance and positive behavior by the adults who are significant in those children's lives. When youngsters have pain, for example, they need to feel that caretakers are available at all times who will respond in a sympathetic, reassuring, and positive manner. This tends to diminish their fear of abandonment, minimizes the development of a sense of isolation, and helps them better to tolerate the pain. The need for psychological support is heightened if the pain is severe enough to require hospitalization. Hospitalization physically separates children from those who love and care for them and thus tends to accentuate the fear of abandonment.

Part of the feeling of helplessness generated in children with sickle cell anemia is related to another aspect of hospitalization, the exposure to painful procedures inherent in medical care. Since hospitalization and the attendant medical procedures are frightening, efforts should be made to minimize the untoward effects by preparing children (and parents) for this experience. If little is done to interpret the world of the hospital to children, particularly to explain when painful procedures are going to occur, hospitalized children can live in constant fear of the unknown. Moreover, resentment of the unpleasant aspects of hospitalization can augment resentment over having the disease.

The provision of support is not the only way to relate to youngsters' fear of helplessness and abandonment. If children can communicate their feelings, they are less likely to develop a sense of isolation. Children with sickle cell anemia should be permitted and encouraged to talk about their fear of pain, fatigue, or helplessness. No areas of the disease or their feelings should be off limits. Any aspects of the condition that are forbidden for discussion will tend to increase the feelings of loneliness and abandonment. Children will quickly sense the adult's reluctance or disinterest in respect to discussing certain areas and may then comply with the adult's desires so that they can continue to remain close even though their needs are not being met.

Parents need to be counseled on how to encourage their child to talk about fears and feelings about being sick. Many parents believe children will be upset if they speak about their illness when, in reality, it is the parents who are disturbed and wish to avoid talking about it. Parents can be told that children always have feelings and thoughts about their illness and that while some of their thoughts and observations are accurate, others are likely to be misconceptions. If parents are advised that their child wishes and needs to communicate thoughts and feelings but that he or she needs their permission and support to do so, most parents will be able to speak with their child.

Parents should be told that among other things, children may cry, express anger, say that they are unloved, express jealousy toward siblings who are not ill, and talk about fears and misconceptions about their illness. Parents should respond by being supportive but not overprotective. If the children are anxious, they should be assured that the parents will care for them. If they are depressed, parents should let them know that the feeling is not unreasonable. If they are angry that fate, often represented by the parents, has dealt them an unfair blow, parents can agree that it is unpleasant, but they should not accept blame for the illness. As the parents hear the children out, they should give verbal approval for what they have been able to say and encourage children about the future.

In these discussions, illness and its manifestations, such as pain, need to be explained in terms of the children's frame of reference. If they are not given clear, honest, simple explanations, they are forced to create answers for themselves. These will often be erroneous. Children will create a cause-and-effect relationship because this is the natural mode of thought in childhood. They may firmly believe that their illness or pain are forms of punishment for "bad" thoughts or past behavior. They may hope or imagine that if they are "good," they will be subjected to fewer symptoms or acute exacerbations of their illness. They may also believe that if they are good and compliant, they will not lose those on whom they depend.

The younger children's concerns are related to pain, helplessness, and abandonment rather than death because they imagine death not as a permanent condition but as one in which they are alone, unprotected, without parents to care for them. Parents can be guided in how to talk to children in a reassuring manner about these issues. School-age children become aware that death is irreversible and perhaps that another child has died of sickle cell anemia. The psychiatrist should provide anticipatory guidance so that parents will acknowledge the children's questions about death but say that death from the illness is not usual or frequent, that the doctors are find new ways of treatment, and that many people live a long life. Hope should never be taken away from the children, and in reality medical advances are being made. Of course adolescents are more aware than children that death is a possibility, but they also are aware that adults who have sickle cell disease live productive lives and that some have lived to be over sixty year old. If the adolescents have had good emotional support as children, they are not preoccupied with the possibility of death. They are concerned with the pain they have during a sickle cell crisis, the possibility of a stroke, and the physical limitations imposed by the disease.

Although no specific time should be set aside to discuss the illness, if parents encourage children to talk there are times when conversation will take such a turn naturally or spontaneously. For example, after a sudden episode of illness has subsided, a child can more easily share feelings and thoughts with those who have been providing supportive care.

If parents say their child has never spoken about the illness, they should be told that he or she may need their permission to do so.

A well-adjusted adult is capable of functioning independently. Sickle cell anemia, like all chronic childhood illnesses, creates longer and more intense psychological dependency on adults and thus makes it more difficult for the child to learn to function independently. Therefore, throughout childhood, it is essential that all areas of functioning that promote autonomy and independence be emphasized and encouraged. Parents of children with sickle cell anemia should be informed that, when the children have severe pain, they will be completely dependent on them psychologically and will need total care. However, when the acute phase has passed, children should be encouraged and expected to do as much as they are capable of doing. For example, depending on the children's age, they should be required to dress themselves, help to straighten up their room, be responsible for specific chores, and be disciplined appropriately and consistently. If children are making a successful adaptation to their illness, they wish to be up and about as much as possible, to engage in activities, to play with friends, and to continue in school. One indication of a poor adjustment is the desire to continue in a dependent role after the pain crisis.

Another essential characteristic of a well-adjusted adult is a sense of self-esteem. This is developed in childhood in part through the concrete mastery of situations. Certain features of sickle cell anemia pose barriers to the development of a sense of mastery over the disease. In a number of chronic illnesses such as diabetes, some of the manifestations can be controlled by acts of the person with the disease. In contrast, victims of sickle cell anemia are powerless to influence the fatigue or the time of onset, frequency, duration, or intensity of pain. Although they cannot control the symptoms, involved children may develop a sense of mastery by becoming less fearful of the illness and by learning to do well in studies, hobbies, or games. We have indicated how parents can help children be less fearful. Parents must also help children with sickle cell anemia to find areas where they can excel.

There is another aspect of chronic illness that can undermine children's ego development; this involves the interruption of critical normal activities. When pain crises occur, children may be unable to attend school. If this occurs frequently enough and home tutoring is not available, children's academic performance can fall below that of classmates and thereby further threaten their sense of self-worth. Absences can be frequent enough to lead to actual failure. To foster children's sense of competence, mastery, and self-esteem, they should continue to study at home. This means that periodic home tutoring is essential. The school should be informed that the children may be absent frequently; a continuance plan should be available, one that can be implemented whenever they have to be out of school for any length of time. If they are absent for a short period of time, parents or others might help with studies, but homebound teaching is critical when children with sickle cell anemia must be out of school for long periods. This is a form of primary prevention. It minimizes the possibility of children becoming so frustrated and discouraged about falling behind peers that they actually drop out of school.

Realistic limitations are imposed by the tendency of these children to tire easily. These limitations can also undermine the development of self-esteem and should be approached via primary prevention. Since the youngsters may not want or be able to engage fully in all of the activities of their playmates, a wide range of activities should be made available that they might perform at a slower pace or while sitting down. For instance, they can be encouraged to develop sedentary hobbies such as crafts, building models, working with wood or metal, photography, sewing or tailoring, and cooking. Tabletop competitive games also should be encouraged. In school, if children do not wish to or cannot engage in gym activities, they should have an opportunity to work with audiovisual materials, help in the library, or serve as an aide in the office. Some older children may enhance their self-esteem by helping younger children who are having difficulty with their studies.

This is not to suggest that these children should not engage in more strenuous physical activities, such as playing ball or riding bicycles. However, it is likely that they will not do as well as their peers in these activities. Many children want to go to gym both because they enjoy it and because they do not want to be treated as though they are different. They can and should be permitted to engage in sports until they tire. In most instances, the children are the best judges of their tolerance; children soon learn their physical limitations and abide by them.

No child likes to be smaller than his or her friends, but many a child must face the fact that growth retardation does occur in sickle cell anemia. The children are not expected to like this feature (or any other aspect of the disease), but if they feel that they are capable in some realm, it will be easier for them to cope. Some of the techniques that can be utilized to develop their sense of competency have already been described. If the emphasis has been on identifying and developing abilities rather than dwelling on the disadvantages of the disabilities, the smaller size becomes less important.

Other children may tease the child who is smaller and fatigues easily, and adults may treat such children as though they are much younger than they are. These practices can be devastating to children's egos. Children should be taught how to use "one-upsmanship" in response to the teasing, and parents must strive not to permit other adults to relate to the children inappropriately. The children should not be allowed to degrade themselves.

PARENTAL RESPONSES

As we have indicated, the parents' responses to children's illness are a major determinant of their adjustment. The parents will have many concerns. They will worry about the future outlook of the children with respect to their ability to achieve social and economic success; they will experience resentment at having children whose care may be demanding and will frequently inconvenience them; there will be disappointment and guilt over being responsible for the children's illness; and there will be recurrent episodes of anxiety about the potential for early death. There may also be anger over economic problems related to frequent hospitalizations as well as feelings of embarrassment, shame, and displeasure because of the children's size. The parents may react by being unduly restrictive and overprotective (not permitting children to be as active and independent as they are capable of being), by pressing for accomplishments beyond the children's abilities, by being unduly permissive, by neglecting the children, or by rejecting them outright.

Most parents require counseling in order to manage so ill a child in an appropriate manner. If their feelings are raised early and discussed in an open, supportive manner, these emotions will exert much less force. In addition to working with their reactions in the counseling sessions, parents should learn the facts of the disease and what to expect on a day-to-day basis. Above all, however, they must be encouraged to express their feelings and communicate their problems. To accomplish this, they need to be made aware that none of these reactions is unusual or forbidden. In time they will then gain confidence that the clinician is there to support them; and this in turn will help them develop coping techniques for specific problems and learn the importance of developing their child's self-esteem.

In addition to the frequent occurrence of pain, the ubiquitous fatigue, and the recurrent need for hospitalizations, parents should be prepared to face a number of additional aspects of the disease. Parents should be alerted in advance that their children may wet the bed frequently, have a poor appetite, exhibit growth retardation, and experience a delay in adolescent development. In this connection, it is important to consider the nature of anticipatory guidance. This should not be thought of as a single session in which questions are asked and all explanations are given or even understood. Instead it must be regarded as a process that extends over time. Through the years, parents may need to have these areas reexplained many times and clarified over and over in ever greater detail. The first time such material is presented, they may not fully understand what is explained, or they may wish to minimize or deny the reality of what they hear. If those events most likely to occur are explained clearly to the parents, they will be less anxious, they can spell out what is happening to the child, and they will be able to plan rather than merely living from crisis to crisis. This increases the parents' feeling of competence, which in turn is transmitted to the child.

ADOLESCENT RESPONSE

Normal adolescent development is characterized by sexual maturation, psychological separation from the parents, and the need to be increasingly independent. This takes place over a span of years. If the children and the family have not related to the illness appropriately by the time the children reach adolescence, they may be afraid to take the steps necessary to become an autonomous individual and may continue to remain in a passive, dependent relationship to their parents. The children's view of life and of their own potential may be constricted, and gradual withdrawal from normal relationships may occur. Their motivation and aspirations to succeed in any area are likely to be limited and their self-esteem inadequate. Emotionally, they would tend to feel depressed, helpless, fearful, and they may be preoccupied with death. Such youngsters are prone to become hypochondriacal and experience more pain and fatigue than can be accounted for by their physical condition. Slight changes in their physical state may evoke a great deal of anxiety. They may lack the dreams and aspirations universal to adolescence. A girl with sickle cell anemia once said: "If you had a stroke, it's like living with a gun at your head because you never know when you will have another one."

Adolescents with sickle cell anemia who have had a stable supportive background may experience adolescence in much the same way as an adolescent without an illness. But it is not unusual for teenagers with a chronic illness, even if they are well adjusted, to find the years from age thirteen to sixteen to be somewhat stressful. During this period of time, they may want to feel that they have no limits or "imperfections." This is typical of all adolescents. However, youths with sickle cell disease may thrust themselves into stressful situations in order to prove that they are like the others. The net result is that for a time they may exacerbate the illness.

During this teenage period, a strong supportive relationship with an adult is often helpful. The relationship may be used only intermittently, and, in fact, these may be more telephone contacts than face-to-face discussions. Nonetheless, the knowledge that the adolescents have someone to turn to is often sufficient.

It is troublesome for many youths to confront the fact that they cannot compete in physical activities. They will probably be disappointed and resent physical limitations; nonetheless, adolescents who are coping with sickle cell anemia in a satisfactory fashion often find pleasure in those things that they can do.

As mentioned, adolescents with this disease may encounter a delay in the onset of puberty. Boys and girls may tease those who are slow to develop and thereby make them feel inferior, resentful, and rejected. All adolescents need to feel accepted by their peers, and if acceptance is not forthcoming, they may withdraw from social relationships. However, for the well-adjusted child, delayed sexual development in adolescence, though it may be a source of unhappiness, does not in itself lead to social isolation.

All teenagers need to ponder career goals, be they vocational or professional. This is especially true for teenagers with chronic illness. Adolescents with sickle cell anemia need not make specific commitments concerning future occupations, but they need to be aware of the wide range of realistic possibilities. They usually have only a vague conception of what specific occupations demand. Such youths will have great hopes and aspirations for the future, and their fantasies may very well be similar to those of adolescents without illness. The realities gradually become apparent to these young people through the ease with which they may become tired. This may serve to direct their interest to occupations that do not require great physical endurance. But the majority will need vocational counseling and guidance, both in terms of their need to select a sedentary type of occupation and in respect to the opportunities that are available.

There has been a rapid expansion of sickle cell centers and programs. These centers offer families a multidisciplinary approach that includes medical treatment; family, individual, and group therapy and counseling; vocational counseling and rehabilitation; and educational sessions and literature. Taken in aggregate, these modalities present the facts of sickle cell anemia accurately and dispel those myths and misinformation that still exist (though they are less prevalent than in the past). As is true with other chronic diseases, when these centers and programs have offered expertise and excellence, they have proven repeatedly to be the best way to treat families and children who have sickle cell anemia.

ACKNOWLEDGMENT

Supported by National Institutes of Health Sickle Cell Center Grant HL16008.

REFERENCES

1. ALLEN, J., et al. "Anxiety, Self-concept, and Personal and Social Adjustments in Children with Sickle Cell Anemia," *Journal of Pediatrics,* 88 (1976):859–863.

2. BEHRMAN, R. E., and VAUGHAM, V. C., III. *Nelson Textbook of Pediatrics,* 12th ed. Philadelphia: W.B. Saunders, 1983.

3. CONYARD, S., DOSIK, H., and KRISHNAMURTHY, M. "Psychosocial Aspects of Sickle Cell Anemia in Adolescents," *Health and Social Work,* 5 (1980):20–26.

4. GOLDBERG, R. T. "Toward an Understanding of the Rehabilitation of the Disabled Adolescent," *Rehabilitation Literature,* 42 (1981):3–4.

5. MCELROY, S. R. *The Handbook of Psychology of Hemoglobin-S: A Perspicacious View of Sickle Cell Anemia.* Baltimore: University Press of America, 1980.

6. MOORE, A., WAUGH, D., and WHITTEN, C. F. "Unmet Needs of Parents of Children with Sickle Cell Anemia," *Proceedings of the First National Symposium on Sickle Cell Disease.* Washington, D.C.: Howard University, 1974, pp. 275–76.

7. NISHIURA, E., and WHITTEN, C. F. "Psychosocial Problems in Families of Children with Sickle Cell Anemia," *Urban Health,* 9 (1980):32–35.

8. ———. "Psychosocial Effects of Sickle Cell Anemia: Employment and Sickle Cell Conditions," Paper presented at the annual Conference on Sickle Cell Disease, St. Louis, 15 June 1981.

9. TETRAULT, S. M. "The Student with Sickle Cell Anemia," *Today's Education, The Journal of the National Education Association,* 70 (1981):52–57.

10. VAVASSUR, J. "A Comprehensive Program for Meeting Psychosocial Needs of Sickle Cell Anemia Patients," *Journal of the National Medical Association,* 69 (1977):335–339.

11. WHITTEN, C. F., and FISCHHOFF, J. "Psychosocial Effects of Sickle Cell Disease," *Archives of Internal Medicine,* 133 (1974):681–689.

12 / Developmental Impacts of Incest

Jean Goodwin

It is currently estimated that the incidence of incest is one thousand times higher than was believed to be the case a generation ago. Developmental thinking about incest is being revised accordingly. Moreover, the incest experience is no longer viewed as a unitary factor with invariable impact; instead it is regarded as a multipotential sequence that must be assessed within the context of family factors, other environmental influences, and the child's constitution and development. Some incest experiences satisfy the criteria for trauma; in keeping with this, some symptomatic children and adolescents can be understood as experiencing a developmentally mediated posttraumatic syndrome secondary to incest. At each developmental stage from infancy to adulthood symptoms of anxiety, reenactment, depression and sleep disturbance, ego constriction, and disturbed discharge of aggression are likely to be expressed differently. The severity of associated environmental and family problems as well as of the trauma and the posttraumatic symptoms will in large measure determine the extent of the developmental impact on the victims. In addition, the child's temperament is always a factor. In the worst cases, these effects can continue into the next generation.

The High Frequency of Incest

In the course of the past twenty years, psychiatry's approach to incest has changed radically. This is largely because our concepts about the frequency of incest has undergone considerable change. At one point Freud postulated that adult reconstructions of childhood incest experiences might be based on developmentally appropriate fantasy rather than on memories of actual events. At the time, he believed that the incidence of actual incest was less than one per million population.[15,18] This figure continued to be quoted over the next fifty years[56] and is cited as recently as 1975 in a standard textbook of psychiatry.[24] This estimated incidence was based on the numbers of incest

cases successfully prosecuted in western nations. However, we now understand that over 90 percent of childhood sexual abuse is never even reported outside of the family[51] and that less than 2 percent of incest cases are reported to the police.[45] Also, legal definitions of incest, which may require genetic relatedness or "criminal sexual penetration," overlap only partially with the psychosocial definition of incest as the sexual exploitation of a child by an adult in a parental role.[18]

When Kinsey and colleagues reported that 4 percent of women had been sexually involved with a family member,[29] the door was opened to the possibility that the actuality of childhood sexuality was more varied, complex, and active than even Freud had dared believe. As Ferenczi[13] noted, "Even children of very respectable, sincerely puritanical families, fall victim to real violence or rape much more often than one had dared to suppose" (p. 227). Surveys by Landis[31] and Finkelhor[14] confirmed that 20 to 30 percent of college women had experienced childhood sexual encounters with adult males. In Finkelhor's total population of 530 women, 9 percent had been sexually abused by some close relative; 1.5 percent reported incest experiences with a father or stepfather. Finkelhor's figures are similar to those found in an Albuquerque, New Mexico, survey of 500 women in church and volunteer groups. One percent of these women reported typical long-term incest experiences with a father or stepfather.[18] Using a random sample of adult women rather than volunteer respondents, Diana Russell[45] found an even higher percentage of father-daughter incest, with 42 (or 4.5 percent) of her 930 subjects reporting such a history. Sixteen percent of the women in her sample reported sexual abuse by a relative.

Incest, or intrafamilial child sexual abuse, usually involves a male perpetrator at least five years older than the female child participant. Seventy to 96 percent of reported perpetrators are male and 75 to 90 percent of reported victims are female. Mother-son incest is rare, with male victims more often involved with fathers, uncles, grandfathers, or other male relatives. Brother-sister incest is common but seems most damaging when it occurs in connection with parent-child sexual abuse.[18]

When incest was believed to be rare, occurring with an incidence of one per million per year, Freud's special explanation was required to account for its frequent mention by psychiatric patients.[18,43] However, the actual incidence appears to be closer to the 1,000 incest cases per million population per year now being prosecuted in Santa Clara County, California, where treatment is a mandated part of the law enforcement process.[17] In the face of such figures, no special explanations are needed to tell us why between 5 and 30 percent of female psychiatric patients report a sexual experience with a family member.[7,32,42] The one-per-thousand-per-year incidence figure multiplied by fifteen childhood years of risk for incest would predict a 1 to 2 percent frequency rate among adult women in the general population; such a calculation does not leave room for too many of the adult reports in the survey studies to be the results of fantasy or confabulation.

Once the belief in the rarity of childhood sexual abuse is abandoned, it becomes apparent how much energy was expended in maintaining this belief. One is reminded of Charcot's comment that theory is good, but it doesn't keep things from existing.[15] One of every 1,000 emergency room visits is a request for examination of a sexually abused child,[11] and one-third of reported rapes occur in prepubertal children.[44] Yet for many years psychiatrists avoided or explained away such cases. The myth of the infrequency of childhood sexual abuse has functioned at once to maintain the image of children as asexual, to maintain overly severe legal penalties for offenders,[18] and to encourage lax enforcement or nonenforcement of these overly severe laws against childhood sexual abuse.[25,39,44] It has fostered professional avoidance of children and families with a sexual abuse complaint[41] and has inclined professionals to join parents in insisting that children maintain silence and secrecy about both their sexual experiences and the associated feelings.[34] Assuming that 1 to 4 percent of women have had prolonged, secret sexual contact with a father figure leads one to approach the question of developmental impact in a new way. No longer do we anticipate some type of automatic and profound harm, as was the assumption of early investigators like Bender.[4,5] It is remarkable how relieved those early workers were to find that the worst they had to deal with among the sexually abused children they evaluated were merely sexual preoccupation, impaired social relations, withdrawal, pessimism, and regression.[60] Yet, in a condition that occurs now more frequently than does tonsillectomy,[44] it is this wide spectrum of responses that assumes therapeutic and research importance. If sexual abuse of children is

as common as it now seems, there must exist patterns of effective coping as well as pathology.

Important Variables Affecting the Impact of Incest on the Child

Many investigators have reported that there are a number of variables which affect the child's response. These include the child's constitutional endowment and previous developmental history; the amount and type of support available to the child at the time of incest; the developmental stage of the child; the degree of parental relatedness of the partner; the duration, frequency, and type of sexual contact; and the degree of violence, force, or coercion used to enforce the contact.[21,50] Nearness in age of the participants and shared affection and pleasure in the relationship are thought to mitigate harmful effects.[36] The complexity of these interacting variables is great; in an Albuquerque study of five hundred adult women, for example, no significant relationship was found between the degree of intrusiveness of the sexual contact and the degree of upset in the adult; the confounding effects of other factors likely obscured the impact of this variable.[18] Finkelhor also found that contacts involving penetration were not invariably more traumatizing than other types of sexual abuse. Age of perpetrator and degree of coercion were the only variables in his study that correlated significantly with the victim's experience of distress.[14]

Although statistical data are inconclusive, therapists have little difficulty in recognizing the extreme "worst-case" examples in which all negative factors combine. Adult multiple personalities, for example, frequently describe this worst-case situation: Initiation into intercourse before age three by a psychotic parent who used objects to penetrate the anus and vagina, causing physical damage with penetration; the use of torture and physical locking up of the child in order to enforce silence; the sexual interaction continuing for years with new intrafamilial and extrafamilial sexual partners being added; and the family having multiple problems and few resources for nurturance.[47]

The question of whether developmental age at the time of sexual abuse influences the quantitative impact, as well as the qualitative nature of the child's response, continues to be fraught with controversy. Talmudic and English Common law established age twelve, or puberty, as the age of sexual consent in females. One might imagine that sexual experiences before this age would be more damaging. However, since the 1930s, some investigators have reported young children to be less disturbed than adolescents by sexual molesta-tion.[1,4,5] Age at onset has been difficult to disentangle from duration because of the general unavailability to the young child of resources that can halt the abuse.

The family environment is critical in mediating the child's response. Typical patterns in cases of incest have been well described.* Families in which incest occurs often have intense shared fears of family disinte-gration. These are dysfunctional families that tend to isolate themselves from the rest of society. In more than 40 percent of cases sexual relations between mother and father are impaired at the time that incest is disclosed. The mother has a distant or troubled rela-tionship with her daughter; she may be clinically de-pressed and has often ceded many of her functions to this child. Superficially, both parents may seem well adjusted; however, careful life histories will reveal early abandonments of these adults by their own par-ents and the presence of extreme, lifelong inhibitions and confusions about sexuality. On psychological test-ing both parents may show signs of paranoia, denial, and rationalization.

Encapsulated paranoia,[19] sociopathy,[2,57] and sub-stance use[35] have each been proposed as explanations for the parent's ability to justify the sexual intrusion on the child. Paranoid and/or sociopathic fathers proba-bly account for many of the worst-case examples of incestuous families—for example, those associated with extreme child abuse and other family violence and with eventual suicide, homicide, or complex suicide.

Early family experiences of deprivation or deviation in sexual development may produce vulnerabilities to unusual sexual experiences in children.[42] In incest vic-tims the normal sexual explorations of the child may be intruded upon, interfered with, or inhibited by fam-ily members.[46] Thus one finds cases in which the child was cross-dressed by a parent,[49] genitally examined by a parent for signs of masturbation,[58] exposed to unusual voyeuristic experiences,[18] or prohibited from interacting with opposite-sex peers.[54] In these cases we may be dealing as much with the absence of usual sexual experiences as with the presence of unusual ones. When the child's normal sexual expression is interfered with, informational and ego lacunae may develop. What kinds of touching are wrong? Do I have a right to stop someone from touching if that makes me feel bad? Or to ask someone about it? Can I get away or say no?

Children who have not had the chance to have these questions answered may be uniquely vulnerable to adults who request genital contact.[41] They may later attempt to find answers in action either by sexual vic-timization or sexual perpetration. Some studies report

*See references 7, 10, 18, 27, and 54.

that 30 percent of women who have been raped three or more times and 74 percent of men incarcerated for sexual perversions have been victims of incest.[18] A paralyzing deficit of normal responses to sexual stimuli characterizes recurrent victims. One adult incest survi-vor reported that she froze when a stranger in a bar put his hand down her blouse and touched her breast. Even much later, in therapy, she could imagine no response she might have made to this interpersonal advance.

Roland Summit[51] attributes many of the sequelae of sexual abuse to the silence about the event forced on the child by the surrounding adults. He describes the "sex-ual abuse accommodation syndrome" as a five-stage process that involves (1) secrecy about the event often enforced by threats from the adult participant; (2) help-lessness to understand or describe, much less to protest, the worrisome touching; (3) entrapment within the sex-ual relationship if it is ongoing, with a number of psy-chological sequelae including: increased dependence on the partner, the development of a sense of altruistic responsibility for keeping the secret, and the structuring of internal mechanisms for self-comforting and self-expression, such as imaginary companions, dissocia-tion, and self-castigation; (4) delayed, unconvincing disclosure that can be easily misinterpreted as a rebel-lious, manipulative attack on the partner; and (5) re-traction of the complaint under family or other adult pressure. It is likely that these very common false re-tractions of sexual complaints have contributed to the myth of the infrequency of childhood sexual abuse.[18] Swift, firm adult support at any step in the accommoda-tion syndrome can help the child escape the assumption of badness, the sense of being out of control, and the sense of loss of touch with reality that can be the legacy of accommodation without support.[6]

In the area of constitutional factors that may affect the impact of childhood sexual experiences, two items seem worthy of further research. First, one must be concerned about the possibility of affective disorder in children who have been sexually abused within the family. As many as 50 percent of the mothers in such families have been reported to be clinically de-pressed[18]; as many as half of the fathers may be al-coholic,[35] a condition that accompanies depression in certain families; in over 5 percent of these families, after the incest secret is revealed, one or more suicide attempts are known to occur.[18] Careful history-taking about the incident may reveal that at the time he ap-proached the child, the adult partner was in a hyper-sexual, manic state.[41] Depression in victims has been described as a sequel to childhood sexual abuse.[13,27,32,37]

Another constitutional area worthy of exploration concerns the relationship between seizure disorders and incest. Several thousand years ago, Galen hypothesized that epilepsy resulted from premature sexual intercourse.[18] A connection between epilepsy and incest continued to be made in medieval Europe, where epileptics were sent on pilgrimage to the shrine of Saint Dymphna, whose legend recounted her attempt to flee from her incestuous father. Navajo folklore echoes this association, asserting that anyone who has seizures must have participated in incest and be a witch. Some investigators, like Freud, have attributed the association between seizures and childhood sexual abuse to the development of pseudoseizures as symptomatic dissociated repetitions of the sexual experience. Other investigators have pointed out that a child with organically based seizures, especially if retarded, may be less protected by the incest taboo than is a normal child.[38] A recent study by Davies[9] reports abnormal electroencephalographic (EEG) findings in seventeen of twenty-two (77 percent) of adult psychiatric inpatients with prior incest (whereas only 20 to 30 percent of psychiatric inpatients in general have such abnormalities). Similarly high percentages of EEG abnormalities have been reported in adults with sexual deviation. Was the EEG abnormality associated in childhood with some idiosyncrasy of sexual expression or of psychosexual development that placed the child at risk for sexual abuse? Whatever the cause, seizure disorder remains high on the list of problems revealed in the course of pediatric screening of sexually abused children.[7,53]

Incest as Trauma

There are those who contend that childhood sexual contact with adults is natural, educational, and beneficial.[23,59] Others feel that childhood sexual abuse is a neutral accidental event that does not weigh heavily in the developmental balance.[29]

What factors suggest that intrafamilial sexual abuse may function as a traumatic incident? First, many studies indicate that sexually abused children are symptomatic. Adams-Tucker[1] found that all of twenty-eight sexually abused children referred for psychiatric care were symptomatic, complaining variously of sleep disturbances, psychosomatic problems, anxiety, withdrawal, behavior problems, depression, school difficulties, and other problems. In a German study of seventy forensically identified incest victims,[33] 31 percent suffered school failure, 25 percent were having behavior problems (of which lying, promiscuity, running away, and truancy were most prominent), 28 percent were depressed, 20 percent had psychosomatic symptoms, and 16 percent were having severe sleep disturbances. Only about one-third of the seventy children were not given a psychiatric diagnosis. Other studies have found

that at the time they report the sexual abuse, depressive symptoms, school problems, or behavior problems are present in almost all victimized children.

In one study of twenty-six forensically identified incest victims followed into adulthood,[32] about 40 percent either became promiscuous or engaged in some other form of acting out. Twenty percent complained of orgasmic dysfunction, 20 percent complained of depression, and 20 percent had a good adjustment. Meiselman[35] found that about three-quarters of those adult psychiatric patients who have histories of incest had suffered some kind of orgasmic dysfunction; this included some who, along with their dysorgasmia, were promiscuous. Pelvic pain syndromes have also been reported in incest victims.[22]

These studies have been criticized on the grounds that sexually abused children who go through a trial process or who are referred to a psychiatrist have been traumatized by more than sexual contact.[36] It is important to recognize, however, that studies that show no effects of sexual abuse also have methodological difficulties, including the use of testing instruments that do not tap posttraumatic symptoms, the mixing of cases of one-time sexual abuse by a nonfamily member with incest cases, and the mixing of consenting nonviolent sexual contacts with peer siblings or cousins with classical coercive incest.

Retrospective studies have also been used to support the hypothesis that incest is traumatic.[18] If one examines runaway girls in a juvenile detention home, on the average about 50 percent are victims of incest. In a study cohort of women with three or more illegitimate pregnancies, 25 percent will have histories of prior incest. In severe drug abusers, over 40 percent of the women have been found to be incest victims. However, these retrospective studies of adolescents and adults are open to even more methodological criticisms than are the controlled studies of symptoms found acutely in sexually abused children.

Is sexual abuse the kind of experience that traumatizes children? Some psychiatrists believe that multiple personality results from early trauma before age four.[30] They have tried to catalogue the kinds of experiences that caused their patients to switch in early childhood to a new personality for the first time. These factors include fear of one's own death; exposure to, or fear of, the death of someone else, especially a parent figure; extreme isolation; illness, pain, fatigue, or other physical factors clouding consciousness; and "brainwashing" or other systematic lies, especially when these have led to moral dilemmas. The kinds of events that cause dissociation in children are not too dissimilar from those associated with posttraumatic stress disorder in soldiers.[55] Symptomatic Viet Nam veterans differ from their asymptomatic fellows in being more likely to have experienced life-threatening intense combat; the death of a close friend or "buddy"; a family environment that does not allow conversation about the war experience; wounds, illnesses, or injuries; and the witnessing or participation in some episode of abusive violence or "atrocity" about which there was a question of right and wrong.

Does sexual abuse provide this kind of experience for a child? One answer to this question is that over 70 percent of the patients with multiple personalities were incestuously abused in childhood.[40] Also, posttraumatic symptoms including dissociation have been well described in adult rape victims.[8] If one sought to assess the potential impact on a child of a particular sexual abuse event, one way would be to assess the degree to which these traumatic factors were present in the sexual incident. Did the child fear for her life? I recall a seven-year-old who did not become symptomatic until more than a year after being sexually abused. At that point she witnessed a fatal accident and became intensely phobic. When confronted with the imminence of death, she began to relieve her memories of the implicit threat in the sexual abuse incident.

Did the child fear for the life of someone close to her? In incest situations, child victims are often terribly concerned about the safety of other family members. One incest victim thought her father was urinating on her when he ejaculated and worried that he had lost control of his bladder. If mother has a reputation for ill health, the perpetrator may be believed absolutely when he tells a child, "Don't tell your mother or she'll die." Child victims are often very much aware of the other children involved in the sexual abuse and may feel quite guilty that something they did led to the sexual involvement of another child.

How isolated is the child victim? One should be most concerned about the child who has few or no other sources of comfort available.

Was the child more vulnerable because of her physical state? Was the child asleep when sexually approached? Did she bleed? Were there longstanding physical sequelae, such as vaginal discharge or dysuria? Kestenberg[28] has hypothesized that for young children the female orgasm itself, with its widespread effects on invisible body parts, may be physically disorganizing.

How many lies has the child been told about the moral implications of the sexual event? It may take years for a child victim to realize that the adult's "explanations" for the sexual abuse were only self-serving rationalizations.[18]

What symptoms would we anticipate in children who have been exposed to a traumatic event? By analogy with the war neuroses, one would expect most reactions to be transient, with only a small percentage of those exposed developing chronic, incapacitating syndromes. We understand little at present about the

mechanisms that allow the majority of combat veterans and abused children to master their traumatic experiences without recourse to formal psychotherapeutic support. Also, by analogy, one might expect that some abused children, albeit initially asymptomatic, might experience a delayed onset of symptoms later under stress, as, for example, the stress of adolescence, pregnancy, parenthood, or success.[16] Kardiner[26] described five kinds of posttraumatic symptoms seen in World War I veterans: fear and startle; reenactment of trauma; sleep disturbances and signs of guilt and depression; constriction of ego functions; and explosive, aggressive behavior. These five symptom areas cover the symptoms outlined in the third revision of the *Diagnostic and Statistical Manual of Mental Disorders* as defining posttraumatic disorder.

The posttraumatic syndrome has been described in children as well as adults. Lenore Terr,[52] a child psychiatrist, interviewed twenty-three of the twenty-six grade school children involved in the 1976 Chowchilla, California, school bus kidnapping. These children had been held by their kidnappers for twenty-seven hours. They spent sixteen hours buried in a truck trailer before two of the older boys dug them out and all the children escaped. Five to thirteen months after the incident, on interview, the children showed symptoms in all five categories described by Kardiner:

1. Fears related to being kidnapped (traumatophobia) (23/23), new phobias (21/23), and anxiety (8/23).
2. Reenactment of the kidnapping attack, with children experiencing daily events as if they were fragments of the trauma or of its "day residues" (14/23), and reexperiencing physiological aspects of the trauma (9/23); reenactment also was seen in "traumatic play" about the event (11/23) and compulsive retelling (5/23) of the story.
3. Terror dreams or playback dreams about the kidnapping (23/23), and depression reflected in personality changes in some children with regression to immobile, dreamy, or clinging behaviors (9/23).
4. Ego deficits manifested by disturbances of cognition that included inaccurate time sequencing (8/23) and hallucinations and misidentifications (8/23); some children showed a decline in school performance (8/23).
5. Aggressive personality change (6/23); revenge fantasies (6/23).

Posttraumatic Symptoms in Incest Victims at Various Developmental Stages

Incest victims also experience a syndrome that includes fears and anxiety, reenactment of the abuse, nightmares and depressive symptoms, ego constriction, and disturbed discharge of aggression. This syndrome can be difficult to recognize because prior deprivation or scapegoating may leave overlapping symptom traces as the child matures and because one sees a developmental transformation of the posttraumatic symptoms.

The preschool incest victim often presents with an expression of "frozen watchfulness" and immobility. The child's fears are often of men, of certain rooms or activities, or of being alone. Fragments of the sexual experience may reappear momentarily in inappropriate undressing or in the form of an inappropriately sexual caress. The event may also be reenacted in driven, stereotyped play in which the sexual partner is repetitively killed or punished. The child may whimper and appear sad. Lost ego functions include exploration, the ability to sleep alone, toilet training, and speech. The child clings to her mother and seeks control through negativism and passive refusal. The child may be diffusely irritable or erupt into tantrums.

The older child, ages four to six, will be more afraid of being punished than the young toddler; she will fear abandonment in a different way, anticipating it as a potential consequence of impending family breakup for which she assumes the blame. The oedipal-stage child is now able to involve others in recreating the sexual abuse. She will be particularly adept at reenacting her experience of the abuse as punishment and may construct for herself a "Cinderella" home situation where external neglect or physical punishment assuages her internal guilt. [18] "Badness" is now a worry, not merely death. Traumatic play now involves punishing both child and partner and repetitive washing and cleaning. To quote Fairbairn [12]: "There has arisen in the child a sense that his own love is rejected because it is bad" (p. 37). The older child may be even less verbal than the toddler about the sexual abuse because of guilt and fear of family dissolution if she discloses. As with younger toddlers, some of these older victims will be carried into the playroom clinging to a parent. Overdocility and lack of initiative make play sessions with children of this age harder work than usual.

The incest victim ages seven to thirteen will have well-differentiated fears of retaliation by the sexually intrusive parent figure if she resists or discloses. She particularly fears threats of retaliation against her mother or siblings. Sexual experiences may be reenacted with peers, younger siblings, or friends in order to attain mastery and control. Reminders of the event may trigger pain or other somatic memories rather than evoking verbally retrievable memory. Plans to escape the situation or to bring the incestuous partner to justice may provide fantasied or acted-out retaliation against the partner. This often backfires into repetitions of the trauma for the child, and in the legal system she may reexperience feeling helpless, not lis-

tened to, and physically and psychologically raped. Latency-age children will often experience nightmares or suicidal thoughts, but they may not complain of these or define them as problems; instead they will continue to cope in the same brave, altruistic, matter-of-fact way that they dealt with the sexual abuse. Ego constriction will be most evident at school where biology, history, and physical education may require skills that the child must repress. Pseudoretardation and conversion symptoms like psychogenic blindness and elective mutism may appear in the service of keeping the child's secret. [18] Inappropriate aggression may also appear at school or may be directed against younger siblings with whom the child is cast in a premature parental role.

In adolescence, the victim's chronic anxiety, her fears of her own expanding emotional understanding and of intimacy, and her inability to relax may lead to acting out or substance abuse. Reenactments include self-mutilation, psychogenic seizures, promiscuity, and illegitimate pregnancy. [18] Flashbacks during sexual activity become a problem at this stage. Compared to adolescent rape victims, incest victims tend to experience more intractable, nonfluctuating sexual difficulties, such as primary or secondary anorgasmia. [3] Now the victim may encounter recurrent nightmares and emotional deadness. As the adolescent deidealizes her parents and experiences herself more as an autonomous entity, guilt about the incest replaces fear of retaliation. The painfulness of the guilt produced by her developing sense of personal responsibility may, in fact, teach the adolescent to withdraw from precisely those developmental tasks that involve viewing herself as equipotent with parents. Another source of pain is the incest victim's grief about the premature despoiling of her sexuality, which is no longer as available to her for use in forming a sexual identity. Searles [48] has likened sexual strivings to the trump card in the game of self-realization; the incest victim no longer has the card of virginity to play, whether with a lover, a husband, a god, or with herself. When she makes her first serious attempts at intimacy, problems with aggression are likely to appear in the form of tormenting victim-aggressor relationships. Continued idealization of the hurting parent leads some adolescents to choose a negative identity; they in turn become aggressor and tormentor. It is as if in living up to the parents' view of the victim as monster, the adolescent is able to salvage some sense of the parents' rightness.

By the time the adult victim seeks treatment, her chronic tension and anxiety may conceal both the underlying fear of being raped again and her continuing fear of being punished or killed by the aggressor-parent. The adult victim may not perceive that her experience of being trapped and helpless in her marriage, or in her job, is a reenacted vestige of the abuse situation. Good sexual experience remains elusive. She may be unaware that her self-destructive thoughts and actions are repetitions of her parents' attitude toward her. Insomnia and nightmares will have become routine. Her defensive refusal to acknowledge the nature and extent of her hurt may exacerbate her frustration, confusion, and self-blame about her anhedonia. Perfectionism may cloak her guilty fear that any error will lead to the unmasking of her badness, to blame, and to rejection. Constriction of affects and of functioning may be the consequence of the massive repression and dissociation employed to keep the abuse out of awareness; she may take this as further evidence of her unworthiness. Revenge fantasies about the parents may be elaborate, but they may coexist with an absolute inability to assert herself effectively enough against them to prevent recurrence of abuse either to herself or to her children.[20] It has been recommended that the mother of an incest victim be asked routinely about sexual abuse in her own childhood.[18,20]

The following case history illustrates how posttraumatic symptoms and their developmental transformations become manifest in the history of an adult incest victim.

Mary, a twenty-eight-year-old married secretary with one child, came to a crisis clinic with concerns about her sanity. She had just come home from the grocery store and thrown all the groceries on the kitchen floor. She had been reading a book of reminiscences by incest survivors for the past two days and had been unable to sleep. Mary could not recall any time in her life when she had felt relaxed, but the tension of the past forty-eight hours had been unbearable. The book had reawakened feelings of rape, guilt, and grief about her incest experiences with her father from age four to twelve. A few weeks previously her father had been diagnosed as having dementia. Mary felt unsure if she had successfully protected her son from her father's sexual advances. She felt trapped both in her marriage and her job. Although Mary forced

herself to participate in martial sexuality, flashbacks to the incest blocked both arousal and orgasm. Her childhood had been complicated by her mother's psychosis as well as by her father's sexual abuse of all siblings. Of Mary's five siblings, one had been convicted for pedophilia, one had been diagnosed as schizophrenic, one was alcoholic, one had numerous suicide attempts, and one was a psychotherapist. Mary had been taken to psychiatrists twice in childhood. At age six, her teacher reported that Mary looked frightened, cried often, was afraid to go to the bathroom, and did not socialize with other children. Tranquilizers were prescribed. At fifteen, Mary was brought to a guidance clinic by her mother because of runaways, drug use, promiscuity, and chronic rule-breaking. She was diagnosed as having a conduct disorder and no further treatment was recommended. Prior incest was not uncovered at either evaluation, even though it was Mary's complaint to her mother about the father's sexual abuse that precipitated the second evaluation.

Developmental perspectives can assist therapists planning treatment both for the adult who is experiencing the later derivative symptoms of childhood incest and for the child victim who awaits the developmental transformations of symptoms. Like the child victim, the victim who presents in adulthood deserves an evaluation of family psychopathology and deficits, a search for additional victims within the family, an assessment of the need for legal protection, or redress, and a reassessment of previous developmental difficulties as possible responses to the incest trauma. The diagnosis of posttraumatic disorder, when appropriate, can be less frightening and less stigmatizing than other labels acquired by incest victims when the therapist is unaware of the prior sexual abuse; conduct disorder, hysterical personality, major depressive disorder, and schizotypal personality are common misdiagnoses.[16] Recognizing troublesome behaviors as learned responses to truly traumatic prior events can make therapeutic interventions more accurate and empathic and can help patient and therapist identify key symptoms for monitoring therapeutic progress.

REFERENCES

1. ADAMS-TUCKER, C. "Proximate Effects of Sexual Abuse in Childhood: A Report on 28 Children," *American Journal of Psychiatry,* 139 (1982):1251–1256.

2. ANDERSON, L., and SHAFER, G. "The Character-disordered Family: A Community Treatment Model for Family Sexual Abuse," *American Journal of Orthopsychiatry,* 49 (1979):436–445.

3. BECKER, J., et al. "Incidence and Types of Sexual Dysfunctions in Rape and Incest Victims," *Journal of Sex and Marital Therapy,* 8 (1982):65–74.

4. BENDER, L., and BLAU, A. "The Reaction of Children to Sexual Relations with Adults," *American Journal of Orthopsychiatry,* 7 (1937):500–518.

5. BENDER, L., and GRUGETTE, A. "A Follow-up report on Children Who Had Atypical Sexual Experience," *American Journal of Orthopsychiatry,* 22 (1952):825–837.

6. BERLINER, L., and STEVENS, D. "Special Techniques for Child Witnesses," in L. G. Schultz, ed., *The Sexual Victimology of Youth.* Springfield, Ill.: Charles C Thomas, 1979, pp. 32–42.

7. BROWNING, D. H., and BOATMAN, B. "Incest: Children at Risk," *American Journal of Psychiatry,* 134 (1977):69–72.

8. BURGESS, A., and HOLMSTROM, L. "Rape Trauma Syndrome," *American Journal of Psychiatry,* 131 (1974):981–986.

9. DAVIES, R. "Incest: Some Neuropsychiatric Findings,"

International Journal of Psychiatry in Medicine 9 (1978–79): 117–119.

10. DEFRANCIS, V. *Protecting the Child Victim of Sex Crimes.* Denver: American Humane Association, 1969.

11. EATON, A. P., and VASTBINDER, E. "The Sexually Misused Child. A Plan of Management," *Clinical Pediatrics,* 8 (1969):438–441.

12. FAIRBAIRN, W. R. *Psychoanalytic Studies of the Personality.* London: Tavistock, 1952.

13. FERENCZI, S. "Confusion of Tongues Between the Adult and the Child (The Language of Tenderness and of Passion)," *International Journal of Psycho-Analysis,* 30 (1949):225–230. (Originally published 1932.)

14. FINKELHOR, D. *Sexually Victimized Children.* New York: Free Press, 1979.

15. FREUD, S. "An Autobiographical Study," in J. Strachey, ed., *The Standard Edition of the Complete Psychological Works of Sigmund Freud,* vol. 20. London: Hogarth Press, 1960, p. 13.

16. GELINAS, D. "The Persisting Negative Effects of Incest," *Psychiatry,* 46 (1983):312–332.

17. GIARETTO, H. "Humanistic Treatment of Father-Daughter Incest," in R. Helfer and C. H. Kempe, eds., *Child Abuse and Neglect: The Family and the Community.* Cambridge, Mass.: Ballinger, 1976, pp. 143–162.

18. GOODWIN, J. *Sexual Abuse: Incest Victims and Their Families.* Boston: Wright/PSG, 1982.

19. ———. "Persecution and Grandiosity in Incest Fathers," in P. Pichot et al., eds., *Psychiatry: The State of the Art.* New York: Plenum Press, 1985, pp. 309–322.

20. GOODWIN, J., CORMIER, L. and OWEN, J. "Grandfather-Granddaughter Incest: A Trigenerational View," *Child Abuse and Neglect,* 7 (1983):163–170.

21. GREENE, A. H. *Child Maltreatment: A Handbook for Mental Health Professionals.* New York: Jason Aronson, 1980.

22. GROSS, R., et al. "Borderline Syndrome and Incest in Chronic Pelvic Pain Patients," *International Journal of Psychiatry in Medicine,* 10 (1981):79–96.

23. GUYON, R. *The Ethics of Sexual Acts.* New York: Octagon Books, 1974. (Originally published 1941.)

24. HENDERSON, D. J. "Incest," in A. M. Freedman, H. I. Kaplan, and B. J. Sadock, eds., *Comprehensive Textbook of Psychiatry.* Baltimore: Williams & Wilkins, 1975, pp. 1530–1538.

25. HERMAN, J. *Father-Daughter Incest.* Cambridge, Mass.: Harvard University Press, 1981.

26. KARDINER, A. "Traumatic Neuroses of War," in S. Arieti, ed., *American Handbook of Psychiatry,* vol. 1. New York: Basic Books, 1959, pp. 245–257.

27. KAUFMAN, I., PECK A. L., and TAGIURI, C. K. "The Family Constellation and Overt Incestuous Relations Between Father and Daughter," *American Journal of Orthopsychiatry,* 24 (1954):266 279.

28. KESTENBERG, J. "Outside and Inside, Male and Female," *Journal of The American Psychoanalytic Association,* 16 (1968):456–520.

29. KINSEY, A., et al. *Sexual Behavior in the Female.* Philadelphia: W. B. Saunders, 1953.

30. KLUFT, R. "Treatment of Multiple Personality Disorder: A Study of 33 Cases," *Psychiatric Clinics of North America,* 7 (1984):9–30.

31. LANDIS, J. "Experiences of 500 Children with Adult Sexual Deviants," *Psychiatric Quarterly Supplement,* 30 (1956):91–109.

32. LUKIANOWICZ, N. "Incest," *British Journal of Psychiatry,* 120 (1972):301–313.

33. MAISCH, H. *Incest.* London: Andre Deutsch, 1973.

34. MASSON, J. M. *The Assault on Truth: Freud's Suppression of the Seduction Theory.* New York: Farrar, Straus & Giroux, 1984.

35. MEISELMAN, K. *Incest: A Psychologic Study of Causes and Effects with Treatment Recommendations.* San Francisco: Jossey-Bass, 1978.

36. MRAZEK, P., and KEMPE, C. H. *Sexually Abused Children and Their Families.* New York: Pergamon Press, 1981.

37. NAKASHIMA, I., and ZAKUS, G. E. "Incest: Review and Clinical Experience," *Pediatrics,* 60 (1977): 696–701.

38. NEUTRA, R., LEVY, J., and PARKER, D. "Cultural Expectations Versus Reality in Navajo Seizure Patterns and Sick Roles," *Culture, Medicine and Psychiatry,* 1 (1977): 255–275.

39. PETERS, J. "Children Who Are Victims of Sexual Assault," *American Journal of Psychotherapy,* 30 (1976):398–421.

40. PUTNAM, F. "The Psychophysiologic Investigation of Multiple Personality Disorder," *Psychiatric Clinics of North America,* 7 (1984):31–40.

41. RENSHAW, D. *Incest: Understanding and Treatment.* Boston: Little, Brown, 1982.

42. ROSENFELD, A. A. "Incidence of a History of Incest Among 18 Female Psychiatric Patients," *American Journal of Psychiatry,* 136 (1979):791–795.

43. ROSENFELD, A. A., NADELSON, C., and KRIEGER, M. "Incest and the Sexual Abuse of Children," *Journal of the American Academy of Child Psychiatry,* 16 (1977):327–339.

44. RUSH, F. *The Best Kept Secret.* Englewood Cliffs, N.J.: Prentice-Hall, 1980.

45. RUSSELL, D. "The Incidence and Prevalence of Intrafamilial and Extrafamilial Sexual Abuse of Female Children," *Child Abuse and Neglect,* 7 (1983):133–146.

46. RUTTER, M. "Normal Psychosexual Development," *Journal of Child Psychology and Psychiatry,* 11 (1971): 259–283.

47. SALTMAN, V., and SOLOMON, R. S. "Incest and the Multiple Personality," *Psychological Reports,* 50 (1982): 1127–1141.

48. SEARLES, H. "The Effort to Drive the Other Person Crazy—An Element in the Etiology and Psychotherapy of Schizophrenia," *British Journal of Medical Psychology,* 32 (1959):1–18.

49. SHENGOLD, L. "Some Reflections on a Case of Consummated Mother/Adolescent Son Incest," *International Journal of Psycho-Analysis,* 61 (1980): 461–476.

50. STEELE, B. F. "The Effect of Abuse and Neglect on Psychological Development," in J. D. Call, E. Galenson, and R. L. Tyson, eds., *Frontiers of Infant Psychiatry,* New York: Basic Books, 1983, pp. 235–244.

51. SUMMIT, R. "Beyond Belief: The Reluctant Discovery of Incest," in M. Kirkpatricks, ed., *Women's Sexual Experience: Explorations of the Dark Continent.* New York: Plenum Press, 1982, pp. 110–122.

52. TERR, L. "Children of Chowchilla: A Study of Psychic Trauma," *Psychoanalytic Study of the Child,* 34 (1979):552–623.

53. TILELLI, J., TUREK, D., and JAFFE, A. "Sexual Abuse of Children," *New England Journal of Medicine,* 302 (1980): 319–323.

54. TORMES, Y. *Child Victims of Incest.* Englewood, Col.: American Humane Association, 1968.

55. VAN DER KOLK, B. A. *Post-traumatic Stress Disorder: Psychological and Biological Sequelae.* Washington, D.C.: American Psychiatric Press, 1984.

56. WEINBERG, S. *Incest Behavior.* New York: Citadel, 1955.

57. WELLS, L. "Family Pathology and Father-Daughter Incest: Restricted Psychopathy," *Journal of Clinical Psychiatry,* 42 (1981):197–202.

58. WILLIAMS, G. J., and MONEY, J. *Traumatic Abuse and Neglect of Children at Home.* Baltimore: Johns Hopkins University Press, 1980.

59. YATES, A. *Sex Without Shame.* New York: William Morrow, 1978.

60. YORUKOGLU, A., and KEMPH, J. "Children Not Severely Damaged by Incest with a Parent," *Journal of the American Academy of Child Psychiatry,* 5 (1966):111–124.

13 / Violent Youth

Charles R. Keith

Introduction

In the past five years there has been a surge of interest in violent youth, especially in the search for psychobiological vulnerabilities to delinquency. [82] Early pioneers such as William Healy raised many of the same questions that are being addressed today. However, our modern tools—such as powerful statistical methodologies, the burgeoning knowledge of neurotransmitters, and sophisticated longitudinal and early child developmental studies—allow us to probe the questions more deeply, to find hitherto unsuspected correlations, and to integrate the distal and proximate causes of violence into an interactional, homeostatic system.

This chapter reviews recent developments in the areas of neurobiology, neuropsychiatry, early child development, forensics, treatment, and psychopharmacology as they apply to violence and delinquency in youth, particularly adolescents.

Neurobiology of Aggression

Numerous laboratory and ethological animal studies are defining types of aggression and correlating these behavioral modes with central nervous system pathways, hormonal stimuli, and neurotransmitter families. [49,119,158,182] These animal models allow investigators of violence to control variables, perform pharmacodynamic interventions, and obtain brain tissue that would be impossible and unethical in humans.

For example, Alpert and associates [3,4] destroyed dopaminergic terminals in rat pups with 6-hydrox-

ydopamine. These rats became hyperactive and impulsive; as adults they were deficient mothers. These behaviors reverted to normal upon the administration of methylphenidate. Subsequently, Rogeness and co-workers [149] found that boys with undersocialized conduct disorder had low blood levels of dopamine-beta-hydroxylase (DBH) and elevated serotonin (5HT) levels, whereas boys with socialized conduct disorder had the opposite, namely elevated DBH and below-normal 5HT. Though the meaning of these levels is uncertain, they suggest that there may be biological differences between these two diagnostic subgroups that could further be clarified through both animal and human studies.

Brown and others [16] found that 5-hydroxyindoleacetic acid (5-HIAA), the metabolite of 5HT, was decreased in the cerebrospinal fluid (CSF) of young servicemen who manifested high levels of aggressive behavior. The lowest levels of 5-HIAA were found in men with both aggressive behavior and suicide attempts.

Genetic factors continue to be explored. There are a small number of offenders in whom disorders of the Y chromosome may be linked to aggressive behavior, body height, and CSF 5-HIAA. [15] However, a closer look at the crimes of XYY individuals has revealed little evidence of violence toward persons. The overrepresentation of XYY males in prison populations may be more related to their low IQ and social ineptitude than to any special inclination toward destructiveness. [110]

Monozygotic twins have a 36 percent concordance rate for criminality as compared to 12.5 percent for dizygotic twins. [111] Danish adoptee studies indicate that if a male adoptee's biological father were criminal, the adoptee has a 20 percent chance of becoming criminal in turn. In contrast to this, if his biological father (and his adoptive father) were not criminal, then the adoptee had only a 10 percent chance of following a criminal course.[12] A more recent study of Swedish adoptees failed to fully confirm the Danish findings.[13,14] Instead, the criminality of the Swedish adoptees was more alcohol-related, and the genetic link between biological fathers and their adopted-away sons appeared to be an alcohol-abuse diathesis.

Low autonomic nervous system arousal can be manifested by slow pulse rate[185] and slow recovery of skin conductance responses.[52,111] These responses have been found in aggressive children and adolescents and may be genetically linked.

Endogenous fetal androgens play a role in male aggressiveness in adolescence. Exogenous androgen-based compounds administered during pregnancy appear to increase physically aggressive behavior in childhood and adolescence.[112,142] Postpubertal testosterone levels in delinquent populations are slightly elevated over those of normals. In extremely violent delinquents, testosterone levels are sometimes much higher than normal.[54,108,109] For many youths, as they enter puberty, their normal testosterone levels may be "too high" relative to the weakness of their available ego controls over impulses.

Studies continue to suggest that exposure of the young child's brain to environmental insults, such as low-level lead exposure,[122] food additives,[186] malnutrition,[44,137] and even artificial lighting[53] may contribute to aggressivity.

The role of neurobiological factors in the biopsychosocial complexities of youthful violence has recently been summarized by Alpert and associates,[4] Brown and Goodwin,[15] and Shaffer, Meyer-Bahlburg, and Stokeman.[164]

Neuropsychiatric Aspects of Delinquency and Violence

In the last five years there has been a renewed emphasis on neuropsychiatric studies of violent and delinquent youths. Such studies are aimed at increasing diagnostic precision[113] in order to facilitate the search for specific treatments, biological markers, and correlations with other diagnostic entities.

To place these neuropsychiatric studies into context, some definitional issues should first be addressed. Delinquency is not synonymous with violence. A delinquent is a youth who has been legally charged in court. Only 10 to 13 percent have committed violence against persons.[171,174] The remainder are usually charged

with property crimes. Of those charged with violent offenses, only 3 to 5 percent will be charged with two or more violent crimes. Thus, of all the youths receiving charges in court, the majority will be nonviolent and nonrepeaters. Most recent studies have more carefully described these youths by type of crime and degree of violence, in contrast to earlier studies, which often did not carefully delineate these issues.

It is estimated that only 10 percent of criminal activities are detected and end up with legal charges. Given that, the scope of the problem is highlighted by the fact that by the age of twenty, 25 to 35 percent of all youths have a nontraffic-related court record.[174,192] In addition, many youths with delinquent behavior are diverted to mental health facilities prior to legal charging.[101] Most authors believe that increases in reported juvenile crimes over the past twenty years are real and are not statistical artifacts[152]; some, however, remain skeptical.[123] Historical evidence indicates rampant adolescent violence in the 1800s and earlier eras. The most extreme form of violence and the most easily measured is murder. Murders committed by youths do not appear to have increased significantly in recent years.[47]

The psychobiological and neuropsychiatric perspective is epitomized by the recent studies of Lewis and her coworkers.* Most of their findings come from intensive study of seriously violent, incarcerated, or hospitalized youths. (Other corroborating studies will also be noted.) Compared with nonviolent populations, they found that violent, delinquent adolescents displayed an increased frequency of (1) abuse, injuries, and head trauma in early childhood[12,72]; (2) early hospitalization and emergency room visits; (3) psychopathology, alcoholism and criminality with concomitant familial violence in one or both parents†; (4) general learning problems and specific learning disabilities[144]; (5) psychotic thought disorder[58]; (6) neuropsychological disabilities[184, 194]; (7) abnormal electroencephalograms especially indicative of psychomotor seizures[177]; (8) hard and soft neurological signs[193]; (9) previous history of psychiatric hospitalizations (with psychiatric diagnoses often being changed at adolescence to facilitate entry into correctional systems); (10) drug and alcohol abuse[73]; and (11) suicidal behavior.[2]

These multiple, psychobiological vulnerabilities are found with increasing frequency in the more violent end of the spectrum of delinquencies. One hoped-for outcome of the preceding studies involving these most disturbed and hard-to-treat youths is that interest in treatment may be rekindled and that thought will be given to the utilization of modern psychopharmacologic agents.

*See references 58, 83, 84, 85, 86, 87, 89, 91, 92, and 167.
†See references 50, 51, 57, 96, 125, and 172.

Lower socioeconomic status (SES) continues to be associated with higher levels of delinquency and youth violence,[179] though some researchers maintain that overrepresentation of the poor may be strongly influenced by arrest patterns and court procedures. Self-report studies of crime suggest that there may be little difference in middle and lower SES crime rates.[180] Poverty appears to have little direct effect on the occurrence of violence. The common stereotypes associating crime, violence, poverty, and social class belie the complexities involved.[153,155] In reality, most of the children who grow up in criminogenic, violence-prone environments turn out to be nonviolent, law-abiding citizens. Once again this reminds us that individual vulnerabilities are crucial.[151]

High levels of major depression are now being found in delinquent populations, usually among those who are incarcerated.[2,26,67] This correlates with much clinical experience which suggests that acting out impulsive behavior is often a defense against depression.[143] In clinical and correctional settings, it is known that when acting out is controlled by external restrictions through the use of lock-up or a quiet room, there is an increase in both the appearance of depression and the risk of suicide. Shaffer[162,163] studied successful suicides in early adolescence and found that many occurred in the context of a disciplinary crisis that had resulted from a period of escalating antisocial activity. Puig-Antich[139] found that one-third of a group of pre-pubertal boys with major depressive disorders also had conduct disorders. When these boys were treated with imipramine, the conduct disorder usually remitted, along with the depression, at least temporarily.

Hyperactivity and attention deficit disorder have been viewed as childhood precursors of adolescent delinquency and sociopathy. However, recent studies indicate that many diagnoses of hyperactivity in preadolescence are probably picking up on the faulty behavioral controls of conduct-disordered children. The small number of children with pure hyperactivity (i.e., without concomitant conduct disorder) probably do not turn out to have an increase in behavioral problems in adolescence. This may explain why hyperactivity is so infrequently diagnosed in Great Britain; British clinicians often view hyperactive symptomatology as a manifestation of conduct disorder.*

In 1976 Murray[120] criticized studies that up to then had purported to show an increase in learning disabilities in delinquent populations. Delinquents frequently manifested learning problems, such as lack of interest in school and underachievement, but whether they had a high level of true, narrowly defined, specific learning disabilities was not clear. Subsequent studies have delineated more clearly the different subtypes of learning problems and have found some increase in specific learning disability in delinquent populations.[76] Those youngsters whose history of conduct disorder includes a learning disability tend to be more violent than do those with a history of only hyperactivity (as noted earlier).[90]

Haizlip[47] found that adolescents who murdered a parent had less evident psychopathology and fewer previous court contacts than did those who murdered a stranger; they also remained in prison for shorter periods and were usually accepted back into their immediate family. McCarthy[97] described the narcissistic rage and attempts to restore the self that fueled the murders committed by a group of early adolescents.

Latency-age children who murdered and/or who were hospitalized for violent behavior were found to have essentially the same familial and development background factors as those described earlier for the more violent adolescents.*

Prospective longitudinal studies continue to confirm the findings of the retrospective clinical investigations so far described. Most of the prospective studies begin with male cohorts in early elementary school and follow them into adolescence and adulthood.† All studies conclude that childhood aggression is one of the most stable personality traits to persist through adolescence, and that parental discord, harshness, and violence are the strongest predictors of aggression in children. Aggression in childhood may be variously identified through negative peer or teacher ratings or psychiatric diagnosis of conduct disorder; in any case, it strongly predicts future violence and delinquency. This correlation is so strong that if violence is demonstrated for the first time in adolescence, the clinician must immediately suspect an organic or psychotic process.[136] Robins[147] found a common developmental sequence of deviancy that tended to repeat in case after case. It began with early school truancy, then led on to school failure, then to alcohol use and sexual promiscuity, and finally to drugs, dropping out of school, and entrance into delinquency.

The vast majority of studies have focused on male delinquency because males at all developmental levels, cross-culturally (and in most species of higher-level animals as well), demonstrate more aggressiveness than do females.[98,178] In recent years, however, as a result of an increase in female arrests and violent crimes[67] and through the stimulus of the feminist movement, there has been a reexamination of female delinquency. The results have challenged the stereo-

*See references 24, 25, 78, 127, 138, 159, 161, 173, and 187.

*See references 74, 93, 130, 132, 134, 135, and 181.
†See references 8, 34, 55, 69, 80, 116, 118, 129, 145, 146, 147, 148, and 185.

types and sexist biases in this area.* With rapidly changing sexual norms, earlier clinical views concerning the meaning of sexual promiscuity in the female delinquent are being revised.[11] Research in this area remains scant, however. Recently Offord and associates[126] studied a group of female delinquents and found that the strongest factor distinguishing delinquents from controls was a higher frequency of broken homes, a factor that had not been found to be powerful in male delinquency. The question this raises is whether girls are more vulnerable to broken homes than are boys.

Common sense would indicate that if harsh punitive parental behavior and marital discord are powerful predictors of aggressive behavior in children, then most likely these parent-child interactions were present from infancy. Indeed, earlier longitudinal studies have suggested that aggression at age three is predictive of adolescent aggression. However, some investigators believe that behavior problems among preschool children are too variable and not sufficiently stable and predictive. In any case, the longitudinal studies just cited begin with latency-age children because by that age, aggressive behavior has become an identifiable persistent pattern and it is easy to obtain cohorts in school populations.

In recent years several investigators have described the varieties of hostility and aggression that appear within the context of the early mother-infant relationship. The most comprehensive has been Parens's[131] typology of aggression in early childhood. He distinguishes three basic categories of aggressive behavior: *non destructive aggression* which fuels assertiveness, *non affective destructiveness* which fuels prey aggression e.g. in alimentation, and *hostile destructiveness* which aims at inflicting pain or harm on an object. Hostile destructiveness is fueled primarily by excessive unpleasure. All these, he holds, influence each other in the course of development and constitute the "aggressive drive."

Paren's work provides a conceptual bridge between animal studies of aggression and the current interest in early maternal and parental psychopathology, for example, the abusing, depressed, avoidant, and abandoning caretaker and his or her impact on the child's development through the arousal of excessive unpleasure which, in turn, may result in repetitive hostile destructiveness.[20,45,63]

In a currently ongoing study, Galenson[43] has observed sadistic mothers teasing their infants to the point of rage. At around eight months of age, this rage sometimes transforms into "hollow" masochisticlike pleasure so that the infant appears to be smiling and laughing at the mother's provocations. In the second year of life, these toddlers are disruptive. They tease other children and exhibit learning problems.

In their studies of abusing and avoidant mothers, Main and Stadtman[99] and Fraiberg[40] described how nine to twelve-month-old infants rage and strike aggressively at their mothers. Though these studies focused on the maternal caretaker, the early presence of the father is now receiving increasing emphasis.[88,170] Cross-cultural studies indicate that societies which keep boys with mothers and away from fathers for lengthy periods have high levels of personal crime, violence, and mistrust toward other members of the community.[6,42]

Legal Issues Concerning Delinquency and Youthful Violence

The introduction of adversarial proceedings into the juvenile justice system[64] and of hospitalization procedures for adolescents[5,94] have corrected certain abuses. But they have also created a host of problems that will call for continued dialogue between the mental health and legal systems. All agree that if clinicians and lawyers work together, the adversarial proceedings can result in support of the adolescents' need for treatment and behavioral controls.[48]

Another recent thorny issue has been the nationwide movement to remove status offenders (youths who run away, stay out late, or do not attend school) from training schools and, ultimately, from the jurisdiction of the juvenile justice system.* Some workers feel that when youthful status offenders fall under court jurisdiction, it is often because they and their families have not been able to use community social service and mental health resources. Hence it follows that the court should continue to play a role in such instances in order to enforce the utilization of resources. Others feel strongly that only those who commit a crime should be under court jurisdiction. From this vantage point it is then up to the community to find alternatives for these status offenders.

Of particular interest is a recent class action suit in North Carolina where the decision requires the state to provide necessary educational, medical, and psychiatric treatment to rehabilitate violent children and youths. An oversight process was set up to ensure the state's compliance.[17,18,19] As of 1984, 1,300 youths have been designated members of this class, and the state is spending over 20 million per year to set up a wide array of community services.

Currently, psychiatrists are reluctant to make any predictions about violence. However, by their very na-

---

*See references 7, 32, 101, 104, and 116.

*See references 60, 102, 157, 166, 190, and 198.

ture, most clinical and legal decisions concerning violent youths involve some prediction about future behavior.[75,189] Monahan[117] and Fisher[38] describe some of the parameters that may be employed in making predictive decisions concerning violence, and they suggest ways in which the available extensive data base can be used to improve predictive success.

In 1979 a law went into effect in Sweden prohibiting parents from hitting or humiliating their children. This is landmark legislation in that it attempts to limit violence at its sources.[37]

Treatment of Violent, Aggressive Youth

During the 1970s, pessimism pervaded the treatment and rehabilitative efforts aimed at violent, antisocial youths.* Programs that had begun with optimism appeared to end up having no effect.[61] However, over the past five years a more hopeful and positive atmosphere is developing.

One source of encouragement is the current intensive study of violent youths from a biopsychosocial perspective, an avenue of approach that may open up new treatment possibilities, as described earlier in this chapter.

Another optimistic note has been sounded from an unexpected source, namely, a new look at the statistical methodologies applied to treatment outcome studies. Murray and Cox[121] discovered that up until very recently, virtually all program evaluations in juvenile corrections have used recidivism rates as the criterion for success. This meant that youths committing even one crime during the follow-up period were counted as a treatment failure. This "absolutist" criterion has doomed all programs to appear as failures with high recidivism rates, and it has been a major factor in maintaining the pervasive gloom about treatment efficacy. If, however, this form of symptomatic change is compared with the level of relief achieved for other symptoms, then youths with major antisocial pathology who commit crimes repeatedly would not be expected to cease their criminality entirely as a result of a treatment program. Murray and Cox then evaluated the treatment results of a program designed to provide case managers and community services for chronically offending, violent inner-city delinquents. If the delinquents could not utilize the community programs and continued to commit crimes, they were sent to a training school for short stays. The community program resulted in a 60 percent reduction in crime and training

school, a 70 percent reduction! These dramatic figures resulted from comparing crime rates before and after treatment. In sum, Murray and Cox found that using before-and-after crime rates, the only programs that resulted in crime reduction were those that provided strict controls and threatened actual loss of freedom. Appearances in court or the usual probationary supervision had no impact on crime rates.

During the past five years, two inpatient treatment programs for violent youth stand out as prototypes in their respective fields of juvenile corrections and adolescent psychiatry.

The first is the Closed Adolescent Treatment Center in Denver, Colorado. This is a twenty-six-bed secure facility for violent youthful male offenders, many of whom have murdered or committed violent sexual crimes.[1,41,77] The program utilizes behavioral, social learning, and psychodynamic principles. The patients stay an average of two years and must participate actively in intensive daily group therapy, a tightly structured milieu therapy program, and constant peer and staff feedback concerning disruptive behavior. The basic philosophy, which is stated explicitly to patients is that there is "no way out" except through therapeutic change and that the staff and the patients' peers are prepared to go "all the way" to set whatever limits necessary. Only 2 percent of those admitted are dismissed early as unsuitable or unresponsive to the program. Using the "absolutist" criterion of post-treatment crime rate since the program's inception in the middle 1970s, the rate of recidivism has been only 33 percent; it may now be in the upper 20 percent range.* This program is exciting in that it addresses the depth of violent delinquents' psychopathology with a long-term, intensive treatment program geared toward their areas of developmental failure; moreover, it is being carried out within a corrections framework. Other states are considering inaugurating similar programs.

Marohn and associates,[104,105] at the Illinois State Psychiatric Institute, have described in detail the crucial dynamic components of their intensive inpatient program for violent, chronically offending youths. They developed a diagnostic typology[123] consisting of four categories: impulsive; narcissistic; empty borderline; and depressive borderline (which some clinicians might designate as a severe neurotic character). Although there was some overlap, each delinquent's ego structure and defenses tended to place him or her in one of these categories. Typical treatment processes and transferences evolved with patients from each of these diagnostic categories. (It should be noted that both Agee's and Marohn's programs concentrate heavily on deepening therapeutic relationships with staff

---

*See references 27, 33, 140, 154, and 165.

*V. Agee, personal communication, 1984.

and peers as a primary means of treatment. As a result, openly psychotic youths were generally excluded from each.) The psychodynamic understanding of the use of physical space and moment-by-moment daily activities follows the rich tradition of Bettleheim.[10] Though many of the patients remained in the program for only six months, follow-up studies have shown considerable reduction in crime rate and drug and alcohol use.

In a five-year follow-up of borderline adolescents treated in his inpatient unit, Masterson[107] also reported significant improvement. Many of these youths were violent and had criminal records prior to treatment.

In many instances psychotherapy with more violent youths can begin only on an inpatient unit that provides the necessary behavioral controls.* Those youths with more ego controls and a supportive family milieu and those who are brought to treatment prior to adolescence can often be treated initially in outpatient psychotherapy.[9,95,150,168] A recent trend in the psychotherapeutic literature is the study of adolescent violence within the framework of narcissism and disturbances of the self.[97,105,191] To place these recent psychotherapeutic trends into context, the reader is referred to Marshall's excellent review.[106]

Behavior therapy continues to play a central role in many inpatient units, treatment-oriented correctional facilities, and community programs.† Behavior therapists are attacking the problem of lack of generalization by moving treatment programs into the family and onto the streets.[176] Humanistic behavioral approaches not only reduce aggressive behavior but can also provide the consistency, immediate feedback, and attention to details of everyday life that were often lacking in the family milieu of the delinquent.

Family therapy is becoming increasingly incorporated into inpatient and outpatient treatment programs for delinquent youths.[21,29] Group therapy remains a central treatment modality for violent youths in both mental health and correctional facilities.[79] With the current emphasis on deinstitutionalization, community programs[124] and day programs[59,196] will become increasingly important.

Violent behavior in school remains a vexing issue.[128] Evidence is now accumulating that school organization can make a difference. Rutter and associates[156] studied twelve English secondary schools. Those schools with a solid administration, communicative school staff, and positive educational milieu were found to be effective in reducing the predicted delinquency rate, whereas schools with low morale, weak administration, and noncommunicative staff had greater than expected delinquency. (Entrance variables were controlled in this study so that the delinquency rates reflected in-school effects.)

Psychopharmacologic Treatment of Violent Youth

Psychoactive drugs are becoming increasingly important in the treatment of violence in the adolescent and preadolescent.[22,81] It is of critical importance that such drugs be used only within the context of an overall treatment program, with continual scrutiny for side effects.[46] Establishing an accurate diagnosis is as important for selecting the proper drug as it is for the establishment of other facets of the treatment program. Butyrophenones, eg. Haldol, and phenothiazines may be indicated when violence arises as a consequence of a psychotic thought disorder. Stimulants may reduce aggressiveness if there are signs of accompanying hyperactivity and distractibility. Antidepressants may reduce aggression arising in the context of a major depressive disorder.[139] Lithium carbonate may be used when aggressive overactivity is part of a juvenile manic-depressive illness.[23,195] Anticonvulsants are used when violence is clearly connected with a seizure disorder.

Indications for medication are less clear when aggression is not linked with a specific syndrome or when it is an expression of a conduct disorder. Phenothiazines are probably most likely resorted to in this situation.[114] It is estimated that currently over 100,000 brain-damaged and/or mentally retarded children in institutions are receiving long-term phenothiazines in order to control aggressive, disruptive behaviors.[197] In recent years, lithium and propranolol hydrochloride have been used increasingly for aggression not clearly linked to a specific disorder, such as depression or psychosis. So far, these two drugs have had fewer long-term side effects than the phenothiazines and appear to be as effective in reducing violence.[30,141,169,188] Carbamazepine and other anticonvulsants may be helpful in alleviating aggressive outbursts that are part of the episodic dyscontrol syndrome.[160]

There is no firm evidence yet that illicit street drugs directly cause violence. Though phencyclidine (PCP) may lead to violent, psychoticlike outbursts in some susceptible individuals,[35] a recent study showed no difference in aggressive behavior between those who chronically abuse PCP and other groups of drug abusers.[71] When adolescent violence is associated with drug use, the mechanism is usually removal of inhibiting controls through intoxication. The most common offending drug by far is alcohol.[81]

*See references 28, 62, 68, 133, and 160.
†See references 31, 36, 39, 56, 65, 70, 175, and 183.

REFERENCES

1. AGEE, V. *Treatment of the Violent Incorrigible Adolescent.* Lexington, Mass.: Lexington Books, 1979.

2. ALESSI, N. E., et al. "Suicidal Behavior Among Serious Juvenile Offenders," *American Journal of Psychiatry,* 141 (1984):286–287.

3. ALPERT, J. A., et al. "Animal Models and Childhood Behavioral Disturbances," *Journal of the American Academy of Child Psychiatry,* 17 (1978):239–251.

4. ALPERT, J. A., et al. "Neurochemical and Behavioral Organization: Disorders of Attention, Activity and Aggression," in D. O. Lewis, ed., *Vulnerabilities to Delinquency.* New York. SP Medical and Scientific Books, 1981, pp. 109 171.

5. AMAYA, M., and BURLINGAME, W. V. "Judicial Review of Psychiatric Admissions," *Journal of the American Academy of Child Psychiatry,* 20 (1981):761–776.

6. BACON, M. K., CHILD, I. L., and BARRY, H. "A Cross-Cultural Study of Correlates of Crime," *Journal of Abnormal and Social Psychology,* 66 (1963):291–300.

7. BENEDEK, E. "Female Delinquency: Fantasies, Facts and Future," in S. C. Feinstein, and P. L. Giovacchini, eds., *Adolescent Psychiatry,* vol. 7. Chicago: University of Chicago Press, 1979, pp. 524–437.

8. BERG, I. "When Truants and School Refusers Grow Up," *British Journal of Psychiatry,* 141 (1982):208–210.

9. BERSE, P. "Psychotherapy with Severely Deprived Children," *Journal of Child Psychotherapy,* 6 (1980):49–55.

10. BETTLEHEIM, B. *The Empty Fortress.* New York: Free Press, 1967.

11. BLOS, P. "Postscript 1976" (postscript to "Etiology of Female Delinquency," pp. 207–214), in E. N. Rexford, ed., *A Developmental Approach to Problems of Acting Out,* rev. ed. New York: International Universities Press, 1978, pp. 183–206.

12. BLOUNT, H. R., and CHANDLER, T. A. "Relationship Between Childhood Abuse and Assaultive Behavior in Adolescent Male Psychiatric Patients," *Psychological Reports,* 44 (1979):1126.

13. BOHMAN, M., et al. "Predisposition to Petty Criminality in Swedish Adoptees: 1. Genetic and Environmental Heterogeneity," *Archives of General Psychiatry,* 39 (1982):1233–1241.

14. BOHMAN, M., et al. "Gene-Environment Interaction in the Psychopathology of Swedish Adoptees: Studies of the Origins of Alcoholism and Criminality," in S. B. Guze, F. J. Earls, and J. E. Barrett, eds., *Childhood Psychopathology and Development.* New York: Raven Press, 1983, pp. 265–278.

15. BROWN, G. L., and GOODWIN, F. K. "Aggression, Adolescence and Psychobiology," in C. R. Keith, ed., *The Aggressive Adolescent.* New York: Free Press, 1984, pp. 63–97.

16. BROWN, G. L., et al. "Aggression, Suicide, and Serotonin: Relationships of CSF Amine Metabolites," *American Journal of Psychiatry,* 139 (1982):741–746.

17. BURLINGAME, W. V. "Political and Legal Issues Involving the Aggressive Adolescent," in C. R. Keith, ed., *The Aggressive Adolescent.* New York: Free Press, 1984, pp. 168–188.

18. BURLINGAME, W. V., and AMAYA, M. "The North Carolina Class Action Suit on Behalf of Violent and Assaultive Youth," *North Carolina Journal of Mental Health,* 10 (1983):11–17.

19. ———. "The North Carolina Class Action Suit on Behalf of Violent and Assaultive Youth: Treatment Dilemmas and Programmatic Repercussions," Paper presented at the American Academy of Child Psychiatry Annual Meeting, San Francisco, 1983.

20. BURNSTEIN, M. H. "Child Abandonment: Historical, Sociological, and Psychological Perspectives," *Child Psychiatry and Human Development,* 11 (1981):213–221.

21. BURQUEST, B. "Severe Female Delinquency: When to Involve the Family in Treatment," in S. C. Feinstein, and P. L. Giovacchini, eds., *Adolescent Psychiatry,* vol. 7. Chicago: University of Chicago Press, 1979, pp. 516–523.

22. CAMPBELL, M., COHEN, I. L., and SMALL, A. M. "Drugs in Aggressive Behavior," *Journal of the American Academy of Child Psychiatry,* 21 (1982):107–117.

23. CAMPBELL, M., PERRY, R., and GREEN, W. H. "Use of Lithium in Children and Adolescents," *Psychosomatics,* 25 (1984):95–109.

24. CANTWELL, D. P. "Hyperactivity and Antisocial Behavior," *Journal of the American Academy of Child Psychiatry,* 17 (1978):252–262.

25. CANTWELL, D. P. "Hyperactivity and Antisocial Behavior Revisited: A Critical Review of the Literature," in D. O. Lewis, ed., *Vulnerabilities to Delinquency.* New York: SP Medical and Scientific Books, 1981, pp. 21–38.

26. CHILES, J. A., MILLER, M. L., and COX, G. B. "Depression in an Adolescent Delinquent Population," *Archives of General Psychiatry,* 37 (1980):1179–1186.

27. CLARKE, R.V.G., and CORNISH, D. B. "The Effectiveness of Residential Treatment for Delinquents," in L. A. Hersov, M. Berger, and D. Shaffer, eds., *Aggression and Antisocial Behavior in Childhood and Adolescence* (Book Supplement to the *Journal of Child Psychology and Psychiatry*). Oxford: Pergamon Press, 1978, pp. 143–159.

28. CRABTREE, L. H. "Hospitalized Adolescents Who Act Out: A Treatment Approach," *Psychiatry,* 45 (1982):147–158.

29. CURRY, J. F., WEINCROT, S. I., and KOEHLER, F. "Family Therapy with Aggressive and Delinquent Adolescents," in C. R. Keith, ed., *The Aggressive Adolescent.* New York: Free Press, 1984, pp. 209–239.

30. DALE, P. G. "Lithium Therapy in Aggressive Mentally Subnormal Patients," *British Journal of Psychiatry,* 137 (1980):469–474.

31. ELDER, J. P., EDELSTEIN, B. A., and NARICK, M. M. "Adolescent Psychiatric Patients: Modifying Aggressive Behavior with Social Skills Training," *Behavior Modification,* 3 (1979):161–178.

32. ERSKINE, C. "Female Delinquency, Feminism and Psychoanalysis," in C. R. Keith, ed., *The Aggressive Adolescent.* New York: Free Press, 1984, pp. 403–451.

33. FARETRA, G. "A Profile of Aggression from Adolescence to Adulthood: An 18-year Follow-up of Psychiatrically Disturbed and Violent Adolescents," *American Journal of Orthopsychiatry,* 51 (1981):439–453.

34. FARRINGTON, D. P. "The Family Backgrounds of Aggressive Youth," in L. A. Hersov, M. Berger, and D. Shaffer, eds., *Aggression and Antisocial Behavior in Childhood and Adolescence* (Book Supplement to the *Journal of Child Psychology and Psychiatry*). Oxford: Pergamon Press, 1978, pp. 73–93.

35. FAUMAN, B., and FAUMAN, M. "Phencyclidine Abuse and Crime: A Psychiatric Perspective," *Bulletin of the American Academy of Psychiatry and Law,* 10 (1982):171–176.

36. FEHRENBACH, P. A., and THELEN, M. H. "Behavioral

Approaches to the Treatment of Aggressive Disorders," *Behavior Modification,* 6 (1982):465–497.

37. FESHBACH, N. D. "Tomorrow Is Here Today in Sweden," *Journal of Clinical Child Psychology,* 9 (1980):109–112.

38. FISHER, R. B. "Predicting Adolescent Violence," in C. R. Keith, ed., *The Aggressive Adolescent.* New York: Free Press, 1984, pp. 151–165.

39. FIXSEN, D. L., et al. "Preventing Violence in Residential Programs for Adolescents," in R. B. Stuart, ed., *Violent Behavior: Social Learning Approaches to Prediction, Management and Treatment.* New York: Brunner/Mazel, 1981, pp. 203–226.

40. FRAIBERG, S. "Pathologic Defenses in Infancy," *Psychoanalytic Quarterly,* 51 (1982):612–635.

41. GADOW, D., and MCKIBBON, J. "Discipline and the Institutionalized Violent Delinquent," in *The Violent Juvenile Offender Anthology.* San Francisco: The National Council of Crime and Delinquency, 1984, pp. 311–325.

42. GADPAILLE, W. J. "Adolescent Aggression from the Perspective of Cultural Anthropology," in C. R. Keith, ed., *The Aggressive Adolescent.* New York: Free Press, 1984, pp. 432–454.

43. GALENSON, E. "A Pain-Pleasure Behavioral Complex in Mothers and Infants," Paper presented at the Vulnerable Child Discussion Group, American Psychoanalytic Association, New York, 1983.

44. GALLER, J. R., et al., "The Influence of Early Malnutrition on Subsequent Behavioral Development: II. Classroom Behavior," *Journal of the American Academy of Child Psychiatry,* 22 (1983):16–22.

45. GEORGE, C., and MAIN, M. "Social Interactions of Young Abused Children: Approach, Avoidance, and Aggression," *Child Development,* 50 (1979):306–318.

46. GUALTIERI, C. T., et al. "Tardive Dyskinesia and Other Movement Disorders in Children Treated with Psychotropic Drugs," *Journal of the American Academy of Child Psychiatry,* 19 (1980):491–510.

47. HAIZLIP, T. M., CORDER, B. F., and BALL, B. C. "The Adolescent Murderer," in C. R. Keith, ed., *The Aggressive Adolescent.* New York: Free Press, 1984, pp. 126–148.

48. HALLER, L. E., DUBIN, L. A., and BUXTON, M. "The Use of the Legal System as a Mental Health Service for Children," *Journal of Psychiatry and Law,* 7 (1979):7–48.

49. HAMBURG, D. A., and TRUDEAU, M. D., eds., *Biobehavioral Aspects of Aggression.* New York: Alan R. Liss, 1981.

50. HARBIN, H. T., and MADDEN, D. J. "Battered Parents: A New Syndrome," *American Journal of Psychiatry,* 136 (1979):1288–1291.

51. ———. "Assaultive Adolescents: Family Decision-making Parameters," *Family Process,* 22 (1983):109–118.

52. HARE, R. D. "Electrodermal and Cardiovascular Correlates of Psychopathy," in R. D. Hare, and D. Schalling, eds., *Psychopathic Behavior: Approaches to Research.* New York: John Wiley & Sons, 1978, pp. 107–144.

53. HARTUNG, J. "Light, Puberty, and Aggression: A Proximal Mechanism Hypothesis," *Human Ecology,* 6 (1978):273–297.

54. HAYS, S. E. "The Psychoendocrinology of Puberty and Adolescent Aggression," in D. A. Hamburg and M. D. Trudeau, eds., *Biobehavioral Aspects of Aggression.* New York: Alan R. Liss, 1981, pp. 107–120.

55. HENN, F., BARDWELL, R., and JENKINS, R. L. "Juvenile Delinquents Revisited," *Archives of General Psychiatry,* 37 (1980):1160–1163.

56. HERBERT, M. *Conduct Disorders of Childhood and Adolescence: A Behavioral Approach to Assessment and Treatment.* New York: John Wiley & Sons, 1978.

57. HETHERINGTON, E. M., and MARTIN, B. "Family Interaction," in H. C. Quay and J. S. Werry, eds., *Psychopathological Disorders in Childhood,* 2nd ed., New York: John Wiley & Sons, 1979, pp. 257–276.

58. INAMDAR, S. C., et al. "Violent and Suicidal Behavior in Psychotic Adolescents," *American Journal of Psychiatry,* 139 (1982):932–935.

59. JACOBS, B. J., and SCHWEITZER, R. "Conceptualizing Structure in a Day Treatment Program for Delinquent Adolescents," *American Journal of Orthopsychiatry,* 49 (1979):246–251.

60. JENKINS, R. L. "Status Offenders," *Journal of the American Academy of Child Psychiatry,* 19 (1980):320–325.

61. JOHNSON, V. S. "An Environment for Treating Youthful Offenders: The Robert F. Kennedy Youth Center," *Offender Rehabilitation,* 2 (1977):159–171.

62. JONES, J. D. "Principles of Hospital Treatment of the Aggressive Adolescent," in C. R. Keith, ed., *The Aggressive Adolescent.* New York: Free Press, 1984, pp. 359–400.

63. JONES, N. B., et al. "Aggression, Crying and Physical Contact in One- to Three-Year-Old Children," *Aggressive Behavior,* 5 (1979):121–133.

64. KALOGERAKIS, M. "Due Process in Family Court," in S. C. Feinstein and R. L. Giovacchini, eds., *Adolescent Psychiatry,* vol. 7. Chicago: University of Chicago Press, 1979, pp. 497–502.

65. KAPLAN, S. "Behavior Modification as a Limit-Setting Task in Family Psychotherapy of a Disruptive Boy," *Journal of the American Academy of Child Psychiatry,* 18 (1979): 492–504.

66. KASHANI, J. H., et al. "Patterns of Delinquency in Girls and Boys," *Journal of the American Academy of Child Psychiatry,* 19 (1980):300–310.

67. KASHANI, J. H., et al. "Depression in Diagnostic Subtypes of Delinquent Boys," *Adolescence,* 17 (1982):943–949.

68. KEITH, C. R. "Individual Psychotherapy and Psychoanalysis with the Aggressive Adolescent," in C. R. Keith, ed., *The Aggressive Adolescent.* New York: Free Press, 1984, pp. 191–208.

69. KELLAM, S. G., BROWN, C. H., and FLEMING, J. P. "Developmental Epidemiological Studies of Substance Use in Woodlawn: Implications for Prevention Research Strategy" (National Institute on Drug Abuse: Research Monograph Series), 41 (1982):21–33.

70. KENDALL, P. C., and WILCOX, L. E. "Cognitive-behavioral Treatment for Impulsivity: Concrete Versus Conceptual Training in Non-Self-Controlled Problem Children," *Journal of Consulting Clinical Psychology,* 48 (1980):80–91.

71. KHAJAWALI, A. M., ERICKSON, T. B., and SIMPSON, G. M. "Chronic Phencyclidine Abuse and Physical Assault," *American Journal of Psychiatry,* 139 (1982):1604–1606.

72. KINARD, E. M. "Emotional Development in Physically Abused Children," *American Journal of Orthopsychiatry,* 50 (1980):686–696.

73. KRAUSS, J. "Juvenile Drug Abuse and Delinquency: Some Differential Associations," *British Journal of Psychiatry,* 139 (1981):422–430.

74. KUHNLEY, E. J., HENDREN, R. L., and QUINLAN, D. M. "Fire-setting by Children," *Journal of the American Academy of Child Psychiatry,* 21 (1982):560–563.

75. LAMIELL, J. T. "Discretion in Juvenile Justice, A Framework for Systematic Study," *Criminal Justice and Behavior,* 6 (1979):76–101.

76. LANE, B. A. "The Relationship of Learning Disabilities to Juvenile Delinquency: Current Status," *Journal of Learning Disabilities,* 13 (1980):20–29.

77. LANE, S., and ZAMORA, P. "A Method for Treating the Adolescent Sex Offender," in *The Violent Juvenile Offender Anthology.* San Francisco: The National Council of Crime and Delinquency, 1984, pp. 347–362.

78. LANGHORNE, J. E., LONEY, J., and PATERNITE, E. "Childhood Hyperkinesis: A Return to the Source," *Journal of Abnormal Psychology,* 85 (1976):201–209.

79. LAVIN, G. K., TRABKA, S., and KAHN, E. M. "Group Therapy with Aggressive and Delinquent Adolescents," in C. R. Keith, ed., *The Aggressive Adolescent.* New York: Free Press, 1984, pp. 240–267.

80. LEFKOWITZ, M. M., et al. *Growing Up to be Violent: A Longitudinal Study of the Development of Aggression.* New York: Pergamon Press, 1977.

81. LEVENTHAL, B. L. "The Neuropharmacology of Violent and Aggressive Behavior in Children and Adolescents," in C. R. Keith, ed., *The Aggressive Adolescent.* New York: Free Press, 1984, pp. 299–358.

82. LEWIS, D. O. "Psychobiologic Vulnerabilities to Delinquency," *Journal of the American Academy of Child Psychiatry,* 17 (1978):193–196.

83. ———. "Diagnostic Evaluation of the Delinquent Child: Psychiatric, Psychological, Neurological and Educational Components," in D. H. Schetsky and E. P. Benedek, *Child Psychiatry and the Law.* New York: Brunner/Mazel, 1980, pp. 139–155.

84. LEWIS, D. O., ed., *Vulnerabilities to Delinquency.* New York: SP Medical and Scientific Books, 1981.

85. LEWIS, D. O., and SHANOK, S. S. "Delinquency and the Schizophrenic Spectrum," *Journal of the American Academy of Child Psychiatry,* 17 (1978):263–276.

86. ———. "A Comparison of the Medical Histories of Incarcerated Delinquent Children and a Matched Sample of Nondelinquent Children," *Child Psychiatry and Human Development,* 9 (1979):210–214.

87. ———. "The Use of a Correctional Setting for Follow-up Care of Psychiatrically Disturbed Adolescents," *American Journal of Psychiatry,* 137 (1980):953–955.

88. LEWIS, D. O., SHANOK, S. S., and BALLA, D. A. "Toward Understanding the Fathers of Delinquents: Psychodynamic, Medical and Genetic Perspectives," in E. N. Rexford, ed., *A Developmental Approach to Problems of Acting Out,* rev. ed. New York: International Universities Press, 1978, pp. 137–152.

89. LEWIS, D. O., SHANOK, S. S., and PINCUS, J. H. "A Comparison of the Neuropsychiatric Status of Female and Male Incarcerated Delinquents: Some Evidence of Sex and Race Bias," *Journal of the American Academy of Child Psychiatry,* 21 (1982):190–196.

90. LEWIS, D. O., et al. "Psychiatric Correlates of Severe Reading Disabilities in an Incarcerated Delinquent Population," *Journal of the American Academy of Child Psychiatry,* 19 (1980):611–622.

91. LEWIS, D. O., et al. "Race Bias in the Diagnosis and Disposition of Violent Adolescents," *American Journal of Psychiatry,* 137 (1980):1211–1216.

92. LEWIS, D. O., et al. "Psychomotor Epilepsy and Violence in a Group of Incarcerated Adolescent Boys," *American Journal of Psychiatry,* 139 (1982):882–887.

93. LEWIS, D. O., et al. "Homicidally Aggressive Young Children: Neuropsychiatric and Experiential Correlates," *American Journal of Psychiatry,* 140 (1983):148–153.

94. LEWIS, M. "Comments on Some Ethical, Legal and Clinical Issues Affecting Consent in Treatment, Organ Transplants and Research in Children," *Journal of the American Academy of Child Psychiatry,* 20 (1981):581–596.

95. LIMENTANI, A. "From Denial to Self Awareness: A Twenty-Year Study of A Case of Childhood Delinquency Evolving into Adult Neurosis," *British Journal of Medical Psychology,* 54 (1981):175–186.

96. LOEBER, R., WEISSMAN, W., and REID, J. B. "Family Interactions of Assaultive Adolescents, Stealers, and Nondelinquents," *Journal of Abnormal Child Psychology,* 11 (1983):1–14.

97. MCCARTHY, J. B. "Narcissism and the Self in Homicidal Adolescents," *American Journal of Psychoanalysis,* 38 (1978):19–29.

98. MACCOBY, E. E., and JACKLIN, C. N. "Sex Differences in Aggression: A Rejoinder and Reprise," *Child Development,* 51 (1980):964–980.

99. MAIN, M., and STADTMAN, J. "Infant Response to Rejection of Physical Contact by the Mother," *Journal of the American Academy of Child Psychiatry,* 20 (1981):292–307.

100. MAIURO, R. D., TURPIN, E., and JAMES, J. "Sex Role Differentiation in a Female Juvenile Delinquent Population," *American Journal of Orthopsychiatry,* 53 (1983):345–352.

101. MALMQUIST, C. P. *Handbook of Adolescence.* New York: Jason Aronson, 1978.

102. ———. "Juveniles in Adult Courts: Unresolved Ambivalence," in S. C. Feinstein and P. L. Giovacchini, eds., *Adolescent Psychiatry,* vol. 7. Chicago: University of Chicago Press, 1979, pp. 444–456.

103. MANNARINO, A. P., and MARSH, W. E. "The Relationship Between Sex Role Identity and Juvenile Delinquency in Adolescent Girls," *Adolescence,* 13 (1978):643–652.

104. MAROHN, R. C. "Adolescent Violence: Causes and Treatment," *Journal of the American Academy of Child Psychiatry,* 21 (1982):354–360.

105. MAROHN, R. C., et al., *Juvenile Delinquents: Psychodynamic Assessment and Hospital Treatment.* New York: Brunner/Mazel, 1980.

106. MARSHALL, R. J. "Antisocial Youth," in J. D. Noshpitz, ed., *Basic Handbook of Child Psychiatry,* vol. 3 New York: Basic Books, 1979, pp. 536–554.

107. MASTERSON, J. F. *From Borderline Adolescent to Functioning Adult: The Test of Time.* New York: Brunner/Mazel, 1980.

108. MATTSSON, A. "Psychoendocrine Aspects of Male Delinquency and Aggression," in D. O. Lewis, ed., *Vulnerabilities to Delinquency.* New York: SP Medical and Scientific Books, 1981, pp. 205–219.

109. MATTSSON, A., et al. "Plasma Testosterone, Aggressive Behavior and Personality Dimensions in Young Male Delinquents," *Journal of the American Academy of Child Psychiatry,* 19 (1980):476–490.

110. MAZUR, A. "Hormones, Aggression and Dominance in Humans," in B. B. Svare, ed., *Hormones and Aggressive Behavior.* New York: Plenum Press, 1983, pp. 563–576.

111. MEDNICK, S. A., and HUTCHINGS, B. "Genetic and Psychophysiological Factors in Asocial Behavior," *Journal of the American Academy of Child Psychiatry,* 17 (1978):209–223.

112. MEYER-BAHLBURG, H. F., and EHRHARDT, A. A. "Prenatal Sex Hormones and Human Aggression: A Review, and New Data on Progestogen Effects," *Aggressive Behavior,* 8 (1982):39–62.

113. MEZZICH, A. "Exploring Diagnostic Formulations for Violent Delinquent Adolescents," *Bulletin of the American Academy of Psychiatry and Law,* 10 (1982):61–67.

114. MIKKELSEN, E. J. "Efficacy of Neuroleptic Medica-

tion in Pervasive Developmental Disorders of Childhood," *Schizophrenia Bulletin,* 8 (1982):320–332.

115. MILLER, P. Y. "Female Delinquency: Fact and Fiction," in M. Sugar, ed., *Female Adolescent Development.* New York: Brunner/Mazel, 1979, pp. 115–140.

116. MITCHELL, S., and ROSA, P. "Boyhood Behavior Problems as Precursors of Criminality: A Fifteen-year Follow-up Study," *Journal of Child Psychology and Psychiatry,* 22 (1981):19–33.

117. MONAHAN, J. "The Prediction of Violent Behavior: Toward a Second Generation of Theory and Policy," *American Journal of Psychiatry,* 141 (1984):10–15.

118. MOORE, D. R., CHAMBERLAIN, P., and MUKAI, L. H. "Children at Risk for Delinquency: A Follow-up Comparison of Aggressive Children and Children Who Steal," *Journal of Abnormal Child Psychology,* 17 (1979):345–355.

119. MOYER, K. E. *The Psychobiology of Aggression.* New York: Harper & Row, 1976.

120. MURRAY, C. A. *The Link between Learning Disabilities and Juvenile Delinquency.* Washington, D.C.: National Institute for Juvenile Justice and Delinquency Prevention, U.S. Department of Justice, 1976.

121. MURRAY, C. A., and COX, L. A. *Beyond Probation,* Beverly Hills, Calif.: Sage Publications, 1979.

122. NEEDLEMAN, H. L., and BELLINGER, D. C. "The Epidemiology of Low-level Lead Exposure in Childhood," *Journal of the American Academy of Child Psychiatry,* 20 (1981):496–512.

123. OFFER, D., MAROHN, R. C., and OSTOV, E., *The Psychological World of the Juvenile Delinquent.* New York: Basic Books, 1979.

124. OFFORD, D. R., and JONES, M. B. "Skill Development: A Community Intervention Program for the Prevention of Antisocial Behavior," in S. B. Guze, F. J. Earls, and J. E. Barrett, eds., *Child Psychopathology and Development.* New York: Raven Press, 1983, pp. 165–188.

125. OFFORD, D. R., ALLEN, N., and ABRAMS, N. "Parental Psychiatric Illness, Broken Homes and Delinquency," *Journal of the American Academy of Child Psychiatry,* 17 (1978):224–238.

126. OFFORD, D. R., et al. "Broken Homes, Parental Psychiatric Illness, and Female Delinquency," *American Journal of Orthopsychiatry,* 49 (1979):252–264.

127. OFFORD, D. R., et al. "Delinquency and Hyperactivity," *Journal of Nervous and Mental Disease,* 167 (1979): 734–741.

128. OLWEUS, D. "Antisocial Behavior in the School Setting," in R. D. Hare and D. Schalling, *Psychopathic Behavior: Approaches to Research.* New York: John Wiley & Sons, 1978, pp. 319–327.

129. ———. "Familial and Temperamental Determinants of Aggressive Behavior in Adolescent Boys: A Causal Analysis," *Developmental Psychology,* 16 (1980):644–660.

130. PALUSZNY, M., and McNABB, M. "Therapy of a Six-Year-Old Who Committed Fratricide," *Journal of the American Academy of Child Psychiatry,* 14 (1975):319–336.

131. PARENS, H. *The Development of Aggression in Early Childhood.* New York: Jason Aronson, 1979.

132. PETTI, T. "The Juvenile Murderer," in D. H. Schedsky, and E. P. Benedek, eds., *Child Psychiatry and the Law.* New York: Brunner/Mazel, 1980, pp. 194–203.

133. PFEFFER, C. "Psychiatric Hospital Treatment of Assaultive Homicidal Children," *American Journal of Psychotherapy,* 34 (1980):197–207.

134. PFEFFER, C. R., PLUTCHIK, R., and MIZRUCHI, M. S. "Predictors of Assaultiveness in Latency Age Children," *American Journal of Psychiatry,* 140 (1983):31–35.

135. ———. "Suicidal and Assaultive Behavior in Children: Classification, Measurement, and Interrelations," *American Journal of Psychiatry,* 140 (1983):154–157.

136. PINCUS, J. H., and TUCKER, G. J. "Violence in Children and Adults: A Neurological View," *Journal of the American Academy of Child Psychiatry,* 17 (1978):277–288.

137. POLLIT, E. "Nutrition, Cognition, and Behavioral Adjustment: In Search of a Connection," in D. O. Lewis, ed., *Vulnerabilities to Delinquency.* New York: SP Medical and Scientific Books, 1981, pp. 241–266.

138. PRINZ, R. J., CONNOR, P. A., and WILSON, C. C. "Hyperactive and Aggressive Behaviors in Childhood: Intertwined Dimensions," *Journal of Abnormal Child Psychology,* 9 (1981):191–202.

139. PUIG-ANTICH, J. "Major Depression and Conduct Disorder in Prepuberty," *Journal of the American Academy of Child Psychiatry,* 21 (1982):118–128.

140. QUAY, H. C. "Residential Treatment," in H. C. Quay and J. S. Werry, eds., *Psychopathological Disorders of Childhood,* 2nd ed., New York: John Wiley & Sons, 1979, pp. 387–410.

141. RATEY, J. J., MORRILL, R., and OXENKRUG, G. "Use of Propranolol for Provoked and Unprovoked Episodes of Rage," *American Journal of Psychiatry,* 140 (1983):1356–1357.

142. REINISCH, J. M. "Prenatal Exposure to Synthetic Progestins Increases Potential for Aggression in Humans," *Science,* 211 (1981):1171–1173.

143. REXFORD, E. N. "A Selective Review of the Literature," in E. N. Rexford, ed., *A Developmental Approach to Problems of Acting Out,* rev. ed. New York: International Universities Press, 1978, pp. 249–326.

144. ROBBINS, D. M., et al. "Learning Disability and Neuropsychological Impairment in Adjudicated Unincarcerated Male Delinquents," *Journal of the American Academy of Child Psychiatry,* 22 (1983):40–46.

145. ROBINS, L. N. "Follow-up Studies," in H. C. Quay, and J. S. Werry, eds., *Psychopathological Disorders of Childhood,* 2nd ed. New York: John Wiley & Sons, 1979, pp. 483–513.

146. ———. "Epidemiological Approaches to Natural History Research: Antisocial Disorders in Children," *Journal of the American Academy of Child Psychiatry,* 20 (1981): 556–580.

147. ROBINS, L. N. and WISH, E. "Childhood Deviance as a Developmental Process," *Social Forces,* 56 (1977):448–471.

148. ROFF, M. "Long-term Follow-up of Juvenile and Adult Delinquency with Samples Differing in Some Important Respects: Cross-validation Within the Same Program," in J. Strauss, H. M. Babigian, and M. Roff, eds., *The Origins and Course of Psychopathology.* New York: Plenum Press, 1977, pp. 323–343.

149. ROGENESS, G. A., et al. "Biochemical Differences in Children with Conduct Disorder Socialized and Undersocialized," *American Journal of Psychiatry,* 139 (1982):307–311.

150. RUDOLPH, J. "Aggression in the Service of the Ego and the Self," *Journal of the American Psychoanalytic Association,* 29 (1981):559–579.

151. RUTTER, M. "Invulnerability, or Why Some Children Are Not Damaged by Stress," in J. J. Shamsie, ed., *New Directions in Children's Mental Health.* New York: SP Medical and Scientific Books, 1979, pp. 53–75.

152. ———. *Changing Youth in a Changing Society.* Cambridge, Mass.: Harvard University Press, 1980.

153. ———. "The City and the Child," *American Journal of Orthopsychiatry,* 51 (1981):610–625.

154. ———. "Psychological Therapies: Issues and Pros-

pects," in S. B. Guze, F. J. Earls, and J. E. Barrett, eds., *Child Psychopathology and Development.* New York: Raven Press, 1983, pp. 139–164.

155. RUTTER, M., and GILLER, H. *Juvenile Delinquency: Trends and Perspectives.* Harmondsworth, U.K.: Penguin Press, 1983.

156. RUTTER, M., et al. *Fifteen Thousand Hours.* Cambridge, Mass.: Harvard University Press, 1979.

157. SACKS, H. S., and SACKS, H. L. "Status Offenders: Emerging Issues and New Approaches," in D. H. Schetky and E. P. Benedek, *Child Psychiatry and the Law.* New York: Brunner/Mazel, 1980, pp. 156–193.

158. SANDER, M. *Psychopharmacology of Aggression.* New York: Raven Press, 1979.

159. SATTERFIELD, J. H. "The Hyperactive Child Syndrome: A Precursor of Adult Psychopathy?" in R. D. Hare and D. Schalling eds., *Psychopathic Behavior: Approaches to Research.* New York: John Wiley & Sons, 1978, pp. 329–346.

160. SCHMIDEBERG, M. "The Treatment of a Juvenile 'Psychopath,' " *International Journal of Offender Therapy and Comparative Criminology,* 22 (1978):21–28.

161. SCHUCKIT, M. A., PETRICH, J., and CHILES, J. "Hyperactivity: Diagnostic Confusion," Journal of Nervous and Mental Disease, 166 (1978):79–87.

162. SHAFFER, D. "Diagnostic Considerations in Suicidal Behavior in Children and Adolescents," *Journal of the American Academy of Child Psychiatry,* 21 (1982):414–416.

163. SHAFFER, D., and FISHER, P. "The Epidemiology of Suicide in Children and Young Adolescents," *Journal of the American Academy of Child Psychiatry,* 20 (1981):545–565.

164. SHAFFER, D., MEYER-BAHLBURG, H.F.L., and STOKMAN, C.L.J. "The Development of Aggression," in N. Rutter, ed., *Scientific Foundations of Developmental Psychiatry.* Baltimore, Md.: University Park Press, 1981.

165. SHAMSIE, J. J. "Antisocial Adolescents: Our Treatments Do Not Work—Where Do We Go From Here?" in S. Chess and A. Thomas, eds., *Annual Progress in Child Psychiatry and Child Development.* New York: Brunner/Mazel, 1982, pp. 631–647.

166. SHANOK, S. S. "On Protecting the Status Offender from the Juvenile Justice System," *Journal of the American Academy of Child Psychiatry,* 19 (1980):326–327.

167. SHANOK, S. S., et al. "A Comparison of Delinquent and Nondelinquent Adolescent Psychiatric Inpatients," *American Journal of Psychiatry,* 140 (1983):582–585.

168. SHERICK, I. "Adoption and Disturbed Narcissism: A Case Illustration of a Latency Boy," *Journal of the American Psychoanalytic Association,* 31 (1983):487–514.

169. SIASSI, I. J. "Lithium Treatment of Impulsive Behavior in Children," *Journal of Clinical Psychiatry,* 43 (1982): 482–484.

170. SMITH, R. M., and WALTERS, J. "Delinquent and Nondelinquent Males' Perceptions of Their Fathers," *Adolescence,* 13 (1978):21–28.

171. SONIS, M. "Aicchorn Revisited: A Report on Acting Out Behavior," in S. C. Feinstein and P. L. Giovacchini, eds., *Adolescent Psychiatry,* vol. 7. Chicago: University of Chicago Press, 1979, pp. 484–496.

172. STEWART, M. A., and LEONE, L. "A Family Study of Unsocialized Aggressive Boys," *Biological Psychiatry,* 13 (1978):107–117.

173. STEWART, M. A., et al. "The Overlap Between Hyperactive and Unsocialized, Aggressive Children," *Journal of Child Psychology and Psychiatry,* 22 (1981):35–45.

174. STRASBURG, P. A. *Violent Delinquents* (report to the Ford Foundation from the Vera Institute of Justice). New York: Sovereign Books, 1978.

175. STUMPHAUZER, J. S., ed. *Progress in Behavior Therapy with Delinquents.* Springfield, Ill.: Charles C Thomas, 1979.

176. STUMPHAUZER, J. S., VELOZ, E. V., and AIKEN, T. W. "Violence by Street Gangs: East Side Story?" in R. B. Stuart, ed., *Violent Behavior: Social Learning Approaches to Prediction, Management and Treatment.* New York: Brunner/Mazel, 1981, pp. 68–82.

177. SURWILLO, W. W. "The Electroencephalogram and Childhood Aggression," *Aggressive Behavior,* 6 (1980):9–18.

178. TIEGER, T. "On the Biological Basis of Sex Differences in Aggression," *Child Development,* 51 (1980):943–963.

179. TINKLENBERG, J. R., and OCHBERG, F. M. "Patterns of Adolescent Violence: A California Sample," in D. A. Hamburg and M. D. Trudeau, eds., *Biobehavioral Aspects of Aggression.* New York: Adam R. Liss, 1981, pp. 121–140.

180. TITTLE, C. R., and VILLEMEZ, W. J. "Social Class and Criminality," *Social Forces,* 56 (1977):474–502.

181. TOOLEY, K. "The Small Assassins: Clinical Notes on a Subgroup of Murderous Children," *Journal of the Academy of Child Psychiatry,* 14 (1975):306–318.

182. VALZELLI, L. *Psychobiology of Aggression and Violence.* New York: Raven Press, 1981.

183. VARLEY, W. H. "Behavior Modification Approaches to the Aggressive Adolescent," in C. R. Keith, ed., *The Aggressive Adolescent.* New York: Free Press, 1984, pp. 268–298.

184. VOORHEES, J. "Neuropsychological Differences Between Juvenile Delinquents and Functional Adolescents: A Preliminary Study," *Adolescence,* 16 (1981):57–66.

185. WADSWORTH, M. *Roots of Delinquency,* Oxford: Martin Robertson and Company, 1979.

186. WEISS, B. "Food Additives and Environmental Chemicals as Sources of Childhood Behavior Disorders," *Journal of the American Academy of Child Psychiatry,* 21 (1982):144–152.

187. WEISS, G., et al. "Hyperactives as Young Adults," *Archives of General Psychiatry,* 36 (1979):657–687.

188. WILLIAMS, D. T., et al. "The Effect of Propranolol on Uncontrolled Rage Outbursts in Children and Adolescents with Organic Brain Dysfunction," *Journal of the American Academy of Child Psychiatry,* 21 (1982):129–135.

189. WILSON, J. Q. *Thinking about Crime.* New York: Basic Books, 1983.

190. WIZNER, S. "Punishing the Innocent," *Journal of the American Academy of Child Psychiatry,* 19 (1980):328–333.

191. WOLF, E. S. "Tomorrow's Self: Heinz Kohut's Contribution to Adolescent Psychiatry," *Adolescent Psychiatry,* 8 (1980):41–50.

192. WOLFGANG, M. E. "Real and Perceived Changes of Crime and Punishment," *Daedalus,* 108 (1978):143–157.

193. WOODS, B. T., and EBY, M. D. "Excessive Mirror Movements and Aggression," *Biological Psychiatry,* 17 (1982):23–32.

194. YEUDALL, L. T. "Neuropsychological Concomitants of Persistent Criminal Behavior," Paper presented at the annual meeting of the Ontario Psychological Association, 1979.

195. YOUNGERMAN, J. K., and CANINO, I. A. "Violent Kids, Violent Parents: Family Pharmacotherapy," *American Journal of Orthopsychiatry,* 53 (1983):152–156.

196. ZANG, L. E. "The Antisocial Aggressive School-Age Child: Day Hospitals," in B. Wolman, J. Egan, and A. Ross, eds., *Handbook of Treatment of Mental Disorders in Childhood and Adolescence.* Englewood Cliffs, N.J.: Prentice-Hall, 1978, pp. 317–329.

197. ZIMMERMAN, R. L., and HEISTAD, G. T. "Studies of the Long Term Efficacy of Anti-psychotic Drugs in Control-

ling the Behavior of Institutionalized Retardates," *Journal of the American Academy of Child Psychiatry,* 21 (1982):136–143.

198. ZINN, D. "Therapeutic and Preventive Interventions

in Juvenile Delinquency," in G. P. Sholevar, R. M. Benson, and B. S. Blinder, eds., *Treatment of Emotional Disorders in Children and Adolescents.* New York: Spectrum Publications, 1980, pp. 535–539.

14 / The Chronically Ill or Disabled Child

Carl Feinstein and Karen Berger

Introduction

The presence of a childhood disability or chronic illness constitutes a substantial and unique stress on both the development of the child and on the life course and adaptation of the parents and other family members. For the child, possible adverse consequences include both direct emotional/behavioral symptomatology and secondary psychosocially based limitations in adaptive functioning. The family members face similar risks. In addition, successful adaptation by the parents requires the development of exceptional resources for coping. To begin with, the parents must incorporate the demands of caring for a disabled child into the family routines, without overly disrupting their personal and vocational lives. More than that, however, they must cope with personal grief, negative attitudes on the part of society toward their child, and, often enough, limited future opportunities as the child moves toward adulthood.

The Disabled Child: Recent Trends

Prior to 1970, the literature emphasized psychological features of children with various specific disabilities. Most of these studies suffered from serious methodological problems, including lack of standardized assessment procedures and absence of control groups. The last decade has seen much improvement in the way such studies have been conducted. Considerable progress has been made regarding the issue of whether many specific disabilities or chronic illnesses in childhood are correlated with psychopathology. This approach, however, fails to provide a theoretical model that indicates either the mechanisms of action by

which psychopathology develops or the nature of any protective psychosocial factors that could promote mental health. Only such a conceptual approach can provide the structure for either rational clinical intervention or primary prevention.

In this chapter, advances in the sociology of disabling conditions, studies of the educational environment of the disabled child, family responses to disability, and both parental and child coping responses are integrated with recent data regarding psychopathology and other outcome measures. The goal is to achieve a first approximation of a much-needed developmental theory of disabling conditions. The principle question may be stated as follows: How does the development of disabled or chronically ill children differ from that of nondisabled ones? A subsidiary but clinically crucial question is: In the course of the psychiatric evaluation of the chronically ill child, what specific additional information related to chronic illness or disability must be obtained?

The theoretical approach we have found most helpful in organizing this highly complex topic is that embodied in the literature on stress, vulnerability, and coping. This approach postulates "vulnerability factors" and "protective factors" residing in individuals or groups that, in the presence of a stressor, serve either to increase or to decrease the likelihood that those subject to the stressor will suffer an unfavorable outcome. [83] Due to the absence of prospective longitudinal studies of chronically ill or disabled children, reference will be made to research done on children at risk from other psychosocial factors. It is understood that such analogies are partial at best and must also be confirmed by further research on the population in question.

For the chronically ill or disabled child, the specific biological deficit constitutes the primary stressor. However, the presence of this biological deficit sets off a complex chain of secondary stressors. Proceeding from the more general to the more specific, these stressors may originate in the overall social environment, the educational environment, or the family. Individually or in concert, they greatly increase the risk of impaired adaptation by the child. In particular, the social situation of the family, the personality structure of the parents, and the temperamental characteristics of the child are critical sites where the presence or absence of protective factors may determine whether psychopathology or poor adaptation results.

Disability, Chronic Illness, and Handicap: Definitions

Chronic illness may be defined as a medical disorder with a protracted course. The disorder may be progressive and ultimately fatal, or it may be stable in character but lifelong in duration and result in impaired physical or cognitive functioning. The more stable form of impairment is referred to as a disability. Pless and Pinkerton,[75] defined the *illness* as the biological substrate of the disability. The *disability* represents the direct behaviorial manifestations of the biological problem—that is, the limitation of functioning imposed directly by the illness.

In the more recent literature,[33,57,75] *handicap* has been conceptualized as an amalgamation of the disability with the chronic effect of adverse psychosocial influences. For example, by the time severely disabled children reach adolescence, many aspects of their rehabilitation have been made more difficult by the immense practical and emotional stress that these conditions, and the ensuing difficulty in coping, have thrust upon the youngsters, their parents, and their educators. Thus the disability may be compounded by maladaptive emotional and behavioral sequelae.

DEMOGRAPHICS

It has proven quite difficult to obtain an accurate count of the number of chronically ill or disabled children and adolescents in the United States. Based on data and projections from Kakalik,[50] Pless and Roghmann,[76] and the United Kingdom National Survey of Children and the Isle of Wight Study,[16] it can be estimated that, by using a broad definition, between 10 and 12 percent (or approximately 9.5 million) of American youths may be considered handicapped. Reynolds[82] reviews the effect of the Education for All Handicapped Children Act (Public Law 94–142) on current knowledge of the prevalence of handicapping conditions in childhood. According to this study, of

the 10 to 12 percent of children thus classified, a large majority have diagnoses of learning disability, speech impairment, mental retardation, and emotional disturbance. Approximately 3 percent of all children may be considered to have distinct chronic physical handicaps or illnesses not in the just-cited categories. Prior to Public Law 94–142 and its mandated seeking out of all handicapped children, large numbers of children, especially adolescents, remained outside the educational and health care delivery systems and were not reliably included in any statistics. These youngsters have subsequently been identified by state child-find programs.[82]

The Social Matrix of the Chronically Ill or Disabled Child

There has been a steady and massive accumulation of evidence that the psychosocial matrix in which the chronically ill child develops is distinctly and unfavorably different from that of the nonhandicapped child. Negative social attitudes permeate the daily lives of disabled persons. Goffman, in 1963,[31] described the social stigma attached to disability. Kleck, Ono, and Hastorf[53] delineated the characteristic behavioral responses of normal individuals in social encounter with disabled persons. These responses include: a constricted range of interactions, less openness and spontaneity, and a strong pressure to terminate the social engagement. This social response is further complicated by superficial efforts on the part of the nondisabled individual to deny awareness of either the disability or the disfigurement.[80]

Many authors have reported that the social interactions between disabled and nondisabled individuals are frequently accompanied by uncertainty, anxiety, and discomfort.[39,40] These repetitive, shallow, and uncomfortable interpersonal experiences profoundly affect the self-image and self-esteem of the disabled child and adolescent.

Children's attitudes toward disabled individuals have been studied by a number of researchers.[86,100,103,104] In these studies, children consistently indicate a preference for interacting with able-bodied peers rather than with disabled children. Furthermore, negative attitudes toward the disabled child increase with age; older children show greater bias than younger ones.[104] Facially disfigured children constituted the most rejected category. Wheelchair users are also among the most rejected.[27] The disfigured or crippled adolescent is particularly likely to experience avoidance and exclusion by peers.[94]

With regard to the nonpeer school environment, many authors have documented negative attitudes and expectations of teachers,[34,63] rehabilitation workers,[93] and medical providers.[24] Breslau and Mortimer[10] established that continuity of care is a critical factor that must be present in order to provide useful medical support for chronically ill adolescents and their families. Unfortunately, a large proportion of chronically ill adolescents receive *less,* and *less consistent,* care during these years than they did as younger children.[15,67,74]

From a future-oriented perspective, Gliedman and Roth[30] have described "the sociological destiny of the disabled," which includes a greater probability of unemployment, lower wages, lower educational attainments, more frequent divorces, more frequent hospitalizations, and a greater likelihood of social isolation than is true for their able-bodied peers.

Educational Issues Regarding Disabled Children

During the last decade, the dominant educational issue for the handicapped child has been the impact of PL 94-142, the Education for All Handicapped Children Act, which was passed by Congress in 1975 and became fully effective in the fall of 1978. This law mandates that public schools provide free, appropriate, public education to all handicapped children in the "least restrictive environment." Local school districts must search out all handicapped children, make a multidisciplinary assessment of each, and formulate an Individualized Educational Plan (IEP). The principles of due process are guaranteed. These stipulate the right of parents to participate in placement decisions and to appeal decisions for their disabled children.[82] In practice, the school district's IEP responsibilities include planning for necessary medical services and arranging for diagnostic studies. Thus this legislation represents a major loss of initiative and influence for the medical profession.[82]

The provision of PL 94-142 mandating "appropriate education" has greatly expanded the range of instructional requirements for the schools, requiring them, in addition to the traditional "three R's," to teach severely handicapped students to walk, feed themselves, use the toilet on their own, and develop other basic skills in the "activities of daily living."[82] Another consequence of this "child-find" policy has been the entrance of approximately one million previously unserved severely disabled children into the public school system.[110]

The provision of PL 94-142 mandating "the least restrictive environment" has been interpreted generally to mean that, whenever possible, special education and related services should be delivered in regular education classrooms, a practice frequently referred to as "mainstreaming."[82] The handicapped student may be placed in special classes or separate schools only for a limited time when the placement can be justified, and then only to achieve clearly stated objectives.

Underlying the mainstreaming provision in PL 94-142 is the philosophical position that placement in special institutions or in special educational classrooms stigmatizes the handicapped child and results in a vicious cycle of lower expectations and lower performance, which prevents him or her from developing the social skills necessary to function as an adult in the real world.[82,110] However, there are serious unanswered questions regarding whether or not mainstreaming is truly advantageous for all these children.* Research is lacking that would enable rational decisions to be made regarding just which children with which handicaps actually do benefit from mainstreaming.[18]

Unfortunately, many school districts, facing financial shortages, have interpreted "least restrictive" as "least expensive."[110] As a result, vulnerable children are being placed in regular classrooms without support services or special teacher training. Social stigmatization and social isolation, with consequent damage to already precarious self-esteem, are major problems for these children.[71,87,108]

Given a critical lack of research in this area, it can only be said that the choice of classroom placement of a child with visible or severe disabilities must take into account a wide range of psychological and emotional factors. Where mainstreaming is the best alternative, some form of psychological support may well be necessary.

The Families of Disabled Children

In order to understand the development of the disabled child, it is first necessary to comprehend how the disability affects the family milieu within which the child develops. Numerous factors influence the way parents respond to the chronically ill child. These include general parental coping styles, the parents' social support system, possible vulnerability factors predisposing toward parental psychopathology, and the marital relationship. The parental response is also influenced by the disability characteristics of the child and the child's

*See references 14, 35, 36, 48, 102, and 110.

stage of development. Thus "goodness of fit" may be different as each parent interacts with the chronically ill child at different ages. Unsolved problems in the parental or family adjustment to the chronically ill child may result in overt psychopathology. Of equal importance, however, are the ways in which these problems may alter the general pattern of adaptation for the child, particularly with regard to the development of skills necessary for self-care, independent functioning, and social competence as an adult.

GENERAL FAMILY VULNERABILITY FACTORS

Recent research [12,83] has shown that certain parental attributes are highly significant in determining whether vulnerable children successfully adapt or whether they develop serious social and behavior maladjustments. The Island of Kauai longitudinal study has revealed that chronic poverty, low educational level in the mother, and parental psychopathology are the major parental risk factors in infancy. [105] Parental risk factors in childhood and adolescence include prolonged separations from the infant during the first year of life, paternal mental illness, chronic discord, changes in employment or of residence, divorce of parents, remarriage, and entry of a stepparent into the household. Major parental protective factors include much attention paid to the infant during the first year, a positive parent-child relationship during early childhood, the availability of additional caregivers besides the mother, care by siblings and grandparents, mother having some steady employment outside of the household, availability of kin and neighbors for emotional support, and the presence of structure and rules in the household.

SPECIFIC PARENTAL VULNERABILITY FACTORS

Recent research indicates that having a disabled child both exacerbates the effects of preexisting parent vulnerabilities and creates new ones. Holroyd [44] found that mothers of handicapped children are less able to experience personal development or freedom, are more limited in the use of their time, have poorer health and mood, are more sensitive to how the child fits into the community, and report more family discord. Single mothers experienced these problems to a greater degree than married mothers.

Tavormina and associates [98] found that parents of disabled or chronically ill children have a particular constellation of problems. They, especially the fathers, experience less parenting confidence, feel less influential in their child's behavior, and are less accepting of their child than normal parents. The mothers appeared more "neurotic." Both parents were found to be less extroverted (sociable) than parents without a disabled child. They experience many special problems, including extra demands on their time and energy, a tense home atmosphere, pressure to do "the right thing," and the centering of their lives around their ill child's needs. More recently Friedrich and Friedrich [26] have confirmed that families with handicapped children experience more stress and less marital satisfaction, psychological well-being, and social support.

Problems of depression and "chronic sorrow" have long been attributed to parents of handicapped children. [107] Recently Breslau, Staruch, and Mortimer [11] have confirmed that mothers of disabled children with cystic fibrosis, cerebral palsy, myelodysplasia, or multiple physical handicaps suffer from considerable emotional distress. This study also found that the daily care of the disabled child depletes the parents' energy and time, causing withdrawal from social and cultural activities. Frequent visits to physicians and the many hospitalizations disrupt family life and the parents' employment. They experience financial problems, worries about the future, guilt, isolation, increased marital tension, and parent-child conflicts. The mothers of these disabled children showed significantly more depression and anxiety than randomly selected normal controls. White mothers with handicapped children showed significantly more severe problems with depression, anxiety, and "maternal distress" than black mothers in like circumstances. The critical factor affecting maternal response was not so much the specific illness as it was the level of daily care the child required.

Cummings, Bayley, and Rie [19] have also found that both mothers and fathers of handicapped children suffer from lowered self-esteem and depressive feelings. This is most pronounced for mothers of retarded children, who were found to be more preoccupied with their children and enjoying them less than other mothers. They confirmed Poznanski's [79] observation that parents of chronically ill children were likely to retreat from their own relationships with their neighbors and to discourage socializing by the disabled son or daughter.

This impressive evidence for an increased rate of depression in the mothers of chronically disabled children is of considerable theoretical importance. Recent research by Ferguson and coworkers [23] has addressed the relationship between family life events, maternal depression, and child-rearing problems. They found that the presence or absence of a maternal depressive response, rather than the number of adverse life events, determine whether behavior problems develop in the child.

One may therefore conclude that mothers of chronically ill children are highly vulnerable to depression. This, in turn, heavily predisposes their children to various problems in adjustment. Vulnerability to depression or the absence of protective psychosocial factors against parental depression are therefore critical variables in understanding the development of the chronically ill child.[68]

Specific Factors Affecting Child Rearing

Many lines of research highlight the importance of the parental response to the disabled infant. Bell and Harper[5] have summarized a considerable body of research documenting that infants are powerful elicitors and shapers of parenting behavior. Sameroff and Abbe state[89] that, when confronted with a deviant infant, normal parents behave nonadaptively.

Parents may create risk factors for their disabled infants by means of altered forms of social response. Mintzer and associates[68] found that parents of infants with visible birth defects experience a series of assaults to their self-esteem that compromise their capacity to interact with their new offspring.

A frequently overlooked parenting vulnerability factor is the increased risk of abuse or neglect of the impaired infant. Hunter and coworkers[47] did a prospective study of families of premature and ill newborns and found that approximately 20 percent were at high risk for maltreatment. Of these, 24.4 percent were later abused during the first year of life. This represents a 3.9 percent incidence of abuse or neglect, an eightfold increase of risk in comparison to normal infants. The high-risk families in this study showed a number of vulnerability factors, including severe isolation, inadequate social support, marital maladjustments, financial problems, poor use of medical services, and inadequate child-care arrangements. The abusing parents were found to be impulsive, apathetic, childishly dependent, and often retarded or illiterate.

A major vulnerability factor in the parenting of disabled children is parental overprotectiveness. Poznanski[79] found parental overprotectiveness to be a frequent cause or correlate of passivity and immaturity in disabled children. Resnick[80] reports that for children with cerebral palsy, the degree of parental overprotection is directly correlated with a number of unfavorable psychological outcomes, including unhappiness, poor self-esteem, high anxiety, lower popularity, and greater self-consciousness. It seems likely that parental overprotectiveness is correlated with poor self-help skills and other aspects of independent functioning.[58,66,90] This has never been systematically studied, however.

It is important to note that "overprotectiveness" of the disabled child is not necessarily indicative of psychopathology. A more apt way of viewing this phenomenon is to acknowledge that for such children to learn to cope independently, their parents must develop unusual fortitude in allowing them to encounter an increased measure of pain, failure, or disappointment.

Another parenting issue of the disabled child involves the concept of "goodness of fit." Chess, Fernandez, and Korn[17] found that at different child developmental stages, the parenting response to the disabled child can be quite different. The personality of the parents, the nature of the disability, and the child's personality characteristics at a given age may elicit more or less supportive parenting. Beckman[4] found four behavioral characteristics of the young handicapped child that increase the stress experienced by their mothers. These were difficult temperament, low social responsiveness, repetitive behavior, and quantity of demands on maternal caregiving. These stress-inducing characteristics would all increase the difficulty of caring for these babies and could lead to a compromised quality of mothering.

GENERAL PARENTAL COPING FACTORS

Protective parenting factors have also been the subject of recent research, particularly with regard to styles of coping. Assessments of parental coping compare different adaptive mechanisms and their relative utility for the raising of the handicapped child. McCubbin[60] developed the Coping Health Inventory for Parents (CHIP) to assess parents' coping strategies regarding the management of family life with a chronically ill child. Employing factor analytic techniques, McCubbin found three coping patterns used by the parents of handicapped children: maintaining family integration and cooperation using an optimistic definition of the situation; maintaining social support, self-esteem, and psychological stability; and understanding the medical situation through communication with other parents and consultation with the medical staff.

Intuitively, this method of assessing parents is helpful in understanding the way they organize their lives in response to a handicapped child. It may also shed light on how, through identification with their parents, handicapped children develop various coping styles to deal with their disability. More research is needed in this area to ascertain the relationship between parental coping styles and measures of both psychopathology and adaptation in chronically ill children.

SPECIFIC PARENTAL COPING FACTORS

Family systems theorists have reported the frequent occurrence of a distinctive pattern of relationships in families with a chronically ill child.* In such a family system, the primary caretaker (usually the mother) and

*See references 6, 38, 69, 72, and 101.

the handicapped child develop an exclusive dyad within the family that tends to relegate other family members to the periphery of family life. This family organization may, in turn, have harmful consequences for the marital relationship, limit family coping strategies, and even provoke or exacerbate medical symptomatology.[69]

Studies of Psychopathology

Earlier research tended to show that chronic illness predisposes children to psychopathology.* Rutter, Tizard, and Whitmore,[84] for example, found a twofold increase of psychiatric disorder among chronically ill or disabled children. This group also found that the incidence of psychopathology for chronically ill children with brain involvement was markedly higher than for those without it. Rutter, Dorner, and Sullivan have all reported the high incidence of depression among physically disabled adolescents.[21, 84, 95, 96]

More recently, however, a number of studies have contradicted these findings and have failed to find marked differences in the rate of psychopathology between children with several chronic diseases and normals.[22, 29, 54, 97] According to Breslau,[9] "the belief that chronic illness in children is associated with psychopathology has been replaced by uncertainty."

Breslau[9] has recently reported on the incidence of psychopathology in children suffering from a variety of disabling conditions, including several disorders affecting the central nervous system (CNS), cystic fibrosis, and a normal control group. She confirmed that children with these chronic physical conditions were at increased risk for severe psychiatric impairment. Where the physical conditions involved brain abnormality, the youngsters were more pervasively disturbed. All the disabled groups showed increased psychopathology in two categories: conflict with parents and regressive anxiety. Those CNS-disabled children with mental retardation showed a higher incidence of mentation problems. Isolation was more common in children with CNS problems, even in the absence of mental retardation. These findings, however, are compromised by Breslau's use of a screening psychiatric rating instrument that is nonspecific for psychopathology according to modern diagnostic criteria and that relies entirely on parent ratings. In addition, the inclusion of large numbers of mentally retarded children, for whom a high rate of psychopathology would be expected, introduces additional elements of uncertainty.

*See references 42, 55, 56, 61, 75, and 99.

Emotional problems associated with chronic illness or disability in children have been widely reported. These have included anxiety, resistance to medical treatment, depression, low self-esteem, poor body image, increased emotional dependency, and deficits in social skills.[64, 106] In particular, social isolation has been a common characteristic of children with visible or disfiguring disabilities.[80] More general maladaptive traits such as passivity and immaturity have been widely described as well.[80] Simonds[92] identified a particular pattern of maladaptive coping behaviors in children with poor acceptance of their condition; these behaviors included denial, poor frustration tolerance, rebellion, depression, and self-destructive behavior. However, many of these studies are not well controlled and describe children with widely disparate medical conditions.

Remarkably, there has been almost no research on whether or not important areas of adaptation such as school achievement, vocational competence, or the capacity to function independently are compromised by the general effects of chronic illness or disability. It has recently been observed by Havens[41] that psychiatry in general does not include tests of healthy adaptation.

DISABILITY CHARACTERISTICS

The relationship between illness characteristics and psychological functioning is very complex. Research to date indicates no simple linear relationship between such factors as severity of disability and degree of psychosocial disturbance. Hughes[45] and Levy and Nir[57] recommend that four factors should be considered: (1) whether the condition is visible or nonvisible, (2) the degree of restriction of the child's activities, (3) age of onset of the disease, and (4) severity of the illness. Mattson[65, 66] observed that attempts to derive distinct personality types from different disease entities have been fruitless. However, factors such as conspicuousness of the illness, degree of physical restriction, severity, and the stability or life-threatening aspect of chronic illness may all play an important role in the psychosocial functioning of the chronically ill child.

It has been noted that a fluctuating course of illness or a heightened degree of severity may have a negative impact on psychosocial functioning.[73] Other authors, however, have found that the most severely disabled children may in fact suffer fewer psychiatric disorders than those with milder disabilities.* According to this view, the more mildly disabled suffer more because they are competing with able-bodied peers, but on unequal terms. The most severely disabled individuals have fewer and different expectations and are not competing directly with their able-bodied peers.

*See references 13, 21, 49, 59, 75, and 85.

Several investigators have found that the conspicuousness of the disability is a major consideration, especially during adolescence, when body image, physical appearance, and peer group conformity are important sources of self-esteem.*

The work of Rutter and associates[85] recently confirmed by Breslau,[9] has established that disabilities involving brain damage are at very high risk for severe psychopathology. Sensory deficits also exert a characteristic effect on the psychosocial development of those afflicted with these conditions by limiting important sources of information and experience.[3, 25, 28] Mattson found[65] that illnesses which require strict adherence to a regular treatment regimen, rigid therapeutic schedules, or strict precautionary routines tend to elicit rebellious behavior in some children and adolescents.

In summary, the current state of knowledge indicates that visibility or conspicuousness of the disability, brain damage, and perceptual deficits are associated with distinctive types of psychological problems. Other factors seem to play a part in some children's course of adaptation and not in that of others, perhaps because of additional intervening variables.

OTHER CHILD CHARACTERISTICS AS
COVARIABLES

The role of temperament as a source of either vulnerability or protection has also been noted.[17] Rutter[83] has identified certain protective factors that decrease the vulnerable child's risk status. These included "positive personality dispositions" such as "positive mood" and "flexibility of response." Along a similar vein, Neuchterlein and Garmezy[83] have reported studies of competent black children in the urban ghettos who were at risk as a consequence of chronic poverty and prejudice. Significant personality traits related to the success of these children were strong social skills, social responsiveness, interpersonal sensitivity, cooperation, participation, and emotional stability. These students also had an internal locus of control and a dominant cognitive style of reflectiveness and controlled impulses.

The Island of Kauai study[105] identified temperamental factors that were protective of the at-risk child. These included high activity level, goodnaturedness, an affectionate disposition, social responsiveness, positive social orientation, advanced self-help skills, age-appropriate sensorimotor and perceptual skills, ability to focus attention and control impulses, and internal locus of control.[105]

In summary, it appears that an outgoing, social, and flexible temperament complemented by good impulse

control and sound perceptual and sensorimotor functioning constitute powerful protective factors in vulnerable children. It seems quite likely that these attributes, when present, would be significantly supportive of the chronically ill child as well, although little direct research exists to support this hypothesis.

The issue of social skills is a particularly complicated one in respect to the adjustment of the disabled child. It would seem that a "positive" outgoing temperament would be a protective factor but that this advantage could be undone by repeated harmful social interactions. Evidence for this point is particularly strong in the case of children suffering from disfiguring disabilities. Dorner,[21] Minde,[67] Podeneau-Czehofski,[77] Boyle and associates,[8] Schloss,[91] Blum,[7] and Resnick[81] have all observed that visibly disabled children or adolescents—for example, those with spina bifida, cerebral palsy, and even cystic fibrosis (when obvious physical differences were evident)—all suffer from extreme social isolation. Although it is possible that a primary self-esteem problem related to the disability could inhibit these children socially, it is probably more likely that repeated painful avoidance, rejection, and other problematic social responses on the part of both peers and adults drive them into social isolation. A child or adolescent with a disfiguring condition would have to have an exceptionally outgoing and resilient temperament to avoid succumbing to the tremendous social obstacles interfering with peer relations.

Many researchers have reported a high rate of depression and poor self-esteem in disabled children.* It has been generally assumed that this depression is purely reactive to the disability. Only slight evidence from the work of Kashani[51] or, by extension, from adult studies such as those by Akiskal[1] supports this assumption. Vulnerability or resistance to depression is as likely to be an innate factor for the disabled child, as it is for other individuals. Depression in disabled children could well be influenced by constitutional factors as well as by the psychosocial stress of disability.

Several authors have noted that peer support in the form of friendships and confidant relationships is tremendously helpful to disabled children.[2,43,80,109] Findings now available from psychotherapeutic work utilizing peer support groups give credence to the notion that communication and regular social interaction with peers promote psychological adaptation.[46,62,88]

Minde[67] has documented the fact that disabled children who associate with both handicapped and healthy individuals have a better psychological outcome. Subsequently, several authors have advocated social skills training for these at-risk children.[37,67,78]

---

*See references 8, 32, 43, 52, 64, and 71.

*See references 7, 20, 85, 95, and 96.

Conclusion

In summary, research into the emotional problems of children with chronic illness or disability provides ample confirmation that a sizable subset of these children are suffering emotionally and experiencing diagnosable psychiatric disorder. Conspicuousness of the disability, whether it involves brain damage or perceptual deficits, and whether the disabled child has certain protective temperamental qualities are the most likely intervening variables that interact with the disability and the family, the school, and environmental influences to determine the quality of psychological adaptation.

REFERENCES

1. AKISKAL, H. S. "Dysthymic Disorder: Psychopathology of Proposed Chronic Depressive Subtypes," *American Journal of Psychiatry,* 140 (1983):11–20.
2. ANDERSON, E. M., and KLARKE, L. *Disability in Adolescence.* London: Methuen, 1982.
3. BALIKOV, H., and FEINSTEIN, C. "The Blind Child," in J. D. Noshpitz, ed., *Basic Handbook of Child Psychiatry,* vol. 1. New York: Basic Books, 1979, pp. 413–420.
4. BECKMAN, P. J. "Influence of Selected Child Characteristics on Stress in Families of Handicapped Infants," *American Journal of Mental Deficiency,* 88 (1983): 150–156.
5. BELL, R. Q., and HARPER, L. V. *Child Effects on Adults.* New York: Halsted Press, 1977.
6. BERGER, N., and FOWLKES, M. "Family Intervention Project: A Family Network Model for Serving Young Handicapped Children," *Young Children,* 51 (1980):22–32.
7. BLUM, R. W. *Chronic Illness and Disabilities in Children and Adolescents.* Orlando, Fla.: Grune & Stratton, 1984.
8. BOYLE, I. R., et al. "Emotional Adjustment of Adolescents and Young Adults with Cystic Fibrosis," *Journal of Pediatrics,* 88 (1976):318–326.
9. BRESLAU, N. "Psychiatric Disorder in Children with Physical Disabilities," *Journal of the American Academy of Child Psychiatry,* 24 (1985):87–94.
10. BRESLAU, N., and MORTIMER, E. A. "Seeing the Same Doctor: Determinants of Satisfaction with Speciality Care for Disabled Children," *Medical Care,* 19 (1981):741–758.
11. BRESLAU, N., STARUCH, K., and MORTIMER, E. "Psychological Distress in Mothers of Disabled Children," *American Journal of Diseases of Children,* 136 (1982):682–686.
12. BRISTOL, M. M. "Maternal Coping with Autistic Children: Adequacy of Interpersonal Support and Effects of Child's Characteristics." (Ph.D. diss., University of North Carolina, Chapel Hill, 1979).
13. BRUHN, J. G. "Self-concept and the Control of Diabetes," *American Family Physician,* 15 (1977):93–97.
14. BUDOFF, M., and GOTTLIEB, J. "Special Class Students Mainstreamed: A Study of an Aptitude (Learning Potential) × Treatment Interaction," *American Journal of Mental Deficiency,* 81 (1976):1–11.
15. CARROLL, G., et al. "Adolescents with Chronic Disease," *Journal of Adolescent Health Care,* 4 (1983):261–263.
16. CHARLES, M. "Stark Reality," *Nursing Mirror,* 14 October 1981.
17. CHESS, S., FERNANDEZ, P., and KORN, S. "The Handicapped Child and His Family: Consonance and Dissonance," *Journal of the American Academy of Child Psychiatry,* 19 (1980):56–67.
18. CRUICKSHANK, W. M. "Least Restrictive Placement: Administrative Wishful Thinking," *Journal of Learning Disabilities,* 10 (1977):193–194.
19. CUMMINGS, S. T., BAYLEY, H. C., and RIE, H. E. "The Impact of the Child's Deficiency on the Father: A Study of Fathers of Mentally Retarded and of Chronically Ill Children," *American Journal of Orthopsychiatry,* 46 (1976):246–255.
20. DORNER, S. "The Relationship of Physical Handicap to Stress in Families with an Adolescent with Spina Bifida," *Developmental Medicine and Child Neurology,* 17 (1975):765–776.
21. ———. "Adolescents with Spina Bifida," *Archives of Disease in Childhood,* 51 (1976):439–444.
22. DROTAR, D., et al. "Psychosocial Functioning of Children with Cystic Fibrosis," *Pediatrics,* 67 (1981):338–343.
23. FERGUSSON, D.M., et al. "Relationship of Family Life Events, Maternal Depression, and Child-Rearing Problems," *Pediatrics,* 73 (1984):773–776.
24. FINKLESTEIN, V. *Attitudes and Disabled People: Issues for Discussion.* New York: World Rehabilitation Fund, 1980.
25. FRAIBERG, S. *Insights from the Blind.* New York: New American Library, 1977.
26. FRIEDERICH, W. N., and FRIEDERICH, W. L. "Psychosocial Assets of Parents of Handicapped and Nonhandicapped Children," *American Journal of Mental Deficiency,* 85 (1981):551–553.
27. FRIEDMAN, R.S. "Modeling Behavior of Nondisabled and Disabled Adolescents Based Upon Social Preference for and Similarity to Nondisabled and Disabled Models" (Ph.D. diss., Hofstra University, Hempstead, Long Island, N.Y., 1974).
28. FURTH, H. *Thinking Without Language: Psychological Implications of Deafness.* New York: Free Press, 1966.
29. GAYTON, W. F., et al. "Children with Cystic Fibrosis: Psychological Test Findings of Patients, Siblings, and Parents," *Pediatrics,* 59 (1977):888–894.
30. GLIEDMAN, J., and ROTH, W. *The Unexpected Minority: Handicapped Children in America.* New York: Harcourt Brace Jovanovich, 1980.
31. GOFFMAN, E. *Stigma: Notes on the Management of Spoiled Identity.* Englewood Cliffs, N.J.: Prentice-Hall, 1963.
32. GOLDBERT, R. T. "Adjustment of Children with Invisible and Visible Handicaps: Congenital Heart Disease and Facial Burn," *Journal of Counseling Psychology,* 21 (1974):428–432.
33. GOLDENSON, R. M., ed. *Disability and Rehabilitation Handbook.* New York: McGraw-Hill, 1978.
34. GOOD, T., and BROPHY, J. *Looking in Classrooms.* New York: Holt, Rinehart, & Winston, 1978.

35. GOODMAN, H., GOTTLIEB, J., and HARRISON, R. H. "Social Acceptance of EMR's Integrated into a Nongraded Elementary School," *American Journal of Mental Deficiency,* 76 (1972):412–417.

36. GOTTLIEB, J., and DOOLITTLE, G. "Social Acceptance of Retarded Children in Nongraded Schools Differing in Architecture," *American Journal of Mental Deficiency,* 78 (1973):15–19.

37. GRESHAM, F. "Misguided Mainstreaming: The Case for Social Skills Training with Handicapped Children," *Exceptional Children,* 48 (1982):422.

38. HALEY, J. *Problem-Solving Therapy.* San Francisco: Jossey-Bass, 1976.

39. HALEY, S. *Strategies of Psychotherapy.* New York: Grune & Stratton, 1963.

40. HASTORF, A. H., WILDFOGEL, J., and CASSMAN, T. "Acknowledgement of Handicap as a Tactic in Social Interaction," *Journal of Personality and Social Psychology,* 37 (1979): 1790–1797.

41. HAVENS, L. L. "The Need for Tests of Normal Functioning in the Psychiatric Interview," *American Journal of Psychiatry,* 141 (1984):1208–1211.

42. HOFMAN, A. D. "The Impact of Illness in Adolescence and Coping Behavior," *Acta Paediatrica Scandinavica,* 256 (Supplement), (1975):29–33.

43. ———. "Managing Handicapped Adolescents with Impaired Body Image," *Feelings and Their Medical Significance,* 22 (1980):13–18.

44. HOLROYD, J. "The Questionnaire on Resources and Stress: An Instrument to Measure Family Response to a Handicapped Family Member," *Journal of Community Psychology,* 2 (1974):92–94.

45. HUGHES, J. G. "The Emotional Impact of Chronic Disease," *American Journal of Diseases of Children,* 130 (1976):1199–1203.

46. HUGHES, M. "Chronically Ill Children in Groups: Recurrent Issues and Adaptations," *American Journal of Orthopsychiatry,* 52 (1982):704–711.

47. HUNTER, R. S., et al. "Antecedents of Child Abuse and Neglect in Premature Infants: A Prospective Study in a Newborn Intensive Care Unit," *Pediatrics,* 61 (1978):629–635.

48. IANO, R. P., et al. "Sociometric Status of Retarded Children in an Integrative Program," *Exceptional Children,* 40 (1974):267–271.

49. IRWIN, C., MILLSTEIN, S., and SHAFER, M. "Appointment-Keeping Behavior in Adolescents," *Journal of Pediatrics,* 99 (1981):799–802.

50. KAKALIK, J. S., et al. *Services for Handicapped Youth: A Program Overview.* Santa Monica, Calif.: Rand Corporation, 1973.

51. KASHANI, J. H., BARBERO, G. J., and BOLANDER, F. D. "Depression in Hospitalized Pediatric Patients," *Journal of the American Academy of Child Psychiatry,* 20 (1981): 123–134.

52. KLECK, R. E. "Physical Stigma and Nonverbal Cues Emitted in Face-to-Face Interaction," *Human Relations,* 21 (1968): 19–28.

53. KLECK, R. E., ONO, H., and HASTORF, A. H. "The Effects of Physical Deviance Upon Face-to-Face Interactions," *Human Relations,* 21 (1966): 425–436.

54. KLEIN, S. D., and SIMMONS, R. G. "Chronic Disease and Childhood Development: Kidney Disease and Transplantation," in R. G. Simmons, ed., *Research in Community and Mental Health,* vol. 1, Greenwich, Conn.: Jai Press, 1979.

55. KNOWLES, H. C., JR. "Diabetes Mellitus in Childhood and Adolescence," *Medical Clinics of North America,* 55 (1966): 1007–1018.

56. LAWLER, R., NAKIELNY, W., and WRIGHT, N. "Psychological Implications of Cystic Fibrosis," *Canadian Medical Association Journal,* 94 (1966):1043–1052.

57. LEVY, A. M., and NIR, Y. "Chronic Illness in Children," in J. Bemporad, ed., *Child Development in Normality and Pathology.* New York: Brunner/Mazel, 1980.

58. LINKOWSKI, D. C. "A Study of the Relationship Between Acceptance of Disability and Response to Rehabilitation" (Ph.D. Diss., State University of New York at Buffalo, 1969).

59. MCANARNEY, E., et al. "Psychological Problems of Children with Chronic Juvenile Arthritis," *Pediatrics,* 53 (1974):523–528.

60. MCCUBBIN, H. *Coping Health Inventory for Parents.* St. Paul: University of Minnesota Press, 1981.

61. MCCULLUM, A. T., and GIBSON, L. E. "Family Adaptation to the Child with Cystic Fibrosis," *Journal of Pediatrics,* 75 (1970):571–578.

62. MAGRAB, P. R. "Psychological Management and Renal Dialysis," *Journal of Clinical Child Psychology,* 4 (1975):38–40.

63. MARTINEK, T. J., and KARPER, W. B. "Teachers' Expectations for Handicapped and Non-Handicapped Children in Mainstreamed Physical Education Classes," *Perceptual Motor Skills,* 53 (1981):327–330.

64. MATTAR, M. G., and YAFFE, S. J. "Compliance of Pediatric Patients with Therapeutic Regimens," *Pediatrics,* 54 (1974).

65. MATTSON, A. "The Chronically Ill Child: A Challenge to the Family," *Medical College of Virginia Quarterly,* 8 (1972):171.

66. ———. "Long-term Physical Illness in Childhood: A Challenge to Psychosocial Adaptation," *Pediatrics,* 50 (1972):801–809.

67. MINDE, K. K. "Coping Styles of 34 Adolescents with Cerebral Palsy," *American Journal of Psychiatry,* 35 (1978): 1355–1359.

68. MINTZER, D., et al. "Parenting an Infant with a Birth Defect," *Psychoanalytic Study of the Child,* 39 (1984): 561–89.

69. MINUCHIN, S., ROSSMAN, B., and BAKER, L. *Psychosomatic Families.* Cambridge, Mass.: Harvard University Press, 1978.

70. O'MALLEY, J. E., et al. "Adjustment Among Pediatric Cancer Survivors," *American Journal of Psychiatry,* 137 (1980):94–96.

71. PALMER, D. J. "Factors to Be Considered in Placing Handicapped Children in Regular Education Classes," *Journal of School Psychology,* 18 (1980): 163–171.

72. PENN, P. "Coalitions and Binding Interactions in Families with Chronic Illness," *Family Systems Medicine,* 1 (1983):6–25.

73. PINKERTON, P. "Psychological Problems of Children with Chronic Illness," in *The Case of Children with Chronic Illness.* Columbus, Ohio: Ross Laboratories, 1974.

74. PLESS, I. B. "Practical Problems and Their Management," in A. P. Scheiner and I. F. Abrug, eds., *The Practical Management of the Developmentally Disturbed Child.* St. Louis: C.V. Mosby, 1980.

75. PLESS, I. B., and PINKERTON, P. *Chronic Childhood Disorder: Promoting Patterns of Adjustment.* Chicago: Year Book Medical Publishers, 1975.

76. PLESS, I. B., and ROGHMANN, K. J. "Chronic Illness and Its Consequences: Observations Based on Three Epidemiologic Surveys," *Journal of Pediatrics,* 79 (1971):351–359.

77. PODENEAU-CZEHOFSKI, I. "Is It Only a Child's Guilt?

Aspects of Family Life of Cerebral Palsied Children," *Rehabilitation Literature,* 36 (1975): 308–311.

78. POLSGROVE, L., and NELSON C. "Curriculum Intervention According to the Behavioral Model," in R. McDowell, G. Adamson, and F. Woods, eds., *Teaching Emotionally Disturbed Children.* Boston, Little Brown, 1982.

79. POZNANSKI, E. O. "Emotional Issues in Raising Handicapped Children," *Rehabilitation Literature,* 34 (1973):322–326.

80. RESNICK, M. "The Social Construction of Disability and Handicap in America," in R. W. Blum, ed., *Chronic Illness and Disabilities in Childhood and Adolescence.* Orlando, Fla.: Grune & Stratton, 1984, pp. 29–46.

81. ———. "The Teenager with Cerebral Palsy," in R. W. Blum, ed., *Chronic Illness and Disabilities in Children and Adolescents.* Orlando, Fla.: Grune & Stratton, 1984, pp. 299–326.

82. REYNOLDS, M. C. "The Educational Needs of Disabled Children and Youths," in R. W. Blum, ed., *Chronic Illness and Disabilities in Childhood and Adolescence.* Orlando, Fla.: Grune & Stratton, 1984, pp. 75–95.

83. RUTTER, M. "Stress, Coping, and Development: Some Issues and Some Questions," in N. Garmezy and M. Rutter, eds., *Stress, Coping, and Development in Children.* New York: McGraw-Hill, 1983, pp. 1–42.

84. RUTTER, M., TIZARD, J., and WHITMORE, E. *Education, Health, and Behavior.* London: Longman, 1970.

85. RUTTER, M., et al. "Adolescent Turmoil: Fact or Fiction," *Journal of Child Psychology and Psychiatry,* 17 (1976): 35–56.

86. RYAN, K. M. "Developmental Differences in Reactions to the Physically Disabled," *Human Development,* 24 (1981): 240–256.

87. SALEND, S., and LUTZ, G. "Mainstreaming or Mainlining: A Competency Based Approach to Mainstreaming," *Journal of Learning Disabilities,* 17 (1984):27–29.

88. SALHOOT, J. T. "The Use of Two Group Methods with Severely Disabled Persons," in R. E. Hardy, and J. C. Cull, eds., *Group Counseling and Therapy Techniques in Special Settings.* Springfield, Ill.: Charles C Thomas, 1974.

89. SAMEROFF, A. J., and ABBE, L. C. "The Consequences of Prematurity: Understanding and Therapy," in H. L. Pick, ed., *Psychology: From Research to Practice.* New York: Plenum Press, 1978.

90. SANDOWSKI, C. L. "The Handicapped Adolescent," *School of Social Work Journal,* 4 (1979):3–13.

91. SCHLOSS, A. L. "The Adolescent with Myelomeningocele," *Developmental Medicine and Child Neurology 15,* Supplement 29 (1973).

92. SIMONDS, J. F. "Emotions and Compliance in Diabetic Children," *Psychometrics,* 20 (1979):544–551.

93. SINGLETON, G., COLE, J., and LONG, M. "The Attitudes of Rehabilitation Professional, Their Colleagues and Other Disciplines," Paper presented at the 56th Annual Session of American Congress of Rehabilitation Medicine, Honolulu, Hawaii, 1979.

94. STRAX, T., and WOLFSON, S. "Life Cycle Crises of the Disabeled Adolescent and Young Adult: Implications for Public Policy," in R. Blum, ed., *Chronic Illness and Disabilities in Childhood and Adolescence.* Orlando, Fla.: Grune & Stratton, 1984.

95. SULLIVAN, B. J. "Self-Esteem and Depression in Adolescent Diabetic Girls," *Diabetes Care,* 1 (1978):18–22.

96. ———. "Adjustment in Diabetic Adolescent Girls: I. Development of the Diabetic Adjustment Scale. II. Adjustment, Self-Esteem, and Depression in Diabetic Girls," *Psychosomatic Medicine,* 41 (1979):119–138.

97. TAVORMINA, J. B., et al. "Chronically Ill Children— A Psychologically Deviant Population," *Journal of Abnormal Child Psychology,* 4 (1976):99–110.

98. TAVORMINA, J. B., et al. "Psychosocial Effects on Parents of Raising a Physically Handicapped Child," *Journal of Abnormal Child Psychology,* 9 (1981):121–131.

99. TROPAUER, A., FRANZ, M., and DILGARD, V. "Psychological Aspects of Care of Children with Cystic Fibrosis," *American Journal of the Diseases of Childhood,* 119 (1970): 424–432.

100. VOELTZ, L. M. "Children's Attitudes Toward Handicapped Peers," *American Journal of Mental Deficiencies,* 84 (1980):455–464.

101. WALKER, G. "The Pact: The Caretaker Parent/Ill-Child Coalition in Families with Chronic Illness," *Family Systems Medicine,* 1 (1983):6–29.

102. WALKER, V. S. "The Efficacy of the Resource Room for Educating Retarded Children," *Exceptional Children,* 40 (1974):288–289.

103. WEINBERG, N. "Social Stereotyping of the Physically Handicapped," *Rehabilitation Psychology,* 23 (1976):115–124.

104. WEINBERG, N., and SANTANA, R. "Comic Books: Champions of the Disabled Stereotype," *Rehabilitation Literature,* 39 (1978):327–331.

105. WERNER, E. E., and SMITH, R. S. *Vulnerable but Invincible: A Study of Resilient Children.* New York: McGraw-Hill, 1982.

106. WERTHEIM, E. S. "Developmental Genesis of Human Vulnerability: Conceptual Re-evaluation," in E. J. Anthony, C. Koupernik, and C. Chiland, eds., *The Child in His Family: Vulnerable Children,* vol. 4. New York: John Wiley & Sons, 1978, pp. 17–36.

107. WIKLER, L., WASOW, M., and HATFIELD, E. "Chronic Sorrow Revisited: Parent vs. Professional Depiction of the Adjustments of Parents of Mentally Retarded Children," *American Journal of Orthopsychiatry,* 51 (1981):63–70.

108. WILKES, H. H., BIRELEY, J. K., and SCHULTZ, J. J. "Criteria for Mainstreaming the Learning Disabled Child into the Regular Classroom," *Journal of Learning Disabilities,* 12 (1979):46–51.

109. ZELTLER, L., et al. "Psychologic Effects of Illness in Adolescence. II. Impact of Illness in Adolescents—Crucial Issues and Coping Styles," *Journal of Pediatrics,* 97 (1980): 132–138.

110. ZIGLER, E., and MUENCHOW, S., "Mainstreaming: The Proof is in the Implementation," *American Psychologist,* 34 (1979):993–996.

SECTION III

Assessment

Richard L. Cohen / Editor

Introduction

Richard L. Cohen

In the Assessment section of volume 1 of the *Basic Handbook of Child Psychiatry,* published in 1979, the contributors attempted a comprehensive overview and analysis of the state of our knowledge about assessment and diagnosis of child and adolescent psychiatric disorders. As might be expected, two things became clear as a result of that effort. First, during the first half century of child psychiatry's growth as a medical discipline, we had already developed a considerable body of theory and clinical procedures. Second, to any discerning reader, an array of significant knowledge and skill deficits emerged in bold relief. For instance, one area in which there is inadequate data to draw firm conclusions has to do with the best method of conducting a developmental interview. In volume 1, I stated that a developmental interview is conducted best with the adult who had been the primary caretaker of the child. This statement engendered a two-year correspondence with one prominent child psychiatrist who is strongly convinced that the quality of such interviews is higher if conducted with both parents present. In fact, despite the fact that workers hold deep convictions on both sides of the question, there remains little empirical evidence to support either position. This is but one example of the many questions that still require intensive study.

In this update, the contributors have attempted to provide a progress report on our efforts to address some of these deficits. Clearly, we have made some progress. At the same time, however, I wish to express my admiration for the candor and forthrightness with which the contributors freely acknowledge our continued limitations and the vexing problems that continue to confront us.

Briefly stated, the major areas that receive attention by the contributors to this section and that continue to be the central issues for ongoing investigation in assessment and diagnosis include:

1. The development of a nosological system for child psychiatry that is sufficiently specific for each clinical entity to permit uniformity of data collection among clinicians and clinical centers. It is a classification system in which each syndrome may be characterized by the biological, behavioral, and developmental phenomena specific to that particular disorder, allowing for maximum discrimination between pathological entities.
2. The development of data collection techniques that are most efficient and cost effective to arrive at a specific diagnosis.
3. Correlative to this, the identification of instruments that are at once specific and sensitive along both psychosocial and biomedical parameters for syndrome identification.
4. The experimentation with new technologies to elicit, organize, store, and retrieve information, as required by both the volume and the heterogeneity of clinical data now being identified.

Of course, the reader will quickly perceive that within their specialized areas, most of the contributions to this section address not one but several of these questions. Chapters 15, 17, and 23 are concerned with an up-to-date understanding of the progress and problems we continue to encounter in developing a clinically relevant nosology for child and adolescent psychiatry.

At the same time, chapters 17 and 23 also concern themselves with our need to develop a data collection system that is uniform and that addresses the need for efficient use of staff time, as does chapter 16. In this connection, particular attention should be paid to the caveats mentioned by all authors around the use of highly structured instruments. These question sets should be seen as aids in diagnosis and in communication between clinicians and investigators. They cannot, at this writing, take the place of sensitive clinical interviewing.

It is evident from several of the contributions that child psychiatrists are becoming ever more aware that their assessment procedures must be increasingly sensitive and syndrome-specific. Chapters 18, 20, and 21 are examples of progress in that direction.

Finally, elegant illustrations of the state-of-the-art use of high technology for assessment can be found in chapters 19, 20, and 22. As we go to press, large numbers of children and adolescents are being studied by new brain imaging techniques such as nuclear magnetic resonance. There is reason to hope that these procedures will tell us more about the etiology of some of the major disorders and provide sensitive diagnostic markers for their identification.

This is a rapidly developing "territory" in the discipline of child psychiatry. Insights and tools are available that five years ago were only in the planning stages. It should become apparent from a review of the following chapters that the next five years may bring together even more definitive ideas along with the tools to implement them.

15 / Issues in the Use of DSM-III

David Shaffer and Madelyn S. Gould

Historical Background

Lists of diseases have been in existence for just over one hundred years. In 1923, an international classification, confined to causes of mortality, became the responsibility of the then League of Nations and, after World War II, of the World Health Organization. Psychiatric conditions were first included in 1938, although only as causes of death. The first list of *morbidity* was issued in 1947 as the sixth version of the *International Classification of Diseases* (ICD-6), with psychiatric conditions occupying the fifth section of that list.

In 1952 the American Psychiatric Association (APA) issued its first *Diagnostic and Statistical Manual* (DSM-I) separately from with the ICD listings.[1] DSM-II followed in 1968.[2] Both included a glossary and embodied diagnoses with etiological implications. Influenced by the theories of Adolf Meyer, most conditions were termed reactions. Relatively few categories were used, particularly in the field of child psychiatry, which resulted in widespread dissatisfaction with the system. This, in turn, led to the development of rival listings, such as the classification of child psychiatric disorders issued by the Group for the Advancement of Psychiatry.[11]

In 1974 the APA established a committee to prepare the third version of the DSM, which would be released at the same time as ICD-9.[3] The committee was led by Robert Spitzer, a research psychiatrist with expertise in psychiatric measurement and definition. Specialist subcommittees were set up to advise on the classification and description of different diseases. Among these was a subcommittee charged with developing a classification system for disorders that usually have their onset in childhood. Although criticized by some,[28] the contribution of "committees" in creating DSM-III was intended to ensure that the new system not only took advantage of advances in knowledge but that it did not run too far ahead of accepted clinical practice. Inevitably this resulted in some measure of compromise. Some decisions were made that were not based entirely on scientific information, in part because such information did not exist and in part to facilitate accommodation to established clinical practice by different schools of thought.

After its release in 1980, DSM-III was variously hailed as a "turning point in the history of American psychiatry"[14] and as a scourge whose "disadvantages outweighed its advantages."[28] The judgments (see also Garmezy,[10] Quay[18] and Zubin[29]) need to be evaluated in the context of criticisms that have long been leveled against the process of psychiatric classification as well as against the specifics of DSM-III. The remainder of this chapter reviews criticisms of psychiatric classification in general, describes the special characteristics of DSM-III, reviews research of the system that has been undertaken, and summarizes those criticisms that seem well founded.

Objections to Psychiatric Classification

Classification systems order and group information, a process basic to all scientific activity. They enable professionals to communicate with each other and are essential for education and research. Curiously, however, in the field of mental disorders, psychiatrists have often opposed diagnostic classifications.[24] It seems appropriate to explore why this should have been the case.

One common complaint is this: Diagnoses, such as those found in the various DSM's or ICD's, do not convey the idiosyncratic and complex features of the cases psychiatrists see in their practice; they therefore cannot be used as a basis for psychological or psychosocial treatment. In some ways this is a reasonable concern. Any psychiatrist who responded to all children with the same diagnosis by dispensing a given psychological treatment without taking into account the circumstances under which the condition first arose, family and school factors, the intelligence of the child, and the mental and economic resources of the parents, among many other variables, would be a poor clinician. However, to levy this criticism is to misunderstand the function of diagnostic systems like DSM-III. The classical psychiatric formulation is "idiographic," that is to say, it sets out to describe features that are *unique* to the patient. In order to draw up a detailed treatment plan, a formulation of this kind is indeed necessary. Such formulations, however, can only be communicated to others in full, as, for example, in the form of the classical case history. They do not help to deal with classes of patients or conditions. Nomothetic diagnoses, on the other hand, such as those found in DSM-III or ICD-9, convey information not about the characteristics unique to a given patient but rather about the characteristics a patient shares *in common* with certain others.

As a consequence, diagnoses do have clear limitations for treatment planning. To some extent this problem is addressed by the use of multiple dimensions or axes (e.g., as are employed in DSM-III). These axes code different aspects of a patient's condition (associated medical problem, precipitating event, etc.) without requiring that one dimension be regarded as more salient than any other.

A second objection has been that psychiatric diagnoses are often *unreliable* and that given the risks of labeling, for example, their dubious advantages are outweighed by their more certain disadvantages. To address this criticism sensibly, one needs to examine the different sources of unreliability. One reason for disagreement among psychiatrists is that, for the most part, the precise cause of most psychiatric conditions is unknown. As a result, different etiological theories have emerged that seek to explain the same phenomenon. To some extent this is understandable, and perhaps even desirable. However, clinicians who have different theories about the cause of a condition may also interpret clinical phenomena quite differently. The psychoanalyst may see antisocial behavior as the "acting out" of an unconscious conflict, while the behavior

therapist may see the same behavior as one that has been too successfully reinforced by parental response. In viewing the same case, the clinicians' theoretical orientations will influence the phenomena on which they put the greatest emphasis and, therefore, the diagnostic formulation they will use. DSM-III acknowledges this source of disagreement and seeks to bypass any terminology that has theoretical implications, relying solely on observable phenomena. Its success in doing this has been shown by finding comparable reliabilities from behavioral psychologists and analytic psychiatrists that have been found in a large case history study.[17]

Other sources of unreliability include the use of criteria that are ambiguously worded or require inference. Here again DSM-III has sought to diminish disagreement wherever possible by using operationalized criteria, written clearly, and backed by ample definition in an accompanying glossary.

There is, however, one other source of unreliability, and this one has not been addressed satisfactorily by DSM-III. Diagnostic systems can become unreliable if they are too long or too complex. The more choice given to the user, the more opportunity there is for variation. If the choice is set out in a rather complicated format, or if the choices are not all mutually incompatible (so that the same clinical phenomena could be grouped with subtle differences of emphasis in different places), then opportunities for disagreement are created.

Another criticism voiced against diagnostic classification systems is that they encourage the use of the "medical model." Since the term medical model means different things to different people, a single rejoinder to this concern may not suffice. To some, the medical model seems to imply that only a professional with a medical qualification should treat the patient; in respect to psychiatric therapy, this is clearly not the case. Psychologists and social workers treat countless child patients, applying DSM-III diagnoses with equal reliability to psychiatrists.[17] To others the medical model implies that only biological causes are to be considered at the expense of a patient's psychological experiences or environment. As DSM-III makes no etiological assumptions, this too cannot be a valid perspective.

Still others view the medical model in a more positive light, as a way of organizing information about physical or mental dysfunction, one that enables the mental health clinician to make predictions about natural history and treatment and that may, depending on the state of knowledge, carry information about cause. Such predictive criteria should apply to any valid diagnostic entity, and, insofar as they are encompassed by a classification system, they are welcome.

The process of diagnosis has also been criticized

because it carries with it a risk of *labeling* and stigmatizing the individual. There can be no doubt that being assigned a diagnosis of, for example, schizophrenia will carry with it implications of poor prognosis and serious dysfunction. Inevitably, diagnosis will at times be applied inaccurately and inappropriately, and when that happens, it may have damaging consequences for the patient. However, it is unreasonable to generalize from bad practice or imperfect knowledge. To say that a diagnosis is dangerous because it carries a poor prognosis is not unlike attacking the messenger who comes with bad tidings. Nevertheless, all who use diagnoses should be aware of their power for both helping and harming the patient. DSM-III has, in fact, taken one step toward ameliorating the stigmatizing effect of labeling by not using diagnostic terms as descriptive nouns.

At a more technical level, categorical diagnoses, such as those used in DSM-III, have been criticized by some psychologists who suggest that it is wrong to conceive of psychiatric disorders as being categorically different from normal behavior; that many psychiatric symptoms represent more severe or extreme variations of thoughts, feelings, or behaviors which occur normally, and that it is more appropriate to think of psychiatric disturbance as being *quantitatively* different but on the same dimension as normal behavior.[18] This view may or may not be correct; certainly there is evidence that some psychiatric conditions may find expression on a spectrum of severity that ranges from the normal to the most deviant. However, at this time relatively few clinicians think about psychopathology in this way, and it is important for the success of any classification system that it both take into account the most knowledge and be in accord with reasonable clinical practice.

Special Features of DSM-III

What then are the special features of DSM-III that have led it to be greeted with both enthusiasm or criticism?

First, DSM-III defines what is meant by a mental disorder. It must be a *clinically significant* condition, that is to say, it must cause distress or interfere with function, and it should not be merely a transient, "understandable" distress response to some adverse experience. Similarly, it should not be applied to behaviors that may only represent a difference in values between the individual and society. Behavior that characterizes a cult or sect should not be regarded as a manifestation of mental illness.

Second, as indicated earlier, the basis of DSM-III is generally *atheoretical* and *nonetiological*. As far as possible, the symptoms referred to are behaviorally descriptive and do not require interpretation in respect to any covert psychological meaning they may possess. Exceptions to the behaviorally descriptive categories are found in the adjustment disorder and organic diagnoses. Although both imply an etiology, both are categorized behaviorally. Thus adjustment reactions are classified according to their predominant symptomatology—for example, antisocial behavior, affective disturbance, and so forth. Furthermore, stringent criteria have been written for the adjustment disorders. For one thing, they are a "residual diagnosis"—they should only be used if no other diagnosis applies. For another, adjustment reactions should be diagnosed only when the onset of the disorder has been in close temporal proximity to the experience of a stress event, and the clinician making the diagnosis should be able to predict that the condition will diminish in severity as adaptation to the stressor occurs or if the stressor is removed. Despite these stringent demands, currently the diagnosis is made very frequently, probably in the absence of good evidence of reactivity. It may be that clinicians who had become used to the Meyerian "reactive" disorders of DSM-I and DSM-II have not yet adapted to the changing rules for similar terminology.

Third, DSM-III provides codes that can be applied in a *multiaxial fashion*. That is to say, different features of an individual's functioning or health can be coded simultaneously without the rater having to decide on the primacy of one or the other. Axis I is for the clinical psychiatric diagnosis. Axis II, in children and adolescents under age eighteen, is for coding associated developmental delays (not including mental retardation, which is listed as a psychiatric disorder on Axis I). Axis III covers associated physical disorders or disease, and under usual circumstances the listing in ICD-9 (Clinical Modification) would be used for this purpose. Axis IV codes associated psychosocial stressors. The rater using this axis quantifies the severity of the stress to which the onset of the disorder was related; this is estimated by comparing the case to a range of examples. Axis V codes the highest level of adaptive functioning in the recent past. There is empirical evidence that the presence of a multiaxial classification system is not only popular with users,[5,16,23] but results in a significant increase in the amount of information that is coded.[21]

Fourth, and perhaps of greatest importance, is the fact that DSM-III uses specific *diagnostic criteria*. These were modeled on the Research Diagnostic Criteria (RDC) developed by Spitzer, Endicott, and Robins based on the criteria developed by Feighner and others[9] at Washington University in St. Louis. The development of specific criteria originates from the researcher's need to be able to study comparable groups. One way of doing this is to specify patient characteristics with a high degree of precision. DSM-III has adapted this procedure to clinical practice. Criteria are differentiated into those that are *necessary* for a given diagnosis to be made (essential criteria) and associated features that are found commonly but not invariably and/or that may not be specific for the diagnosis. Heretofore, clinicians tended to vary in the criteria they used for making a given diagnosis; this introduced an inevitable element of unreliability. The clear rules for the use of specific criteria along with the definitions that appear in DSM-III should reduce this quality of uncertainty.

Fifth, diagnoses can be coded at different degrees of *specificity*. The first three digits of a diagnostic code usually describe a general category of disorders —for example, 314 refers to the attention deficit disorders. The code numbers for these first three digits have been designed to be as nearly compatible with ICD-9 codes as possible;[27] hence they are presented in the list of codes and in the manual *out* of numerical sequence.

The fourth and fifth digits are used inconsistently to code variations of the first 3 digits—for example, attention deficit disorder with (314.01) or without (314.00) hyperactivity—*or* to indicate a stage in the natural history of a condition (e.g., infantile autism is 299.00; infantile autism, residual syndrome, is 299.01) or type of natural history, such as remitting or continuous or both (see the 296.xx subcodes for the affective disorders).

Sixth, except for the personality disorders on Axis II (which can only be given to a child under age eighteen if the disorder has been markedly chronic), there are *no age-restricted codes*. If a child presents with a psychiatric condition that is similar in form to that found in adults and that usually has its onset in adulthood—for example, a major depressive disorder —then the child will be diagnosed with the same diagnostic code as an adult. Conversely, if an adult is seen with a disorder that nearly always arises in childhood but that may persist on into adulthood— such as the residual form of infantile autism—then the diagnostic code will be drawn from the section dealing with disorders usually first evident in infancy, childhood, or adolescence.

Seventh, DSM-III is much more *comprehensive* than its predecessors or than ICD-9, particularly regarding the codes for child psychiatric disorders. Most of the entities that have been described in recent years—such as infantile autism, the various movement disorders, and so forth—now find their place in the classification system. Indeed one of the criticisms of DSM-III is that

some conditions that have *not* been adequately described, such as oppositional disorder,[26] have also found their way into the system.

The addition of new categories, coupled with their increased level of specificity, has had the predictable effect of increasing the formulation of *multiple diagnoses*. Clearly there are many different ways of ordering multiple diagnoses. For example, the primary diagnosis could be either the one that is causing the most disability or the one that has been present for the longest time. However, DSM-III indicates that the primary diagnosis should be the one for which treatment is *currently* being sought. Clinically, this is perhaps the easiest to apply, but arguably, it may be the least appropriate for purposes of research communication among clinical investigators.

Finally, DSM-III clearly sets out to be an *educational* document. Its 300-page manual reads much like a textbook, and its tone is by and large authoritative.

DSM-III and Research

A number of studies have examined the properties of DSM-III. Most of these have addressed the issue of reliability rather than validity. Although reliability is necessary for validity, it does not provide validity. For example, clinicians may indeed agree with each other as to whether or not a child meets the criteria for oppositional disorder. In itself, however, agreement on such a label will not indicate whether the children so diagnosed have a significant mental illness, nor will it allow prediction about the natural history of the condition or its response to treatment.

Research can be grouped into those studies that have tested interrater reliability on the basis of written case history reports and those that have arranged for patients with various clinical syndromes to be examined by more than one psychiatrist. So far there has been relatively little research into the discriminant validity of the codes—that is, whether children diagnosed with one particular variant of a general type of disorder differ in background or prognosis from those diagnosed with another.

Some of the earliest reliability studies that employed case histories were carried out by Cantwell and his colleagues[5,15,22] on a preliminary version of DSM-III. These investigators found that relatively high reliability could be obtained with cases of pervasive developmental disorder, autism, and mental retardation, and for psychotic conditions like schizophrenia. Agreement was not as good for affective and anxiety disorders.

Using the final version of DSM-III, Mezzich, Mezzich, and Coffman [17] undertook a case-history study with seventy-two psychologists (who had a predominantly behavioral orientation) and sixty-two psychiatrists (with a predominantly analytic background). Despite differences in training and orientation, reliabilities from the psychologists and the psychiatrists were similar, a finding that confirmed the value of the atheoretical approach. Reliability was generally modest, however, being highest for mental retardation, enuresis, pervasive developmental disorder, and conduct disorder.

Strober, Green, and Carlson [25] studied ninety-five consecutive adolescent cases who had been admitted to an adolescent inpatient unit for the first time. The investigators restricted their reliability assessment to a single diagnosis, used a standardized assessment form, and shared access to the patients' clinical records. They also confined their choices of diagnoses to a list of fourteen diagnostic entities. All of these factors would tend to promote agreement. They used a statistical technique that took account of chance agreement and reported high reliability for most categories except for the anxiety, socialized conduct, and dissociative disorders.

Werry and associates [26] undertook a reliability study on consecutive inpatients. Diagnoses were made on the basis of a weekly ward round at which intake histories were provided. Each of the raters therefore had available the same information base. The statistical measures they employed have been subject to criticism (see Cantwell [4]). Raters were allowed to make multiple diagnoses, and the criterion they checked against was agreement with the diagnostic profile assigned by the most senior psychiatrist. Good reliability was found for enuresis, encopresis, schizophrenia, anxiety, and attention deficit disorders. Moderate reliability was found for the conduct and somatiform disorders, and poor agreement for the oppositional disorders. Indeed, disagreement on oppositional disorder tended to lower agreement on many of the diagnostic profiles. As in Cantwell's original study, [5] reliability tended to be better for diagnoses made at the general three-digit level (particularly among the conduct disorders) than at the more specific four-digit levels.

In a different type of study, Earls [8] applied DSM-III criteria to a group of three-year-olds identified in an epidemiological survey as having significant problems. With respect to DSM-III, the most significant finding was that all of the cases identified as being problematic could be given a DSM-III diagnosis. This settled some of the concerns expressed by critics of DSM-III that the rigid criteria requirements would lead to a large number of unclassifiable cases.

Criticisms of DSM-III

The most common target of criticism has been the use of explicit diagnostic criteria. It is, of course, recognized that such a requirement should increase reliability or agreement among different users. In fact, for many of the criteria, there is an empirical basis. However, because of the authoritative tone of DSM-III, criteria that may initially have been intended as suggestions or mere indicators are in practice being treated as if their accuracy and appropriateness has been demonstrated by adequate research. For most conditions, we do not yet know which are the necessary or sufficient criteria, whether it makes a difference to have three, four, or five items on the list of criteria, and so forth.

Another criticism is that some of the conditions described in DSM-III may not meet the manual's own criterion for what is a significant mental disorder. Examples are oppositional disorder and separation anxiety disorders, which can be identified in a high proportion of children who are not being seen at a psychiatric clinic and who do not in other respects appear to be patients. [6,7]

Other criticisms have focused on individual details of different criteria (see Rutter and Shaffer [20] for a review). An example would be that the criteria for the attention deficit disorder diagnosis include certain antisocial behaviors that will actively increase confusion around these two commonly associated conditions.

The complexity and length of the system are likely to lower reliability. Under ideal circumstances, a diagnostic system should be capable of being scanned systematically and with ease, all diagnostic possibilities reviewed, and the case then assigned the diagnosis that offers the best fit. When the diagnostic system is too long or excessively complex, it becomes difficult to review, and unreliability is likely to increase. The problem is made even greater in DSM-III because the system is not mutually exclusive. That is to say, it is sometimes possible to code a case with given characteristics in more than one category. Reliability studies (discussed earlier) indicate that even for some of the more common psychiatric conditions, such as the conduct and anxiety disorders, unreliability is a major problem, at least at the four-digit level. In general, reliability at the three-digit level is considerably more satisfactory.

Research findings point to problems of length and complexitity of DSM-III. In the course of a comparative diagnostic study, Cohen [6] noted that although clinicians identified and recorded symptoms that would qualify individuals for a number of diagnoses, they did not necessarily assign these diagnoses. This may be either because of a mechanical failure to match

15 / *Issues in the Use of DSM-III*

the presence of symptoms to diagnostic requirements (a reflection of length and complexity), or because clinicians use criteria that differ from those prescribed by DSM-III (so that when they do assign a diagnosis they are selective in which criteria they apply). This potential for variable application of DSM-III rules may actually make the system's reliability worse than if it had fewer criterion rules.

As indicated earlier, the organization of codes in DSM-III permits diagnoses to be made at two and sometimes at three degrees of specificity or generality. For example, conduct disorders can be coded using only the three-digit formula, 312, or they can be coded more specifically with respect to the presence or absence of aggression or evidence of socialization, in which case four digits are used.

The problem of multiple diagnoses has been referred to. Multiple diagnoses also act to reduce reliability because the guidelines provided in DSM-III for designating one diagnosis as primary (i.e., that it should be the diagnosis that led to referral for treatment) could result in the same patient legitimately receiving quite different diagnoses for the same episode of illness from different subspecialists.

There are two major criticisms of the multiaxial system for children. First, mental retardation is currently listed on Axis I, yet retardation can occur in a variety of different types, and with or without another psychiatric disorder. In a systematic study Rutter, Shaffer, and Shepherd[21] demonstrated that the institution of a separate axis for intellectual level markedly improved the accuracy with which it was reported. Second, Axis IV (psychosocial stressors) has been held to be inappropriate for children. The axis was originally designed to differentiate psychiatric disorders into those that had an unprecipitated onset and those that had an onset after the occurrence of a stress event (when the conditions were presumed to have a better prognosis). The list of adult stressors has been adapted to convey events more likely to occur in childhood. However, this revealed a misunderstanding of the nature of stressor effects on children. By and large (see Rutter and Shaffer[20]), chronic stress appears to have a more noxious effect on children than does acute, unrepeated stress. Thus the death of a parent, which is listed at the most extreme pole of childhood stressors, may actually be a less severe stressor than chronic marital disharmony. Not only is this axis inappropriate for child psychiatric disorder, but it is also unreliable.[17]

Finally, the authorative, didactic tone of DSM-III has been criticized despite the disclaimer noted in the introduction. The manual rarely qualifies its descriptions by stating that evidence to demonstrate criteria are not available, which may lead users to believe that there is more evidence to support the criteria than in fact exists. Its emphasis on hard and fast rules for diagnostic criteria conveys to users that if DSM-III says it is so, it must be so. However, the same authoritative tone may have provided a stimulus to the researcher promoting studies of the described entities. This heuristic value has been considerable. DSM-III's well-specified hypothetical diagnoses are currently the subject of a sizable body of research, with publications appearing in almost every issue of the most important scientific journals. Examples of research that has examined the discriminant validity of the diagnostic entities themselves include studies into the difference between socialized and unsocialized conduct disorder[12] and the differences between attention deficit disordered children with and without hyperactivity,[13] and so forth. These studies have led to insights and information that might not have emerged had DSM-III not been so provocative an instrument.

The Future of DSM-III

At this writing, change is already upon us. The American Psychiatric Association has set up advisory committees to develop a revised version of DSM-III (DSM-III R). Unsatisfactory categories such as oppositional disorder and diagnoses about which there is a considerable disagreement among experts (such as the differentiation between socialized and unsocialized conduct disorder) have been the subjects of conferences. Decisions have been made about new criteria that take new findings and diverse opinions into account. Criteria that have been subject to criticism because of their poor definition or ambiguous wording have been revised and additional listings have been added. Although one welcomes the responsiveness of the designers of DSM-III to criticism, in many ways the very exciting impact that DSM-III has had in promoting research into classification will inevitably be curtailed as, almost before the initial version has been subjected to adequate study, a new version emerges.

Another development has been the establishment of diagnostic instruments specifically oriented to DSM-III criteria. The childhood version of the Schedule for Affective Diseases and Schizophrenia (K-SADS) has been based on DSM-III and Research Diagnostic Criteria. The National Institute of Mental Health has sponsored the development of a new instrument, the Diagnostic Interview Schedule for Children (DISC), to be used in epidemiological surveys; it is designed specifically to elicit the diagnostic criteria which appear in DSM-III. DSM-III has also established new standards of objectivity and has

SECTION III / ASSESSMENT

probably eroded some of the implicit influence of untested theories that were fundamental to earlier classification systems. There may or may not be a causal relationship, but all of this has coincided with a great increase in the amount of research in the area of child psychiatry. For all of its faults, in general, one must regard the first five years of DSM-III as having been an outstanding success.

ACKNOWLEDGMENT

This work has been made possible by NIMH Research Training Grant #MH 16434, Clinical Training Grant #MH 17344, Study of Completed and Attempted Suicides in Adolescents Grant #MH 39818, and by Dr. Gould's William T. Grant Foundation Scholars Award #84095484.

REFERENCES

1. AMERICAN PSYCHIATRIC ASSOCIATION. *Diagnostic and Statistical Manual of Mental Disorders,* 1st ed. (DSM-I). Washington, D.C.: American Psychiatric Association, 1952.

2. AMERICAN PSYCHIATRIC ASSOCIATION. *Diagnostic and Statistical Manual of Mental Disorders,* 2nd ed. (DSM-II). Washington, D.C.: American Psychiatric Association, 1968.

3. AMERICAN PSYCHIATRIC ASSOCIATION. *Diagnostic and Statistical Manual of Mental Disorders,* 3rd ed. (DSM-III). Washington, D.C.: American Psychiatric Association, 1980.

4. CANTWELL, D. P. "Clinical Child Psychopathology: DSM-III Research," Paper presented at a conference on assessment, diagnosis, and classification in child psychopathology at the National Institute of Mental Health, Washington, D.C., September 1984.

5. CANTWELL, D. P., et al. "A Comparison of DSM-II and DSM-III in the Diagnosis of Childhood Psychiatric Disorder. I. Agreement with Expected Diagnosis," *Archives of General Psychiatry,* 36 (1979):1208–1213.

6. COHEN, P. "A Comparison of Lay and Clinician Administered Psychiatric Diagnostic Interviews of an Epidemiological Sample of Children," Paper presented at the 31st Annual Meeting of the American Academy of Child Psychiatry, Toronto, October 1984.

7. COSTELLO, E. J., COSTELLO, A. J. and EDELBROCK, C. "Validity of the NIMH Diagnostic Interview Schedule for Children: A Comparison of Psychiatric and Pediatric Referrals," Paper presented at the 31st Annual Meeting of the American Academy of Child Psychiatry, Toronto, October 1984.

8. EARLS, F. "Application of DSM-III in an Epidemiological Study of Preschool Children," *American Journal of Psychiatry,* 139 (1982):142–243.

9. FEIGHNER, J. P., et al. "Diagnostic Criteria for Use in Psychiatric Research," *Archives of General Psychiatry,* 26 (1972):57–63.

10. GARMEZY, N. "DSM-III. Never Mind the Psychologist, Is It Good for the Children?" *Clinical Psychologist,* 31 (1978):1, 4–6.

11. GROUP FOR THE ADVANCEMENT OF PSYCHIATRY. *Psychopathological Disorders in Childhood* (Report #62). New York: Group for the Advancement of Psychiatry, 1966.

12. HENN, R. A., BARDWELL, R., and JENKINS, R. L. "Juvenile Delinquents Revisited: Adult Criminal Activities," *Archives of General Psychiatry,* 37 (1980):1160–1163.

13. KING, C., and YOUNG, R. D. "Attentional Deficits With and Without Hyperactivity: Teacher and Peer Perceptions," *Journal of Abnormal Child Psychology,* 10 (1982): 483–496.

14. KLERMAN, G. L. "The Advantages of DSM-III," *American Journal of Psychiatry,* 141 (1984):539–542.

15. MATTISON, R., et al. "A Comparison of DSM-II and DSM-III in the Diagnosis of Childhood Psychiatric Disorders. II. Inter-rater Agreement," *Archives of General Psychiatry,* 36 (1979):1217–1222.

16. MEZZICH, A. C., and MEZZICH, J. E. "Perceived Suitability and Usefulness of DSM-III vs. DSM-II in Child Psychopathology," *Journal of the American Academy of Child Psychiatry,* 1985, 25:281–285.

17. MEZZICH, A. C., MEZZICH, J. E. and COFFMAN, G. A. "Reliability for DSM-II vs. DSM-III in Child Psychopathology," *Journal of the American Academy of Child Psychiatry,* 24 (1985):273–280.

18. QUAY, H. C. "A Critical Analysis of DSM-III as a Taxonomy of Psychopathology in Childhood and Adolescence," in T. Millon and G. Klerman, eds., *Contemporary Issues in Psychopathology.* New York: Guilford Press, forthcoming.

19. RUTTER, M. "Classification and Categorization in Child Psychiatry," *Journal of Child Psychology and Psychiatry,* 6 (1965):71–83.

20. RUTTER, M., and SHAFFER, D. (1980) "DSM-III: A Step Forward or Back in Terms of the Classification of Child Psychiatric Disorders?" *Journal of the American Academy of Child Psychiatry,* 19 (1980):371–394.

21. RUTTER, M., SHAFFER, D., and SHEPHERD, M. *A Multiaxial Classification of Child Psychiatric Disorder.* Geneva: World Health Organization, 1975.

22. RUSSELL, A. T., et al. "A Comparison of DSM-II and DSM-III in the Diagnosis of Childhood Psychiatric Disorders. III. Multiaxial Features," *Archives of General Psychiatry,* 36 (1979):1223–1226.

23. SPITZER, R. L., and FORMAN, J.B.W. "DSM-III Field Trials: II. Initial Experience with the Multiaxial System," *American Journal of Psychiatry,* 136 (1979):818–820.

24. STENGEL, E. "Classification of Mental Disorders," *Bulletin of the World Health Organization,* 21 (1959):601 663.

25. STROBER, M., GREEN, J., and CARLSON, G. "Reliability of Psychiatric Diagnosis in Hospitalized Adolescents," *Archives of General Psychiatry,* 38 (1981):141–145.

26. WERRY, J. S., et al. "The Inter-rater Reliability of DSM-III in Children," *Journal of Abnormal Child Psychology,* 11 (1983):341–354.

27. WORLD HEALTH ORGANIZATION. *Manual of the International Classification of Diseases,* 8th rev. (ICD-8). Geneva: World Health Organization, 1978.

28. VAILLANT, G. E. "The Disadvantages of DSM-III Outweigh Its Advantages," *American Journal of Psychiatry,* 141 (1984):542–545.

29. ZUBIN, J. "But Is It Good for Science?" *Clinical Psychologist,* 31 (1977):5–7.

16 / Structured Interviewing for the Assessment of Child Psychopathology

Anthony J. Costello

The last few years have seen considerable growth in all forms of systematic assessment of child psychopathology. Though checklists and rating scales have been most popular, that bastion of the clinical method, the clinical interview, has also been the subject of energetic attempts to improve it, to make it more useful for research purposes, and to improve on its usually mediocre diagnostic reliability. The demand for more accurate diagnostic discrimination has lead to successive refinements of the nosological system[2] (and see the introduction to this section). With the advent of the third edition of the *Diagnostic and Statistical Manual of Mental Disorders* (DSM-III) and its categories that better reflected current beliefs, together with its introduction of definitions rather than descriptions of diagnoses, it had been hoped that the reliability of psychiatric diagnosis would improve. So far it has been hard to find proof that this hope has been realized. Indeed there is some evidence that the simpler categories of DSM-II, despite their lack of definitions, were more reliable.[32,33] The larger number of diagnostic categories now available has made it even more important to use great care in defining the criteria on which the categories depend. This in turn has focused attention on how to elicit the information needed to decide if a child meets these criteria.

Another reason for seeking better interview data arises from the inherent limitations of the usual alternatives to clinical interviewing such as checklists, questionnaires, and ratings. Instruments of this type depend on a fixed set of questions that are posed either directly to the informant or indirectly by asking a trained rater to evaluate the informant's response. A child, or an unsophisticated adult, may not see the relevance of these devices to the problems he or she experiences, and may resent what appears to be an impersonal and mechanical approach. The questions may include some that are obviously inappropriate for a particular case and ignore variations in behavior that both clinician and patient consider important. Self-response instruments depend on a standard of literacy that most younger children and some parents do not

have, and the use of rating systems introduce the same difficulties of variation between raters that have plagued clinical diagnosis. In return for these sacrifices, the fixed format provides substantial gains in analytic power and reliability. A more systematic approach to interviewing could thus effect a useful compromise between checklists or rating scales and the traditional interview, while retaining the merits of both.

Merits of Structured Interviews

Structured interviews can engage and maintain the interest of the respondent better than questionnaires; this is particularly true if a child is being interviewed. The interviewer can press for clarification of unclear replies in a way that is impossible with questionnaires. It is possible to elucidate meaning when the reply is ambiguous or has insufficient detail, and the reply can be recorded for coding more easily than is the case with either unstructured interviewing or questionnaires. In an interview it is easier to cope with the unexpected response, and it is easier to avoid redundancy and repetition. The onus of understanding the questions always lies with the interviewer, and so whenever the subject is handicapped by emotional, developmental, or other limitations, an interview is likely to be preferable to a questionnaire.

Another reason for preferring the interview is the recognition that the child's own view of his or her behavior deserves more attention than it usually receives. Children's reports may not be more valid or reliable than those of other informants, but they can add information that is not accessible in any other way. The dominant mode of interviewing younger children in psychiatric assessment has been some variant of a play interview. The belief underlying this technique is that a child may not be able to understand the concepts contained in direct questions about his or her own behavior and feelings, but if engaged in play will reveal behavior and feelings indirectly. Much of the information thus obtained rests on interpretations of play themes whose meaning and significance may often be ambiguous. Even if interpretation of behavior is not thought to be necessary, the play interview provides a somewhat standardized context in which the child's behavior can be observed. Though this approach should not be dismissed lightly, for there are indeed certain developmental limitations to a child's understanding of behavior and feelings,[5] recent experience suggests that a child has many feelings that are often not shared with parents but that may be discovered by careful direct interviewing.[23,28]

The Impact on Nosology

So far the recognition that a child may experience feelings that go unrecognized by the adults in his or her life has not had much impact on the diagnostic framework, but this must come soon. For example, suicidal ideation had been thought to be relatively uncommon in childhood, but when referred children were asked about their thoughts on unhappiness, death, and dying, as many as 52 percent reported having had ideas of suicide in the last year.[7] Similarly, I have found concerns over separation sufficient, by self-report, to meet DSM-III criteria for separation anxiety disorder in as many as 28 percent of a representative sample of children referred for psychiatric assessment. In contrast, clinicians made the diagnosis in only 6.5 percent of this sample. Interestingly, a similar rate was found in a study of pediatric patients whose behavior ostensibly was normal. Many of these children saw the pediatrician only for routine care.[12] The diagnostic criteria are based mainly on traditional parental reporting, but since parents are aware of few of these feelings of their children, only direct interviewing with the child could elicit the data. Even if an adult informant is used, the information may be far from perfect. Feasibility dictates that the evidence about social interactions for most children seen is obtained from the adults who see the child in the family or at school rather than from direct observation of the children themselves. Practical considerations often force us to collect most of our information about the child's interpersonal behavior from the parents, thus introducing some inevitable distortions.[3] One such distortion is that adults, not unreasonably, emphasize that which is most important to an adult—the impact the child's behavior has on themselves. Structured interviewing emphasizes but provides no solution to this conceptual problem in diagnosis.

Choice of Interviewing Method

The question still remains of how best to obtain that information needed to make a diagnosis which can only be obtained by interview, and how to determine which method or instrument will give the best information. The ultimate criterion is, of course, diagnostic validity, but the process of improving clinical diagnosis has to proceed step by step, and the steps necessary to producing replicable diagnoses must be taken before much can be done to increase their validity. Table 16–1 shows the major sources of variation in diagnosis. Categorical and criterion variance are still quite large in clinical practice, for the publication of a system such as DSM-III does not guarantee either that it will be used or used well.

When diagnoses are made on the basis of independent examinations with unstructured interviews, the variance in the kind of questions asked is enormous, and is probably the largest single source of diagnostic disagreements. It is this source of variance that structured interviewing attempts to reduce. By having prescribed the questions to ask, the investigator can at

TABLE 16–1

Sources of Variation in Diagnosis

Clinician	
Categorical variance	Different clinicians use differing categories
Criterion variance	
a. Overt	Clinicians use different criteria for same diagnoses
b. Concealed	Clinicians interpret the same criteria in different ways
Question variance	Interviewers (clinicians) ask different questions to elicit same criteria
Respondent or patient	
Informant variance	Each informant (parent, child, teacher) reports different behavior or symptoms
Temporal variance	Behavior and symptoms change over time
Practice effect	Repeated questioning induces change in reports
Interaction	
Therapeutic effect	Interview induces positive change (reassurance, catharsis, etc.)
Rapport	Quality of interaction between interviewer and interviewee modifies report

least be confident that negative information is based on specific inquiries and does not merely mean that the appropriate questions were never asked. A range of strategies can be used to reduce question variance. At one end of the range the investigator can require the interviewer to complete a checklist that reviews the diagnostic criteria but does not specify the questions that must be used to obtain this information. Such an "interview" can at best be described as only loosely structured. Many phrases can be used to express the same concept, and they may be understood (or misunderstood) in many more ways.

If the questions are prepared beforehand for the interviewer, one major source of variation (and hence disagreement) is reduced, even though the fidelity with which they are administered may vary.

Most investigators who have constructed such interviews have been reluctant to phrase their questions so that they only require a "yes" or a "no" reply, since such questions may inhibit the detail more open-ended questions elicit. To overcome the difficulties of recording a lengthy answer, it has been customary to distinguish between alternatives that are diagnostically significant. For example, if a child has answered yes to the question "Do you ever lie to your parents about important things?" the interviewer might ask "How long have you been telling lies about important things to your parents?" The answer might simply be coded as more or less than six months, since this is the critical duration for a diagnosis of conduct disorder in DSM-III. However, a child will commonly give a vague answer to this question, such as "Quite a long time." In the case of duration, a sequence of probes can obviously be constructed without too much difficulty, though it may be clumsy if every question in the sequence has to be written down in the interview. Other details of symptomatology may be more difficult to elicit and suitable questions harder to anticipate and prepare beforehand. It may be necessary either to accept some imprecision for the sake of uniformity in interviewing or to train the interviewer to exercise judgment, and allow him or her some liberty in choosing an appropriate phrase or in deciding if a response meets criterion or not. This strategy is best described as semistructured interviewing.

The alternative, in which all questions are prepared beforehand and the interviewer is not allowed to deviate from them, has rarely been attempted in psychiatric interviews. The National Institute of Mental Health (NIMH) Diagnostic Interview Schedule[11] for Children, which is the most highly structured interview for child psychiatric disorders now available, allows and indeed encourages the interviewer to devise unstructured prompts to elicit the duration of symptoms (which of all the information needed for psychiatric diagnosis is the most difficult to elicit reliably from children). The most widely used schedule, the schedule for Affective Disorders and Schizophrenia for School-Age Children (K-SADS),[37] not only gives the interviewer much more latitude, but allows the questions asked of the child to be modified by the information the interviewer has already obtained from the parent, who must therefore be seen first. This method of interviewing is believed to give the interviewer more chance of eliminating errors in the child's report that arise from misunderstanding or from the child's inability to recall spontaneously problems of the past. Unfortunately, it also means that it is impossible to obtain and evaluate a truly independent report from the child. If an independent interview is necessary, it is preferable to have the child interview given by someone who has not heard the parent interview, since the probability of interviewer bias is very high.

Validation

Though structured interviewing is theoretically desirable in some circumstances, there are many difficulties in evaluating its merits. The central problem is the lack of a criterion against which to validate the diagnoses thus generated. Clinical diagnosis has been shown repeatedly to have very poor reliability.[4,5,44] No validating criterion can be satisfactory if it is not itself reliable, and since clinical diagnosis is so flawed, even a perfect diagnostic instrument could not correlate better with a clinician than two independent clinicians would with each other.[21] To some extent checklist assessments may be helpful measures against which concurrent validation may be obtained. Obvious circularities arise if information from the same informant is used to validate a diagnosis. This is true even if the data are analyzed in a different way (e.g., a checklist completed by the parent may be used to "validate" a parent's interview). However, if it can be shown that children diagnosed by an interview with the parent or child as having aggressive conduct disorder receive higher scores for aggression and delinquency on an independant assessment such as a teacher checklist, then there is some *prima facie* evidence to support the diagnosis. There have been few attempts to validate either clinical or structured interview diagnoses in this way, perhaps because the generally accepted belief is that differences between the teacher's and the child's or the parent's report are to be expected.

Reliability

The argument that limits the usefulness of clinical diagnosis as a criterion can also be applied to the structured interview itself. If it is not reliable, it cannot be valid. The question is, which sort of reliability should be assessed? As noted, there are differences between children's and parents' reports. Children are less reliable reporters but do report symptoms parents have not recognized, so it should be expected that diagnoses generated from the reports of parents and children will disagree. Thus interinformant agreement in this case is a poor criterion. Reliability between independent interviews on different occasions also has some problems. If good agreement can be obtained, then the interview is reliable, but poor agreement does not necessarily mean that the interview is unsatisfactory.[36] Children change some symptomatology very rapidly, and the reliable interview may simply be insensitive to such changes. Clinicians claim that the interview process may itself bring some symptomatic relief, and it is possible that structured interviews may have the same effect. On the other hand, the process of being interviewed may be frankly aversive or may train the child in strategies he or she can use on the second occasion to shorten the interview. Conversely, it could be argued that an interview with high test-retest reliability may have introduced spurious reliability by reifying the symptoms or by suggesting to the child syndromic associations that do not really exist. Issues such as these are familiar in psychological testing and were solved by the device of alternate forms, each version having similar performance on a matched sample of children, which could be compared with one another. Further research using this design would undoubtedly resolve some of these difficulties.

Unless clinicians are allowed to explore the meaning of replies, a structured interview and associated diagnostic rules may award some children diagnoses clinicians themselves would not make. However, if clinicians *are* given this freedom, more variability in diagnosis is inevitable. The most popular solution has been to train clinicians so rigorously that all use similar diagnostic constructs and even when given some latitude adopt a very similar interviewing technique. For example, Chambers and associates[8] trained seven clinicians but did not use three who did not meet their criteria after training. This solution is probably the best when small numbers of children have to be diagnosed accurately, but it is still not totally satisfactory. Rigorous training is difficult to define operationally, and others may find it difficult to replicate the original procedures. The inconvenience and cost of using selected, highly trained clinicians may make this approach impracticable. Moreover, experience with the much simpler judgments involved in direct observation suggests other problems. Even when simple behaviors are operationally defined and observers trained to criterion, it has been found that without repeated reliability checks observers' decisions tend to drift.[39] The problem is even greater when diagnostic decisions are in question, and repeated reliability checks on diagnosticians present a daunting task.

Criteria for a Review Assessment

The basic criteria for assessing an instrument derive from the preceding discussion. The recording of answers must be reliable, which can be tested by comparing the scores of independent raters rating a videotape. If it is not to be a limiting factor, the investigator should seek interrater reliability correlation coefficients of about 0.9 for symptom scores. Second, the raw data on which diagnostic decisions are based (symptom scores or symptom ratings) must have reasonable reliability when two independent interviews are compared. Product moment or intraclass correlations of the order of 0.75 to 0.85 are acceptable and comparable with the performance of many symptom-specific scales that have proven heuristic value. Third, the classificatory rules used to make diagnoses must give reliable results. Fourth, the instrument must have reasonable specificity and sensitivity. Specificity is the number correctly identified as healthy, divided by the actual number of healthy individuals in the population. Sensitivity is the number of cases identified as abnormal divided by the number of true cases in the population studied.[21] These two properties conflict, so the instrument should either have specificity and sensitivity suitable for the application or the method of scoring be such that specificity and sensitivity can be adjusted.

Finally, there must be evidence of validity. The instrument can be inspected for face validity—that is, the questions should correspond to the diagnostic concepts being used. Though a perfect correspondence should not be expected, there should be correlations with other instruments measuring the same constructs—thus a depression score from an interview might be correlated with other measures of depression. There should be some correspondence with clinical diagnosis. Though it will not be high, for the reasons reviewed earlier, in particular there should be no evidence of systematic disagreement. Better criteria than these involve validating the diagnostic constructs as well, which is clearly a long-term task.

Reviews of Specific Instruments

One difficulty in making a choice of instrument is that basic information on performance is often not available. Such comparisons as can be made are shown in table 16–2, but, as Orvaschel's more extensive review [34] showed, crucial aspects of performance are often not reported. Given this lack of evaluative data, it is not unreasonable to select an interview on the basis of practical considerations such as the information generated, the time taken, the ease of training interviewers, and the like. Several instruments developed in recent years are described in the next sections. Inevitably most are still undergoing development, and would-be users of structured interviews should keep abreast of current revisions.

THE BEHAVIOR SCREENING QUESTIONNAIRE

The Behavior Screening Questionnaire (BSQ) instrument was developed by Richman and Graham [40] to identify disturbed preschool children and is the only interview available for this age range. It contains approximately sixty questions, most of which focus on current behavior, but a few cover the last month or year. Questions can be read verbatim or can also be supplemented until the interviewer feels confident about the rating, so the interview is best described as semistructured. Responses are coded on a 0–1–2 scale, where 0 indicates that the behavior is absent, 1 indicates that the behavior occurs sometimes or to a mild degree, and 2 indicates that the behavior occurs frequently or to a marked degree. Because of the unstructured format and the level of judgment required, a trained, preferably clinically experienced, interviewer is needed. Diagnoses are not generated.

The behavior scale consists of only twelve items, which were chosen because they discriminated between clinically referred and nonreferred children. Since few children this age are referred to psychiatrists, this criterion may have led to the omission of behaviors that might be of interest in longitudinal studies. Interrater reliability on taped interviews was 0.94, falling to 0.77 for independent interviews, but the reliability for individual items only averaged 0.44, with a range of 0.15 to 0.77 (product-moment correlation). Validity was tested by comparing twenty children referred for services with fifty-seven normal controls, and a cut-off score of 11 out of a possible 24 points gave good separation. At this cut-off sensitivity was 70 percent and specificity 91.2 percent.

A number of epidemiological studies* support the

*See references 13, 14, 15, 16, 17, and 41.

instrument's validity. A four-year longitudinal study by Richman, Stevenson, and Graham [42] offers further evidence to support its usefulness. Earls and associates [17] reported a correlation of 0.74 between scores on the BSQ behavior scale and clinicians' ratings of psychiatric impairment, which were based on observations of the child's behavior in the home, parent ratings, and a summary of the entire interview with the parent. Using clinicians' ratings as the criterion of psychiatric disorder, a cut-off score of 11 gave a sensitivity of 64 percent and a specificity of 98 percent. Dropping the cut-off score to 8 gave a sensitivity of 100 percent, but at the expense of reducing specificity to 70 percent, so that although all cases were detected, out of every one hundred normal children thirty would be mistakenly identified as abnormal. Given the difficulties of psychiatric nosology in the preschool child, this instrument is as useful a tool as could reasonably be expected at the time. As more knowledge of symptomatology in this age range is acquired, a more detailed interview will probably be needed.

THE DIAGNOSTIC INTERVIEW FOR CHILDREN AND ADOLESCENTS

The Diagnostic Interview for Children and Adolescents (DICA) is the result of research begun in 1975 by Herjanic and her colleagues. [22,23,39] This is a highly structured interview in which the order and wording of questions are specified and the responses precoded. Lay interviewers have used it successfully. The organization of the interview is a compromise between themes such as behavior at home, behavior at school, and friendships, and diagnostic syndromes such as the affective disorders. A "skip" structure allows many questions to be omitted if initial screening questions elicit a negative response. Most questions can be answered yes or no. The interview covers the ages six through sixteen and lasts sixty to ninety minutes. Alternative versions for parent and child are available, with virtually the same wording apart from the changes of grammar involved. Interrater agreement on two videotaped interviews was of the order of 85 percent. No data have been published so far on test-retest reliability, but there is extensive information on agreement between mother and child interviews conducted independently by different interviewers. Agreement between mother and child averaged 80 percent for the 207 items in the questionnaire, but this largely reflects agreement that the behavior was *absent*. When kappa, [9] a coefficient of agreement that corrects for chance agreement, is used, the average coefficient of agreement is only 0.22. [23] Agreement on diagnoses based on information from mother and child is fair, with kappas ranging from 0.14 for neurotic disorder to 0.59 for

TABLE 16–2

Comparison of Selected Interviews

Attribute	BSQ[40]	DICA[22,23]	K-SADS[8]	CAS[26]	ISC[30]	DISC[11,12]	
Age range	3–5	6–16	6–17	7–12	8–17	6–17	
Informant	Parent	Parent and child	Parent and child	Child	Parent and child	Parent and child	
Format	Semistructured	Structured	Semistructured	Semistructured	Semistructured	Structured	
Interviewer training	Clinical and specific training needed	Specific (interview) training only	Clinical and specific training needed	Clinical and specific training needed	Clinical and specific training needed	Specific (interview) training only	
End product	Symptom score, specific symptomatology	Symptom scores, ICD-9 diagnoses	Symptom scores, DSM-III diagnoses	Symptom scores	Symptom scores	Symptom scores, DSM-III diagnoses	
Processing	Computer or manual	Computer	Clinical judgment	Computer or manual	Clinical judgment	Computer	
Inter-rater reliability: range	Not reported	80–90%	0.86 (parent), 0.89 (child)	0.44–0.82	0.50–1.0	0.94–1.0 (child)	
average	0.94 (total score)	85%	Not reported	0.74	0.91	0.98 (child)	
median	Not reported	Not reported	Not reported	0.70	0.87	0.99 (child)	
						Parent	**Child**
Test-retest reliability: range	0.15–0.77	Not reported	0.09–0.89	Not reported	Not reported	0.40–0.86	0.26–0.77
average	0.44	Not reported	0.57	Not reported	Not reported	0.80	0.69
median	0.48	Not reported	0.56	Not reported	Not reported	0.83	0.74
Sensitivity	64–100%	72%	Not reported	78%	Not reported	60–92.5% (parent)	
Specificity	98–70%	76%	Not reported	83.8%	Not reported	95–30% (parent)	
Study sample size	18 patients, 39 controls	257 patients, 50 controls	52 patients	50 patients, 37 controls	75 patients	316 patients, 40 controls	
Validation criteria	Referred vs. nonreferred, Follow up data	Referred vs. nonreferred	Biological studies, Follow-up data	CBCL and other scales, Referred vs. nonreferred	Follow-up data	CBCL (teacher, parent), Referred vs. nonreferred, Clinical comparison	

enuresis, the majority falling below 0.40.[39] Younger children agreed less well with their mothers, and diagnoses related to overt behavior, such as "antisocial personality," tended to be more reliable.

Despite these difficulties, the total symptom score discriminated significantly between fifty children referred to a psychiatric clinic and fifty matched controls taken from a pediatric clinic.[23] Items relating to problems of relationships and adjustment at school gave the best discrimination. More obviously psychiatric symptoms were not so effective, with neurotic and somatic symptoms yielding the poorest discrimination. Screening efficiency for the total score cannot be calculated from the data provided, but from the data on relationship problems it appears that sensitivity was 72 percent and specificity 76 percent.

THE SCHEDULE FOR AFFECTIVE DISORDERS AND SCHIZOPHRENIA FOR SCHOOL-AGE CHILDREN

The K-SADS was developed by Puig-Antich and his colleagues[37] from the SADS (Schedule for Affective Disorders and Schizophrenia), a structured interview for adults.[20] It is a semistructured interview that, despite the title, is designed to provide information for a broad range of DSM-III diagnoses. It can also generate the information needed for diagnoses made using the Research Diagnostic Criteria (RDC),[45] where these can be applied to children ages six to seventeen. The interview should be administered by an interviewer with clinical training who has also received specific training on the instrument. Performance may be poor if interviewers are not selected carefully and trained rigorously.[8] To make best use of the interview, they must be familiar with DSM-III and RDC criteria.

The parent and child are interviewed separately, but the parent is interviewed first and this interview establishes the broad framework of the symptomatology. If there are discrepancies between parent and child in the subsequent report from the child, the child can be asked about the differences, before the interviewer makes final ratings. Each interview begins with an unstructured section lasting fifteen to twenty minutes, which the interviewer uses to establish rapport, to determine the child's general functioning, and to obtain an outline of presenting complaints, their duration and frequency. This done, the interviewer moves on to structured segments, each covering a specific diagnostic area, and starts with a set of screening questions. If the replies to these are negative, the remainder of the segment can be skipped. Though suggested questions are provided, these are not intended to be used as structured probes. Younger children may need simpler wording, and the authors recommend that if there is

doubt about the answer, the question should be rephrased to verify that the child understood. The interview takes about one hour each for the parent and for the child, but may take longer for children under eight years old. The interviewer rates the response to each question or set of questions eliciting a symptom (either present or absent or present, suspected, or absent) and also completes summary ratings of the criteria, which are used to make formal diagnoses. Two versions are available: one focuses on the present episode (K-SADS-P), the other on past illness (K-SADS-E). The latter is somewhat more structured and was designed for epidemiological work.[35]

Preliminary studies, which were inspired by the need to diagnose depression reliably in children, gave interrater reliabilities of 0.86 for the parent section and 0.89 for the child on the component criteria of depression (intraclass correlation coefficients). Subsequent interinterview reliability was assessed in a design in which two evaluations were done one to three days apart. For summary ratings of symptom scores, combining parent and child information, the intraclass correlations between the two sets of interviews ranged from 0.09 to 0.89, with a mean of 0.57 and a median of 0.56.[8] The poorer correlations were all for internalizing symptoms; the scales for hypochondria, panic attacks, and obsessions/compulsions were particularly unreliable. Some of the subscales for depression were also poor, though the summary ratings all had acceptable reliability (mean $r = 0.70$). Reliability (kappa) for diagnosis ranged from 0.24 for nondepressed neurotic disorder to 0.70 for minor and chronic intermittent depression.

THE CHILD ASSESSMENT SCHEDULE

The Child Assessment Schedule (CAS) was developed by Hodges and associates[25,26,27] to remedy what these investigators saw as defects of the K-SADS and its predecessors. Specifically, the CAS was designed to have structured content, to be easy to use, and to maintain rapport by making only modest demands on the child. It is organized by topics related to a child's ideas and interests rather than to diagnostic syndromes. It is designed for seven- to twelve-year-olds, though with additions it would be suitable for adolescents. The authors emphasize a clinical orientation; they suggest that it can be used in a clinical setting and may be helpful in training novice clinicians in interviewing skills. No parent version is available. Clinical judgment is required in coding responses and in rating behavioral observations, but the exact wording of the questions to be asked is provided, with alternate wording for some questions that may not be understood. Despite this, the authors describe it as a semistructured interview, so it is not clear how far an interviewer may deviate from the prescribed questions. Some disorders that are rarely diagnosed in children (e.g., manic disorder) are covered by some preliminary questions, but probes to establish the diagnosis are not provided, and if the child gives a positive reply to one of these screening questions, then the clinician would have to pursue the diagnosis further with additional questions.

Three sections cover (1) the direct interview with the child, which contains approximately seventy-five questions; (2) the observer's ratings of the child's behavior, which has fifty-three items; and (3) questions dealing with onset and duration of symptoms, when these are needed to make a DSM-III diagnosis. The interview is reasonably concise, taking forty-five minutes to an hour to administer. Children's replies are rated as yes/no/ambiguous/no response/not applicable. Symptom scales are provided that are related to DSM-III diagnoses, but the authors argue that many criteria cannot be elicited in a child interview, and so clinical judgment must be used to make a diagnosis. Interrater reliability was tested on videotaped interviews and averaged 0.9 for the total score. Mean kappas for individual items ranged from 0.47 to 0.61. Correlations for subscales ranged from 0.44 for socialized conduct problems to 0.82 for depression. In another study[26] using a smaller sample, raters rating live interviews independently through a one-way mirror achieved much higher reliability on symptom scales, with an average reliability of 0.93. No test-retest reliability data have been published.

Concurrent validity was assessed by comparing CAS scores with the Child Behavior Checklist (CBCL),[1] the Children's Depression Inventory,[29] and the State-Trait Anxiety Inventory for Children.[43] Correlations between corresponding scales in the CAS and these instruments were adequate. A discriminant analysis was used to compare the CAS with these instruments in their ability to discriminate between inpatients, outpatients, and normal controls. For this review the data has been recalculated to test the discrimination between patients and nonpatients, though differences between inpatients and outpatients were also detectable. Sensitivity for the CAS was 78 percent and specificity 83.78 percent. Corresponding figures for the CBCL on the same subjects were 86.9 percent and 94.6 percent. Combining the CAS and the CBCL in one discriminant function gave a sensitivity of 93.6 percent and specificity of 100 percent. Of course the categorization by patient status reflects the parents' and clinicians' evaluation of similar information, but this is perhaps the strongest support available to validate the use of a structured diagnostic interview as an element in a case-finding procedure.

THE INTERVIEW SCHEDULE FOR CHILDREN

The Interview Schedule for Children (ISC) is a semistructured research interview for children ages eight to seventeen that was developed for a study of depression in childhood by Kovacs and her colleagues.[30] Since the main interest of this study was temporal change in symptomatology, the instrument is unique in that parallel forms are available for initial assessment and for follow-up interviews. It has undergone several revisions and expansions since initial construction in 1974. Though the emphasis is on affective diagnoses, the range of symptoms explored is broad. Parent and child are interviewed separately, the parent first. The initial assessment generally requires 90 to 150 minutes with the parent and 45 to 90 minutes with the child. The interview is organized by symptom areas. Symptoms are rated separately for each informant, and an overall summary rating is provided. Clinical judgment is required both in the choice of phraseology and in rating; however, an extensive set of questions that the interviewer should use is provided. Interviewers need both clinical training and extensive specific training in the use of the ISC.

Interrater reliability was studied by having pairs of interviewers conduct joint interviews in which one interviewer gave the questions and the other observed; each rated the answers independently.[30] Intraclass correlations on overall ratings ranged from 0.50 for the clinician's rating of psychomotor retardation to 1.0 for some psychotic symptoms, encopresis, and dating behavior. The median correlation was 0.87 and the average was 0.91. Parent and child symptom scores correlations varied from 0.02 (pessimism) to 0.95 (truancy); the median correlation was 0.62 and the mean 0.66. As in other studies, there was a tendency for children to report more internalizing symptoms such as anxiety or depressed feelings than their parents had noted. Test-retest data are not available, and although the instrument has strong content validity, its ability to discriminate between normals and abnormals is unknown. Kovac's longitudinal data support the construct validity of the diagnostic scales.[31]

THE DIAGNOSTIC INTERVIEW SCHEDULE FOR CHILDREN

The Diagnostic Interview Schedule for Children (DISC) is the most recently developed structured interview. Initially written by Conners, Herjanic, and Puig-Antich, the earliest version was based closely on the DICA, though subsequent revision by Costello and associates[10,11] introduced many changes. The DISC, a highly structured interview, was designed as an epidemiological instrument to be administered by lay interviewers. Virtually all the wording of questions is predetermined, and responses are precoded. No training, other than on the use of the DISC itself, is required to administer it, and scoring is by computer. It can be given to children from six to seventeen years of age, and covers nearly all the DSM-III diagnoses that can be applied to children of this age range. An equivalent form for the parent (the DISC-P) covers the same questions but adds some additional items a child could not answer. The child interview takes forty-five minutes, the parent interview about seventy-five minutes; because there are many skip structures children with many symptoms may take longer. Answers are coded on the conventional three-point scale. Symptom scores are derived by summing the answer codes for questions addressing the same symptom area and are grouped hierarchically using DSM-III criteria as organizing principles. Diagnoses are derived by applying algorithms that operationalize DSM-III criteria.

The interrater reliability of coding from videotapes was tested using lay interviewers as raters. The reliability of symptom scores ranged from 0.94 to 1.0 (product-moment correlations); the average reliability of all scores for all raters was 0.98. Test-retest reliability was studied in a balanced, crossover design in which one set of interviews were conducted by lay interviewers and another by trained clinicians. The lay interviewers proved virtually identical in performance to the trained clinicians. Correlations between the first and second parent interview ranged from 0.40 (mania) to 0.86 (all conduct problems), with a mean of 0.80 and a median of 0.83. For children the range was from 0.26 (mania) to 0.77 (nonaggressive conduct disorder); the mean correlation for all symptom scores was 0.69 and the median was 0.74. Younger children were the least reliable; the reliability of children over ten approached, and by fourteen equaled, that of the parents.

All children tended to report far fewer symptoms in the second interview, with a reduction in symptom scores of the order of 20 percent, though again the effect was most marked for younger children. Parents showed a much smaller reduction, on the order of 5 percent. Given the reliability of the symptom scores and this tendency for fewer symptoms to be reported on the second occasion, the poor test-retest reliability of diagnoses made by computer was disappointing but hardly surprising. When the criteria were stiffened by requiring that a child not only meet DSM-III criteria but also pass a cutoff point on the relevant symptom scale, reliability improved. Kappas for the parent interview ranged from 0.21 (overanxious disorder) to 0.73 (major depression), with a mean of 0.50. For the child interview the range was 0.21 (attention deficit disorder and oppositional disorder) to 0.47 (conduct disorder), with a mean of 0.34.

Sensitivity and specificity were measured by comparing pediatric and psychiatric samples of children ages seven to eleven. Predictably, the parent interview was more powerful; using any DSM diagnosis generated by the DISC-P as a criterion, sensitivity ranged from 60 percent for severe diagnoses to 92.5 percent for all diagnoses. Coresponding specificities were 95 percent and 30 percent, which illustrates the tradeoff between these two characteristics. For the child interview, although a sensitivity of 95 percent could be achieved with a specificity of 25 percent, restricting the analysis to severe diagnoses improved specificity to only 80 percent, while sensitivity fell to 45 percent. Total symptom scores were highly effective in discriminating the two groups ($t = 7.5, p < 0.001$ for the DISC-P; $t = 3.2, p < 0.01$ for the DISC).[12] A discriminant function using symptom scores from the two interviews gave a sensitivity of 95 percent and specificity of 97.5 percent with more weight given, as might be expected, to the parent report.

Concurrent validity was studied by comparing the DISC and DISC-P scores with the CBCL parent and teacher forms.[1] The correlations of the parent interview with the parent CBCL were greater than 0.70. The correlation for the child interview total score with CBCL was only of the order of 0.30. There were significant correlations between relevant symptom scales on the DISC-P and these instruments for all but neurotic symptoms. There were some associations between the DISC subscales and the two sets of CBCL scores, but they were weaker and less consistent. Finally, though exact agreement with clinical diagnosis was poor, which is not surprising given the known unreliability of clinical diagnosis, the patterns of symptom scores distinguished consistently between different clinical diagnostic groups.

Summary

It is not easy at this time to make a choice of interview instrument. No single instrument emerges as superior for all purposes, and each has some strengths and some weaknesses. In research applications, it will be necessary to make a choice that will depend on the nature of the research question. More work is obviously needed on the comparative merits of the different approaches displayed here, and it is regrettable that so little of the performance data is comparable from one instrument to another.

Though the current state of the field is in many ways perplexing, clinicians who have attempted structured interviewing have found that asking questions that are not prompted by the presenting complaints or clinical intuition can reveal extensive psychopathology. The experience is salutary and instructive. Although when making a clinical assessment it may not always be feasible, and is sometimes undesirable, to give an exhaustive interview, experience with structured interviewing shows that many questions must be asked routinely. Many clinicians who have used structured interviews acknowledge that the experience has improved their interviewing technique. Though the ultimate validity of diagnoses depends on other data, such as consistency in etiology or prognosis, if the fundamental symptomatology cannot be reliably defined then validity will remain elusive. It seems inevitable that reliable definition will have to depend on good structured interviews.

These approaches are clearly more suitable for research than for clinical practice. However, clinicians who wish to calibrate their diagnostic skills and to discover if cases of depression or other major disorder match those described in the research literature should consider using an instrument designed with high specificity for this purpose, such as the ISC or the K-SADS. Clinicians who wish to improve their interviewing skills with young children might consider the CAS. Someone wanting to survey a population at risk should consider an instrument that can be used by less skilled interviewers and that can have high sensitivity, such as the DISC. All are worth reading and using, if only to help the reader understand current research literature and its limitations. All must be used with care, for none can give an authoritative diagnosis and none elicit the complementary information on family life, background, and development that is so essential to the planning of treatment.

ACKNOWLEDGMENT

Preparation of this chapter was supported in part by contract #278-81-0027 from the National Institute of Mental Health.

REFERENCES

1. ACHENBACH, T. M., and EDELBROCK, C. *Manual for the Child Behavior Checklist.* Burlington: University of Vermont, 1983.

2. AMERICAN PSYCHIATRIC ASSOCIATION. *Diagnostic and Statistical Manual of Mental Disorders,* 3rd ed. Washington, D.C.: American Psychiatric Association, 1980.

3. BECKER, W. "Parental Ratings and Behavior of Children," *Journal of Consulting Psychology,* 24 (1960):507–527.

4. BEITCHMAN, J. H., et al. "Reliability of the Group for Advancement of Psychiatry Diagnostic Categories in Child Psychiatry," *Archives of General Psychiatry,* 35 (1978):1461–1466.

5. BIERMAN, K. L. "Cognitive Development and Clinical Interviews with Children," in B. Lahey and A. E. Kazdin, eds., *Advances in Clinical Child Psychology,* vol. 6. New York: Plenum Press, 1984, pp. 217–250.

6. CANTWELL, P., et al. "A Comparison of DSM-II and DSM-III in the Diagnosis of Childhood Psychiatric Disorders: I. Agreement with Expected Diagnosis," *Archives of General Psychiatry,* 36 (1979):1208–1213.

7. CARLSON, G. A., and CANTWELL, D. P. "A Survey of Depressive Symptoms in a Child and Adolescent Psychiatric Population," *Journal of the American Academy of Child Psychiatry,* 18 (1979):587–599.

8. CHAMBERS, W. J., et al. "The Assessment of Affective Disorders in Children and Adolescents by Semi-structured Interview: Test-retest Reliability of the K-SADS-P," *Archives of General Psychiatry,* 42 (1985):696–702.

9. COHEN, J. "A Coefficient of Agreement for Nominal Scales," *Educational and Psychological Measurement,* 20 (1974):37–46.

10. COSTELLO, A. J., et al. "The Development of the Diagnostic Interview Schedule for Children," Paper presented at the Annual Meeting of the American Academy of Child Psychiatry, Washington D.C., 1982.

11. COSTELLO, A. J., et al. "Report to NIMH on the Diagnostic Interview for Children," Unpublished manuscript, University of Pittsburgh, 1984.

12. COSTELLO, E. J., EDELBROCK, C. S., and COSTELLO, A. J. "Validity of the NIMH Diagnostic Interview Schedule for Children: A Comparison Between Psychiatric and Pediatric Referrals," *Journal of Abnormal Child Psychology,* 13 (1985):579–595.

13. EARLS, F. "The Prevalence of Behavior Problems in Three-year-old Children: Comparison of Reports of Mothers and Fathers," *Journal of the American Academy of Child Psychiatry,* 19 (1980):439–452.

14. ———. "The Prevalence of Behavior Problems in Three-year-old Children: A Cross-national Replication," *Archives of General Psychiatry,* 37 (1980):1153–1157.

15. EARLS, F., and RICHMAN, N. "The Prevalence of Behaviour Problems in Three-year-old Children of West Indian–born Parents." *Journal of Child Psychology and Psychiatry,* 21 (1980):99–107.

16. ———. "Behaviour Problems of Preschool Children of West Indian–born parents: A Re-examination of Family and Social Factors," *Journal of Child Psychology and Psychiatry,* 21 (1980):108–117.

17. EARLS, F., et al. "Concurrent Validation of a Behavior Problems Scale for Use with 3-year-olds," *Journal of the American Academy of Child Psychiatry,* 21 (1982):47–57.

18. EDELBROCK, C. S., et al. "Age Differences in the Reliability of the Psychiatric Interview of the Child," *Child Development,* 56 (1985):265–275.

19. ENDICOTT, J., and SPITZER, R. L. "A Diagnostic Interview: The Schedule for Affective Disorders and Schizophrenia," *Archives of General Psychiatry,* 35 (1978):837–844.

20. GALEN, R. S., and GAMBINO, S. R. *Beyond Normality: The Predictive Value and Efficiency of Medical Diagnoses.* New York: John Wiley & Sons, 1975.

21. GROVE, W. M., et al. "Reliability Studies of Psychiatric Diagnosis," *Archives of General Psychiatry,* 38 (1981):408–413.

22. HERJANIC, B., and CAMPBELL, W. "Differentiating Psychiatrically Disturbed Children on the Basis of a Structured Interview," *Journal of Abnormal Child Psychology,* 5 (1977):127–134.

23. HERJANIC, B., and REICH, W. "Development of a Structured Interview for Children: Agreement Between Child and Parent on Individual Symptoms," *Journal of Abnormal Child Psychology,* 10 (1982):307–324.

24. HERJANIC, B., et al. "Are Children Reliable Reporters?" *Journal of Abnormal Child Psychology,* 3 (1975):41–48.

25. HODGES, K. "The Child Assessment Schedule (CAS)," Unpublished interview, University of Missouri, 1982.

26. HODGES, K., et al. "The Child Assessment Schedule (CAS) Diagnostic Interview: A Report on Reliability and Validity," *Journal of the American Academy of Child Psychiatry,* 21 (1982):468–473.

27. HODGES, K., et al. "The Development of a Child Assessment Interview for Research and Clinical Use," *Journal of Abnormal Child Psychology,* 10 (1982):173–189.

28. KAZDIN, A. E., et al. "Assessment of Childhood Depression: Correspondence of Child and Parent Ratings," *Journal of the American Academy of Child Psychiatry,* 22 (1983):157–164.

29. KOVACS, M. "Children's Depression Inventory (CDI)," Unpublished manuscript, University of Pittsburgh, 1978.

30. ———. "The Interview Schedule for Children (ISC): Inter-rater and Parent-child Agreement," Unpublished manuscript, University of Pittsburgh, 1984.

31. KOVACS, M., et al. "Depressive Disorders in Childhood," *Archives of General Psychiatry,* 41 (1984):229–237.

32. MATTISON, R., et al. "A Comparison of DSM-II and DSM-III in the Diagnosis of Childhood Psychiatric Disorders," *Archives of General Psychiatry,* 36 (1979):1217–1222.

33. MEZZICH, A. C., and MEZZICH, J. E. "Diagnostic Reliability of Childhood and Adolescent Behavior Disorders," Paper presented at the Annual Meeting of the American Psychological Association, New York, 1979.

34. ORVASCHEL, H. *The Assessment of Psychopathology and Behavioral Problems in Children: A Review of Scales Suitable for Epidemiological and Clinical Research (1967–1979).* Rockville, Md.: National Institute of Mental Health, 1979.

35. ORVASCHEL, H., et al. "Retrospective Assessment of Child Psychopathology with the K-SADS-E," *Journal of the American Academy of Child Psychiatry,* 4 (1982):392–397.

36. PLATT, S. "On Establishing the Validity of 'Objective' Data: Can We Rely on Cross-interview Agreement?" *Psychological Medicine,* 10 (1980):573–581.

37. PUIG-ANTICH, J., et al. "Prepubertal Major Depressive Disorders," *Journal of the American Academy of Child Psychiatry,* 17 (1978):695–707.

38. REICH, W., et al. "Development of a Structured Psychiatric Interview for Children: Agreement on Diagnosis Comparing Parent and Child," *Journal of Abnormal Child Psychology,* 10 (1982):325–336.

39. REID, J. B. "Reliability Assessment of Observation Data: A Possible Methodological Problem," *Child Development,* 41 (1970):1143–1150.

40. RICHMAN, N., and GRAHAM, P. "A Behavioural Screening Questionnaire for Use with Three-year-old Children: Preliminary Findings," *Journal of Child Psychology and Psychiatry,* 16 (1968):277–287.

41. RICHMAN, N., STEVENSON, J., and GRAHAM, P. "Prevalence of Behaviour Problems in Three-year-old Children: An Epidemiological Study in a London Borough," *Journal of Child Psychology and Psychiatry,* 16 (1975):277–287.

42. ———. *Pre-school to School: A Behavioural Study.* London: Academic Press, 1983.

43. SPIELBERGER, C. D. *Test Manual for the State-Trait Anxiety Inventory for Children.* Palo Alto, Calif.: Consulting Psychologist Press, 1973.

44. SPITZER, R. L., and FLEISS, J. F. "A Re-analysis of the Reliability of Psychiatric Diagnosis," *British Journal of Psychiatry,* 125 (1974):341–347.

45. SPITZER, R. L., ENDICOTT, J., and ROBINS, E. "Research Diagnostic Criteria: Rationale and Reliability," *Archives of General Psychiatry,* 35 (1978):773–782.

---

17 / **Behavioral Checklists and Rating Scales**

Craig Edelbrock

Introduction

Behavioral checklists and rating scales play a central role in many clinical and research efforts in child psychiatry. Their importance is due in part to the nature of childhood psychopathology and the way in which mental health services are provided to children. Few children refer themselves for mental health services, and clinical decisions about children depend heavily on reports and ratings by adults. Many childhood disorders (e.g., oppositional disorder, attention deficit disorder, separation anxiety) are defined by deviations in fairly common behaviors that occur sometimes or to some degree in most children. Moreover, behaviors of clinical significance occur primarily in natural settings such as home and school and are not always observable in the clinic. Parents' and teachers' perceptions of children's behavioral functioning are therefore crucial to the detection and diagnosis of childhood disorders. Standard ways of describing children's emotional and behavioral functioning and of comparing such data to normative baselines are essential. Rating scales represent one means of fulfilling this need.

As assessment and taxonomic tools, checklists and rating scales have numerous assets. Compared to other assessment methods, such as direct observation, clinical interviewing, and psychological testing, paper-and-pencil questionnaires are simple, economical, and efficient in terms of professional time. They also yield a wealth of descriptive information. Rating scales increase the objectivity of adult's descriptions of children's behavior, and they require the informant to rate specific behaviors rather than making a global judgment of normality or deviance. Rating scales are standard tools for describing children's behavior, and they provide operational rules for capturing, combining, scaling, and interpreting such data. Scales with age-graded norms provide a basis for determining whether reported behaviors are age-appropriate or are deviant relative to normal agemates. This is crucial because the prevalence and severity of many problem behaviors vary with age, and definitions of behavioral deviance must be developmentally oriented.[2,22] Ratings scales also yield quantitative indices that are useful for plotting changes in behavior over time and in response to interventions.

The goals of this chapter are to review selected checklists and rating scales, discuss issues related to their use, and illustrate their applications. Considerable progress has been made since Conners's review in the first edition of this *Handbook*.[18] There has been increasing sophistication in the scaling and standardization of behavioral ratings and greater attention to reliability and validity issues, normative-developmental considerations,[22] and technical and methodological problems.[21] There has also been a move toward viewing the child as a valuable informant regarding his or her own behaviors and feelings. Self-report measures for children are becoming much more commonly used in research and clinical practice.[24,28]

Hundreds of rating scales have been developed, but most represent ad hoc efforts employed in only one setting or study. Few rating scales have acceptable reliability and validity, and fewer still have been standardized on representative samples of normal children. Not suprisingly, the more psychometrically sound measures, and those with age-graded norms, have been more widely used. In fact, the research literature is dominated by a handful of measures, which will be the focus of this review.

These measures are scorable in terms of empirically derived scales instead of traditional or *a priori* syndromes or disorders. Informants rate the presence, frequency, or severity of selected behavior problems. Responses are then factor-analyzed to identify behavior problem syndromes. Factor analysis is a multivariate statistical procedure that summarizes correlations among several variables in terms of a few dimensions or factors. Each factor represents a subset of behaviors that cooccur and form a distinct syndrome. Almost all rating scales yield scores on two or more factor-based scales. Factor analysis thus provides a basis for multidimensional assessment. Taken together, scores portray how much of each type of behavior the child manifests.

Overview of Selected Rating Scales

The focus of this review is on the most reliable, valid, and widely used measures and on recent progress in the development and use of rating scales. As a framework for discussing specific instruments, I distinguish between instruments designed for *adult informants* such as parents and teachers and *self-report measures* for children and adolescents.

RATINGS BY ADULTS

Most child behavior rating scales are designed to capture adults' perceptions. A recent trend has been toward developing parallel rating scales for different informants. This seems desirable in that no one informant—whether it is a parent, teacher, clinician, trained observer, or child—can provide a comprehensive and veridical picture of a child's behavior. Each type of informant embodies unique perspectives, qualifications, and biases. By tailoring rating scales to different informants, one can capitalize on the predictive and discriminative power each affords. Data from different sources must be combined to elucidate differences in children's behavior across settings and to construct a more comprehensive description of a child's overall functioning.

Two multi-informant assessment systems have been widely used in research on child psychopathology: the Parent and Teacher Rating Scales developed by Conners and his colleagues[31] and the Child Behavior Checklist and Profile developed by Achenbach and Edelbrock.[2,3]

Conners' Rating Scales. The rating scales developed by Conners are among the most widely used assessment tools in child psychiatric research. His original teacher rating scale [16] comprised thirty-nine behaviors, the presence of each being rated on a four-step scale corresponding to *not at all, just a little, quite a bit,* and *very much.* Scales labeled Aggressive Conduct Disorder, Daydreaming-Inattentive, Anxious-Fearful, Hyperactivity, and Sociable-Cooperative were developed by factor analysis of teachers' ratings of 103 disturbed children. Conners' original parent rating scale comprised seventy-three items grouped into twenty-four categories (e.g., fears and worries, restless, problems in school). [17] Factor analysis of ratings on 316 referred children revealed five factors that were dubbed Aggressive Conduct Disorder, Anxious-Inhibited, Antisocial Reaction, Enuresis, and Psychosomatic Problems. In terms of syndrome identification, these results suggest that teachers are a better source of information about inattention and hyperactivity, whereas parents are better informants about antisocial behavior, enuresis, and somatic complaints.

An Abbreviated Parent-Teacher Questionnaire has also been developed, which includes the ten most commonly checked items common to the two measures. It takes little time to complete, so it can be readministered repeatedly to plot changes in behavior over time and in response to interventions.

Conners' Parent and Teacher Rating Scales were recently revised and restandardized. [31] The parent and teacher versions were shortened to forty-eight and twenty-eight items, respectively, and subjected to separate factor analyses. Analyses of parent ratings yielded factors labeled Learning Problem, Psychosomatic, Impulsive Hyperactive, and Anxiety. Additionally, two Conduct Problem factors were derived, one comprising destructiveness and fighting, the other disobedience, talking back, and moodiness. Factor analyses of teacher ratings revealed three factors dubbed Conduct Problem, Hyperactivity, and Inattentive Passive. Both parent and teacher measures are scorable in terms of a Hyperkinesis Index, which includes the ten items on the Abbreviated Questionnaire. Norms for the revised scales have been computed for boys and girls ages three through seventeen. Several studies indicate that Conners' scales are reliable and valid indices of child psychopathology. [6]

Child Behavior Checklist and Profile. Parallel versions of the Child Behavior Checklist and Child Behavior Profile are being developed for different informants, including parents, teachers, trained observers, and children ages eleven to eighteen. Each instrument is designed to tap a broad range of children's behavioral problems and adaptive competencies. To account for age and sex differences in the prevalence and patterning of children's behaviors, separate editions of the parent and teacher measures are being developed and standardized for boys and girls ages four to five, six to eleven, and twelve to sixteen.

The checklist designed for parents includes twenty social competence items reflecting school performance, social relations, and participation in activities. It also includes 118 behavior problem items, each rated 0, 1, or 2 reflecting Not true, Somewhat or sometimes true, and Very or often true, respectively. The checklist requires a fifth-grade reading level, is self-administered, and takes about seventeen minutes to complete. Responses are scored on the Child Behavior Profile, which includes three social competence scales labeled Activities, Social, and School, and behavior problem scales based on factor analyses of checklists completed on large samples of clinically referred children. Factor analyses were performed separately for each age/sex group.

Scales are not identical for each edition of the profile, but there is considerable overlap. Most or all of the editions of the profile include scales labeled Schizoid, Depressed, Somatic Complaints, Social Withdrawal, Hyperactive, Aggressive, and Delinquent. Some syndromes were identified for certain age or sex groups. Syndromes characterizing Immature and Uncommunicative behavior, for example, were identified only for boys, whereas a Cruel syndrome was identified only for girls. This may seem contradictory in that behaviors that form the Cruel syndrome, such as cruelty to animals and destructiveness, are more common among boys than girls. However, a syndrome reflects the *patterning* of behaviors, not their *prevalence.* Among girls, cruel behaviors tend to occur together and form a distinct syndrome, whereas among boys they occur in association with other behaviors such as aggression and delinquency.

The teacher version of the checklist and profile has been completed for boys ages six to eleven. [23] The teacher checklist parallels that developed for parents, but includes problems teachers are more qualified to rate, such as "difficulty following directions," "disrupts class," and "doesn't complete tasks." It is scorable in terms of scales reflecting school performance, adaptive functioning, and problem behavior. Eight behavior problem scales have been constructed via factor analysis: Anxious, Social Withdrawal, Unpopular, Self-Destructive, Obsessive-Compulsive, Inattentive, Nervous-Overactive, and Aggressive. As in Conners' earlier work, teachers' ratings did not yield syndromes characterizing delinquency or somatic complaints but did reveal more specific patterns of inattention and overactivity.

An example of the behavior problem portion of the teacher profile is shown in figure 17–1. The profile scored from parent reports is similar in format, but the items, scales, and norms differ. The figure shows the eight behavior problem scales, their items, and summary labels. The first two scales correlate positively with one another and form a broad-band grouping labeled Internalizing. The the last three scales correlate with one another and form the broad-band Externalizing grouping. Mixed scales, labeled Unpopular, Self-Destructive, and Obsessive-Compulsive, do not align exclusively with either the Internalizing or Externalizing groups.

After the responses to each item (i.e., 0, 1, or 2) are filled in, the raw sum for each scale is computed. For example, the raw score for the Social Withdrawal scale was 5. Raw scores are entered on the graphic display and translated into T-scores, which are comparable across scales having different numbers of items. T-scores are standardized so as to correspond to percentile ranks based on a large sample of non-referred children. A raw score of 5 on the Social Withdrawal scale, for example, corresponds to a T-score of 64 and percentile rank of 90. In other words, this score is at or above that obtained by 90 percent of normal boys ages six to eleven. Lines connecting scores can be drawn in to yield a visual profile depicting the pattern and severity of scores across the eight scales.

As an interpretive guide, the "normal range" of scores—defined as up to and including the ninety-eighth percentile for normal boys—is indicated on the left side of the profile. T-scores greater than 70 exceed the ninety-eighth percentile and represent clinically significant deviations. A perfectly "normal" child would obtain T-scores of 55 on each scale, giving a flat profile along the bottom of the display. Most disturbed children score outside the normal range on one or more scales.

The teacher profile yields a great deal of information. It summarizes what problems were reported, indicates the severity of each on the 0–1–2 scale, shows how problems are concentrated in different areas, and permits comparisons with normal agemates. Studies of the reliability and validity of the checklist and profile have been summarized recently.[3] Clinical and research applications of the profile will be discussed in a subsequent section.

Behavior Problem Checklist. The Behavior Problem Checklist (BPC), developed by Quay and Peterson,[53,55] was one of the first rating scales to be widely used in research on child psychopathology. The original version, introduced in 1967, comprised fifty-five items covering a broad range of problem behaviors. It was designed primarily for parents or teachers of school-age children but has been expanded to other informants, such as child-care workers and residential treatment staff; other age groups including preschoolers, adolescents, and young adults; and a variety of

special populations such as deaf, blind, and developmentally disabled children. The BPC has been subject to numerous factor analyses, all of which yield two broad-band factors labeled Personality Problem and Conduct Problem, which correspond to the global Internalizing/Externalizing dichotomy. Two additional factors, labeled Inadequacy-Immaturity and Socialized Aggression, emerged in some analyses. Quay has reviewed a large body of literature supporting the reliability and validity of the BPC.[54]

A revision of the BPC was undertaken in 1980. It was expanded to 150 items and subject to several factor analyses on diverse clinical samples.[57] Six robust factors were identified: Conduct Disorder, Socialized Aggression, Attention Problems-Immaturity, Anxiety-Withdrawal, Psychotic Behavior, and Motor Excess. The Revised BPC was reduced to eighty-nine items: seventy-seven scored on six factor-based scales and twelve considered useful when rating very young children (e.g., separation anxiety, poor language skills).

Other Measures. The research literature is dominated by the three measures just described, but other instruments deserve mention. Several rating scales have been developed for tapping specific syndromes or disorders. The Child Behavior Inventory developed by Eyberg, for example, focuses on conduct disorders.[27] It is designed to be completed by parents of children and youth ages two to sixteen and employs unique response scaling. Parents indicate the frequency of each behavior on a seven-point intensity scale, then rate the degree to which each behavior is a problem on a two-point problem scale. This is advantageous in that some high-frequency behaviors (e.g., arguing) may not be viewed as problematic, whereas some low-frequency behaviors (e.g., firesetting) may be serious problems. Children's fears can be assessed using the Louisville Fear Survey,[50] which includes eighty-one items covering a broad range of potentially fear-provoking places, situations, and objects. Several parent and teacher rating scales have been developed for assessing childhood hyperactivity, including the Werry-Weiss-Peters Activity Scale,[59] the Hyperkinesis Index,[19] the Hyperactivity Rating Scale,[63] and the Home and School Situations Questionnaires.[6]

Additional measures have been developed for obtaining teachers' reports and ratings. Two measures are designed for preschoolers. The Symptom Checklist and Social Competence Scale developed by Kohn and Rosman yield scores on two scales labeled Interest-Participation vs. Apathy-Withdrawal and Cooperation-Compliance vs. Anger-Defiance.[38] Scores were moderately stable in a longitudinal follow-up for preschoolers into first grade and have been useful for identifying disturbed children in the general population.[38,39,40] The thirty-six-item Preschool Behavior Questionnaire

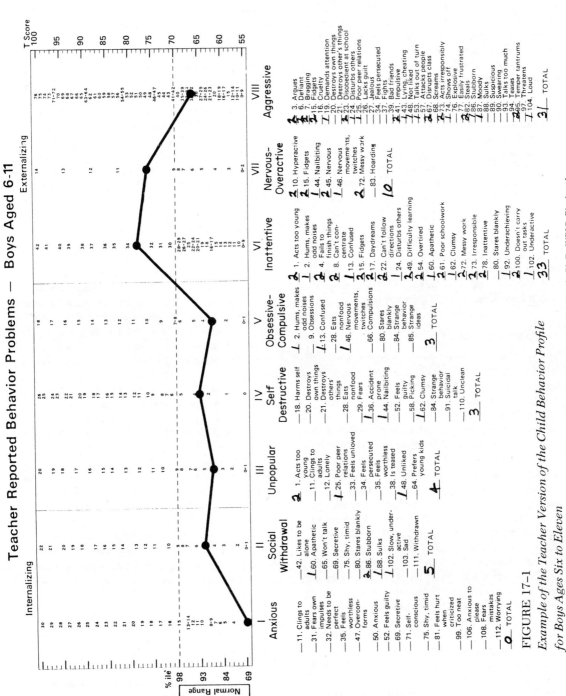

Teacher Reported Behavior Problems — Boys Aged 6-11

FIGURE 17–1

Example of the Teacher Version of the Child Behavior Profile for Boys Ages Six to Eleven

NOTE: Copyright © 1982 Craig S. Edelbrock and Thomas M. Achenbach. Craig S. Edelbrock, Ph.D. WPIC, Pittsburgh, PA 15213 and Thomas M. Achenbach, Ph.D. Dept. Psychiatry, University of Vermont, Burlington, VT 05401.

yields scores on three factor-based scales labeled Hostile-Aggressive, Anxious-Fearful, and Hyperactive-Distractible.[9] Scores on the latter scale have been shown to correlate significantly with other indices of hyperactive behavior and to be useful in identifying hyperactive toddlers.[11,12]

Additional scales have been developed for grade-school children. The School Behavior Checklist covers both prosocial and deviant behaviors.[48,49] Six factor-based scales have been developed for children ages seven to thirteen: Low Need Achievement, Aggression, Anxiety, Academic Disability, Hostile Isolation, and Extraversion. Norms have been constructed based on teacher ratings of more than five thousand randomly selected school pupils. The forty-nine-item Teacher Referral Form was developed to evaluate children referred to a school-based mental health program.[15] It yields scores on three empirically derived scales labeled Learning Problem, Acting Out, and Shy Anxious. Last, Walker's Checklist[66] covers fifty common classroom behavior problems, which are scored on five factors: Acting Out, Withdrawal, Distractibility, Disturbed Peer Relations, and Immaturity.

CHILDREN'S SELF-REPORTS

A major trend in recent years has been toward viewing the child as a valuable informant regarding his or her own feelings and behaviors. Several self-report measures have been developed or revised recently.[28] Most focus on specific types of behavior, particularly "private" phenomena. Considerable progress has been made in the areas of anxiety, depression, social behavior, and self-control.

Anxiety. The Children's Manifest Anxiety Scale was developed more than twenty-five years ago[14] and was recently revised and standardized on a large normative sample.[58] The revised version includes twenty-eight anxiety items and is scored on three factor-based scales labeled Physiological, Worry-Oversensitivity, and Concentration. The State-Trait Anxiety Inventory for Children[62] was designed for children ages nine to twelve and consists of parallel forms for measuring state anxiety assumed to be situational and temporary and trait anxiety assumed to reflect more persistent anxious tendencies. Several studies support the reliability and validity of these two anxiety measures.[28]

Depression. Increasing interest in childhood depression has spawned several self-report measures.[37] The Beck Depression Inventory (BDI) was designed for adults,[8] but can be used with adolescents.[64] The twenty-seven-item Child Depression Inventory, modeled after the BDI, focuses on depressive symptoms such as sadness, anhedonia, and sleep and appetite disturbance. It yields a single depression score, which

has been shown to be stable over a one-month period and to discriminate significantly between pediatric and psychiatric referrals.[41] The thirteen-item Short Children's Depression Inventory, also modeled after the BDI, has been useful in identifying children with major affective disorders.[13] Other adult depression inventories have been adapted for use with children.[42,67] Additionally, Birleson has developed a new self-report depression scale for children ages seven to thirteen.[10]

Social Behavior. Two self-report measures for assessing children's social behavior have been recently developed. The Children's Action Tendency Scale measures children's assertive, aggressive, and submissive responses to hypothetical social situations.[10] Each item describes a conflict situation (e.g., someone shoves you out of line). Children respond by choosing between submissive, assertive, or aggressive courses of action. Scores have correlated significantly with teacher and peer ratings of children's behavior and have been shown to discriminate between hyperactive/aggressive boys and normal controls. A similar measure is the Children's Assertive Behavior Scale, which comprises twenty-seven multiple-choice items reflecting common social situations such as giving and receiving compliments, handling complaints, and making requests.[46] It yields assertive, passive, and aggressive scores that correlate with classroom observations and teachers' ratings of children's social behavior. Additionally, scores have been shown to be sensitive to a social skills training program for elementary school children.[45]

Self-Control. The Children's Perceived Self-Control Scale was designed to tap children's ability to delay, tolerate frustration, plan ahead, and resist temptation.[34] Children respond either "Usually Yes" or "Usually No" to eleven items (e.g., It is hard to wait for something I want). Four factor-based scales have been constructed: Personal Self Control, Interpersonal Self Control, Self Evaluation, and Consequential Thinking. Children's self-ratings have been found to correlate with teachers' ratings of children's self-control, school adjustment, aggression, frustration tolerance, and shy/anxious behavior.

Problems and Issues

Numerous problems and issues arise when developing and using child behavior rating scales. These include (1) agreement between studies aimed at identifying behavioral syndromes, (2) the reliability and validity of specific measures, (3) the use of multiple informants, and (4) the influence of informant characteristics on behavioral ratings.

SYNDROME IDENTIFICATION

Multivariate analyses of behavior ratings have yielded very heterogeneous results. However, differences in the number and nature of empirically derived syndromes are largely due to differences in the measures, subject samples, and methods of analysis. In general, large item pools yield more syndromes than do small item pools, and more syndromes are identified when the researcher uses lenient criteria for minimum number and size of item loadings.[1] Moreover, extremely rare behavioral patterns may be missed due to lack of relevant items or underrepresentation of such disorders in the subject sample. The prevalence and patterning of problem behaviors also varies according to sex and age. It follows that analyses must be conducted separately for sex and age groups in order to detect specific patterns of covariation. Only one measure, the Child Behavior Profile, has been developed separately for boys and girls of different ages.

A major difference among studies is whether they identify a few global "broad-band" syndromes or many circumscribed "narrow-band" syndromes. However, second-order factor analyses, which involve analyzing correlations among narrow-band scales, have shown that scores on aggressive, hyperactive, and delinquent scales correlate positively with one another and form a broad-band "undercontrolled" or "externalizing" syndrome. Alternatively, scores on anxious, withdrawn, somatic, depressed, and obsessive-compulsive scales correlate positively and form a broad-band "overcontrolled" or "internalizing" syndrome. Studies may differ, therefore, in their ability to resolve global syndromes into more circumscribed behavioral patterns.

Despite differences in methods, measures, and subject samples, there is considerable consistency in identifying certain syndromes.[1,55] Agreement between studies is obscured by differences in summary labels applied to factors. A syndrome encompassing behaviors such as truancy, vandalism, stealing, running away, and drug abuse, for example, has been labeled Delinquent,[3] Antisocial Reaction,[17] and Socialized Aggression.[56] Although summary labels vary, most studies have identified two broad-band syndromes characterizing depression, withdrawal, and anxiety on one hand and aggression, hyperactivity, and delinquency on the other. There is also consensus regarding the existence of narrow-band aggressive, delinquent, hyperactive, schizoid, anxious, depressed, somatic, and withdrawn syndromes. Additionally, syndromes characterizing immaturity, obsessions-compulsions, sex problems, sleep problems, and uncommunicativeness have been identified in two or more analyses.

RELIABILITY AND VALIDITY

A reliable rating scale yields scores that are accurate and dependable indices of behavior, whereas an unreliable one yields scores that are highly contaminated with error and are therefore inaccurate and unstable. *Test-retest reliability* reflects stability of scores over time. Most parent and teacher rating scales yield high test-retest reliabilities (ranging from $r = 0.80$ to 0.90) over a one-week to one-month interval.[3,15,16] From one to six months, reliabilities are generally lower and average 0.50 to 0.70, but this may be due to true change in behavior over time. Self-ratings by children and adolescents are less reliable than ratings by adults, but are still moderately high ($r = 0.60$ to 0.70). *Interrater reliability,* which reflects similarity between scores derived from different raters, depends on similar exposure to the target child's behavior. Raters who observe and interact with the child in similar settings and situations, such as mothers and fathers, tend to agree fairly well ($r = 0.60$ to 0.80). Parent-teacher agreement is generally low ($r = 0.30$ to 0.40), but this may reflect differences in children's behavior at home and at school. Children's self-ratings do not correlate highly with adults' ratings, but this may reflect differences in awareness and tolerance of different problems. Parent-child agreement on child symptoms is low, but there is a clear pattern of disagreement.[33] Parents report more overt, annoying problems such as hyperactivity and aggression, while children report more emotional and affective symptoms, such as fears, anxiety, and depression. Overall, most rating scales designed for adult informants are highly reliable. Those designed for children and adolescents are less reliable but are still acceptable for clinical and research purposes.

Validity concerns *what* is being measured. A valid rating scale is one that reflects what it purports to measure. Establishing the validity of a behavioral measure is a formidable task involving a vast network of findings. Moreover, there are different kinds of validity, and a given rating scale may be valid for some purposes but not others. The rating scales reviewed here all have *face* or *content validity*. In other words, they look as if they measure what they were designed to measure. The items reflect problem behaviors and the scales are intuitively reasonable. The *criterion-related* validity of most rating scales is supported by their ability to discriminate between criterion groups, such as clinically referred and nonreferred samples. Most rating scales, including self-report measures for children, also discriminate between diagnostic subgroups such as depressed, aggressive, hyperactive, and anxious children. The *concurrent validity* of rating scales is supported by significant relations between instruments designed to measure similar phenomena.

The Child Behavior Profile scored from parent reports, for example, has been shown to correlate significantly with Conners' Parent Rating Scale and the Revised Behavior Problem Checklist.[3] In this case, the convergent relations between measures supports the validity of both. *Predictive validity* is perhaps most important. Several parent and teacher rating scales have been shown to predict clinically important criteria such as the course, prognosis, treatment responsiveness, and outcome of childhood disorders. Conners' scales, for example, have been shown in many studies to identify hyperactive children who are candidates for drug treatment, predict drug response, and reflect drug-mediated behavioral change. Less is known about the predictive power of children's self-reports, but this is the focus of several ongoing studies.

MULTIPLE INFORMANTS

It is highly advisable to obtain ratings from more than one informant. However, only a few assessment systems include parallel forms for different informants, and there is often low correspondence between raters —especially parents and teachers. Children's behavior is recognized as highly situation specific,[36] so different raters may provide perfectly valid and reliable data but still disagree about the nature, patterning, and severity of a child's problems. Arguing about who is right or wrong is pointless, and it is probably not worthwhile for researchers to seek ways to boost agreement between informants. Two courses of action seem more profitable. The first involves determining *what data,* from *which type of informant,* is maximally useful and predictive. Teacher ratings of inattention, overactivity, and peer acceptance, for example, may prove more valuable than ratings by parents, clinicians, or children. Conversely, parent-reported somatic complaints, family relations, and behavior in the community may be more valuable than such information from teachers.

The second approach involves optimally combining information from different informants. One way to do this is to identify the subgroup of children about whom informants agree. This idea underlies the distinction between *situational* and *pervasive* hyperactivity.[60] Situationally hyperactive children are described as hyperactive by *either* parents or teachers, whereas pervasively hyperactive children are described as hyperactive by *both.* This combination of ratings has been shown to have discriminative and predictive power over and above that derived from a single source.

INFORMANT CHARACTERISTICS

To some extent, behavioral ratings reflect the personalities, perceptions, biases, and expectations of the informant rather than the actual behavior of the child. Simply telling a teacher that a child is "disturbed" or "learning disabled," for example, results in higher behavior problem ratings.[29] Professional training and experience also influence ratings. Sonis and Costello, for instance, found that teachers rated videotaped behavioral episodes more severely than child psychiatrists, child psychologists, and pediatricians.[61] Less experienced professionals also tended toward more extreme ratings. Further research is needed to elucidate the nature and size of such effects. In the meantime, it is important to realize that ratings reflect both the true behavior of the child and diverse and complex aspects of the rater.

Although adults' perceptions of children's behavior are not perfectly accurate, they are important in their own right. Adults' impressions of children's behavioral functioning are usually crucial to the referral and diagnosis of disturbed children, and they are vital to the implementation, monitoring, and evaluation of treatments. Changes in subjectively reported behavior, for example, can provide "social validation" of treatment effects detected by more objective methods such as direct observation.[35] Whether valid or not, adult perceptions of children's behaviors and abilities are likely to influence children's ongoing development.

Applications of Rating Scales

CLINICAL USES

Rating scales have many clinical applications. Omnibus rating scales, such as the Child Behavior Profile, are well suited to initial assessment of children referred for mental health services, and they provide an economical means of identifying salient problems. They can also reveal areas of greatest concern and can pinpoint areas of behavioral deviance. Information from an initial assessment is a natural springboard for clinical interviews in which the history and context of specific problems are addressed. In terms of treatment selection, standardized ratings can reveal whether the child's behavior is deviant and/or in need of treatment. They also indicate degree of deviance in various areas, which can be valuable when prioritizing treatment goals. Periodic assessments can be used for treatment monitoring and evaluation.

Ratings scales also have diagnostic applications. Few rating scales tap diagnostic criteria per se, but almost all tap diagnostically relevant behaviors and syndromes. Moreover, several measures[17,26,57] have been shown to discriminate among diagnostic groups.

Rating scales that tap a broad range of behaviors, such as the Child Behavior Profile, can be used *heuristically* to identify areas of deviance that may be diagnostically significant. More focused rating scales—such as Conners', which focus on hyperactivity, and Eyberg's, which focuses on conduct disorder—can be used in a *confirmatory* manner to verify or reject a diagnostic hypothesis.

Last, rating scales embody a common data language for professional communication and training. They provide a common ground for discussing individual cases and for linking experience with other cases having similar or different behavioral patterns.

CASE EXAMPLE

These clinical applications can be illustrated by a case example of Billy, an eight-year-old boy referred primarily for behavior problems at school. On intake, Billy's mother completed the parent version of the Child Behavior Checklist. She reported few internalizing problems related to anxiety, depression, obsessions-compulsions, somatic complaints, or social withdrawal, but indicated some externalizing problems in the areas of hyperactivity and aggression. Billy had relatively high scores on the Hyperactive and Aggressive scales of the Child Behavior Profile, but these were within the normal range for boys his age. Clinical interview with the mother revealed that she did not feel Billy was a big problem at home, although he was rather active and impulsive. Her main concern was his poor school performance. His teacher had also pressured her to seek professional help because Billy was difficult to manage in the classroom, disturbed other pupils, disrupted the class, and was failing many subjects.

Billy's teacher completed the teacher version of the checklist. She reported many behavior problems and said that he was not behaving appropriately in class, working hard, or learning much. The behavior problem portion of the teacher profile is shown in figure 17–1. According to his teacher, Billy had few internalizing problems. His scores on the Anxious and Social Withdrawal scales were low and were typical of normal boys his age. He had a few problems related to the mixed scales labeled Unpopular, Self-Destructive, and Obsessive-Compulsive but was well within the normal range. Billy had several externalizing problems, many of which were rated "2," corresponding to "very or often true." These problems were concentrated on the scales labeled Inattentive and Nervous-Overactive, where his scores were far above the normal range. His score on the Aggressive scale was technically within normal bounds but was relatively high and exceeded the ninety-third percentile for normal boys. His

teacher did not report overt aggressive behaviors such as fighting, attacking people, stealing, or cruelty, but reported many oppositional behaviors such as arguing, disobedience, stubbornness, and temper tantrums.

Billy was diagnosed attention deficit disorder with hyperactivity and oppositional disorder. The teacher ratings supported this diagnosis, in that many of Billy's reported problems correspond to DSM criteria for these disorders. Billy's profile pattern is also very similar to that obtained by other hyperactive boys.[26] Both parent and teacher ratings were useful in formulating a treatment plan. The decision was made to focus primarily on modifying Billy's behavior at school. He seemed to have difficulties adjusting to structured situations during class, and his mother did not feel he was a problem at home. The teacher ratings were also useful in prioritizing treatment goals. The primary focus was on reducing his inattentiveness, distractibility, and overactivity. A secondary goal was to reduce oppositional behavior and foster cooperation and compliance with adults.

Billy was put on a trial of stimulant medication for his hyperactivity, and his teacher implemented a behavioral program wherein he could earn points for cooperation and compliance during class. If he earned enough points during the week, the whole class received a special reward. To chart changes in Billy's behavior, his teacher agreed to complete Conners' ten-item Abbreviated Questionnaire every week during the drug trial. In order to assess his behavior in several areas, she also completed the teacher checklist three times a year when report cards come out. At the time of this writing only two months have elapsed, but Billy has already shown marked improvement. Teacher ratings show that he is less active and distractible and more able to concentrate. He is also becoming more cooperative and less oppositional at school.

RESEARCH APPLICATIONS

The research applications of checklists and rating scales are numerous and diverse. They are well suited to epidemiological applications in that they provide a simple, reliable, and efficient way to survey large populations and they do not depend on complex inferences by highly trained clinical personnel.[65] Rating instruments are also useful for constructing behaviorally homogeneous comparison groups for research purposes. Scores on Conners' scales, for example, are widely used as selection criteria for studies of childhood hyperactivity.[6] Age and developmental differences in children's problem behaviors have been widely studied using rating scales. Cross-sectional studies have documented age differences in the prevalence and severity of children's behavioral problems,[2] and longitudinal follow-up studies have revealed differences in the stability of child symptoms over time.[30]

The etiology, course, prognosis, and outcome of childhood disorders have also been studied using both quantitative and categorical indices derived from rating scales. Behavioral ratings have also been widely used in evaluations of treatment effects, particularly in the area of childhood hyperactivity.[25]

Conclusions

Behavioral checklists and rating scales represent a simple, efficient, and reliable means of describing and differentiating among disturbed children. They require little professional time or expertise to administer or score, and they yield a wealth of information that is useful in the detection, diagnosis, and treatment of childhood disorders and in research. The focus here has been on measures that have been widely used in child psychiatry and on new self-report measures for children and adolescents. There are several excellent sources of further information on child behavior assessment in general and the use of rating scales in particular. These include recent textbooks[44,51] and scholarly reviews.[4,28,43] Additionally, reviews of specific measures are available in the areas of children's adaptive functioning,[52] social skills,[32,47] fears,[7] depression,[37] hyperactivity,[6,25] and conduct disorder.[5]

ACKNOWLEDGMENTS

Preparation of this chapter was supported by NIMH grant #MH37372, NIMH Research Scientist Development Award #MH00403, and a Faculty Scholar's Award from the William T. Grant Foundation.

REFERENCES

1. ACHENBACH, T. M., and EDELBROCK, C. S. "The Classification of Child Psychopathology: A Review and Analysis of Empirical Efforts," *Psychological Bulletin,* 85 (1978):1275–1301.

2. ———. "Behavior Problems and Competencies Reported by Parents of Normal and Disturbed Children Aged 4 Through 16," *Monographs of the Society for Research in Child Development* 46:(1, Serial No. 188).

3. ———. *Manual for the Child Behavior Checklist and Revised Child Behavior Profile.* Burlington, Vt.: University Associates in Psychiatry, 1983.

4. ———. "Psychopathology of Childhood," *Annual Review of Psychology,* 35 (1984):227–256.

5. ATKESON, B. M., and FOREHAND, R. "Conduct Disorders," in E. J. Mash and L. Terdal, eds., *Behavioral Assessment of Childhood Disorders.* New York: Guilford Press, 1982, pp. 185–220.

6. BARKLEY, R. A. *Hyperactive Children: A Handbook for Diagnosis and Treatment.* New York: Guilford Press, 1981.

7. BARRIOS, B. A., HARTMANN, D. P., and SHIGETOMI, C. "Fears and Anxieties in Children," in E. J. Mash and L. Terdal, eds., *Behavioral Assessment of Childhood Disorders.* New York: Guildford Press, 1982, pp. 259–304.

8. BECK, A. T. *Depression: Causes and Treatment.* Philadelphia: University of Pennsylvania Press, 1967.

9. BEHAR, L. B., and STRINGFIELD, S. "A Behavior Rating Scale for the Preschool Child," *Developmental Psychology,* 10 (1974):601–610.

10. BIRLESON, P. "The Validity of Depressive Disorder in Childhood and the Development of a Self-rating Scale: A Research Report," *Journal of Child Psychology and Psychiatry,* 22 (1981):73–88.

11. CAMPBELL, S. B., and BREAUX, A. M. "Maternal Ratings of Activity Level and Symptomatic Behaviors in a Nonclinical Sample of Young Children," *Journal of Pediatric Psychology,* 8 (1983):73–82.

12. CAMPBELL, S. B., et al. "A Multidimensional Assessment of Parent-identified Behavior Problem Toddlers," *Journal of Abnormal Child Psychology,* 10 (1982):569–592.

13. CARLSON, G. A., and CANTWELL, D. P. "A Survey of Depressive Symptoms in a Child and Adolescent Psychiatric Population," *Journal of the American Academy of Child Psychiatry,* 18 (1979):587–599.

14. CASTANEDA, A., McCANDLESS, B., and PALERMO, D. "The Children's Form of the Manifest Anxiety Scale," *Child Development,* 27 (1956):317–326.

15. CLARFIELD, S. P. "The Development of a Teacher Referral Form for Identifying Early School Maladaption," *American Journal of Community Psychology,* 2 (1974):199–210.

16. CONNERS, C. K. "A Teacher Rating Scale for Use in Drug Studies with Children," *American Journal of Psychiatry,* 126 (1969):884–888.

17. ———. "Symptom Patterns in Hyperkinetic, Neurotic, and Normal Children," *Child Development,* 4 (1970):667–682.

18. ———. "Rating Scales," in J. D. Noshpitz et al., eds., *Basic Handbook of Child Psychiatry,* vol. 1. New York: Basic Books, 1979, pp. 675–689.

19. DAVIDS, A. "An Objective Instrument for Assessing Hyperkinesis in Children," *Journal of Learning Disabilities,* 4 (1971):499–501.

20. DELUTY, R. H, "Children's Action Tendency Scale: A Self-report Measure of Aggression, Assertiveness, and Submissiveness in Children," *Journal of Consulting and Clinical Psychology,* 47 (1979):1061–1071.

21. EDELBROCK, C. "Problems and Issues in Using Rating Scales to Assess Child Personality and Psychopathology," *School Psychology Review,* 12 (1983):293–299.

22. ———. "Developmental Considerations," in T. H. Ollendick and M. Hersen, eds., *Child Behavioral Assessment: Principles and Procedures.* New York: Pergamon Press, 1984, pp. 20–37.

23. EDELBROCK, C., and ACHENBACH, T. M. "The Teacher Version of the Child Behavior Profile: I. Boys Aged 6–11," *Journal of Consulting and Clinical Psychology,* 52 (1984):207–217.

24. EDELBROCK, C., and COSTELLO, A. J. "Structured Psychiatric Interviews for Children and Adolescents," in G. Goldstein and M. Hersen, eds., *Handbook of Psychological Assessment.* New York: Pergamon Press, 1984, pp. 276–290.

25. EDELBROCK, C., and RANCURELLO, M. "Childhood Hyperactivity: An Overview of Rating Scales and Their Applications," *Clinical Psychology Review,* 5 (1985):429–445.

26. EDELBROCK, C., COSTELLO, A. J., and KESSLER, M. D. "Empirical Corroboration of Attention Deficit Disorder," *Journal of the American Academy of Child Psychiatry,* 23 (1984):285–290.

27. EYBERG, S. "The Eyberg Child Behavior Inventory," *Journal of Clinical Child Psychology,* 9 (1980):29.

28. FINCH, A. J., and ROGERS, T. R. "Self-report Instruments," in T. H. Ollendick and M. Hersen, eds., *Child Behavioral Assessment: Principles and Procedures.* New York: Pergamon Press, 1984, pp. 106–123.

29. FOSTER, G. G., and SALVIA, J. "Teacher Response to the Label of Learning Disabled as a Function of Demand Characteristics," *Exceptional Children,* 43 (1977):533–534.

30. GLOW, R. A., GLOW, P. H., and RUMP, E. E. "The Stability of Child Behavior Disorders: A One-year Test-retest Study of the Adelaide Versions of the Conners Parent and Teacher Rating Scales," *Journal of Abnormal Child Psychology,* 10 (1982):33–60.

31. GOYETTE, C. H., CONNERS, C. K., and ULRICH, R. F. "Normative Data on Revised Conners Parent and Teacher Rating Scales," *Journal of Abnormal Child Psychology,* 6 (1978):221–236.

32. GREEN, K., et al. "Assessment of Children's Social Skills," Unpublished manuscript, 1979.

33. HERJANIC, B., and REICH, W. "Development of a Structured Psychiatric Interview for Children: Agreement Between Child and Parent on Individual Symptoms," *Journal of Abnormal Child Psychology,* 10 (1982):307–324.

34. HUMPHREY, L. L. "Children's and Teachers' Perspectives on Children's Self-control: The Development of Two Rating Scales," *Journal of Consulting and Clinical Psychology,* 50 (1982):624–633.

35. KAZDIN, A. E. "Assessing the Clinical or Applied Significance of Behavioral Change Through Social Validation," *Behavior Modification,* 1 (1977):427–452.

36. ———. "Situation Specificity: The Two-edged Sword of Behavioral Assessment," *Behavioral Assessment,* 1 (1979):57–59.

37. KAZDIN, A. E., and PETTI, T. A. "Self-report and Interview Measures of Childhood and Adolescent Depression," *Journal of Child Psychology and Psychiatry,* 23 (1982):437–457.

38. KOHN, M., and ROSMAN, B. L. "A Social Competence Scale and Symptom Checklist for the Preschool Child: Factor Dimensions, Their Cross-instrument Generality, and Longitudinal Persistence," *Developmental Psychology,* 6 (1972):430–444.

39. ———. "Cross-situational and Longitudinal Stability of Social-emotional Functioning in Young Children," *Child Development,* 44 (1973):721–727.

40. ———. "A Two-factor Model of Emotional Disturbance in the Young Child: Validity and Screening Efficiency," *Journal of Child Psychology and Psychiatry,* 14 (1973):31–56.

41. KOVACS, M. "Rating Scales to Assess Depression in School-age Children," *Acta Paedopsychiatry,* 46 (1981):305–315.

42. LEFKOWITZ, M. M., and TESINY, E. P. "Assessment of Childhood Depression," *Journal of Consulting and Clinical Psychology,* 48 (1980):43–50.

43. MCMAHON, R. J. "Behavioral Checklists and Rating Scales," in T. H. Ollendick and M. Hersen, eds., *Child Behavioral Assessment: Principles and Procedures.* New York: Pergamon Press, 1984, pp. 80–105.

44. MASH, E. J., and TERDAL, L., eds. *Behavioral Assessment of Childhood Disorders.* New York: Guilford Press, 1981.

45. MICHELSON, L., and WOOD, R. "A Group Assertive Training Program for Elementary School Children," *Child Behavior Therapy,* 2 (1980):1–9.

46. ———. "Development and Psychometric Properties of the Children's Assertive Behavior Scale," *Journal of Behavioral Assessment,* 4 (1982):3–13.

47. MICHELSON, L., FOSTER, S., and RITCHEY, W. L. "Social-skills Assessment of Children," in B. Lahey and A. E. Kazdin, eds., *Advances in Child Clinical Psychology, vol. 4.* New York: Plenum Press, 1981, pp. 119–166.

48. MILLER, L. C. "School Behavior Checklist: An Inventory of Deviant Behavior for Elementary School Children," *Journal of Consulting and Clinical Psychology,* 38 (1972):134–144.

49. ———. *Louisville Behavior Checklist Manual.* Los Angeles: Western Psychological Services, 1977.

50. MILLER, L. C., et al. "Factor Structure of Childhood Fears," *Journal of Consulting and Clinical Psychology,* 39 (1972):264–268.

51. OLLENDICK, T. H., and HERSEN, M., eds. *Child Behavior Assessment: Principles and Procedures.* New York: Pergamon Press, 1984.

52. ORVASCHEL, H., and WALSH, G. *A Review of Existing Measures of Adaptive Functioning for Children,* final report (Contract #82-M087020801D). Rockville, Md.: Center for Epidemiologic Studies, National Institute of Mental Health, 1983.

53. PETERSON, D. R. "Behavior Problems of Middle Childhood," *Journal of Consulting Psychology,* 25 (1961):205–209.

54. QUAY, H. C. "Measuring Dimensions of Deviant Behavior: The Behavior Problem Checklist," *Journal of Abnormal Child Psychology,* 5 (1977):277–289.

55. ———. "Classification," in H. C. Quay and J. S. Werry, eds., *Psychopathological Disorders of Childhood,* 2nd ed. New York: John Wiley & Sons, 1979, pp. 1–42.

56. QUAY, H. C., and PETERSON, D. *Manual for the Behavior Problem Checklist.* Champaign, Il.: Author, 1967.

57. ———. *Manual for the Revised Behavior Problem Checklist.* Coral Gables, Fla.: Author, 1983.

58. REYNOLDS, C. R., and PAGET, K. D. "Factor Analysis of the Revised Children's Manifest Anxiety Scale for Blacks, Whites, Males and Females with a National Normative Sample," *Journal of Consulting and Clinical Psychology,* 44 (1981):352–359.

59. ROUTH, D. K., SCHROEDER, C. S., and O'TAUMA, L. "Development of Activity Level in Children," *Developmental Psychology,* 10 (1974):163–168.

60. SCHACHAR, R., RUTTER, M., and SMITH, A. "The Characteristics of Situationally and Pervasively Hyperactive Children: Implications for Syndrome Definition," *Journal of Child Psychology and Psychiatry,* 22 (1981):375–392.

61. SONIS, W. A., and COSTELLO, A. J. "Evaluation of Different Data Sources: Application of the Diagnostic Process

in Child Psychiatry," *Journal of the American Academy of Child Psychiatry,* 20 (1981):597–610.

62. SPIELBERGER, C. D. *Manual for the State-Triat Anxiety Scale for Children.* Palo Alto, Calif.: Consulting Psychological Press.

63. SPRING, C., et al. "Validity and Norms of a Hyperactivity Rating Scale," *Exceptional Children,* 11 (1977):313–321.

64. TERI, L. "The Use of the Beck Depression Inventory with Adolescents," *Journal of Abnormal Child Psychology,* 10 (1982):277–284.

65. TRITES, R. L., et al. "Prevalence of Hyperactivity," *Journal of Pediatric Psychology,* 4 (1979):179–188.

66. WALKER, H. M. *Walker Behavior Problem Identification Checklist.* Los Angeles: Western Psychological Services, 1976.

67. WEISSMAN, M. M., ORVASCHEL, H., and PADIAN, N. "Children's Symptom and Social Functioning Self-report Scales: Comparisons of Mothers' and Children's Reports. *Journal of Nervous and Mental Disease,* 168 (1980):736–740.

18 / Advances in Neuropsychological Assessment

Maureen Dennis

In the first edition of the *Basic Handbook of Child Psychiatry,* I discussed neuropsychological assessment as a form of statistical decision making about a child's behavior in a test situation, one that also involves an inference about the brain bases of the observed test behavior.[2] Decision making was considered to involve several steps: establishing the *level* of test performances; describing the skill *configuration* or skill *pattern* of which broadly characterized behavioral functions like intelligence, language, or visual perception are constituted; and making hypotheses about the *processing impairments* that underlie a set of deficient test performances. Some rules to guide decision making about level, pattern, and process were discussed. The task in child assessment was considered to involve separating cognitive impairment from normal but immature function.

Neuropsychological assessment of the child aims to draw implications from aberrant test performances about the nature of the child's impaired cognitive processing. Assessment of this kind points the way to effective and well-directed remediation. The remedial task involves isolating critical aspects of cognitive processing and giving their control back to the child. This can be accomplished either by retraining specific target behaviors (perhaps along the lines suggested by Goldstein[14] for adults) or by teaching compensatory strategies.

This account of child neuropsychological assessment is still an adequate program description. In the five years since it was written, however, material has been published that, in various ways, amplifies, alters, or extends the 1979 discussion. Some provides additional information of the kind available earlier; some offers a novel basis for considering what tests mean, in both the narrow and the broad sense; and some has called into question the theoretical and conceptual bases on which tests have traditionally been constructed and used. Each of these new developments will be considered.

New Approaches to Decision Making with Old Assessment Techniques

Since 1979 the formal aspects of decision making with existing psychometric tests have been considerably expanded. This trend can best be illustrated by new approaches to the most widely used individual child intelligence test, the Wechsler Intelligence Scale for Children-Revised (WISC-R).

The administration and interpretation of intelligence tests was once regarded as the province of the clinician. The older clinical manuals provided statements about defective performance based on a clinical impression of what the subject was doing during the test, together with a combined clinical and empirical judgment about what the test measured. The mix of statistical decision making and clinical judgment was sometimes an uncertain one.

Statistical decision making for the WISC-R has been expanded of late in a variety of ways. In addition to earlier procedures for deciding whether differences within and between parts of a test are abnormal (i.e., so large as to occur infrequently in a population of normal children), reliable (larger than the variability arising from errors of test measurement), or oddly patterned (see Field[11] and Rhodes[24,25], several new procedures have been developed.

The Tardor Interpretation Scoring System for the WISC-R[29] provides an objective summary of the WISC-R based on accepted statistical interpretation, without entering into clinical, educational, behavioral, or other inferences. Statements in the Tardor report are based on scaled score equivalents of raw scores, reliability coefficients of the tests, IQ scores, the intercorrelation of the tests by age level, and the differences between scaled scores required for statistical significance. The aim of the system is to allow the clinician to simultaneously take all these factors into account in a consistent and standardized manner when scoring the test and describing the test results.

Decision making has also been formalized as a series of interpretive strategies with corresponding remedial implications. Profile handbooks such as the one by Nicholson and Alcorn[23] provide worksheets that systematically examine a number of factors influencing test performance. The value of such handbooks is that they address both predictive and remedial issues within the framework of the psychometric properties of the test. The Nicholson and Alcorn system integrates statistical issues, quality of responses, and descriptions of test behavior into a series of predictions about both current level of school achievement and theoretical achievement by age sixteen. Along with these predictions, it offers suggestions for specific educational remediation. Such systems greatly increase the coherence with which the clinician can link a defective pattern of test performance to particular remedial suggestions.

Recent user manuals for the WISC-R[16] stress the logic of decision making rather than either purely quantitative or remedial issues. They encourage the tester to use simple psychometric guidelines and then go beyond the statistics to formulate useful hypotheses about the child's strengths and weaknesses. The idea behind such manuals is that the results of a WISC-R interpretation can be meaningful if interpreted in the context of test statistics, clinical observation, and a variety of aspects of research in cognition, intelligence, and brain function.

These new approaches to the WISC-R vary along a number of dimensions. One involves how closely interpretation is tied to the statistical aspects of decision making and another relates to how much extra-test information is incorporated into the interpretations. In no case is the value of the clinician's observational experience downplayed. Instead, clinical skill is placed in the context of a coherent treatment of the test statistics. There are features of test performance that should

be decided on statistical rather than observational grounds. The effect of the new approaches has not been to deny clinical skills so much as to allow them to be exercised against an adequate understanding of these features. A decision about whether any two WISC-R subtest scores differ from each other, for example, requires the evaluation of the test error associated with each subtest, rather than a clinical impression. Each of these systems provides new and useful guidelines for the practicing clinician. At the same time, they quantify the statistical issues associated with test performance and sharpen the clinical questions that the test performance addresses.

Sourcebooks and New Tests

Two trends are evident in the area of sourcebooks and new tests. One is the grouping of old tests into sourcebooks or compendia. The other is the development in the neuropsychological research literature of test instruments that have considerable potential for use in a clinical neuropsychological assessment.

Although their focus is not specifically on children, Lezak's books[20,21] on neuropsychological assessment are examples of sourcebooks that catalogue existing test instruments. The practical utility of a test sourcebook is obvious. Less obvious is the fact that a neuropsychological assessment based only on a test compendium will not necessarily sample in an adequate fashion all those aspects of behavior that might need to be tapped in a thorough neuropsychological assessment.

Test behaviors may be considered as signs of other behaviors that they do not ordinarily resemble and as indicative of underlying traits (as, e.g., when a low score on the Coding subtest of the WISC-R is viewed as a sign of distractibility) or, alternately, as samples of behavior essentially similar to those for which predictions are to be made (as, e.g., when a low score on the WISC-R Arithmetic subtest is used to predict difficulties in this academic skill). The distinction concerns whether test performance is regarded as a sign of underlying psychological structures or as a sample of response classes.[22] Neuropsychological tests are a mixture of both types: In general, tests rooted in the history of neurology are viewed as signs of underlying neurofunctional disruption, while tests derived from mainstream psychology are behavior samples. The heterogeneity of tests with respect to this dimension often makes it difficult for the clinician basing a neuropsychological assessment only on a compendium to make inferences about test behavior in a coherent manner.

The fact that a compendium features several different tests for a given psychological function is no guarantee that the function will be adequately assessed. In fact, a large number of different tests of a function may be less desirable than one well-studied procedure whose scope and psychometric properties have been systematically explored. [1]

Mainstream research in the psychology of memory, reading, and language has considerably advanced understanding of these cognitive processes. Research neuropsychology has recently begun to exploit these developments and to apply test instruments based on this research to the elucidation of cognitive impairment in clinical populations. Examples of this trend are studies of head-injured children using a process analysis of memory [18,19] and research in brain-damaged children that considers reading within the framework of cognitive analyses of automaticity and text reading [3,8] or that studies language processes, such as the understanding of grammar, the production of surface structure syntactic forms, and the mechanisms of word finding, within a framework of developmental psycholinguistics. [7,9,31] These techniques could be adapted, most likely with profit, to the neuropsychological assessment of children.

Test compendia assemble old tests; research neuropsychology explores new tests. Both are necessary. But a proper neuropsychological assessment requires, in addition, the demonstration of the scope and utility of tests it uses, whether old or new. The clinician needs not just a test description but illustrations of a test's operation in its target clinical populations (see Rourke et al. [27]), and demonstrations of a test's ability to perform the predictive and/or discrimination tasks for which it was designed (see Satz and Fletcher [28]).

New Approaches to the Broader Questions of Statistical Decision Making

The approaches discussed earlier formalize statistical issues around particular test results and integrate these with clinical observations and remedial implications. The use of tests in assessment, however, involves other, broader, issues. Recently attempts have been made to reflect upon these more general questions.

There has been a growing dissatisfaction with interpretations of test results based purely on single figures or summary scores. In one such view:

It is of greater interest to know what children can do well, relative to their own level of ability, than to know how well they did. Finding out that a girl with a Full Scale IQ of 63 did poorly, compared to other children her age, in all abilities tapped by the WISC-R leads to a dead end. Discovering that she has strengths in nonverbal reasoning and short-term memory, relative to her own level of functioning, provides information that can be used to help write her individualized education program. (P. 14) [16]

Ideally, of course, a neuropsychological assessment considers two kinds of issues: the test scores (and the statistical questions on which they are predicated) as well as the strengths and problem-solving tactics that indicate the way in which the scores were obtained. Skilled clinicians have always attempted to consider both. Recently there have been attempts to reconsider the assessment of children in relation to each of these issues.

Messick's review [22] of child assessment considers a wide variety of questions. It discusses sources of variation in the test performance of children. It lists and compares various facets of measurement, such as trait versus response class and state; signs versus samples; structures versus processes; normative (allowing comparison between individuals) versus ipsative (comparison within an individual) structures; nomothetic (procedures designed to discover general laws) versus ideographic (attempts to characterize particular individuals) methods; norm-referenced (constructed to discriminate among individuals, and interpreted in terms of the relationship to others on the same measures) versus criterion-referenced (yielding measurements that are interpretable in terms of performance standards) interpretations; competence versus performance; maximal versus typical performance; correctness versus goodness of response; and content versus style. In addition, it considers different assessment media (questions, objective performance tests, behavioral observations, and the questions of typologies and tradeoffs in measurement) and it reviews various systems of variables (the child as context, the assessment of context, and assessment in context). It analyses a variety of psychometric issues such as reliability and dependability of measurements; measurement error; regression and confidence intervals; the estimation of stability, equivalence, and internal consistency; the question of group heterogeneity; the theory of generalizability; and the theory of latent trait measurement.

The Messick review provides a comprehensive coverage of many significant issues relating to the assessment of children. It demonstrates clearly that recent research in assessment theory can incorporate not only the statistical manipulation of test performance measures but also the context in which these measures were obtained and the characteristics of the children obtaining them.

The growth of the computer has also affected the broad direction of psychological and educational measurement. Two developments in testing—latent trait test theory (item-response theory) and computerized adaptive testing—reflect this influence directly.[30] Although full application of these developments to neuropsychological assessment still remains to be made, it is likely that they will eventually help the clinician with such tasks as measuring individuals using more than ability levels, obtaining measurements with equal precision across individuals differing in clinical symptomatology (some of which may create problems in test administration); and making decisions about what constitutes mastery of a cognitive task.

New Approaches to the Brain Bases of Child Assessment

Neuropsychologists wishing to make inferences about the child's brain from test behavior must do so against a background of concern about the nature and purpose of assessment itself. The concept of intelligence and the application of tests for its measurement have been most particularly criticized. Intelligence testing has been called a form of bourgeois rationalization in which tests can serve as instruments of social or racial discrimination[10]; it is alleged that the idea of intelligence as a reified entity cannot be supported[15]; and it is argued that intelligence tests fail to capture a variety of other mental and physical talents that might be termed intelligences.[13]

Of most concern to child neuropsychology is the claim that the brain basis of IQ test performance has not been convincingly demonstrated (see Gould[15]). Although in adults the evidence for focal brain representation is better for cognitive functions other than psychometric intelligence (see Gardner[13]), intelligence in brain-damaged children has been shown to be related to variables related to the brain insult, even though it cannot be localized in any simple manner[5,6]: It is brain-related but not brain-localized.

The question, then, is not simply one of localizing neuropsychological test performance in the young damaged brain but one of developing and explicating the process by which inferences about brain function are made on the basis of neuropsychological test results. Child neuropsychologists have lately begun to consider this core problem from a variety of perspectives. In children with known or suspected brain pa-

thology, attempts are underway at integrating existing test methods with new multivariate statistical procedures; there are ongoing reflections concerning the process by which inferences are made about the brains of exceptional children; and systems are being developed for using test behavior itself as a possible basis for selecting relevant from irrelevant facts about the young damaged brain.

Of late, there has been a recognition that, with children, certain issues require their own assessment techniques and procedures. Rourke and associates[27] provide an integrated view of the methods of child assessment and treatment, and they employ illustrative case histories to show how neuropsychological methods work with exceptional children. The same laboratory has also provided a review of what a modern quantitative approach to neuropsychological assessment of children might involve.[26]

It is important to reflect upon how we make inferences about central nervous system pathology and to consider what kind of brain-behavior relationships would validate these inferences (see Fletcher and Taylor[12]). The kinds of tests we design and the interpretations we make with them depend on our views about these core questions. If the basis for a test is a brain variable such as the left brain–right brain dichotomy, then particular test measures will be interpreted as representing types of mental functioning identified on the basis of the variable of interest, lateral cerebral specialization (see Kaufman and Kaufman[17]). Alternatively, tests might be designed based on current knowledge of psychological processes like language or memory; then different patterns of test performance might be viewed as more or less brain-based to the extent that they can be predicted from constellations of brain variables, variables that were not the basis on which the tests were constructed (see Dennis[4,5,6]).

Discussion

The task of child neuropsychological assessment is one of evaluating samples of test behavior in relation to recent methods of statistical decision making and current views about brain-behavior inferencing.

We need, first, to know which behavioral functions to assess. The child's history and previous test results may provide some indication about the abilities that should be tested, but how a cognitive skill like memory might be evaluated must be continually refined. In light of new research into the features of normal and aberrant memory, the use of items like serial digit repetition to make inferences about the nature of memory in children referred for neuropsychological assessment is clearly inadequate. Neuropsychological assessment must continue to reflect developments in mainstream psychology: Good neuropsychology, in effect, must be good psychology.

Second, we need a wider variety of assessment tools. The tendency to catalogue existing tests perhaps causes us to be overly impressed with the number of tests available. At the same time, we tend to be insufficiently critical of their quality. The research literature is replete with well-developed test instruments for a wide range of cognitive skills. By and large, these have yet to be incorporated into child assessment. Effective assessment involves continually updating test instruments in light of new research.

Third, we need to know how to analyze and interpret test figures. In the past, clinical decisions have sometimes been used in contexts that, more properly, required statistical address. In using the new statistical aids to test interpretation, the child neuropsychologist need not fear becoming wedded to test statistics at the expense of clinical skills. Emerging concepts of the analysis and interpretation of test scores incorporate both statistical decision making and a rich observational base.

Finally, we need to know how to formulate hypotheses about the brain bases of observed test behavior. Understanding the nature of the inferences we make about the young brain on the basis of neuropsychological test results (in effect, being able to explicate how we reason from test scores to normal or aberrant brain function) is probably the most important task facing those involved in child neuropsychological assessment.

ACKNOWLEDGMENTS

Preparation of this chapter was supported by an Ontario Mental Health Foundation Associateship.

REFERENCES

1. DENNIS, M. "Epilogue: Research Applications and Directions," in F. Boller and M. Dennis, eds., *Auditory Comprehension: Clinical and Experimental Studies with the Token Test.* New York: Academic Press, 1979, pp. 171–180.

2. ———. "Neuropsychological Assessment," in J. Noshpitz, et al., eds., *Basic Handbook of Child Psychiatry,* vol. 1. New York: Basic Books, 1979, pp. 574–583.

3. ———. "The Developmentally Dyslexic Brain and the Written Language Skills of Children With One Hemisphere," in U. Kirk, ed., *Neuropsychology of Language, Reading, and Spelling.* New York: Academic Press, 1983, pp. 185–208.

4. ———. "Syntax in Brain-Injured Children," in M. Studdert-Kennedy, ed., *Psychobiology of Language,* Cambridge, Mass.: MIT Press, 1983, pp. 195–202.

5. ———. "Intelligence After Early Brain Injury. I: Predicting IQ Scores from Medical Variables," *Journal of Clinical and Experimental Neuropsychology,* 7 (1985):526–554.

6. ———. "Intelligence after Early Brain Injury. II: IQ Scores of Subjects Classified on the Basis of Medical History Variables," *Journal of Clinical and Experimental Neuropsychology,* 7 (1985):555–576.

7. DENNIS, M., and KOHN, B. "The Active-Passive Test: An Age-Referenced Clinical Test of Syntactic Discrimination," *Developmental Neuropsychology,* 1 (1985):113–137.

8. DENNIS, M., LOVETT, M., and WIEGEL-CRUMP, C. A. "Written Language Acquisition After Left or Right Hemidecortication in Infancy," *Brain and Language,* 12 (1981):54–91.

9. DENNIS, M., SUGAR, J., and WHITAKER, H. A. "The Acquisition of Tag Questions," *Child Development,* 53 (1982):1254–1257.

10. EVANS, B., and WAITES, B. *IQ and Mental Testing.* London: Macmillan, 1981.

11. FIELD, J. G. "Two Types of Tables for Use with Wechsler's Intelligence Scales," *Journal of Clinical Psychology,* 16 (1960):3–7.

12. FLETCHER, J. M., and TAYLOR, H. G. "Neuropsychological Approaches to Children: Towards a Developmental Neuropsychology," *Journal of Clinical Neuropsychology,* 6 (1984):39–56.

13. GARDNER, H. *Frames of Mind.* New York: Basic Books, 1983.

14. GOLDSTEIN, G. "Methodological and Theoretical Issues in Neuropsychological Assessment," *Journal of Behavioral Assessment,* 1 (1979):23–41.

15. GOULD, S. J. *The Mismeasure of Man.* New York: W. W. Norton, 1981.

16. KAUFMAN, A. S. *Intelligent Testing with the WISC-R.* New York: John Wiley & Sons, 1979.

17. KAUFMAN, A. S., and KAUFMAN, N. L. *Kaufman Assessment Battery for Children.* Circle Pines, Minn.: American Guidance Service, 1983.

18. LEVIN, H., BENTON, A. L., and GROSSMAN, R. G. *Neurobehavioral Consequences of Closed Head Injury.* New York: Oxford University Press, 1982.

19. LEVIN, H. S., et al. "Memory and Intellectual Ability After Head Injury in Children and Adolescents," *Neurosurgery,* 11 (1982):668–672.

20. LEZAK, M. *Neuropsychological Assessment.* New York: Oxford University Press, 1979.

21. ———. *Neuropsychological Assessment,* 2nd ed. New York: Oxford University Press, 1983.

22. MESSICK, S. "Assessment of Children," in P. H. Mussen, ed., *Handbook of Child Psychology,* vol. 1, *History, Theory, and Methods.* New York: John Wiley & Sons, 1983, pp. 477–526.

23. NICHOLSON, C. L., and ALCORN, C. L. *Educational Applications of the WISC-R: A Handbook of Interpretive*

Strategies and Remedial Recommendations. Los Angeles: Western Psychological Services, 1980.

24. RHODES, F. *Manual for the Rhodes WISC Scatter Profile.* San Diego: Educational and Industrial Testing Service, 1969.

25. ———. *Manual for the WISC-R Scatter Profile.* San Diego: Educational and Industrial Testing Service, 1975.

26. ROURKE, B. P., and ADAMS, K. M. "Quantitative Approaches to the Neuropsychological Assessment of Children," in R. Tarter and G. Goldstein, eds., *The Neuropsychology of Childhood.* New York: Plenum Press, 1984.

27. ROURKE, B. P. et al. *Child Neuropsychology: An Intro-*

duction to Theory, Research, and Clinical Practice.* New York: Guilford Press, 1983.

28. SATZ, P., and FLETCHER, J. *The Florida Kindergarten Screening Battery.* Odessa, Fla.: Psychological Assessment Resources, 1982.

29. VITELLI, R. J., and GOLDBLATT, R. B. *Tardor Interpretive Scoring System for the WISC-R.* Manchester, Conn.: Tardor Corporation, 1979.

30. WEISS, D. J. *New Horizons in Testing.* New York: Academic Press, 1983.

31. WIEGEL-CRUMP, C. A., and DENNIS, M. "Development of Word-Finding," *Brain and Language,* 27 (1986):1–23.

19 / Brain Imaging Techniques: Relevance to Child Psychiatry

Carl Feinstein and Daniel Weinberger

Introduction

The advent of technologies for the visualization of the living human brain has generated new interest in the relationship between brain structure and physiology on the one hand and mental functioning on the other. The images and related information generated by these procedures offer hope of bridging the gap between the clinical observation of functional aspects of psychiatric disorders and direct visualization of structural, electrophysiological, metabolic, or neurochemical processes in the brain. While the vast majority of research in this area has been done with adults, recently there has been increased interest in applying brain visualization techniques to children.

The involvement of child psychiatry in research utilizing these new imaging techniques is of critical importance for two reasons. In the first place, the documentation of structural or physiological abnormalities in adult psychiatric patients raises the question of when and how in development these abnormalities make their appearance. At present, however, it is not known whether early evidence of brain abnormalities would be found if children known to be vulnerable to major psychiatric disorder in adulthood were subjected to these brain visualization techniques prior to the manifestation of psychopathology. Second, although a growing body of evidence indicates that brain dysfunction may be associated with many types of childhood psychiatric disorders, the utilization of brain visualiza-

tion procedures has barely begun to be applied to the understanding of these conditions.

In this chapter, the technical aspects of the major brain visualization procedures are summarized briefly. The data generated by the different techniques are compared according to four criteria: (1) what the image represents, (2) the spatial resolution capacities of the technique, (3) the temporal resolution capacities of the technique, and (4) technical requirements necessary to obtain the image, particularly invasiveness and expense.

Significant trends in their applications to both research and clinical practice with adult psychiatric patients are summarized. Finally, where a technique has been applied to child psychiatry research, findings to date are summarized. In this brief review it is impossible to present all the data or major arguments concerning each of these techniques. The aim, rather, is to outline the various opportunities and limitations each technique offers both to clinical practice and to research in child psychiatry.

Computerized Axial Tomography

Of the current techniques for brain visualization, computerized axial tomography is the most widely used. This computer-enhanced x-ray technique mathematically reconstructs images of the internal structure of the brain in the form of anatomical cross-sections. The data processed by the computer to generate these images consist of the quatity of x-rays, which arrive at a series of sensors circling the head, after having been beamed through the brain. The image, therefore, is based on localized differences in radiodensity. Anatomically distinct structures that have similar radiodensities are thus poorly delineated using this methodology. An example of this limitation would be the fact that gray and white matter differ relatively little in their transmission of x-rays and, therefore, are not as readily distinguished in the CT image as ventricular spaces are from brain substance. The use of intravenously injected radio-opaque contrast media can aid in the delineation of structures with close but different densities. Nonetheless, this fundamental limitation of CT scans for distinguishing many central nervous system (CNS) structures remains, despite recent improvements in spatial resolution.[25] Currently, lesions or structural defects larger than 5 mm can be detected by CT scan if the difference in radiodensity is sufficiently great.

As a consequence of these factors, CT scanning in clinical psychiatry and research has been most useful in detecting many types of gross pathological lesions and in identifying various signs of cortical atrophy or structural abnormality, such as enlarged ventricles or cortical sulci.[34] Diagnostically, the CT scan is indicated to rule out neurological disease in patients referred for emotional, behavioral, or acute cognitive disorders.[34] It can also be used to monitor the severity of brain involvement in certain disorders such as anorexia nervosa and alcohol abuse and in high-dose steroid administration. These conditions are associated with CT images of cortical atrophy, which are reversible with clinical improvement.[34]

In research, the principal application of the CT scan has been in the search for evidence of structural brain pathology in various psychiatric disorders. In this regard, there have been many studies focusing on enlarged cerebral ventricles, dilated cortical fissures and sulci, and atrophy of the cerebellar vermis.[35] Several different measurement techniques have been developed to discern and measure structural abnormalities. These may be subdivided into techniques employing various two-dimensional measurements, such as the ventricular brain ratio (VBR), and other techniques that use computer algorithms to calculate overall cerebrospinal fluid volumes.[35] More recently, techniques for comparing tissue radiodensity at comparable brain sites in different subjects have been used.[35]

CT scan research in schizophrenic adults has produced a long series of findings, that, with a few exceptions, indicate the existence of a clinically distinct subgroup of schizophrenic patients who manifest one or more of the just-cited evidences of cerebral atrophy.[35] These patients are characterized by a preponderance of negative symptomatology, poor premorbid social history, poor prognosis, and both historical and current evidence of "soft" neurological signs, including cognitive deficits. This finding is not an artifact of pharmacological treatment and apparently is not progressive from the time of the first CT scan.[35]

Ventricular size abnormalities have also been reported in other psychiatric conditions, particularly affective disorders.[35] In the case of affective disorders, however, unlike schizophrenia, ventricular size may correlate with age and/or length of illness.[29] This body of work seems to suggest that structural brain pathology is associated with major categories of psychiatric disorder; however, CT scan data have produced only nonspecific findings for these disorders. In none of these cases have CT scan findings been correlated with specific pathological processes. Along these lines, Larson, Mack, and Watts,[19] in a retrospective study of 123 diagnostically heterogeneous patients scanned to rule out CNS disorder, found that 35 percent had cortical atrophy and 10 percent had focal CNS disease. While this finding lends itself to more than one interpretation, it certainly supports the hypothesis that structural brain abnormalities detected by CT scan are indicative of a nonspecific vulnerability factor present in a variety of psychiatric disorders.

Both clinical and research applications of the CT scan in child psychiatry have been impeded by the fact that radiation exposure is involved and by the relative expense and inconvenience of the procedure. Using the most current generation of equipment, radiation dosage to the head is 2 to 3 rads, a level so low that the CT scan is properly used in all clinical situations where acute, progressive, or reversible CNS pathology is a diagnostic issue. However, insufficient normative developmental data for children is available, since, ethically, even this low radiation dosage has been unacceptable for research purposes in children. At present, the only normative data available consists of series by Barron, Jacobs, and Kinkel,[1] Fukuyama and associates,[12] and Pederson, Gyldensted, and Gyldensted.[21] All CT scan research on childhood psychiatric disorders that has attempted age- and sex-matched controls has resorted to the use of children being evaluated for head injury or various possible CNS pathology (seizure disorder, headaches, etc.) as a control group.

The procedure itself is somewhat arduous. It involves placing the subject within the head scanner for at least ten to fifteen minutes, during which time the head must be absolutely immobile in a precisely defined position for a series of approximately ten intervals of sixty to ninety seconds. In most cases, especially with younger children or children with a more severe type of psychiatric disorder, sedation in advance and general anesthesia is required.

Autism has been the subject of considerable CT scan research in child psychiatry. A significant precursor of this was the work of Hauser, DeLong, and Rosman,[15] utilizing pneumoencephalograpy. They reported increased left ventricular size in a group of autistic patients. Hier, Rosenberger, and colleagues,[16,17] using the CT scan, found reversals of normal cerebral lobar asymmetry in a significant number of children with early-onset developmental disorders, including autism, developmental language disorder, dyslexia, and mental retardation. Since then investigators have reported a variety of structural brain abnormalities in some of the autistic children studied, using the CT scan.[6,7,8]

Caparulo and associates[7] reported on CT scan findings for eighty-five patients with childhood-onset pervasive developmental disorders, including infantile autism, pervasive developmental disorder, developmental language disorders, severe attention deficit disorders with learning disabilities, and Tourette's syndrome. Unfortunately, their method of analyzing of the scans was subjective, and they lacked a normal control group; however, their finding of differential rates of abnormal CT scans in the different diagnostic categories and their demonstration of a highly significant correlation between abnormal scans and abnormal electroencephalograms (EEGs) are important contributions. The most common structural defect they found was left ventricular enlargement; however, a heterogeneous group of other abnormalities was also observed. In their population, children with pervasive developmental disorder had a 59 percent incidence of abnormal scans, followed by developmental language disorders (43.5 percent), Tourette's syndrome (37.5 percent), severe attention deficit disorder with learning disabilities (28 percent), and infantile autism (18 percent).

Two major methodological issues cited in the Caparulo and coworkers study are of importance in the evaluation of all other CT scan research in autism, and in other conditions as well. These are, first, the great difficulty defining clinically homogeneous diagnostic groups and, second, the lack of specificity in the type of CT abnormalities found. In the studies of autism cited, there were children with apparently similar psychopathology, some of whom had no identifiable CNS pathology by CT scan and others of whom had a variety of structural abnormalities. Prior and colleagues[22] have recently argued against the tactic of searching for a characteristic CT scan abnormality in autism. This view was based on their findings that, in a group of nine "classically autistic" boys they studied, no CT scan abnormalities were found. However, their subjects were an extremely high functioning group within this diagnostic category; the boys' was mean IQ of 87 (five attended normal school, and four attended special programs for the mildly handicapped). The authors concluded that previous findings of CT scan abnormalities resulted from the presence of a variety of forms of brain damage in the populations studied.

Rosenbloom and others,[25] however, have recently reported a CT scan study of a carefully diagnosed, homogeneous group of young autistic children who had no other evidence of brain damage. They found a minority of these children to have significantly enlarged ventricles compared to a control group. It appears likely, at this point, that a subgroup of autistic children have structural abnormalities by CT scan but that this finding, like that for schizophrenia in adults, is a nonspecific indicator of brain pathology.

Recently the CT scan has been used as a research tool to search for structural brain abnormalities in other childhood psychiatric disorders. Shaywitz and associates[27] used standardized, highly reliable, objective linear measurement to compare thirty-five children with attention deficit disorder and twenty-seven controls (diagnostic CT scans done for "a variety of clinical indications") who were comparable in age, sex, and IQ. They were unable to replicate the earlier Yale finding of CT scan abnormalities in children with severe attention deficit disorder. Comparison of group mean values for measurements made by raters blind to clinical status did not distinguish the attention deficit disorder group from the control group. This method of data analysis, however, did not report data regarding intersubject variability in the two samples and thus did not explore the possibility that subgroups of children might have had significantly different structural brain measurements.

Behar and coworkers[2] studied sixteen obsessive-compulsive adolescents with CT scans, EEGs, and neuropsychological testings, utilizing as scan controls teenagers matched for age, sex, race, handedness, and IQ. The controls had received diagnostic scans for reasons unspecified in the report; however, all cases read as questionable clinically, associated with changes in consciousness or having hard neurological signs or any history of psychiatric problems were excluded. CT scan measurements were done using reliable linear measurement techniques. The obsessive-compulsive group had a mean ventricular brain ratio significantly higher than the controls and also showed significantly more neuropsychological deficits. However, there was no pattern of correlation of these abnormal findings by subject.

All of this research suggests that abnormal CT scan findings suggestive of cerebral atrophy, a nonspecific result of cerebral pathology, are found with greater frequency in association with some childhood psychiatric disorders. The fact that only some members within a diagnostic group have this finding does not rule out the possibility that all patients with this disorder might have a common underlying neurological deficit. In some of these patients, such a deficit might be associated with other brain abnormalities, which, by virtue either of being located at a particular brain site or of being a sufficient magnitude, are detectable by computerized tomography. For other patients with the disorder in question, these associated abnormalities might be absent or of a type not detectable using this technology. In summary, CT scan research involving childhood psychiatric disorders, like similar research in adult psychiatric disorders, has not yet isolated a brain abnormality specifically associated with any diagnosis.

The possibly converging lines of evidence that (1) subgroups of young but chronic adult patients have CT scan evidence of stable structural brain abnormalities, (2) neuropsychological deficits have been found in child psychiatric patients without known brain damage, [31] and (3) subgroups of children with several different psychiatric disorders have CT scan abnormalities have led a few investigators to use the CT scan to examine serious childhood psychiatric disorders in general. Reiss and associates [24] compared CT scan findings from twenty child psychiatry inpatients suffering from a variety of disorders with twenty age and sex-matched controls. The controls consisted of children who had received diagnostic scans for nonpsychiatric complaints and whose scans had been read as normal by an experienced neuroradiologist. All of the inpatient psychiatry group had received diagnostic CT scans based on a suspicion of neurological disorder. The VBR of the psychiatry patients was significantly greater in the patients than in the controls, with sixteen having VBRs greater than the mean for the controls. This finding could not be explained by the presence of later diagnosed neurological disorder in some of the psychiatry patients, since this subgroup, in fact, had (nonsignificantly) smaller VBRs than those psychiatric patients without diagnosable neurologic disorder.

Tramontana and Sherrets [30] recently studied twenty hospitalized child psychiatric patients ages nine to fifteen, for whom there was no suspicion from psychiatric or neurological evaluations of a neurological disorder. The objective was to search for correlations between abnormal neuropsychological test findings and CT scan abnormalities. VBRs and a computerized determination of regional cortical densities were used in the evaluation of the CT scans. Using standard criteria, they found that the Halstead Reitan Neuropsychological Battery classified 60 percent of the patients as impaired. Correlation of these findings with the CT scan data revealed that the neuropsychologically im-

paired group showed significantly less right-hemisphere density relative to left-hemisphere density when compared to the patients classified as nonimpaired. Using the Luria Nebraska Neuropsychological Battery, 70 percent of the patients were classified as impaired. The impaired group displayed significantly lower densities by CT scan in several areas bilaterally when compared to the nonimpaired group. Interestingly, only one of these scans was read as definitely abnormal by a neuroradiologist blind to the children's neuropsychological status.

It should be noted that the method of CT scan analysis employed in the Tramontana and Sherrets study, namely that of calculating brain parenchymal densities using CT numbers, is still controversial. Nevertheless, this report, in addition to finding a high rate of neuropsychological abnormalities in a nonneurologically suspect child psychiatric population, is the first CT study of childhood psychiatric disorder in which CT scan findings were found to be correlated with defined neuropsychological deficits. Replication of these findings would be of obvious significance.

In summary, the current status of CT scan research in child psychiatry is that structural brain abnormalities seem to be more frequent findings in at least the more severe psychiatric disorders; however, these findings lack specificity both with regard to the nature of the brain alteration or damage and with regard to their usefulness in correctly diagnosing any specific psychiatric disorder. Clinically, for children as for adults, computerized tomography has a place in the evaluation of possible CNS pathology. Research aimed at correlating CT scan abnormalities with specific neuropsychological deficits, or at utilizing CT scan findings in conjunction with imaging techniques that do not involve readiation, such as topographic EEG mapping, would seem to be promising. Limitations in the ability of this technology to distinguish components of the brain with similar radiodensities as well as to improve spatial resolution may curtail its long-range applications for both research and clinical practice. These limitations will loom larger as the nuclear magnetic resonance imaging technique becomes increasingly available.

Nuclear Magnetic Resonance Imaging

Nuclear magnetic resonance imaging (NMR) is a revolutionary new technique just becoming available that is certain to have a profound effect on both research and clinical practice in all areas of medicine, including psychiatry. This method exploits the fact that atomic nuclei that have an odd number of nucleons (protons or neutrons) assume different and specific energy states in a magnetic field.[23] Applying an elecromagnetic field at a frequency identical to the natural precessional frequency of the nuclei to be imaged causes them to shift to a different energy state (hence the term resonance). When the electromagnetic field is withdrawn, the nuclei revert to a lower energy state—"relax"—and emit energy in the form of an electromagnetic pulse, which can be detected by a coil surrounding the sample. The distribution of the nuclei in a sample can be mapped by computerized mathematical algorithms.

At present, the hydrogen nucleus (a proton) is the principal one being mapped with this technique, although procedures for mapping others are rapidly being developed. Mapping hydrogen nuclei in the human body with NMR generates an image that represents the density and distribution of hydrogen molecules, principally water but also, to a lesser extent, lipids. The NMR computer can generate images of cross-sectional "slices" of the organs being studied, from many different planes. The image generated is far more sensitive to tissue differences between adjacent biological structures than that generated by the CT scan and, in addition, has better spatial resolution.

Applied to the brain, NMR produces images of far greater detail and delineation of soft tissue structures than the CT scan. As a result, it is already being used in a few centers as a superior technique for detecting CNS lesions. As the technical aspects of mapping other nuclei are developed, biochemical and pharmacological mapping of the brain will become possible. It is of particular importance that the electromagnetic frequencies that NMR utilizes are far below x-rays or even visible light and do not cause damage to biological systems. Thus this technique will be available for research and clinical purposes in child psychiatry. In addition, although the actual procedure somewhat resembles the CT scan technique, the images are generated in a shorter time and therefore should be more convenient for use with children.

Positron Emission Tomography

Positron emission tomography (PET) is a method for the *in vivo* assaying and visualizing of neuronal metabolism and pharmacology.[32] Positron-emitting radioisotopes with short half-lives are incorporated into a substrate such as glucose, or into a drug with known receptor-binding properties, and injected intravenously. The radioisotopes enter and thereby label the biochemical sites being studied and emit positrons that travel within the brain for 1 to 2 mm and then combine with an electron to yield two gamma rays. These gamma rays head in opposite directions (180 degrees) and are detected by means of a circle of radiation sensors that ring the patient's head. Images are then constructed using computer algorithms that calculate the locations of the radioisotope molecules within the brain. Current technology allows for a spatial resolution of 8 mm; however, machines with a resolution of 2 to 3 mm are under construction.

Research in utilizing the PET scan in psychiatry has employed several different strategies. Principle among them are measurements of regional brain metabolic rate and the mapping of neuronal receptor sites or the binding of specific drugs to such sites.[4] PET images of the brain can be generated with the subject at rest, or they can be used to study the biochemical physiology of the brain in response to a variety of cognitive tasks or sensory experiences. This latter makes the PET scan one of the brain imaging techniques capable of studying relationships between different types of mental activity and brain physiology.

PET imaging of regional glucose metabolic rate has been employed fairly extensively as a research tool.[4] The technique, developed by Sokoloff,[28] uses a fluorine-labeled analogue of glucose, 2-deoxyglucose (FDG). This compound, when injected, is taken up by the brain tissue and enters the glycolytic metabolic pathway. Because of its structure, however, metabolism is blocked after an initial step and the cells are thereby labeled in proportion to their glucose uptake. The scan is begun after fifty minutes, when FDG uptake is complete. The PET image, therefore, reflects glucose uptake in the initial period, not during the time of the scan.

During the uptake period, a variety of sensory, cognitive, or emotion-stimulating tasks or even sleep may be introduced, a form of the research strategy referred to as cognitive activation. The PET scan then obtained will reflect the increased metabolic activity of the area(s) of the brain principally involved in the mental activity being studied. This mental task, however, must be sustained throughout the FDG uptake phase. Thus the temporal resolution of this technique is very sluggish (thirty to forty minutes). This procedure has been used to perform classical neuropsychological experiments correlating brain areas with various cognitive activities. More recently the FDG method has been used to compare PET scans from selected patient populations with those of normal controls or to study treatment effects in response to various drugs. Buchsbaum and colleagues,[5] using both resting and pain stimulation paradigms, have reported that both schizophrenic and bipolar affective disorder patients both show a lower anterior-posterior brain metabolism gradient in comparison to normal controls. This pattern of "hypofrontality" for both schizophrenia and major affective disorder has also been found in some studies utilizing regional cerebral blood flow methods (to be discussed).

Use of PET scan technology has resulted in recent breakthroughs in the identification of *in vivo* receptor binding sites in the brain for dopamine, serotonin, opiates, and several psychoactive drugs.[32,33,36] Dopamine and serotonin type 2 receptor sites have been shown to decrease substantially with age in adults. The pathophysiology of psychiatric disorder is being studied by comparing neurotransmitter receptor sites in normals and patients. The mechanisms of action of various psychoactive drugs are now being studied via drug effects on receptor binding of both neurotransmitters and other drugs. This type of research is enabling *in vivo* neuroanatomical, neurochemical, and clinical psychiatric data to be integrated directly for the first time.

Due to the radiation exposure inherent in this technique, PET scan technology has had no significant direct research applications in the study of children with psychiatric disorders. Applications to child psychiatry must be pursued by indirect means, such as the study of adult patients who have a continuous history of a disorder from childhood. Recently Rumsey and coworkers[26] have used this approach in a study of ten adult autistic men. The future of PET scan technology in psychiatric practice is unclear, although many possible clinical applications have been described.[32] The procedure is complex and expensive, and currently requires the presence of a cyclotron on site or very close by to supply the short half-life radioisotopes it employs. Two approaches to this problem currently under exploration are single photon emission tomography (SPECT), a variant of PET technology that does not require the presence of an on-site cyclotron, and the development of various short-lived radioactive tracer compounds that do not require quite such rapid availability.

Regional Cerebral Blood Flow

Regional cerebral blood flow (RCBF) utilizing inhalation of xenon-133, a low-energy gamma-ray-emitting radioisotope, is a brain imaging technique that displays physiological data collected from the cerebral cortex. It has a number of advantages for the study of higher cortical functioning.[3] It is noninvasive, relatively easy to carry out, and involves relatively low doses of radia-

tion. According to this technique, the subject inhales xenon-133, an inert, freely diffusable gas that has no effect on metabolic processes, until brain tissue saturation is achieved. When inhalation of the gas is stopped, the rate at which xenon-133 is washed out of any region of the brain is a function of blood flow to that area. A helmet with radiation detectors monitors the decrease in radiation levels over time. This information is then processed by computer to generate an image that describes blood flow rate (which is proportional to metabolic activity) over the surface of the cortex. Unlike PET, NMR, and CT scan techniques, this method cannot image subcortical structures. RCBF is particularly well suited for cognitive activation studies. The mental activity being studied is performed by the subject during the xenon-133 washout period, which takes about ten minutes. This is a shorter period (temporal resolution) than that required for PET scan studies, and, moreover, the physiological measurements are made simultaneous with the mental activity instead of afterward, as in the PET scan technique. In addition, it is also possible to monitor the EEG simultaneously. A disadvantage of the RCBF technique, however, is its poor spatial resolution—2 to 4 cm of surface cortex.

Ingvar and Franzen, using intravenous xenon-133, found that resting chronic schizophrenic patients had relatively reduced anterior blood flow compared to controls.[18] This finding, however, was not consistently replicated until cognitive activation tasks were introduced into the procedure. Berman and associates[3] compared unmedicated schizophrenic patients with controls utilizing the Wisconsin Card Sort task in conjunction with RCBF. They confirmed that schizophrenics showed a *decrease* in anterior cerebral blood flow relative to posterior flow during cognitive activation, in contrast to normals, who demonstrated the expected increase in frontal flow during the performance of a cognitive task. Using a similar approach, Gur and coworkers[13] found overactivity of the left hemisphere in schizophrenic patients as compared to controls. Neuroleptic medication in these patients resulted in increased relative flow to the right hemisphere for male patients and overall increased and more symmetrical flow in women. Major affective disorders are currently being studied using RCBF,[14] and there is no reason why a variety of other psychiatric disorders could not be explored using this technique.

The noninvasive, relatively nonarduous RCBF procedure would lend itself well to the study of children with various psychiatric disorders. However, ethical constraints regarding radiation exposure (even though this is quite low in RCBF) currently stand in the way of using this procedure with them. It may be that findings from topographic EEG mapping will be sufficiently compelling to warrant RCBF research, which has inherently greater ease of use and less hairtrigger temporal state dependency. In the meantime, applying RCBF in the study of adults with psychiatric disorder continuous from childhood is a likely tactic.

Topographic EEG Mapping

Topographic EEG mapping is a computer-assisted extension of EEG technology by which electrophysiological data collected from a standardized placement of electrodes on the scalp is condensed, organized, and summarized by computer onto a graphic display, which represents the surface of the cerebral cortex. Various forms of electrophysiological data may be displayed in this fashion, including spectral EEG and cortical evoked responses. These two forms of information regarding the electrical activity of the brain are described in detail elsewhere in this volume (see chapter 22) and will not be elaborated upon here. The advantage of this imaging technique is that it assists the researcher or clinician in assimilating the vast amounts of data collected from multiple-lead EEG recordings into either a static graphic image or a dynamic moving video display of the shifting patterns of electrical activity of the brain, detected from its surface.[9]

Compared to the PET scan or RCBF data, EEG data is extremely responsive temporally. Electrophysiological activity, which reflects the processing of sensory input or cognitive activity, is recorded in increments of milliseconds. Using modern computer technology, parameters of this electrophysiological data can be displayed in real-time graphic displays, from which very short segments can be captured for static presentation. It is therefore a powerful medium for studying the correlation between mental phenomena and physiological processes in the brain. As Yingling points out in chapter 22, however, the value of the data presented in graphic images is dependent on the quality and relevance of the data recorded. Normative information is critical for research, as is the study of homogeneous diagnostic groups. Also, since electrophysiological activity is extremely state-dependent, the environmental and technical conditions under which the data are collected must be carefully controlled.

Duffy and others[10,11] have reported on a study comparing eleven dyslexic boys with thirteen normal controls using a twenty-lead topographic EEG mapping technique called brain electrical activity mapping (BEAM). This method includes both spectral EEG and cortical evoked response data. They found four discrete regions of difference between the two groups.

These involved both hemispheres, the left more than the right. For the dyslexic patients, spectral analysis revealed greater alpha activity both at rest and during cognitive activation procedures. The dyslexic boys also differed from the normals in cortical auditory evoked responses in the left temporal and the left parietal areas as well as bifrontally. Using a statistically based technique for diagnostic classification based on EEG data, 90 percent of the subjects and controls were correctly classified.

Morihisa, Duffy, and Wyatt,[20] using the BEAM technology, have studied eleven drug-free and fourteen medicated schizophrenic adult patients contrasted with eleven normal controls. They found a dramatic increase in bifrontal EEG delta activity and more beta activity in the left parietal area in the schizophrenic patients as compared to normal controls. This finding corresponds to both PET scan and RCBF studies showing decreased frontal lobe metabolism in schizophrenic patients. These researchers also reported significant differences in visual and auditory evoked response patterns between the two groups. It is quite likely that this type of research, using topographic EEG mapping techniques to distinguish various psychiatric disorders from each other and from normal controls, will continue.

Topographic EEG mapping is likely to have expanded applications in child psychiatry, because of the great interest in better understanding and diagnosing neuropsychological disorders (learning disabilities, attention deficit disorders, etc). Since no radiation is involved, it is the only one of the currently available brain imaging procedures that both collects physiological information and (pending NMR) is currently available for research with children. It should be mentioned, however, that the time and technical expertise required for the accurate placement of twenty or more scalp EEG leads and the cooperation required on the part of the child for the auditory and visual evoked potentials recordings combine to make the procedure an arduous one, which may be difficult for some children to complete. In addition, both normative data for different ages and a highly standardized testing environment will be necessary if the data collected is to have true scientific or clinical value.

Summary

Recent rapid developments in technology have generated a number of new methods for visualizing physical or physiological dimensions of the living human brain. These techniques offer opportunities for increased understanding of the interconnections between biological and mental processes, including the pathophysiology of mental illness. It is only recently that brain imaging techniques have been applied in child psychiatry. The principal rate-limiting factor has been the radiation dosage involved in several of these procedures. How- ever, research in adult disorders using these techniques is likely to generate new hypotheses and research strategies in child psychiatry. In addition, at least two techniques that do not involve radiation, nuclear magnetic resonance imaging and topographic EEG mapping, are becoming increasingly available.

REFERENCES

1. BARRON, S. A., JACOBS, L., and KINKEL, W. R. "Changes in Size of Normal Lateral Ventricles During Aging Determined by Computerized Tomography," *Neurology*, 26 (1976):1011–1013.

2. BEHAR, D., et al. "Computerized Tomography and Neuropsychological Test Measures in Adolescents with Obsessive-Compulsive Disorder," *American Journal of Psychiatry*, 141 (1984):3.

3. BERMAN, K. F., et al. "Regional Cerebral Blood Flow in Psychiatry: Application to Clinical Research," in J. M. Morihisa, ed., *Brain Imaging in Psychiatry*. Washington, D.C.: American Psychiatric Association Press, 1984, pp. 43–46.

4. BUCHSBAUM, M. S. "Positron Emission Tomography (PET) in Psychiatry," in J. M. Morahisa, ed., *Brain Imaging in Psychiatry*. Washington, D.C.: American Psychiatric Association Press, 1984, pp. 1–25.

5. BUCHSBAUM, M. S., et al. "Anteroposterior Gradients in Cerebral Glucose Use in Schizophrenia and Affective Disorders," *Archives of General Psychiatry*, 41 (1984):1159–1166.

6. CAMPBELL, M., et al. "Computerized Axial Tomography in Young Autistic Children," *American Journal of Psychiatry*, 139 (1982):72–77.

7. CAPARULO, B. K., et al. "Computerized Tomographic Brain Scanning in Children with Developmental Neuropsychiatric Disorders," *Journal of the American Academy of Child Psychiatry*, 20 (1982):338–357.

8. DAMASIO, H., et al. "Computerized Tomographic Brain Scan Findings in Patients with Autistic Behavior," *Archives of Neurology*, 37 (1980):504–510.

9. DUFFY, F. H., BURCHFIEL, J. L., and LOMBROSO, C. "Brain Electrical Activity Mapping (BEAM): A Method for Extending the Clinical Utility of EEG and Evoked Potential Data," *Annals of Neurology*, 5 (1978):309–321.

10. DUFFY, F. H., et al. "Dyslexia: Automated Diagnosis by Computerized Classification of Brain Electrical Activity," *Annals of Neurology*, 7 (1980):421–428.

11. DUFFY, F. H., et al. "Dyslexia: Regional Differences in Brain Electrical Activity by Topographic Mapping," *Annals of Neurology*, 7 (1980):412–420.

12. FUKUYAMA, Y., et al. "Developmental Changes in Normal Cranial Measurements by Computed Tomography," *Developmental Medicine and Child Neurology*, 21 (1979): 425–432.

13. GUR, R. E., et al. "Brain Function in Psychiatric Disorders: #1. Regional Cerebral Blood Flow in Medicated Schizophrenics," *Archives of General Psychiatry*, 40 (1983): 1250–1254.

14. GUR, R. E., et al. "Brain Function in Psychiatric Disorders: #11. Regional Cerebral Blood Flow in Medicated Unipolar Depressives," *Archives of General Psychiatry*, 41 (1984): 695–699.

15. HAUSER, S. L., DeLONG, G. R., and ROSMAN, N. P. "Pneumographic Findings in the Infantile Autism Syndrome," *Brain*, 98 (1975): 667–688.

16. HIER, D. B., LE MAY, M., and ROSENBERGER, P. B., "Autism and Unfavorable Left-Right Asymmetries of the Brain," *Journal of Autism and Developmental Disorders*, 9 (1979):153–159.

17. HIER, D. B., et al. "Developmental Dyslexia: Evidence for a Subgroup with Reversal of Cerebral Assymetry," *Archives of Neurology*, 35 (1978):90–92.

18. INGVAR, D. H., and FRANZEN, G. "Abnormalities of Cerebral Blood Flow Distribution in Patients with Chronic Schizophrenia," *Acta Psychiatrica Scandinavica*, 50 (1974): 425–462.

19. LARSON, E. N., MACK, L. A., and WATTS, B. "Computed Tomography in Patients with Psychiatric Illnesses: Advantage of A Rule-In Approach," *Annals of Internal Medicine*, 95 (1981):360–364.

20. MORIHISA, J. M., DUFFY, F. H., and WYATT, R. J. "Brain Electrical Activity Mapping (BEAM) in Schizophrenic Patients," *Archives of General Psychiatry*, 40 (1983): 719–728.

21. PEDERSON, H., GYLDENSTED, M., and GYLDENSTED, C. "Measurement of the Normal Ventricular System and Supratentorial Subarachnoid Space in Children with Computed Tomography," *Neuroradiology*, 17 (1979): 231–237.

22. PRIOR, M. R., et al. "Computed Tomographic Study of Children with Classic Autism," *Archives of Neurology*, 41 (1984):482–484.

23. PYKETT, I. L. "NMR Imaging in Medicine," *Scientific American*, 246 (1982):78–88.

24. REISS, D., et al. "Ventricular Enlargement in Child Psychiatric Patients: A Controlled Study with Planimetric Measurements," *American Journal of Psychiatry*, 140 (1983): 453–456.

25. ROSENBLOOM, S., et al. "High Resolution CT Scanning in Infantile Autism: A Quantitative Approach," *Journal of the American Academy of Child Psychiatry*, 23 (1984):72–77.

26. RUMSEY, J. M., et al. "Brain Metabolism in Autism," *Archives of General Psychiatry*, 42 (1985):448–457.

27. SHAYWITZ, B. A., et al. "Attention Deficit Disorder: Quantitative Analysis of CT," *Neurology*, 33 (1983):1500–1503.

28. SOKOLOFF, L. "The Radioactive Deoxyglucose Method," in B. W. Agranoff and M. H. Aprison, eds., *Advances in Neurochemistry*, vol. 4. New York: Plenum, 1982, pp. 1–81.

29. STANDISH-BARRY, H. M., et al. "Pneumo-encephalographic and Computerized Axial Tomography Changes in Affective Disorder," *British Journal of Psychiatry*, 141 (1982):614–617.

30. TRAMONTANA, M. G., and SHERRETS, S. D., "Brain

Impairment in Child Psychiatric Disorders: Correspondences Between Neuropsychological and CT Scan Results," *Journal of the American Academy of Child Psychiatry,* in press.

31. TRAMONTANA, M. G., SHERRETS, S. D., and GOLDEN, C. J. "Brain Dysfunction in Youngsters with Psychiatric Disorders," *Clinical Neuropsychology,* 2 (1980):118–123.

32. WAGNER, H. N. "Probing the Chemistry of the Mind," *New England Journal of Medicine,* 312 (1985):44–46.

33. WAGNER, H. N., et al. "Imaging Dopamine Receptors in the Human Brain by Positron Tomography," *Science,* 221 (1983):1264–1266.

34. WEINBERGER, D. R. "Brain Disease and Psychiatric Illness: When Should a Psychiatrist Order a CAT Scan," *American Journal of Psychiatry,* 141 (1984):1521–1527.

35. WEINBERGER, D. R., WAGNER, R. L., and WYATT, R. J. "Neuropathological Studies of Schizophrenia: A Selective Review," *Schizophrenia Bulletin,* 9 (1983):193–212.

36. WONG, D. F., et al. "Effects of Age on Dopamine and Serotonin Receptors Measured by Positron Tomography in the Living Human Brain," *Science,* 226 (1984):1393–1396.

20 / Biological Tests in the Diagnosis of Affective Disorders in Children and Adolescents

Joaquim Puig-Antich

Introduction

At this writing, there is no proven biological test for the diagnosis of affective disorders in children or adolescents. Although the possibility of developing such test(s) in the future is an exciting one, and although some interesting leads do exist, the child psychiatric clinician should be cautious about communicating such a message to the more sophisticated parents and to the patients themselves. Doing so at this juncture is a misrepresentation of reality; it can serve various short-term purposes for the physician or the family, but such gains are only apparent. In fact, they frequently sow the seeds of future disenchantment in the doctor/patient relationship.

The frank sharing of the informed clinical judgment of different possible outcomes, with and without treatment, is the basis on which a trusting physician/patient relationship is built. Of necessity, this involves a sharing of uncertainty[31] about the future. Physicians who feel insecure due to their lack of knowledge, experience, or own psychological reasons can always take refuge in a false feeling of omnipotence, which they can easily obtain by overblowing the powerful significance of the doctor's role in the mind of the patient. Ultimately such a position cannot be maintained, and the patient realizes the lack of substance of the earlier exaggerated claims. As a result, the physician/patient relationship is shaken.

The key issue is not the outcome of treatment itself but the setting of realistic expectations over the nature of the disorder, its natural history, and chances for positive treatment effects.

Child and adolescent patients rarely, if ever, wish for an omnipotent child psychiatrist. But some parents do desire this "magic." In the case of depression, the parental search for a biological test is most frequently a search for reassurance or "moral justification" against the possibility of marital or parental problems having "caused" the child's episode. This issue can be openly discussed with the parents. Their thinking should be explored and their fears realistically contrasted with informed scientific judgment in light of current knowledge.

This chapter evaluates what we know, what we have some evidence for, and what we definitely do not know regarding biological markers and diagnostic tests in the affective disorders in children and adolescents. This is necessary in order to avoid unnecessary and premature claims regarding the diagnostic usefulness of any potential test.

The fact that no clinically useful diagnostic test for the affective disorders of the pediatric age group has emerged does not mean that the field of the psychobiology of these disorders is a wasteland. Instead, given its youth, this has been a very productive field. But the requirements for a diagnostic test are quite different from those of a psychobiological marker. At present, after more than two decades of intensive research on affective disorders in adults, only shortening of rapid-eye-movement [24,40,61,78] (REM) latency could possibly be considered a diagnostic test in that age group. As we will see later, however, it is not yet clear if or when it normalizes upon affective recovery.

Requirements of a Diagnostic Test

By definition, any psychobiological diagnostic test that may be shown useful in the future would be a biological marker. But the converse is not necessarily true: Not all biological markers can be developed into diagnostic tests. *Biological markers* are characteristics that have been shown to be specifically associated with the disorder in question, either during an episode, during the symptom-free intervals, or both. They are likely to reflect, more or less indirectly, limbic/hypothalamic mechanisms that mediate the predisposition to and/or the full expression of depressive disorders.

Biological markers are different from chromosomal markers,[36] which are associated with the *transmission* of particular disorders on the basis of chromosomal geography alone. In and of themselves, chromosomal markers do not have the potential to point toward pathophysiological mechanisms, unless the genes actually involved in the causation of the disorder in question are isolated and identified.

As in adult affective disorders, during the depressive episode and/or during the recovered state, biological abnormalities have been found in children and adolescents with major affective illness. Obviously, the areas investigated first have been some of those shown to be involved in adult affective illness: electroencephalogram (EEG) sleep* and neuroendocrine studies.† Nevertheless, this does not indicate that these are necessarily the only relevant areas. Biochemical [3,66,70,73] and peripheral tissue receptor abnormalities [21,47,51] are likely to be found in the future, as they have been found in adult affective illness.

Studies of sleep have been conducted and neuroendocrine markers explored in prepubertal children both during the depressive episode and after sustained affective recovery. These investigations have yielded several positive findings. To clarify the discussion of these findings, several definitions are necessary. A *state marker* is an abnormality that appears in close temporal relationship to the onset of the depressive episode and that then normalizes with the episode's termination. Finding an abnormality during the depressive episode is not tantamount to defining a state marker. To live up to its definition, a state marker should, in addition, normalize in a loosely parallel, chronological relationship to sustained affective recovery. Biological abnormalities that remain or become abnormal during the sustained recovered state may be markers of trait or markers of a past episode. A *marker of past episode* would not be abnormal before the onset of the first depressive episode, and it would therefore represent a kind of sequela from the episode of depressive illness. A true *trait marker* would be abnormal before the onset of the first affective episode and therefore would be a very sensitive indicator of the child's predisposition to develop affective illness in the future. These distinctions are important as the potential significance of biological markers varies according to their respective type. It should be emphasized that the study of patients during the depressive episode only will not lead to the identification of this type of marker.

Compared to both normal and nondepressed psychiatric groups, any biological characteristic that is significantly associated with affective disorder in youngsters can be considered a marker. But to be useful as a diagnostic test a marker should fulfill additional requirements: first, it should be relatively inexpensive and easy to measure; second, the association should be strong enough as to discriminate clearly between the group in question and *those groups of patients who may present diagnostic problems for the clinician.* Note that the emphasis here is strictly pragmatic: helping the clinician in making a diagnosis. Differential diagnosis of major affective conditions in youngsters is rarely concerned with medical or psychiatric normality; the problem is rather to distinguish depression from other conditions. In this context, in order to determine if a marker can become a diagnostic test, the contrast between the depressed group and the nonaffective psychiatric control group is crucial. Another aspect of this pragmatism is that what underlies the association is very important for understanding the significance of a marker but is irrelevant for a test. Thus there is substantial evidence from child, adolescent, and adult studies that the sleep correlates found in adult depressive patients during a major depressive episode are probably the result of *an* interaction between depression and age.* Although this is an important observation for further hypothesis testing, it is irrelevant to the usefulness of sleep EEG variables as a diagnostic test in adult depressive illness.

No diagnostic test can pass muster unless it can be considered adequately *sensitive* to the disorder it seeks to identify and, within acceptable limits, specific to the disorder. One cannot speak of specificity without addressing the question of which nondepressive population the data represent. Thus in a particular study the dexamethasone suppression test (DST) was found to be 63 percent sensitive to major depression and 90 percent

---

*See references 15, 24, 40, 41, 61, and 78.
†See references 9, 10, 29, 30, 53, 67, 68, and 75.

*See references 15, 25, 55, 77, and 80.

specific compared to nondepressed psychiatric disorders.[52] In another study of conduct disorder children, the test was found to be 89 percent specific.[76] In still other studies, comparisons are being carried out with normal children. The results of the first two studies suggest that this putative marker, if demonstrated, may have potential as a diagnostic test. However, the results of the contrasts with normal subjects will not apply to the issue of the possible diagnostic utility of such a test. Another caveat also made clear by these examples is the lack of replication in a sufficiently large sample that includes enough patients with different nonaffective disorders. Without such replication, the estimates on differential specificities do not have sufficiently narrow confidence limits to serve as guides for solid clinical judgments.

So far, the discussion applies only to potential diagnostic tests evolved from demonstrated state markers. Markers that remain abnormal at recovery could also evolve into diagnostic tests. But these would not necessarily carry the information that the patient was in an active episode of major depression. Instead they would indicate only that the patient had had an episode in the past or was having one currently. Nevertheless, it should be kept in mind that early in the recovery period a state marker may continue to be abnormal simply because its normalization may follow clinical recovery. To avoid this pitfall as well as its mirror image (i.e., a state marker turning positive before the clinical onset of a major depressive episode), it is important that regimens include a sufficiently long period of sustained affective recovery as well as an equally long follow-up period after retesting for all cases. In adult depressive patients there is experimental evidence that both clinical situations do in fact occur.* It is on this basis that state markers have been proposed in the past as prognostic indicators. Such *prognostic tests* may be also found in affective disorders in children.

True trait markers that are evident before the first depressive episode would signify the first preclinical manifestation of the probably genetic predisposition to future depressive episodes independent of their timing. As such, these markers may be useful in the study of familial transmission of these disorders. Ultimately they could serve as a potentially more sensitive indicator of vulnerability than would the clinical episodes themselves.

Biological marker research in the affective disorders in children and youth can help to identify subgroups that may be quite different from each other on a neurobiological basis but not on a syndromic, clinical basis. By identifying the roots of at least some heterogeneity in this population, future research questions can be more focused and analytical.

*See references 7, 8, 18, 26, 28, 38, and 50.

The Effects of Age and Puberty on State and Trait Markers.

SLEEP EEG

During a depressive episode adults will display shortened REM latency, increased REM density, decreased delta sleep, and decreased sleep efficiency. In spite of frequent and persistent sleep complaints reported both by themselves and by their parents, prepubertal children with major depressive disorders do not show the expected polysomnographic abnormalities presented by their adult counterparts.[55,80] Although surprising, these findings are consistent with the influence of age on sleep EEG variables both in normal adults[25] and in adult patients with depressive illness.[15,77] In the Coble and associates[15] study it was shown that, if one controls for severity, the older the patient, the more abnormal the sleep EEG is likely to be. In view of these data, it was proposed that sleep EEG correlates of adult depressive illness arise out of an interaction between depression and age and, therefore, notwithstanding their diagnostic value, may reflect processes less intrinsic to depressive illness than those reflected by age independent markers.[55]

To date, there have been no studies of EEG sleep in depressed adolescents adequate enough to delineate the influence of age in depressive illness in this group. A recent report of a small ($N = 13$) controlled study from Lahmeyer, Poznanski, and Bellur[42] indicated the presence of shortened REM latency and sleep-continuity problems in adolescent endogenous depression. However, these patients were all at least seventeen years old; therefore, the study represented only the late-adolescent/young-adult age group. My associates and I are conducting an ongoing study of children with a mean age of fourteen years, maximal age of seventeen years eleven months. The sample includes forty-nine major depressive adolescents and forty-five normal controls. The midpoint analysis so far has shown that, as a group, adolescent major depressive patients do not show shortened REM latency. They do, however, show sleep-continuity disturbance. Within the adolescent sample, both REM latency and sleep efficiency, as well as delta sleep and REM density, are highly correlated with age in the expected direction. Therefore, it appears that it is not until well into late adolescence that these variables become significantly different from age-matched normal controls. Thus it is unlikely that the standard measures of sleep EEG as currently obtained by manual scoring will become a diagnostic test for children and adolescents suffering from a major depressive episode.

In surprising contrast to the lack of positive findings during the depressive episode, prepubertal children show significantly shortened REM latency after sustained affective recovery, while in a drug-free state.[56] They also show evidence of slight but significant improvement in sleep-continuity measures. This is likely to be related to the marked improvement in sleep complaints from episode to recovery. If so, it would indicate that children's subjective perception of how well they slept is highly sensitive to relatively minor changes in sleep continuity that would go largely unnoticed in an adult patient. Carskadaon and Dement's data [11,12,13] on the massive behavioral effects of sleep deprivation in normal children are in agreement with this hypothesis.

It is too early to come to any conclusions regarding the presence or absence of shortened REM latency in recovered adult major depressive patients. Although there is some evidence to the contrary, most published studies did not find REM latency shortening to persist into the recovered state. Nevertheless, the available studies are small in sample size and suffer from methodological problems. However, at least one ongoing study is likely to provide definitive answers. What already is known is that a tendency toward REM advancement, at least for the second REM period, remains during the recovered state in adult depressive patients and that it can be made apparent by the injection of arecholine, a cholinergic agonist.[74] This advancement is not elicited in never-depressed adult controls. Whether or not this phenomenon is equivalent or related to shortening of REM latency is, at present, an open question.

The REM latency findings in prepubertal children who recovered from major depression suggest that shortened REM latency may be a marker of trait or past episode for prepubertal major depression. Data regarding fully recovered adolescent major depressive patients are not yet available. The recent findings of Coble and Kupfer* comparing sixteen normal prepubertal children with a positive family history for affective illness to sixteen children without such a family history would suggest that this may be more a marker of past episode than of trait. This is likely if the calculated risk in the first group, estimated from the affective density of their pedigrees, were shown to be very high. No differences were found in REM latency or measures of sleep continuity. But children with positive family history showed significantly higher REM densities than those without. Further research in the area of sleep EEG trait markers for very-early-onset depressive illness is warranted and will constitute a focus of future work by Coble and Kupfer. To achieve greater validity, such studies should probably also include offspring of dual affective disorder parental matings, who appear to be at the highest risk for these disorders, in order to maximize the proportion of at-risk children who in fact will develop the disorder at a later date.

The differences in sleep continuity between episode and recovery, although significant, are too small in magnitude to have diagnostic value. More important, they do not reach significance compared to the psychiatric control group. Depending on the data in other age groups and on the final demonstration of this marker's nature (trait versus past episode), shortened REM latency in the recovered state may ultimately be found to have value as a research tool. It will help in sorting out the truly predisposed but still-unaffected children among a high-risk group (i.e., positive family history) or in the retrospective diagnosis of major depressive episodes in prepubertal children. In addition, normalization of REM latency could predict the next major depressive episode. Before an informed judgment can be made regarding the diagnostic and prognostic potential of this and the other markers discussed in this chapter, these findings must be replicated in large enough samples.

Neuroendocrine Markers

GROWTH HORMONE

During a major depressive episode, prepubertal children secrete more growth hormone (GH) during their regular nightly sleep than do both psychiatric and normal controls.[58] No differences were found in delta sleep.[58] In response to insulin-induced hypoglycemia,[57] endogenously depressed prepubertal children have also been shown to hyposecrete GH. This is true as well of their postmenopausal adult counterparts.[29,30] Interestingly, both abnormalities persist in the sustained affectively recovered state, retested under drug-free conditions.[59,60] These findings again raise the possibility of the existence of trait markers in prepubertal major depression, subject to the same considerations and caveats indicated regarding REM latency.

Work carried out by Jarrett and Kupfer* indicates that after controlling for delta sleep, adult endogenous depressive patients hyposecrete GH during sleep. Similar trends are found in this author's ongoing adolescent major depression study, in the absence of significant differences in delta sleep. If these findings are confirmed at the end of the study, it would suggest a strong pubertal effect that reverses the influence of major depression on the amount of GH secreted during sleep. There is also an age effect in the sense that after adolescence, there is a steady decrease of both delta sleep and sleep-related GH secretion. But contrary to

*P. Coble and D. J. Kupfer, personal communications, 1985.

*D. B. Jarrett and D. J. Kupfer, personal communication, 1985.

what was found in sleep EEG variables, these age and pubertal effects reverse the direction of the differences. Data on sleep GH secretion in recovered adolescent and adult depressives is not available as yet.

In contrast, the effects of estrogens on GH response to the insulin tolerance test (ITT) have been known from the time of the first studies on this test in adult depressive patients.[48] In the original study the sample was restricted to postmenopausal women.[30] In some studies[39] patients with insulin resistance are excluded from the protocol because of insufficient hypoglycemic stimulus. It is important to repeat the test the following day with a slightly higher dose of insulin. The results then reflect GH responsivity of non-insulin-resistant patients. This may explain the negative findings of Koslow and associates[39] in adult depressive patients. In this author's ongoing study of adolescent depression, a significant degree of hyposecretion of GH has been found in the second hour among the endogenous group when compared to the nonendogenous depressive patients. But, as expected, the findings in the first hour are negative, as are those of premenopausal women. In the ITT there seems to be no major age effects per se. But there is a strong pubertal effect, probably mediated by the estrogen potentiation of GH responsivity to all stimuli. Thus only during prepuberty and after menopause does the GH response to the ITT seem to reflect the neuroregulatory mechanisms involved in depressive illness. In adolescence and early adulthood the manifestation of these effects is probably blurred by estrogen overstimulation.

There is evidence that the GH response to the ITT normalizes in recovered adult depressive patients.[35] Data from recovered adolescents is not yet available. It would be important to know if age of onset of affective illness influences the findings in adult depressive patients. Regarding the diagnostic potential of these markers, it should be stated both that GH responses are difficult to obtain and that the ITT carries too high an element of risk for routine use even if discrimination were excellent. Other studies that also activate the noradrenergic system and have been found to discriminate adult major depressed patients[14,46,73] are likely to be fruitful. Particularly important would be investigations of other diurnal, short-term GH responses like those to clonidine hydrochloride, which is used routinely in pediatric endocrinology.[23,32,69] In addition, all this work needs to be replicated, probably in larger samples.

CORTISOL SECRETION

When the circadian cortisol patterns of prepubertal children in a major depressive episode are compared to their own values after recovery,* cortisol hypersecretion is found only occasionally (in approximately 10

percent of the sample). Furthermore, no differences were found when cortisol secretion in children with major depression was compared to that of both nondepressed psychiatric and normal control children. Therefore, during and after a major depressive episode the majority of these children have normal cortisol secretion. There is no change in cortisol latency either.[34] Although at variance with the well-known findings among adult endogenous depressive patients,[67] the findings in children are quite consistent with the influence of age on cortisol hypersecretion in adult endogenous major depressive patients.[1] In the latter, the older the patient the more likely he or she is to hypersecrete cortisol. As in the case of sleep EEG variables, in terms of the pathophysiological mechanisms resulting in cortisol hypersecretion in older depressed patients, it appears that age may be at least as important as major depression.

The published data on the DST in depressed children is contradictory. In a small outpatient controlled study of Research Diagnostic Criteria (RDC) endogenous prepubertal depressive patients, the DST showed a sensitivity of 63 percent and a specificity versus nondepressed psychiatric disorders of 90 percent.[52] In an uncontrolled study of ten outpatient children with the same diagnosis, only one escaped suppression.[22] Dosage was fixed (0.5 mg) in the first study and weight-corrected in the second, but in fact dosage differences were minor and unlikely to explain the discrepant results. In a third study, a nonsuppression rate of 70 percent was found in an inpatient sample of twenty children with major depression who received 1 mg dexamethasone.[79] Although the study was not controlled, samples were obtained not only at 4 P.M. but also at 8 A.M. Most 8 A.M. samples were suppressed, providing some indirect evidence that the dexamethasone pill was in fact ingested. Two other studies have addressed mostly specificity questions. Targum, Chastek, and Sullivan[76] found a 1 mg suppression rate of 89 percent among prepubertal inpatient conduct-disorder children, while Livingston, Reis, and Ringdahl[45] found that three of five children with separation anxiety and three of five children with major depression escaped suppression with a dose of 0.5 mg. In a recent study, now in the process of analysis, this author has found a very low rate of nonsuppression among all four groups of prepubertal children: endogenous and nonendogenous depressive patients, nondepressed psychiatric controls, and normal children. The study involved postdexamethasone hourly sampling for a full twenty-four hours through an indwelling catheter. In adolescents the pattern of DST results appears to be quite similar to adults: Among inpatients there is a 30 to 70 percent escape rate,*[,65] while the rate is much lower among outpatients.

*J. Puig-Antich et al., unpublished data.

*M. Strober, personal communication, 1984.

It is too early to come to conclusions regarding the DST in prepubertal and adolescent affective illness. For children as well as for adults many questions are still unanswered regarding mechanisms of cortisol hypersecretion in depression, the role of weight loss,* and specificity.

Conclusion

Psychobiological marker research on very-early-onset affective disorders presents an opportunity to determine separately the full range of effects of age and sexual maturity. I have suggested that age-dependent markers are likely to be associated only peripherally with the neuroregulatory mechanisms intrinsic to affective illness. If depressive illness exists before puberty and cortisol hypersecretion is absent in prepubertal depression, it should follow that the strength of the association between the neuroregulatory mechanisms of depression and cortisol secretion cannot be very firm. On the other hand, markers that continue to be associated with depression through the age spectrum

*See reference 4, 5, 19, 56, and 62.

are thought more likely to be intimately associated with the intrinsic mechanisms of depressive illness and should be the focus of further research. It should be added that there is strong evidence from animal data that maturational changes in the central nervous system are likely to include differential onsets and rates of development for the different neurotransmitter systems.* Thus the strong age and pubertal effects on some biological markers, the rarity of mania,[54] and the lack of euphoric response to dextroamphetamine among prepubertal children[64] may not be as surprising as originally thought. In addition, normative data from experiments on neuroendocrine regulation in adult volunteers cannot be extrapolated to the younger age groups. Findings during the recovered state may reflect neural mechanisms associated with a predisposition to future episodes and could conceivably help to individualize the risk for affective illness in the still-unaffected offspring of pedigrees heavily loaded for affective illness.

Regardless of the interesting potential of some of these findings, clinicians should remain circumspect regarding these tests' current applicability for diagnostic and prognostic purposes and simply inform the patients and parents of their many limitations, when clinically appropriate.

*See references 2, 17, 27, 33, 43, 44, 63, 72, and 81.

REFERENCES

1. ASNIS G. M., et al. "Cortisol Secretion in Relation to Age in Major Depression," *Psychosomatic Medicine,* 43 (1981):235–242.

2. BAKER P. C., and GOODRICH, C. A. "The Effects of the Specific Uptake Inhibitor Citalopram upon Brain Indoleamine Stores in the Maturing Mouse," *General Pharmacology,* 13 (1982):59–61.

3. BECKMAN, H., and GOODWIN, F. K. "Antidepressant Response to Tricyclics and Urinary MHPG in Unipolar Patients: Clinical Response to Imipramine or Amitriptyline," *Archives of General Psychiatry,* 32 (1975):17–21.

4. BERGER, M., KRIEG, C., and PIRKE, K. M. "Is the Positive Dexamethasone Suppression Test in Depressed Patients a Consequence of Weight Loss?" *Neuroendocrinology Letters,* 4 (1982):177.

5. BERGER, M., et al. "Neuroendocrinological and Neurophysiological Studies in Major Depressive Disorders: Are There Biological Markers for the Endogenous Subtype?" *Biological Psychiatry,* 17 (1982):1217–1242.

6. BERGER, M., et al. "Influence of Weight Loss on the Dexamethasone Suppression Test (letter)," *Archives of General Psychiatry,* 40 (1983):187.

7. BOND, P. A., JENNER, F. A., and SAMPSON, G. A. "Daily Variations of the Urine Content of 3-methoxy-4-hydroxyphenylglycol in Two Manic-depressive Patients," *Psychological Medicine,* 2 (1972):81–85.

8. BOND, P. A., et al. "Urinary Excretion of the Sulfate and Glucuronide of 3-methoxy-4-hydroxyphenyl-ethyleneglycol in a Manic-depressive Patient," *Psychological Medicine,* 5 (1975):279–285.

9. CARROLL, B. J., CURTIS, G. C., and MENDELS, J. "Neuroendocrine Regulation in Depression. I: Limbic System Adrenocortisol Dysfunctions," *Archives of General Psychiatry,* 33 (1976):1039–1044.

10. ———. "Neuroendocrine Regulation in Depression. II: Discrimination of Depressed from Nondepressed Patients," *Archives of General Psychiatry,* 33 (1976):1051–1058.

11. CARSKADAN, M. A., HARVEY, K., and DEMENT, W. C. "Acute Restriction of Nocturnal Sleep in Children," *Perceptual and Motor Skills,* 53 (1981):103–112.

12. ———. "Sleep Loss in Young Adolescents," *Sleep,* 4 (1981):299–312.

13. CARSKADAN, M. A., et al. "Pubertal Changes in Daytime Sleepiness," *Sleep,* 2 (1980):5–460.

14. CHECKLEY, S. A., SLADE, A. P., and SHUR, E. "Growth Hormone and Other Responses to Clonidine in Patients with Endogenous Depression," *British Journal of Psychiatry,* 138 (1981):51–55.

15. COBLE, P. A., et al. "EEG Sleep and Clinical Characteristics in Young Primary Depressives," *Sleep Research,* 9 (1980):165.

16. COBLE, P. A., et al. "Automated Delta Wave Analysis

in NREM Sleep: Preliminary Findings in Normal Health Children," *Sleep Research,* 11 (1982): 80.

17. DASZUTA, A., et al. "Endogenous Levels of Trypotophane, Serotonin, and 5-HIAA in the Developing Brain of the Cat," *Neuroscience Letters,* (1979):187–192.

18. DELEON-JONES, F. D., et al. "Urinary Catecholamine Metabolites During Behavioral Changes in a Patient with Manic-depressive Cycles," *Science,* 179 (1973):300–302.

19. EDELSTEIN, C. K., et al. "Effects of Weight Loss on the Dexamethasone Suppression Test," *American Journal of Psychiatry,* 140 (1983):338–341.

20. GALEN, R., and GAMBINO, F. R. *Beyond Normality: The Predictive Value and Efficiency of Medical Diagnosis.* New York: John Wiley & Sons, 1975.

21. GARCIA-SEVILLA, J. A., et al. "Platelet-adrenergic Receptors in Major Depressive Disorder," *Archives of General Psychiatry,* 38 (1981):1327–1333.

22. GELLER, B. et al. "Nortriptyline in Major Depressive Disorder in Children: Response, Steady State Plasma Levels, Predictive Kinetics and Pharmacokinetics," *Psychopharmacology Bulletin,* 19 (1983):62–65.

23. GIL-AD, I., TOPPER, E., and LARON, Z. "Oral Clonadine as a Growth Hormone Stimulation Test," *Lancet,* 1 (1979): 278–280.

24. GILLIN, J. C., et al. "Successful Separation of Depressed, Normal and Insomniac Subjects by EEG Sleep Data," *Archives of General Psychiatry,* 36 (1979):85–90.

25. GILLIN, J. C., et al. "Age Related Changes in Sleep in Depressed and Normal Subjects," *Psychiatry Research,* 4 (1981):73–78.

26. GOLDBERG, I. K. "Dexamethasone Suppression Tests in Depression and Response to Treatment," *Lancet,* 1 (1980):92.

27. GOLDMAN-RABIK, P. S., and BROWN, R. M. "Postnatal Development of Monoamine Content and Synthesis in the Cerebral Cortex of the Rhesus Monkeys," *Brain Research,* 256 (1982):339–349.

28. GREDEN, J. F., et al. "Normalization of Dexamethasone Suppression Tests: A Probable Index of Recovery Among Endogenous Depressives," *Biological Psychiatry,* 15 (1980):449–458.

29. GREGOIRE, F., et al. "Hormone Release in Depressed Patients Before and After Recovery," *Psychoneuroendocrinology,* 2 (1977):303–312.

30. GRUEN, P. H., et al. "Growth Hormone Responses to Hypoglycemia in Postmenopausal Depressed Women," *Archives of General Psychiatry,* 32 (1975):31–33.

31. GUTHEIL, T. G., BURSZTAJN, H., and BRODSKY A. "Malpractice Prevention Through the Sharing of Uncertainty: Informed Consent and the Therapeutic Alliance," *New England Journal of Medicine,* 311 (1984):49–50.

32. HEALTH SERVICES HUMAN GROWTH HORMONE COMMITTEE. "Comparison of the Intravenous and Oral Clonidine Tolerance Tests for Growth Hormone Secretion," *Archives of Diseases in Childhood,* 56 (1981):852.

33. HEDNAR, T., and LUNDBERG, P. "Neurochemical Characteristics of Cerebral Catecholamine Neurons During Post-natal Development in the Rat," *Medical Biology,* 59 (1981):212–223.

34. JARRETT, D. B., COBLE, P. A., and KUPFER, D. J. "Reduced Cortisol Latency in Depressive Illness," *Archives of General Psychiatry,* 40 (1983):506–511.

35. KATHOL, R. G., et al. "Provocative Endocrine Testing in Recovered Depressives," *Psychoneuroendocrinology,* 9 (1984):57–68.

36. KIDD, K. K. "Genetic Linkage Markers in the Study of Psychiatric Disorders," in E. Usdin and I. Hanin, eds., *Biological Markers in Psychiatry and Neurology.* New York: Pergamon Press, 1981, pp. 459–466.

37. KIRKEGAARD, C., et al. "Protirelin Stimulation Test and Thyroid Function During Treatment of Depression," *Archives of General Psychiatry,* 33 (1976):1393–1396.

38. KIRKEGAARD, C., et al. "Studies on the Influence of Biogenic Amines and Psychoactive Drugs on the Prognostic Value of the TRH Stimulation Test in Endogenous Depression," *Psychoneuroendocrinology,* 2 (1977):131–136.

39. KOSLOW, S. H., et al. "Insulin Tolerance Test: Human Growth Hormone Response and Insulin Resistance in Primary Unipolar Depressed Bipolar Depressed and Control Subjects," *Psychological Medicine,* 12 (1982):45–55.

40. KUPFER, D. "REM Latency: A Psychobiological Marker for Primary Depressive Disease," *Biological Psychiatry,* 11 (1976):159–174.

41. KUPFER, D., and FOSTER, F. G. "EEG Sleep and Depression," in R. L. Williams and I. Karacan, eds., *Sleep Disorders: Diagnosis and Treatment.* New York: John Wiley & Sons, 1979, pp. 163–203.

42. LAHMEYER, H. W., POZNANSKI, E. O., and BELLUR, S. N. "EEG Sleep in Depressed Adolescents," *American Journal of Psychiatry,* 140 (1983):1150–1153.

43. LENGVARI, I., BRAUCH, B. J., and TAYLOR, A. N. "Effects of Prenatal Thyroxine and/or Corticosterone Treatment of the Ontogenesis of Hypothalamic and Mesencephalic Norepinephrine and Dopamine Content," *Developmental Neuroscience,* 3 (1980):59–65.

44. LIDOV, H. G., and MOLLIVER, M. E. "An Immunohistochemical Study of Serotonin Neuron Development in the Rat: Ascending Pathways and Terminal Fields," *Brain Research Bulletin,* 8 (1982):389–430.

45. LIVINGSTON, R., REIS, C. J., and RINGDAHL, I. C. "Abnormal Dexamethasone Suppression Test Results in Depressed and Nondepressed Children," *American Journal of Psychiatry,* 141 (1984):106–107.

46. MATUSSEK, N., et al. "Effect of Clonidine on Growth Hormone Release in Psychiatric Patients and Controls," *Psychiatry Research,* 2 (1980):25–36.

47. MELTZER, H. Y., et al. "Serotonin Uptake in Blood Platelets of Psychiatric Patients," *Archives of General Psychiatry,* 38 (1981):1322–1326.

48. MERIMEE, T. J., and FINEBERG, S. E. "Studies of Sex Based Variation of Human Growth Hormone Secretion," *Journal of Clinical Endocrinology and Metabolism,* 33 (1971):896–902.

49. NADI, N. S., NURNBERGER, J. I., and GERSHON, E. S. "Muscarinic Cholinergic Receptors on Skin Fibroblasts in Familial Affective Disorder," *New England Journal of Medicine,* 311 (1984):225–230.

50. PAPAKOSTAS, Y., et al. "Neuroendocrine Measures in Psychiatric Patients: Course and Outcome with ECT," *Psychiatry Research,* 4 (1981):55–64.

51. PAUL, S. M., et al. "Depressed Patients Have Decreased Binding of Tritiated Imipramine to Platelet Serotonin Transporter," *Archives of General Psychiatry,* 38 (1981): 1315–1317.

52. POZNANSKI, E. O., et al. "The Dexamethasone Suppression Test in Prepubertal Depressed Children," *American Journal of Psychiatry,* 139 (1982):321–324.

53. PRANGE, A. J. "Patterns of Pituitary Responses to THR in Depressed Patients," in W. Fann et al., eds., *Phenomenology and Treatment of Depression,* New York: Spectrum Publications, 1977, pp. 1–16.

54. PUIG-ANTICH, J. "Affective Disorders in Childhood: A Review and Perspective," in B. Blinder, ed.,: *Psychiatric Clin-*

ics of North America, Vol. 3. Philadelphia: W. B. Saunders, 1980, pp. 403–424.

55. PUIG-ANTICH, J., et al. "Sleep Architecture and REM Sleep Measures in Prepubertal Major Depressives During an Episode," *Archives of General Psychiatry,* 39 (1982):932–939.

56. PUIG-ANTICH, J., et al. "Sleep Architecture and REM Sleep Measures in Prepubertal Major Depressives: Studies During Recovery from a Major Depressive Episode in a Drug-Free State," *Archives of General Psychiatry,* 40 (1983): 187–192.

57. PUIG-ANTICH, J., et al. "Growth Hormone Secretion in Prepubertal Major Depressive Children: I. Sleep-related Plasma Concentrations During a Depressive Episode," *Archives of General Psychiatry,* 41 (1984):455–460.

58. PUIG-ANTICH, J., et al. "Growth Hormone Secretion in Prepubertal Major Depressive Children: II. Sleep-related Plasma Concentrations During a Depressive Episode," *Archives of General Psychiatry,* 41 (1984):463–466.

59. PUIG-ANTICH, J., et al. "Growth Hormone Secretion in Prepubertal Major Depressive Children. III. Response to Insulin-induced Hypoglycemia in a Drug-free, Fully Recovered Clinical State," *Archives of General Psychiatry,* 41 (1984):471–475.

60. PUIG-ANTICH, J., et al. "Growth Hormone Secretion in Prepubertal Major Depressive Children: IV. Sleep-related Plasma Concentrations in a Drug-free Fully Recovered Clinical State," *Archives of General Psychiatry,* 41 (1984):479–483.

61. QUITKIN, F. M., et al. "Sleep of Atypical Depressives," *Journal of Affective Disorders,* 8 (1985):61–67.

62. RABKIN, J., STEWART, J., and KLEIN, D. "Overview on the Relevance of the Dexamethesone Suppression Test to Differential Diagnosis," in R. Hirshfeld, ed., *Proceedings, Workshop on the Clinical Utility of the Dexamethasone Suppression Test,* DHHS Publication no. (ADM) 85-1318, Washington, D.C.: Government Printing Office, 1985, pp. 12–33.

63. RAMSAY, P. E., KRIGMAN, M. R., and MORELL, P. "Development Studies of the Uptake of Choline, GABA and Dopamine by Crude Synaptosomal Preparations After *in vivo* or *in vitro* Lead Treatment," *Brain Research,* 187 (1980):- 383–402.

64. RAPOPORT, J. L., et al. "Dextro-Amphetamine: Its Cognitive and Behavioral Effects in Normal and Hyperactive Boys and Normal Men," *Archives of General Psychiatry,* 37 (1980):933–943.

65. ROBBINS, D. R., et al. "Preliminary Report on the Dexamethasone Suppression Test in Adolescents," *American Journal of Psychiatry,* 139 (1982):942–943.

66. SABELLI, H. C., et al. "Urinary Phenyl Acetate: A Diagnostic Test for Depression?" *Science,* 220 (1983):1187–1188.

67. SACHAR, E. H., et al. "Disrupted 24-hour Patterns of Cortisol Secretion in Psychotic Depression," *Archives of General Psychiatry,* 28 (1973):19–24.

68. SACHAR, E. J., et al. "Three Tests of Cortisol Secretion in Adult Endogenous Depressives," *Acta Psychiatrica Scandinavica,* 71 (1985):1–8.

69. SALTI, R., et al. "Oral Clonidine: An Effective Provocative Test of Growth Hormone Release," *Helvetica Paediatrica Acta,* 36 (1981):527–531.

70. SCHILDKRAUT, J. J., et al. "Toward a Biochemical Classification of Depressive Disorders. I. Differences in Urinary MHPG and Other Catecholamine Metabolites in Clinically Defined Subtypes of Depressions," *Archives of General Psychiatry,* 35 (1978):1427–1433.

71. SCHILDKRAUT, J. J., et al. Toward a Biochemical Classification of Depressive Disorders. II. Application of Multivariate Discriminant Function Analysis to Data on Urinary Catecholamines and Metabolites," *Archives of General Psychiatry,* 35 (1978):1436–1439.

72. SHELTON, D. L., NADLER, J. V., and COTMAN, C. W. "Development of High Affinity Choline Uptake and Associated Acetylcholine Synthesis in the Rat Fuscia Dentata," *Brain Research,* 164 (1979):263–275.

73. SIEVER, L. J., et al. "The Growth Hormone Response to Clonidine as a Probe of Noradrenergic Receptor Responsiveness in Affective Disorder Patients and Controls," *Psychiatry Research,* 6 (1982):171–183.

74. SITAREM, M., et al. "Faster Cholinergic REM Sleep Induction in Euthymic Patients with Primary Affective Illness," *Science,* 208 (1980):200–201.

75. TAKASHI, S., et al. "Thyrotropin Response to TRH in Depressive Illness," *Folia Psychiatrica Neurologica Japonica,* 28 (1974):355–365.

76. TARGUM, S., CHASTEK, C., and SULLIVAN, A. "Dexamethasone Suppression Test in Prepubertal Conduct Disorder," *Psychiatry Research,* 5 (1981):107–108.

77. ULRICH, R., SHAW, D. H., and KUPFER, D. J. "The Effects of Aging on Sleep," *Sleep,* 3 (1980):31–40.

78. VOGEL, G. W., et al. "Improvement of Depression by REM Sleep Deprivation: New Findings and a Theory," *Archives of General Psychiatry,* 37 (1980):247–253.

79. WELLER, E. B., et al. "The Dexamethasone Suppression Test in Hospitalized Prepubertal Depressed Children," *American Journal of Psychiatry,* 141 (1984):290–291.

80. YOUNG, W., et al. "The Sleep of Childhood Depressives: Comparison with Age-matched Controls," *Biological Psychiatry,* 17 (1982):1163–1168.

81. YUWILER, A., and BRAMMER, G. L. "Neonatal Hormone Treatment and Maturation of the Pineal Noradrenergic System: Hydrocortisone and Thyroxine," *Journal of Neurochemistry,* 37 (1981):985–992.

21 / Assessment Procedures for Diagnosis of Sleep Disorders in Children

Richard Ferber

Introduction

With the establishment of sleep disorders centers, systematic approaches emerged for the evaluation of adult sleep disorders. These strategies were greatly aided by the development of a nosological classification of sleep disorders.[6] It is now clear that similar approaches can and should be applied systematically to the assessment of sleep complaints in the child.*

In the evaluation of the child, however, additional factors require consideration. The nature of a child's complaint and the cause(s) of the disturbance may have no exact adult counterpart. Thus one may encounter a child's unwillingness and "inability" to sleep anywhere but with the parents. Or the problem may be secondary to heightened issues of control during toilet training. In addition, at different ages and developmental levels, the same complaint—for example, sleep terrors, nighttime fears, or headbanging—may have different etiologies and significance. At times, the complaint of a sleep disturbance in a child really expresses the caretakers' distress and not that of the patient. Thus children may yearn to and try to stay awake, when the parents want them to sleep. And finally, children's sleep patterns reflect parent-child interactions since the parents are, or should be, intimately involved in their child's sleep routines, bedtime rituals, and schedule decisions.[14,17,29]

The sleep laboratory plays a much smaller role in the evaluation of the child than it does in assessing the adult. Excessive daytime sleepiness remains a symptom for which laboratory evaluation of sleep is very important; it is, however, an uncommon complaint in childhood. Also, causes of insomnia in adults that require polysomnographic recordings for diagnosis, such as periodic movements of sleep (nocturnal myoclonus)[12] or central sleep apnea, seldom occur in otherwise healthy youngsters.

There are a number of common sleep problems encountered in childhood. These include: sleeplessness, principally in the form of bedtime struggles and nighttime wakings in infants and toddlers; sleepwalking and sleep terrors; enuresis; schedule disorders (most often a sleep phase delay leading to bedtime difficulties in toddlers or sleep-onset "insomnia" and difficulty waking for school in adolescents); and snoring suggestive of obstructive sleep apnea.* For most of these complaints, careful and proper history and developmental and psychological evaluation are usually sufficient to permit accurate diagnosis. The evaluation of the enuretic child, however, requires more careful physical examination and laboratory screening. This is even more true for children with suspected sleep apnea or known excessive daytime sleepiness.

There are too many specific sleep-related complaints and associated diagnoses to discuss each individually in a brief overview. However, in the initial assessment of all sleep disorders, certain areas should be considered. These are: (1) a detailed sleep history, (2) a general medical history, (3) a complete social history, (4) an assessment of the child's psychological/developmental status, and (5) a physical examination. Beyond these, on the basis of the initial findings, a full psychiatric assessment, formal psychological testing, and various laboratory studies may be indicated. The emphasis that should be placed on each of these will vary depending on the type of complaint and the way it presents. Each of these areas are considered in detail in the following sections.

Sleep History

Sleep can be affected by many different factors. Some may be primary, that is, be the initial cause of a sleep disturbance—whereas others may be secondary to al-

*See references 1, 14, 16, 17, 24, 35, 36, and 49.

*See references 1, 4, 8, 10, 13, 16, 17, 19, 21, 24, 26, 32, 33, and 34.

ready existing sleep disturbances. Thus one problem may cause a child to sleep poorly, but the child's sleeplessness may then bring about increased family tensions which, in turn, may give rise to increased nighttime fears and refusal to sleep alone. The initial interview must therefore be far-reaching, with sufficient time allotted to cover all areas. This part of the interview has many components.

PRESENTING COMPLAINT

It is important to start by listening to a description of the problem as it is perceived by the family. If the children are old enough, first let them describe the "problem" as they see it or hear about it: "I won't go to sleep," "I get afraid of monsters at night," "My mother says I do funny things when I am asleep." Children may perceive the problem differently from their parents—for example, a ten-year-old may feel her sleep is fine, it is only her parents who feel she should fall asleep earlier and sleep longer. Children having sleep terrors may know of no one else with the same symptom, and accordingly feel unique and strange. Enuretic children may be teased and embarrassed. They may grossly underestimate the frequency of wetting, or they may be frankly concerned, discuss the problem forthrightly, and ask for help. Latency-age children may claim to lie awake for a whole hour before falling asleep, yet deny tossing and turning. They may admit that the time in bed is not unpleasant (it may be very pleasant, a chance to process daytime events, listen to the radio, or masturbate). The manner in which children describe their nighttime fears may help in estimating their true significance. Furthermore, impressions may be gleaned of the children's willingness to communicate with and relate to the examiner and observations made of their ongoing interactions with the parents during the interview. These will help give a picture of the children's self-confidence, separation difficulties, impulsivity, and degree of enmeshment, as well as of the parents ability to set limits.

Ultimately, most information usually comes from the parents. On listening to them describe the problem, their feelings of anger, frustration, helplessness, and/or empathy, as well as the need they may experience to maintain strict controls, often become quite evident. Sometimes parents are unable to describe a coherent complaint. This may become even more apparent as efforts are made to clarify specific details. Their global comments may imply a severe disorder ("he never sleeps") whereas, on closer questioning, only a minor disturbance may seem present (occasional wakings or minor bedtime struggles but consolidated sleep). This should alert the clinician that the problems may be interactional rather than somnologic. Some families in need of psychological supports may find it easier to ask

for help indirectly by complaining of a sleep disturbance. On the other hand, significant sleep problems may exist and be quite real without any significant dysfunction in family dynamics except for those that are secondary to the disturbance with parents becoming overtired and stressed.

One should ask about the onset, duration, character, frequency, and consistency of the sleep symptom. Circumstances surrounding the onset of symptoms may be particularly important. For instance, sleeplessness may begin after the birth of a sibling, the death of a grandparent and attendance at a wake, a move to a new neighborhood or from crib to bed, or the start of toilet training. Sleep terrors may begin in association with an extended separation and in connection with other events over which children have little control, such as the parents' divorce or a child's hospitalization and surgery. It is important to inquire concerning what remedies have been tried (medication, "letting the child cry," spankings, star charts, "bell and pad") in an effort to improve matters. Also, the parents should describe the responses to these interventions.

The parents should be asked if they can predict problematic nights. For example, do sleepwalking or sleep terror episodes occur more frequently when their child is overtired? Does difficulty falling asleep follow when there has been family conflict or evening excitement? The frequency and intensity of sleepwalking and sleep terrors are particularly important to assess. Do they occur nightly or monthly; is there associated personal injury or property damage; are attempts made to leave the house? Such data are essential, not so much to help make a diagnosis but to help decide on the urgency of therapy. The frequency of wetting is, of course, the most pertinent datum in evaluating nocturnal enuresis. One should also try to distinguish primary enuresis (where there has never been a prolonged period of nighttime continence) from secondary enuresis (in which there is a history of a completely dry period of at least several months, followed by a return of wetting). And, of course it must be determined whether or not the incontinence is confined to sleep.

SLEEP ASSOCIATIONS, CURRENT SLEEP-WAKE SCHEDULE, AND SLEEP RHYTHM

Sleep associations are those conditions that precede and are present during children's transition to sleep at bedtimes, naptimes, and after nighttime wakings. Learning about these is usually the most important part of the interview when assessing the complaint of nighttime wakings in infants or toddlers.* It is not sufficient to hear from parents that "our child wakes four times every night." The clinician must determine

*See references 14, 16, 17, 22, 23, 25, 36, and 49.

the precise nature of their pattern of interaction with the child at these times. Do they hand the children a bottle or pick the children up and rock them? Do they take them into their bed? Do they get up and play with them? Children who are always rocked to sleep at bed and naptimes may be unable to fall back to sleep without being rocked after normal wakings during the night.[14,22] When the parents "treat" the wakings with rocking, the disturbance may only be perpetuated.

The *sleep-wake schedule* is the specific timing of bed and naptimes, the actual hours of sleeping and waking, and the pattern of meals and other daytime activities. The *sleep rhythm* represents the current pattern of circadian functioning—that is, the time children are ready and able to fall asleep, the time they would wake naturally, the time during the day when they are unlikely to be able to fall asleep (during their "second wind" after dinner), and the amount of sleep they require. Sleep cannot be viewed simply as an independently functioning biological process. It must be evaluated as a state carefully integrated with circadian and psychological functioning, behavior, and social and environmental requirements throughout the day. The clinician must know not only that children fall asleep early or late but also what time they awaken in the morning (both on weekdays and on weekends) and what time they nap during the day. It is especially important to have a clear understanding of children's schedules and underlying circadian rhythms when evaluating youngsters with bedtime difficulties but no nighttime wakings, children with the morning problems of either early or difficult waking, or toddlers and preschoolers with sleepwalking or sleep terrors.

Sleep associations and circadian factors are discussed together because the easiest and most efficient way to learn about both of them is to take a twenty-four-hour history of the child's day. One might start by inquiring about the timing and regularity of dinner, which family members are present, and what activities take place afterward. Next are the prebedtime activities (bath, pajamas) and bedtime rituals (story, bottle, song). It should be learned when the child goes to bed, if bedtime is consistent, and how this time is set. Do the parents decide when they feel their child "should" go to bed, is it after a certain television show, or do they wait "until he gets tired"? Are both parents involved? In some households there may be no formal bedtime at all; the children simply fall asleep "whenever and wherever."

The actual "bedtime ritual" should be described in detail since this routine is so important in helping children separate and go to sleep. For instance, the assessment is aided by knowing that children are abruptly sent to bed when the father comes home for supper without any other bedtime ritual to help them deal with the separation. Most children have difficulty making such a transition smoothly. Bedtime struggles and stalling techniques should also be carefully described ("I want a drink of water," "Please, just one more story," "I have to go to the bathroom") as well as the ways these are handled by the parents.

The conditions present when children actually fall asleep must be identified through careful questioning.[14,16,17] What exactly is happening when children fall asleep? Are they in their own room and bed, are they in the parents' bed, or are they on someone's lap? Are they rocked or nursed, and do they use a pacifier? Do they have a transitional object or does someone have to be in their room, on their bed, touching them or being rubbed or stroked by them? Is the radio or television on, a bright light, a nightlight? Are the patterns of falling asleep the same each night, or do they vary? Do the children fall asleep quickly, or do they keep waking as if checking to be sure the parent has not left? Do they wake if nursing is stopped or if they are transferred from lap to crib, or if their mother or father simply tries to leave the room before sleep is sufficiently deep? If children "insist" that a parent be present, how do they do this—by crying, claiming to be afraid, screaming, throwing a tantrum, coming out of the room? If there is a complaint of "fear," is it convincing —that is, do the children really seem frightened, or does it sound more manipulative? And what fears do they describe (monsters, robbers, shadows, the dark)?

Daytime patterns should also be explored. For the morning, the timing, regularity, and spontaneity of waking should be examined. Do children always come into the parents' bed at that time? Does this happen after one parent leaves for work, and do the children go back to sleep there? A brief description of activities during the day is helpful in order to get an overall picture of the children's life. To what extent do they play alone or with peers, inside or outside, in structured or unstructured activities, and in front of the television? And, if mealtimes are too varied or inappropriately timed, they may interfere with circadian function. Thus, feedings too early in the morning may reinforce early wakings from nighttime sleep, and lunch postponed until after a nap may shorten daytime sleep in a similar fashion.

It is important to learn about the occurrence, timing, and regularity of naps as well as the circumstances under which they occur. Late-afternoon naps may interfere with bedtime. Lack of an early-afternoon nap may leave children overtired and cause increased bedtime difficulties and nighttime wakings, whereas early-morning naps may reinforce early wakings.[16,17,35] Nap routines may be similar to those at bedtime along with the associated rocking, nursing, story, and use of the crib, or they may be structured quite differently in a cot at a day-care center or in the car or living room. Some children do best if all sleep transitions are handled in the same manner. When different caretakers such as a parent, childcare worker, or sitter are involved at different times, they may manage naptimes in diverse ways with quite different results. Understanding who has the most success and why may be quite helpful in trying to understand the nature of the overall disturbance. The differences in management may range among better limit setting, more appropriate transitional routines, a more structured milieu, and a less intense relationship.

Assessment of children's sleep rhythm should follow. It is important to determine not only the time children go, are sent, or are put to bed but also what time they actually fall asleep. Moreover, one should ascertain whether the time of sleep onset is independent of bedtime and whether bedtime struggles occur only at the earlier bedtimes. For example, do the children fall asleep at 11:00 P.M. regardless of the time they go to bed, 8:00, 9:30, or 10:45, and whether or not limits are firmly set at the earlier bedtimes? One should also inquire as to what happens when the children are allowed to wake spontaneously. What time do they wake in the morning? Is there much difficulty waking them earlier? The answers to these questions help to clarify whether a delay in sleep onset is secondary to a lack of limit setting (in which case the children would fall asleep if kept in bed); whether there is some primary interference with sleep initiation so that falling asleep is affected at both early and late bedtimes; or whether the problem is due mainly to a shift in the underlying circadian sleep phase, with the children operating as if they had just arrived from a more western time zone.[16,17,21,57] If they fall asleep at 11:00, wake spontaneously at 10:00 on weekends, and are difficult to wake at 7:00 for school or day care, it suggests that they need eleven hours of sleep at night, that they are not getting enough sleep during the week, and that on their current sleep rhythm, they are not ready either to fall asleep or to wake until a late hour.

NIGHTTIME WAKINGS

It is important to elicit a description of events that occur throughout the night. This usually is the most important part of the twenty-four-hour history, at least when evaluating complaints of sleeplessness. What time do children wake during the night and what do they do: call out, cry, or come out of the room? What do the parents do: let the children cry, go right in, comfort them, take them into their bed, or threaten or punish them? What conditions have children come to associate with falling back to sleep after waking? If their parents settle them quickly, is this done by reestablishing those conditions that were present when the children fell asleep at bedtime, such as rocking, using

a bottle or pacifier, nursing, or back rubbing? If they are fed, how long are they nursed or how many ounces of fluid do they take (excess fluid at night is often associated with frequent wakings[14,20])? As an indication of the degree of such excess fluid, how often must the diaper be changed? Is the waking prolonged and, if so, does a parent play with the children, thus positively reinforcing the waking? Do the children seem frightened at the time and reach up to the parents, and clutch them tightly? Such behavior might be expected after a true nightmare or a full waking with scary fantasies. Does the pattern of intervention change throughout the night? At some point are the children allowed into the parents' bed? Do both parents deal with the child at night? Does each parent handle matters in the same way?

Another type of arousal must be distinguished from the one just discussed. This is a partial waking from stage 4 non-rapid-eye-movement (NREM) sleep[10,27] and may take many forms. Confused thrashing is seen mainly in young children,[18] sleepwalking occurs at all ages, and sleep terrors with real terrorlike behavior (as opposed simply to marked confusion, bizarre thrashing, and upset without the appearance of panic or fear) is not often seen before latency and is most common in adolescence.

The distinction between these partial stage 4 arousals and other wakings is crucial since partial wakings are not behavioral in nature, and parents' rapid and empathetic responses to them are neither reinforcing nor necessary.

A full description of the timing and characteristics of these events usually makes the diagnosis certain. Most episodes of partial stage 4 arousal occur within the first few hours of sleep. If these arousal symptoms happen more than once a night, the first (when sleep is deepest) should be the most intense. Memory of the events themselves, after full waking or in the morning, should be absent or, at best, fragmentary and without complex dream detail.[10,18,27,28]

In one form young children "wake" crying, thrashing, and confused within a few hours of sleep onset but do not respond to the parents when they come into the room.[16,17,18] Instead of reaching up to them for comfort and reassurance as the children would after a bad dream or full waking, they only arch their back and pull away. Even vigorous attempts to wake these children are unsuccessful. After one to thirty minutes there is a rapid calming and a return to sleep *unless* the parents persist in trying to wake the children at that time. If they do finally awaken, they do not seem frightened and have no memory of the preceding event. Since, at best, toddlers' ability to describe a dream is limited, parents may decide incorrectly that a child had a bad dream; or, if the confused phase is brief and the parents successfully wake the child when it is over, the parents may describe a waking but forget about the initial component.

In the more familiar patterns of sleepwalking or sleep terrors, youngsters, especially older children or adolescents, may show a range of symptoms. During a mild arousal they may get out of bed, walk about calmly as if looking for something, and possibly urinate inappropriately. If the arousal is more intense, they may move about in an agitated manner as if trying to get away from something. During a maximally intense arousal children will issue forth with a "blood-curdling scream," and they may even jump out of bed and run, knock over furniture, break glass, or try to get out of the front door or window.

If the characteristics of stage 4 arousals are well understood, seizures should not be confused with these nonictal events (even though the possibility should be considered). One should check whether or not similar events ever occurred during the waking state, and if there are other accompanying behaviors such as tonic stiffening and/or clonic jerking, which suggest seizures or are at least atypical for sleep terrors or sleepwalking (perhaps with the children waking before the event and realizing that something is about to happen, or with events happening mainly near morning).

Although enuresis is not confined to arousals from stage 4, it does usually happen during a partial waking from sleep. Unlike the more obvious states of arousal, enuretic episodes are not ordinarily witnessed by the family. The children should be asked if they are ever aware of wetting the bed—for example, in the morning when they are too cold to get out of bed to go to the bathroom. The timing of the wetting should be clarified if possible. Are the children already wet before the parents retire? If the children wake up, it is important to know whether the parents are then wakened, if sheets must be changed, and who takes on this responsibility.

SLEEP ENVIRONMENT

It is often helpful to learn about the physical setting in the children's home at night. This includes the number of bedrooms, their location, and who sleeps where. Is the parents' bedroom far from the children's, is it on the same level of the house and can the parents hear their children easily when they call out? If the parents' bedroom is nearby, can the children see directly into it and can they overhear or witness nighttime arguments or sexual activity? It may be important simply to learn that the children's door is open at bedtime and closed later during the night or that there is not enough light in their room to let them orient themselves on waking during the

night after a dream. Even discovering that the landlord or other complaining neighbor lives in the next apartment may help explain current difficulties.

DEVELOPMENT OF SLEEP PATTERNS AND PROBLEMS

If the current problem has been longlasting, its full evolution should now be traced. For example, continued nighttime wakings in three-year-olds may be a direct extension of a problem that has been present all their life.[50] The development of children's sleep patterns, the presence of other sleep abnormalities, and relevant behavioral milestones should all be reviewed.

If the children were already considered to be poor sleepers in infancy, the parents may have allowed their early impressions to become a self-fulfilling prophesy. Discover when the children first began sleeping through the night, and if and when they later began to wake. Find out when they moved out of the parents' room to their own and from a crib to a bed. Was this decision made because they were climbing out of the crib or because they were evicted by the arrival of a new sibling? Ask what the children's hours of sleep have been over the years, when they stopped napping, if they are restless in bed, and whether they seem to be "deep sleepers" or wake at the slightest noise. Check if there have been any episodes of rocking or headbanging, or any occurrences of sleepwalking, sleep terrors, confused thrashing, or bedwetting. If the children snore, ask about its frequency (every night, all night?), its intensity (can it be heard in other rooms?), and about any apparent struggling to breathe, retractions, cyanosis, and possible apneic pauses. Finally, find out about nursing (breast or bottle), weaning, finger sucking, pacifier use, and toilet training.

CURRENT SYMPTOMS OF EXCESSIVE DAYTIME SLEEPINESS

Clarification of any symptoms of excessive daytime sleepiness is most important when sleepiness is the chief complaint, but it is also important when assessing children who supposedly are not sleeping well at night and even those the parents have decided "only need very little sleep." First of all, there are the obvious symptoms of sleepiness, namely the children look sleepy and, of greatest importance, fall asleep at inappropriate times.[5] If the children do nap inappropriately, then the frequency and timing of the naps should be determined as well as the circumstances in which they occur (do they take place when the children are bored, in or after school, or during physical activity?), the suddenness and irresistibility of onset, their length and refreshing value, the ease with which children may be wakened from such sleep, and their mood on waking. Hypersomnolence, in the form of excessively long nocturnal sleep, should already be clear from other parts of the history.

It is also important to keep in mind that symptoms of sleepiness in children are not always obvious. Sleepy children do not necessarily yawn, complain of being sleepy, or even nap. Instead they may appear overactive, impulsive, distractible, and irritable with attentional difficulties and tantrums.[16,45] Daily behavior should therefore be described carefully. Although occasional behavioral deterioration caused by temporarily excessive sleepiness is usually recognized as such by parents ("He is just overtired" or "It is past her bedtime"), longstanding behavioral effects of chronic daytime sleepiness are often misinterpreted, at least until behavior improves after the sleepiness resolves.

With any complaint of daytime sleepiness, the other symptoms of narcolepsy should be explored. Young children (in whom narcolepsy is rare anyway) may be unable to report the symptoms of cataplexy, hypnagogic hallucinations, or sleep paralysis, even if they are present. Older children or teenagers may be able to verbalize such symptoms but they may have been afraid to do so. Although cataplexy ought to be observable by parents, milder forms are often difficult for others to notice. Furthermore, young children, and even some older children, will fall to the ground when laughing very hard and feeling silly. Hence it is important to learn whether children simply continue laughing and rolling about when on the ground or if they quiet immediately on falling and seem frightened or upset.

Finally, an attempt should be made to distinguish lethargy, tiredness, and sluggishness from true sleepiness. Although these symptoms may go together, they are different. Sleepiness means an increased tendency to fall asleep. Physical activity or inactivity, boredom, illness, preoccupation, and affective illness may lead to tiredness or lethargy without necessarily causing sleepiness.

FAMILY HISTORY OF SLEEP PROBLEMS

Some sleep disorders clearly are more common in children whose parents suffer or suffered from the same disorder; this is true of both narcolepsy and enuresis. In others, such as insomnia and sleep apnea, the familial tendency is less clear. In any case, it is important to ask about any familial tendencies toward excessive sleepiness, cataplexy, hypnagogic hallucination, sleep paralysis, snoring, headbanging or rocking, sleepwalking or sleep terrors, enuresis, bruxism, insomnia, and the sudden infant death syndrome.

Past History and Review of Systems

The format for the medical review segment of the history is standard and should include prenatal and birth history, neonatal course, developmental milestones, hospitalizations, operations, ongoing illnesses and medications, and general systems review. By learning that a child barely survived after a premature birth, one may better understand some of the parents' difficulties in setting limits. Knowledge of a long history of recurrent middle ear infections may raise concerns that chronic serous otitis media is responsible for nighttime wakings, or that adenoidal hypertrophy may explain the snoring and possible apnea. Or the discovery that sleepless children have nocturnal asthma attacks should make one consider that the children may be afraid of dying in their sleep, or that the insomnia may be secondary to the asthmatic medications.

Social History

The taking of the social history, a complex and often time-consuming component of the evaluation, should not be overlooked even if the sleep problem seems "straightforward." Despite how positive matters may seem on the surface, some probing is necessary. Although a family may come without any concern about possible "emotional" problems ("It's just that he doesn't sleep"), examiners should be prepared to carry out a family interview in the same manner as would be done in the evaluation of a child with behavioral or affective disorders. This should include a general family history and a detailed assessment of the social situation, parent-child and marital relationships, school performance, behavior, and peer interactions.

Psychological, Developmental, and Psychiatric Assessment

The tactics employed for the direct psychological assessment of children will vary considerably depending on youngsters' ages and the nature of the problem. In young children it may be enough to observe a sample of the ongoing interactions between parents and children and to have the children engage in some limited interactions with the examiner. A general evaluation of youngsters' developmental/cognitive status should be made using tests appropriate for age. The use of a direct interview becomes progressively more important with increasing age. It is essential to evaluate children's thought processes; affective state; fears, worries, and concerns; manner of dealing with feelings of anger and aggression; and mode of coping with control issues, separation, individuation, and autonomy. Toddlers will be able to communicate through play if they are not ready to do so verbally, and school-age children should be able to verbalize much that is relevant.

Full psychiatric assessment and formal psychological testing is usually not necessary. However, it may be indicated after the initial evaluation if there is reasonable suspicion of psychiatric or cognitive disorder (e.g., learning disabilities, school refusal, attentional deficits, depression, or phobic behaviors).

Physical Examination

A general physical examination is desirable, but unless the history is suggestive, it is unlikely that unsuspected positive physical findings of diagnostic character will emerge. Certainly a careful examination of facial features, ears, nose, and throat, auscultation of the heart and lungs, abdominal palpation, and sphygmomanometry should be conducted on all children with major snoring or suspected apnea. A neurological assessment should be carried out if there is any question of seizures or a complaint of excessive sleepiness. In enuretic children, the examination should include inspection of the lower spine and urethral meatus, possibly along with assessment of sphincter tone and perineal sensation. In infants and toddlers with poor sleep, even if there is no history of recurrent infections, the ears should be carefully checked.

Laboratory Studies Including Polysomnographic Recordings

No studies are mandatory for all children with sleep problems. Depending on the complaint and the initial findings, however, various studies may be indicated. If there is a question of systemic illness, then a complete blood count, sedimentation rate, and other screening tests are required as indicated from history and physical examination. Enuretic children should have a baseline urinalysis and possibly a urine culture. Full urological assessment is necessary only occasionally.

Children with sleep apnea should always have an electrocardiogram, and radiological assessment of the airway should be considered. Although glucose and thyroid levels are frequently obtained in sleepy individuals, in the absence of other symptoms of diabetes or hypothyroidism they are rarely abnormal. When seizures are suspected, routine electroencephalography should be performed.

Polysomnography[11] is the all-night recording of the various physiological parameters necessary for identification of sleep stages and the assessment of sleep pathology. This includes, as a minimum, electroencephalogram, chin muscle tone, eye movements, respiration, and electrocardiogram. Respiration monitors include thermosters, thermocouples, or carbon dioxide sensors to record nasal and oral airflow, an impedance plethysmograph (or similar device) and intercostal electromyography to measure chest and abdominal excursion and to estimate tidal volume and inspiratory effort, and an oximeter that clips onto the ear, finger, or foot to measure oxygen saturation. The monitoring of leg movements is via anterior tibial electromyogram, to recognize nocturnal myoclonus. And, most studies now include closed-circuit video monitoring with low-light-sensitive television cameras.

A multiple sleep latency test (MSLT)[43] is a similar study but one carried out five times *during the day* at two-hourly intervals. Each study continues for twenty minutes, or until the child has obtained ten uninterrupted minutes of sleep, whichever occurs first. Sleepiness is quantified by measuring the number of times sleep is achieved and the average latency to sleep onset. In addition, sleep-onset REM periods (REM onsets or SOREMPs) are scored, with two or more usually being diagnostic of narcolepsy.

There are three principle situations in which polysomnographic recordings are indicated in the child: (1) Any child with unexplained excessive daytime sleepiness should have a nighttime sleep recording to determine the actual amount and quality of sleep and an MSLT to objectively estimate sleepiness and to look for the presence of the sleep-onset REM periods characteristic of narcolepsy. (2) Children with snoring suggestive of obstructive apnea should be evaluated in the sleep laboratory.[9,31] Only in this way can the severity of the syndrome be known. This information should be available before decisions are made as to surgery and follow-up. If facilities are not locally available, such children should be referred to appropriate centers. (3) Finally, for certain children in whom sleep-associated seizures are known or suspected, including epileptics with sleep-terrorlike behavior or enuresis, or any child with paroxysmal nocturnal behavior of unclear etiology, polysomnographic studies with simultaneous video monitoring are important.[53]

In addition, polysomnographic study should be considered in a number of other situations. In a child with frequent sleepwalking or sleep terrors, polysomnography may show that all of NREM sleep is severely disrupted, with only some of the disruption associated with clinically apparent events. Such study may also help remove any lingering doubts that the arousals are epileptic in nature. The study may clarify the nature of nocturnal headbanging or body rocking (jactatio capitus) by showing either that it occurs only in waking and drowsiness (states in which it would be under semivoluntary control and, therefore, possibly responsive to behavioral intervention) or within well-formed sleep (which would probably imply resistance to such modes of therapy). Some children with poor daytime seizure control, and possibly sleepiness blamed on their anticonvulsant medications, may be shown to have very poor nonrestorative sleep at night due to the sleep-disrupting effects of frequent clinical or subclinical epileptiform activity. [15,53] Eventually the recognition of certain sleep parameter abnormalities, such as shortened REM latency, increased REM density, increased arousals and decreased delta sleep, and the identification of various circadian rhythm dysfunctions, such as increased sleep-wake cycle length, blunted circadian rhythm amplitudes, and phase advance of a rhythm influencing the timing of morning waking, may prove as useful in the diagnosis, treatment, and understanding of depression in children as it has in adults.* Some preliminary studies in prepubertal and adolescent youngsters have in fact found some similar abnormalities. [40,46,47,58] Finally, even children for whom sleep disturbances seem behavioral and interactional in nature should be considered for study if the expected response to intervention is not forthcoming. During the study, the usual pattern of nocturnal parent-child interaction should be allowed to continue and be carefully observed and recorded on videotape. In-home telemetry and video monitoring probably provides more accurate assessment of certain parameters, especially interactional ones, [2,3] but few centers yet can provide this service on a regular, clinical, and nonresearch basis.

*See references 30, 38, 39, 40, 54, 55, 56.

REFERENCES

1. ABLON, S. L. and MACK, J. E. "Sleep Disorders," in J. D. Noshpitz, ed., *Basic Handbook of Child Psychiatry,* vol. 2. New York: Basic Books, 1979, pp. 643–660.

2. ANDERS, T. F. "Night-waking in Infants During the First Year of Life," *Pediatrics,* 63 (1979):860–864.

3. ANDERS, T., and SOSTEK, A. "The Use of Time Lapse Video Recording of Sleep-Wake Behavior in Human Infants," *Psychophysiology,* 13 (1976):155–158.

4. ANDERS, T. F., and WEINSTEIN, P. "Sleep and Its Disorders in Infants and Young Children: A Review," *Pediatrics,* 50 (1972):312–324.

5. ANDERS, T. F., et al. "Sleep Habits of Children and the Identification of Pathologically Sleepy Children," *Child Psychiatry and Human Development,* 9 (1978):56–63.

6. ASSOCIATION OF SLEEP DISORDERS CENTERS. *Diagnostic Classification of Sleep and Arousal Disorders,* prepared by the Sleep Disorders Classification Committee. *Sleep* 2 (1979): 1–137.

7. BAKWIN, H. "The Genetics of Enuresis," in I. Kolvin, R. C. Mac Keith, and S. R. Meadow, eds., *Bladder Control and Enuresis.* Philadelphia: J. B. Lippincott, 1973, pp. 73–77.

8. BAX, M.C.O. "Sleep Disturbance in the Young Child," *British Medical Journal,* 280 (1980):1177–1179.

9. BORNSTEIN, S. K. "Respiratory Monitoring During Sleep," in C. Guilleminault, ed., *Sleeping and Waking Disorders: Indications and Techniques.* Menlo Park, Calif.: Addison-Wesley, 1982, pp. 183–212.

10. BROUGHTON, R. "Sleep Disorders: Disorders of Arousal?" *Science,* 159 (1968):1070–1078.

11. CARSKADON, M. "Basics for Polygraphic Monitoring of Sleep," in C. Guilleminault, ed., *Sleeping and Waking Disorders: Indications and Techniques.* Menlo Park, Calif.: Addison-Wesley, 1982, pp. 1–16.

12. COLEMAN, R. "Periodic Movements in Sleep (Nocturnal Myoclonus) and Restless Legs Syndrome," in C. Guilleminault, ed., *Sleeping and Waking Disorders: Indications and Techniques.* Menlo Park, Calif.: Addison-Wesley, 1982, pp. 265–295.

13. DE JONGE, G. A. "Epidemiology of Enuresis: A Survey of the Literature," in I. Kolvin, R. C. Mac Keith, and S. R. Meadow, eds., *Bladder Control and Enuresis.* Philadelphia: J. B. Lippincott, 1973, pp. 39–46.

14. DOUGLAS, J., and RICHMAN, N. *Sleep Management Manual.* London: Great Ormond Street Children's Hospital In-House Publication, 1982.

15. ERBA, G., and FERBER, R. "Sleep Disruption by Subclinical Seizure Activity as a Cause of Increased Waking Seizures and Decreased Daytime Function," *Sleep Research,* 12 (1983):307.

16. FERBER, R. A. "Sleep Disorders in Infants and Children" in T. Riley, ed., *Clinical Aspects of Sleep and Sleep Disturbance.* Boston: Butterworths, 1985, pp. 113–157.

17. ———. *Solve Your Child's Sleep Problem.* New York: Simon & Schuster, 1985.

18. FERBER, R., and BOYLE, M. P. "Confusional Arousals in Infants and Toddlers (Not Quite Pavor Nocturnus)," *Sleep Research,* 12 (1983):241.

19. ———. "Delayed Sleep Phase Syndrome versus Motivated Sleep Phase Delay in Adolescents," *Sleep Research,* 12 (1983):239.

20. ———. "Nocturnal Fluid Intake: A Cause of, Not Treatment for, Sleep Disruption in Infants and Toddlers," *Sleep Research,* 12 (1983):243.

21. ———. "Phase Shift Dysomnia of Early Childhood," *Sleep Research,* 12 (1983):242.

22. ———. "Sleeplessness in Infants and Toddlers: Sleep

Initiation Difficulty Masquerading as a Sleep Maintenance Insomnia," *Sleep Research,* 12 (1983):240.

23. ———. "Sleeplessness in Infants Up to the Age of 12 Months: Diagnosis and Treatment," *Sleep Research,* 13 (1984):79.

24. FERBER, R., BOYLE, M. P., and BELFER, M. "Initial Experience of a Pediatric Sleep Disorders Clinic," *Sleep Research,* 10 (1981):194.

25. ———. " 'Insomnia' in Toddlers Seen in a Pediatric Sleep Disorders Clinic," *Sleep Research,* 10 (1981):195.

26. FERBER, R., FRIEDMAN, E., and DIETZ, W. "Obstructive Sleep Apnea in Childhood: 80 Cases," *Sleep Research,* 12 (1983):245.

27. FISHER, C., et al. "A Psychophysiological Study of Nightmares and Night Terrors. I. Physiological Aspects of the Stage 4 Night Terror," *Journal of Nervous and Mental Disease,* 157 (1973):75–98.

28. FISHER, C., et al. "A Psychophysiological Study of Nightmares and Night Terrors. III. Mental Content and Recall of Stage 4 Night Terrors," *Journal of Nervous and Mental Disease,* 158 (1974):174–188.

29. FRAIBERG, S. "On the Sleep Disturbances of Early Childhood," *Psychoanalytic Study of the Child,* 5 (1950): 285–309.

30. GILLIN, J. C., et al. "Successful Separation of Depressed, Normal, and Insomniac Subjects by Sleep EEG Data," *Archives of General Psychiatry,* 36 (1979):85–90.

31. GUILLEMINAULT, C. "Sleep and Breathing," in C. Guilleminault, ed., *Sleeping and Waking Disorders: Indications and Techniques.* Menlo Park, Calif.: Addison-Wesley, 1982, pp. 155–182.

32. GUILLEMINAULT, C., and ANDERS, T. F. "Sleep Disorders in Children," *Advances in Pediatrics,* 22 (1976):151–174.

33. GUILLEMINAULT, C., KOROBKIN, R., and WINKLE, R. "A Review of 50 Children with Obstructive Sleep Apnea Syndrome," *Lung,* 159 (1981):275–287.

34. ILLINGWORTH, R. S. "Sleep Problems in the First Three Years," *British Medical Journal,* 1 (1951):722–728.

35. ———. "Sleep Problems of Children," *Clinical Pediatrics,* 5 (1966):45–48.

36. JONES, D.P.H., and VERDUYN, C. M. "Behavioural Management of Sleep Problems," *Archives of Diseases in Childhood,* 58 (1983):442–444.

37. KESSLER, S. "Genetic Factors in Narcolepsy," in C. Guilleminault, W. C. Dement, and P. Passouant, eds., *Narcolepsy.* New York: Spectrum Publications, 1976, pp. 285–302.

38. KRIPKE, D. F., et al. "Circadian Rhythm Disorders in Manic-Depressives," *Biological Psychiatry,* 13 (1978):335–351.

39. KUPFER, D. J. "REM Latency: A Psychobiologic Marker for Primary Depressive Disease," *Biological Psychiatry,* 11 (1976):159–174.

40. KUPFER, D. J., and THASE, M. E. "The Use of the Sleep Laboratory in the Diagnosis of Affective Disorders," *Psychiatric Clinics of North America,* 6 (1983):3–25.

41. LAHMEYER, H. W., POZNANSKI, E. O., and BELLUR, S. N. "EEG Sleep in Depressed Adolescents," *American Journal of Psychiatry,* 140 (1983):1150–1153.

42. MILLER, F.J.W. "Children Who Wet the Bed," in I. Kolvin, R. C. Mac Keith, and S. R. Meadow, eds., *Bladder Control and Enuresis.* Philadelphia: J. B. Lippincott, 1973, pp. 47–52.

43. MITLER, M. M. "The Multiple Sleep Latency Test as an Evaluation for Excessive Somnolence," in C. Guilleminault, ed., *Sleeping and Waking Disorders: Indications and Techniques.* Menlo Park, Calif.: Addison-Wesley, 1982, pp. 145–153.

44. MOORE, T., and UCKO, L. E. "Nightwaking in Early Infancy: Part 1," *Archives of Disease in Childhood,* 32 (1957): 333–342.

45. NAVELET, Y., ANDERS, T., and GUILLEMINAULT, C. "Narcolepsy in Children," in C. Guilleminault, W. C. Dement, and P. Passouant, eds., *Narcolepsy.* New York: Spectrum Publications, 1976, pp. 171–177.

46. PUIG-ANTICH, J., and WESTON, B. "The Diagnosis and Treatment of Major Depressive Disorder in Childhood," *Annual Review of Medicine,* 34 (1983):231–245.

47. PUIG-ANTICH, J., et al. "Sleep Architecture and REM Sleep Measures in Prepubertal Major Depressives. Studies During Recovery From the Depressive Episode in a Drug-free State," *Archives of General Psychiatry,* 40 (1983):187–192.

48. RICHMAN, N. "A Community Survey of Characteristics of One- to Two-Year-Olds with Sleep Disruptions," *Journal of the American Academy of Child Psychiatry,* 20 (1981): 281–291.

49. RICHMAN, N., et al. "Sleep Problems in Young Children," *Archives of Disease in Childhood,* 56 (1984):491–493.

50. SALZARULO, P., and CHEVALIER, A. "Sleep Problems in Children and Their Relationship with Early Disturbances of the Waking-Sleeping Rhythms," *Sleep,* 6 (1983):47–51.

51. SHIRLEY, H. F., and KAHN, J. P. "Sleep Disturbances in Children," *Pediatric Clinics of North America,* 5 (1958): 629–643.

52. SIMONDS, J. F., and PARRAGA, H. "Prevalence of Sleep Disorders and Sleep Behaviors in Children and Adolescents," *Journal of the American Academy of Child Psychiatry,* 21 (1982):383–388.

53. THARP, B. R. "Epilepsy and Sleep," in C. Guilleminault, ed., *Sleeping and Waking Disorders: Indications and Techniques.* Menlo Park, Calif.: Addison-Wesley, 1982, pp. 373–381.

54. VOGEL, G. W., et al. "Improvement of Depression by REM Sleep Deprivation: New Findings and a Theory," *Archives of General Psychiatry,* 37 (1980):247–253.

55. WEHR, T. A., GILLIN, J. C., and GOODWIN, F. K. "Sleep and Circadian Rhythms in Depression," in M. Chase and E. D. Weitzman, eds., *Sleep Disorders, Basic and Clinical Research.* New York: Spectrum Publications, 1983, pp. 195–225.

56. WEHR, T. A., et al. "Circadian Rhythm Disturbances in Manic-Depressive Illness," *Federation Proceedings,* 42 (1983):2809.

57. WEITZMAN, E. D., et al. "Delayed Sleep Phase Syndrome," *Archives of General Psychiatry,* 38 (1981):737–746.

58. YOUNG, W., et al. "The Sleep of Childhood Depressives: Comparison with Age-Matched Controls," *Biological Psychiatry,* 17 (1982):1163–1168.

22 / Applications of Computerized EEG in Child Psychiatry

Charles D. Yingling

Introduction

In 1929 psychiatrist Hans Berger first described the human electroencephalogram (EEG).[2] Since that time many researchers and clinicians have hoped that it would prove to offer, as Berger had suggested, a window on the mind. In fact, a half century of effort into probing the electrical potentials of the brain has yet to produce such a clear-cut understanding. However, there has been substantial progress in using the EEG to index brain activities associated with sensation and cognition. This chapter provides an overview of the current state of the art in the use of computer techniques for the analysis of EEG phenomena, the uses and limitations of current methodologies, and the likely directions for future progress.

At the present time, computerized analysis of spontaneous EEG, and especially of evoked potentials, has been solidly established as a useful diagnostic tool in neurology, neurosurgery, audiology, opthalmology, and other fields where there is a primary concern in assessing gross pathology of the nervous system or integrity of the sensory pathways.[5,14] These techniques may be useful in discerning the presence or absence of various neurological conditions that can masquerade as, or complicate, psychiatric symptoms. On the other hand, progress in the use of EEG techniques in psychiatry and child psychiatry per se has been slower, and these methods are not yet routinely used to make diagnostic decisions or assess prognosis in individual cases. Given the subtle nature of the cognitive and affective disturbances that are the domain of psychiatry, this is not surprising. Yet it would be incorrect to conclude that EEG approaches have proven unfruitful and should be abandoned. Much research suggests that measures of brain electrical activity can index several aspects of human information processing and that these indices may differ significantly between normal subjects and those with various psychiatric disorders. Clinical application of these findings awaits (1) better understanding of the neural generators of cognitively determined potentials, (2) greater precision in the delineation of the psychological processes associated with specific brain activities, and (3) specification of the similarities and differences in the electrophysiological profiles of different diagnostic categories. We are dealing with a field that, if no longer in its infancy, has yet to reach full maturity.

EEG Spectral Analysis

There are two basically different uses for computers in connection with the EEG. The first is in the quantification of spectral power values in the spontaneous EEG. Using either digital filters or the fast Fourier transform (FFT), it is possible to ascertain the power content of the EEG as a function of frequency. This method quantifies the process of visual interpretation of clinical EEGs and allows easier comparison of an individual with group means, assessment of drug effects or changes over time, and similar determinations. Typically, power values are summed into discrete bands representing the classical frequency components—delta (0–3 Hz), theta (4–7 Hz), alpha (8–12 Hz), and beta (13–30 Hz). The power values in each band can be printed or plotted in graphic form. A useful representation is the compressed spectral display, pioneered by Bickford and colleagues,[3] where successive spectra are plotted in a pseudo-three-dimensional graph that allows one to see changes over time in the shape and amplitude of the spectra.

Event-Related Potentials

The second major application of computers is to obtain averaged evoked potentials, also termed event-related potentials (ERPs). These are obtained by summing many samples of EEG time-locked to the presentation of a sensory stimulus or other discrete event. The spontaneous EEG, which varies randomly in relation to the time of stimulus presentation, is suppressed; the ERPs, which have a constant phase relation with the stimulus, are augmented. In this manner a great enhancement of signal/noise ratio is obtained, and it is possible to obtain clear ERPs of a few tenths of a microvolt even in the presence of spontaneous EEG activity hundreds of times larger. Averaged ERP waveforms are composed of two categories of components: exogenous, those waves that represent the brain's reception of the stimulus, and endogenous, waves that reflect the cognitive processes of stimulus evaluation.[9]

The exogenous components occur in the earlier portion of the waveform (roughly within the first 200 msec poststimulus) and are largely determined by the physical characteristics of the stimulus—that is, intensity, duration, modality, and so forth. For example, brief auditory clicks elicit a series of seven waves within the first 10 msec; these waves are generated by the structures of the auditory pathways within the brain stem. Auditory brain stem responses are routinely used in audiometry, especially with infants or small children with suspected hearing loss where conventional audiometry cannot be employed. Similarly, a series of early somatosensory components are generated by brainstem pathways and the primary somatosensory cortex, where the response is seen approximately 20 msec following electrical stimulation of the median nerve at the contralateral wrist. These early responses are routinely used to assess the integrity of the somatosensory pathways or assist in localization of subcortical lesions. In the visual modality, responses can be recorded quite readily from occipital electrodes following presentation of a flash or of a reversing checkerboard. These responses are useful in the diagnosis of diseases affecting the retina or optic pathways. For example, a significant difference in the visual ERP latency between left- and right-eye stimulation is immediately suggestive since it is often one of the defining clinical signs of multiple sclerosis.

In contrast, the endogenous components occur later in the averaged response (roughly 200 msec and beyond). They are determined primarily by cognitive rather than by stimulus factors. For example, a sequence of brief auditory tones can be presented to a subject, with a small percentage of the tones being slightly different in pitch. If the subject is asked to detect the rare tones by pressing a button or maintaining a mental count, the responses to the rare (but not to the frequent) tones will contain a complex of later components, including a prominent positive wave at approximately 300 msec latency, which is thus termed P300. That this component is cognitive rather than sensory in origin can be clearly demonstrated by a slight modification of the paradigm: Instead of chang-

ing the pitch of certain tones, a random percentage of an otherwise regular series of tones is omitted, and the subject is asked to detect the omissions.[28,33] If the EEG is averaged from the time of the expected, but missing, stimuli, a P300 is still present, even though the earlier components (which depend on activation of sensory pathways) are completely absent! Since endogenous components reflect cognitive processes, many researchers hope they will ultimately produce insights into the mechanisms underlying cognitive disorders.

Brain Electrical Activity Mapping

A recent application of computers to EEG is the production of graphical displays of EEG or ERPs. Rather than display the waveforms directly, selected parameters are converted into a topographical image representing a view down onto the top of the head. Such displays can be much easier to interpret than are the traditional arrays of waveforms, particularly where changes in the scalp distribution of activity are important. Duffy, Burchfield, and Lombroso[10] have combined these display techniques with statistical transformations of the original data in a technique they term BEAM (brain electrical activity mapping). For example, a group of normal subjects can be used to define a mean and normal range for any measured parameter, such as power in a given frequency band or amplitude of the visual ERP at a given latency. Data from individual subjects with a specific diagnosis, such as dyslexia, are transformed into z scores and then plotted in color maps. The z scores represent the degree to which the selected feature(s) diverges from the normative range. For each feature selected, the maps will display the scalp regions exhibiting abnormal values and whether they are above or below the mean of the normal group. Different colors are used to represent degrees of deviance. It is thus possible to tell at a glance the location and nature of EEG or ERP abnormalities, either in an individual subject or in the average of a given diagnostic group.[10]

Neurometrics

Of course, whether it results in a graphic display or simply yields columns of numbers, the validity of any such statistical method depends on the appropriateness of the measures chosen for analysis and the definition of the normative reference group. The most ambiguous effort along these lines is the "neurometrics" approach, developed by E. Roy John and his colleagues at New York University (NYU).[17] John's group has developed a standardized protocol for EEG and ERP data collection and over the last ten years has tested several thousand children and adults. Since this is the first computerized EEG diagnostic system that has been commercially available, I will consider it in some detail. The protocol consists of an individual calibration for automatic artifact rejection, at least one minute of eyes-closed EEG, and a series of visual and auditory ERP conditions: blank flash, coarse and fine checkerboard flash, regular and irregular clicks, the lower-case letter "b," and the lower-case letter "d."

A normative data base has been assembled consisting of several hundred cases collected at NYU and other collaborating institutions. The EEG data are analyzed by comparing each individual's EEG power spectrum at each lead with the values predicted for his or her age by developmental equations based on the normative data base.[18] Z scores are then calculated, representing the degree to which each value deviates from the predicted value. Z scores are calculated for eight bipolar lead derivations (bilateral fronto-temporal, temporal, central, and parieto-occipital) for each of four frequency bands (delta, theta, alpha, and beta); the result is a total of thirty-two values. Conservative criteria for abnormality are used: A given case is deemed abnormal if four of thirty-two values are significantly deviant at $p < 0.05$, or alternately two of thirty-two at $p < 0.01$, more than twice the number of significant values expected by chance.

Using these criteria, Ahn and associates[1] reported a false-positive rate in their normal population of 10 percent (at $p < 0.05$) or 4 percent (at $p < 0.01$). In an independent normal sample from Barbados, the false-positive rates were 9 percent and 2 percent, respectively. Three clinical groups were also studied: a neurological group consisting of patients examined in a pediatric neurology service who were considered at risk for neurological disorders; a group of children with borderline intelligence who had exhibited generalized learning disabilities and poor achievement in one or more areas; and a group of children of normal intelligence who had exhibited specific learning difficulties, with poor achievement in at least one area. The true positive rates obtained in these three groups were 58 percent, 57 percent, and 54 percent (at $p < 0.05$), or 48 percent, 46 percent, and 47 percent (at $p < 0.01$). Neurometrics thus produces low false-positive rates, shown to be stable both within and across cultures. In addition, it is able to detect a substantial number of significant deviations from normal values in various groups of children at risk for neurological problems or learning disabilities. Together, these findings suggest

that neurometrics may be useful as a screening technique in populations at risk for a variety of neurological diseases or learning disabilities.

However, these results do not clearly establish that neurometric abnormalities are associated with cognitive dysfunction per se. In the studies just cited, candidates for the normative group were excluded on the basis of any history of neurological problems. Screening criteria for the learning-disabled groups were not specified, but John* has stated that the learning-disabled groups did in fact contain subjects with neurological and/or sensory deficits. This raises the possibility that the abnormalities reported in the learning-disabled groups may reflect overt neurological dysfunction rather than their cognitive disabilities. My group at the University of California at San Francisco has recently addressed this issue by using the neurometrics protocol and equipment to evaluate a group of severely dyslexic boys, and an age and performance-IQ matched group of normal readers.[36] In contrast to those just described, *all* subjects in our study—control and dyslexic alike —underwent rigorous screening to ensure freedom from any overt neurological, sensory, or emotional dysfunction. Neurological screening was carried out utilizing the examination methods of Touwen and Prechtl.[35] The criteria for exclusion from the study were the presence of moderate disabilities in three or more motor categories or a consistent pattern of disability in the sensory-perceptual area. No child was included who demonstrated major neurological signs, such as clearly impaired motor coordination or seizures. Pure-tone audiometry, visual acuity, refraction, and binocular function examinations were performed. All subjects had clinically normal hearing and vision and full-scale IQs of greater than eighty-eight on the revised Weschler Intelligence Scale for Children. The dyslexic children were severely impaired in both oral reading (average grade level was 2.0) and silent reading (average grade level was 3.0), while the controls were at the 8.5 grade level in both oral and silent reading.

When we compared these two groups with neurometric criteria for the EEG, we obtained "hit rates" of two of thirty-eight (5.3 percent) in the control group and four of thirty-eight (10.5 percent) in the dyslexic children. These are not significantly different (chi-square $= 0.18$, $p < 0.10$). To increase the sensitivity, we also examined the "hit rate" at the 0.05 significance level; this resulted in increases in the abnormality rates to five of thirty-eight controls (13.2 percent) and eight of thirty-eight dyslexic children (21.0 percent), again not significantly different (chi-square $= 0.37$, $p >$

*E. R. John, personal communication, 1984.

0.50). We also used our control group rather than the NYU data to define the norms, and recomputed the z scores with essentially identical results: Three of thirty-eight controls met the criteria of two of thirty-two values differing from the norms at $p < 0.01$, and six of thirty-eight dyslexic children (chi-square = 0.50, $p > 0.10$). Evaluation of the ERP data similarly failed to discriminate the groups.

We thus concluded that when neurological status is normal in both groups, neurometric evaluation of the resting EEG does not discriminate severe dyslexic children from normal readers. In fact, the abnormality rates we found in both groups were roughly comparable to the false-positive rate obtained by John's group in their normative population. These findings suggest that the high true positive rates found in the NYU learning-disabled samples[1] were probably due to the presence of overt neurological dysfunction rather than because of any association with learning disabilities per se. Thus neurometrics may be appropriate for screening learning-disabled populations in order to determine which cases should be referred for a thorough neurological examination; however, the technique does not appear to tap those brain processes associated with learning problems as such.

Methodological Considerations

Over the years there have been numerous reports in the literature that claimed to find significant differences between dyslexic patients and normals on one measure or another. As a result, this failure to find consistent EEG or ERP correlates of dyslexia may seem puzzling. It is worth noting Conner's interesting calculation,[6] in which he observed that the correlation between the incidence of reported EEG abnormalities in dyslexia and the year of publication was -0.91! Clearly, as selection criteria have been refined to produce groups with more pure learning disabilities, the incidence of reported EEG abnormalities has dropped. Furthermore, among the different studies there has been little consistency in the exact abnormalities reported: Thus some studies of dyslexic individuals have reported a deficit in alpha power, others an increase. Virtually no studies have employed a replication component as part of the design; in electrophysiological studies where the number of variables obtained can easily outnumber the subjects several times over, this is particularly crucial. Since 5 percent of a totally random data set will show significant differences between groups at the $p < 0.05$ level (by definition!), the importance of replication cannot be overstated.

The studies described thus far have employed EEG and ERPs recorded under passive conditions that require no active involvement of the subject. Such techniques are necessary in recording from young and/or uncooperative subjects but provide limited information. It seems reasonable that physiological correlates of disturbed information processing would be best obtained by recording during active tasks. A sizable literature documents the fact that both spontaneous EEG and ERPs are quite sensitive to concomitant task involvement and can index cognitive processing as well as stimulus reception.

ERPs in Attention Deficit Disorder

An example of a study using ERPs recorded during active task involvement is that of Roy Halliday and associates,[15,16] who have demonstrated that visual ERPs can predict clinical response to methylphenidate hydrochloride (Ritalin) in children with attention deficit disorder with hyperactivity. This study is also noteworthy in that it is one of the few studies in the literature that have included a replication. Children detected a rare dim flash embedded in a series of brighter flashes and responded with a button press when the dim target was detected. A passive task was also employed, in which there were no dim flashes and the subjects simply watched the display. Recordings were obtained after administration of 0.33 mg per kg methylphenidate or a matching placebo. Subsequently, in a double-blind clinical trial with methylphenidate and placebo using a within-subjects crossover design, the children were classified as responders or nonresponders by the referring pediatrician.

The initial retrospective study[16] had identified two visual ERP measures that conjointly predicted clinical response to methylphenidate, and cross-validated the findings on an independent sample. The prospective follow-up study[15] employed the same predictors and correctly identified 91 percent of the responders and 56 percent of the nonresponders. Across all three experiments, the percent of correct predictions was 81 percent for responders and 70 percent for nonresponders. It is noteworthy that the criteria included both a comparison of the response to the active versus passive conditions and an assessment of the effect of methylphenidate on the response. In other words, the ability to predict clinical reponse to medication in children with attention deficits required recording brain activity both in a task demanding attention and during administration of the drug.

ERP Studies in Autism

Courchesne and coworkers[8] used ERP methods to study information processing in autistic subjects. Three intermixed stimuli were employed: frequent (the spoken word "me"); infrequent targets (the word "you," which required a button-press response); and infrequent novels (bizarre concoctions of human, mechanical, and computer sounds, which the subjects did not expect). When only the "me" and "you" stimuli were presented, with no active detection task required of the subjects, there were no ERP differences between autistic individuals and age-matched controls. When all three types of stimuli were presented, with subjects required to detect the target "yous," both autistic persons and controls produced different responses to the target and novel stimuli than to frequent stimuli. Targets evoked enhanced P300 and slow wave (SW) responses in both groups, and novel stimuli produced a P300 component that was more frontal in its scalp distribution than that to targets, and a late negativity peaking at 800 msec poststimulus. These responses are similar to those obtained in a previous study of normal subjects ages four to forty-four,[7] and suggest that the autistic group did *not* misperceive novel information as nonnovel and were able to make simple classification decisions as accurately as normal controls. However, the amplitude of the P300 component to target stimuli and of both the P300 and late negativity to novel stimuli were significantly smaller in autistic than normal subjects, suggesting that these stimuli elicited less processing in autistic subjects than in normals. Once again, it is noteworthy that the differences were elicited only during tasks requiring active information processing and not during passive conditions requiring no task involvement by the subjects.

ERPs in Schizophrenia

Many studies have consistently demonstrated smaller P300 amplitudes in schizophrenic patients compared to controls. In particular, two recent studies have suggested that P300 may be abnormal in children who are either schizophrenic or genetically at risk for schizophrenia. Strandburg and associates[32] employed the Span of Apprehension Task, which has been shown to discriminate between schizophrenic and normal individuals. This task involves the detection of a randomly placed target letter among an array of distractors. In Strandburg and coworkers' task, the letter

arrays were preceded 500 msec earlier by a warning tone. This paradigm causes the appearance of an anticipatory negative shift, termed the contingent negative variation (CNV), prior to the appearance of the visual array. The investigators recorded ERPs from ten schizophrenic and thirteen normal children during performance of this test. The schizophrenic children were found to have a small CNV that was slow to develop and resolve, as well as diminished amplitudes for several visual ERP components, including P300. Early (exogenous) visual components were smaller and less lateralized in the schizophrenic children, and P300 was significantly smaller at all electrode sites over the left hemisphere or midline. According to this study, the effects on the ERP of increasing task difficulty were seen only in the normal children. The authors concluded that "underlying the impaired performance of the schizophrenic children are very different patterns of both general and selective CNS activation related to the control of information acquisition and subsequent processing" (p. 250).

In an ongoing longitudinal study, Friedman, Vaughan, and Erlenmeyer-Kimling[12] studied a group of normal control children and a group of children with schizophrenic parents, who are thus at risk for the development of schizophrenia.[11] The investigators recorded P300 to both pitch changes and missing auditory stimuli. The high-risk group showed significantly smaller P300 amplitudes, but only when the eliciting event was relevant. Reaction time means and variances were not different between the two groups. Two factors suggest that the finding represents a true amplitude difference, even though the authors did not assess single trial latency variability of P300. These are, first, the similar variability in reaction time in both groups and, second, the finding that reduced P300 amplitude in adult schizophrenic patients is not due to increased latency variability.[25] Friedman, Vaughan, and Erlenmeyer-Kimling[12] conclude that "the reduced P300 amplitudes found in high risk children are due to a defect in the basic cognitive mechanisms that are indexed by these late positive waveforms and may reflect dysfunctions in the neural structures responsible for their generation" (p. 527).

However, it must be pointed out that these differences are not specific to schizophrenia. Reduced P300 amplitudes have also been reported in hyperactive children[19,24] and in dyslexic subjects.[21] In adults, reduced and/or delayed P300s have been reported in dementia* and depression.[20,26,27,31] In a comprehensive study of P300 in normal aging and various clinical syndromes in adults, Pfefferbaum and associates[22,23] concluded that "the P300 amplitude and latency ab-

---

*See references 4, 13, 29, 30, and 34.

normalities observed reflect a common, rather than a diagnostically specific deficit" (p. 122). They also reported that, in contrast to earlier studies, the magnitude of the observed differences was not great enough to be useful in diagnosis of individual cases. At the present time, this caveat certainly also applies to the use of P300 or other ERP measures in children.

Conclusion

In conclusion, this brief survey of applications of computer analysis of EEG and ERP in child psychiatry has made the following points: (1) in clinical diagnosis, computerized EEG and ERP measures can be used to help confirm and/or rule out overt neurological dysfunction that can complicate the diagnosis of psychiatric disturbances; (2) these measures are not yet sensitive and specific enough to contribute to psychiatric diagnoses per se; and (3) a growing body of research results suggests that many psychiatric disorders do have significant electrophysiological correlates, some of which will undoubtedly develop into diagnostically useful measures as knowledge in the field advances. Future progress is likely to result from the use of larger and more carefully characterized subject populations and standardized data collection protocols that emphasize the recording of brain activity during behavioral conditions that activate brain systems involved in cognitive and affective disturbances.

REFERENCES

1. AHN, H., et al. "Developmental Equations Reflect Brain Dysfunctions," *Science,* 210 (1980):1259–1262.
2. BERGER, H. "Uber das Elektrenkephalogramm des Menschen," *Archiv fuer Psychiatrie und Nervenkrankheiten,* 87 (1929):527–570.
3. BICKFORD, R. G., FLEMING, N. I., and BILLINGER, T. W. "Compression of EEG Data by Isometric Power Spectral Plots," *Electroencephalography and Clinical Neurophysiology,* 31 (1971):631–636.
4. BROWN, W. S., MARSH, J. T., and LaRUE, A. "Event-related Potentials in Psychiatry: Differentiating Depression and Dementia in the Elderly," *Bulletin of the Los Angeles Neurological Society,* 47 (1982):91–107.
5. CHIAPPA, K. H. *Evoked Potentials in Clinical Medicine.* New York: Raven Press, 1983.
6. CONNERS, C. K. "Critical Review of 'Electroencephalographic and Neurophysiological Studies in Dyslexia,' " in A. L. Benton and D. Pearl, eds., *Dyslexia: An Appraisal of Current Knowledge.* New York: Oxford University Press, 1978, pp. 251–261.
7. COURCHESNE, E. "Cognitive Components of the Event-related Brain Potential: Changes Associated with Development," in A.W.K. Gaillard and W. Ritter, eds., *Tutorials in ERP Research: Endogenous Components.* Amsterdam: Elsevier/North Holland, 1983, pp. 329–344.
8. COURCHESNE, E., et al. "Autism: Processing of Novel Auditory Information Assessed by Event-related Brain Potentials," *Electroencephalography and Clinical Neurophysiology,* 59 (1984):238–248.
9. DONCHIN, E., RITTER, W., and McCALLUM, W. C. "Cognitive Psychophysiology: The Endogenous Components of the ERP," in E. Callaway, P. Tueting, and S. H. Koslow, eds., *Event-Related Brain Potentials in Man.* New York: Academic Press, 1978, pp. 349–441.
10. DUFFY, F. H., BURCHFIEL, J. L., and LOMBROSO, C. T. "Brain Electrical Activity Mapping (BEAM): A Method for Extending the Clinical Utility of EEG and Evoked Potential Data," *Annals of Neurology,* 5 (1979):309–321.
11. ERLENMEYER-KIMLING, L. "Studies of the Offspring of Two Schizophrenic Parents," in D. Rosenthal and S. S.

Kety, eds., *The Transmission of Schizophrenia.* New York: Pergamon Press, 1968, pp. 65–83.
12. FRIEDMAN, D., VAUGHAN H. G., JR., and ERLENMEYER-KIMLING, L. "Cognitive Brain Potentials in Children at Risk for Schizophrenia: Preliminary Findings," *Schizophrenia Bulletin,* 8 (1982):514–531.
13. GOODIN, D. S., SQUIRES, K. C., and STARR, A. "Long Latency Event-related Components of the Auditory Evoked Potential in Dementia," *Brain,* 101 (1978):635–648.
14. HALLIDAY, A. M. *Evoked Potentials in Clinical Testing.* Edinburgh: Churchill Livingstone, 1982.
15. HALLIDAY, R., CALLAWAY, E., and ROSENTHAL, J. H. "The Visual ERP Predicts Response to Methylphenidate in Hyperactive Children," *Psychophysiology,* 21 (1984):114–121.
16. HALLIDAY, R., et al. "Averaged Evoked Potential Predictors of Clinical Improvement in Hyperactive Children Treated with Methylphenidate: An Initial Study and Replication," *Psychophysiology,* 13 (1976):429–440.
17. JOHN, E. R., et al. "Neurometrics," *Science,* 196 (1977):1393–1410.
18. JOHN, E. R., et al. "Developmental Equations for the Electroencephalogram," *Science,* 210 (1980):1255–1258.
19. KLORMAN, R., et al. "Effects of Methylphenidate on Hyperactive Children's Evoked Responses During Passive and Active Attention," *Psychophysiology,* 16 (1979):23–39.
20. LEVIT, R. A., SUTTON, S., and ZUBIN, J. "Evoked Potential Correlates of Information Processing in Psychiatric Patients," *Psychological Medicine,* 3 (1973):487–494.
21. LOVRICH, D., and STAMM, J. S. "Event-related Potential and Behavioral Correlates of Attention in Reading Retardation," *Journal of Clinical Neuropsychology,* 5 (1983):13–37.
22. PFEFFERBAUM, A., et al. "Clinical Application of the P3 Component of Event-related potentials. I. Normal Aging," *Electroencephalography and Clinical Neurophysiology,* 59 (1984):85–103.
23. PFEFFERBAUM, A., et al. "Clinical Application of the P3 Component of Event-related Potentials. II. Dementia, Depression and Schizophrenia," *Electroencephalography and Clinical Neurophysiology,* 59 (1984):104–124.

24. PRICHEP, L. S., SUTTON, S., and HAKEREM, G. "Evoked Potentials in Hyperkinetic and Normal Children Under Certainty and Uncertainty: A Placebo and Methylphenidate Study," *Psychophysiology,* 13 (1976):419–428.

25. ROTH, W. T., et al. "P3 Reduction in Auditory Evoked Potentials of Schizophrenics," *Electroencephalography and Clinical Neurophysiology,* 49 (1980):497–505.

26. ROTH, W. T., et al. "Auditory Event-related Potentials in Schizophrenia and Depression," *Biological Psychiatry,* 4 (1981):199–212.

27. SHAGASS, C., et al. "Evoked Potential Correlates of Psychosis," *Biological Psychiatry,* 13 (1978):163–184.

28. SIMSON, R., VAUGHAN, H. G., JR., and RITTER, W. "The Scalp Topography of Potentials Associated with Missing Visual and Auditory Stimuli," *Electroencephalography and Clinical Neurophysiology,* 40 (1976):33–42.

29. SQUIRES, K., GOODIN, D. S., and STARR, A. "Event Related Potentials in Development, Aging and Dementia," in D. Lehmann and E. Callaway, eds., *Human Evoked Potentials.* New York: Plenum Press, 1979, pp. 383–396.

30. SQUIRES, K. C., et al. "Electrophysiological Assessment of Mental Function in Aging and Dementia," in L. Poon, ed., *Aging in the 1980s.* Washington, D.C.: American Psychological Association, 1980, pp. 125–134.

31. STEINHAUER, S., and ZUBIN, J. "Vulnerability to Schizophrenia: Information Processing in the Pupil and Event-related Potential," in I. Hanin and E. Usdin, eds., *Biological Markers in Psychiatry and Neurology.* Oxford: Pergamon Press, 1982, pp. 371–385.

32. STRANDBURG, R. J., et al. "Event-related Potential Concomitants of Information Processing Dysfunction in Schizophrenic Children," *Electroencephalography and Clinical Neurophysiology,* 57 (1984):236–253.

33. SUTTON, S., et al. "Information Delivery and the Sensory Evoked Potentials," *Science,* 155 (1967):1436–1439.

34. SYNDULKO, K., et al. "Long-latency Event Related Potentials in Normal Aging and Dementia," in J. Courjon, F. Mauguiere, and M. Revol, eds., *Clinical Applications of Evoked Potentials in Neurology.* New York: Raven Press, 1981, pp. 279–286.

35. TOUWEN, B.C.L., and PRECHTL, H.F.R. "The Neurological Examination of the Child with Minor Nervous Dysfunction," *Topics in Developmental Medicine,* 30 (1970):1–105.

36. YINGLING, C. D., et al. "Neurometrics Does Not Detect 'Pure' Dyslexics," *Electroencephalography and Clinical Neurophysiology,* 1986, in Press.

23 / Single-Case Research: Assessment and Evaluation Strategies

Alan E. Kazdin

The individual case study has long been recognized as an important method of inquiry; it has served as a means of generating hypotheses about the nature of clinical problems and their treatment.[10] Indeed, it is not difficult to pinpoint individual case studies that have played a pivotal role in a number of scientific realms. These include the elaboration of particular theories such as psychoanalysis; the achievement of important insights about rare clinical phenomena (such as multiple personalities)[15]; and the differentiation of clinical disorders.[9] The case study has enjoyed special attention for yet another reason. Alternative theories and research findings must ultimately be translated in practice into the treatment of a particular patient at a specific point in time. In clinical practice, the question is not simply whether one treatment works better than another in general but rather what treatment will work for this particular patient now. The questions are obviously related, but the answers are not invariably the same. The case study provides the opportunity to test concretely the generality and applicability of theoretical notions and research findings. In turn, the information obtained from such applications may have important implications for revising theory or for future research.

Notwithstanding their contributions, case studies have been relegated to secondary status in the overall scheme of scientific knowledge. By their very nature, case studies have been largely uncontrolled and have relied upon anecdotal information, clinical impression, and judgments. The knowledge they yield is not at all commensurate with their persuasive impact and dramatic appeal.

Recently, alternative strategies have emerged that permit intensive investigation of individual cases. The strategies are referred to as *single-case research designs.* The designs incorporate methodological features that permit valid inferences to be drawn about the impact of treatment. As such, they greatly improve the scientific yield over traditional approaches. Perhaps as important, they are somewhat flexible so they can be applied in such a way as to meet many of the exigencies

23 / *Single-Case Research: Assessment and Evaluation Strategies*

of clinical work. This chapter highlights salient features of single-case designs, the assessment strategies they embrace, and their use in clinical work.

Since the usual requirements of research are often seen as incompatible with clinical work, introducing the notion of research design in order to enhance practice can raise a number of concerns. In daily practice, the clinician is confronted with the individual case, such as a child or family. Treatment needs to be individually tailored and flexible enough to satisfy clinical and management issues. In research, treatment usually is administered in a standardized albeit not necessarily rigid manner. The standardization is dictated by the protocol and may affect who provides this treatment and when and how much treatment is provided. Other features of clinical research may not be appropriate for clinical work. These include such requirements as the need to accumulate homogeneous groups of patients, their assignment to alternative conditions on a random basis, and the administration of a standardized assessment battery that may or may not evaluate relevant domains.

In any attempt to study therapies, there are always extraneous factors that might explain those changes the investigator wishes to attribute to the treatment. In outcome research, the purpose is to rule out or make implausible the impact of such factors. The evaluation of groups of patients who receive alternative treatment and control conditions, who are randomly assigned to conditions, and whose symptoms are assessed before and after treatment all contribute to the validity of the inferences that can be drawn. For the practicing clinician, there has been no analogous way to obtain scientifically acceptable information from the treatment of individual patients. Single-case research strategies represent a methodology that can evaluate alternative treatments and can rule out the impact of extraneous factors that may serve as rival explanations of the results. The methodology is currently in use in experimental research in diverse areas with both human and infrahuman subjects.[8] However, the special feature of the methodology is that it can be used in clinical work. The method provides a flexible approach to evaluation that is consistent with many of the priorities and demands of clinical practice. In order to use single-case methodology, there are, of course, a number of requirements regarding assessment and design considerations.

Assessment Prerequisites

SPECIFICATION OF THE TREATMENT FOCUS

An essential prerequisite of single-case designs is careful specification of the goals of treatment. The specific symptoms and areas of functioning that will reflect the effects of treatment must be made as explicit as possible. A specific measure or several measures need to be selected well before treatment begins. The measure serves to operationalize the clinical problems brought to treatment and is used to evaluate the changes that occur during treatment. The fact that the treatment focus must be specified in objective terms does not in any way limit the types of symptoms or problems that can be studied. The investigator/therapist can focus on cognitive, affective, behavioral, physiological, or psychological functioning. All have been used alone or in combination in single-case designs in diverse clinical applications.[6]

In addition to specifying the focus of treatment, it may also be important to state the situations or circumstances in which the changes would be expected. Whether the hoped-for changes should become evident at home, at school, on a hospital unit, or in the clinician's office are all implicitly incorporated into the specification of the focus. It may be that broad effects of treatment are expected (e.g., that depression will be lifted or psychosis dissipated) and that assessment in many different situations would reflect this progress of treatment. Alternatively, changes may be anticipated only at certain times (e.g., within a particular time frame after a single dose of medication) but not at other times. Specification of treatment requires noting what symptoms are to be focused on and are likely to change, how they are measured, and under what circumstances.

CONTINUOUS ASSESSMENT

The inferences drawn in single-case designs depend on the observation of performance over time. Thus, once the treatment focus is specified, the measure selected to evaluate treatment progress is administered on several occasions. The first measurement is taken before treatment is initiated and the procedure is then continued over the course of therapy. Ideally the measure is administered on a daily basis or on several occasions each week. However, there is room for flexibility here as long as the purposes of repeated assessment are achieved.

Before treatment is initiated, continuous assessment permits the clinician to examine the pattern and stability of performance. The pretreatment information provides a baseline from which judgments about the effects of treatment can subsequently be made. One or two assessments of performance before treatment may not be sufficient to delineate the pattern of symptoms or to evaluate the extent of their variability. It is likely that there will be some fluctuation as a function of several variables: processes within the child, day-to-day changes in the environment, and the imperfect reliability of the instrument. Optimally, there would be repeated observations of the symptoms on multiple occasions before treatment is administered; this would provide a more reliable basis for judging treatment effects at a later date. Since assessment continues over the course of treatment, comparisons can be made of the child's performance before and during treatment. In comparison to the tactic of making assessments at single points before and after treatment, the conclusions that can be drawn about the effects of a given intervention and the factors responsible for therapeutic change are greatly enhanced by continuous assessment.

METHODS OF ASSESSMENT

The key requirement of single-case research, namely continuous assessment, raises questions about what should be measured and with what instruments. Actually, there are no inherent restrictions on the range of measurement options. Various clinical ratings, self-report and interview measures, checklists and rating scales—methods that are frequently used in group research—can be employed in single-case research as well. However, the more commonly used techniques are those that sample problematic behavior directly.

The emergence of single-case designs in clinical work has been part of a larger movement that entails an empirical approach toward treatment and evaluation of clinical problems.[11] As part of this movement, efforts have focused increasingly on identifying and assessing clinical problems in descriptive and objective terms. In varying degrees such measures as global clinical ratings, interviews, and checklists obviously reflect clinical problems and therapeutic change. Yet they are often removed from the direct symptoms of the child. There is evidence that the less well grounded the measure might be in specific or concrete definitions of the symptoms or dysfunction, the more subject the measure is to extraneous influences. For example, by their very nature global ratings do not specify precisely what is being assessed. Scores on such ratings can be very vulnerable to other influences, such as biases and expectancies on the part of the rater; often they bear no relation to measures of the child's actual behavior. Similarly, parent checklist information, with criteria somewhat more well specified than global ratings, obviously can reflect the child's symptoms. Yet several studies have shown that parent ratings of deviant child behavior are often inaccurate in their reflection of how the child behaves.[3] Moreover, parental ratings vary considerably as a function of psychiatric problems (especially depression) on the part of the parent rather than in response to the child's behavior.

Coincident with the emergence of single-case designs has been the attempt to define in concrete and observable terms those areas that need to be focused on in treatment. The degree of inferential leap from the assessment measure to the child's problems should be minimal. The direct assessment of observable symptoms is by no means free from its own assessment problems and biases; however, it has been less subject to the impact of rater expectancies and biases.[4]

Precisely what is to be assessed and how assessment is conducted obviously depend on the nature of the clinical problem. When possible, clinical problems are often translated into overt behaviors that can be observed reliably. Examples of undesirable or maladaptive behaviors that have been assessed in clinical applications include fighting, truancy, self-stimulation, stuttering, fear and anxiety, excessive activity, and not complying with requests. Examples of prosocial behaviors include initiating and maintaining appropriate social interaction, completing schoolwork, and engaging in cooperative play. Not all clinical problems involve publicly observable behaviors. Private events have often been assessed by having the patients report on such events as obsessions, intrusive thoughts, and headaches. In many applications, there are objective signs that correlate with reports of private or subjective experience. Such signs can then be recorded and used as a basis of evaluating treatment. For example, facial expressions and verbal statements have been assessed to reflect such subjective experiences as sad affect, hallucinations, and physical pain.

A given measurement technique often relies on persons in the child's everyday life to provide critical information. Frequently parents are relied on to report information about oppositional or aggressive behaviors at home. For example, parents can be telephoned on a daily or almost daily basis, and they can report reliably on concrete and well-defined behaviors that may have occurred at home. Teachers also are utilized to tally particular problems at school. Parent and teacher information can be used to evaluate the impact of treatment. Such data have the advantage of conveying the extent to which improvement has occurred in particular areas that may have served as the basis of referral. A large number of measurement strategies have been enumerated for single-case designs; these approaches are based on specifying clinical problems in concrete terms and assessing their frequency, duration, or occurrence within particular time intervals.[7,12]

Design Prerequisites

The design refers to the specific plan that will be used to evaluate the intervention. As with assessment, there are a few features that are crucial to single-case studies.

SEPARATE PHASES

Assessment is conducted continuously before and during treatment. Different phases or assessment periods need to be delineated. Usually the design begins with a pretreatment phase (referred to as baseline). Baseline data serve separate purposes that are essential for drawing inferences about treatment. The data *describe* the existing level of the problem; they also *predict* the likely level of performance in the immediate future. To a considerable extent the logic of single-case research depends on the fact that continuous data serve descriptive and predictive functions. Because there are multiple data points before treatment, one can extrapolate to what would happen if treatment were not implemented—that is, to what the likely course of symptoms would be in the very immediate future. There is an inherent measure of uncertainty in identifying the level of the symptoms and in any projection about their likely course over the next several days or weeks. In order to increase the confidence in these conclusions, multiple data points are needed. On most measures, performance is likely to fluctuate. Symptoms may improve or deteriorate over time. Even without treatment, baseline data are needed to provide a picture of performance and to note the direction of change, if any.

After a period of baseline observations, a treatment phase is initiated. Data continue to be collected. During the treatment phase the data obtained on performance also serve a number of functions. Again, the data describe the level of current performance. In addition, that level of performance is compared with the level of performance projected from the initial baseline phase. If the patient's actual performance departs markedly from that which would have been expected from an extrapolation of the baseline level, this is consistent with the view that treatment has produced an effect. Basically, then, the projected level of performance serves as a criterion that allows one to evaluate whether or not treatment produced change. From the standpoint of traditional methods of research and experimental design, baseline data include an implicit prediction that there will be no change (i.e., that performance will continue at the level of baseline even if treatment is begun). A test of this prediction is made when treatment begins, and treatment and baseline data are compared. Presumably, if treatment is effective, performance during the treatment phase will depart from the projected baseline level.

Such a comparison of data across baseline and treatment phases provides critical information about whether change has been achieved and whether or not the change is sufficiently great to be clinically useful. Yet single-case designs usually consist of more than initial baseline and treatment phases. With only these two phases, one cannot discern whether therapeutic changes are due to treatment or are the consequence of other influences in the patient's life that are unrelated to treatment. The goal of clinical research in general is to rule out alternative explanations of the data. Single-case studies include special arrangements (i.e., experimental designs) to help rule out the influence of extraneous factors that might explain the changes from baseline to treatment phases.

STABILITY OF PERFORMANCE

As already noted, the baseline data are used to predict the level of the patient's symptoms in the immediate future. Consequently, it is important to sample behavior on several occasions in order to discern the pattern of performance and to obtain a relatively stable rate. A stable rate refers to the absence of trend and to the fact that little variability or fluctuation is present in the data. A trend refers to a systematic increase or decrease in symptoms over time. For example, even in the absence of a special treatment, the symptoms of depression may systematically decrease over time. A trend toward improvement during baseline may make evaluation of treatment difficult because the anticipated treatment effect is in the same direction as baseline performance. Under such circumstances a veridical treatment effect might be difficult to distinguish from the projected course of change obtained from the baseline data. Ideally, baseline data show little or no trend or a trend in the direction opposite from what would be expected during treatment.

Excessive variability during baseline or other phases may also interfere with any conclusions that might be drawn about treatment effects. The data may reflect no symptoms on one day, severe symptoms on another day, and continue to oscillate in this fashion over time. With such extreme fluctuations it may be difficult to predict a stable level of performance in the immediate future. The extreme fluctuations may be clinically significant in their own right, and may then be focused on as part of treatment. However, from the standpoint of evaluation, extreme fluctuations may raise problems. As a general rule, the greater the variability in the data, the more difficult it is to draw conclusions about the effects of treatment. Alternatively, the greater the variability, the greater the change that is needed in the patient's behavior to produce a clear effect.

Trend and variability in the data are relative notions; whether they raise problems depends both on their degree and on other considerations, such as the number of assessment occasions and the strength of treatment effects. In practice, obtaining stable rates of performance is usually not a problem. The designs can tolerate a considerable degree of trend and instability because, as a rule, these parameters are affected by treatment and phase changes and hence are part of the treatment evaluation. In special instances where there are problems with trend or variability, several design options and statistical techniques can be readily applied to clarify the data and to draw inferences about the effects of the intervention.[6]

Selected Design Options

A large number of designs are available in clinical work. Two commonly used designs are illustrated here to convey the logic and application of single-case research. In addition, in order to convey their flexibility, an illustration is offered of the use of single-case designs in an improvised way.

ABAB DESIGNS

One sequence commonly used in research is referred to as the ABAB or reversal design. The approach is organized into separate phases, where *A* refers to the baseline (or no intervention) phase and *B* refers to the intervention (or treatment) phase. Each phase is implemented for a period of time (e.g., a specified number of days) in order to obtain a good sampling of the patient's behavior. The phases are alternated for the purpose of showing that it was the intervention (in the B phase) rather than any other influences that probably accounted for a given change.

As an illustration, Rosen and Rosen[14] treated a seven-year-old male, named Steve, for his frequent stealing of other children's property at school. To record the number of items Steve stole in class, his personal possessions and school items were marked. Periodically throughout the day (every fifteen minutes), a check was made to see what he had on his person, at his desk, and with his supplies. These observations were made throughout the project and used as the measure of stealing in class. After baseline observations, Steve was told he could earn points for having just his own items when checked and that he would lose points if someone else's possessions were discovered. The points he earned could be redeemed for class breaks, extra reading time, and items from a classroom "store."

The point system was evaluated in an ABAB design in which baseline (A) phases were alternated with intervention (B) phases. As evident in figure 23–1, when the point system was introduced, stealing dropped considerably. The effects can be seen by comparing the first two phases of the figure. Of course, it is possible that stealing would have decreased anyway as a result of extraneous factors that coincided with the onset of treatment. To examine this possibility, in a reversal or return-to-baseline phase, the point system was temporarily suspended for a few days. Stealing increased, which suggested that the intervention was indeed responsible for the change. The point system was then reinstated and stealing once again decreased, thus completing the requirements of the ABAB design. In the penultimate phase, the procedures were gradually withdrawn (faded) to reduce Steve's dependence on checking. He was checked only once every two hours but still earned points. In the follow-up phase, Steve's possessions were no longer marked and all points and fines were discontinued. Stealing other children's possessions remained at a near-zero rate over the thirty-one-day follow-up period. Overall, the effects of the intervention were clearly demonstrated. In explaining the results, the pattern in the data makes it implausible to ascribe the changes to the effects of extraneous factors (e.g., spontaneous improvements over time).

The essential feature of an ABAB design is the alternation of phases over time in order to assess whether treatment produces change. Inferences may be drawn about the effects of treatment both by comparing performance in adjacent phases and from the overall pattern of data across all phases. If a child's performance changes when the intervention is introduced, reverts back to baseline levels when treatment is briefly suspended, and improves once again when the intervention is reintroduced, then the case for the impact of the intervention is very strong. Although from the standpoint of research the design is very clear, it bears an obvious liability for clinical work. Temporarily suspending the intervention is tantamount to making the child worse. Many alternative single-case designs that avoid this problem are available for use in clinical work.

MULTIPLE-BASELINE DESIGNS

One such possibility is a multiple-baseline design. This includes a number of variations, each of which demonstrates the effects of treatment without reverting to baseline conditions. The special feature of the multiple-baseline design is that treatment is introduced sequentially across different aspects of performance. Two or more baselines are assessed and may include different symptoms (e.g., aggressive acts, noncompliance) or the same problem in several different situations (e.g., at home and at school). The effects of treatment are demonstrated if changes occur when treatment is applied and these changes occur in sequence as treatment is extended to each symptom or situation.

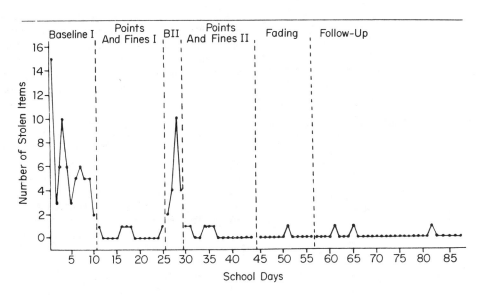

FIGURE 23-1

Number of Items Stolen Each School Day by Steve During Baseline (A), Intervention (B), Fading, and Follow-up Conditions

NOTE: Reprinted from p. 60, H. S. Rosen and L. A. Rosen, "Eliminating Stealing: Use of Stimulus Control with an Elementary Student," in *Behavior Modification,* 7 (1983):56–63. Reprinted by permission of Sage Publications.

As an illustration, Frame and her colleagues[2] evaluated hospital treatment with a ten-year old boy with a DSM-III diagnosis of major depression. Evaluation of the child revealed several prominent features, including avoidance of social interaction with others. This was evident in the form of poor eye contact, bodily positions that turned away from others, inaudible and constricted speech, and bland affect. These areas in turn served as the focus of a treatment plan. The intervention was provided in individual sessions five times per week over a five-week period. Before and during treatment, interviews were conducted with the child in order to assess the specific social behaviors just noted. The interviews were videotaped and evaluated by blind raters who scored each of the behaviors. The treatment was conducted individually by a therapist; it consisted of training the child to interact in a variety of interpersonal situations. The therapist modeled specific social behaviors, encouraged the child to practice what was modeled, and provided praise and feedback as needed to improve socially appropriate interaction. The training procedure was introduced across the different social behaviors at different points in time in order to meet the requirements of a multiple-baseline design.

As evident in figure 23–2, treatment began with the first two behaviors (eye contact and body position), each of which served as the focus of the sessions. The figure reveals that marked changes occurred in both behaviors when treatment was introduced. The other behaviors that were not focused on at this time remained at baseline levels. When training was extended to these other behaviors, they changed as well. In general, the pattern of change indicated that each behavior changed when the intervention was introduced, and not before. The sequence suggests that it was the intervention which accounted for the change rather than any extraneous factors such as contact with the therapist, repeated assessment, or exposure to social situations in training. Follow-up assessment twelve weeks after all training had been terminated indicated that the gains were maintained.

IMPROVISED DESIGNS FOR CLINICAL WORK

The preceding examples were chosen for illustrative purposes in order to convey basic features of the designs. However, it may be that this was accomplished at the expense of noting how the designs may be appropriate in actual practice. In the course of clinical work, the clinician may be unable to identify the maximally effective intervention. Implementation of a given treatment may produce no change or only a small change. A particular treatment may need to be supplemented, augmented, or simply discarded. The important feature of single-case designs is that they can be improvised readily in response to the effects that treatment exerts on the individual patient. Treatments can be implemented and altered in separate phases until thera-

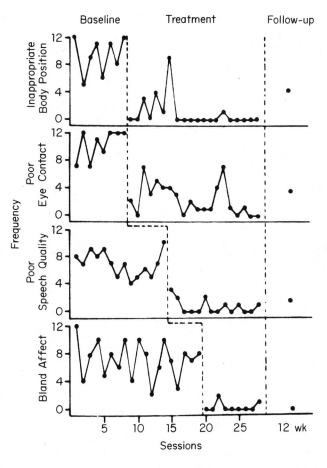

FIGURE 23–2

Frequency of Social Behaviors of a Depressed Boy as Measured During Assessment Interviews

NOTE: Reprinted with permission from p. 241 in C. Frame, et al, in Behavioral Treatment of Depression in a Prepubertal Child. *Journal of Behavior Therapy and Experimental Psychiatry,* 13 (1982):239–243, Pergamon Press, Inc.

peutic change is achieved. The clinician can add new interventions or bolster the one currently in place. Each change denotes a separate phase and can be evaluated as such.

An illustration of an improved design with multiple phases is provided by Wells and associates,[16] who evaluated the effects of medication and self-control procedures on the hyperactive behavior of a nine-year-old hospitalized boy. The basis for the referral included poor concentration and unmanageable and aggressive behavior. In a variation of an ABAB design, the effects of dextroamphetamine sulfate (Dexedrine) and methylphenidate hydrochloride (Ritalin) on classroom performance were evaluated in the hospital. Two of the measures (off-task behavior and inappropriate gross motor behavior) are illustrated in figure 23–3. It is

clear that relative to baseline (phases 1 and 3), Dexedrine (phase 2) did not yield improvements in behavior. The use of Ritalin may have led to some improvement, but clearly further intervention was needed. The investigators added a self-control procedure in which the child was trained to monitor his own behavior and to provide himself with tokens if he was on task. The combined self-control and medication regimen had a marked impact on behavior. To evaluate the impact of the combined procedure, the child was switched to placebo and then to medication again, all the time retaining the self-control procedure. The pattern of change suggests that the combination of medication with the self-control procedure accounted for the change. The design illustrates the importance of continuous assessment and the utility of altering treatment in response to the data.

GENERAL COMMENTS

The preceding designs convey only a small fraction of the options available in clinical applications of single-case research.[1,6] Each of the designs is characterized by continuous assessment of the symptoms or dysfunction over time. As with any empirical research, the designs make comparisons of some sort, usually between ratings of performance with and without treatment or with alternative forms of treatment. In ABAB designs, comparisons involve performance under baseline (or return-to-baseline) and treatment conditions or multiple treatment conditions. In multiple-baseline designs, either untreated symptoms or performance in situations where treatment has yet to be introduced serves as the comparison conditions. With both designs, the effects of the intervention are judged in part on the basis of comparing treatment either with no treatment, with placebo, or with alternative treatment conditions.

Special Considerations

FEASIBILITY IN CLINICAL SETTINGS

The assessment and design prerequisites may raise questions about whether single-case strategies are feasible for clinical work. In many cases, it may be possible only to approximate certain features of such designs. Even so, approximations are likely to increase the validity of the inferences that can be drawn about the effects of intervention on child dysfunction.[5]

Both the designs and the assessment strategies that they embrace are flexible, a feature that makes their

Single-Subject Methodology and Hyperactivity

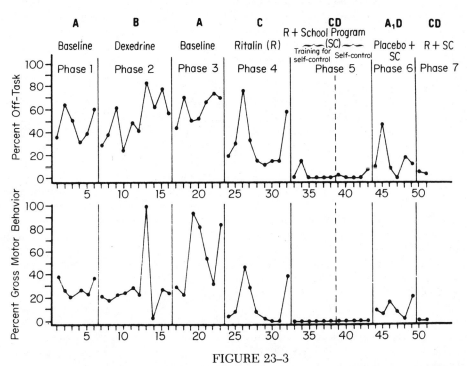

FIGURE 23–3

Percent occurrence in the classroom of off-task and gross motor behavior. The data were obtained in a variation of an ABAB design with baseline (A phase) and alternative treatment (B, C, D alone and in combination) phases. SC and R refer to self-control and Ritalin, respectively.

NOTE: Reprinted with permission from K.C. Wells et al., in "Use of Single-Subject Methodology in Clinical Decision-Making with a Hyperactive Child on the Psychiatric Inpatient Unit," *Behavioral Assessment*, 3 (1981):359–369, Pergamon Press, Inc.

clinical use quite feasible. There are options available to the clinician that permit approximations of the designs even under the usual constraints and exigencies of clinical work. For example, it may not be possible for a therapist to assess the child's symptoms daily in outpatient treatment. Yet it may be feasible daily, or almost daily, for a parent or teacher to complete a brief rating form or checklist that defines the child's problems concretely. In some instances, a parent may be called and interviewed briefly in order to obtain daily information on selected clinical problems in the home.[13] Assessment information is needed to clarify the pattern of performance over time and to determine whether a particular form of treatment affects that pattern. Even if daily assessment is not feasible, this goal can still be achieved.

Implementation of particular single-case designs may also not be feasible for a given clinical case. For example, ABAB designs may require temporarily withdrawing the intervention after clinical improvements have been achieved; obviously, in most clinical situations this is unacceptable. Analogously, multiple-baseline designs may require producing highly specific effects with an intervention so that one can see changes only in selected symptoms or only in respect to performance in selected situations. Yet many interventions (e.g., medication, psychotherapy) either tend to produce or are intended to produce broad effects that might not be identified by the design. These concerns need not be ignored in the use of single-case design strategies. It is feasible to utilize features of the designs by beginning with baseline phases and then assessing performance in separate phases where different treatments (e.g., medication, psychotherapy) or variations of a single treatment (e.g., different medication doses) are administered. The resulting information greatly strengthens any conclusions about therapeutic change and the factors to which such change might be attributed.

Rather than present obstacles, single-case designs may introduce benefits into clinical work. Continuous assessment provides ongoing data about treatment progress and yields critical information to the clinician. The data provide feedback regarding whether treatment is producing change or enough change to be clinically important. If the effects need to be augmented, changes can be made in treatment or alternative treatments can be applied. The use of data to monitor change and to make decisions about treatment can enhance the quality of clinical care in the same way that medical assessment (e.g., urine glucose tests) can provide feedback regarding the adequacy of a particular treatment regimen (e.g., regulation of insulin, diet, and exercise). The assessment data provide the basis of judging the adequacy of treatment and whether changes are needed.

GENERALITY OF RESULTS

A salient concern with single-case research is that the results demonstrated in a particular case may not be generalizable to other persons. The issue is usually raised in the context of between-group research where an intervention (e.g., medication) is evaluated by comparing groups of subjects who receive alternative conditions. The concern over generality can be addressed at the level of both research and clinical work.

At the level of research, group studies do not necessarily produce more generalizable results than single-case research. In most between-group studies, results are evaluated on the basis of average (mean) group performance. That one group produces an *average effect* greater than another group does not say anything about how many persons were affected by the intervention or affected to a clinically significant degree. Individual data need to be scrutinized in order to determine how generalizable treatment effects were within the study. Even so, until additional research is conducted, the question of generalizability to samples not included in the study remains open.

In clinical work, the immediate goal is to ameliorate the conditions and dysfunction that brought the patient to treatment. It is quite possible the effects of treatment may not be generalizable to other patients. This is not a special problem or prospect raised by single-case research; it is evident in clinical applications of medical or psychiatric treatment that focus on one or a few cases. The traditional uncontrolled case study has the same problem. The unique benefit of single-case designs is that they permit much more to be said about the effects of treatment for that case, and they provide evidence that the patient's problem has indeed been altered as intended.

Although individual differences always need to be recognized, the efficacy of alternative treatments is not entirely idiosyncratic. Generality of treatment effects is likely to vary as a function of many things, including strength, dose, duration, and other parameters of treatment in addition to the characteristics of patients and the nature of their disorders. Treatments demonstrated to be effective in single-case research are not less generalizable than those identified in group research. Indeed, important parameters of treatment can often be intensively studied and best identified with individual cases in order to determine the most potent way to implement treatment.

Both in clinical work and research, the ultimate test of generality of findings is replication—that is, repeated demonstration of treatment effects across patient samples. Replications help examine the extent to which results obtained in one demonstration extend to other realms such as cases, populations, settings, measures, disorders, clinicians, and treatment sites. Thus the way to answer questions of generality of single-case research is the same as it is for group research—through independent replications of treatment effects. For clinical work, the important feature of single-case designs is that they provide objective information about the effects of treatment. The information can be accumulated across cases so that the generality of treatment effects can be examined with a basis in data rather than on the authority of an anecdotal record of what seems to have worked.

ETHICAL ISSUES

Research desiderata are often seen as competing with the exigencies of clinical care. As a result, integration of assessment and research into clinical work can raise important ethical issues. For example, in a between-group research treatment protocol, patients may be randomly assigned to medication, placebo, or no-treatment conditions. Ethical and professional concerns obviously are raised if a patient in need of treatment is assigned to a condition that is not likely to improve functioning. In single-case research, the demands of the design could also raise problems and might indeed be difficult to justify in a given case. For example, the urgency of clinical intervention (e.g., medication for a depressed and suicidal patient) may preclude obtaining baseline data over an extended period prior to intervening. Yet this would not interfere with continuous assessment over the course of the treatment and subsequent evaluation after treatment is altered (e.g., withdrawn or reduced).

Not all clinical problems will require immediate clinical intervention without the opportunity for collecting adequate baseline data. Baseline assessment should not be viewed as an obstacle that delays treatment but rather as part of a careful clinical work-up. Baseline data provide important information about how, where, and whether to intervene. Continuous assessment before and during treatment further offers the clinician an objective and operational basis for evaluating ongoing treatment and for making decisions about how to proceed.

Final Comments

Single-case designs are important because they increase the prospect of evaluating treatment for the individual patient and they take advantage of the tremendous potential of clinical work for generating knowledge about treatments. The special function of the methodology is that it may serve to reduce the hiatus between clinical research and clinical practice. The designs permit an ongoing evaluation of patient progress over time; hence they provide an empirically based means for making decisions about treatment. In many ways, single-case designs do not add new features to clinical work; continuous evaluation and decision making about treatment are inherent in any therapeutic endeavor. What the methodology offers is a systematic way of evaluating dysfunction and obtaining a clearer basis for decision making. In addition, the designs permit the clinician to evaluate whether it was the treatment instead of some extraneous factors that was responsible for a particular therapeutic change. Thus the strength of the inferences that can be drawn is much greater than would be achieved from the usual uncontrolled case study.

Single-case designs do not replace other methods of research such as between-group trials of alternative treatments. The strategies are quite complementary and mutually interdependent. Findings from large-scale research need to be evaluated at the level of the individual case in clinical practice where the most demanding conditions of treatment exist. Use of single-case methodology may be valuable not only as a way of increasing the scientific knowledge base that emerges from clinical work but also as a proving ground for findings obtained from large-scale clinical trials.

ACKNOWLEDGMENT

Completion of this manuscript was facilitated by a Research Scientist Development Award (MH00353) from the National Institute of Mental Health.

REFERENCES

1. BARLOW, D. H., and HERSEN, M. *Single-case Experimental Designs: Strategies for Studying Behavior Change,* 2nd ed. New York: Pergamon Press, 1984.

2. FRAME, C., et al. "Behavioral Treatment of Depression in a Prepubertal Child," *Journal of Behavior Therapy and Experimental Psychiatry,* 13 (1982):239–243.

3. GRIEST, D. L., and WELLS, K. C. "Behavioral Family Therapy with Conduct Disorders in Children," *Behavior Therapy,* 14 (1983):37–53.

4. KAZDIN, A. E. *Research Design in Clinical Psychology.* New York: Harper & Row, 1980.

5. ———. "Drawing Valid Inferences from Case Studies," *Journal of Consulting and Clinical Psychology,* 41 (1981): 183–192.

6. ———. *Single-case Research Designs: Methods for Clinical and Applied Settings.* New York: Oxford University Press, 1982.

7. ———. *Behavior Modification in Applied Settings,* 3rd ed. Homewood, Ill.: Dorsey Press, 1984.

8. KAZDIN, A. E., and TUMA, A. H., eds. *New Directions for Methodology of Social and Behavioral Sciences: Single-case Research Designs.* San Francisco: Jossey-Bass, 1982.

9. KRAEPELIN, E. *Compendium der Psychiatrie.* Leipzig: Abel, 1883.

10. LAZARUS, A. A., and DAVIDSON, G. C. "Clinical Innovation in Research and Practice," in A. E. Bergin and S. L. Garfield, eds., *Handbook of Psychotherapy and Behavior Change: An Empirical Analysis,* New York: John Wiley & Sons, 1971, pp. 196–213.

11. MASH, E. J., and TERDAL, L. E., eds. *Behavioral Assessment of Childhood Disorders.* New York: Guilford Press, 1981.

12. NELSON, R. O. "Realistic Dependent Measures for Clinical Use," *Journal of Consulting and Clinical Psychology,* 49 (1981):168–182.

13. PATTERSON, G. R. *Coercive Family Process.* Eugene, Ore.: Castalia, 1982.

14. ROSEN, H. S., and ROSEN, L. A. "Eliminating Stealing: Use of Stimulus Control with an Elementary Student," *Behavior Modification,* 7 (1983):56–63.

15. THIGPEN, C. H., and CLECKLEY, H. M. *Three Faces of Eve.* New York: McGraw-Hill, 1957.

16. WELLS, K. C., et al. "Use of Single-subject Methodology in Clinical Decision-making with a Hyperactive Child on the Psychiatric Inpatient Unit," *Behavioral Assessment,* 3 (1981):359–369.

SECTION IV

Deviations of Development: Etiology, Nosology, and Syndromes

Joseph D. Noshpitz and Saul I. Harrison / Editors

Introduction / Child and Adolescent Psychiatric Syndromes: Status and Prospects

Saul I. Harrison

In the years since the publication of volume II of this *Handbook* in 1979, the delineation of child psychiatric syndromes has been influenced significantly by the publication in 1980 of the *Diagnostic and Statistical Manual of Mental Disorders,* 3rd edition (DSM-III), by the American Psychiatric Association (APA). The preparation of this manual represents progress in nosologic striving for objective phenomenologic rigor.

When the first such manual, DSM-I, appeared in 1952,[2] it was comprised of presumably etiological dynamic "reactions." Comparison with the more reliably replicable descriptive behavioral criteria inherent in DSM-III's syndromes highlights the explicit effort on the part of DSM-III's framers to exclude etiological and theoretical considerations. Each classificatory system parallels its time and reflects the prevailing American psychiatric zeitgeist. Lacking special attention to children, DSM-I represented a blending of Adolph Meyer's psychobiology with the psychodynamic ferment and fervor following World War II. In contrast to this, DSM-III is intertwined with diagnostic criteria evolved in the course of investigations with a biological emphasis.

Despite DSM-III's imperfections and the fact that precise behavioral criteria sometimes call for subjective judgments, its appearance places us on the threshold of an era in which rational, publicly documentable, replicable strategies will replace some of those aspects of our clinical traditions that have bordered on folklore and mythology. As these words are being written, DSM-III R (revision) is in preparation and there are expectations that laboratory criteria might enrich and further objectify DSM-IV.

It is vital to remember, however, that despite the fact that these diagnostic classificatory systems convey a sense of scientific truth, they are not the result of empirical research (as is Achenbach and Edelbrock's[1] system, which is derived from cluster and factor analysis). Instead, DSM-III was developed by committee compromise and consensus, following which it had to be approved by majority vote of additional APA bodies. In short, the data on which it is based are largely uncontrolled and their validity remains uncertain. Nevertheless, the operational diagnostic criteria in

DSM-III may suggest a degree of precision and certainty that lends itself to misuse by reinforcing a spurious black-and-white clinical assessment mindset. Such a reification of diagnostic categories can sabotage clinical evaluations, which, at our current level of knowledge, inevitably entail a probabilistic approach. All of us have observed efforts to force clinical data that do not fit into any of the delineated diagnostic categories into procrustean conformity. The risk of such enforced conformity is enhanced with children and adolescents because DSM-III devotes minimal attention to developmental considerations.

To some extent DSM-III reflects the growing employment of rating scales in clinical research activities. In turn, the manual has spawned still more such instruments and has generated increasing use of structured interviews and rating scales in clinical practice as well as in clinical research. There are both advantages and potential pitfalls inherent in this interplay between DSM-III and rating scales.

It cannot be emphasized too strongly that using such systematic methods to handle uncertainty requires meticulous care lest we lose sight of the human being codified in the rating scale. This risk exists not only in clinical practice but also in those clinical research activities whose refinement has been so enhanced by the employment of rating scales.

On the other hand, the predetermined question format of structured interviews entails an advantage that is highlighted by recalling the epistemology of the concept of childhood depression. Clearly, there are a multitude of reasons why the field took so long to acknowledge the existence of this syndrome. One of the delaying factors stems from the longstanding tradition in child psychiatric assessment of deriving factual data from interviews with the parents or other caretakers; the evaluative interview with the child was designed primarily to illuminate dynamic themes expressed in play. For years, clinicians asked parents about depressive affect and elicited negative responses while neglecting to ask the child directly. Today we know that if the rapport and the phrasing of the inquiry are appropriate, youngsters do respond affirmatively. (It cannot be underscored too strongly that highlighting this particular factor contributing to delay in recognition of childhood depression in no way diminishes the influence of other factors. These include the prevailing adult bias that childhood should be a joyful, carefree time and sometimes appears to be so even in the face of misery and devastation. Also, there were presumed to be theoretical obstacles to the existence of sustained depression prior to certain developmental achievements. In fact, due to developmental modifications in the expression of affect, children's manifestations of depression, grief, and bereavement differ from those of adults.)

The adaptation and extension by DSM-III of the multiaxial system inherent in the World Health Organization's child psychiatric classificatory proposals[4] represent an encouraging advance. But much more progress is required before we can leave behind all remnants of the sense that current psychiatric diagnoses are conceptually comparable to the medical diagnoses employed earlier in this century—for example, fever, rheumatism, and pleurisy. At that time it was possible, for instance, to diagnose pleural inflammation reliably and with validity; however, that precise categorization contained no information regarding etiology and treatment. The chapters that follow catalogue the progress our field is making in outgrowing such analogies.

REFERENCES

1. ACHENBACH, T. M., and EDELBROCK, C. S. "The Classification of Child Psychopathology: A Review and Analysis of Empirical Efforts," *Psychological Bulletin,* 85 (1978):1275–1301.

2. AMERICAN PSYCHIATRIC ASSOCIATION. *Diagnostic and Statistical Manual of Mental Disorders,* 1st ed. (DSM-I). Washington, D.C.: American Psychiatric Association, 1952.

3. ———. *Diagnostic and Statistical Manual of Mental Disorders,* 3rd ed. (DSM-III). Washington, D.C.: American Psychiatric Association, 1980.

4. RUTTER, M., SHAFFER, D., and SHEPHERD, M. *A Multiaxial Classification of Child Psychiatric Disorders.* Geneva: World Health Organization, 1975.

PART A
Etiology

24 / Stress and Its Implications for Child Mental Health

R. Dean Coddington

Whatsoever therefore makes the blood to boyl, or raises it into an effervescence, as violent motion of the body or minde, the drinking of wine, venery, yea sometimes mere heat of the Bed doth cause asthmatical assults to such as are predisposed.

—THOMAS WILLIS, 1679

Introduction

The necessity of maintaining a homeostatic balance within the body was articulated by the great French physiologist Claude Bernard[7] over one hundred years ago and by Walter Cannon[11] in the early part of this century. In his life table, Adolf Meyer[47] focused attention on specific life events that in essence amounted to a graphic developmental history. Many psychiatrists had previously emphasized the importance of traumatic events; Meyer, however, was the first to consider positive, desirable events to be significant. In 1950 Selye[59] formulated his General-Adaptation-Syndrome (G-A-S) and suggested that any agent—a change in occupation, for instance—capable of eliciting an alarm reaction should be termed a stressor. In the face of any given stress, he postulated a transient emotional "adaptational crisis" that was followed by a systemic resistance to the stressor. If the stress persisted the G-A-S ensued and continued until a state of exhaustion set in.

At this point some form of maladaptation or disease would appear. In the mid-1960s, Holmes and his colleagues[34,46] set forth a list of stressful events. They used a psychophysical method to determine a weight to be assigned to each item in the list. In order to measure the amount of readjustment required of an individual, they summed the weights of the events that had occurred over a year's time. These investigators contended that it was not the positive or negative valence ordinarily attached to the particular event that made the difference. Rather the crucial factor was change from the status quo. Using the same methodology, Coddington[13,14] developed life-event scales for children and adolescents, scales that were later modified when data from adolescent raters were taken into account.[16] Several other scales have since been proposed for work with this age group, and preliminary work[23,69,71] supports their use as valid instruments. For a more thorough discussion of historical events, the reader is referred to Henry and Stephens' well-written monograph.[32]

Change as a Stressor

The concept that change itself can be stressful was suggested by Meyer[47] and by Selye[59] and articulated clearly by Holmes and Rahe.[34] Several authors have questioned this assumption, arguing that negative events are more highly correlated with illness than are positive events.* Tennant, Bebbington, and Hurry[63] have pointed out the beneficial effect of *neutralizing events,* that is, positive events following and apparently ameliorating the effect of negative events. Brown and Harris[9] and Rutter[56] have emphasized the need to have the subject define the event as positive or negative. Though each of these approaches is valid, none really resolves the problem of either true ambivalence regarding some event or the likelihood of an event carrying opposite valences at different times. A divorce may at first end the fighting but somewhat later result in loneliness and despair. Holmes and Rahe's argument seems most logical; any event requires an adjustment, and adjustments require emotional and physical energy in order to maintain homeostasis. Although couched in endocrinological terms, this is precisely the same formulation presented by Selye. There are empirical data on both sides of the debate and considerable anecdotal evidence.† [16,50]

General systems theory encourages the use of cross-level analogies. Since the maintainance of homeostasis is a biological function, we should be able to find other living systems at lower and higher organizational levels in which the effect of positive as well as negative events can be observed.

LOWER-LEVEL SYSTEMS

Jennings[38] made extensive studies of the responses of unicellular organisms (e.g., amoeba, paramecium, infusoria) and other lower life forms to a number of changes, none of which was particularly adverse or injurious to the organism. These included alterations in temperature, salinity, nutrients, oxygen, water currents, and light. He found that it was a change in the concentration or intensity of the agent that seemed important, and this led him to conclude that *change simply as change may produce reaction.*

During his work with cultures of cardiac muscle cells, Kasten‡ discovered that they contracted rhythmically while under a microscope but that the contractions ceased when new medium was added. The rate at which the medium was added seemed critical. If the flow were slow enough, the cells continued to contract,

but as the flow increased to what appeared to be too great a rate, the cells ceased contracting, although, after a period of time, they began once again.

An interesting hypothesis has been put forward by Schmid[58] to explain the high incidence of cancer reported among top athletes in later life. He suggested that whereas exercise was beneficial, the cells being flushed with abundant oxygen, the common practice of twice-daily training to the point of exhaustion resulted in repetitive disturbances of homeostasis. In his view it was this frequent positive event of increased oxygen that may have altered cellular metabolism in a way that led to an activation of oncogenic genes.

It would seem that positive as well as negative events occurring in a cell's environment produce a reaction and that either the reaction may be temporarily detrimental (e.g., the cessation of contraction of myocardial cells) or the cells may be permanently altered (as Schmid hypothesizes).

HIGHER-LEVEL SYSTEMS

In the business world it is well known that a company that finds itself in a very favorable economic climate encounters a particular kind of hazard. It may be tempted to expand too rapidly and exceed its credit rating because it has underestimated the time required for money to flow back. The result of this positive economic situation may therefore be bankruptcy.

Henry and Cassel[31] have reviewed the socioanthropological literature in search of genealogically similar but geographically distinct groups that differ in their propensity for developing hypertension with advancing age. These investigators concluded that a stable society, well equipped with a cultural background to deal with a familiar world, will not be conducive to the development of hypertension among its aged members. However, when radical cultural changes of seemingly positive character disrupt the familiar environment, age-related hypertension may eventuate.

In his analysis of the effects of socioeconomic change, Brenner[8] matched the unemployment rate and changes in per-capita income over time against a number of indicators of pathology in the population: cardiovascular mortality, death from cirrhosis of the liver, first admissions to mental institutions, homicide, suicide, and criminal activity. Although the response to unemployment was more intense and occurred over a five-year period, the desirable change of rapid economic growth had a similar effect, although only for about one year.

Thus, although an undesirable event may be more detrimental to most people than an equally weighted desirable event, it would be a mistake at this point to disregard the fact that desirable events do function as potential stressors. In brief, it appears that change itself

---

*See references 9, 19, 25, 49, 53, and 57.

†Tennessee Williams wrote an eloquent essay that appeared in the New York *Times* Drama Section, 30 November 1947—four days before the New York opening of *A Streetcar Named Desire.* The essay, entitled *On A Streetcar Named Success,* describes the traumatic transformation of his life following the successful production three years earlier of *The Glass Menagerie.* Williams became significantly depressed as the royalty checks, which eliminated his need to struggle for bare existence, began rolling in. This essay is reproduced as the introduction to *A Streetcar Named Desire,* published as a Signet Book by New American Library, New York, 1947.

‡F. Kasten, personal communication, 1984.

is at once growth promoting and potentially dangerous.

Stress and Childhood Morbidity

In 1973 a retrospective investigation of several groups of ill children was carried out by Coddington's group.[29] Children with juvenile rheumatoid arthritis, general pediatric patients, surgical patients, and psychiatric patients had all experienced more frequent and/or more distressing life events in the year preceding the onset of their illnesses than did same-aged children in a separately studied healthy population.[14] This work was later confirmed by Kashani and coworkers[40] and by Beautrais, Fergusson and Shannon[5,6] in an extensive prospective study of a birth cohort of 1,082 New Zealand children. Family life events were associated with increased risk; this was expressed in the form of medical consultation and hospital attendance for illness of the lower respiratory tract, gastroenteritis, accidents, burns, scalds, and accidental poisoning. In a smaller prospective investigation,[44] Margolis and Farran followed children of recently unemployed parents. They reported that over the first few months there was a greater risk for episodes of illness in general and for infectious diseases in particular.

In young children either specific stressors or high life-event scores have been reported to be associated with infectious disease,[27] chest pain,[3] burn accidents,[43] pica,[60] speech problems[67] and behavioral problems.[6] In older children and adolescents the connection has been with peptic ulcer disease[1] and juvenile rheumatoid arthritis.[28,30] Among adolescents, high life-event scores have been implicated as contributing factors to psychiatric hospitalization,[4,29,65] suicide,[36] delinquency,[4] substance abuse,[20,64] automobile accidents,[35,36] pregnancy,[15] and football injuries.[17]

Vulnerability Versus Invulnerability

A number of studies have been cited that suggest that in both children and adolescents, stressors are sometimes followed by accidents, illnesses, and emotional problems. The associations are statistically significant but their correlations are ordinarily low, 0.2 to 0.4. That is to say, following stressful life events, some children do develop physical or behavioral symptoms that might allow a casual relationship to be inferred, but many children do not. Why are not all children equally susceptible?

We know from the work of Hinkle[33] that the presence of disease is not equally distributed among all adults; 25 percent of the population in fact experiences 50 percent of the illnesses. Starfield and associates[62] have shown that in a large prepaid medical plan, about 37 percent of the children account for 50 percent of the illness episodes (though it is possible that emotional problems were not reported as reliably as were physical illnesses). Gottschalk[26] asserts that these epidemiological studies have been adequately confirmed. The fact that some adults remain relatively free of disease is particularly well demonstrated by the work of Stewart Wolf and his group.[10] These investigators studied the town of Roseto, Pennsylvania, and the neighboring town of Bangor. Residents of Roseto were remarkably healthy, a condition attributed to their group cohesiveness and the maintenance of their cultural heritage with clearly defined male and female roles.

However, notwithstanding the work of Starfield's group, the situation may be quite different in children. Kessler[42] says, for instance, "that the incidence of reactive disorders is universal; it is difficult to conceive of a human being progressing from infancy through adolescence without trauma sufficient to interfere, at least temporarily, with psychosocial development" (p. 177). Likewise, Wallerstein and Kelly[66] have found very few, if any, children or adolescents to come through a divorce completely unscathed. Murphy and Moriarty[50] also concluded that no child was invulnerable. At one time or another, when confronted with threatening or stressful experiences all children exhibited some loss of their best functioning.

Nevertheless, Garmezy[24] has pointed out that certain children from chaotic families seem *invulnerable.* He cites the work of Mary Engel,[22] who described children from impoverished and broken homes who had apparently learned to cope surprisingly well. These children may have still suffered a significant loss of their *potential* functioning, but we know there is tremendous individual variation and Garmezy's opinion cannot be taken lightly. It is imperative to learn to what degree genetic factors, temperament, and early experiences account for variations in children's responses to stressors. What determines the limits of the homeostatic plateau within which a child can adjust to change without distress? What circumstances lower the threshold, sensitizing the child to stressor effect, and what circumstances raise it?

While it is unlikely that any child is invulnerable to the effect of change, some seem relatively so. Under certain conditions involving sociopsychological and intrapsychic support systems, growth into adulthood seems to carry with it an increase or decrease in one's sensitivity to stressors. This accounts for the well-established epidemiological fact that throughout their lives some people remain remark-

able healthy, while others suffer from a disproportionate amount of illness.

Coping with Stress

In a review of his own work and that of his colleagues
at Harvard and the Hebrew University of Jerusalem,
Caplan[12] divided the process of mastery into four in-
terdigitating phases. Phase 1 is behavior that changes
the stressful environment or enables the individual to
escape from it. This involves goal-directed, problem-
solving behavior in the world of reality. The individual's capacity for effective problem solving is felt to be
influenced by previous successes or failures. Caplan
also asserted that perseverance in problem solving is
dependent on both the *individual's* expectation of a
certain amount of pain and suffering and the belief that
other similar persons are capable of tolerating the discomfort.

Phase 2 is behavior devoted to acquiring new
capabilities for action in order to change the external
circumstances and their aftermath. Individuals may be
capable of developing more effective problem-solving
skills through generic educational and training programs. They may also be taught to endure more discomfort than they had previously been able to tolerate.
This has been accomplished in educational programs
for children[51,61] and in the Outward Bound program
for adolescents.[37] In this context Caplan also emphasizes the capacity to be able to recognize when one is
approaching his or her limits and the need for skill in
initiating the mobilization of a support system. Similarly, workshops on stress management have been
found to be effective in preventing maladaptive responses in adults.[39,55]

The third and fourth phases involve intrapsychic
processes, first the response to emotional arousal and
dysphoria that calls forth ego defenses and second,
grief work, which may take a long time to resolve.
Throughout Caplan's formulation is the emphasis that
support groups are needed at every phase: family,
friends, and the fellow members of small (e.g., athletic
team) and large (e.g., religious) groups.

Parker and Brown[52] demonstrated the value of
thinking through a problem and discussing it with
warm friends or relatives. These serve as coping mechanisms that mediate effectively between stressful events
and the development of depression.

The cognitive aspects of Caplan's formulation (i.e.,
Phases 1 and 2) are undoubtedly correct, and they raise
some interesting questions for child psychiatrists, particularly in view of the suggestion of relative invulnerability discussed earlier. Are we preparing children to

cope with the modern world, or are our child-rearing
practices and advice more appropriate for encountering the world of a generation ago? A stimulating environment enhances language, motor, and cognitive development. Are there other coping skills we could
teach by challenging children to deal with age-appropriate stressors?

The Outward Bound program mentioned earlier had
its roots in World War II. At the time, it was discovered that when adrift on a life raft after their boat was
torpedoed, young, inexperienced but physically fit mer-
chant seamen did not survive as long as did their older,
more experienced shipmates who were, in general, in
poorer physical condition. Kurt Hahn built a training
program that taught men that they could do more than
they thought they could do, both physically and mentally. One objective was to demonstrate that they could
survive for a few days even if alone on a life raft. A
similar *solo experience* became part of all subsequent
traditional Outward Bound programs. To be alone on
a tiny island with no sounds except for the occasional
chatter of a red squirrel, no task to accomplish except
to exist, and no food except for what can be found or
caught is for most people both unique and at least
mildly stressful. But it is also challenging and seems to
be growth promoting. As Miller[48] put it, "If I can stop
the roller coaster, I don't want to get off," meaning, of
course, that if one has control of a situation, it is less
stressful.

Can similar stressors be designed for younger children and yet be morally acceptable? In every culture
within which an attempt has been made to measure
relative stressfulness, the loss of a love object is far and
away the most significant life event. Marital separations and divorces are becoming ever more frequent.
Can or should we prepare children to cope with such
an eventuality by designing a graded series of brief
separations from first one and then both parents? Is
silence—that is, lack of stimulation—a stressor with
which children should learn to cope? Boredom seems
to plague many latency-age children and adolescents.
Is it possible that this is a consequence of our earlier
efforts to provide stimulating environments combined
with the youngsters' own inability to maintain that
level of stimulation as they begin to fend for themselves? Would life seem less boring to individuals who
had had a solo experience?

Clinical Implications

We know that children and adolescents are constantly
adjusting to changes in the environment. We know too
that change is both growth promoting and at times

detrimental. Given those verities, the need for child psychiatrists to have a firm understanding of the complexities in the field becomes obvious. Such knowledge requires further scientific research.

Life-event lists used as screening devices can help in either longitudinal prospective studies or short, retrospective studies. However, to depend on them as valid indicators of stressors that occurred more than six months earlier is unwise. There are two reasons for this: The effect of a stressor seems to diminish rapidly as intrapsychic mechanisms come into play,[16] and there is a tendency for people to recall stressful events as chronologically related to the onset of an illness when, in fact, they were not. No life-event list should ever be viewed as a substitute for a good interview. The two methods can, however, be combined nicely into a semistructured interview. Child psychiatrists who use such a technique routinely in clinical practice would soon come across children who seemed to cope surprisingly well in some situations but not in others. Careful study of the child's coping mechanisms would be very helpful. Even more helpful would be longitudinal studies of healthy, nonreferred children in which life-event data were collected regularly at three- or four-month intervals. If some children are indeed invulnerable, we have much to learn from them.

The development of a child's coping style has not been systematically studied. We know that newborn infants vary in terms of their autonomic reactivity. We know too that young children vary in terms of temperament. These facts may represent a genetic contribution to the ability to master, at a later age, environmental stressors. The impulsive child, for instance, may escape from the stressor or may immediately lash out aggressively but, in so doing, miss the opportunity to learn from the experience. Caplan's formulation regarding the coping process suggests the importance of thought as well as action and also includes the fact one must expect to tolerate a certain amount of discomfort. The impulsive child learns relatively little about either; everything happens too fast. The personality traits of the parents also undoubtedly contribute to the development of the child's coping skills. Both by example and by precept the parent teaches the tolerance of pain. Children see their parents' reactions to physical and emotional pain and learn much from the manner in which the parents respond to their own problems.

It would seem wise, therefore, to include in family and developmental histories data regarding the coping mechanisms employed both by parents and by the child along with personality and temperamental traits. This would give the child psychiatrist a better understanding of the manner in which the child's coping skills have developed and a clue as to why he or she is having difficulty with current, age-related stressors that demand new coping mechanisms if they are to be mastered.

Notwithstanding the need for further research, the child psychiatrist has an opportunity to teach principles of preventive psychiatry when speaking to lay groups. One can point out, for instance, that the sick child must cope with at least three stressors: the physical stress of the illness, the anxiety associated with previous experience with similar illnesses, and the anxiety emanating from the parents. If hospitalization is necessary, the child faces a fourth stressor. The child can be helped to cope with the medical problem and its treatment through open and honest discussions. Teaching the importance of cooperation and balance between parents can reduce anxiety caused by them. Anxiety regarding hospitalization can be minimized by describing as much as we know about the procedures to be performed. Other opportunities accompany the occurrence of untoward events such as the death of a family member. Children can be participants in religious rituals and in the grieving process. The pain of unfortunate negative events can be partially ameliorated by trying to convert them into learning experiences and by sharing one's grief with the child.

Many books are appearing that profess to aid people in handling stress, and a number of high schools offer courses on the subject. Several studies [18,21,27,70] have shown that people tend to seek help first from nonpsychiatric physicians and only later from mental health professionals. If one accepts the tenet that a number of psychiatric disorders present first as adjustment reactions, the place for secondary prevention is here, limiting symptomatology by aiding the coping processes. The investigation of adjustment mechanisms and the effect of various child-rearing practices on these mechanisms is a valid approach to the formulation of primary preventative efforts. There is a great need for child psychiatrists to be active in this developing field.

A discussion of the pathogenic pathways by which stressors bring about maladaptive behavior or illness is beyond the scope of this chapter. The reader is referred to two reviews in earlier volumes of this work [41,54] and to a very useful monograph by Henry and Stephens.[32] Robert Ader[2] had edited a book on the immunological system, John Mason[45] has reviewed endocrinological mechanisms, and Harold Wolff[68] has summarized his many years of work in the field. Although almost all of the research on pathogenesis has utilized adult subjects, perusal of these contributions may well stimulate new investigations by child psychiatrists.

REFERENCES

1. ACKERMAN, S. H., MANAKER, S., and COHEN, M. I. "Recent Separation and the Onset of Peptic Ulcer Disease in Older Children and Adolescents," *Psychosomatic Medicine*, 43 (1981):305–310.

2. ADER, R., ed. *Psychoneuroimmunology*. New York: Academic Press, 1981.

3. ASNES, R. S., SANTULLI, R., and BEMPORAD, J. R. "Psychogenic Chest Pain in Children," *Clinical Pediatrics*, 20 (1981):788–791.

4. BARBEE, L., LUQUET, W., and WENCK, M. B. "A Study of Adolescent Life Events Prior to Psychiatric Hospitalization and First-time Involvement in the Juvenile Court System" (Unpublished paper).

5. BEAUTRAIS, A. L., FERGUSSON, D. M., and SHANNON, F. T. "Life Events and Childhood Morbidity: A Prospective Study," *Pediatrics*, 70 (1982):935–940.

6. ———. "Family Life Events and Behavioral Problems in Preschool-aged Children," *Pediatrics*, 70 (1982):774–779.

7. BERNARD, C. L. *Rapport sur less Progrès et la Marche de la Physiologic Generale*. Paris: Bailliere, 1867.

8. BRENNER, M. H. "Influence of the Social Environment on Psychopathology: The Historic Perspective," in J. E. Barrett, R. M. Rose, and G. L. Klerman, eds., *Stress and Mental Disorder*. New York: Raven Press, 1979, pp. 161–177.

9. BROWN, G. W., and HARRIS, T. *Social Origins of Depression: A Study of Psychiatric Disorder in Women*. London: Tavistock Publications, 1978.

10. BRUHN, J. G., et al. "Social Aspects of Coronary Heart Disease in Two Adjacent, Ethnically Different Communities," *American Journal of Public Health*, 56 (1966):1493–1506.

11. CANNON, W. B. "New Evidence for Sympathetic Control of Some Internal Secretions," *American Journal of Psychiatry*, 2 (1922):15.

12. CAPLAN, G. "Mastery of Stress: Psychosocial Aspects," *American Journal of Psychiatry*, 138 (1981):413–420.

13. CODDINGTON, R. D. "The Significance of Life Events as Etiologic Factors in Diseases of Children: I: A Survey of Professional Workers," *Journal of Psychosomatic Research*. 16 (1972):7–18.

14. ———. "The Significance of Life Events as Etiologic Factors in the Diseases of Children: II: A Study of a Normal Population," *Journal of Psychosomatic Research*, 16 (1972): 205–213.

15. ———. "Life Events Associated with Adolescent Pregnancies," *Journal of Clinical Psychiatry*, 40 (1979):180–185.

16. ———. "Measuring the Stressfulness of a Child's Environment," in J. H. Humphrey, ed., *Stress in Childhood*. New York: AMS Press, 1984, pp. 97–126.

17. CODDINGTON, R. D., and TROXELL, J. R. "Stress and Football Injury Rates—A Pilot Study," *Journal of Human Stress*, 6 (1980):3–5.

18. DICKMAN, D. L., and STEINHAUER, P. D. "Role of the Family Physician in the Management of Psychologic Crises in Children and Their Families," *Canadian Medical Association Journal*, 124 (1981):1566–1570.

19. DOHRENWEND, B. P. "Problems in Defining and Sampling the Relevent Population of Stressful Life Events," in B. S. Dohrenwend and B. P. Dohrenwend, eds., *Stressful Life Events: Their Nature and Effects*. New York: John Wiley & Sons, 1974, pp. 275–310.

20. DUNCAN, D. F. "Life Stress as a Precursor to Adolescent Drug Dependence," *International Journal of Addictions*, 12 (1977):1047–1056.

21. DZEGEDE, S. A., PIKE, S. W., and HACKWORTH, J. R. "The Relationship Between Health-related Stressful Life Events and Anxiety: An Analysis of a Florida Metropolitan Community," *Community Mental Health Journal*, 17 (1981):294–305.

22. ENGEL, M. "Children Who Work," *Archives of General Psychiatry*, 17 (1967):291–297.

23. FORMAN, B. D., EIDSON, K., and HAGAN, B. J. "Measuring Perceived Stress in Adolescents: A Cross Validation," *Adolescence*, 18 (1983):573–576.

24. GARMEZY, N. "Vulnerability Research and the Issue of Primary Prevention," *American Journal of Orthopsychiatry*, 41 (1971):101–116.

25. GERSTEN, J. C., et al. "Child Behavior and Life Events: Undesirable Change or Change Per Se?" in B. S. Dohrenwend and B. P. Dohrenwend, eds., *Stressful Life Events: Their Nature and Effects*. New York: John Wiley & Sons, 1974, pp. 159–170.

26. GOTTSCHALK, L. A. "Vulnerability to Stress," *American Journal of Psychotherapy*, 37 (1983):5–23.

27. HAGGERTY, R. J. "Breaking the Link Between Stress and Illness in Children: What Role Can Physicians Play?" *Postgraduate Medicine*, 74 (1983):287–291.

28. HEISEL, J. S. "Life Changes as Etiologic Factors in Juvenile Rheumatoid Arthritis," *Journal of Psychosomatic Research*, 16 (1972):411–420.

29. HEISEL, J. S., et al. "The Significance of Life Events as Contributing Factors in the Diseases of Children: III: A Study of Pediatric Patients," *Journal of Pediatrics*, 83 (1973): 119–123.

30. HENOCH, M. J., BATSON, J. W., and BAUM, J. "Psychosocial Factors in Juvenile Rheumatoid Arthritis," *Arthritis and Rheumatism*, 21 (1978):229–233.

31. HENRY, J. P. and CASSEL, J. C. "Psychosocial Factors in Essential Hypertension, Recent Epidemiologic and Animal Experimental Evidence," *American Journal of Epidemiology*, 90 (1969):171–200.

32. HENRY, J. P., and STEPHENS, P. M. *Stress, Health and the Social Environment: A Sociobiologic Approach to Medicine*. New York: Springer-Verlag, 1977.

33. HINKLE, L. E. "Ecological Observations of the Relations of Physical Illness, Mental Illness and the Social Environment," *Psychosomatic Medicine*, 23 (1961):289–296.

34. HOLMES, T. H., and RAHE, R. H. "The Social Readjustment Rating Scale," *Journal of Psychosomatic Research*, 11 (1967):213–218.

35. HOLT, P. L. "Stressful Life Events Preceding Road Traffic Accidents," *Injury*, 13 (1981):111–115.

36. ISHERWOOD, J., ADAM, K. S., and HORNBLOW, A. R. "Life Event Stress, Psychosocial Factors, Suicide Attempt and Auto-accident Proclivity," *Journal of Psychosomatic Research*, 26 (1982):371–383.

37. JAMES, D., ed. *Outward Bound*. London: Routledge and Kegan Paul, 1957.

38. JENNINGS, H. S. *Behavior of the Lower Organisms*. Bloomington, Ind.: Indiana University Press, 1976.

39. JOHNSON, J. W. "More About Stress and Some Management Techniques," *Journal of School Health*, 5 (1981): 36–42.

40. KASHANI, J. H., et al. "Life Events and Hospitalization in Children: A Comparison with a General Population," *British Journal of Psychiatry*, 139 (1981):221–225.

41. KAVANAUGH, J. G., JR., and MATTSON, A. "Psychophysiologic Disorders," in J. D. Noshpitz, ed., *Basic Hand-

book of Child Psychiatry, vol. 2. New York: Basic Books, 1979, pp. 341–380.

42. KESSLER, E. S. "Reactive Disorders," in J. D. Noshpitz, ed., *Basic Handbook of Child Psychiatry,* vol. 2. New York: Basic Books, 1979, pp. 173–184.

43. KNUDSON-COOPER, M. S., and LEUCHTAG, A. K. "The Stress of a Family Move as a Precipitating Factor in Children's Burn Accidents," *Journal of Human Stress,* 8 (1982):32–38.

44. MARGOLIS, L. H., and FARRAN, D. "Unemployment: The Health Consequences in Children," *North Carolina Medical Journal,* 42 (1981):849–850.

45. MASON, J. W. "Emotion as Reflected in Patterns of Endocrine Integration," in L. Levi, ed., *Emotions—Their Parameters and Measurement.* New York: Raven Press, 1975

46. MASUDA, M., and HOLMES, T. H. "Magnitude Estimations of Social Readjustment," *Journal of Psychosomatic Research,* 11 (1967):219–225.

47. MEYER, A. "The Life Chart and the Obligation of Specifying Positive Data in Psychopathological Diagnosis," in E. E. Winters, ed., *The Collected Papers of Adolf Meyer,* vol. 3, *Medical Teaching.* Baltimore: Johns Hopkins University Press, 1951, pp. 52–56.

48. MILLER, S. M. "Why Having Control Reduces Stress: If I Can Stop the Roller Coaster, I Don't Want to Get Off," in J. Garber and M.E.P. Siliquan, eds., *Human Helplessness: Theory and Application.* New York: Academic Press, 1980.

49. MUELLER, D. P., EDWARDS, D. W., and YARVIS, R. M. "Stressful Life Events and Psychiatric Symptomatology: Change or Undesirability," *Journal of Health and Social Behavior,* 18 (1977):307–317.

50. MURPHY, L. B., and MORIARTY, A. E. *Vulnerability, Coping and Growth: From Infancy to Adolescence.* New Haven: Yale University Press, 1976.

51. OJEMANN, R. H. "Investigation of the Effects of Teaching an Understanding and Appreciation of Behavior Dynamics," in G. Caplan, ed., *Prevention of Mental Disorders in Children.* New York: Basic Books, 1961, pp.

52. PARKER, G. B., and BROWN, L. B. "Coping Behaviors that Mediate Between Life Events and Depression," *Archives of General Psychiatry,* 39 (1982):1386–1391.

53. PAYKEL, E. S., PRUSOFF, B. A., and UHLENHUTH, E. H. "Scaling of Life Events," *Archives of General Psychiatry,* 25 (1971):340–347.

54. PRUGH, D. G., and ECKHARDT, L. O. "Psychophysiological Disorders," in J. D. Noshpitz, ed., *Basic Handbook of Child Psychiatry,* vol. 3, New York: Basic Books, 1979, pp. 578–604.

55. RICHARDSON, M., and WEST, P. "Motivational Management: Coping with Burnout," *Hospital and Community Psychiatry,* 33 (1982):837–840.

56. RUTTER, M. "Stress, Coping and Development: Some Issues and Questions," *Journal of Child Psychology and Psychiatry,* 22 (1981):323–356.

57. SANDLER, I. N., and RAMSAY, T. B. "Dimensional Analysis of Children's Stressful Life Events," *American Journal of Community Psychology,* 8 (1980):285–305.

58. SCHMID, L. "Malignant Tumours as Causes of Death of Former Athletes," *Journal of Sports Medicine and Physical Fitness,* 15 (1975):117–124.

59. SELYE, H. *The Physiology and Pathology of Exposure to Stress.* Montreal: Acta, Inc., 1950.

60. SINGHI, S., SINGHI, P., and ADWANI, G. B. "Role of Psychosocial Stress in the Cause of Pica," *Clinical Pediatrics,* 20 (1981):783–785.

61. SPIVACK, G., PLATT, J. J., and SHURE, M. B. *The Problem-Solving Approach to Adjustment: A Guide to Research and Intervention.* San Francisco: Jossey-Bass, 1976.

62. STARFIELD, B., et al. "Morbidity in Childhood—A Longitudinal View," *New England Journal of Medicine,* 319 (1984):824–829.

63. TENNANT, C., BEBBINGTON, P., and HURRY, J. "The Short-term Outcome of Neurotic Disorders in the Community: The Relation of Remission to Clinical Factors and to 'Neutralizing' Life Events," *British Journal of Psychiatry,* 139 (1981):213–220.

64. VAN HOUTEN, T., and GOLEMBIEWSKI, G, *Adolescent Life Stress as a Predictor of Alcohol Abuse and/or Runaway Behavior.* Washington, D.C.: National Youth Alternatives Project, 1978.

65. VINCENT, K. R., and ROSENSTOCK, H. A. "The Relationship Between Stressful Life Events and Hospitalized Adolescent Psychiatric Patients," *Journal of Clinical Psychiatry,* 40 (1979):262–264.

66. WALLERSTEIN, J., and KELLY, J. *Surviving the Breakup: How Children and Parents Cope with Divorce.* New York: Basic Books, 1980.

67. WEXLER, K. B. "Developmental Disfluency in 2-, 4-, and 6-year-old Boys in Neutral and Stress Situations," *Journal of Speech and Hearing Research,* 25 (1982):229–234.

68. WOLFF, H. G. "Life Stress and Bodily Disease—A Formulation," in H. G. Wolff, S. G. Wolf, Jr., and C. C. Hare, eds., *Life Stress and Bodily Disease.* Baltimore: Williams & Wilkins, 1950, pp. 1059–1094.

69. YAMAMOTO, K., and FELSENTHAL, H. M. "Stressful Experiences of Children: Professional Judgments," *Psychological Reports,* 50 (1982):1087–1093.

70. YATES, A. "Stress Management in Childhood," *Clinical Pediatrics,* 22 (1983):131–135.

71. YEAWORTH, R. C., et al. "The Development of an Adolescent Life Change Event Scale," *Adolescence,* 15 (1980):91–97.

25 / Cognition and Psychopathology

Peter E. Tanguay

Introduction

Cognition is the act of knowing, of understanding, of intellectually wrestling with ideas and concepts. In its widest sense, cognition implies not only the manipulation and linkage of ideas but the unconscious and conscious activities involved in these processes, including perception, learning, memory, reasoning, and judgment. Extending the concept further, less tangible mental activities such as "grasping" what had formerly been an affect or an "action experience" could also be included in the definition. Together with the study of affect, investigation of cognitive function is an important part of the psychiatric examination of children, especially if they are suspected of having schizophrenia, attention deficit disorder, or a specific learning disorder involving language or reading handicap. Child psychiatrists should have a good understanding of the many ways in which formal and informal clinical assessment of cognitive function may be carried out. Above all, however, they need a solid grasp on the theoretical framework that links function to specific pathology.

Cognitive Development

There is but one comprehensive model of cognitive development available today, the system worked out by Swiss psychologist Jean Piaget. Although the model does not concern itself with important questions such as the relationship between emotional factors and cognitive development, it is relatively comprehensive in scope and provides a good theoretical framework for understanding this aspect of human functioning. Not all psychologists have interested themselves in Piaget's ideas, however, and for some, notably the behaviorists, his work has been totally irrelevant. In the past two decades, psychologists of the Genevan tradition have continued to study and refine Piaget's theory. Their

findings have generally validated Piaget's description of the universality of the stages in cognitive development, at least insofar as he described children between age three years and adolescence (see Appleton, Clifton, and Goldberg[2]; Haith and Campos[16]; and Niemark[24] for a review of the more recent work). This chapter discusses Piaget's model very briefly and only from the viewpoint of the stages of development. Those wishing to pursue Piaget's contributions further may consult a general review of his work,[13] an edited anthology of his writings,[15] or his original books, many of which are now available in English translations. A particularly good synthesis of Piaget's ideas with those of psychoanalysis has been provided by Basch.[4]

Piaget described development as taking place over several major "periods." As with most neuropsychological phenomena, the onset of each is gradual, so that the several epochs sequentially merge into one another. There is considerable variation as to the age at which each new phase appears; this variation becomes progressively broader as later periods are reached. It must be emphasized, however, that differences between periods are not simply quantitative but qualitative. Children are not merely ignorant adults. They are persons who see and understand the world from a unique perspective and who use reasoning processes that are quite different from those employed by adults. Without such qualitative differences, there would be no basis for distinguishing specific "periods" in development.

THE SENSORIMOTOR PERIOD

The sensorimotor period extends from birth to approximately eighteen to twenty-four months of age. Initially neonatal behavior is largely reflexive, molded by innate capacities and tendencies that orient the responses of newborn infants to specific stimuli in their environment. As a result, these innate propensities to respond are profoundly influenced by contact with caretakers and physical surroundings and soon adapt and interconnect to form behavioral schemata capable of acting or reacting to an ever greater variety of events. These schemata of the sensorimotor period differ from those of later periods in that they are what Piaget termed "external" operations. External operations, as distinguished from the "internal" operations of imagination and thought, are motor actions aimed at dealing with physical objects under the guidance and control of sensory input. Faced with a "problem," children will attempt to find a solution in a trial-and-error fashion using such sensorimotor schemata as are already in their repertory. If the problem is solvable by one of these existing schemata, they will be successful; if not, they may go on trying until, by chance, they happen upon an approach that is successful. This approach is then likely to be incorporated into their future problem-solving tactics through addition to, or modification of, existing behavioral schemata. An example is the story of a nine-month-old girl who sees an elongated toy outside of her playpen and wishes to bring it into the playpen with her. She has already learned to reach out between the bars, and she can easily grasp the object. Her behavioral competencies do not, however, include a schemata for "bringing elongated objects through narrow spaces." In attempting to do this new task, she repeatedly, and unsuccessfully, tries to pull the toy through, only to find each time that she is blocked by the bars. However, by chance, she discovers that in order to succeed, it is necessary to line up the long axis of the toy parallel with the bars of the crib. The operation is *external* in that it did not involve an internal "thinking out" of the solution.

PERIOD OF CONCRETE OPERATIONS

In Piaget's developmental scheme, the period of concrete operations extends from approximately the end of the sensorimotor period to eleven or twelve years of age. Children's cognitive operations differ from those of the sensorimotor period in that more and more they are "internal"—that is, carried out in thought. An example of the early use of internal operations is given by Piaget.[26] His sixteen-month-old daughter, Lucienne, is shown a matchbox, of the sort that is operated by sliding a container in and out of a cover that is open at each end. Into the box, where the matches belong, Piaget placed a gold chain. Lucienne has not seen him do this and is not aware of how the box is opened and closed. When the box is only half closed, she can very easily retrieve the chain by using any of her existing sensorimotor operations: dumping it out of the opening, pulling it out with her finger, and so forth. But this time Piaget presents the box to her almost fully closed, so that the slit is too small to admit her finger. At an earlier age she would have attempted to extract the chain by exercising, in "external" trial-and-error fashion, all of her repertory of sensorimotor operations and, short of destroying the box in the process,

would probably have failed. But now she behaves very differently. She pauses and looks at the slit with close attention. Then, several times in succession, she opens and shuts her mouth, at first slightly, then wider and wider. Suddenly, with no hesitation, she puts her finger in the slit and, instead of trying to reach the chain as she had before, she pulls so as to enlarge the opening fully and open the box. Piaget suggested that, lacking language, Lucienne may have been employing a type of body-oriented visual imagery to express the idea of opening up a cavity adjacent to a slit. Whatever the meaning of her oral movements, she clearly solved the problem without having to resort to a series of manual trial-and-error operations, though it is possible that she did rehearse such operations in her imagination before opening the box.

The period of concrete operations is remarkable in that two qualitatively different types of cognitive operations appear to unfold side by side on a staggered schedule. The first type of cognitive operation is clearly in evidence by three or four years of age, whereas the second does not begin to appear in thought until five or six years of age and is not fully developed until ten years of age or later. Having observed this fact, Piaget divided the period of concrete operations into two parts: a "preoperational" subperiod that ends around age six years and a later subperiod extending to age eleven or twelve years.

From our present vantage point, the division of the period of concrete operations into subperiods may be misleading. As was already mentioned, what we may be seeing is the parallel development of two sets of quite different cognitive operations rather than the sequential development of one set and its replacement by a better one. Adults continue to use both types of cognitive operations, depending on the task before them.

What cognitive operations predominate in children before age five years? Piaget noted that children's thought in the preoperational subperiod was markedly "egocentric," a term denoting that children see the world from one point of view only—their own—without being at all aware that other viewpoints or perspectives might exist. Presented with a three-dimensional toy landscape on which there are three mountains and asked what several observers sitting at different vantage points might see, four-year-old children will readily draw the various perspectives of the observers, but, *mirabile dictu,* each and every one is the same, namely the view seen by the children themselves.

Piaget also noted that the thought of preoperational children is action-oriented and imagistic rather than expressed in language-based terms. Furthermore, he noted that children are also animistic in their understanding of the world (e.g., stones and rocks are alive and have feelings) and that they reason backward with great difficulty, if at all. And finally, he noted, young children do not reason in a cause-and-effect manner, they fail to understand logical relationships, and they cannot use inductive or deductive thought.

There is one descriptor of preoperational thinking that, while it was not given a particular preeminence by Piaget, may capture the fundamental nature of the cognitive strategies employed by three- to five-year-old children. The term is "syncretic." An important characteristic of syncretic preoperational reasoning is that relationships are explained in terms of some accidental juxtaposition of attributes and events. Asked "Why does the moon stay up in the sky?" children will reply, seemingly filled with confidence because they know they are right, "Because it is dark outside (or night, or cold, etc.)." Water rises in a glass when a stone is added because the stone is heavy or because the stone "wants the water to rise."

Faced with a transformation in the shape of an object, very young children reason on the basis of their perceptual impressions alone. Thus water poured from a tall, narrow container to a short, squat one not only "appears" to younger children to have been transformed to a larger or smaller amount but, to their way of thinking, actually *has* been transformed. In contrast, older children have a more logical and flexible reasoning capacity: Nothing has been added to the quantity of water, nothing has been taken away, hence the amount of water has remained the same.

It is through observation of how children go about solving problems that we can observe their developing cognitive skills. Piaget chose to study this development using a method that is closely akin to the clinical interview in psychiatry. He would present various tasks to children in a flexible and nonstandardized manner, listening to their answers, puzzling out why children might be answering in a particular way, requestioning the children with the goal of learning whether his hypotheses were true, and, above all, allowing children free rein to demonstrate, through their word and actions, how they sought the solution to the task in question. The tasks were chosen to explore children's understanding of such concepts as causation, quantity, number, space, time, geometrical relationships, movement and velocity, laws of chance, classification, and even concepts of moral judgment.

Although it is beyond the scope of this chapter to present a detailed account of Piaget's findings, the development of children's cognitive skills in three areas will be briefly described. The areas are "the conservations," seriation, and classification.

Conservation. "Conservation" refers to the fact that changes in certain properties of an object (quantity, number, length, etc.) may be conserved (remain unchanged) in the face of certain transformations (change in shape, displacements in space, being cut into pieces, etc.). The conservations, Piaget discovered, are generally acquired in a particular order. The youngest children learn conservation of number: of two lines of marbles, each may have the same number of marbles even while one line may be longer; conversely, a shorter line may contain more marbles than a longer line, depending on how closely spaced the marbles are in each line. Prior to age five, children may insist that the longer line always has more marbles, even when this is not true. Around the age of seven or eight years children learn conservation of mass: that changes in shape do not lead to changes in quantity. The method of assessing children's comprehension of conservation of mass was illustrated earlier in the example of water poured from a tall, narrow jar into a low, wide one. It can also be tested in the well-known transformation of a tall pillar of clay into a flat pancake. Having witnessed this transformation, younger children very often believe that the pancake now contains more clay or less clay than did the pillar.

Around age nine children begin to understand both conservation of weight (an object that changes in shape does not become heavier or lighter) and conservation of area. Children's understanding of the conservation of area can be tested using the two meadow's task.[27] Children are presented with two pieces of green tracing paper, representing meadows, upon each of which is placed a toy cow and an identical number of houses. The task can be put to the children in many different ways, but the prototypic moment of truth comes at the point when the houses on one meadow are arranged in a neat row along one edge, while those on the other are scattered about. Children are asked if one cow has more, less, or the same amount of grass to eat as the other. When they have chosen, they are asked to justify their answer. The task is perceptually very compelling: At first glance it would appear that one cow (the one standing on the expanse of uncluttered grass) clearly has more grass to eat than the other, even though logically we "know" this is not true.

The last conservation to be achieved (generally not before eleven or twelve years of age) is conservation of volume: Even though the shape of an object may change, the volume of water it will displace in a container remains constant.

Seriation. "Seriation" is the act of arranging a series of different size objects in ascending or descending order. While children can draw what such a series would look like at age six or seven, it is not until one or two years later that they become adept at carrying out the task using the actual objects. The difficulty appears to lie in the three- and four-way comparisons that are required: Children have little difficulty in comparing one object with another, but they experience difficulty in comparing results of that first comparison to the admixture of sizes represented in the remaining objects. Given sufficient time, five- or six-year-old children may eventually accomplish the task, in a trial-and-error sensorimotor way, but they do not use the more rapid sorting methods of older children.

Classification. In Piaget's view, solving problems involving sorting and classification is difficult because it requires an understanding of logical hierarchical systems. Piaget employed many types of classification problems in his studies of how children think. One example addressed the question of inclusionary classes. Children are shown a number of small objects, such as ten small wooden blocks of two different colors. There might, for instance, be seven red blocks and three blue blocks. After the children have been allowed to handle the blocks and familiarize themselves with them, ascertaining they are all made of wood, they are asked: Are there more red blocks or more wooden blocks? It is always surprising to inexperienced examiners how difficult it is for children, even at age eight and nine, to accept that one class may include another. Even when they are carefully led to the correct answer by appropriate coaching, they have great difficulty accepting that a concrete object may belong to two classes at one and the same time. Perhaps the problem lies with an inability of children of this age to understand abstract concepts, an ability they will not possess for another one or two years.

PERIOD OF FORMAL OPERATIONS

The final period of development, the period of formal operations, which begins around eleven or twelve years, is characterized by children's increasing ability to deal with *abstract* reality. This ability is manifested both as a capacity to reason and a more ordered approach to solving problems. At this time children begin to be able to "abstract" meaning from proverbs and to understand and solve problems involving the laws of chance. Faced with the requirement that they make a pendulum they are holding swing faster, eight-year-olds will rush haphazardly into random experimentation with such factors as the weight of the bob, the length of the pendulum, or the magnitude of the push to start it into motion. In the process they will confound all three variables, and usually they will fail to find an answer. In contrast, fifteen-year-olds may stand back and begin the search by hypothesizing what factors could be important and then, in an orderly and complete manner, test each hypothesis in turn.

As was true in all previous periods, learning occurs in the context of a variety of experiences: exploration of the everyday world, play, interactions with friends, and schooling. Mastery of the more complex problem-solving strategies of the type acquired after age nine or ten are particularly dependent on formal didactic instruction. But one important point must be kept in mind, and that is that no amount of schooling will teach children to use logical or abstract operations until they are ready to learn.

Having reached the level of formal operations, children begin to be able to learn to solve more complex or abstract problems, such as those involving the laws of chance. The following is an example of a task involving the laws of chance. Six red, five blue, three green, and two white marbles are put into a cloth bag, and children, who have observed this action, are told that they may blindly withdraw one marble, but before they do so, they are asked what color they think they are likely to get. Prior to age ten or eleven, children may respond with the correct answer, but when asked to justify their choice they may reply with such statements as "Because red is my favorite color" or "Because the red one was the last you put in." Only when children have entered the period of formal operations can they learn to do this and other similar tasks.

Cognitive Operations— A Neuropsychological Viewpoint

Let us turn at this point to a very different model for understanding cognitive operations, specifically the model of "hemispheric specialization" derived from the work of Roger Sperry and his colleagues and continued by a large number of investigators since the early 1970s (see Benson and Zaidel[5] for a review of recent work). There are two basic premises to the model. The first is that humans use two quite different types of cognitive operations in their everyday interactions with the world: holistic operations and sequential operations. The second premise, and one that is largely irrelevant to this chapter, is that the neural substrates underlying holistic cognitive operations are to be found to a greater extent in the right hemisphere than the left, while the opposite relationship exists for sequential operations.

HOLISTIC AND SEQUENTIAL OPERATIONS

Although scientists have only recently postulated a duality in information processing systems in man, the notion that such a duality might exist has been expressed for many hundred years. Bogen[7] has identified nineteen such references. In each instance, the dichotomy (often "newly discovered") is announced under yet another set of names: atomistic-gross, digital-analogic, abstract-maplike, rational-metaphoric, buddhi-manas, and so forth. In the current literature the terms parallel and serial are also used instead of holistic and sequential.

"Sequential" processing refers to the coding and decoding of meaning in terms of the relationship of elements within a sequence, as represented by the semantic relationship of words within a sentence, the problem-solving sequences of syllogistic reasoning, or the order of steps in cause-and-effect reasoning. It is a form of cognition that resembles the "concrete" operations Piaget described as developing largely after age six or seven, or that is characteristic of language development in a four- or five-year-old child. In contrast, "holistic" thinking is nonverbal, presumably carried out by means of visual, kinesthetic, tactile, and auditory images, with multiple parallel information inputs being synthesized and compared. It has often been related to such behavioral tasks as facial recognition or recognizing the auditory gestalt of familiar words or phrases. It is a type of reasoning referred to earlier in the Piagetian model as "syncretic" thought, typical of the preoperational stage in cognitive development. Various psychoanalysts[20,23] have noted the similarity between holistic cognitive operations and primary process thought and between sequential cognitive operations and secondary process thinking.

Cognition and Psychopathology

If the analogy between the Piagetian and the neuropsychological models are correct, one could postulate that in addition to the fundamental cognitive differences between holistic and sequential operations just outlined, they differ in another important way: They mature at different ages and, perhaps, independently from one another. This speculation raises an important hypothesis: that the cognitive and language symptoms of certain serious psychiatric disorders in childhood are a direct result of a failure to learn sequential and/or holistic cognitive operations. This failure could be a result of biological abnormalities or a lack of adequate learning experience, or both. The syndromes in question would include early infantile autism, schizophrenia, nonautistic forms of mental retardation, and specific language and reading disorders.

While this hypothesis may not have much immediate clinical application (except perhaps as a way of intellectually understanding symptomatology), it is nonetheless interesting from a research viewpoint.

Studies based on the hypothesis could lead to a more precise understanding of the nature of psychotic syndromes in childhood and provide a method of classifying childhood psychiatric disorders in terms of specific factors that would cut across current DSM-III categories. And should the neural substrate underlying holistic and sequential operations ever become understood, it could be an important step in the direction of finding more effective methods of treatment for serious psychopathology in childhood.

Evidence for the hypothesis has come from the analysis and interpretation of symptoms seen in various psychiatric disorders[10,11,31] and by indirect and direct experimental means. Indirect studies have employed Piagetian or neuropsychological approaches, while the very few direct studies have relied on techniques derived from perceptual psychology. The results of these investigations suggest that while the hypothesis may have merit, it cannot account for all of the symptoms seen in the major psychiatric disorders of children, including early infantile autism and schizophrenia.

INDIRECT PIAGETIAN STUDIES

Although it was initially reported[1,12] that autistic children were unable to reach the highest stage of sensorimotor operations (the stage in which children are capable of understanding object permanence), more recent investigations have demonstrated that most autistic persons, except perhaps profoundly retarded ones, possess remarkably good sensorimotor skills[22,30] and are quite capable of understanding object permanence. Carrying the investigations further, several authors have attempted to assess the degree to which autistic children can carry out cognitive operations characteristic of the concrete stage. Lancy and Goldstein[22] studied four- to nine-year-old autistic children, all of whom were in an intense treatment program aimed at increasing their social relationships. Because some of the twelve children did not understand language, the investigators profoundly modified the manner in which the Piagetian tasks were administered, which made interpretation of the results difficult. Fifty-three percent of the children were found to have some seriation skills, 36 percent understood a simple type of number conservation, and 92 percent were able to classify objects along one dimension. While the children's performance was impaired in contrast to what one would have expected given their ages, their capacity to use rudimentary cognitive operations of the concrete period was not entirely deficient. In a study that employed more traditional Piagetian tasks, Hobson[18] studied twelve autistic children from nine to sixteen years of age whose IQs ranged from moderately retarded to normal. Several children with higher IQs were capable of understanding number conservation and were able to carry out a seriation task. The results served to emphasize that a relatively wide range of cognitive levels, from the preoperational to the early concrete, are found among children diagnosed as autistic.

Breslow and Cowan[9] have reported an investigation of fourteen children, whose ages ranged from 6.4 to 11.10 years, with a mean age of 9.2 years. All had thought disorder, severely impaired social relationships, and flatness of affect, and all had been diagnosed as having schizophrenia. Three children had some autistic features but did not meet the usual Kannerian criteria for the diagnosis of autism. No IQ scores were given but it was noted that eleven of the children had fluent speech. Tests included "classification along multiple dimensions" and seriation. Eight of the fourteen children were found to be preoperational in their classification level. The remaining six psychotic subjects had either transitional to concrete operations or had clearly reached that stage. Based on these results, it would appear that many schizophrenic children are impaired in their ability to use concrete cognitive operations, some not even reaching the level of seven- or eight-year-old children.

INDIRECT NEUROPSYCHOLOGICAL APPROACHES

Neuropsychological and similar experimental approaches to the study of the holistic/sequential hypothesis must begin with the same rigorous goal: to identify tasks or experimental paradigms that represent, in as pure a form as possible, sequential or holistic cognitive acts and to use these tasks or paradigms to study individuals having various psychiatric disorders.

Almost all of the pertinent neuropsychological studies derive from the model of hemispheric specialization. In this model, holistic cognitive processing is attributed primarily to neural systems in the right hemisphere and sequential processing to systems in the left hemisphere. In most of these experiments various auditory or visual stimuli are presented to one hemisphere at a time. The results are then interpreted in terms of right- or left-hemisphere impairment or impairment in communication between the hemispheres. In some experiments, stimuli are chosen on the basis of their linguistic or spatial content, with the implication that right- or left-hemisphere impairment also implies holistic or sequential processing deficits. While very popular in the recent literature, this approach suffers from a number of shortcomings. First, our understanding of the relationship of left- and right-hemisphere functioning to holistic and sequential processing skills is really quite poor. That there is some relation-ship is undoubtedly true,[14] but what it is, and how it varies among individuals, is not well understood. A second difficulty is that at this time there is still much to be learned about the manner in which rather small changes in task or procedure can bias information processing to favor use of holistic or sequential strategies.[29] A number of findings have been reported that variously implicate left-hemisphere, right-hemisphere, or corpus callosal dysfunction in schizophrenia and other psychiatric disorders.[32] Unfortunately, the literature is replete with studies that contradict each other. It might be preferable if such work were confined to careful studies of normal individuals, with the goal of first defining in a clear manner the variables that control the results. Only when this is achieved could one approach psychiatric populations with any degree of confidence.

DIRECT STUDIES

Direct studies focus on tasks that are thought to measure holistic or sequential cognitive operations directly. Finding such tasks is, in fact, extremely difficult, since many tasks require an admixture of both holistic and sequential operations, and even minor changes in task demand may lead to changes in the holistic/sequential ratio. The most promising tasks may be those whose performance requires brief periods of time, on the order of 100 milliseconds or less. Under these conditions several investigators[6,8,33] have developed experimental tasks that seem specifically to measure parallel and serial processing, or at least measure tasks having a preponderance of one or the other type of processing activity. The specific method of processing can be validated by examining the degree to which subject reaction time changes with task complexity: Reaction time increases with serial processing or fails to increase if the task truly involves parallel processing. This approach has been applied to studying children with childhood-onset schizophrenia.[3] In comparison to normal age-matched controls, schizophrenic children were markedly impaired in serial information-processing strategies. Where the task appeared to involve a relatively greater degree of parallel as compared to serial processing, however, it was noted that the schizophrenic children had normal information-processing capacity. Such studies have promise and should be replicated and extended to other populations of psychiatrically impaired children.

DISCUSSION

The preceding studies suggest that both autistic and schizophrenic children appear to suffer from a range of serious impairments in the ability to use cognitive operations of a concrete type, with many children remaining at a preoperational level and some reaching the lower levels of the concrete subperiod. Insofar as these operations may require the ability to use sequential cognitive processing, one could postulate that both autistic and schizophrenic children often fail to develop such skills. In the one experiment in which serial (sequential) operations were directly studied in schizophrenic children, they were indeed found to have difficulty with this specific skill.[3]

In regard to holistic operations, we have less information. Many previous investigators have remarked on the large number of autistic children who have some skills on such perceptual-spatial tasks as the block design test of the Weschler Intelligence Scale for Children. Perhaps this is an indication that when autistic children do learn some skills, they are likely to do better in holistic than in sequential processing. In a similar vein, Asarnow and Sherman's data[3] would indicate that some schizophrenic subjects may learn advanced holistic operations, even when they remain seriously handicapped in sequential processing skills.

It must be emphasized that this discussion is germane to only the cognitive and language deficits of autistic and schizophrenic children. Within the past few years, even the more cognitively and language-oriented investigators have come to recognize the degree to which other "social" or "emotional" dysfunctions are crucial features of early infantile autism[25,28] in children and schizophrenia in adults.[17] Occasionally autistic children develop relatively good language, and their IQ scores fall within the normal range, but even these children usually remain profoundly impaired in social relationships.[28] Their syntactic and semantic language skills may be good, but their pragmatic language skills are grossly impaired. They lack the knowledge of how to open and sustain a conversation, how to take turns in a conversation, and how to phrase their communications in such a way as to "tune in" to the listener's point of view. It is as if they have an almost total lack of "empathy"[19] and of the ability to sense another's emotional and social viewpoint. Concomitantly, they are often equally handicapped in their production of affectual and social cues—in the use of gesture and facial communication and in the prosodic melody of speech. In his original report Kanner[21] emphasized autistic children's "affective" disturbance in addition to their cognitive and language handicaps. Future investigators may find it scientifically profitable not only to study cognitive and linguistic disorders of psychosis in children, but to investigate the range of "affective" disorders in these individuals, including disorders in empathy and prosodic expression of affect.

Summary

In Piaget's stage model of cognitive development, three- to five-year-old preoperational children reason in a manner that is action-oriented, image-dominated, and syncretic. Older children, in comparison, learn to use cognitive operations that are logical and that permit them to understand problems in classification, conservation, cause and effect, and, eventually, those requiring inductive and deductive reasoning. Looking at cognition from a different point of view, neuropsychologists have postulated two types of fundamental information-processing strategies in man: holistic and sequential operations. Holistic operations resemble what Piaget called syncretic thought, while the cognitive operations Piaget described as characteristic of older children may require sequential processing strategies. It is postulated that children who have serious psychopathology (including infantile autism and schizophrenia) may suffer from varying degrees of holistic and/or sequential processing impairments, and that this may result in their cognitive and linguistic impairments, though not their social and affectual handicaps.

REFERENCES

1. ALPERN, G. D. "Measurement of 'Untestable' Autistic Children," *Journal of Abnormal Psychology,* 72 (1967): 478–496.

2. APPLETON, T., CLIFTON, R., and GOLDBERG, S. "The Development of Behavioral Competency in Infancy," in D. Horowitz, ed., *Review of Child Development Research,* vol. 4. Chicago: University of Chicago Press, 1975, pp. 101–186.

3. ASARNOW, R., and SHERMAN, T. "Studies of Visual Information Processing in Schizophrenic Children," *Child Development,* 55 (1984): 249–261.

4. BASCH, M. F., "Psychoanalytic Interpretation and Cognitive Transformation," *International Journal of Psycho-Analysis,* 62 (1981):151.

5. BENSON, F., and ZAIDEL, E., eds. *The Dual Brain: Hemispheric Specialization in the Human,* New York: Guilford Press, 1985.

6. BERGEN, J. R., and JULESZ, B. "Parallel Versus Serial Processing in Rapid Pattern Discrimination," *Nature,* 303 (1983):697–698.

7. BOGEN, J. E. "The Other Side of the Brain. II: An

Appositional Mind," *Bulletin of the Los Angeles Neurological Society,* 34 (1969):135–162.

8. BRADSHAW, J. L., and SHERLOCK, D., "Bugs and Faces in Two Visual Fields: The Analytic/holistic Processing Dichotomy and Task Sequencing," *Cortex,* 18 (1982):211–216.

9. BRESLOW, L., and COWAN, P. A. "Structural and Functional Perspectives on Classification and Seriation in Psychotic and Normal Children," *Child Development,* 55 (1984):226–235.

10. BROWN, T. A. "The Microgenesis of Schizophrenic Thought," *Archives de Psychologie,* 48 (1980):215–237.

11. CALLAWAY, E., and NAGHDI, S. "An Information Processing Model for Schizophrenia," *Archives of General Psychiatry,* 39 (1982):339–347.

12. CURCIO, F. "Sensorimotor Functioning and Communication in Mute Autistic Children," *Journal of Autism and Childhood Schizophrenia,* 8 (1978):281–292.

13. FLAVEL, J. *The Developmental Psychology of Jean Piaget.* Princeton, N.J.: Van Nostrand Rheinhold, 1963.

14. GALIN, D. "Lateral Specialization and Psychiatric Issues: Speculations on Development and the Evolution of Consciousness," *Annals of the New York Academy of Sciences,* 299 (1977):222–232.

15. GRUBER, H., and VONECHE, J. *The Essential Piaget.* New York: Basic Books, 1977.

16. HAITH, M., and CAMPOS, J. "Human Infancy," *Annual Review of Psychology,* 28 (1977):251–293.

17. HARROW, M., and MILLER, J. G. "Schizophrenic Thought Disorders and Impaired Perspective," *Journal of Abnormal Psychology,* 89 (1980):717–727.

18. HOBSON, R. P. "Early Childhood Autism and the Question of Egocentrism," *Journal of Autism and Developmental Disorders,* 14 (1984):85–104.

19. HOBSON, R. P. "The Autistic Child's Concept of Person," in D. Park, ed., *Proceedings of the 1981 International Conference on Autism in Boston.* Washington, D.C.: National Society for Children and Adults with Autism, 1982.

20. HOROWITZ, M. J. "Modes of Representation of Thought," *Journal of the American Psychoanalytic Association,* 20 (1972):793–819.

21. KANNER, L. "Autistic Disturbances of Affective Contact," *The Nervous Child,* 2 (1943):217–250.

22. LANCY, D. F., and GOLDSTEIN, G. I. "The Use of Nonverbal Piagetian Tasks to Assess the Cognitive Development of Autistic Children," *Child Development,* 53 (1982): 1233–1241.

23. MCLAUGHLIN, J. T. "Primary and Secondary Process in the Context of Cerebral Hemispheric Specialization," *Psychoanalytic Quarterly,* 67 (1978):237–266.

24. NIEMARK, E. "Intellectual Development During Adolescence," in D. Horowitz, ed., *Review of Child Developmental Research,* vol. 4. Chicago: University of Chicago Press, 1975, pp. 541–594.

25. PAUL, R., and COHEN, D. J. "Communication Development and Its Disorders: A Psycholinguistic Perspective," *Schizophrenia Bulletin,* 8 (1982):279–293.

26. PIAGET, J. *The Origins of Intelligence in Children,* M. Cook, trans. New York: International Universities Press, 1952.

27. PIAGET, J., INHELDER, B., and SZEMINSKA, A. *The Child's Conception of Geometry.* New York: Basic Books, 1960, pp. 261–273.

28. RUTTER, M. "Cognitive Deficits in the Pathogenesis of Autism," *Journal of Child Psychology and Psychiatry,* 24 (1983):513–531.

29. SERGENT, J. "Inferences from Unilateral Brain Damage About Normal Hemispheric Functions in Visual Pattern Recognition," *Psychological Bulletin,* 96 (1984):99–115.

30. SIGMAN, M., and UNGERER, J. "Sensorimotor Skills and Language Comprehension in Autistic Children," *Journal of Abnormal Child Psychology,* 9 (1981):149–165.

31. TANGUAY, P. E. "Toward a New Classification of Serious Psychopathology in Children," *Journal of the American Academy of Child Psychiatry,* 23 (1984):373–384.

32. ———. "Implications of Hemispheric Specialization for Psychiatry," in F. Benson and E. Zaidel, eds., *The Dual Brain: Hemispheric Specialization in the Human.* New York: Guilford Press, 1985, pp. 375–382.

33. TREISMAN, A. M., and GELADE, G. "A Feature-integration of Attention," *Cognitive Psychology,* 12 (1980):97–136.

PART B
Nosology

26 / DSM-III and Child Psychiatry

J. Gary May

Introduction

Issues of classification of psychiatric disorders in infancy, childhood, and adolescence are current, controversial, and relevant. Attention to diagnosis has been heightened by the introduction in 1980 of the third edition of the *Diagnostic and Statistical Manual of Mental Disorders* (DSM-III)[1] and the upcoming revision that is now in progress. The manual gave the young more attention and prominence than had any previous official classification, and as such it was a landmark in diagnostic classification of the psychiatric problems of the young.

The issues of nosology for children and adolescents have been extremely controversial. Major questions remain regarding the separation of adult categories from those of children and adolescents. This is particularly true of childhood depression—is it the same disorder as adult depression? What remains in question is the continuity of child and adolescent disorders with adult conditions, particularly in respect to antisocial, affective, borderline, and narcissistic personality disorders. Similar questions can be asked regarding psychosexual, schizophrenic, paranoid, and other psychotic disorders. Controversy continues regarding the use of the word neurosis, the classification of specific developmental disorders, attention deficit disorders (particularly with hyperactivity), of infant and adolescent disorders, and of numerous other conditions both listed and not listed in DSM-III.

The relevance of nosology for today's practitioner of child psychiatry is clear. The classification becomes the foundation upon which, for many, the field of child psychiatry is based. Teaching of child psychiatry, third-party reimbursement, court testimony, development of treatment approaches, and clinical communication are based increasingly on DSM-III. Much of the current research in child psychiatry uses DSM-III criteria as its diagnostic benchmark for comparison with other research work. In child psychiatry it appears that never has nosology been more relevant.

We can debate among ourselves the merits of which diagnostic system we prefer. Earls[6] states that there are at least four nosological systems in current use: DSM-III, the Group for the Advancement of Psychiatry (GAP),[10] Rutter,[21] and Eissler.[7] In fact, there is at least one other, the ninth edition of the *International Classification of Diseases* (ICD-9).[27] Earls expresses hope that a consensus will be reached as to which system is most accurate. As will be discussed throughout this chapter, over the next several decades the approach to the diagnosis of young people is expected to change greatly. What is clear is that currently the only offical classifications are ICD-9 and DSM-III (which is a special case of ICD-9). In this chapter DSM-III therefore will receive most of our attention.

This chapter is designed to be an extension of the original chapter on nosology in the second volume of the *Basic Handbook of Child Psychiatry*.[17] A number of topics discussed there will not be reviewed here in depth, including the history of classification in child psychiatry, the rationale of classification (why classify?), the hazards of classification, and a detailed comparison of earlier classification systems. The reader is referred to that chapter for that material. At some points, however, it will be necessary to quote extensively from DSM-III. Again, this chapter is not intended to replace a thorough acquaintance with DSM-III.

Finally, it is important to repeat a warning made in the original chapter—diagnosis is a shorthand, symbolic means of communication and only one small step toward understanding and working with the child. Diagnosis does not replace the necessity for in-depth understanding of the development, dynamics, and familial social aspects of the child's life. Nor does diagnosis alone dictate the treatment of the child; it is not a substitute for solid clinical judgment and acumen.

DSM-III

By the time DSM-III was published in 1980, it represented the intense efforts of hundreds of professionals for six years. The work was done under the auspices of the American Psychiatric Association. The final document was the result of intense advisory committee work, passed upon by the Task Force, and tested in extensive field trials. Most of the original drafts for DSM-III came from the fourteen advisory committees, including the advisory committee on infancy, childhood, and adolescent disorders. The chairperson of the Task Force was Robert Spitzer, M.D., who met with numerous groups, including with the Committee on Diagnostic Categories of the American Acadamy of Child Psychiatry at an annual meeting. At that meeting many differences were aired, much discussion occurred, and several important changes and additions were made to DSM-III.

The basic concepts of DSM-III were clearly outlined in its introduction. It was stated that the DSM-III was designed to be "atheoretical with regard to etiology or pathophysiological process" (p. 7). Spitzer outlined the process in detail and spoke of the achievements associated with the section regarding infants, children, and adolescents. He pointed out that there are four times as many categories in this section as there were in DSM-II's childhood section. In spite of the best efforts of Spitzer and the Task Force, there remained much controversy and disagreement. Many believed that much could have been added. The more traditional nomenclature, particularly the neurotic disorders, could have been maintained. Nonetheless, the document did advance the awareness and prominence of child psychiatric disorders.

Many advances in nosology are reflected in DSM-III. The positives include: (1) criteria have been codified and expanded and are usable and testable; (2) child and adolescent diagnoses are prominent; (3) much of the current thinking in child psychiatry is reflected; (4) room is left for change; and (5) it is a descriptive, nonetiological document. The problems include the fact that DSM-III: (1) is a descriptive, nonetiological document; (2) is nondynamic; (3) lacks a comprehensive developmental dimension; (4) lacks any systematic diagnoses for infants and adolescents; (5) has no system for family diagnosis; (6) provides an uneven transition to adult diagnoses; and (7) equates learning disorders with developmental disorders.

At issue throughout is the fact that DSM-III offers a descriptive system, not one based on etiology and/or development.

A very promising new area of technology offers the hope of making a major impact on the diagnosis of infants, children, and adolescents. That hope arises in the area of biological markers. Several chapters in this volume deal with these developments, including brain visualization techniques, the use of automated electroencephalogram (EEG) techniques, some of the newer screening devices and rating scales, and neuropsychological assessment. In discussing research directions in child psychiatry, Phillips[19] mentions the use of biochemical determinations (3-methoxy-4-hydroxy-phenylglycol, serotonin, norepinephrine breakdown products), and goes on to speak of the use of extensive population studies and the ongoing quest to quantify transactional relationships. There is also considerable promise in the recognition of temperament in infancy and its implications for disorders seen later in life. Several investigators have looked at the use of the dexamethasone suppression test to evaluate depression in children and adolescents. Robert Freedman and his associates[22] studied the relatives of schizophrenic patients by measuring deficits in the sensory gating of auditory evoked responses coupled with measurement of pursuit eye movement (a technique developed by Holzman).[12] Investigators have thus begun to identify the existence and transmission of these defects in families. The impact of a measurable deficit that is seen with regularity in any of a variety of conditions will do much to change our diagnostic thinking and systems.

One aspect of DSM-III has been a particularly valuable contribution. The multiaxial system, known in child psychiatric literature as the tri-axial system, was originally developed by Rutter.[21] That system was expanded into the five axes of DSM-III and is used for all cases, adult as well as child and adolescent.

Most of the major diagnostic categories are discussed at length in the original four volumes of the *Basic Handbook of Child Psychiatry* as well as in this volume. Instead of reiterating that material, the focus of this chapter is on particular diagnostic topics.

Diagnostic Topics

DEPRESSION IN CHILDHOOD

While there is no longer any controversy over the existence of childhood depression, there has been considerable discussion in the current literature regarding its nature. The issue is whether or not depression in infants and children is the same as in adults. One can argue for or against this in the areas of clinical manifestations, etiological (including genetic) factors, diagnostic criteria, and implications for treatment. The diagnostic question is whether infant and/or childhood depressions require categories separate and different from those of adult (general) affective disorders.

In volume 2 of this *Handbook* Cytryn and McKnew[5] reviewed, in detail, the issues of childhood depression. They made a strong case for the existence of depression in childhood, and most authorities now agree that childhood depression does exist. At the time of that writing (1979), the authors left open these questions:

(1) Are adult and childhood depression part of a limited spectrum of depressive disorders?; (2) Does childhood depression lead to or predispose to depression in later life?; and (3) Because of their disparity in etiology and course, despite clinical similarities, can childhood and adult depressions best be thought of as representing separate, independent entities? (p. 337).

In 1983 Cantwell and Carlson[4] published an update on affective disorders in childhood and adolescence. Cantwell summarized his finding that childhood depression does exist and manifests itself in essential features similar to depression in adult life. He did grant that children may have associated and age-specific symptoms. Others, although acknowledging the need for a unified classification like the DSM-III, also emphasize the importance of developmental considerations in the study of childhood depression.[19] Childhood depression reflects the concept that formal diagnosis is only the beginning, not the end, of understanding disorders of young people.

MENTAL RETARDATION

Mental retardation was particularly well integrated into DSM-III. This was brought about with the assistance of the American Association on Mental Deficiency; four major diagnostic points need to be underlined.

Mental retardation, the first diagnostic category listed in DSM-III, illustrates the concept that the heading "Disorders Usually First Evident in Infancy, Childhood, or Adolescence" may be utilized in later life (adulthood). Of course, as will be discussed later, adult (general) diagnoses may be used with young people as well. The Task Force decided that it made developmental sense to place the disorders of infancy, children, and adolescents at the beginning of the manual. The prominent location of mental retardation also reflects the importance given to these diagnoses by Spitzer and the Task Force on Nomenclature and Statistics.

Second, the diagnosis of lowered IQ must be made by individually administered general intelligence tests. The importance of individual assessment cannot be overstated. Appropriate concern has been expressed regarding the stigmatizing consequence of labeling a young person as retarded on the basis of group IQ testing (or by appearance or behavior alone). The criteria also rule out making the diagnosis of mental retardation for anyone with an IQ of over 70 (which is generally considered to represent a spread of plus or minus five points, that is, 65 to 75).

Third, it is not enough that IQ should be lowered on individual testing, but adaptive behavior must be impaired as well. Although at the time DSM-III was developed, no scales of adaptive behavior were available that offered acceptable validity and reliability, the diagnosis requires the clinical finding that the individual is not functioning well in areas of social responsibility, personal independence, or education, in comparison to others of similar age and cultural group.

Fourth, the DSM-III category eliminates the old, pejorative, and often misused category of "borderline mental retardation." That category was not reflective of a statistically significant deviation in IQ and was usually of unknown, idiopathic etiology. The condition was frequently seen in ethnic minority, socially deprived, or "understimulated" children, and making the diagnosis often resulted in negatively labeling children whose long-term outcome for independent living and self-sufficiency was not necessarily impaired.

FRAGILE X SYNDROME

One of the most exciting recent developments in the etiology of disorders of children has been the discovery of the fragile X syndrome. Although this syndrome is not included in DSM-III, it is a major diagnostic addition to the literature. The disorder is commonly associated with mental retardation, however, it also has been found in a number of children who have been diagnosed as autistic. Fragile X syndrome may be the second most common cause of mental retardation, second only to Down's syndrome. It is an X-linked disorder, characterized by an aberrant gene or locus on the long arm of the X-chromosome where a fragile site exists. [25]

Upon physical examination, 80 percent of the boys display enlarged testicles (macroorchidism). [11] There are some common facial features, including large or prominent ears (in over 80 percent of cases) and a highly arched palate with or without dental malocclusion. Less frequently there may be a high forehead, mild supraorbital ridging, and mild prognathism. In one study all eleven of the children had hyperextensibility of at least two finger joints. Over 80 percent of the patients with the disorder had mitral valve prolapse. There were also unusual dermatoglyphic (fingerprint) findings.

Most fragile X syndrome patients have moderate mental retardation, with some indication that IQ drops with age. Rarely there can be a "normal" male with the syndrome. A significant number have abnormal EEGs, with 20 percent having clinical seizures.

Most children with the syndrome have behavioral problems ranging from hyperactivity to severely autistic or violent behavior. Fragile X syndrome has many features in common with autism. These features have been extensively reviewed by Levitas, McBogg, and Hagerman. [15] Hand biting, hyperactivity, and characteristic language deficits seen in autistic children are seen as suggestive of fragile X syndrome. Rarely or not seen in fragile X syndrome are pronominal language, metaphorical language, hyperacute memory, or prodigious skills.

Many questions remain regarding the effect of the chromosomal disorder in heterozygous females. Some affected females have either learning disorders or mental retardation.

It appears certain that there will be rapid advances in our understanding of the fragile X syndrome over the next few years, and these advances will have a major effect on our approach to diagnosis of autistic-like children.

MAJOR BIPOLAR DISORDER (MANIC-DEPRESSIVE DISORDER) IN YOUNG PEOPLE

Increasingly, major bipolar disorder has been established as a disorder with familial-genetic underpinnings. As that fact has been increasingly well established in adults, it is a bit surprising that the expression of this genetic syndrome is not as clearly established in children and young people. A number of papers, particularly case studies, have demonstrated the existence of lithium-responsive adolescents. While occasional papers study the children of major bipolar disorder adults, very little information is available regarding genetic aspects of major bipolar disorder in childhood.

If a genetic factor is necessary for major bipolar disorder to exist in adults, then it would appear likely that the affected chromosomal-enzymatic defect would be present in early childhood. Indeed it should be there at the time of birth, even if it did not yet demonstrate its full biochemical effect. A finding that major bipolar disorder does not exist in childhood, or is only rarely found, might imply that: (1) an enzymatic trigger, presumably biochemical but perhaps psychogenic, is required to set off the clinical manifestations; (2) the disorder is triggered by a developmental change, such as puberty; or (3) all genetically marked children are subtly affected but do not exhibit clear clinical manifestations.

In the future there may be offered other explanations. Major bipolar disorder represents an intriguing mystery whose solution may bridge adult psychopathology. Hopefully a biochemical marker will emerge that may be observed in early childhood or even *in utero*.

Many clinicians are finding adolescents with family and/or clinical symptoms of major bipolar disorder who are lithium responsive. Nonetheless, it is still generally felt that major bipolar disorder is not routinely seen in adolescence, and especially not in childhood. DSM-III states that "the first manic episode of Bipolar Disorder typically occurs after the age of 30" (p. 215). It is important to note, however, that DSM-III does not rule out the diagnosis in young people. In my clinical experience, many young people with positive family histories and/or some clinical manifestations of major bipolar disorder who have not responded well to other forms of treatment have responded to lithium. To miss such a diagnosis would be to deprive a young patient of a specific treatment.

CHILDHOOD SCHIZOPHRENIA

When Fish and Ritvo [8] wrote their chapter "Psychosis of Childhood" in volume 2 of the *Basic Handbook of Child Psychiatry* in 1979, they assumed that childhood schizophrenia would have to be included in the DSM-III category of schizophrenia as defined for adults. Fish and Ritvo stated, "unfortunately, they [the criteria for adult schizophrenia] represent a compromise which is ill-adapted to the facts of development in childhood" (p. 263). Since the decision was made to *not* include a separate category of childhood schizophrenia in DSM-III, there has been considerable discussion in the literature regarding children and this issue. In "Childhood Schizophrenia: Present But Not Accounted For," Cantor and Associates [3] studied thirty young people who had been psychotic since childhood and met DSM-III criteria for schizophrenia except for "deterioration from a previous level of functioning." The authors felt that psychiatry has been resistant to the idea that an illness as serious as schizophrenia can occur in childhood, and refer back to the psychiatric literature of 1906 to illustrate their statement. They argue, "If we insist that symptoms which occur at age two are part of a different disease process than the same symptoms which occur at age 12, we are conceptualizing a disease unlike any other." They conclude that "early-onset Schizophrenia is at the severest end of the schizophrenic spectrum," and that childhood schizophenia belongs within the general spectrum of schizophrenia. They do note that many of the children studied did show some variation from adults in their clinical presentation, a variation that likely reflected developmental issues. Those who presented before age four had delayed speech; those between three and seven had temper tantrums, hyperactivity, and negativism; the authors found, in general, a rarity of echolalia, neologisms, and hallucinations. Other classic symptoms such as paranoia and ambivalence increased with age—that is, in adolescence.

The issue of continuity in childhood onset of schizophrenia is particularly interesting. Howells and Guirguis[13] examined in later life some twenty patients who had been diagnosed as being schizophrenic more than twenty years earlier as children (age twelve or younger). They found that all of the patients "remained unchanged in adulthood, retaining most of the cardinal signs of childhood schizophrenia" (p. 125). However, whether they would be seen as having schizophrenia in adult life varied. Using Schneider's first-rank symptoms, none would be seen as adult schizophrenics; however, using Feigner criteria, all were "schizophrenic." The outcome of the group reflected the prognostic pessimism for childhood schizophrenia —60 percent were hospitalized. The other eight (40 percent) were at home, and only two of them were taking medication.

Petty and associates[18] looked at the issue of autistic children who become schizophrenic. They describe three children and examine the literature to conclude that schizophrenia may develop in some autistic children. Marcus and coworkers[16] established the Jerusalem Infant Development Study and reported in 1981 on infants at risk for schizophrenia. To accomplish this they studied infants in their first year of life who were born to parents with serious mental disorders. They found a subgroup of thirteen out of nineteen children born to schizophrenic parents who had poor performance in sensorimotor areas of development. These infants were especially vulnerable to external insults. These findings were repeated in a study of older children by the same authors.

The question remains whether the nosology of children would be better served by a separate category "childhood schizophrenia." Although opinions differ, one can make a case for the fact that there is a continu-ity of pathology for some schizophrenic patients from childhood to adulthood and, less frequently, from adulthood back to childhood. The principal limitation of the current DSM-III designation of schizophrenia is the potential for underdiagnosis of a serious condition of childhood because all of the criteria cannot be fulfilled. The current diagnosis also carries the implication that the childhood schizophrenic patient will be schizophrenic in adult life. However, the failure to include a separate classification of childhood schizophrenia contradicts the underlying approach utilized in the section on disorders usually first evident in infancy, childhood, or adolescence. In that section are included conditions that often begin in childhood and are frequently seen in adolescence. The nosological issue remains one of confusion and controversy.

FAMILY DIAGNOSIS

At the time DSM-III was finalized, there was interest in including a family diagnostic system. However, no system examined was inclusive enough for consideration. The inclusion of such a group (nonindividual) classification system would also have been a departure from the format of DSM-III. Solomon[23] has developed a useful model regarding one dimension of families, the minimally distant family and the maximally distant family, referring to the pattern of emotional distance maintained by family members with one another. Joan Farley* has developed a system of family diagnosis that assesses the family's affect tolerance, ability to relate, impulse control, and ability to observe. However, as useful as this system may be, it still does not offer a nosological classification analagous to that utilized for individuals—that is, a specific named diagnostic categorization of specific family (versus individual) disorders. Fleck[8] felt that the DSM-III diagnoses were an "insufficient, an incomplete reflection of the total situation" (p. 125). He offered an elaborate grid for an approach to "Family Typology," but it does not present specific classic diagnostic categories. Family diagnosis remains an area for future nosological efforts.

Use of DSM-III

DISORDERS USUALLY FIRST EVIDENT IN
INFANCY, CHILDHOOD, OR ADOLESCENCE

The DSM-III separates diagnoses of young people by having a separate section for childhood disorders and then allows (requires) the use of adult (general) diagnoses for a wide variety of other disorders.

*J. Farley, personal communication, 1984.

The cross-over of DSM-III sections does not go in just one direction, as adults may be given a diagnosis from the child section if a condition beginning in youth persists into adult life.

This section includes five broad, major categories for disorders of intellect, behavior, emotion, physical (somatic) conditions, and development. DSM-III recognizes that its categories may not fit all the disorders seen in young people and suggests the use of "Unspecified Mental Disorder" (nonpsychotic) (300.90) for "problems in development that are not subsumed within the specific DSM-III diagnostic categories" (p. 36). However, this suggestion has some serious limitations. The unspecified mental disorder is defined as ". . . a residual category to be used when enough information is available to rule out a psychotic disorder, but further specification is not possible" (p. 335). The use of this category may imply a more individualized, idiosyncratic expression of an individual clinician's judgment, which, in turn may lessen its effectiveness as a "valid" category. In general, because of the problems with insurance and other official standards, its use is not recommended.

Most of the existing categories are subject to controversy. Other classification systems offer other approaches to the diagnosis of young people. While they are interesting, they are also controversial.

The specific categories discussed are intended to highlight features, controversy, and reflections regarding each category.

MENTAL RETARDATION

This category was discussed earlier.

ATTENTION DEFICIT DISORDER

Few diagnostic categories create as much disagreement, opinion, or controversy as does attention deficit disorder (ADD) (and hyperactivity). Even the name used for the category is problematic. DSM-III lists seven of the many names that have been used for this condition—"Hyperkinetic Reaction of Childhood, Hyperkinetic Syndrome, Hyperactive Child Syndrome, Minimal Brain Damage, Minimal Brain Dysfunction, Minimal Cerebral Dysfunction, and Minor Cerebral Dysfunction" (p. 611). It is apparent that these nosological titles are used for children who are in many ways similiar to one another. However, the way in which an individually affected child is regarded, along with the associated speculations as to the cause and the essential features of the condition, varies markedly with the observing professional. Few disorders of childhood have had as much written about them, have had the benefit of as much research, or have received as much professional attention.

DSM-III rather cleverly sidesteps many of the problems by avoiding speculation as to etiology. It identifies the disorder by an important aspect of its manifestations (i.e., its "developmentally inappropriate inattentions") and by dividing the disorder into three types: ADD with hyperactivity, ADD without hyperactivity, and ADD residual type. This allows for a category broad enough to encompass nearly all opinions, although perhaps not behaviorally specific enough for some uses. For example, by means of computer-assisted polygraphic analysis along with EEG records, Callaway, Holleday, and Naylor found "robust electrophysiological differences between [hyperactive children] and [normal children]."[2] They felt that the DSM-III criteria were not based on standardized norms and therefore were not sufficient for research (at least their research). However, all of their research subjects did meet DSM-III criteria for ADD.

Despite the many uncertainties, the category is clinically useful. Even if it does not presume a specific, known etiology, it often does lead to a specific treatment approach. (See chapters 38 and 56.)

CONDUCT DISORDERS

The conduct disorders have been of special interest, in part because the young people suffering from them are difficult patients who present many problems in theoretical understanding as well as in management and in part because the disorders are so common. In essence, this is a diagnosis of the patient's actions, not his or her words. It is a category that falls between a psychiatric diagnosis and a sociological/criminological conceptualization. Sometimes it seems to be a matter of which professional sees the young person first, someone from the mental health system or someone from the criminal justice system.

Thus it is a diagnostic category that is strictly behaviorally defined, where the basic criterion is a repetitive and persistent disturbance of conduct. Such an approach is far removed from dynamic and etiological considerations. The subcategories are also behaviorally defined. The DSM-III Childhood and Adolescence Committee decided on this approach because of the number of differing opinions and the lack of any consistent outcome for these conditions.

One useful differentiation did not find its way into DSM-III. The GAP report on the psychopathology of childhood included in its nosological approach to these conditions a category of tension-discharge disorders (under a broader classification of personality disorders), and divided them into three subcategories, which allowed for a more dynamic evaluation. The categories include impulse-ridden disorder, neurotic personality disorder, and sociosyntonic personality disorder.

ANXIETY DISORDERS OF CHILDHOOD OR ADOLESCENCE

In DSM-III the category of anxiety disorders of childhood or adolescence consists of three diagnoses: separation anxiety disorder, avoidant disorder of childhood or adolescence, and overanxious disorder. These are differentiated from the general DSM-III categories of anxiety disorders, which include phobias, anxiety states (anxiety neuroses), and posttraumatic stress disorders.

In the earlier GAP classification there was a more limited classification of psychoneurosis—anxiety type and phobic type—and personality disorder—anxiety type. By markedly expanding the range of anxiety disorders that can be used with children, DSM-III has served a useful clinical need. The specific disturbances have long been recognized as occurring in children and adolescents. Indeed, one of the prominent early journals dedicated to child psychiatry was entitled *The Nervous Child,* a designation reflective of the frequency of anxiety in this age group.

Separation anxiety disorder has been a common problem in the practice of child psychiatry. It encompasses the earlier diagnoses of school phobia and school refusal, and its predominant feature is "excessive anxiety on separation from major attachment figures, or from home or other familiar surroundings"[1] (p. 50).

Avoidant disorder of childhood or adolescence usually begins in the preschool years; it may be severe enough to interfere markedly with social and functioning and therefore require treatment. Even though it may border on several other disorders, such as schizoid disorders or adjustment disorder with withdrawal, it describes a significant and important group of children.

The third category of this section, overanxious disorder, is a common condition. Although they are very common in childhood, in DSM-III phobias do not have a separate listing among childhood conditions. Instead, they are included as part of the general classification of anxiety disorders where they are divided into three categories—agoraphobia (a diagnosis seldom made in childhood), social phobia, and simple phobia. There are some problems with these subdivisions, particularly in relationship to the developmental and etiological aspects of anxiety and phobia. These again are examples of the difficulties of developing a comprehensive nosology. DSM-III is designed as a descriptive document, and it has maintained that approach. The "basic science" of child psychiatry is child development, and it is perhaps inevitable that there will be some incongruity between a nosology based on description (signs and symptoms) and an approach so rooted in development.

There follows an interesting mixture of common conditions all placed under the rubric of anxiety states (or anxiety neuroses). These include: panic disorder; generalized anxiety disorder (must be eighteen years of age or older for this diagnosis); obsessive-compulsive disorder (or obsessive-compulsive neurosis); posttraumatic stress disorder, acute, chronic, or delayed; and atypical anxiety disorder. It was clearly the intent of DSM-III not to have duplicate diagnoses. For example, it was not seen as appropriate to include a separate diagnostic category of obsessive-compulsive disorder for young people as well as one for adults. (In this and a number of other conditions, a case can be made for the absence of sufficient data clearly to distinguish between the disorder in adults and children.) Yet children and adolescents may present somewhat differently than adults with similiar disorders; should that fact lead to separate diagnostic categories? DSM-III thought not.

With the exception of generalized anxiety disorder (which by DSM-III definition cannot be used before the age of eighteen), all of the disorders listed under anxiety states are common problems of children and adolescents; when seen, they require the use of the general category.

OTHER DISORDERS OF INFANCY, CHILDHOOD, OR ADOLESCENCE

In the diverse category of "other disorders" are included some diagnoses of special interest. These are reactive attachment disorder of infancy, Schizoid disorder of childhood or adolescence, elective mutism, oppositional disorder, and identity disorder.

Two of these diagnoses are age specific: reactive attachment disorder of infancy and identity disorder. This categorization represents an advance in diagnostic thinking; for the first time specific diagnoses for infancy and adolescence appear within the offical psychiatric classification system. Their appearance is seen by many as a major breakthrough.

The use of the term schizoid in the diagnosis schizoid disorders of childhood or adolescence is problematic. Under the rubric personality disorders, the GAP classification listed isolated and mistrustful types, which are now presumably encompassed by the schizoid diagnosis. Although clinically useful, the schizoid category overstates the condition for many young people, and they may end up being lumped into this diagnosis in the absence of some other, more suitable category.

Elective mutism is a disorder seen with varying frequency; it tends to occur more frequently in rural areas, such as Appalachia. It is specifically a disorder of children. General psychiatrists who have not had occasion to see children with the disorder may be skeptical of its existence, particularly as a discrete condition. However, it does exist and is a significant form of disturbance requiring a separate diagnosis.

Oppositional disorder is the one specific diagnosis that was transferred to DSM-III directly from the GAP classification. It represents a form of disorder that is common in children and adolescents; it can be very difficult to deal with but does not involve the type or degree of antisocial behavior characteristic of patients with conduct disorders. It is an important diagnosis in that it offers an alternative to the stigmatization of both the conduct disorders of young people and the adult diagnoses of antisocial and passive aggressive personality disorders.

A common and often a serious problem during adolescence is the severe stress occasioned by uncertainties about identity. By including the category of identity disorder, DSM-III for the first time recognized a psychiatric disorder of adolescence in an official classification. It is also an important alternative to adult personality diagnoses. The associated DSM-III text suggests that after eighteen years of age the appropriate diagnosis may be borderline personality disorder; this suggestion seems particularly dubious and lacking in support.

EATING DISORDERS, STEREOTYPED MOVEMENT DISORDERS, AND OTHER DISORDERS WITH PHYSICAL MANIFESTATIONS

Concurrent physical and psychiatric disorders are common in patients seen by the child psychiatrist. In one study by Kashani and Cantwell,[14] 17 percent of psychiatric outpatients and 29 percent of inpatient children (ages seven to twelve years) had physical problems. DSM-III added Axis III, physical disorders or conditions, but eliminated the DSM-II category of psychophysiologic disorders. DSM-III also offers the category of psychological factors affecting physical condition. In the course of discussing the major achievements of DSM-III, Spitzer, Williams, and Skodol[24] observed that the DSM-II classification of psychophysiologic disorders was rarely employed and that "the differentiation of these disorders from physical illnesses tended to be made idiosyncratically by clinicians." Yet many patients of child psychiatrists suffer from a wide variety of what may be classic psychophysiological problems, such as asthma, migraine and tension headaches, obesity, bulimia, anorexia, hypertension, arthritis, neurodermatitis, a wide variety of gastrointestinal disorders, and many others. These may present as primary (Axis I) conditions that would require the use of the rather convoluted and unfamiliar classification of psychological factors affecting physical condition.

For disorders usually first evident in infancy, DSM-III includes a group of conditions expressed, for the most part, by means of physical symptoms. These are divided into three groups, beginning with the eating disorders. Five specific diagnoses are included in this group: anorexia nervosa, bulimia, pica, rumination disorder of infancy, and atypical eating disorder.

Anorexia nervosa and bulimia have received enormous media attention. Anorexia is an important category that may need additional subclassification. By definition, bulimia involves episodic binges of overeating. DSM-III's description is accurate. However, the popular media have picked up the term bulimia and use it to mean bulimia-purge; they see it as a variation of anorexia nervosa (which it may be), and it therefore loses some of its precise definition.

Pica is a well-recognized, specific disorder in children and is an important addition to DSM-III.

Rumination disorder of infancy is the second infant disorder to be included in DSM-III, and, although it is "very rare," it can be fatal. Its representation in DSM-III may aid clinicians in recognizing this disorder when it does occur.

The atypical eating disorders classification is reserved for those eating disorders that cannot be classified with other DSM-III categories.

Stereotyped movement disorders is a new group of classifications in the third edition of the manual. All of these disorders include tics as their principal sign. This group includes transient tic disorder, chronic motor tic disorder, Tourette's disorder, atypical tic disorder, and atypical stereotyped movement disorder.

This is an interesting group of disturbances about which little is known. There is a question as to whether all are part of the same general condition with variations in the ways in which they manifest themselves and/or perhaps in their severity. It also may be asked whether or not the condition is a symptom of some other, more global and significant childhood disorder, such as organic brain disease or one of the anxiety disorders.

Within the category of atypical stereotyped movement disorders, an interesting hodgepodge of movements is to be found that seems as a rule to occur in association with a variety of primary diagnoses, any of which may include a pattern of nonspasmodic, repetitious, rhythmic motions. They may be associated either with such conditions as developmental disabilities (mental retardation, organic brain syndrome, pervasive developmental disorders) or with acute states such grief, depression, anxiety, fear, deprivation, and abuse.

The next group is other disorders with physical manifestations. These include stuttering, functional enuresis, functional encopresis, sleepwalking disorder, and sleep terror disorder.

All of these disorders share in common the overriding importance of developmental concerns. All may be normal and expected; and except for night terrors, all are statistically normal variants of behaviors regularly encountered at various stages of childhood. Clearly all infants are "enuretic" and "encopretic" before bladder and bowel training. Diagnosis requires not only consideration of chronological age but also overall evaluation of the several lines of development. Symptoms may occur as a result of psychological regression in the face of stress. When these conditions are signs of regression, they should not be regarded as evidence of the "disorder" per se but rather as a manifestation of the more basic condition. This group again reflects the problem of using signs and symptoms as if they were synonymous with a diagnostic category. That is not to say that these are not useful listings as disorders, but their limitations as primary conditions, particularly vis-à-vis developmental considerations, must be noted.

Enuresis is a common finding, yet the condition involves so many variations that subclassification seems in order. Subclasses may include: chronic/acute, intermittent/continuous, dribble/flood, nocturnal/diurnal, and rapid-eye-movement (REM)/non-REM sleep occurrence. DSM-III implies a distinction between primary and secondary functional enuresis, but it does not define the terms. In the section on encopresis, the word primary is used to refer to a child who "has reached the age of four and [where the condition] has not been preceded by fecal continence for at least one year" (p. 81). This is congruent with the usual use of "primary" to represent a child who has been continuously incontinent and "secondary" to describe the child who once had achieved control but who later becomes incontinent. These definitions are important. Confusion could arise over the use of "primary" as equivalent to a functional but isolated symptom or disorder versus "secondary" as representing a condition caused by or seen in association with another, more primary condition.

The two major sleep disorders are sleepwalking disorder and sleep terror disorder. With the abundance of research being done on sleep, it will soon be necessary to expand this group. DSM-III describes psychogenic fugue, sleep drunkenness, REM sleep nightmares, and hypnagogic hallucinations, but it does not include them as specific disorders. There appears to be a need for, at least, an atypical sleep disorder of infancy, childhood, and adolescence category that would include these and other related conditions. DSM-III does offer a discussion of "classification of sleep and arousal disorders" (appendix E), which divides sleep disorders along symptom lines of insomnias (which includes a designation of childhood-onset disorder of initiating and maintaining sleep (DIMS) without further elaboration), excessive somnolence, disorders of sleep-wake schedule, and parasomnias, but does not divide the conditions along age and developmental lines. All these conditions will receive much more attention over the next several decades.

PERVASIVE DEVELOPMENTAL DISORDERS

Since the inception of child psychiatry, the category of pervasive developmental disorders (PDDs) has been a nosological thorn in the side of neat and orderly diagnostic systems. Much debate and discussion continue regarding the nature of these conditions, and until more is known about them, particularly about their etiology, the diagnosis will evoke controversy and differences among professionals. Included in this category of PDDs are three diagnoses: infantile autism, childhood-onset pervasive developmental disorder, and atypical.

The current status of research and professional thinking is examined in detail in chapter 39. Diagnostically, PDD has long been seen as a syndrome that encompasses a wide spectrum of variants. DSM-III makes an important and logical step forward by moving the classification away from the term autistic into a broader framework. It does so by acknowledging the differences between the classic autistic child, whose signs appear before eighteen months, and the later-onset PDD (after eighteen months). In addition, the description uses markers that are more or less objective, such as the onset of speech.

As is true for a number of the infant, childhood, and adolescent DSM-III classifications, a decision was made not to include certain categories that had achieved some acceptance in other childhood diagnostic systems, terms that have been useful for a small but significant group of patients. These include the atypical child,[20] schizophreniform psychosis, and childhood schizophrenia (discussed earler in this chapter). In addition, it will be of great interest to see what impact our increasing knowledge of the genetic disorder, fragile X syndrome will have on the way we regard these PDDs. Nonetheless, it seems as if the DSM-III diagnostic approach to the PDDs will be useful until there are other research developments in this rapidly changing area.

The Use of General Adult Diagnoses with Infants, Children, and Adolescents

DSM-III mandates that many conditions seen in the young must use the same title of a disorder from the general section. This offers a more parsimonious arrangement overall but presents some problems for the child psychiatrist. We will look briefly at each category and its relationship to infants, children, and adolescents.

ORGANIC MENTAL DISORDERS

Many of the organic mental disorders listed do occur with some frequency in young people. For example, DSM-III states that "delirium can occur at any age, but is especially common in children and after the age of 60" (p. 105). Dementia, on the other hand, is found predominantly in the elderly, but the diagnosis can be made "any time after the intellectual quotient is fairly stable (usually by age 3 or 4)" (p. 109).

SUBSTANCE USE DISORDERS

A long list of substances can induce organic brain syndromes. Many of these conditions can be encountered in young people, particularly in adolescents. Indeed, these conditions are all too often seen in adolescents and even, on occasion, in children. When they are the primary problem, they are to be diagnosed as the Axis I condition.

SCHIZOPHRENIC DISORDERS, PARANOID DISORDERS, AND PSYCHOTIC DISORDERS NOT ELSEWHERE CLASSIFIED

The diagnosis of schizophrenia can be made in adolescence (or even in childhood), but, as discussed before, a case can be made for a separate category of childhood schizophrenia. The paranoid disorders do not appear to be disorders of young people, or, if they do occur this early, they are rather rare. The remaining group of DSM-III psychoses may all apply to young people. Schizophreniform disorder is a condition identical to schizophrenia but with a duration of less then six months. Brief reactive psychosis is a disorder most often seen in adolescents and young adults. It is possible but seems unlikely that schizoaffective disorder will be seen in young people. Of course, the listing atypical psychosis may have occasional use with children or adolescents.

AFFECTIVE DISORDERS AND ANXIETY DISORDERS

These disorders have been discussed earlier.

Somatoform Disorders and Dissociative Disorders

The entire group of somatoform disorders—somatization disorder, conversion disorder (hysterical neurosis), psychogenic pain disorder, hypocondriasis, and atypical somatoform disorder—can be diagnosed in young people. Psychogenic amnesia, multiple personality, and depersonalization disorder may begin in childhood and adolescence; psychogenic fugue is less typically seen in the young.

Psychosexual Disorders

The psychosexual disorders are a large group of disorders that are first manifested in adolescence, although many begin in childhood. These are discussed in part in chapter 6.

Factitious Disorders and Disorders of Impulse Control Not Elsewhere Classified

The factitious disorders may occur in childhood and adolescence, but there is little written about them in respect to young people. Kleptomania and pyromania often begin in childhood, pathological gambling may begin in adolescence, and the explosive disorders are described as beginning in the second and third decades. The usefulness of these classifications in work with young people remains to be seen. Certainly the behaviors may occur, but they are often associated with other more primary conditions.

Adjustment Disorders

The category of adjustment disorders is used frequently with children and adolescents. By definition, the diagnosis can be made only where there is a known source of stress and when the reaction has occurred within three months of that stress. The stress may be discrete or continuous, and the severity of the symptoms may not be dependent on the severity of the stress. Clearly, in the assessment of these conditions in young people, developmental considerations will be of overriding concern. DSM-III states, "for example, the stress of losing a parent is different for a child and an adult" (p. 299).

Personality Disorders

The personality disorders are a group of conditions that present particular problems. Several personality disorders diagnoses may be used with young people, but it is of critical importance to be vigilant as to the potential for stigma that can come with this group of diagnoses. The hallmark of personality disorders is the enduring quality of the identifying behavioral patterns. These patterns cause significant impairment that, without effective treatment, may be expected to continue throughout adult life. DSM-III sees certain disorders of children and adolescents as corresponding to certain personality disorders. It recommends changing the child or adolescent diagnosis to the adult equivalent at age eighteen. There is little evidence for the one-to-one correlation of adult personality disorder with each of these conditions, a fact DSM-III recognizes. The intent of the authors of DSM-III was to help avoid the stigmatization and the expectation of a negative outcome. The adult personality disorder diagnoses, which are not generally made before age eighteen, include schizoid, avoidant, antisocial, passive-aggressive, and borderline.

In spite of the common clinical use of the terms narcissistic and borderline, no separate category for young people makes use of them. The criteria for such conditions during childhood and adolescence would be difficult to develop without a strong inference that these conditions would extend into adulthood. This is an area wherein the nosologist must tread carefully.

Specific Developmental Disorders (Axis II)

The limitations of the specific developmental disorders category of Axis II have received considerable attention and criticism. The classification allows no category for psychosexual, maturational, psychosocial, affective, or general cognitive disorders, even though these are conditions seen by clinicians. The category's narrow focus is difficult to understand and appears to represent only one limited view of development. Some aspects of this problem were discussed in volume 2 of this *Handbook*. [17]

Conclusion

DSM-III may be the latest word in nosology, but it is certainly not the final word. As nosology is the beginning step in the understanding of the patient, DSM-III

represents an important beginning step in the understanding of the role of infants, children, and adolescents in the general nosology of psychiatry.

In my view, there are two major limitations in using DSM-III in the diagnosis of young people. The first is the compartmentalization between disorders of infants, children, and adolescents as a group and disorders of "grownups." The rationale for that division is clear, defensible, and perhaps necessary for a general, "official," diagnostic system. However, a strong case can be made for the value of a separate diagnostic document for young people. This separate nosology could be an extension of DSM-III in the same way that DSM-III is an extension (special case) of ICD-9. Continuity should be maintained by keeping as much of the codes and terminology as is possible from both current official classifications.

The second major limitation is the lack of a developmental, dynamic focus, which is essential to an understanding of young people. But, although important, such an orientation is not a substitute for a solid descriptive nosological approach, and in those descriptive areas DSM-III represents a major advance.

These two limitations are, in part, reflective of our greatest weakness in psychiatric nosology: the lack of solid etiological data upon which to base our diagnoses. Most of the conditions encountered in adult life must have a beginning in earlier life. The underlying causes of these conditions and how they present themselves in childhood and adolescence may be an important future key to our understanding of psychiatric disorders in general.

Many specific as well as general criticisms can be made of DSM-III. Vaillant [26] saw many disadvantages, including what he considered its parochial, reductionistic, and adynamic qualities. There are some additional concerns not mentioned earlier. In my view, there is a need for an additional axis for severity of condition. There is a need for developmental considerations and recognition of the change in presentation of symptoms which may vary by age. There may also come a time when some of the criteria that are now defined by their presence or absence may well be quantified or scaled in severity and persistance. Future DSM's may hold many exciting, useful, and creative changes with each new edition. One can hope that what was begun in DSM-III by creating a separate section for the disorders of young people and by including the beginnings of categories for infants and adolescents will be extended and improved upon.

The future of infant, childhood, and adolescent nosology seems bright. Throughout the rest of the twentieth century, we can anticipate major advances in our ability to measure, observe, and understand our patients. Each major advance will surely add to the richness of our knowledge. But undoubtedly, for each question answered by our advancing technology, a dozen more will be presented. It is inevitable that in nosology, as in any other scientific field, we will be increasingly challenged and stimulated by that which is to come. It will help to continue to expand nosology beyond the simple study of dry lists and classifications and form it into an increasingly vital and dynamic tool in the practice of child psychiatry.

REFERENCES

1. AMERICAN PSYCHIATRIC ASSOCIATION. *Diagnostic and Statistical Manual of Mental Disorders*, 3rd ed. Washington D.C.: American Psychiatric Association, 1980.

2. CALLAWAY, E., HALLIDAY, R., and NAYLOR, H. "Hyperactive Children's Event-Related Potentials Fail to Support Underarousal and Maturational-Lag Theories," *Archives of General Psychiatry*, 40 (1983):1243–1248.

3. CANTOR, S., et al. "Childhood Schizophrenia: Present But Not Accounted For," *American Journal of Psychiatry*, 139 (1982):758–762.

4. CANTWELL, D. P., and CARLSON, G. A. *Affective Disorders in Childhood and Adolescence*. New York: SP Medical and Scientific Books, 1983.

5. CYTRYN, L., and MCKNEW, D. H. "Affective Disorders," in J. D. Noshpitz, ed., *Basic Handbook of Child Psychiatry*, vol. 2. New York: Basic Books, 1979, pp. 321–340.

6. EARLS, F. "The Future of Child Psychiatry as a Medical Discipline," *American Journal of Psychiatry*, 139 (1982):1158–1161.

7. EISSLER, R. S., FREUD, A., and KRIS, M. *Psychoanalytic Assessment: the Diagnostic Profile*. New Haven, Conn.: Yale University Press, 1977.

8. FISH, B., and RITVO, E. R. "Psychoses of Childhood," in J. D. Noshpitz, ed., *Basic Handbook of Child Psychiatry*, vol. 2. New York: Basic Books, 1979, pp. 249–304.

9. FLECK, S. "A Holistic Approach to Family Typology and the Axes of DSM-III," *Archives of General Psychiatry*, 40 (1983):901–906.

10. GROUP FOR THE ADVANCEMENT OF PSYCHIATRY, Committee on Child Psychiatry. *Psychopathological Disorders in Childhood: Theoretical Considerations and a Proposed Classification*, vol. 6, Report no. 62. New York: Group for the Advancement of Psychiatry, 1966.

11. HAGERMAN, R., SMITH, A.C.M., and MARINER, R. "Clinical Features of the Fragile X Syndrome," in R. J. Hagerman and P. M. McBogg, *The Fragile X Syndrome*. Dillon, Col.: Spectra, 1983, pp. 17–53.

12. HOLZMAN, P. S., et al. "Pursuit Eye Movement Dysfunctions in Schizophrenia," *Archives of General Psychiatry*, 41 (1984):136–139.

13. HOWELLS, J. G., and GUIRGUIS, W. R. "Childhood Schizophrenia 20 Years Later," *Archives of General Psychiatry*, 41 (1984):123–128.

14. KASHANI, J. H., and CANTWELL, D. P. "Characteristics of Children Admitted to Inpatient Community Mental Health Center," *Archives of General Psychiatry*, 40 (1983):397–400.

15. LEVITAS, A., MCBOGG, P., and HAGERMAN, R. "Behavioral Dysfunction in the Fragile X Syndrome," in R. J. Hagerman and P. M. McBogg, *The Fragile X Syndrome*. Dillon, Col.: Spectra, 1983, pp. 103–173.

16. MARCUS, J., et al. "Infants at Risk for Schizophrenia," *Archives of General Psychiatry*, 38 (1981):703–713.

17. MAY, J. G. "Nosology and Diagnosis," in J. D. Noshpitz, ed., *Basic Handbook of Child Psychiatry*, vol. 2. New York: Basic Books, 1979, pp. 111–143.

18. PETTY, L. K., et al. "Autistic Children Who Become Schizophrenic," *Archives of General Psychiatry*, 41 (1984):129–135.

19. PHILLIPS, I. "Research Directions in Child Psychiatry," *American Journal of Psychiatry*, 137 (1980):1436–1439.

20. RANK, B. "Intensive Study and Treatment of Preschool Children Who Show Marked Personality Deviations or 'Atypical Development' and Their Parents," in G. Caplan, ed., *Emotional Problems of Early Childhood*. New York: Basic Books, 1955, pp. 491–502.

21. RUTTER, M., et al. "A Tri-Axial Classification of Mental Disorders in Childhood," *Journal of Child Psychology and Psychiatry*, 10 (1969):41–61.

22. SIEGEL, C., et al. "Deficits in Sensory Gating in Schizophrenic Patients and Their Relatives," *Archives of General Psychiatry*, 41 (1984):607–612.

23. SOLOMON, M. A. "Typologies of Family Homeostasis: Implications for Diagnosis and Treatment," *Family Therapy*, 1:9–18.

24. SPITZER, R. L., WILLIAMS, J. B. W., and SKODOL, A. E. "DSM-III: The Major Achievements and an Overview," *American Journal of Psychiatry*, 137 (1980):151–163.

25. TURNER, G. "Historical Overview of X-Linked Mental Retardation," in R. J. Hagerman and P. M. McBogg, *The Fragile X Syndrome*. Dillon Col.: Spectra, 1983.

26. VAILLANT, G. E. "The Disadvantages of DSM-III Outweigh Its Advantages," *American Journal of Psychiatry*, 141 (1984):542–545.

27. WORLD HEALTH ORGANIZATION. *Manual of the International Classification of Diseases, Injuries, and Causes of Death*, 9th ed. Geneva, Switzerland, 1977.

PART C
Syndromes

27 / Psychiatric Syndromes of Infancy*

Justin D. Call

Introduction

Diagnosable, maladaptive disorders in the infant or in the patterns of interaction between the infant and other caring persons centering around the mother and/or the father that place the parent/child unit at risk constitute a significant but as yet little recognized series of specific disturbances in the infant which may have both immediate and far-reaching affects upon the course of the infant's development.

In most instances, beginning with conception, but certainly by the end of gestation, the appearance of a baby induces a special state of mind in the prospective parents and in the rest of the family, including siblings and others, who become psychologically involved with the infant. The term infancy refers not only to the first stage of postnatal life but also to this special state of mind induced in the parents and others by the fetus and the infant. This state of mind consists of both positive and negative thoughts and feelings derived from a lifetime of conscious and unconscious memories, experiences, and fantasies centering around a baby, including oneself as a baby and those who care for the baby, such as one's parents. These thoughts and feelings include the strongest of loving and hateful fantasies and the defenses erected against them. The infant is conceived in the mind of the parent long before actual conception takes place. Conception and approaching delivery evokes this past in the preconscious mental state of the parent. Birth and early infant care induce a new set of thoughts and feelings based on the meanings created in the interactional field between the baby and the mother and father. I have purposely avoided the use of the term caretakers because it does not convey the inner psychological attitudes that can occur only with individuals who develop a full sense of being a parent regardless of biological connections.

EXAMPLE:

Mrs. B had been an operating room nurse and, at the time she became pregnant, had consciously negative feelings about having and caring for babies. When she discovered at the fifth month that she would give birth to twins, she was downright negative. Very soon after the birth of the twins, however, she found herself entranced and devoted to her beautiful little girls. She became an excellent mother, quite willing to stay at home and quite confident in relying upon her intuitive convictions about how to proceed with the challenging task of caring for twins. She successfully nursed them and went on to have three additional children. Her negative feelings about pregnancy were based on a conscious concern she had regarding the loss and interruption of her career. Her more powerful unconscious, positive feelings about babies and being a mother, which took her by surprise, were based on a strong positive identification with her own nurturant, loving mother, who was devoted to and entranced by her.

The burgeoning study of normal infancy has made it possible to identify more clearly the landmarks of normal development and to determine the context in which maladaptive behavior occurs. Conversely, the

*Parts of this chapter are reprinted by permission of the publisher from J. D. Call, "Toward a Nosology of Psychiatric Disorders in Infancy," in J. D. Call, E. Galenson, and R. L. Tyson, eds; *Frontiers of Infant Psychiatry.* New York, Basic Books, 1983, pp. 117–128.

study of maladaptive behavior and development in infancy is providing a more dramatic and precise knowledge of these landmarks of normal development. Thus the fields of normal and psychopathological development are codetermined. Infant psychiatry is a newly consolidating, transdisciplinary field, the main thrust of which is the art and science of diagnosing and treating the maladaptive disorders of infancy.

The Earliest Stages of Psychological Development

The human baby is prepared during fetal life and arrives on the scene ready to participate actively as a partner with the parent in structuring its own development. In all likelihood the stage is set for this participant activity by hormonal changes during pregnancy and by the associated psychophysiological regression in the mother. These neuroendocrine changes provide the context for the mother's regressively organized narcissistic identification with the infant, which adds specific psychological content to this underlying physiology. This identification brings about a state of empathy in the mother whereby the infant's helplessness, needs, peculiarities of communication can be met. As this occurs the possibility of mother and infant sharing and modifying each other's feelings states is possible. Trevarhan[44] and Papousek and Papousek[32] have referred to this as intersubjectivity. We now know that this psychophysiological narcissistic regression serves the mother's adaptation; it prepares her physiologically and psychologically for the birth of the infant and for empathically organized care and devotion. The regression allows communication at the affective level[8] and makes it possible for the mother to intuit the meaning of the infant's behavior, patterns of communication, and need states as well as to monitor the infant's actual physiological behavior (i.e., breathing patterns, movement patterns, responses to stimuli) and thus its survival. The infant sets in motion a psychological state in the mother, and the mother, through her responsiveness to the baby, confers upon the infant the validity of its own experiences and collaborates with the infant in becoming the architect of what both of them subjectively experience. This induced psychophysiological regression also renders the mother vulnerable to serious psychiatric disorders, especially schizophrenia and major depression.

Both normal and psychopathological development can be understood in their most fundamental sense as a disturbance in the evolution of infancy as just described. Infancy is considered to have its beginning at conception and its termination at about the age of three, when the child is fully capable of syntactically organized communication, has achieved a high degree of object constancy, and is more able to negotiate psychosocial territory using conventional language. Until this advent the infant remains dependent on others to intuit the meanings of its behavior and moods. It follows then that in most instances psychopathology during this period is dyadic and interactional. All psychiatric disturbances of infancy, even those with known organic causes, should be viewed in the context of this beginning.

Infancy as Viewed by Darwin, Freud, and Piaget

The theories of Darwin,[13,14] Freud,[17] and Piaget[35] have contributed significantly to a developmental view of man. Each of these pioneers actually observed infants, drew significant theoretical inferences, and developed heuristically powerful theories about man's early development. Darwin linked his theory of biological evolution with the observation of emotional expressions in his firstborn son (1844) from birth to about two and one-half by simply recording in a diary his observations of the infant's expressive behavior under various conditions. He concluded that emotional expressions in man emerged from a biological matrix not unlike that of other primates and that such expressions were an essential aspect of the adaptive capacity of social mammals, including man, serving as communicative signals to others of one's own species. These insights, together with his general theory of evolution, the grandest of all developmental theories, have inspired and continue to inspire many infancy studies. The experimental work on primates and other mammals, especially the chimpanzee and the rat, can be linked meaningfully with the developmental studies of normal and pathological development in human babies. This linkage is shown in the development of the field of ethology[29,43] as it relates to human attachments[1,4] and continues to inspire more recent work concerning language development, learning in infancy during the long period of dependency, sociobiology, infancy sleep research, and the significance and implications of breast versus bottle feeding. The psychoanalytic concept of the mother as an auxiliary ego borrows its meanings from Darwin's theory.

Sigmund Freud, always the biologist, moved the focus of concern in adult psychopathology to infancy by linking adult sexuality, character, and the neuroses to infantile sexuality and to phase-specific developmental conflicts leading to fixation. Freud also showed that normal character structure emerges from constitutional givens and from the conflicts of infancy that have become ego syntonic as character traits. He clearly identified the drives as having their origin within biological evolution. Less known is the fact that Freud considered primary ego constituents (choice of defenses) also to have their origin in biological evolution.[18] He even suggested the possibility that superego structures were structured biologically. Current sociobiological theories of altruism support this seemingly outlandish idea.

The modern pioneers in infant development, especially Winnicott, Erikson, Spitz, Mahler, and Bowlby, built upon Freud's scaffolding. It is indeed difficult to find a recent article in the psychoanalytic literature that is not concerned either with the genetic propositions of psychoanalytic theory or with theory and observation coming directly from some aspect of current infancy research. Thus psychoanalysis continues to thrive as a developmental science. Many psychoanalysts are currently in the forefront of psychobiological infancy research.

Jean Piaget, another biologist, who was inspired early in his career[34] by Freud, achieved monumental insights into the child's cognitive development during the sensorimotor phase of infancy by observing his own children from birth. Piaget defined adaptation as the process of assimilation and accommodation—that is, the ways in which children took in stimuli from the outside and modified mental schema by accommodation as they incorporated more and more of the novel stimuli into the schema. Based on Piaget's conception of adaptation, a cognitive view of psychic trauma resulting in psychopathology would be the failure to achieve an equilibrium between the process of assimilation and accommodation. Piaget's studies on the development of object permanence—the stage at which the infant is able to establish a steady mental representation of an inanimate object, usually achieved around eighteen months*—contrasts with the psychoanalytic conception of object constancy—the process by which the human infant can maintain a mental representation of the libidinal object even in the presence of powerful affects and destructive urges toward that object.

Margaret Mahler† suggested that the achievement of relative object constancy was a process of such central importance that a complete nosology of psychiatric disorder could be based on particular deficits relating to developmental problems encountered on the way to achieving it. Much of the ferment in the field of infant psychiatry and much of what it has to offer to an understanding of normal and psychopathological development later on can be traced to the ways in which researchers are currently engaged in attempts to integrate the theories and conceptions of infancy as defined by Darwin, Freud, and Piaget. The theories of all three have provided a rich heuristic network of grand- and small-scale theory that continues to provoke and inspire modern workers.

The Modern Era of Infancy Research

In 1959 Peter Wolff[45] made a very important but, in retrospect, rather mundane discovery that changed the face of infant psychiatry; he showed a correlation between the infant's state of arousal during sleep and wakefulness with specific state-related observable behaviors in the newborn infant. This brought order and predictability to infant behaviors that were previously considered random or reflexive in nature and made possible the rapid development of meaningful infant observational and experimental studies from many viewpoints. Having operational definitions of the state variable in the observational field was like being able to hold the slide steady while viewing it under the microscope. The study of anticipatory approach behavior in the first four days of life,[6] which showed that the newborn infant rapidly learns to anticipate the appearance of the breast or bottle during feeding, would not have been possible had the state variable—that is, the conditions under which this early sensorimotor adaptation occurred—not been defined. Defining the state variable in infancy also made possible the redefinition of what the infant was capable of perceiving in all sensory modalities. The fact that the newborn infant shows a rapid increase in attentive ability and can see objects clearly and follow them in space and the fact that the visual and auditory apparatus are so well developed at birth and continue a rapid development thereafter led to more sophisticated learning experiments utilizing both classical and operant conditioning. Such experiments showed that the infant was indeed a very competent human being even at birth and that the baby, in fact, operates as an architect of its own experience with the mother in its early extrauterine adaptation.

Margaret Mahler's longitudinal studies of normal infants beginning in the early months of life and con-

---

*Shown by the infant's capacity to find a missing object previously within its view or hearing even after sleight-of-hand and other manipulative maneuvers designed to disguise its whereabouts.

†M. Mahler, personal communication, 1985.

tinuing through the second and third year led her to the important conception that the infant and mother develop a symbiotic relationship in the early months. The infant slowly emerges from this symbiotic envelope during the last half of the first year of life and then goes on to further separate him- or herself from the mother through the stages of separation-individuation, finally achieving a state of relative object constancy at around the age of two after proceeding through the treacherous territory of the rapprochement subphase of development. This emergence of independent status takes place as the infant is able to establish a representation of the mother in his or her own mind. Recent studies by McDevitt (see Chapter 5) have shown that the infant's mirroring experience with the mother during the rapprochement subphase contributes to the development of the sense of self in the latter half of the second year of life. Mahler suggests that much of later psychopathology that grows out of a poor sense of coherence about one's sense of self has its origin within the rapprochement subphase where splitting of good and bad and projective mechanisms operate (eighteen months to two years of age) rather than during the first few months of life, the period at which Melanie Klein postulated[27] that the paranoid position develops.

Many other themes and subthemes have evolved very rapidly from this rich matrix of observation and theory. Two world congresses on infant psychiatry sponsored by the World Association for Infant Psychiatry and Allied Disciplines have now been held and a third will take place in Stockholm later this year (1986).

The world view of infant psychiatry is bringing into focus transcultural perspectives, universality of certain forms of psychopathology within the mother/infant dyad, the problems of developing an acceptable nosology that can apply throughout the world, and the need for additional training and research in this transdisciplinary field.

Conception to Birth: Risk Factors and Prevention of Prematurity

Keeping in mind the fact that pregnancy and delivery impose significant risk to the mother and to the infant (and to the father?) and that pregnancy causes lifelong consequences for each, our developmental sciences, education, health care systems, and religious and other value orientations have all attempted to impress upon the about-to-conceive couple the need to consciously consider, rather than passively allow, conception to occur.

Risk factors affecting the development of the central nervous system (CNS) of the fetus are summarized in table 27–1. Examples of inherited CNS diseases include such things as phenylketonuria, cri du chat syndrome, Rh and ABO blood incompatibilities, and certain brain malformations, including inherited neurotransmitter deficiencies. Examples of inherited predisposition toward CNS malfunctioning refer to manic-depressive illness, schizophrenia, attention deficit disorder, and inheritance of neurosensory deficits, including deafness. Recent information[5] suggests that older mothers in good health who elect to have their first infants after the age of thirty and who receive high-quality medical care and supervision during pregnancy as well as relief from psychosocial and physical stressors do much better than previously thought. Health of the mother and low risk for prematurity (to be discussed later) play an important affect in ameliorating the risk factors operating in mothers less than eighteen years of age. It has been shown in the multicenter long-term collaborative studies of infants[33] that bleeding during the first trimester of pregnancy as, for example, with threatened abortion, is a significant variable associated with increased risk for various forms of cerebral palsy,[33] a group of conditions often unrecognized as a source of developmental deviation in the first year and one-half of life if it occurs in milder forms. The study of viral infections, including herpes and the "slow viruses" of AIDS and Jakob-Creutzfeldt disease, is shedding considerable light on the risk factors to the fetus due to these infections. While it is now recognized that the fetal alcohol syndrome is specifically related to the amount of alcohol the mother consumes during pregnancy (more than one ounce of alcohol, 70 percent by weight, per night) in the first trimester, it is becoming clear that the full manifestations of fetal alcohol syndrome as originally described may be only one of several less obvious forms of damage to the fetal CNS. Thus the term alcohol-related abnormalities is preferable to the earlier "fetal alcohol syndrome." A ten-year follow-up of the eleven children with fetal alcohol syndrome first reported by K. L. Jones and D. W. Smith in 1973 has shown that the degree of mental retardation in these children was related to the degree of cranial facial abnormality seen at birth and to the degree of microcephaly and shortness of stature.[40]

Psychosocial stress factors affecting the mother have recently come again into focus as important and verifiable risk factors to the fetus,[33] precipitating premature onset of labor due to hyperirritable uterus and also predisposing to hypertrophic pyloric stenosis,[36] which occurs after birth. The incidence of psychosocial stress during the third trimester of pregnancy has been di-

TABLE 27–1

Risk Factors Adversely Affecting the Development of the Central Nervous System of the Fetus

1. Inherited disease affecting the central nervous system (e.g., phenylketonuria).
2. Inherited predispositions affecting central nervous system malfunctioning (e.g., manic-depressive disorder).
3. Mother younger than eighteen or older than thirty-five with first pregnancy.
4. Prior history of stillbirth, spontaneous abortion, prematurity, or placental insufficiency.
5. Threatened abortion.
6. Use of progestins or estrogens during pregnancy.
7. Exposure of the fetus to ionizing radiation.
8. Exposure of the fetus or placenta to viral or bacterial infection (e.g., German measles).
9. Transmissible venereal disease—herpes, AIDS, syphilis.
10. Exposure of the fetus to alcohol—acetaldehyde, heroin, cocaine, or other addicting substances and harmful medications.
11. Exposure of the fetus to long-term nutritional deficiency due to chronic maternal nutritional deficiency.
12. Psychosocial stress affecting the mother and fetus.
13. Physical injury to fetus, uterus, or placenta and its attachments.

rectly correlated with the onset of hypertrophic pyloric stenosis in the infant after birth. Stress factors, however, are not the only factors to consider in this condition. A genetic predisposition toward hypertrophic pyloric stenosis is also apparent, as is the style of feeding after birth. In ten infants consecutively diagnosed and referred to one surgeon, all were breast-fed and showed an anxiously close relationship with the mother that was engendered by loss and stress factors during the third trimester.[10] Physical injury to the fetus, the uterus, and the placenta are indeed real stress factors to the development of the CNS of the fetus. There is now incontrovertible evidence that cigarette smoking during pregnancy results in babies that are small for their gestational age. The psychosocial history of the mother, including her interpersonal history, a history of having been abused as a child, and traumatic separation experience as a child predisposes the mother toward similar behavior with her own child.

PREVENTION OF PREMATURE BIRTH

It has been recognized for decades that babies that are small for gestational age, "premature babies" (less than 2,500 grams), especially *very* small babies (less than 1,500 grams), are at much greater risk for later neurological, behavioral, learning, developmental, and psychiatric disturbance. It has, therefore, become expedient in any preventive program that risk factors for prematurity be clearly identified and that appropriate intervention be offered to ameliorate those risk factors that can be ameliorated. In recently published studies from Hageneau, France, and Martinique, in the Caribbean, by Papiernik and associates,[31] and by Cole[12] and by Herron, Katz, and Creasy[26] in the United States, it has been possible to reduce the incidence of premature birth by introducing appropriate preventive measures.

A 31 percent reduction in premature birth (from 5.4 to 3.7 percent) has been shown in the French study (less than 16,000 live births), which lasted for twelve years (1971–1982) and was organized and paid for by the French National Social Security System. Herron, Katz, and Creasy,[26] in a preliminary study of 1,150 live births, reported a reduction in premature births from 6.7 to 2.4 percent. A multicenter preterm birth prevention trial is currently (1985) underway sponsored by the March of Dimes.[12] Factors determining premature birth are shown in table 27–2. Those modifiable after the diagnosis of pregnancy are marked with an asterisk. The incidence of premature birth in mothers known to be at risk for premature birth by the basis of cervical examination, poor socioeconomic conditions, age, excessive physical exertion and a history of poor medical care can be significantly reduced when these at-risk mothers are provided with education geared toward explaining the risk factors involved, reduction of physical exertion and of psychosocial and economic stress factors together with good medical care and home care (once-a-week visits by midwives during pregnancy). The incidence of very-low-birth-weight infants (less than 1,500 grams) is reduced by 67 percent. This French study is the first very large scale controlled study to demonstrate such dramatic effects and has inspired similar programs specifically directed toward mothers at risk for premature birth in this country and elsewhere. The implementation of such a program, however, is a problem not only for physicians and mental health workers but for public policy as well. Its cost effectiveness is immediately apparent when one considers the cost savings involved in caring for very-low-birth-weight babies in intensive care nurseries and later medical and mental health care as contrasted with the cost of the preventive program instituted during pregnancy. The specific intervention

TABLE 27–2

Risk Factors for Premature Births

---

*1. Poor general education, including poor information regarding physiology and risk factors of pregnancy and delivery.

*2. Poor understanding of optimal life style for promoting general health, good nutritional health during pregnancy, and infant care.

3. Young age (less than age twenty-two in the french study).

*4. Presence of psychosocial stress factors (economic, psychological, environmental, and disruptive family life, including moves during pregnancy).

5. Hyperirritability of the uterus (can be reduced by reducing strenuous physical activity).

6. Premature ripening of the cervix during pregnancy.

*7. Poor health care and health supervision during pregnancy.

8. High rating of risk factors utilizing standard rating scale developed by Papiernik and associates[31] regarding factors 1, 3, 4, and 7 above.

---

*Modifiable after diagnosis of pregnancy has been made.

techniques utilized in the prevention of prematurity are summarized in table 27–3.

In general, it is safe to conclude that anything that significantly interferes with the biological predisposition of the mother toward creating a warm, secure, nontoxic, nonstressful, nurturant, and nesting environment for the infant in utero and afterward offers significant risk to the infant and the mother. Thus these studies seriously challenge the commonly held attitude of only two or three decades ago that mothers can continue strenuous work, physical activity, disruption in place of residence, and psychosocial stress. The somewhat old-fashioned notion that pregnant women and mothers should be protected and taken care of is ripe for another cycle of popularity. Continued research and demonstration projects are strongly indicated in order to extend current knowledge.

Healthy Responses in Infancy

A significant number of children are brought to various health care and mental health care agencies and practitioners by parents and other concerned adults because the child is behaving, developing, or reacting to situations in ways that are either puzzling or anxiety provoking to parents or others. Often such behaviors in children are age-appropriate developmental markers or appropriate adaptative responses to environmental circumstances and hence can be designated as *healthy responses.*

Two types of crises are included within this general designation:

1. *Developmental crises* may be seen as a part of the infant's healthy responses. They are transient in nature and include such phenomena as eighth-month anxiety, infantile separation anxiety (six months to age two and one-half), infantile stranger anxiety (four months to eighteen months), and the normal infantile rapprochement crisis (eighteen months to twenty-four months), each stemming largely from internal maturational changes in the infant. Also included within this category would be such conditions as teething, thumb and finger sucking, infantile colic, changes in appetite with age, changing food preferences, transient sleep disturbances, occasional breath holding and occasional temper tantrums in the second and third year of life, masturbation beginning in the second year and continuing thereafter in various forms, and transient stuttering during the onset of speech.

2. *Situational crises* may also occur in the course of normal development during infancy as, for example, in the in-

TABLE 27–3

Intervention Strategy for Preventing Premature Birth in Mothers At-Risk

---

1. Determination of mothers at risk as outlined in table 27–2, utilizing risk scores developed by Papiernik and associates[32] (includes cervical examination).

2. Education of at-risk mothers concerning risk factors for premature birth and its implications for the infant.

3. Education toward changing high-risk life style during pregnancy and infant care.

4. Improved health care and health supervision during pregnancy, including supportive mental health care, home visits, and clinic visits by personnel trained to deal with high-risk mothers.

5. Decreased work schedule and decreased level of physical exertion during pregnancy.

6. Compensatory pay for work reduction.

---

fant's anxious response in relation to overanxious parents and to being moved from crib to bed, negative affective reactions to baby sitters, to brief separations, to weaning, and to the birth of a sibling.

Developmental Deviations

Developmental deviations consist of those unusual patterns of neuropsychological development that are either caused by known organic defect of the CNS or of bodily organs or functions or are associated with such deficit. Such deviations include:

1. Deviation in maturational patterns: developmental disturbance without demonstrable deficit in brain or bodily functions. Examples: slow motor and language development, environmental retardation, language delay, infantile-onset pervasive developmental disorder, inappropriate gender orientation, and autism (as described in DSM-III). For a systematic review of the earliest symptoms of autism during the preverbal phase of development from birth to age two, see appendix 27–1.
2. Developmental disturbance associated with impairment of brain structure or function. Example: Down's syndrome, seizure disorder.
3. Developmental disturbance associated with bodily illness or physical defect without deficit in structure or functioning of the CNS. Examples: developmental disturbance associated with blindness, deafness, arthrogryposis, congenital heart disease, or kidney disease.

Psychophysiological Disturbances

By psychophysiological disturbance is meant those disturbances in bodily functions that are associated with psychologically stressful events in either the infant or members of the caring environment. Such stresses need not be the primary etiology for the disorder but are known to be important as precipitating causes. Examples include bronchial asthma, eczema, peptic ulcer, rumination, nervous vomiting, and hypertrophic pyloric stenosis.

Attachment Disorders of Infancy

Perhaps the most significant and most fundamental psychopathological developments during infancy (conception to age three) include various forms of attachment disorder. There are three main varieties: (1) the failure of the infant to form attachments; (2) the disruption of attachments once they are formed (anaclitic depression); and (3) the persistence of or regression to the infantile form of attachments at an age (eighteen months and older) when the healthy infant is heading toward higher degrees of competence and capability of coping with separation from the primary, caring, maternal figure.

REACTIVE ATTACHMENT DISORDER

The term reactive attachment disorder found in DSM-III[2] and the proposals for a broader inclusion of psychopathology under this designation in DSM-III-R refer[3] to attachment disorders of the first type, situations in which the infant has not been able to form adequate attachments to caretaking figures and vice versa due to disruptive environmental circumstances. The criteria for the diagnosis of reactive attachment disorder of infancy given under the evolving DSM-III-R proposal include:

A. Inadequate or disturbed social relatedness in most contexts beginning before the age of five, as evidenced by at least one of the following:
 (1) Persistent failure to initiate or respond to most social interactions.
 (2) Fearfulness and hypervigilance that does not respond to comforting by caregivers.
 (3) Indiscriminate sociability, for example, excessive familiarity with relative strangers by making requests and displaying affection.
B. Grossly inadequate care that includes at least one of the following:
 (1) Psychological abuse or neglect, that is, persistent disregard for child's basic emotional needs for comfort, stimulation, and affection. Examples include: overly harsh punishment by caregiver; withdrawn mother ignores child; overanxious mother keeps trying to soothe tired baby by jostling and loud, fast talking (overstimulation).
 (2) Physical abuse or neglect, that is, persistent disregard for child's basic physical needs, including nutrition, adequate housing, and protection from physical danger and assault.
 (3) Repeated change of primary caregiver so that stable attachments are not possible, for example, frequently changing foster care.
C. It is presumed that the grossly inadequate care of level B is responsible for the disturbed behavior in level A. The presumption of the relationship is warranted if the disturbance in level B began following the inadequate care level of A.
D. The problem does not occur only during the course of a pervasive developmental disorder, such as autistic disorder.

According to these criteria, it is apparent that the term reactive attachment disorder of infancy refers to situations where there has been evidence of gross neglect and/or abuse or other grossly adverse environmental influences affecting the infant. This has led to the failure of or disruption of the process of making an attachment. It should be noted that failures to make attachments are not always due to such circumstances. For example, such failures may come on the heels of illness in the baby necessitating hospitalization at the time the infant is in the process of forming a primary attachment, a series of foster care placements necessitated by serious illness including personality disorder, substance abuse, schizophrenia, and postpartum depression in the mother, the death or absence of the mothering figure and/or the absence of a substitute caring figure in the home environment, or other unavoidable circumstances in the family life of the infant such as disruption of family life from divorce, natural catastrophes such as war, and so forth.

Green[22] has included psychosocial dwarfism as a special category under reactive attachment disorder of infancy. Psychosocial dwarfism is a condition—growth is stunted in association with psychosocial retardation, affective disorder, and low growth hormone levels—that improves rapidly when the child is removed from the noxious nonsupportive environment of his or her own home.

Failure to thrive without organic cause is commonly associated with attachment failure in infancy and can best be diagnosed and treated by evaluating the nature of the child's tie to the mothering figure[8] and providing psychosocial and nutritional care to mother and infant when deficits in attachment are identified. Organic causes for failure to thrive are found in very few cases.[25] The remaining cases are associated with attachment deficits. Since evaluation of attachment is usually accomplished easily, quietly, nonobtrusively, and inexpensively outside of a hospital by a well-trained observer, it is not unreasonable to recommend such evaluation as a first rather than last diagnostic step in all cases of failure to thrive and to begin a psychosocial support program when indicated. Such early diagnosis and management of the most frequent primary cause of the disorder is in the best tradition of pediatric care and would spare most infants the frequently traumatic experience of numerous intrusive diagnostic procedures performed in the hospital. This is not to say that hospitalization of infants with failure to thrive due to attachment failure cannot be helpful in difficult cases. Hospitalization can afford a good opportunity to observe feeding, social play, separation, and reunion by the primary mothering figure and others.

It is important to recognize that the term reactive attachment disorder of infancy now described in DSM-III[2] does *not* refer to the circumstance in which the infant has made a firm attachment to the primary mothering figure and then is suddenly deprived of that attachment. In this circumstance the infant develops the classic syndrome anaclitic depression.

ANACLITIC DEPRESSION

Anaclitic depression in infants was first described by René Spitz[39] in 1946 as one of the psychiatric conditions of early infancy. Spitz credits M. R. Kaufman with having suggested the term. The syndrome usually first appears in the second half of the first year of life, but may be seen as early as age four or five months.[19] During infancy it is characterized by apprehension, sadness, rejection of the environment, withdrawal, retardation of development, retarded responses to stimuli, slowing of movement, dejection, stupor, loss of appetite, refusal to eat, loss of weight, and insomnia. The syndrome was found fully developed in 19 infants and less fully developed in 26 infants from a total of 123 unselected previously healthy infants observed during the first year of life in a nursery for well children by Spitz. He noted that the children who developed the syndrome were those who had been placed in the nursery *after* having developed a very good relationship with the mother. The syndrome began to appear immediately on placement in the nursery and continued to develop in worsening degree through the first month of the illness following placement. Developmental tests showed a definite retardation of development. Spitz reviewed the literature on depression available at that time, noting that both Freud and Abraham had described a similar syndrome in adults (melancholia and major depression with regression to the oral sadistic stage).

In addition, Spitz made some other extremely interesting observations, namely that the expression of "sadness" was one "mixed with worry" and "a searching expression" on the face with "weeping." He related this with his then new observations of eight-month anxiety occurring at eight months in normal infants, which he felt resulted from the infant's increasing capacity for diacritic discrimination between a friend and a stranger. He noted that the "pathognomic dejected expression" of anaclitic depression did not brighten after the observer was "accepted." The afflicted infant played without any expression of happiness, possessing the toy but not playing meaningfully with it. Spitz observed that infants showing this severe degree of psychiatric disturbance improved rather suddenly when their mothers were restored to them if such restoration took place before the passage of one month. He noted that this sudden improvement was often associated with a rapid acceleration in the developmental quotient to high levels followed soon thereafter by a drop of the developmental quotient. He suggested that such a dramatic improvement in developmental quotient could be equated with a "manic episode."

This "manic episode" in young infants is similar to the sudden occurrence of self-assertive and aggressive behavior that is often seen in infants, children, and adults during the first stage of convalescence from physical illness or injury. More detailed psychobiological study and follow-up of such episodes could determine whether or not such episodes are analogous to or precursors of manic-depressive illness.

Spitz[39] noted that as in melancholia, infants afflicted with anaclitic depression attempted to find new love objects and that in the more severe forms of the illness locomotion was severely impaired. In these cases substitution of the love object did not take place. In cases where a substitute mother *was* accepted, depression did not develop. This would, however, require first that the attachment to the original mother was not an exclusive or strong one and also that the substitute mother was an unusually loving, giving, and devoted mothering figure. He stated, "evidently it is more difficult to replace a satisfactory love object than an unsatisfactory one" (p. 336). In addition to recommending the restitution of the original mother, Spitz recommended stimulating the baby's locomotor activities.

Since the original description of this syndrome by Spitz, numerous other articles have been written substantiating its existence, asking additional questions, and more recently attempting to determine the long-term consequences of the syndrome.

At the present time the major criteria for the diagnosis of anaclitic depression consist of:

1. Loss of the primary mothering figure with whom the infant had developed a strong specific attachment from four months of age onward resulting in:
   a. Sadness and weepiness combined with the expression of apprehension.
   b. Rejection of and withdrawal from the environment.
   c. Psychomotor retardation leading to stupor.
   d. Loss of appetite, food refusal, and weight loss or sudden decrease in weight percentile rating.
   e. Disturbance of sleep pattern, insomnia, and unpredictable sleep and wakeful patterns day and night.
   f. Absence of a history of physical illness immediately prior to the loss of the primary mothering figure.
   g. Occurrence of infections after the onset of primary symptoms (*a.* through *e.* above)—for example, upper and lower respiratory illness, eczema, and other allergenic phenomena.
2. No major physical illness prior to loss of primary mothering figure that could account for symptoms.
3. Rapid improvement of clinical picture when the primary mothering figure is restored if such restoration occurs soon enough.

It is readily observed that this list of symptoms corresponds almost exactly with the criteria for major depression set forth for adults in DSM-III and DSM-III-R. It is worth noting, however, that these symptoms all have occurred in infancy in response to a specific *environmental change*—that is, loss of the mothering figure to which the infant had become attached—and that such symptom patterns are responsive to restoration of the mothering figure. The same symptoms (*a.* through *e.*) in adults are considered of endogenous or "vegetative" origin and not specifically related to environmental conditions nor relieved by a change in such conditions. Other symptoms of major depression in adults—feelings of worthlessness, self-reproach, and guilt, which may be delusional—together with complaints of diminished capacity for thought, concentration, indecisiveness, and a marked loosening of associations or incoherence as well as preoccupations about death and suicide are dependent on more advanced cognitive processes and capacity of adults to communicate subjective feeling states, fears, and fantasy not possible for the young infant. There is some evidence to suggest that individuals who have undergone significant losses early in their lives are indeed predisposed toward later depressive episodes of more serious variety. Why is it that these symptoms in infancy are so similar to those we designate as vegetative in the seriously depressed adult? Perhaps it is not too adventurous to suggest that symptoms of endogenous depression in older individuals are manifestations of latent phenomena derived from infancy. A period of depression in infancy due to loss of the mothering figure may have been responsible for establishing the basic physiological and biochemical basis for later depression, requiring only relatively minor precipitating events in adult life to uncover such a predisposition. Such a hypothesis would not negate the importance of genetic factors underlying unipolar and bipolar depressive illness.

The increased susceptibility of infants to gastrointestinal, respiratory, skin, and other infections and allergic responses can be explained on the basis of the suppression of the immune response by traumatic influence, particularly the suppression of B-lymphocytes, which produce antibodies against the disease-producing agents and participate in the autoimmune response.[38]

The outcome for infants showing anaclitic depression may be observed over the short and the long term. *Short-term* consequences include depressive mood, physical illness, accidents, an increased disposition toward infectious disease, continued regression in affectomotor and intellectual functioning as well as increased susceptibility to subsequent trauma, including separation from substitute caretakers or changes in the nonhuman environment. *Long-term* complications include subnormal intellectual functioning, apathy, inability to form meaningful relationships, predisposition toward depressive illness, psychophysiological regression in response to loss or threat of loss or disruption of object relations, and later learning and characterological problems. Difficulties in adaptation to changes to the nonhuman environment may also occur. Harmon, Wagonfeld, and Emde[24] have recently reviewed the literature on the syndrome and have described a seven-year-old boy with repeated depressive episodes from infancy. A constitutional feature of the infant identified before the onset of the first anaclitic depressive episodes seems to have had long-term positive influence, namely the infant's predilection for reaching for new relationships. This child, when of school age, showed the same tendency during a depressive illness, which suggests a biological origin of this ameliorating influence.

ATTACHMENT DISORDER WITH FOOD REFUSAL

Kreisler[28] in France and Egan, Chatoor, and Rosen in the United States[15] have described infants who, during the second half of the first year and on into the second year of life, lose weight, refuse food that is given to them, and often end up in the hospital due to severe malnutrition. No physical cause for the disorder is found and it is soon discovered that a very serious battle has been taking place between the infant and the mother around the issue of food intake. The mothers of these children have been attempting to take control of the infant's eating process and have engaged in traumatic forced feeding. The infants have responded by food refusal even to the point of starvation threatening death. In addition, the mothers of the infants are shown to have severe character disorders and borderline personality disturbance in which they have projected hostile impulses to the child, have felt persecuted by the child, and feel the need to defend themselves against that which they have projected. Thus the battleground around food is endowed with serious psychological conflict. These cases have proved to be extremely difficult to treat. Kreisler has suggested that this is the infantile form of anorexia nervosa. Often a change of caretakers and homes is indicated since treatment cannot proceed successfully and rapidly enough to reverse the infants' downhill course. This syndrome is included as a form of attachment disorder because the onset occurs when the infant is attempting to separate from the primary caretaking figure through self-feeding during the last half of the first year of life. The feeding battle ensues when the mother attempts to reverse the infant's forward movement toward individuation, thus attempting to forcefully reestablish the child within a controlling pathological symbiosis with the mother. These dynamics place the syndrome within the attachment disorder category with food refusal as the major symptom. Such a designation leads to a better understanding of the problem than "feeding problem."

ATTACHMENT DISORDER, SYMBIOTIC TYPE

Various forms of the symbiotic type of attachment disorder are identifiable, including the circumstance where the mother/infant symbiosis persists into late infancy (eighteen months and beyond). This may be due to maternal pathology characterized by the mother's use of the infant as a libidinal object in the absence of other such objects in her life, or where the mother becomes depressed and clings to the child as the only good object available to her and/or as an extension of herself. In this circumstance neither mother nor infant can function adequately outside of that symbiotic relationship. A secondary form of symbiotic attachment disorder can also be identified. In this situation the separation-individuation process has proceeded quite normally at the usual time; from eighteen months onward, however, the symbiotic phase of the mother/infant relationship is reinstituted because of some problem in either the mother or the infant such as illness, operation, failure to convalesce from physical illness, depression in the mother, or other traumatic events affecting both mother and infant such as death, divorce, or the diagnosis of malignancy in the mother or a chronic handicap in the child. *A focal form* of symbiotic attachment disorder can be seen in children with psychogenic megacolon or in situations where a function or a part of the body (vision, walking, oral activity, anal functioning) remains within the symbiotic union of mother and infant for various reasons. This focal form of disorder was described by Greenacre in 1959[23] and Mahler in 1952.[30]

Another form of attachment disorder, symbiotic type, has recently been described[20] by Eleanor Galenson as a sadomasochistic union of mother and child. Galenson studied a number of children who had been physically abused and were living in single-parent families. During the second year of life, these children became more active in actually provoking the abusing parent to acts of physical abuse. Detailed studies of these children showed that such actions were based on earlier trauma in which the child had changed from passive recipient of the trauma to active provoker of the trauma, thus bringing some degree of active mastery to the repeated traumatic episodes. The consequence of the child's provocation was to induce further physical attacks. Hence cycles of traumatic attack followed by quiescence followed by subsequent episodes of attack provoked by the child were established and became a major means by which the child could secure attachment to and control of the abusing parent. These cases were extremely difficult to treat.

Some of the conditions listed under symbiotic attachment disorder could possibly qualify for the diagnosis of separation anxiety disorder described in DSM-

III and DSM-III-R. However, separation anxiety disorder as currently proposed for DSM-III-R does not include specific criteria for diagnosing this condition in children less than age three. This may be modified as DSM-III-R undergoes further revision.

Posttraumatic Stress Disorder of Infancy—Acute, Chronic, and Delayed Forms

The criteria listed for posttraumatic stress disorder in DSM-III do not include symptoms that can be identified in infancy since most of the symptoms involve a high degree of cognition and capacity for communication. For example, such criteria include recurrent and intrusive recollections of the event, recurring dreams of the event, sudden acting or feeling as if the traumatic event were reoccurring, markedly diminished interest in one or more significant activities, and feelings of detachment. In fact, the only two symptoms that could apply to infancy are constricted affect and speech disturbance. Thus it becomes necessary to present criteria for establishing this diagnosis in preverbal children less than age three who undoubtedly suffer from it. An extensive review of this problem is available in the work of Eth and Pynoos,[16] and the traumatic situation and its sequelae are thoroughly explored in the psychoanalytic literature, some of which will be described here and has been referred to in the earlier Group for the Advancement of Psychiatry diagnostic scheme for childhood as reactive disorders. Detailed descriptions of children undergoing such traumatic stress reactions are found in children who have suffered both sexual and physical child abuse[41], or dog bite,[21] the children of Chowchilla,[12] and children who have been severely burned or who have witnessed murder of a parent.[37] In situations of this kind, the infant or small child is overwhelmed with stimuli that cannot be cognitively or affectively organized. Symptoms include:

1. A freezing of capacities to adapt to environmental change.
2. Disturbances at the physiological level in terms of eating, sleeping, and toileting problems.
3. A regression in psychosocial functioning.
4. Regression to the symbiotic union in relation to the parent.
5. Repetitive play patterns (in clinical interview), often including the traumatic event.

Long-term consequences include a tendency to maintain close contact with the parent figure, a frozen affective development and inability to experience pleasure (anhedonia), and an extreme degree of cautiousness regarding new experiences.

Disturbed Parent/Child Relationships

Disturbed parent/child relationships may include (1) dyadic dyssynchrony of infancy, (2) power struggle around issues of control and discipline, (3) parental exploitation of the child, (4) parental neglect, (5) parental abuse, and (6) parental sexual abuse.

Sadomasochistic relationships and severe feeding and toileting have been described earlier as variations of attachment disorder.

Behavioral Disturbances

The category of behavioral disturbances in infancy includes the irritable, colicky infant syndrome, the hyperactive child syndrome as it appears in children less than age three, a child who is accident prone without other evident pathology, and severe discipline problems often reflecting parent/child problems.

Communication Disorders

The communication disorders include: (1) delayed onset of speech, (2) regression of language functioning, (3) syntactic problems, (4) idiosyncratic speech (e.g., twin speech), (5) withholding of speech, (6) retardation of symbolic language functioning, and (7) elective mutism.

Psychoneuroses

The proposed system of classification of psychiatric disorders of infancy as just outlined does not provide for the designation psychoneurotic reaction of infancy or of personality disorder. The main reason for this is that both of these disorders presume the presence of a stable, relatively unchanging, underlying mental structure including the structuralization of defensive operations and of character. Nevertheless, infants do become specifically fearful about certain situations as shown in behavior and play and as is seen in older infants and adults with "traumatic neuroses." Infants may show overwhelming anxiety by withdrawal, profound sleep, bodily symptoms, disturbances of eating and elimination, or by hyperalert paralysis of action —that is, severe inhibition of functioning. Infants may also show various forms of "depression," including somatic disturbances as so-called depressive equivalents. In addition, certain infants, even as early as the second year of life, may show obsessional and phobic features in their functioning. If such disturbances were observed in older children, they might well be diagnosed as psychoneurotic reactions. Such a diagnosis, however, would depend on a clear assessment of the extent to which such symptom patterns evolved from well-established intrapsychic conflicts. In light of current limits of knowledge regarding the infant's psychic structure and capacity for establishing relatively enduring defensive operations, it seems prudent not to designate such problems as full-fledged psychoneurotic reactions.

Most of the reactions described earlier can be subsumed under the diagnostic categories as developmental crises or as transitional stress reactions, modified in each case by specification of symptoms. Investigation into the transition between these early forms of protoneurotic disturbances and full-fledged psychoneurotic disturbances remains a challenge to psychoanalytically oriented infant researchers.

In reviewing the criteria for these disorders, it is apparent that some degree of overlap is possible—for example, between the various forms of attachment disorders and traumatic stress reactions, parent/child problems, behavior disorders, and developmental problems. This is not unusual for any system of classification. The choice of which diagnosis to use when there are indications of other diagnoses is one that should depend on the clinician's judgment as to which diagnostic designation more accurately describes the *"primary"* disturbance at the time the diagnosis is made. This primary diagnosis should be listed, followed by qualifying elements, including other diagnoses. Also, it is readily apparent that a child may have a combination of psychiatric disturbances in relationship to psychophysiological disturbances and medical illnesses. In that case, all diagnoses should be included with the primary diagnosis being given first.

Conclusions

The early pioneers in the field of infant psychiatry provided the theory that liberated infancy from ignorance and prejudice and generated new hypotheses that gave rise to new observations and new theory about both normal and psychopathological development. The field is moving rapidly. Many disciplines are at work and have begun collaboration. There is still need for short-term and long-term detailed case studies that can provide important clues as to what kinds of inherent tendencies persist throughout life and what environmental events are most influential at particular times during infancy. Infancy spans at least seven different epochs of development from birth to age three (see appendix 27–2). There are probably more major shifts in development during infancy than in the remaining sixty-five or so years of the life span.

What we know of psychiatric syndromes during infancy has always been defined by studies of normal development. This summary of psychiatric syndromes would have astonished most infant observers in the 1930s and 1940s. Not all babies who start out poorly end up poorly. There is a high degree of neuroplasticity that makes it possible for babies to recover with second and third chances available for reaching their ultimate potential. Not all infantile traumas are likely to result in unstable psychopathology throughout life. Much further clinical and developmental research needs to be done. An updated summary ten years from now could prove to be even more startling.

APPENDIX 27–1

Early Signs of Possible Autism from Birth to Age Two

Birth to Age 1 Month

1. Failure of the infant to establish eye contact with the mother.
2. Difficulty between the infant and the mother in achieving a comfortable and effective holding position during feeding.
3. Failure of the infant to demonstrate anticipatory behavior when picked up for feeding.
[a]4. Failure to establish reciprocal auditory and visual engagements with mother.

Age 2 to 3 Months

1. Indifference of the infant to the human face, voice, and play overtures when fully awake and calm.
2. Failure to demonstrate anticipatory behavior during play, holding, and dressing.
[a]3. Failure to establish reciprocal auditory and visual engagements with mother.

Age 3 to 4 Months

1. Failure to show the social smile (exchange of smiles with mother) that is present in normal infants at 2 months.
2. Inability to engage in social games or playful activity with mother.
3. Avoidance of direct visual contact with other humans, or appearing to look through them.
4. Turning away with head extended and back arched, making holding difficult.
[a]5. Failure to establish reciprocal auditory and visual engagements with mother.

Age 4 to 6 Months

1. Indifference to humans, whether familiar or not.
2. Excessive bodily rocking.
3. Inexpressive face or facial grimacing without making social contact.
[a]4. Failure to establish reciprocal auditory and visual engagements with mother.

Age 6 Months to 1 Year

1. Failure to show distress or anxiety in response to strangers as opposed to familiar persons, seen normally at 4 to 6 months.
2. Increased interest in inanimate objects and sources of stimulation such as light and noise, rather than people.
3. Failure to show interest in self-care such as dressing and in feeding self by holding bits of food between thumb and forefinger.
4. Unusual repertoire of a few mechanical sounds, consisting usually of single tones occurring in bursts, rather than the use of voice inflection in babbling and beginning word formation.
5. Failure to accept new foods. This is based on child's preference for a few familiar oral textures. Often the child will limit himself to only one or two foods such as crackers or pudding; nutritional and dental problems often result from this.
6. Repetitious, nonfunctional fingering of certain objects. This, like choice of food, is based on limited textural preference rather than function.
7. Showing no evidence of separation distress and appearing to have built a wall around himself which does not permit entry from the outside.
8. Showing either excessive mouthing, sucking, and biting behavior, or holding mouth in a fixed, semiclosed position with no sucking or biting.
[a]9. Failure to establish reciprocal auditory and visual engagements with mother.

Age 1 to 2 Years

1. Very limited, uneven, and unusual speech development. Speech sounds are hollow and without voice inflection.
2. Repeating TV commercials or a few phrases.
3. Failure to establish meaningful eye contact, appearing to look through and beyond the face of the other person.
4. Appearing to be uninterested in social contact with other children.
5. Obsession with ritualized physical activity such as rocking, hand flapping, finger flipping, and visual and sound games with inanimate objects.
6. Self-mutilating behavior such as biting self.
7. Extreme preoccupation with turning and whirling objects and round, shiny surfaces, i.e., making objects spin and whirl and observing them as if in a trance.
8. Showing minimal facial expression on contact with humans—no appropriate smile.

APPENDIX 27–1 *(Continued)*

9. Having favorite rituals such as touching shoes or knees of self and others: flicking fingers against table; smelling, licking, or touching objects; or beginning to do these things and then not doing them.
10. Excessive concern for sameness in the arrangement of inanimate objects, in life-space, and in feeding.
11. Use of objects for self-stimulation rather than for play.
12. Following bizarre play patterns, e.g., in use of string and hard objects in hand or applied to face.
13. Highly idiosyncratic sleep and feeding patterns.
14. Usually not achieving toilet training—excessive smearing. May show panic regarding toilet, tub, or hair washing.
[a]15. Failure to establish reciprocal auditory and visual engagements with mother.

SOURCE: Reprinted, by permission of the publisher, from J. D. Call, "Autistic Behavior in Infants," in V. C. Kelley, ed., *Practice of Pediatrics*, vol. I, rev. ed. (Philadelphia: J. B. Lippincott, 1982–83), pp. 6–7.
[a]Note that failure of reciprocity is a constant deficit across all ages. A child may look at another person without mutually organized visual, vocal, or other sensorimotor engagements. Such failure is one of the central features of autism in young children and distinguishes autism from depression, mental retardation, and other developmental disorders.

APPENDIX 27–2

*Behavioral Differences and Developmental
Milestones According to Age*

Birth–1 Month

Areas for Routine Observation and Inquiry
1. Feeding, anticipatory behavior, visual reciprocity, holding position and play with mother.
2. Spontaneous visual activity, i.e., following an object.
3. Reflexes: rooting, grasp, head prone, startle, suck, and hand-mouth.
4. General activity level and hand-mouth activity.
5. Response to auditory and visual stimuli when alert.
6. Sleep pattern and state transitions, i.e., from sleep to waking.

Landmarks of Normal Psychological Development
1. Holds head up in prone position.
[a]2. Anticipatory behavior at feeding (opening mouth, turning head, and bringing hand up to bottle or breast when feeding position is assumed).
3. Visual fixation and visual following beyond the midline.
4. Stops crying with presentation of novel stimulus, holding, or rocking.
5. Intact vigorous sucking activity occurring with regular bursts of sucking with rest periods between sucking bursts.
6. Responds with alertness to light and sound.
7. Begins to play after feeding.
8. Holds on with hands to whatever is available when hungry and during early part of feeding.

Common Parental Concerns Usually Not Problems
1. Prefers eating every 2 hours.
2. Prickly heat rash.
3. "Not satisfied" with feeding.
4. Wants to be held "all the time."
5. Grunts with red face during bowel movements.
6. Sucking fingers or thumb.

Typical Signs of Psychological Disturbance
1. Failure to gain weight.
2. Excessive spitting up.
3. No eye contact.
4. Failure to hold head up.
5. Failure to show anticipatory behavior at feeding.
6. Failure to hold on with hands.
7. Ticlike movements of face and head.
8. Reciprocity disturbance.

2–3 Months

Areas for Routine Observation and Inquiry

1. Play with mother.
2. Smiling response with mother, with strangers.
3. Sleep and activity patterns.
4. Feeding.
5. Response to social stimuli.
6. Hand use.

Landmarks of Normal Psychological Development

[b]1. Social smile with mother, with stranger, and with face mask.
2. Social games ending with smile.
3. Oral imitation (cough game).
4. Controls breast or bottle with hands.
5. Midline hand use.
6. Prolonged visual tracking and visual reciprocity.

Common Parental Concerns Usually Not Problems

1. Irritable crying.
2. "Colic."
3. "Constipation."
4. Not sleeping through night.
5. Sucking finger or thumb.

Typical Signs of Psychological Disturbance

1. Failure to thrive.
2. Attachment disorder.
3. Indifference to social stimuli, e.g., human face, voice, and play overtures.
4. Persistent hyperactivity and sleep disturbance.
5. Vomiting and diarrhea without physical illness.
6. Hyperresponsiveness or hyporesponsiveness to stimuli.

4–6 Months

Areas for Routine Observation and Inquiry

1. Play with mother.
2. Smiling response with mother, with strangers.
3. Sleep and activity patterns.
4. Feeding.
5. Response to stimuli.
6. Hand use.

Landmarks of Normal Psychological Development

1. Social smile with mother.
[c]2. Many social games with mother and other family members.
3. Quietness, immobile face, and subdued affectomotor responses to stranger.
4. Voluntary hand use.
5. Overtures actively inviting reciprocity with mother.
6. Sleeps through night.
7. Patterned meal time.

Common Parental Concerns Usually Not Problems

1. "Constipation."
2. Demands for attention.
3. Prefers to be propped up.
4. "Spoiled."
5. Teething—biting.
6. Sucking fingers or thumb.

Typical Signs of Psychological Disturbance

1. Persistent sleep problem.
2. Hyperactivity and hyperresponsiveness.

3. Wheezing without infection.
4. Lack of interest in social stimuli.
5. Attachment disorder.
6. Indifference toward feeding.
7. Does not enjoy upright position.
8. Excessive rocking of self (other than at night or when alone).
9. Rumination (swallowing of regurgitated food).

7–9 Months

Areas for Routine Observation and Inquiry

1. Play with mother.
2. Smiling response with mother, not with strangers.
3. Sleep and activity patterns.
4. Feeding.
5. Response to stimuli.
6. Hand use.
7. Response to solid food.
8. Self-feeding.
9. Negative affectomotor response to separation from mother.
10. Response to strange places.
11. Relationship with siblings.

Landmarks of Normal Psychological Development

d_1. Mild separation anxiety.
2. Subtlety in affectomotor responses and in smile.
3. "Dada" or "Mama."
4. Hand use.
5. Use of "executive finger" (extended index finger in touching and exploring objects).

Common Parental Concerns Usually Not Problems

1. Dropping things.
2. Messy feeding.
3. Disrupted sleep associated with teething, move to new home, or illness.
4. "Temper."

Typical Signs of Psychological Disturbance

1. Persistent sleep problems.
2. Eating problems, e.g., refusing to use hands or hold glass, very limited diet, i.e., idiosyncratic food preferences.
3. Unpatterned sleep and eating (lack of predictability).
4. Failure to imitate simple vocal sounds and gestures.
5. Lack of specific affective communication, failure to show and respond to a variety of recognizable affective signals such as joy, surprise, fear, curiosity.
6. Bizarre play.
7. Low socialization.
8. Lack of distress with stranger.
9. Excessive self-stimulation and self-destructive behavior.
10. Rumination.
11. Withholding of bowel movements.
12. Apathy.
13. Attachment disorder, anaclitic type.

10–16 Months

Areas for Routine Observation and Inquiry

1. Play with mother.
2. Smiling response with mother, with strangers.
3. Sleep and activity patterns.

4. Feeding.
5. Response to stimuli.
6. Response to solid food.
7. Self-feeding.
8. Response to separation from mother and reunion.
9. Response to strange places.
10. Relationship with siblings.
11. Interest in exploratory behavior.
12. Manipulative behavior.
13. Behavior limits.
14. Speech: words, sounds, and response to words, sounds, and name.
15. Plans for trips and separation: babysitters.

Landmarks of Normal Psychological Development

1. Walks.
2. Reaches out for, grasps, and manipulates familiar and strange objects.
3. Attentive to parent.
4. Stops and then goes ahead while saying "no."
e5. Play and imitation increase.
6. Problem solving and investigation increase.
7. Points at objects as reference in communication with parents.
8. Genital play begins.

Common Parental Concerns Usually Not Problems

1. Getting into things: climbing.
2. "Constipation."
3. Declining appetite.
4. Self-feeding and being fed.
5. Screaming.
6. Mild tantrums.
7. Attachment to transitional object.

Typical Signs of Psychological Disturbance

1. No words.
2. Sleep problem.
3. Withdrawn behavior.
4. Excessively rocking, posturing.
5. Bizarre play.
6. No separation distress.
7. Night wandering.
8. Excessive distractibility.
9. Bowel disturbances.

16 Months–2 Years

Areas for Routine Observation and Inquiry

1. Speech development.
2. Play.
3. Eating, sleeping, and toilet training.
4. Response to strangers.
5. Response to separation.
6. Limits for mobility and aggressive behavior.
7. Interest in sexual differences.

Landmarks of Normal Psychological Development

1. Says "no" and responds to "no."
2. Use of approximately 20 words.
3. Primary feminine identification, both girls and boys (e.g., interest in dress, shoes, baby).
f4. Separates from parents and reports back (rapprochement).
5. Microcosmic play (solitary play with small objects)—symbolic of real experience.
6. Imitation of vocal inflection.

APPENDIX 27–2 *(Continued)*

7. Enjoys and makes use of new experience when conditions are optimal.
8. Masturbation (early phase).

Common Parental Concerns Usually Not Problems

1. Getting into things: climbing.
2. Stubbornness.
3. Temper outbursts.
4. Upset easily.
5. "Stuttering."
6. Sibling rivalry.

Typical Signs of Psychological Disturbance

1. No speech.
2. Excessive body rocking.
3. No play or toy preferences.
4. Inappropriate play.
5. Withholding and other bowel problems.
6. Sleep disturbance.
7. Retarded development or persistent regression.
8. Attachment disorder, symbiotic type.

25 Months–3 Years

Areas for Routine Observation and Inquiry

1. Sibling and peer relations.
2. Capacity to separate from parents.
3. Different behavior with each parent.
4. Speech and language development.
5. Nursery school.
6. Toileting.
7. Play preferences.
8. Limits, discipline, and daily routine.
9. Dreams and night terrors, fears.
10. Areas of interest and skill.

Landmarks of Normal Psychological Development

g1. Parallel play (appropriate play alongside of peers: 2½ years).
2. Collateral peer play (3 years).
3. Bedtime ritual (including transitional object).
h4. Two- and three-word speech (use of speech as a tool to make things happen: 2 years).
5. Creative use of speech (for reflection and organization: 3–4 years).
6. Successful toilet training (2–2½ years).
7. Accepts reasonable limits (2–2½ years).
8. Special skills and talents (3–4 years).
9. Talks to self (2½ years).
10. "What's this?" (in reference to new objects).

Common Parental Concerns Usually Not Problems

1. Messy play.
2. "Stuttering."
3. Won't put things away.
4. Aggressive and possessive play.
5. Occasional soiling or wetting.
6. Stubbornness.
7. Reluctance to try new foods.
8. Regressive behavior with illness or stress.
9. Wants own way and fusses, screams briefly and cries if doesn't get own way.
10. Occasional temper tantrums (one/week).
11. Short-lived (1–2 weeks) unreasonable fears.

Typical Signs of Psychological Disturbance

1. Persistent disturbed sleep with wild animal dreams.
2. Persistent soiling and wetting or withholding of stool or urine.

3. Persistent eating problems.
4. Nonspeaking (beyond 18 months).
5. Inappropriate play.
6. Fears of dark, ghosts, burglars; shyness.
7. Persistent shyness, withdrawn behavior or excessive independence with children.
8. Excessive body rocking, finger sucking, and tics.
9. Attachment disorder, symbiotic type.

SOURCE: Reprinted, by permission of the publisher, from J. D. Call, "Psychologic and Behavioral Development of Infants and Children," in V. C. Kelley, ed., *Practice of Pediatrics*, vol. 1, rev. ed. (Philadelphia: Harper & Row, 1982–83), pp. 7–10.
[a]Most significant psychological achievement for this age period.
[b]Most significant psychological achievement for this age period.
[c]Most significant psychological achievement for this age period.
[d]Most significant psychological achievement for this age period.
[e]Most significant psychological achievement for this age period.
[f]Most significant psychological achievement for this age period.
[g]Most significant psychological achievement for this age period.
[h]Clear indication of understanding speech (i.e., receptive speech) is as important as expressive speech.

APPENDIX 27–3

Psychiatric Diagnoses Applicable to Children Less Than Age Three

I. Healthy Responses.
  1. Developmental crises, e.g., eighth-month anxiety—DSM-III Phase of Life Problem V62.89.
  2. Situational crises, e.g., birth of sibling—DSM-III Phase of Life Problem V62.89.
II. Developmental Deviations—DSM-III Mental Retardation 317.1, 318.0, 318.1, 318.2, 319.0—DSM-III Pervasive Developmental Disturbances 399, 399.0, 399.8, 399.9.
  1. Deviation of maturational patterns without demonstrable brain deficit, e.g., environmental retardation.
  2. Deviation of maturational patterns with demonstrable brain defect, e.g., Down's Syndrome DSM-III Organic Mental Disorders.
  3. Deviation of maturational patterns due to bodily illness or defect and with no central nervous system defect, e.g., Muscular Dystrophy.
III. Psychophysiological Disorders. Psychological factors affecting physical condition DSM-III 316.00. Specify physical disorder on Axis III.
IV. Attachment Disorders of Infancy.
  1. Reactive Attachment Disorder of Infancy DSM-III-R 313.89.
  2. Attachment Disorder, Anaclitic Type, Major Depression DSM-III and DSM-III-R 296.2.
  3. Attachment Disorder with Food Refusal. Atypical Eating Disorder DSM-III and DSM-III-R 307.5.
  4. Attachment Disorder, Symbiotic Type. Separation Anxiety Disorder as presently defined in DSM-III and DSM-III-R 309.21, but DSM-III does not include criteria applicable to infants less than age 3.
    a. Primary (child and primary parent remain in symbiotic union throughout second year of life).
    b. Secondary (child and parent regress to symbiotic union).
    c. Focal (involving one bodily area or function).
    d. Infantile sadomasochism.
V. Post-Traumatic Stress Disorder of Infancy. Criteria for diagnosis of Post-Traumatic Stress Disorder set forth in DSM-III and DSM-III-R do not include criteria applicable to infants less than age 3.
VI. Disturbed Parent/Child Relationships—DSM-III Parent/Child Problems V61.20.
  1. Dyadic dissynchrony in infancy.
  2. Power struggle around issues of control and discipline.
  3. Parental exploitation of the child.
  4. Parental neglect of child.
  5. Parental abuse of child.
VII. Behavioral Disturbances of Infancy.
  1. Irritable infant.
  2. Hyperactive child.
  3. Attention Deficit Disorder.

APPENDIX 27–3 *(Continued)*

VIII. Communication Disorders.
  1. Developmental Language Disorder—DSM-III 315.31.
  2. Delayed onset of speech.
  3. Regression of language functions.
  4. Syntactic problems.
  5. Idiosyncratic speech, e.g., twin speech.
  6. Withholding of speech.
  7. Retardation of symbolic language functioning.
  8. Elective Mutism—DSM-III 313.23.
IX. Other DSM-III diagnoses which are applicable to children less than age 3.
  1. Eating Disorders.
     a. Pica 207.52.
     b. Rumination 307.53.
     c. Atypical Eating Disorder 307.3.
  2. Sleep Terror Disorder 307.49.
  3. Infantile Autism 299.0.
  4. Organic Mental Disorders 290.00 to 294.80.
  5. Substance Induced Organic Mental Disorders.
  6. Fetal Alcohol Syndrome.
  7. Organic Brain Syndrome.
  8. Overanxious Disorder 313.00.
  9. Gender Identity Disorder 302.6.
  10. Psychological Factors Affecting Physical Disorder 316.00.

SOURCE: Reprinted by permission of the publisher from J. D. Call, "Psychologic and Behavioral Development of Infants and Children," pp. 7–10, and "Autistic Behavior in Infants," pp. 6–7, in V. C. Kelley, ed, *Practice of Pediatrics*, vol. I, rev. ed. (Philadelphia: J. B. Lippincott, 1985).

REFERENCES

1. AINSWORTH, M.D.S., et al. *Patterns of Attachment.* Hillsdale, N.J.: Lawrence Erlbaum Associates, 1978.

2. American Psychiatric Association. *Diagnostic and Statistical Manual of Mental Disorders,* 3rd ed. (DSM-III). Washington, D.C.: American Psychiatric Association, 1980.

3. ———. *Diagnostic and Statistical Manual of Mental Disorders,* 3rd ed., revised—draft; (DSM-III-R). Washington, D.C.: American Psychiatric Association, 1985.

4. BOWLBY, J. "The Nature of the Child's Tie to His Mother, *International Journal of Psycho-Analysis,* 39 (1958): 350–373.

5. BUEHLER, J. W., et al. "Maternal Mortality in Women Aged 35 Years or Older: United States," *Journal of the American Medical Association,* 255 (1986):53–57.

6. CALL, J. D. "Newborn Approach Behavior and Early Ego Development," *International Journal of Psycho-Analysis,* 45: (1964):286–294.

7. ———. "Attachment Disorders of Infancy," in H. L. Kaplan, A. M. Freedman, and B. J. Sadock, eds., *Comprehensive Textbook of Psychiatry,* vol. 3. New York: Williams & Wilkins, 1980, pp. 2586–2597.

8. ———. "Some Prelinguistic Aspects of Language Development," *Journal of the American Psychoanaltic Association,* 28 (1980):259–289.

9. ———. "Autistic Behavior in Infants," in V. C. Kelley, ed., *Practice of Pediatrics,* vol. 1, rev. ed. Philadelphia: Harper & Row, 1982–83, pp. 6–7.

10. CALL, J. D. "Toward a Nosology of Psychiatric Disorders in Infancy," in J. D. Call, E. Galenson, and R. L. Tyson, eds., *Frontiers of Infant Psychiatry.* New York: Basic Books, 1983, pp. 117–128.

11. CALL, J. D. and METZNER, L. "Mother/infant Interaction in 10 Infants with Pyloric Stenosis." Ph. D. diss. by Linda Metzner, unpublished.

12. COLE, C. H. "Prevention of Prematurity: Can We Do It in America?" *Pediatrics,* 76 (1985):310–312.

13. DARWIN, C. *On the Origin of Species by Means of Natural Selection,* London: John Murray, 1859.

14. ———. A biographical sketch of an infant. *Mind,* no. 7, 1877.

15. EGAN, J., CHATOOR, I., and ROSEN, G. "Nonorganic Failure to Thrive: Pathogenesis and Classification," *Clinical Proceedings, Children's Hospital Medical Center,* 36 (1980): 173–182.

16. ETH, S., and PYNOOS, R. S. "Developmental Perspective on Psychic Trauma in Childhood," in: C. Figley, ed., *Trauma and its Wake.* New York: Brunner/Mazel, 1985, pp. 36–52.

17. FREUD, S. "Three Essays on the Theory of Sexuality," in J. Strachey, ed., *The Standard Edition of the Complete Psychological Works of Sigmund Freud* (hereinafter *Standard Edition*), vol. 7. London: Hogarth Press, 1953, pp. 135–243. (Originally published in J. Strachey, ed., 1905.)

18. ———. "Analysis terminable and interminable," in J. Strachey, ed., *Standard Edition,* vol. 23. London: Hogarth Press, 1964, pp. 211–253. (Originally published 1937.)

19. GAENSBAUER, T. J. "Differentiation of Discrete Affects: A Case Report," *Journal of the Psychoanalytic Study of the Child,* 37 (1982): 29–66.

20. GALENSON, E. "Precursors of Masochism: Protomasochism," Paper presented at a panel on sadomasochism in

children, annual meeting of the American Psychoanalytic Association, New York, December 1985.

21. GISLASON, I. L., and CALL, J. D. "Dogbite in Infancy: Trauma and Personality Development, A Case Report," *Journal of the American Academy of Child Psychiatry,* 21 (1982):203–207.

22. GREEN, W. H. "Attachment Disorders of Infancy and Early Childhood," in H. I. Kaplan, A. M. Freedman, and B. J. Sadock, eds., *Comprehensive Textbook of Psychiatry,* vol. 4. New York: Williams & Wilkins, 1985, pp. 1722–1731.

23. GREENACRE, P. "On Focal Symbiosis," in L. Jenner and E. Pavensedt, eds., *Dynamic Psychopathology in Childhood.* New York: Grune & Stratton, 1959, pp. 257–292.

24. HARMON, R. J., WAGONFELD, S., and EMDE, R. N. "Anaclitic Depression: A Follow-up from Infancy to Puberty," *Psychoanalytic Study of the Child,* 37 (1982):67–94.

25. HAYNES, C. F., et al. "Hospitalized Cases of Nonorganic Failure to Thrive: The Scope of the Problem and Short-term Lay Health Visitor Intervention," *Child Abuse and Neglect,* 8 (1984):229–242.

26. HERRON, M. A., KATZ, M., and CREASY, R. K. "Evaluation of a Preterm Birth Prevention Program: Preliminary Report," *Obstetrics and Gynecology,* 59 (1982):452–456.

27. KLEIN, M. *The Psychoanalysis of Children.* London: Hogarth Press, 1932.

28. KREISLER, L. "Depression, A Factor in Psychosomatic Vulnerability in the Infant," manuscript, 1981.

29. LORENZ, K. "The Past 12 Years in the Comparative Study of Behavior," in C. H. Schiller, trans. and ed., *Instinctive Behavior,* vol. 2. New York: International Universities Press, 1957.

30. MAHLER, M. S. "On Child Psychosis and Schizophrenia: Autistic and Symbiotic Infantile Psychoses," *Psychoanalytic Study of the Child,* 7 (1952): 286–305.

31. PAPIERNIK, E., et al. "Prevention of Preterm Births: A Perinatal Study in Haguenau, France," *Pediatrics,* 76 (1985): 154–158.

32. PAPOUSEK, H., and PAPOUSEK, M. "Interactional Failures: Their Origins and Significance in Child Psychiatry," in J. D. Call, E. Galenson, and R. L. Tyson, eds., *Frontiers of Infant Psychiatry.* New York: Basic Books, 1983, pp. 30–37.

33. PASAMANICK, B., ROGERS, M., and LILLIENFIELD, A. "Pregnancy Experience and the Development of Behavior Disorders," *American Journal of Psychiatry,* 112 (1956):613–618.

34. PIAGET, J. *The Language and Thought of the Child,* trans. M. Gabain. New York: Harcourt, 1926. (Originally published 1923.)

35. ———. *The Origins of Intelligence in Children,* 2nd ed. New York: International Universities Press, 1953. (Originally published 1936).

36. PRUGH, D. G., et al. "Hypertrophic Pyloric Stenosis in Infancy: Innate and Experiential Factors," in J. D. Call, E. Galenson, and R. L. Tyson, eds., *Frontiers of Infant Psychiatry,* New York: Basic Books, 1983, pp. 301–323.

37. PYNOOS, R. S., and ETH, S. "Child as Criminal Witness to Homicide," *Journal of Social Issues,* 40 (1984):87–108.

38. REITE, M., and FIELD, T., eds. *The Psychobiology of Attachment and Separation.* New York: Academic Press, 1985.

39. SPITZ, R. "Anaclitic Depression," *Psychoanalytic Study of the Child,* 2 (1946):313–342.

40. STREISSGUTH, A. P., et al. "Ten-year Follow-up of the Original Fetal Alcohol Syndrome Patients," *Lancet,* 2 (1985):85–91.

41. SUMMIT, R. C. "The Child Sexual Abuse Accommodation Syndrome," *Child Abuse and neglect,* 7 (1983):177–192.

42. TERR, L. C. "Children of Chowchilla: A Study of Psychic Trauma," *Psychoanalytic Study of the Child,* 34 (1979):547–623.

43. TINBERGEN, N. *The Study of Instinct.* Oxford: Oxford University Press, 1951.

44. TREVARTHAN, C. "Foundations of Intersubjectivity; Development of Interpersonal and Cooperative Understanding in Infants," in D. R. Olson, ed., *Social Foundation of Language and Thought, Essays in Honor of Jerome S. Bruner.* New York: W. W. Norton, 1977, pp. 316–342.

45. WOLFF, P. "Observations on Newborn Infants," 1977, *Psychosomatic Medicine,* 21 (1959):110–118.

28 / Childhood Psychic Trauma

Lenore Cagen Terr

Introduction and Definitions

So often do the lay public and the psychiatric profession employ such expressions as "he was traumatized when he was young" that they have become clichés. Nonetheless, until recent times scientific studies of the effects of overwhelming childhood experiences have been quite rare. In fact, before the mid-1970s, although we talked about it frequently enough, we knew very little about childhood trauma.

In 1920 Freud[21] had proposed a clear definition for psychic trauma: "a breach in an otherwise efficacious barrier against stimuli" (p. 29). Over the ensuing years, however, ideas about trauma, including those originating with Freud himself, became increasingly fuzzy. Terms such as retrospective trauma,[27] retroactive trauma,[69] strain trauma,[45,70] cumulative trauma,[44] screen trauma,[32] and constructive trauma[95] gradually seeped into the medical and psychoanalytic literature, obscuring Freud's earlier, more clearly delineated concepts. After Freud's death, the "protective shield" idea also came to be variously interpreted, further obscuring the definitions of this concept.[14]

In 1967 Anna Freud recognized this widespread deterioration of the psychic trauma terminology and sought "to rescue it from the widening and overuse that are the present-day fate of many other technical terms in psychoanalysis and, in the course of time, lead inevitably to a blurring of meaning and finally to the abandonment and loss of valuable concepts" (p. 235).[15] She urged a return to Freud's 1920 definition and pointed out a year later, in a paper otherwise unrelated to this area, that in order for there to be a trauma, an external event must take place.[16]

Taking Miss Freud's momentous "rescue" into account, one may now update Freud's 1920[21] and 1926[23] definitions of psychic trauma in the following way: "Psychic trauma occurs when a sudden, unexpected, intense external experience overwhelms the individual's coping and defensive operations, creating the feeling of utter helplessness." As defined in DSM-III[1] the traumatic event is "generally outside the range of usual human experience" (p. 236) and must be of sufficient magnitude that it "would evoke significant symptoms of distress in most individuals, and is generally outside the range of such common experiences as simple bereavement, chronic illness, business losses, or marital conflicts" (p. 236)[13] These new updated definitions virtually eliminate from the "list" of common traumatic events such previously designated childhood "traumas" as the birth of a sibling, a frightening threat from a parent,[76] a bad case of communicable disease, or a cold harsh upbringing.

"Trauma" is thus the psychiatric condition and the "traumatic event" is its external precipitant. The psychiatric diagnosis may be elaborated with such additions as psychic trauma with severe anxiety, psychic trauma with depression or pathological mourning, and psychic trauma with accompanying psychotic thinking (see "Reactive psychosis" in ICD-9[37]). Massive psychic trauma[46] and the cumulative and horribly stressful experiences of childhood physical and/or sexual abuse may lead to conditions closely related, but not the same as, single-blow unexpected psychic trauma. Posttraumatic stress disorder is the current DSM-III terminology for psychic trauma, replacing the old term, traumatic neurosis. DSM-III has attempted to separate acute from chronic posttraumatic disorders, but, in children at least, a distinction based on how soon symptoms appear may not be particularly useful. Childhood symptoms tend to appear immediately upon exposure to a surprising and intense shock.

In this chapter the literature on childhood trauma from Sigmund Freud up to the present is discussed. A set of signs and symptoms of childhood trauma, several of which have not yet been incorporated into the standard diagnostic criteria, is proposed. Those special symptoms and signs of "childhood trauma" that distinguish it from its adult counterpart are described,

and, finally, some of the research areas currently under investigation is noted.

The Literature on Childhood Psychic Trauma

During his lifetime Sigmund Freud wavered in his emphasis on actual events as they affected the developing human mind. Early in his career Freud proposed that real seductions in childhood lie behind the adult neuroses,[24,25] but shortly thereafter he revamped this theory in favor of childhood sexual experience that existed entirely in the realm of fantasy (the Oedipus complex).[19,20] A recent controversy featured in the lay press has centered around Freud's possible motives for shifting directions in 1897–98 from real to imagined youthful seductions.[57,58,59] Whatever Freud's motives, there was considerable validity to his newfound emphasis on sexual fantasy in childhood, and over the ensuing years child psychiatrists have regularly found confirmatory evidence for these imagined oedipal events in the statements and the play of their young patients.

The problem, however, became one of emphasis. Psychoanalysis was so enamoured with the power of the inner life that it tended to ignore real events as they affected young people. During and after World War I, Freud again turned his interest to the traumatic event and its internal aftereffects,[21,26] but somehow the main body of analysis and psychodynamic psychiatry did not follow suit. In 1960 Robert Waelder, one of the pioneers of psychoanalysis, commented that Freud

looked forward to later investigations by psychoanalysts of the traumatic neuroses, and of the possible relationship between shock, anxiety and narcissism.

But there was little follow-up along this line. The war neuroses disappeared with the war, and the interest of psychoanalysts was concentrated on the psychoneuroses from there to expand, later, to character neuroses, behavior disorders and . . . the psychoses, rather than to the traumatic neuroses. (P. 166)[94]

During the ensuing forty years of relative neglect, there were a few bright spots for the study of childhood trauma. Anna Freud and her Hampstead group made some outstanding contributions during World War II. She and Dorothy Burlingham wrote up their wartime experiences with British children who had been evacuated from London during the bombings.[17] They concluded that the presence or absence of parents was more crucial to how children fared during the war than were the bombings themselves. The Hampstead group also made many observations of young European Holocaust survivors brought back after the war to London.[18] Even here, however, the group's attention centered upon how the children fared without their parents. Despite the brilliantly observant case descriptions of traumatically overwhelmed youngsters (see "Bertie," p. 197 of "Report 12"[17]), separation, not single-blow childhood trauma, commanded most of Anna Freud's and her colleagues' interest.

There is one very important piece of work from the Hampstead Nurseries that bears significantly upon current studies in progress; this is Hansi Kennedy's description of how "cover memories" (screen memories) were constructed after a war-generated separation of a nine-month-old girl from her parents.[42] Employing very careful observations after the five-year-old girl returned home, Kennedy followed the development of "Bridget's" wartime remembrances prospectively for two and one-half years. Kennedy remarked that children's memories "are much nearer the surface and distortions much less elaborate and complicated than in the case of an adult" (p. 280). Twenty-one years later Kennedy criticized the psychoanalytic tendency to discount real psychic trauma.[43] She stated that analysts often are led "into analyzing what the child is experiencing predominantly in terms of his defenses and his projections of wishes, fantasies, and conflicts without acknowledging sufficiently that in certain cases, what the child brings is shaped by the fact that he lived in a 'crazy world' which has become internalized" (p. 391).

For the most part, however, during and after World War II, individual children were not sufficiently studied in respect to posttraumatic effects. Youngsters' reactions to frightening events were seen largely as reflections of parent-child interactions. For instance, after a threatened Japanese air raid on San Francisco, J. Solomon considered institutionalized children's behaviors as indications of how calmly or with how much panic the children's house parents and teachers had reacted.[77] Carey-Trefzger saw both exposure to bombings and separation from mothers as the precipitants of wartime emotional disturbances in European children, but she strongly emphasized that "nervous mothers" harmfully influenced their young charges.[9] She stated that once the frightening events were over, such upset mothers would prevent youngsters from settling down. Like that of the other wartime child psychiatric authors, Carey-Trefzger's emphasis fell solidly upon the parents. During the build-up phase of World War II, Mercier and Despert described a few French families and concluded that children "temporarily reflect the attitudes of the surrounding adults" (p. 269).[60]

Upon reading the wartime childhood trauma literature, one could not escape the impression that children, like marionettes, simply reflected the coaxings of their master puppeteers. Despite the obvious fact that par-

ents were important, the question arises: Did the youngsters' display any personal and unique styles of response, and if so, where did these figure in? In papers written by the Hampstead group and by Marie Helen Mercier, there were beautiful case descriptions of children's individual behaviors; nonetheless, these articles did not integrate the important observations into any substantial conclusions or into a comprehensive theory about childhood trauma.

One prominent American author, however, did focus entirely on the frightened children themselves. Though he wrote during the war, David Levy was interested primarily in hospitalized youngsters[49] and in child outpatients who had suffered frights or shocks.[48] From his work he drew the important inference that children could suffer individual psychic traumas, much as adults do. Levy set forth a number of ideas about the origin of psychic traumas in the hospital operating room; eventually these became the focus of a large body of child psychiatric-pediatric research and brought new medical interest to the individual frightened child. Levy's concept of "trauma" was too broad to fit into the current definitions, and many of the cases he described were moderately frightened, transiently anxious, or somewhat depressed youngsters and not those who were overwhelmed. Nonetheless, his concern for the hospitalized youngster and his strong warnings about the hospital as the setting for a "traumatic event" inspired a new humanism in pediatrics.

The first large-scale peacetime study of children's reactions to disaster was conducted in Vicksburg, Mississippi, by a group from the National Institute of Mental Health (NIMH).[5] A large number of youngsters had been at the local movie house watching the Saturday matinee when a "killer-tornado" struck the theater. The investigators personally interviewed eighty-eight parents and issued questionnaires to the students at one Vicksburg school. (Again the old wartime bias toward studying the parents was reflected here. Supposedly the children were the focus of the research, but, in fact, Block and Silber, the two interviewers, did not interview the youngsters and instead worked personally with a number of the parents.) The NIMH group concluded that those children who were physically injured, who were present at the impact zone, and/or who had a family member who was injured or had died were most likely to suffer "overt anxiety, anxiety equivalents, symptom formation or intensification of pathological character traits" (p. 418). They found further that there was "a relationship between a history of parental psychopathology and the child's emotional disturbance" (p. 420). Block, Silber, and Perry commented that researchers cannot "approach parents for information about their children unless [they are] prepared to deal with the parents' problems first" (p. 421). There remains considerable wisdom to this observation today, especially in clinical practice.

For the next twenty-five years, a curious quality of inactivity fell over the field of childhood trauma. To be sure, some psychoanalysts were retrospectively reconstructing childhood traumas from the analyses of their adult patients[6,39] and some psychoanalysts were, perhaps overzealously, "finding" old traumas in accounts from the early lives of famous artists[63,78] or from the published works of writers.[40,41] Despite this interest in retrospective reconstruction, however, few, if any, clinical field studies of psychic trauma in childhood or infancy were being done. It was recognized from the psychotherapies of adults that the reconstruction of childhood frights would be quite useful. Before retrospective adult remembrances could be thoroughly appreciated and optimally utilized in therapy, however, the formation of childhood memories of traumatic events required prospective study, bearing in mind Emanuel Peterfreund's warning that such observations of youngsters must *not* be "adultomorphic."[66] Although no single large-scale prospective study of traumatic memory in formation has yet been achieved, observations such as those of Loftus[55] or of this author[85,92] may eventually offer new insights that can be utilized in the psychodynamic therapies of both adults and young people.

During the 1960s stress researchers took up the slack in the field of psychic trauma. Lois Murphy's studies of coping styles in preschoolers[62] set the tone for a generation of "coping" studies that followed. After John Kennedy was assassinated, Murphy's associate, Moriarty,[61] sent questionnaires to the group of teenagers whom these researchers had been studying over the years. The adolescents' responses were in total agreement with the character assessments that had originally been made of these children many years previously. More recent work of this type has been done by Anthony[2] in a long-term study of the child from a schizophrenic family and by Garmezy[30] in his follow-up work with schoolchildren at risk for mental disorders.

A body of work began to appear during the 1960s describing children who had been exposed to massive, prolonged, and overwhelming fright, degradation, and the hideous deaths of loved ones and strangers. These accounts emerged from both the European Holocaust and Hiroshima. The findings in these studies were not identical to those that followed the simpler traumas (the more "classic" ones by the 1920 and 1967 definitions); there were nonetheless some similarities between massive psychic trauma and single-blow trauma. E. Sterba, for example, found that children who had survived the Holocaust developed emotional disorders as soon as they were settled in this country, which was

unlike surviving adults, who experienced a symptom-free period.[79] This finding was later confirmed by the author of this chapter at Chowchilla, California, following a schoolbus kidnapping.[80] Several Holocaust studies determined that depression and guilt could be "caught" like a contagious disease by the second generation of concentration camp survivors.[7,13] Although these Holocaust studies have been severely criticized for their methodologies,[75] "contagion" of posttraumatic symptomatology has been confirmed in my more recent studies of pure psychic trauma in children.[85]

Lifton's book on the survivors of Hiroshima included some accounts from persons who had been children when the atomic bomb hit.[50] When Lifton interviewed them in the 1960s, these individuals were continuing to suffer the emotional effects of the 1945 explosion; thus Lifton was able to demonstrate how long the effects of massive childhood trauma could last. Lifton developed ideas concerning "psychic numbing" and "survivor's guilt," and he and Olson described how a "shattering of the illusion of invulnerability" may affect traumatized persons.[53] Psychic numbing has not been observed in children who suffer pure single-blow trauma,[83] but when others die during their traumatic experience, the surviving youngsters do experience survivor's guilt. Lifton's concept of "shattering the illusion of invulnerability," however, does not apply directly to classic childhood trauma because it is not at all clear when, developmentally, an "illusion of invulnerability" is established—if ever. For youngsters, Erikson's "basic trust" concept[13] seems a far more useful conception than is the "illusion of invulnerability" idea; in traumatized children, fears of further trauma and chronic fears of the mundane may lead to a destruction of this basic trust.[80]

The first on-site studies devoted exclusively to interviews of traumatized children occurred in the 1970s following the 1966 Aberfan, Wales, mining tragedy[47] and the 1972 Buffalo Creek, West Virginia, flood disaster.[64] These studies broke new ground because they emphasized direct observations of the traumatized children themselves. At Aberfan, over a five-year period during which he worked with the local child guidance center, Gaynor Lacey psychiatrically evaluated the fifty-six children who came to him voluntarily following the slag avalanche that had engulfed their primary school. Although he could reach no conclusions about the incidence of posttraumatic symptoms (the group was already self-selected for chronic family and childhood disturbances), Lacey found that the most severely affected youngsters originated from backgrounds marked by "anxiety creating situations" or by "grief situations in the past . . . [making] them and their parents more vulnerable" (p. 259) to the trauma. The old emphasis on parents still existed at Aberfan, but

Lacey did make some very clear, albeit undefined, observations of childhood posttraumatic play and posttraumatic fears.

C. Janet Newman, a University of Cincinnati child psychiatrist, personally interviewed eleven child survivors of the 1972 Buffalo Creek dam collapse and valley flood, using such projective techniques as the youngsters' on-the-spot drawings, their wishes, and their stories.[64] Newman found that these children shared "a modified sense of reality, increased vulnerability to future stresses, an altered sense of powers within the self, and a precocious awareness of fragmentation and death" (p. 312). Newman did not follow her child patients over an extended period of time, nor did she conclude what symptoms, signs, and psychodynamic mechanisms would be expected in childhood trauma, but her work greatly influenced studies that followed, particularly those that rely on artwork as expressions of emotionally overwhelmed youngsters' posttraumatic fantasies.[28,68]

On July 15, 1976, twenty-six Chowchilla, California, schoolchildren ages five to fourteen and their bus driver, a stranger to most of them, were kidnapped at gunpoint and subjected to twenty-seven hours of unremitting terror. Eventually the group was freed through the efforts of two boys who dug the children out of the buried truck trailer, where all of them had been incarcerated for the final sixteen hours of their ordeal. There were no deaths, and the entire group emerged physically unharmed.

Chowchilla presented an ideal opportunity for clinical field studies of both the short- and longer-term effects of psychic trauma in previously "normal" schoolage children. During the shocking event, the youngsters had been totally separated from their parents. They could be studied prospectively. The children ranged from the oedipal through midadolescent developmental stages, and the group included youngsters of Caucasian, Hispanic, and American Indian background. The first Chowchilla research project involved all twenty-three youngsters and families who had remained in town, and it extended from the fifth to the thirteenth month after the kidnapping.[80,83] The second study was a four- to five-year follow-up of the same group, plus two additional children who had been abducted, and one who had left the bus just prior to its capture.[85] Ongoing clinical psychiatric work with individually traumatized youngsters took place in tandem with the Chowchilla project,[82,87] and a group of twenty-five normal schoolchildren from McFarland and Porterville, California, were interviewed as a matched control population for the four- to five-year follow-up study at Chowchilla.[86]

Through the Chowchilla study and its related projects, the full spectrum of symptoms and signs of psychic trauma in the schoolage child could be observed.

Signs and Symptoms of Childhood Psychic Trauma Based on the Chowchilla Studies

IMMEDIATE EFFECTS

With the initial shock of a trauma, children fear separation from parent(s), death, and/or further fright —"fear itself." Castration fears as such appear very rarely. An immediate cautiousness is established in the child victim. The traumatized child balks and hesitates in the face of new situations or unknown ventures. Misperceptions and/or hallucinations indicate that the child's coping devices have been overwhelmed. Visual distortions are the most common of these perceptual disturbances; however, auditory, smell, and touch misperceptions may also occur. Among the immediate manifestations of psychic trauma are disturbances in time sense. From the first impact, traumatized children will retrospectively search for omens, often mispositioning current or even posttraumatic events into revised or reemphasized sequences originating before the trauma. Children (and also adults) tend to perceive short traumatic occurrences as prolonged and particularly long ordeals as condensed.[87] Children have not been observed to employ massive denial of external reality (though this has been reported in adults[38]) nor do they forget the details of their terrible experience once it is concluded.

EARLY EFFECTS

Fears, both of trauma-related and mundane items (with panic attacks and/or anniversary reactions), repetitive phenomena (dreams, play, and reenactment), and extensions in memory of misperceptions through such secondarily reparative attempts as overgeneralizations and time skew are the most important early posttraumatic symptoms and signs. Posttraumatic dreams may appear in various guises: (1) unremembered terror dreams accompanied at times by sleepwalking or sleeptalking; (2) exact repetitions of the traumatic events or of thoughts during the event; (3) modified repetitions; or (4) deeply disguised versions of the trauma. Shortly after the traumatic event two unique types of posttraumatic dreams—dreams in which the child allows him- or herself to die and dreams that the child believes to be predictive—begin to appear. Another repetitive phenomenon, posttraumatic play, can be recognized by its: (1) failure to relieve anxiety; (2) incessant repetition; (3) literalness; (4) unconscious linkage to the trauma; (5) varying lag times prior to inception; (6) contagiousness to other youngsters and to new generations; (7) dangerousness;

(8) tendency to employ art, storytelling, or audio duplication; (9) secretiveness; and (10) unusually wide age range of players.[82] Reenactments—behaviors repeating the original traumatic experience—may manifest themselves as a single episode or as a personality change based on multiple behaviors. Another type of reenactment—the repetition of a psychophysiological experience originally precipitated during the traumatic event—also occurs. After the event, memories of misperceptions tend to extend and to distort further for months and years. Time distortions are particularly striking in this regard. Memories of the traumatic circumstances become modified, in part, through these increasingly distorted memories of sights, sounds, and sequences.

LONG-LASTING EFFECTS

Longer term findings[85] in childhood psychic trauma include continuing elaborations and extensions of omens, fears, and misperceptions, with the children tending to indulge further in the repetitive phenomena that had originated earlier.

Relatively late in the course of the disorder some new yet very important posttraumatic manifestations appear for the first time. First, the child commonly developes a very pessimistic, foreshortened sense of the future. Second, a tendency toward screen or cover memory formation emerges, and some of these memories can be relatively devoid of emotionality. Though still fully detailed, the posttraumatic remembrances lose affective power because of: (1) a displacement of the trauma-generated affects away from the original perpetrators or the natural causes to specific persons nearer at hand; (2) the narrowing down of an originally wide range of affects to one or two of the fears that were initially stirred up by the traumatic event rather than to the actual memories of the entire event; (3) expression of the affects through recurrent physical sensations identical to those that were in fact brought on by the event; or (4) an experiencing of the memories as leisurely dreamlike visualizations or elaborately visual metaphors.[85] Posttraumatic memories further change through continuing time distortions such as: (1) time confusion, (2) durational prolongation or shortening, (3) missequencing, (4) condensation, (5) omens, (6) time skew, (7) sense of prediction, and (8) future foreshortening.[89] All of these are changes in the quality of late memories of the traumatic event. Though chillingly detailed, they do not seem to inspire the appropriate concomitant horror and dread in the child telling the memory.

When interviewed four to five years after an overwhelming fright, children tend to be ashamed and mortified about their past helplessness during the event. Even though they can still fully recall it, they consistently try to suppress the embarrassing and frightening "story." Their loss of autonomy at the time looms as a particularly upsetting aspect of the entire affair. Many traumatized children begin to develop a deeply entrenched conviction that they are clairvoyant. This, in addition to an oppressive feeling of guilt, may at least partly ward off the trauma-inspired feeling of utter helplessness.

Most traumatized children tend to narrow their worries away from the world at large to far more immediate concerns, like their own bedrooms at night or the local disasters in their own hometowns. Contrary to the powerful wishes of the public at large, child victims are not toughened through their horrible experiences.

MODIFYING FACTORS

The severity of youngsters' responses to psychic trauma have some relationship to their developmental phases, their prior vulnerabilities, and the quality of their family life or the strength of their family-community bonding.[85] Children's internal affective and ideational response combines with their remembrances of the actual external events. Together these become the focus of their subsequent posttraumatic dreams, play, and, in certain instances, even their perceptual distortions. Despite differences in symptom severity from child to child, there is an amazing uniformity of posttraumatic symptoms and signs across a wide range of childhood stages.[85]

If the event they experience is sufficiently shocking and intense, no children can escape psychic trauma. (For a complete review of the adult stress and sensory deprivation literature that makes this same point, see Hocking.[35] The mental health or lack of such health within the family can make a quantitative difference— that is, it can influence the severity of the posttraumatic condition—but it will not make the qualitative determination as to whether or not posttraumatic symptoms will arise. However, each child's developmental stage, past experiences, and fantasy life do paint an individual pattern upon the rather literal posttraumatic canvas.[92]

Childhood versus Adult Psychic Trauma

The literature on psychic trauma in adults has stressed that denial and repression of traumatic events may occur immediately.[36] A sense of psychic numbing may appear in those adults who have lived through some particularly dehumanizing disasters.[46] These three findings—denial, repression, and numbing—are not evident in school-age children who have experienced single-blow psychic trauma. Prior to age two or three, upsetting life events may not be remembered in words, yet they may be played out in imaginative games or partly recaptured in dreams. In children who were traumatized as preschoolers, some particularly shocking, unexpected, and intense single episodes will still be verbally recalled.[64] The data on preschool repression or lack of repression are not yet fully gathered. We do know, however, that latency-age traumatic events are remembered fully and in detail.[85] A recent case report of three toddlers attacked by dogs showed that several years afterward these preschoolers, too, could remember the details of their traumatic experiences.[31]

Traumatized adults have been observed to experience sudden, intrusive dysphoric "flashbacks" of the events they had endured.[36] In contrast to this, children are known to browse leisurely or daydream through the recalled scenes of their externally generated horrors. Children are not suddenly taken by surprise with striking, intrusive visualizations.[83] Perhaps because they do not alternate massive denial with sudden flashbacks as adults reportedly do,[36] traumatized children also do not exhibit the tendency toward decline in work productivity (school performance)[83] that some traumatized adults manifest.

On the other hand, youngsters exhibit far more frequent and striking behavioral repetitions than do adults who have been psychically traumatized. Posttraumatic play and reenactments are particularly important in children, and these may influence their later personality development. Time skew, the mixing up of what came after a traumatic event with what preceded it, is much more common in children than it is in adults. Time condensation, the merging together of two memories that were originally separated in time, is also more common in very young trauma victims[89] (as is the condensation of symbols—"symbolic condensation"[64]). Although it certainly affects psychically overwhelmed adults as well, the sense of a limited future is particularly striking in traumatized children because it is so discrepant with their young years and unlimited horizons.[89]

Current Investigations

THE TRAUMATIZED CHILD AND THE LAW

Beginning with Elizabeth Loftus's fascinating psychological experiments concerning children's memories,[55] the use of children as legal witnesses has become a popular area of inquiry. I outlined how psychically traumatized youngsters might function as courtroom witnesses,[81] and subsequently Pynoos and Eth, in their work with children who had witnessed parental homocide or suicide, studied how traumatized youngsters at various developmental stages function in the criminal process.[67] Pynoos and Eth have also worked out a ninety-minute psychiatric interview procedure for such child witnesses.[68] Similar to the overall trends in the study of psychic trauma, as more is learned about older children in the courtroom, the age spans under investigation seem to grow younger. I have written two quite preliminary, theoretical accounts of how infants and nonverbal toddlers (or their representatives) may function as witnesses in the legal system.[88,90]

PSYCHIC TRAUMA IN SEXUAL ASSAULT, PHYSICAL ATTACK, SUDDEN INJURY, PARENTAL SNATCHING, AND CHILDHOOD GRIEF

The psychically traumatic components in well-known childhood injuries, abuses, and losses are slowly coming under investigation. It is becoming apparent that the major and direct emotional responses to these conditions (depression, excitement, agitation, withdrawal, etc.) may partly cover the more specifically posttraumatic effects. Such psychological necessities for the child as handling radical changes in body image, accommodating to adult-demanded sexual behaviors, coping with diminished physiological capacities, facing surgeries, expecting parental attacks and rejections, and undergoing profound grief and mourning may override and obscure concurrent posttraumatic symptoms and signs. An injured child may suffer repeated nightmares and experience strange omens without ever mentioning this to parents or doctors. The child psychiatrist and pediatrician must be aware that the untreated psychological effects of trauma may partly block the child's eventual physical and emotional recovery from an injury.

Currently, psychic trauma is not a major focus of the literature dealing with childhood injury, assault, and loss; but eventually it will have to be.*

The battered child syndrome and childhood sexual abuse have recently been connected with psychic trauma by such authors as Yates,[96] Goodwin,[33] and Green.[34] Goodwin believes that incest *is* psychic trauma, and therefore does not consider surprise and lack of preparation as crucial to her conception of trauma. It should be noted that most trauma research-

*Excellent works deal with the more specific psychological problems generated by these conditions; Galdston[29] and Bernstein[4] have written articles describing the psychological problems of burned children, Earle[11] has described what youngsters undergoing mutilating surgery endure, and Lipton and Roth[54] have written about children raped by strangers.

ers do consider surprise a key to the subsequent reactions. Green would link the battered child syndrome with psychic trauma; his ideas are, however, not entirely convincing because his theory rests upon the currently out-of-favor "cumulative trauma"[44] concept. It is clear that some elements of psychic trauma *do* lurk behind the repetitive behaviors and the nightmares of battered children, but a few symptoms and signs alone do not make a disorder. Eventually it may be necessary to develop a nosological spectrum of stress-trauma disorders including incest, sexual abuse, and battered child syndrome as well as single-blow trauma.

The new literature on children snatched by their own parents[71,74,84] indicates that along with grief for the lost parent and anger regarding imagined rejection from that parent, snatched children may also be significantly traumatized by that parent—or even traumatized upon rekidnapping by the "legal" parent or by an entirely abortive attempt on the part of the noncustodial parent. I found that of a group of eight children "successfully" snatched, and of ten abortively snatched by one parent, eleven exhibited signs of psychic trauma or severe fright. Seven of the eighteen were mentally indoctrinated ("brainwashed") by the snatching parent, seven were suffering chronic grief for the absent parent, nine were enraged at a parent, and two were exhibiting exaggerated identifications with or wish fulfillment about a snatching parent.[84]

In a study of child pornography participants, Burgess, Groth, and McCausland[8] described a tendency of such sexually misused youngsters to be traumatized when discovered by police or parents. Such findings relating psychic trauma to discovery and "rescue" will require more detailed confirmatory observations before being fully integrated into the general "picture" of psychic trauma.

PSYCHIC TRAUMA IN OTHER CULTURES

At the end of World War II, Tulchin and Levy[93] tried out the newly developed Rorschach test on two groups of refugee children, British and Spanish. The little Spaniards had been subjected to far greater wartime stresses, and the American authors said they could tell from the testing that "the more intense and more traumatic experience of the Spanish group of refugee children has made its mark" (p. 368). They concluded that psychic trauma "plays a part in the dynamic personality structure, as disclosed in the Rorschach findings" (p. 368).

In the first volume of the *Basic Handbook of Child Psychiatry,* Carlin[10] described work she had done with catastrophically uprooted Southeast Asian children. She found that one Korean youngster adopted at age one year was still experiencing night terrors at age

thirteen, and that one year after his evacuation, another patient, a two and one-half-year-old Vietnamese boy, still believed that any loud sounds he heard in the United States represented Viet Cong soldiers coming to get him. Considerable investigation is now underway on the status of displaced and traumatized Central American and Southeast Asian children recently emigrated to the United States. In the next few years, we may expect interesting data from these studies.

VICARIOUS TRAUMA

Robert Lifton[51,52] states that all dwellers in today's world are unwittingly victims of psychic trauma, prone to both psychic numbing and survivor's guilt. Lifton's proposals are theoretical, not clinical; before they can be accepted as "psychiatry" or "science" they probably require acceptance of certain beliefs systems.

A similar problem affects the recent studies that have been done on children's abilities to be traumatized vicariously by the nuclear threat. Some of these studies came about at times of loud public outcry against nuclear escalation and were conducted by researchers who held strong political convictions as well as worthwhile scientific aims. Beardslee and Mack's survey of Boston schoolchildren,[3] Mack's anecdotal account of New England schoolchildren's attitudes,[56] and Schwebel and Schwebel's questionnaire surveys of normal youngsters at school[72,73] were conducted during periods when doctors and public alike were outraged about nuclear threats. The times themselves easily may have influenced the design and the outcome of these studies.

One recent study, which may have some bearing on the question of vicarious nuclear traumatization in children, actually was conducted for other purposes.[86] Twenty-five normal schoolchildren ages nine to seventeen in two rural districts of California were selected as a matched control group for the four to five year Chowchilla kidnapping follow-up study. During a relatively quiet historical period in 1981 just prior to the worldwide antinuclear demonstrations, these youngsters were interviewed in two separate fifteen-minute sessions about their life attitudes, future expectations, and dreams. Although the McFarland-Porterville youngsters were not asked any specific questions about nuclear war, pollution, the economy, or cancer, several of the children spontaneously brought up personal worries about these issues (nuclear war, 7; the economy, 2; crime, 2; world population expansion, 3). Although the topic of life planning was central to all the interviews, none of these McFarland-Porterville children had considered altering his or her own life plans because of the concerns that were mentioned. Despite deep concern about worldwide catastrophe, these California Valley youngsters were still going along making their future plans, tacitly believing that they themselves would be safe. Thus, in the McFarland and Porterville student groups, there was no evidence for "vicarious traumatization" by threatened nuclear war.

Although it appears that the nuclear traumatization question is far from resolved, the issue of vicarious traumatization remains a fascinating one. Indeed, it may have influenced some of the recent investigation of the effects of television on children. Any "answers" in this area will have to come from data collected with the same sense of scientific purpose and rigorous attention to methodology as would be required by any other, albeit less timely or passionately arguable, inquiry.

If we temporarily eliminate from our consideration the very difficult to assess contemporary worries about children's responses to threats of nuclear war and to violence on television, there are some aspects of individual psychic trauma that *do* appear fairly easily transmissible into unaffected populations of children. Posttraumatic play moves so easily from one child to another and from one generation to the next [82] that this

contagion may account for some common rituals, such as the playing of the medieval Black Plague game, Ring Around the Rosie, in twentieth-century nursery schools. Posttraumatic visual and time distortions, such as "ghosts,"[91] and "omens,"[89] also are highly contagious. Traumatic anxiety can be so compelling that it invites those not directly traumatized to try to dissipate the feelings too. It is conceivable that fright transmitted from the traumatized to the nontraumatized may be hidden in our tales of the supernatural, in those philosophies that espouse "living day to day," in our prophesies, and in the songs and games that children play. Whether the contemporary concern is nuclear war, television, world hunger, or cancer, vicarious traumatization would probably not break out like a generalized and rampant epidemic. It is likely that it would behave more like an endemic condition that is contracted as games are taught by one child to the next, as stories are told by one child to another, and as old wives' tales are passed from one grandfather to a two-generations-removed future grandmother.

REFERENCES

1. AMERICAN PSYCHIATRIC ASSOCIATION. *Diagnostic and Statistical Manual of Mental Disorders* 3rd ed. (DSM-III). Washington, D.C.: American Psychiatric Association, 1980.

2. ANTHONY, E. J. "From Birth to Breakdown: A Prospective Study of Vulnerability," in E. J. Anthony, C. Koupernick, and C. Chiland, eds., *The Child and His Family,* vol. 4. New York: John Wiley & Sons, 1978, pp. 273–285.

3. BEARDSLEE, W., and MACK, J. "The Impact on Children and Adolescents of Nuclear Development," in R. Rogers, ed., *Psychosocial Aspects of Nuclear Development,* Task Force Report #20. Washington, D.C.: American Psychiatric Association, 1982.

4. BERNSTEIN, N. "The Child with Severe Burns," in J. D. Noshpitz, ed., *Basic Handbook of Child Psychiatry,* vol. 1. New York: Basic Books, 1979, pp. 465–474.

5. BLOCK, D., SILBER, E., and PERRY, S. "Some Factors in the Emotional Reaction of Children to Disaster," *American Journal of Psychiatry,* 113 (1956): 416–422.

6. BONAPARTE, M. "Notes on the Analytic Discovery of a Primal Scene," *Psychoanalytic Study of the Child,* 1 (1945): 119 125.

7. BOROCAS, C., and BOROCAS, H. "Manifestations of Concentration Camp Effects on the Second Generation," *American Journal of Psychiatry,* 130 (1973): 820–821.

8. BURGESS, A. W., GROTH, A. N., and McCAUSLAND, M. P. "Child Sex Initation Rings," *American Journal of Orthopsychiatry,* 51 (1981): 110–119.

9. CAREY-TREFZGER, C. "The Results of a Clinical Study of War-Damaged Children Who Attended the Child Guidance Clinic, the Hospital for Sick Children, Great Ormand Street, London," *Journal of Mental Science,* 95 (1949): 535–559.

10. CARLIN, J. "The Catastrophically Uprooted Child: Southeast Asian Refugee Children," in J. D. Noshpitz, ed.,

Basic Handbook of Child Psychiatry, vol. 1. New York: Basic Books, 1979, pp. 290–300.

11. EARLE, E. "The Psychological Effects of Mutilating Surgery in Children and Adolescents," *Psychoanalytic Study of the Child,* 34 (1979): 527–546.

12. EPSTEIN, H. *Children of the Holocaust.* New York: G. P. Putnam's, 1979.

13. ERIKSON, E. *Childhood and Society.* New York: W. W. Norton, 1950.

14. ESMAN, A. "The 'Stimulus Barrier'—A Review and Reconsideration," *Psychoanalytic Study of the Child,* 38 (1983): 193–207.

15. FREUD, A. "Comments on Trauma," in S. Furst, ed., *Psychic Trauma.* New York: Basic Books, 1967, pp. 235–245.

16. ———. "Acting Out," *International Journal of Psycho-Analysis,* 49 (1968): 165–170.

17. FREUD, A., and BURLINGHAM, D. "Report 12," *The Writings of Anna Freud,* vol. 3. New York: International Universities Press, pp. 142–211. (Originally published 1942.)

18. FREUD, A., and DANN, S. "An Experiment in Group Upbringing," *Psychoanalytic Study of the Child,* 6 (1951): 127–168.

19. FREUD, S. "Three Essays on the Theory of Sexuality," in J. Strachey, ed., *The Standard Edition of the Complete Psychological Works of Sigmund Freud* (hereafter *The Standard Edition*), vol. 7. London: Hogarth Press, 1953, pp. 123–245. (Originally published 1905.)

20. ———. *The Origins of Psychoanalysis; Letters to Wilhelm Fliess, Drafts and Notes,* ed. M. Bonaparte, A. Freud, and E. Kris. New York: Basic Books, 1954. (Originally published 1887–1902.)

21. ———. "Beyond the Pleasure Principle," *The Standard Edition,* vol. 18. London: Hogarth Press, 1955, pp. 1–64. (Originally published 1920.)

22. ———. "Remembering, Repeating and Working-Through," *The Standard Edition*, vol. 12. London: Hogarth Press, 1958, pp. 147–156. (Originally published 1914.)

23. ———. "Inhibitions, Symptoms, and Anxiety," *The Standard Edition*, vol. 20. London: Hogarth Press, 1959, pp. 75–175. (Originally published 1926.)

24. ———. "The Aetiology of Hysteria," *The Standard Edition*, vol. 3. London: Hogarth Press, 1962, pp. 189–221. (Originally published 1896).

25. ———. "Heredity and the Aetiology of the Neuroses," *The Standard Edition*, vol. 3. London: Hogarth Press, 1962, pp. 141–156. (Originally published 1896).

26. ———. "Introductory Lectures," *The Standard Edition*, vol. 16. London: Hogarth Press, 1963, pp. 273–276. (Originally published 1917).

27. ———. "Moses and Monotheism," *The Standard Edition*, vol. 23. London: Hogarth Press, 1964, pp. 3–137. (Originally published 1939.)

28. GALANTE, R. Presentation on the Treatment of the Child Earthquake Victims in Italy, part of The Abramson Fund Symposium "Children of Disaster," Paper presented at the annual meeting of the American Academy of Child Psychiatry. Washington, D.C., 1982.

29. GALDSTON, R. "The Burning and Healing of Children," *Psychiatry*, 35 (1972): 57–66.

30. GARMEZY, N., and RUTTER, M., eds., *Stress, Coping, and Development in Children*. New York: McGraw-Hill, 1983.

31. GISLASON, L., and CALL, J. "Dog Bite in Infancy: Trauma and Personality Development," *Journal of the American Academy of Child Psychiatry*, 21 (1982): 203–207.

32. GLOVER, E. "The Screening Function of Traumatic Memories," *International Journal of Psycho-Analysis*, 10 (1929): 90–93.

33. GOODWIN, J. "Posttraumatic Symptoms in Abused Children," Paper presented at the 11th Friends Hospital Clinical Conference, Philadelphia, October 14–15, 1983.

34. GREEN, A. "Dimension of Psychological Trauma in Abused Children," *Journal of the American Academy of Child Psychiatry*, 22 (1983): 231–237.

35. HOCKING, F. "Extreme Environmental Stress and Its Significance for Psychopathology," *American Journal of Psychotherapy*, 24 (1970): 4–26.

36. HOROWITZ, M. *Stress Response Syndromes*. New York: Jason Aronson, 1976.

37. *International Classification of Diseases*, 9th Rev., *Clinical Modification*. vol. 1, Ann Arbor, Mich: Edwards Brothers, 1980.

38. JANIS, I. *Psychological Stress: Psychoanalytic and Behavioral Studies of Surgical Patients*. New York: John Wiley & Sons, 1958.

39. KATAN, A. "Children Who Were Raped," *Psychoanalytic Study of the Child*, 28 (1973): 208–224.

40. KATAN, M. "A Causerie on Henry James's *The Turn of the Screw*," *Psychoanalytic Study of the Child*, 17 (1962): 473–493.

41. ———. "The Origin of *The Turn of the Screw*," *Psychoanalytic Study of the Child*, 21 (1966): 583–635.

42. KENNEDY, H. "Cover Memories in Formation," *Psychoanalytic Study of the Child*, 5 (1950): 275–284.

43. ———. "Problems in Reconstruction in Child Analysis," *Psychoanalytic Study of the Child*, 26: (1971): 386–402.

44. KHAN, M.M.R. "The Concept of Cumulative Trauma," *Psychoanalytic Study of the Child*, 18 (1963): 286–306.

45. KRIS, E. "The Recovery of Childhood Memories in Psychoanalysis," *Psychoanalytic Study of the Child*, 11 (1956): 54–88.

46. KRYSTAL, H., ed. *Massive Psychic Trauma*. New York: International Universities Press, 1968.

47. LACEY, G. "Observations on Aberfan," *Journal of Psychosomatic Research*, 16 (1972): 257–260.

48. LEVY, D. "Release Therapy," *American Journal of Orthopsychiatry*, 9 (1939): 713–736.

49. ———. "Psychic Trauma of Operations in Children," *American Journal of the Diseases of Children*, 69 (1945): 7–25.

50. LIFTON, R. *Death in Life: Survivors of Hiroshima*. New York: Random House, 1967.

51. ———. *The Broken Connection*. New York: Simon and Schuster, 1979.

52. ———. "Beyond Psychic Numbing: A Call to Awareness," *American Journal of Orthopsychiatry*, 52 (1982): 619–629.

53. LIFTON, R., and OLSON, E. "The Human Meaning of Total Disaster," *Psychiatry*, 39 (1976): 1–18.

54. LIPTON, G., and ROTH, E. "Rape: A Complex Management Problem in the Pediatric Emergency Room," *Journal of Pediatrics*, 75 (1969): 859–866.

55. LOFTUS, E. *Memory*. Reading, Mass.: Addison-Wesley, 1980.

56. MACK, J. "The Perception of U.S.–Soviet Intentions and Other Psychological Dimensions of the Nuclear Arms Race," *American Journal of Orthopsychiatry*, 52 (1982): 590–599.

57. MALCOLM, J. "Annals of Scholarship (Psychoanalysis Part I)," *The New Yorker*, 5 December, 1983, p. 59.

58. ———. "Annals of Scholarship (Psychoanalysis Part II)," *The New Yorker*, 12 December 1983, p. 60.

59. MASSON, J. M. "Freud and the Seduction Theory," *The Atlantic*, February 1984, pp. 33–60.

60. MERCIER, M., and DESPERT, J. "Effects of War on French Children," *Psychosomatic Medicine*, 5 (1943): 266–272.

61. MORIARTY, A. "Reactions to the Assassination of a President," in L. Murphy and A. Moriarty, eds., *Vulnerability, Coping and Growth*. New Haven: Yale University Press, 1976, pp. 249–262.

62. MURPHY, L. *The Widening World of Childhood: Paths Towards Mastery*. New York: Basic Books, 1962.

63. NEIDERLAND, W. "Psychoanalytic Approaches to Artistic Creativity," *Psychoanalytic Quarterly*, 45 (1976): 185–212.

64. NEWMAN, C. J. "Children of Disaster: Clinical Observations at Buffalo Creek," *American Journal of Psychiatry*, 133 (1976): 306–312.

65. NEWMAN, L. "Emotional Disturbance in Children of Holocaust Survivors," *Social Casework*, 60 (1979): 43–50.

66. PETERFREUND, E. "Some Criticial Comments on Psychoanalytic Conceptualizations of Infancy," *International Journal of Psycho-Analysis*, 59 (1978): 427–441.

67. PYNOOS, R., and ETH, S. "The Child as Witness to Homicide," *Journal of Social Issues*, 40 (1984): 87–108.

68. ———. "Witness to Violence: The Child Interview," *Journal of the American Academy of Child Psychiatry*, in press.

69. RANGELL, L. "The Metapsychology of Psychic Trauma," in S. Furst, ed., *Psychic Trauma*. New York: Basic Books, 1967, pp. 51–84.

70. SANDLER, J. "Trauma, Strain, and Development," in S. Furst, ed., *Psychic Trauma*. New York: Basic Books, 1967, pp. 154–174.

71. SCHETKY, D., and HALLER, L. "Parental Kidnap-

ping," *Journal of the American Academy of Child Psychiatry,* 22 (1983): 279–285.

72. SCHWEBEL, M. "Nuclear Cold War: Student Opinion and Professional Responsibility," in M. Schwebel, ed., *Behavioral Science and Human Survival.* Palo Alto, Calif.: Behavioral Science Press, 1965, pp. 210–223.

73. SCHWEBEL, M., and SCHWEBEL, B. "Children's Reactions to the Threat of Nuclear Plant Accidents," *American Journal of Orthopsychiatry,* 51 (1981): 260–270.

74. SENIOR, N., GLADSTONE, T., and NURCOMBE, B. "Child Snatching: A Case Report," *Journal of the American Academy of Child Psychiatry,* 20 (1982): 579–583.

75. SOLKOFF, N. "Children of Survivors of the Nazi Holocaust: A Critical Review of the Literature," *American Journal of Orthopsychiatry,* 51 (1981): 29–42.

76. SOLNIT, A., and KRIS, M. "Trauma and Infantile Experiences: A Longitudinal Perspective," in S. Furst, ed., *Psychic Trauma.* New York: Basic Books, 1967, pp. 175–222.

77. SOLOMON, J. "Reactions of Children to Black-Outs," *American Journal of Orthopsychiatry,* 12 (1942): 361–362.

78. STEINBERG, E., and WEISS, J. "The Art of Edvard Munch and Its Function in His Mental Life," *Psychoanalytic Quarterly,* 23 (1954): 408–423.

79. STERBA, E. "The Effects of Persecutions on Adolescents," in H. Krystal, ed., *Massive Psychic Trauma.* New York: International Universities Press, 1968, pp. 51–60.

80. TERR, L. "Children of Chowchilla: A Study of Psychic Trauma," *Psychoanalytic Study of the Child,* 34 (1979): 547–623.

81. ———. "The Child As a Witness," in D. Schetky and E. Benedek, eds., *Child Psychiatry and the Law.* New York: Brunner/Mazel, 1980, pp. 207–221.

82. ———. " 'Forbidden Games': Post-Traumatic Child's Play," *Journal of the American Academy of Child Psychiatry,* 20 (1981): 741–760.

83. ———. "Psychic Trauma in Children: Observations Following the Chowchilla Schoolbus Kidnapping," *American Journal of Psychiatry,* 138 (1981): 14–19.

84. ———. "Child Snatching: A New Epidemic of an Ancient Malady," *Journal of Pediatrics,* 103 (1983): 151–156.

85. ———. "Chowchilla Revisited: The Effects of Psychic Trauma Four Years After a Schoolbus Kidnapping," *American Journal of Psychiatry,* 140 (1983): 1543–1550.

86. ———. "Life Attitudes, Dreams, and Psychic Trauma in a Group of 'Normal' Children," *Journal of the American Academy of Child Psychiatry,* 22 (1983): 221–230.

87. ———. "Time Sense Following Psychic Trauma: A Clinical Study of Ten Adults and Twenty Children," *American Journal of Orthopsychiatry,* 53 (1983): 244–261.

88. ———. "The Baby in Court," in J. D. Call, E. Galenson, and R. L. Tyson, eds., *Frontiers of Infant Psychiatry,* vol. 2. New York: Basic Books, 1984, pp. 490–494.

89. ———. "Time and Trauma," *Psychoanalytic Study of the Child,* 39 (1984): 633–666.

90. ———. "The Baby as a Witness," in D. Schetky and E. Benedek, eds., *Emerging Issues in Child Psychiatry and the Law.* New York: Brunner/Mazel, 1985, pp. 313–323.

91. ———. "Remembered Images and Trauma: A Psychology of the Supernatural," *Psychoanalytic Study of the Child,* 40 (1985): 493–533.

92. ———. "Children Traumatized in Small Groups, in S. Eth and R. Pynoos, *Posttraumatic Stress Disorder in Children.* Washington, D.C.: American Psychiatric Association, 1985, pp. 45–70.

93. TULCHIN, S., and LEVY, D., "Rorschach Test Differences in a Group of Spanish and English Refugee Children," *American Journal of Orthopsychiatry,* 15 (1945): 361–368.

94. WAELDER, R., *Basic Theory of Psychoanalysis.* New York: International Universities Press, 1960.

95. ———. "Trauma and the Variety of Extraordinary Challenges," in S. Furst, ed., *Psychic Trauma.* New York: Basic Books, 1967, pp. 221–234.

96. YATES, A. "Narcissistic Traits in Certain Abused Children," *American Journal of Orthopsychiatry,* 51 (1981): 55–62.

29 / Etiology and Diagnosis of Failure to Thrive and Growth Disorders in Infants and Children

Irene Chatoor and James Egan

Introduction

Failure to thrive (FTT) is a serious, complex disorder of multiple etiologies that afflicts infants and young children. It is a symptom complex or a syndrome rather than a specific disease entity. FTT has been subdivided into two major types: failure to thrive secondary to chronic disease (organic FTT) and functional failure to thrive (nonorganic FTT).

Nonorganic FTT was first recognized by Chapin[10] as a phenomenon associated with poverty and the institutional care of infants and children. Since then other terms have been introduced for nonorganic FTT: psychosocial deprivation,[7] maternal deprivation,[38] environmental failure to thrive,[46] deprivation dwarfism,[21] psychosocial dwarfism,[31] and, in the current DSM-III, reactive attachment disorder of infancy. More recently, Egan, Chatoor, and Rosen[17] have described a different type of FTT due to a disorder of separation.

At the same time that a number of studies explored the psychosocial factors contributing to FTT, it was becoming increasingly evident that the problem may be a sequela of any chronic disease. This may include metabolic, genetic, infectious, and autoimmune diseases or those diseases that affect the gastrointestinal, respiratory, nervous, renal, hepatic, cardiac, or hematopoietic systems.

While there is no consensus about the essential inclusionary or exclusionary criteria, FTT is generally diagnosed when weight is below the third percentile or when there is a sudden decrease in the rate of weight gain (e.g., a precipitous drop from the thirty-fifth to the tenth percentile). Height falling below the third percentile is frequently listed as an additional criterion for making the diagnosis. Some authors consider the presence of developmental lags or a delay in the attaining of developmental milestones as important criteria in establishing the diagnosis of FTT. The achievement of these criteria is so variable, however, that most authors do not regard them as cardinal signs of FTT.

The term failure to thrive is usually applied to infants and toddlers during the first two years of life. Disturbances in linear growth are more common in preschool or older children and are then generally classified as psychosocial or deprivation dwarfism. In such cases of dwarfism there may or may not be a corresponding decrease in weight gain. Because there is no clear-cut definition of the parameters delineating these syndromes in describing such infants or children, we prefer to use the more generic term growth disorders.[13]

Historical Background

While FTT has been recognized for a century, until quite recently it received little attention. It was not until the ninth edition (1969) of Nelson's *Textbook of Pediatrics*[36] that FTT was listed in the index.

In the 1940s the pioneering work of Spitz[50] focused attention on the devastating consequences of maternal deprivation. Spitz suggested that when the mother is withdrawn from a child between six and twelve months of age, there often occurred a syndrome that he called anaclitic depression.[51] It is characterized by apathy, withdrawal, loss of interest in the environment, and a rapidly diminishing developmental quotient. In a similar vein, he noted that institutionally reared children who had received adequate nutrition and physical care nonetheless demonstrated a high mortality rate or, if they survived, they were frequently developmentally impaired and delayed.[51] Thus by the mid-1940s it was established that at least some forms of FTT could be understood in terms of disturbances in the mother/infant dyad and, in particular, as a product of maternal deprivation or loss.

Support for this hypothesis was garnered from the work of Goldfarb,[24] who noted the presence of severe developmental disturbances in adolescents who had been institutionally reared. Spitz's and Goldfarb's views were not totally embraced by the medical, psychological, or scientific communities. Serious criticisms of the relation they postulated between the quality of maternal care and poor outcomes were advanced by Orlansky,[37] Pinneau,[40] and Casler,[9] among others. As Stone, Smith, and Murphy[52] point out, such critics "were inclined to carp at what appeared to them as but sentimental exaltation of motherhood: they suggested that it would not be difficult to replace mothers with suitable electronic and mechanical stimulators" (p. 755).

With the publication of the clinical research by Provence and Lipton,[44] Spitz's[50] and Goldfarb's[24] views were increasingly confirmed. Harlow's work[28] with laboratory animals, in this case rhesus monkeys, finally silenced the critics. When infant monkeys were reared in isolation or by substitute wire or terry-cloth mothers, Harlow[28] demonstrated severe failures in development. Thus from the laboratory came strong and compelling confirmation of the association between the quality of maternal care and the nature of the cognitive, social, sexual, and physical development which ensued.

In recent years investigators have attempted to wrestle with what has been an awkward and, in many cases, not a very useful dichotomy—the differentiation of organic and nonorganic FTT. Homer and Ludwig[30] and Casey[8] suggest that a third category of FTT exists. These are patients who manifest a mixed picture, a combination of organic and nonorganic factors in the etiology of their growth disturbance. Thus a trend has begun that deemphasizes the classical dichotomy between organic and functional FTT.

In a recent review Goldbloom[23] emphasizes the need for a holistic approach to FTT. Instead of laboratory "fishing expeditions," he points to the importance of both the medical and psychosocial history, the physical examination, and the direct observation of parent and child in establishing the etiology of the syndrome. He refers to Sills's review[48] of 185 children admitted to Children's Hospital in Buffalo, New York, which showed that out of 2,067 laboratory tests performed on these children, only 36 (1.4 percent) were of positive diagnostic significance.

In psychiatry, as in medicine generally, a diagnosis is made on the basis of the history and the physical and mental status examinations. The authors agree with Accardo's statement[1] that "the overwhelming majority of organic etiologies for FTT are identified by the history and physical examination; non-organic etiologies should be similarly identified. An overreliance on laboratory procedures to exhaustively 'rule out' organic etiologies needs to be discouraged." (p. 817).

To make a diagnosis of nonorganic FTT, the clinician must have full grasp of the various causes of both organic and nonorganic FTT. As Pasteur said, "In the fields of observation, chance favors only the mind that is prepared." Especially because mixed etiologies are common, the likelihood of making a proper diagnosis is increased when the clinician can look simultaneously for multiple contributing factors.

A Developmental Classification

One feature common to all varieties of FTT is the presence of frequent feeding problems. The variety of feeding problems and at the same time the specificity of certain feeding difficulties at different ages have led a number of authors [12,17,54] to search for a conceptual framework within which to understand these conditions. A current view of eating disorders in infants and toddlers suggests that these can create, coexist with, or appear as sequelae of FTT.

Anna Freud [20] first drew attention to the developmental aspect of feeding disorders; she suggested that there was a developmental line from sucking to rational eating. Recently Greenspan and Lourie [27] have put forward a developmental classification of psychopathology in infancy and childhood that draws heavily on observations of caretaker-child interactions. Building on the pioneering work of A. Freud, [20] Spitz, [50,51] Bowlby, [4,5] Mahler, [35] and Greenspan and Lourie, [27] Egan, Chatoor, and Rosen [17] proposed a developmental typology for eating disorders in infancy and childhood. This approach has been further refined by these authors [12] and by Chatoor and associates. [13] They suggest that feeding disturbances or eating disorders of childhood may arise from disorders of homeostasis, disorders of attachment, and disorders of separation and individuation.

DISORDERS OF HOMEOSTASIS

From birth to two months the task of the infant is to achieve regulation of state. The infant must form basic cycles and rhythms of sleep, wakefulness, alertness, feeding, and elimination. Stabilization of the autonomic and motor systems enables the infant to interact more fully with the outside world. The caretaker attempts to provide an environment within which the infant can achieve a balance between internal state and external involvement. In the feeding situation there is a progression from reflex sucking to autonomously motivated oral feedings. Infants must progress from a

state of nutritional equilibrium *in utero* to one in which they control the onset and termination of feedings by offering signals of hunger and satiation. The infant's cues can be interpreted only by a sensitive caretaker.

At this stage of development feeding problems can stem from the infant's constitutional characteristics or from medical difficulties. For example, infants with a labile autonomic nervous system show more difficulty in regulation of states and are frequently referred to as "colicky." The colicky infant seems particularly vulnerable to overstimulation. It is important for the parents to discover the infant's sensory thresholds and to become aware of the relationship between such stimuli as loud noises or bright lights and the infant's irritability. Once they appreciate the connection between colic and particular patterns of overstimulation, the parents can then modify the environment to facilitate calmer feeding periods.

Another early feeding problem related to constitutional variations is a developmental delay in the coordination of the oral musculature. If the resulting poor suck is recognized, the mother can be taught specific techniques of body positioning and providing oral support for the infant that will facilitate better feeding.

Infants with respiratory problems, especially premature infants with a prolonged course of hyaline membrane disease, may have particular difficulty in achieving homeostasis. In the first weeks or months of life rapid respiration or intubation frequently prohibit oral feedings. Consequently, such infants do not make the usual transition from reflex sucking to autonomously motivated feedings. Bernbaum and coworkers [3] showed that the regular offering of a pacifier during gavage feedings facilitated the infants' learning to suck and swallow. Later these infants learned to feed more quickly and gained weight faster than did a control group.

Another group of infants with difficulties in homeostasis are those with congenital abnormalities of the gastrointestinal tract, such as esophageal atresia. Dowling [15] followed infants with esophageal atresia who had had only gastrostomy feedings for the first months of life. Not only did such children have severe difficulties learning to suck, chew, and swallow, but they also displayed marked delays in motor and speech development. These children lacked motivation and vitality and showed general dullness. Dowling [15] concluded that these sequelae could be prevented by offering sham feedings to the infants while they were receiving gastrostomy feedings.

Because the establishment of homeostasis and of a regular feeding pattern sets the stage for growth in all areas of development, the early diagnosis of feeding difficulties and the initiation of appropriate interventions at this stage of development is particularly important. Feeding problems that develop at this early point of the infant's life not only impede physical growth but interfere with motor and speech development and affective engagement as well. Infants' problems in establishing homeostasis and their difficulty in learning to feed successfully frequently leave the mother in a vulnerable state, and lead her to react with anxiety or depression to even normal variations in the child's eating pattern. Because of the mother's anxiety or depression concerning the child's low food intake, some of these infants add to their difficulties or develop new feeding problems during the next stages of development.

DISORDERS OF ATTACHMENT

Having achieved some capacity for self-regulation, the adaptive infant is able to mobilize and engage caretakers in increasingly complex interactions. Consequently, between two and six months of age the infant is ready for the major psychological and affective task of the first year of life—the task of attachment.

Attachment develops within a reciprocal relationship. Either partner can facilitate or impede the process. Evidence of good attachment behavior includes mutual eye contact and gazing, reciprocal vocalizations, and mutual physical closeness expressed through cuddling and molding.

Since at this point of development much of the infant's interactions with the caretakers occurs around feedings, regulation of food intake is closely linked to the infant's affective engagement with the caretaker. Certain feeding disturbances are characteristic of disorders of attachment. Infants with FTT as a consequence of impaired attachment frequently present with a history of vomiting, diarrhea, and poor weight gain. Observations of these mothers and babies during feeding reveal a general lack of pleasure in the interactions. The mothers appear listless, detached, and apathetic. They hold their babies loosely on their laps without much physical intimacy. They rarely initiate verbal or visual contact, and seem unaware of the infant's signals. The infants also appear listless and apathetic. They often actively avoid eye contact with the mother. Some engage in rumination, which appears to be either a means of self-stimulation or of relieving tension.[11] When scanning the environment, some infants seem to be hypervigilant, a process that has been described as radar gaze. When these babies are picked up they are unable to cuddle and mold to the caretaker's body. They usually show some disturbance in body tone, being floppy or rigid. Many are developmentally delayed.

Much has been written about mothers whose infants suffer from the disorders of attachment. They are frequently described as manifesting character pathology and affective illness.[18,41] The mother's poor parenting, social isolation, and economic hardship are also evident. Glaser and coworkers[22] suggest that the highest risk exists when mother's needs take precedence over those of the infant. Fraiberg, Adelson, and Shapiro[19] emphasize that the needs of parents correlate with the "ghosts," the unmet needs, in their own growing years. Drotar, Malone, and Negray[16] state that a traumatic or deprived childhood experience can influence the mother/infant relationship; the manner in which it does so, however, is affected by the current context of family life. Our clinical experiences have alerted us particularly to the mother's feelings of isolation during pregnancy and birth, to current marital distress or unavailability of the father, and to recent death or other loss.

Certain individual infant characteristics can contribute to or exacerbate an attachment disorder. Infants who have problems with homeostasis, who are irritable and difficult to calm, and whose temperamental attributes are confusing or upsetting to the mother pose a threat to the attachment process. Infants with hypersensitivities to touch, sound, light, or change of position are especially vulnerable to an attachment disorder because their avoidance behavior can easily be misinterpreted by the mothers as rejection. Infantile autism provides an extreme example of avoidance behavior in the infant.

DISORDERS OF SEPARATION AND INDIVIDUATION

Between six months and three years of age, the infant enters a new developmental stage that Mahler, Pine, and Bergman[35] describe as separation and individuation. During this stage both motoric and cognitive maturation go forward, enabling the infant to function with ever more emotional independence. As babies begin to crawl away from the mother, they become increasingly aware of their separateness and must confront the developmental issues of autonomy versus dependency. Cognitively the infants have begun to learn means-end differentiation and to understand basic schemes of causality. Part of this learning process involves somatopsychological differentiation (as defined by Greenspan and Lieberman[26])—that is, the infants begin to distinguish among a variety of somatopsychological states, including the differentiation of hunger, from such emotional needs as affection and dependency, or from anger and frustration. As is true during earlier developmental stages, both partners of the dyad contribute to the successful resolution of the developmental task of somatopsychological differentiation: the infant, by clearly signaling his physiological or emotional needs; the caretaker, by reading his signals correctly and responding appropriately to them.

We[12] have observed an eating disorder that usually begins in the second half of the first year of life and attains a peak incidence around nine months of age. It is characterized by food refusal and appears to represent a disturbance in somatopsychological differentiation arising in the course of the infant's struggle for separation and individuation; we have accordingly labeled it a separation disorder.[12,17] It involves certain typical patterns of behavior both in the infants and the mothers. For example, the infants grab for the spoon to participate in the feeding, but mother ignores this signal and insists on feeding the infant herself. She feels more effective if she is getting the food into the infant's mouth. Frustrated in their attempt at self-feeding, the infants then get angry and refuse to open their mouth. This makes mother anxious, and she tries desperately to get the food into the child, only to meet increasing refusal. The battle of the spoons, so well characterized by Levy,[34] becomes a battle of wills.

Other situations may also trigger a battle of wills. Mother may see it as very important for the infant's nutrition that all the food be eaten, but infants might eat very slowly or reject the food because they do not like the taste. In the face of this, mother begins to coax the infant in every way imaginable to get him or her to eat. Soon the babies learn that the less they eat the more attention they can elicit from mother. Their emotional needs come to dictate their eating behavior. As time goes on mother and infant become increasingly involved in these maladaptive interactions around food and many extreme practices begin to emerge. Ultimately there is no normal feeding and the mother alternates between coaxing and forcing her child to eat.

Initially the child may refuse to eat only for the mother; if the condition persists, however, the oppositional food refusal will be generalized to other caretakers. Not infrequently the concern about the child's not eating pervades all aspects of family life.

Unlike the children suffering from an attachment disorder, these children do not usually show delays in cognitive and speech development. However, gross motor development may indeed be impaired, as their food refusal may lead to chronic undernutrition and poor muscle development. The children's serious oppositional behavior frequently involves other areas of their life, such as bedtime, toilet training, or dressing.

Growth Disorders in Older Children

PSYCHOSOCIAL DWARFISM

In 1967 Powell, Brasel, and Blizzard[43] first described a group of children with emotional deprivation and growth retardation simulating idiopathic hypopituitarism. In the same year Silver and Finkelstein[49] reported on deprivation dwarfism. Since then an ever-clearer picture of psychosocial dwarfism has emerged.

It describes children with marked linear growth retardation below the third percentile for age and with significantly delayed bone age who present a variety of abnormal behaviors suggesting emotional disturbance. Careful studies reveal no organic disease to explain their growth disorder. Despite normal availability and adequate caloric intake, bizarre behaviors around food and water are common signs of this disorder. These children are reported to steal food and hoard it, to eat from garbage cans, and to drink stagnant water, dishwater, and water from toilet bowls. They are described as apathetic, irritable, and prone to accidents and self-injury. Many are developmentally delayed with IQs in the borderline or retarded range.[25] Characteristically, once such children are removed from the home environment, growth promptly resumes. No specific medical, hormonal, or psychiatric treatment is required.

Because of the striking improvement in the children's growth and behavior patterns after removal from the home, much attention has been focused on the family environment. The mothers seem to present a variety of psychopathologies, ranging from anxiety and depression to severe personality disorders. The fathers frequently are absent from the home and many are alcoholics.[2,32,39,42]

The exact mechanism of the growth failure remains unclear. The hormones essential for normal growth (pituitary growth hormone, thyroid hormone, insulin, and somatomedin) have been studied in these children but have not yielded any clear-cut results. In 1961 Patton and Gardner[39] suggested that the production and release of pituitary hormones were deterred by emotional stress. In particular, these hormones are known to be influenced by the hypothalamic centers, which are in turn influenced by the limbic cortex. In a review of the literature on psychosocial dwarfism, Green, Campbell, and David[25] noted that growth hormone levels before growth has accelerated and after stimulation (usually with insulin) are low in about one-half of the case reported.[11] With the overlap between normals and psychosocial dwarfs and the fact that growth proceeds in some psychosocial dwarfs while abnormal growth hormones levels remain, one cannot conclude that a specific casual relationship exists between abnormal growth hormone secretion and retardation of growth" (p. 42). While there is a tendency for psychosocial dwarfs to manifest somewhat lower growth hormone levels than do normals, no single value can be considered diagnostic. Indeed, individual patients with psychosocial dwarfism might present with normal growth hormone levels. Thyroid hormone studies have only occasionally yielded subnormal values and are also inconclusive.[33,42]

There is, however, one suggestive exception. Somatomedin is the only hormone that has shown a consistent correlation with a decrease or increase of growth

276

in psychosocial dwarfs.[14,53] Somatomedin is secreted by the liver and is thought to act directly on growing cartilage. Saenger and associates[47] described a child with a low somatomedin level on admission to the hospital. The somatomedin level normalized during the hospitalization when the child was growing and decreased to low normal on his return home, where he grew minimally. After readmission to the hospital when the child showed remarkable catch-up growth, it peaked to high normal.

Saenger and coworkers'[47] case study also illustrates the fact that growth seemed unrelated to caloric intake. The child consumed more calories during periods of slow growth than during periods of catch-up growth. Rate of growth was much more closely related to the absence or presence of the favorite nurse than to caloric intake or hormone levels. Saenger and colleagues.[47] conclude that there is an "as yet unidentified factor affecting growth during emotional stress" (pp. 1–2).

Although the biochemical factor mediating growth in these children has not been identified, there is general agreement that interactions between the child and caretakers seem to produce the crucial psychological factors that influence growth. Some authors point to the deprivation and the lack of an affectional bond between mother and child.[39,49] Others have described the traumatic, negative influences of the environment and the association of deprivation and growth failure with child abuse.[6,42,43] Green, Campbell, and David[25] suggest that psychosocial dwarfism is the result of both the omission of a necessary good relationship plus the presence of a bad one—that is, "(1) the lack of a satisfactory positive mother-child relationship and superimposed upon this, (2) a highly stressful negative relationship with the mother" (p. 43). They conclude that the combination of these two factors would explain the variations in the endocrine status of the cases reported in the literature and the presence of growth lines[29] in the majority of psychosocial dwarfs as evidence of intermittent growth arrest. Their "two-factor" hypothesis explains the growth that occurs when these children enter the hospital and are thus removed from the stressful home environment and also the observation that their growth subsequently accelerates to catch-up rates of two to three times normal as a consequence of their developing a mutual, fulfilling relationship with a nurse.

DWARFISM SECONDARY TO FOOD REFUSAL

We reported dwarfism secondary to food refusal.[12] We hypothesize that the dwarfism is secondary to a disorder of separation and individuation and distinguish this variety of dwarfism from that due to a disorder of attachment, as in "psychosocial dwarfism." These food-refusal children present with the same physical parameters of lack of weight gain, retarded linear growth, and immature bone age, but they show different behavioral characteristics and have none of the developmental delays observed in psychosocial dwarfs.

These children refuse to eat as part of their oppositional struggle for autonomy. They have little or no awareness of their physiological hunger feelings. Their eating, or refusal to eat, is dictated primarily by their emotional feeling states. They suffer from a severe disturbance in somatopsychological differentiation. These children refuse to eat in order to show their parents that they are autonomous; at the same time, they manage to have their dependency needs met through the increased parental involvement around their meals. These dwarfs usually come from intact middle-class families. The parents are frequently overanxious about the nutritional status of their children and unable to set limits to their tyrannical behavior around food. Some of these children are involved in a struggle for autonomy in other areas of their lives as well and may show similar oppositional behaviors around going to bed at night, toilet training, dressing, or other areas of self-care.

Once the parents change their interactions with their children around food, the children begin to eat more, gain weight, and grow taller. We have not been able to study the endocrine status of these children, but clinical experience suggests that the children's growth or lack of growth is related to caloric intake. It needs to be determined if the conflicting endocrine picture in regard to dwarfism could be explained in whole or in part by a heterogenous mixture of the attachment and separation disorder factors.

SHORT STATURE AND DELAYED PUBERTY DUE TO FEAR OF OBESITY

Delayed growth and short stature as a consequence of caloric undernutrition are not restricted to infants and young children. Pugliese and associates[45] have reported on a group of "fourteen patients with a common pattern of delayed growth and sexual development due to a fear of obesity and its alleged consequences—decreased physical attractiveness, poor health and shortened life span. Because of their fear of obesity, these patients reduced their caloric intake and did not gain weight or grow normally" (p. 514). In contrast to patients with anorexia nervosa, these youngsters showed no disturbance in body image. They did not diet to lose weight but did not allow themselves to gain weight. In this particular sample, all fourteen patients were below the fifth percentile for weight, and eleven were below the fifth percentile for height, with a deficit of weight for height of 5 to 23 percent. Puberty was delayed in seven patients, and the bone age was delayed one-half to five and one-half years. The sample included nine boys and five girls, ages nine years four

SECTION IV / Deviations of Development

months to seventeen years eleven months. Thorough evaluation disclosed no evidence of endocrine or other organic causes for their disorders. A common feature in these families was that they were middle to upper class. Twelve of the fourteen families were intact.

Summary

Serious growth failure in infants and toddlers is usually referred to as failure to thrive. In older children, lack of weight gain is frequently accompanied by retardation of linear growth and is referred to as dwarfism. Multiple organic and nonorganic factors can result in growth failure and frequently combine to bring about feeding disturbances leading to a growth disorder.

This chapter presented a developmental classification for growth disorders in infants and children to provide a diagnostic framework within which to differentiate and better understand the various types of growth disturbances. Disorders of homeostasis, attachment, and separation lead to distinct disturbances of eating behavior and growth, and require different treatment interventions, which are discussed in chapter 45 of this volume.

REFERENCES

1. ACCARDO, P. "Growth and Development: Interactional Context," in P. Accardo, ed., *Failure to Thrive in Infancy and Childhood.* Baltimore: University Park Press, 1982, p. 817.
2. APLEY, J., et al. "Dwarfism Without Apparent Physical Cause," *Proceedings of the Royal Society of Medicine,* 64 (1971): 135–138.
3. BERNBAUM, J., et al. "Nonnutritive Sucking, During Gavage Feeding Enhances Growth and Maturation in Premature Infants," *Pediatrics,* 71 (1983): 41–45.
4. BOWLBY, J. *Attachment.* New York: Basic Books, 1969.
5. ———. *Separation and Loss: Anxiety and Anger.* New York: Basic Books, 1973.
6. BULLARD, D. M., GLASER, H. M., and HEAGERTY, M. D. "Failure to Thrive in the Neglected Child," *American Journal of Orthopsychiatry,* 37 (1967): 680–690.
7. CALDWELL, B. M. "The Effects of Psychosocial Deprivation on Human Development in Infancy," *Annual Progress in Child Development.* New York: Brunner/Mazel, 1971, pp. 3–22.
8. CASEY, P. H., BRADLEY, R. and WORTHAM, B. "Social and Nonsocial Home Environments and Infants with Nonorganic Failure to Thrive," *Pediatrics,* 73 (1984): 348–353.
9. CASLER, L. "Maternal Deprivation: A Critical Review of the Literature," *Monographs of the Society for Research in Child Development,* 26 (1961): 2.
10. CHAPIN, H. D. "A Plan of Dealing with Atropic Infants and Children," *Archives of Pediatrics,* 25 (1908): 491–496.
11. CHATOOR, I., and DICKSON, L. "Rumination: A Maladaptive Attempt at Self-Regulation in Infants and Children," *Clinical Proceedings,* 40 (1984): 106–116.
12. CHATOOR, I., and EGAN, J. "Nonorganic Failure to Thrive and Dwarfism Due to Food Refusal: A Separation Disorder," *Journal of the American Academy of Child Psychiatry,* 22 (1983): 294–301.
13. CHATOOR, I., et al. "Non-organic Failure to Thrive. A Developmental Perspective," *Pediatric Annals,* 13 (1984): 829–843.
14. D'ERCOLE, A. J., UNDERWOOD, L. E., and VAN WYK, J. J. "Serum Somatomedin-C in Hypopituitarism and in Other Disorders of Growth," *Journal of Pediatrics,* 90 (1977): 375–381.
15. DOWLING, S. "Seven Infants with Esophageal Atresia: A Developmental Study," *Psychoanalytic Study of the Child,* 32 (1977): 215–256.
16. DROTAR, D., MALONE, C., and NEGRAY, J. "Psychosocial Intervention with Families of Children Who Fail to Thrive," *Child Abuse and Neglect,* 3 (1979): 927–935.
17. EGAN, J., CHATOOR, I., and ROSEN, G. "Non-organic Failure to Thrive: Pathogenesis and Classification," *Clinical Proceedings,* Children's Hospital National Medical Center, 36 (1980): 173–182.
18. FISCHOFF, J., WHITTEN, C. F., and PETTIT, M. G. "A Psychiatric Study of Mothers of Infants with Growth Failure Secondary to Maternal Deprivation," *Journal of Pediatrics,* 79 (1971): 209–215.
19. FRAIBERG, S., ADELSON, E., and SHAPIRO, V. "Ghosts in the Nursery," *Journal of the American Academy of Psychiatry,* 14 (1975): 387–421.
20. FREUD, A. "The Psychoanalytic Study of Infantile Feeding Disturbances," *Psychoanalytic Study of the Child,* 2 (1946): 119–132.
21. GARDNER, L. I. "Physiopathology of the Human Growth Hormone with Special Reference to Deprivation Dwarfism," in C. LaCauza and A. W. Root, eds., *Problems in Pediatric Endocrinology.* London: Academic Press, 1980, pp. 73–81.
22. GLASER, H. H., et al. "Physical and Psychological Development of Children with Early Failure to Thrive," *Journal of Pediatrics,* 73 (1968): 690–698.
23. GOLDBLOOM, R. B. "Failure to Thrive," *Pediatric Clinics of North America,* 29 (1982): 151–166.
24. GOLDFARB, W. "Psychological Privation in Infancy and Subsequent Adjustment," *American Journal of Orthopsychiatry,* 15 (1945): 247–255.
25. GREEN, W. H., CAMPBELL, M., and DAVID, R. "Psychosocial Dwarfism: A Critical Review of the Evidence," *Journal of the American Academy of Child Psychiatry,* 23 (1984): 39–48.
26. GREENSPAN, S. I., and LIEBERMAN, A. F. "Infants, Mothers, and Their Interaction: A Quantitative Clinical Approach to Developmental Assessment," in S. T. Greenspan and G. H. Pollock, eds., *The Course of Life,* vol. 1; *Infancy*

and *Early Childhood.* Bethesda, Md.: National Institute of Mental Health, 1980, pp. 271–312.

27. GREENSPAN, S., and LOURIE, R. S. "Developmental Structuralist Approach to Classification of Adaptive and Pathologic Personality Organizations: Infancy and Early Childhood," *American Journal of Psychiatry,* 138 (1981): 725–735.

28. HARLOW, H., and ZIMMERMAN, R. R. "The Development of Affectional Responses in Infant Monkeys," *Proceedings of the American Philosophical Society,* 102 (1958): 501–509.

29. HERNANDEZ, R. J., et al. "Incidence of Growth Lines in Psychosocial Dwarfs and Idiopathic Hypopituitarism," *American Journal of Roentgenology,* 131 (1978): 477–479.

30. HOMER, C., and LUDWIG, S. "Categorization of Etiology of Failure to Thrive," *American Journal of Diseases of Children,* 135 (1981): 848–851.

31. HOPWOOD, N. J., and BECKER, D. J. "Psychosocial Dwarfism: Detection, Evaluation and Management," in A. W. Franklin, ed., *Child Abuse and Neglect,* vol. 3, London: Pergamon Press, 1979, pp. 439–447.

32. KRIEGER, I. "Maternal and Psychosocial Deprivation," in J. G. Howells, ed., *Modern Perspectives in the Psychiatry of Infancy.* New York: Brunner/Mazel, 1979, pp. 152–162.

33. KRIEGER, I., and MELLINGER, R. C. "Pituitary Function in the Deprivation Syndrome," *Journal of Pediatrics,* 79 (1971): 216–225.

34. LEVY, D. "Oppositional Syndrome and Oppositional Behavior," in R. H. Hoch and J. Zubin, eds., *Psychopathology of Childhood.* New York: Grune & Stratten, 1955, pp. 204–226.

35. MAHLER, M. S., PINE, F. and BERMAN, A. *The Psychological Birth of the Human Infant.* New York: Basic Books, 1975.

36. NELSON, W. E., VAUGHAN, V. C., and McKAY, R. J., eds., *Textbook of Pediatrics,* 9th ed. Philadelphia: W. B. Saunders, 1969.

37. ORLANSKY, H. "Infant Care and Personality," *Psychological Bulletin,* 46 (1949): 1–49.

38. PATTON, R. G., and GARDNER, L. "Influence of Family Environment on Growth: The Syndrome of 'Maternal Deprivation,'" *Pediatrics,* 30 (1962): 957–962.

39. ———. "Deprivation Dwarfism (Psychosocial Deprivation): Disordered Family Environment as Cause of So-called Idiopathic Hypopituitarism," in L. I. Gardner, ed., *Endocrine and Genetic Diseases of Childhood and Adolescence,* 2nd ed. Philadelphia: W. B. Saunders, 1975, pp. 85–98.

40. PINNEAU, S. R. "A Critique on the Article by Margaret Ribble," *Child Development,* 21 (1950): 203–228.

41. POLLIT, E., WEISEL, E. A., and CHAN, C. K. "Psychosocial Development and Behavior of Mothers of Failure to Thrive Children," *American Journal of Orthopsychiatry,* 45 (1975): 525–537.

42. POWELL, G. F., BRASEL, J. A., and BLIZZARD, R. M. "Emotional Deprivation and Growth Retardation Simulating Idiopathic Hypopituitarism: I. Clinical Evaluation of the Syndrome," *New England Journal of Medicine,* 276 (1967): 1271–1278.

43. POWELL, G. F., RAITI, S., and BLIZZARD, R. M. "Emotional Deprivation and Growth Retardation Simulating Idiopathic Hypopituitarism: II. Endocrinologic Evaluation of the Syndrome," *New England Journal of Medicine,* 276 (1967): 1279–1283.

44. PROVENCE, S., and LIPTON, R. C. *Infants in Institutions.* New York: International Universities Press, 1962.

45. PUGLIESE, M. T., et al. "Fear of Obesity: A Cause of Short Stature and Delayed Puberty," *New England Journal of Medicine,* 309 (1983): 513–518.

46. ROSENN, D., STEIN, L., and BATES, M. "The Differentiation of Organic from Environmental Failure to Thrive," Paper presented at American Pediatric Society Meetings, Denver, Colorado, 19 April 1975.

47. SAENGER, P., et al. "Somatomedin and Growth Hormone in Psychosocial Dwarfism," *Pädiatrische Pädologische Supplement,* 5 (1977): 1–12.

48. SILLS, R. H. "Failure to Thrive: The Role of Clinical and Laboratory Evaluation," *American Journal of Diseases of Children,* 132 (1978): 967–969.

49. SILVER, H., and FINKELSTEIN. M. "Deprivation Dwarfism," *Journal of Pediatrics,* 70 (1967): 317–324, 1967.

50. SPITZ, R., "Hospitalism, An Inquiry into the Psychiatric Conditions of Early Childhood," *Psychoanalytic Study of the Child,* 1 (1945): 53–74.

51. ———. "Anaclitic Depression, An Inquiry into the Psychiatric Conditions of Early Childhood," *Psychoanalytic Study of the Child,* 2 (1946): 313–342.

52. STONE, L. G., SMITH, H. T., and MURPHY, L. B., eds., *The Competent Infant.* New York: Basic Books, 1973.

53. TANNER, J. H. "Charts for the Diagnosis of Short Stature and Low Growth Velocity, Allowance for Height of Parents and Prediction of Adult Height," in D. Bergsma and R. N. Schimke, eds., *Growth Problems and Clinical Advances.* (Birth Defects: Original Articles Series, vol. 12, no. 6.). New York: Alan R. Liss, 1976, pp. 1–13.

54. WOOLSTON, J. L. "Eating Disorders in Infancy and Early Childhood," *Journal of the American Academy of Child Psychiatry,* 22 (1983): 114–21.

30 / Child Sexual Abuse

Ira S. Lourie and Linda Canfield Blick

Overview

Child sexual victimization is a broadly defined phenomenon that may be manifest in different forms. Some are impersonal, such as obscene phone calls, exposure, and voyeurism. Others require dynamic interaction between individuals, including fondling of a child and rape at the hands of strangers, friends of the family, or relatives. Incest involves similar behavior with the interaction being confined to members of the family. Finally, there is the exploitative form of victimization, encompassing child pornography and child prostitution. Victimization may occur as a single incident or continue for years. A child is often "engaged" through coercion, deception, intimidation, or seduction, and may or may not be physically harmed. Some children are psychologically and physically maimed, or even murdered, by sadistic sexual acts. Sexual victimization is traumatic for every involved child, and many of the victims carry deep emotional scars.

While the psychological trauma experienced by child victims may be minimal, as a rule it is not. A variety of emotional symptoms tend to accompany sexual victimization. Nightmares, decreased school performance, poor self-esteem, damaged body image, and withdrawal from peers are a few of the common manifestations. Some presenting problems that often mask the trauma of sexual abuse are depression, suicidal ideation, problems with intimacy, psychosis, and the development of multiple personalities.[15]

Recent research has revealed startling facts about child sexual victimization. Studies have suggested that by the age of eighteen, one of every three girls[14] and one of every eleven boys[4] have been sexually victimized. In a study of prostitutes by Cahill,[2] 75 percent were found to have been sexually victimized as children. Another study of prostitutes[1] reports similar histories of sexual victimization although with a much lower incidence. In another study, 81 percent of the sexual abusers of children were found to have been victimized during their own childhood.* Like physical

*A. N. Groth, personal communication, 1985.

child abuse, sexual child abuse has been found to be an intergenerational problem.

Previously the literature on child victimization contained only scattered uncoordinated reports; only very recently has the phenomenon become the focus of extensive study. It was not until 1968 that Vincent De Francis, Director of the Children's Division of the American Humane Association, published his landmark study, *Protecting the Child Victim of Sex Crimes Committed by Adults.*[3] And only in 1971 did Henry Giarretto, in San Jose, California, begin the country's first comprehensive treatment program for both victims and offenders of incest.

Situational and Etiological Factors

While there is a tendency to view the many different forms of child sexual abuse in aggregate, each case is the result of a unique mixture of etiological factors that require an equally unique intervention strategy. (See chapter 47 for a discussion of intervention.) One set of these factors defines an incident of child sexual abuse as lying somewhere on a continuum between abuse at the hands of a stranger and abuse that takes place in the home.

STRANGER ABUSE VERSUS INCEST

The continuum between stranger abuse and incest describes the relationship between the child and the abuser. The child's reaction to sexual abuse is directly related to this context. When children are abused by a stranger, the situation is usually extremely frightening. The children are caught off guard and find themselves in a helpless position, without hope of support. Even though the event may have involved some flirtatious behavior or poor judgment (going off with a stranger), the guilt these children experience tends to be less than that experienced when similar events occur in familial settings or with acquaintances. When victimized by a

stranger, children usually have not done anything out of the ordinary, and their guilt is more generically related to the fact that something sexual has happened. In addition, it may be provoked because they were touched in a confusing, arousing, and/or frightening way that they did not like or, at any rate, know is wrong.

However, when sexual abuse takes place with a person known to children, several other issues come into play. While children are still in a helpless position, the fact that the abuser is a trusted adult helps make the situation less frightening, albeit more confusing, than it is with a stranger. The children are thrust into a situation that feels wrong and unpleasant; no one is there to help the youngsters out of it. The fear of what is being done to the children is partially mitigated by the closeness of the relationship to the abuser. In those cases of incest where the abuse takes place in the context of a caring familial relationship, the trauma of that abuse can be decreased by the positive interpersonal aspects of the relationship. Nonetheless, *the children still feel betrayed.* Someone upon whom the children have relied and in whom was placed a basic sense of trust has taken advantage of this dependency and trust in a destructive way. In addition, victims of incest and acquaintance abuse feel a sense of having participated in a guilt-ridden act.

On the continuum between stranger abuse and incest lie all degrees of closeness. Acquaintances, distant relatives, uncles and aunts, close neighbors, baby-sitters, clergy, school personnel, and athletic coaches all have a special relationship with children and may become abusers. Yet along with parents and complete strangers, each holds a unique place on the continuum. The nature of the relationship is more accurately described by two sets of interactive factors: interpersonal factors and sexual victimization factors.

INTERPERSONAL AND SEXUAL VICTIMIZATION FACTORS

Two sets of factors are involved in the etiology of child sexual abuse and describe that abuse in terms of the dynamic interaction between the abuser and the victim. One of these is the factor set of sexual victimization, in which infantile sexual and aggressive needs of the abuser directly lead to an act against a child. These factors are very similar to those described in adult rape situations.[7] The second set are the interpersonal factors in which the interaction between family members is conducive to the development of incest. These are much like those factors that have been described as leading to physical child abuse.[11]

Cases in which the child is unknown to the abuser are almost exclusively associated with sexual victimization factors. In contrast to this, interpersonal factors

are more prevalent when incest takes place within a caring relationship. All cases will involve some mixture of victimization and interpersonal factors. Stranger abuse is more likely to be dominated by rape factors and incest by interpersonal factors. Certainly, even in a short time, a stranger and a child can form a relationship that will add some degree of interpersonal force to a purely stranger situation. By the same token, abuse by a parent always includes some measure of sexual victimization of the child.

Interpersonal Factors. Interpersonal factors are found to the greatest degree in cases of incest. Incest is symptomatic of disturbances in both individual and family dynamics occurring simultaneously within the context of a family environment. Since every member of the family has a role within the complex pattern of dynamic family interaction, the interpersonal factors found in incest might also be called "family" factors. One of the more common ways in which this is expressed is in cases where parents bring forward unresolved issues around sexual abuse that occurred during their own childhoods and play out these sequences within their families. Other manifestations of family dynamics leading to sexual abuse are not as directly connected.

The theory of incest based on interpersonal factors is similar, if not identical, to the tripartite theory of physical child abuse described by Kempe and Helfer.[10] In this theory, three forces come together to create the atmosphere in which child abuse can take place; they are an abusive parent, a special or unassertive child, and a trigger situation. In incest, the sexual behavior takes place within the familiar context of a family interaction in which each person has a role. These roles have both normal and abnormal aspects and are acted out in a setting where the family is trying to cope with chronic or acute stress. For the most part, the incest is the result of a complex family situation in which a father demonstrates pathological behavior.* While most obvious in incest, these same factors occur to one degree or another in most cases of child sexual abuse.

Like other sexually abusing adults, incestuous fathers demonstrate an immaturity that impairs their ability to delay gratification and tolerate frustration. They tend to be dependent individuals. Their marked dependency is a reflection of a childlike quality characteristic of their interpersonal relationships. They all too easily interchange roles with other family members so that the personal boundaries between them become confused. Both in and out of the family, this creates an atmosphere in which the abuser can project his needs onto others; in this way he perceives his own need for closeness as the child's need. The abuser becomes con-

*Some "fixated offenders" plan and premeditate sexual abuse before they marry and in fact marry a single parent or plan adoption for the purpose of gaining access to children.

fused and his psychologically immature needs for closeness become fused with his biologically mature sexual drives. As a result, a harmless need for closeness changes into a pernicious, harmful sexual act.

In cases of father-daughter incest, the mother's role is often a passive one. There is no way to generalize as to the specific character of this role; it is different in each case. For some, the passivity is incidental and unavoidable. For example, the mother might be ill and have to be away from home for long periods of time, or she must work a shift that takes her out of the home when the children are not in school. In other cases, the passivity is the result of the mother emotionally absenting herself from the family. This in turn drives the child to the father in order to obtain emotional gratification and, occasionally, in cases of stranger and acquaintance abuse, to an individual who is unknown to the child yet who still offers comfort. Some mothers have been told about the abuse by the victim or may have witnessed it; nonetheless, they still choose to ignore or refuse to believe the disclosures of sexual abuse in the family. Others even go so far as to encourage or participate in the abuse.

Children's role in sexual abuse is more easily understood; they participate because they feel they have no choice. Several factors bring them to this conclusion. Many children are seduced into participation by dint of parents offering them (1) bribes of love or goods, (2) improper information about the appropriateness of the behavior, or (3) the chance of doing something good for the parent. Other children are coerced; they are confronted with threats of physical harm, loss of love, or abandonment. Still others are compelled to participate through direct force. They become fearful as to the possible outcomes of disclosure either for themselves or for their family, and are rendered helpless to effect a proper resolution to the problem by both their age and lack of understanding.

Aspects of the child's developmental needs can also facilitate "participation" in child sexual abuse. Dependency is a major reality of childhood. Even when children reach adolescence, they are still emotionally dependent on their parents in many critical ways. In the service of having one's dependency needs met, many compromises are made; one of these may take the form of participation in incest or other forms of sexual abuse. In particular, when mothers are passive and unresponsive, the children have few or none of their dependency needs met in that relationship. Both consciously and unconsciously they are then forced to turn to an incestuous father or to some other "nurturing" figure, often compromising themselves as a trade-off for care and closeness.

Closely related to the developmental aspects of dependency are trust and security. Young children (and

even adolescents) often become engaged in incest and other forms of sexual abuse because they implicitly trust their parents and other adults: "If Daddy wants me to do it, it must be all right." Even when children begin to question the propriety of what is happening (because they are instructed not to tell, they learn that it is wrong, or they begin to develop confused feelings), they find it difficult to give up on this trust. One of the protective mechanisms of development is idealization of the parent. In order to maintain the ideal in the face of obvious parental wrongdoing, children will accept the parental behavior and subsequently turn against themselves. Additionally, children in our society are poorly prepared to judge the appropriateness of adult sexual behavior; they receive little, if any, education about their right to the privacy of their bodies or their right to refuse almost any request made by an adult, especially if that adult is a parent or trusted friend of the family. When they finally do grasp what has happened to them, the anger at being betrayed is monumental. The parental ideal is shattered and the child responds with rage. Along with trust, the sense of security is also related to dependency. Family integrity is a major component of any child's feeling of emotional well-being. Participation in incest is often both a conscious and an unconscious maneuver for ensuring the stability of the family. It is difficult to refuse participation in incest if it means the child has to give up dependency, trust, or security.

From the earliest moments of life, children require closeness in order to feel secure, to make developmental progress, and to grow in their ability to relate to others. Included in this closeness are touching, holding, caressing, and kissing; later, these become the usual signs of love, and children learn to equate them with caring and security. Incestuous behavior often starts as this kind of hugging and caressing, which is perceived by both the parent and child as normal, pleasurable, and welcome. (Where this kind of experience is not available within the family, the child will often look for it outside.) Only when the behavior becomes overtly sexualized does the child realize how the quality of the behavior has changed. However, by that time it is often too late, as the young child begins to equate the new sexualized touches and feelings with the comfort and caring that are needed and desired, but which now have a new and confusing quality. Through the normal forces of the oedipal drama, young girls learn to flirt, to try to please, and to use their developing sexuality in order to solidify their relationship with their fathers and other male role models. In a family where the real adult participant has unresolved oedipal tensions, this process becomes problematic. In such a context, an incestuous father, to meet his own needs, will misinterpret childhood sexuality and perceive it as

a seductive adult invitation. When a father misunderstands in this way, or is in any case unable to deal with these normal sexual developmental issues, he may then act on his own incestuous drives. The same normal behaviors in young girls can also be misinterpreted by strangers as sexual come-ons, and thus lead to abuse.

Sexual Victimization Factors. The second set of etiological factors are the sexual victimization or "rape" factors. Sexual victimization is defined here as a situation in which one person (usually a male) forces another person (usually a female) into a sexual encounter. (While most reports of sexual abuse involve male offenders, the prevalence of female abusers is felt to be much higher than reported. One of the authors [LB] has observed a high incidence of male perpetrators who, in their own childhood, were abused by females.) This presumes unwillingness on the part of the person who becomes the victim of an act perpetrated by another. The perpetrator's prime gratification is an enhanced feeling of self as a result of aggression and conquest played out sexually.[7] When interpersonal factors predominate, there is a measure of concern for the child (even though her needs are often misinterpreted and distorted). In contrast, however, with sexual victimization there is little or no concern with the needs or well-being of the victim, who is viewed as an object. Sexual victimization factors are directly associated with the intimidation and violence that so frequently occur in the course of child sexual abuse. These are primary components; in stranger abuse they are also present in varying degrees in incest. This kind of victimization arouses feelings of helplessness and fear in the victim and is indicative of greater dysfunction in the perpetrator.

The concept of sexual victimization presupposes the presence of an individual who perpetrates an act on another individual. In cases of child sexual abuse, these perpetrators are usually referred to as "child sex offenders." Groth has delineated three types of offenders by differentiating and categorizing the continuum of victimization factors: the child rapist,[7] the regressed offender, and the fixated offender.[8]

The *child rapist* generally uses force in trying to achieve his goal of sexual penetration. He views the child as an object of contempt. The combination of force, feelings of contempt, and lack of affectional or emotional feelings leaves the child devastated. It is likely that this type of offender will physically injure the child. This type of offender is prone to make one-time attacks on multiple victims, rather than seeking to develop an ongoing emotional/sexual relationship with a given child (as the regressed and fixated offenders do).

The *regressed offender* is usually married and actively involved in adult sexual relationships within the

marriage or through extramarital affairs. The onset of the sexually abusive behavior occurs in adulthood and is caused by some life stress that serves as a triggering event. It is estimated that 90 percent of offenders in this category are incestuous. Marital discord is always present in these families and is often accompanied by severe personal stress. This offender is most often an adult male who victimizes his own child, who is usually female. The regressed offender's behavior typically begins in a spontaneous, perhaps in an inadvertent way: "I was rubbing my daughter's back and then realized I had moved my hand to her front—I was scared." It then changes into a premeditated act: "When nothing happened and I realized I wasn't going to get into trouble, I began planning how to be alone with her." The regressed offender is seeking love and acceptance; he rationalizes this behavior as his way "of showing her that I loved her." Such an individual views himself as an adult but fantasizes the child as also being adult. This viewpoint extends to nonsexual areas as well, and can include offender-victim discussions of the offender's marital relationship, financial problems, or stress of being a parent.

The third category is the *fixated offender,* who presents a most pervasive problem. This individual is usually *not* married and usually *not* involved in any adult sexual relationships. The onset of his pedophilia begins in his teen years and becomes a compulsive, repetitive, premeditated behavior pattern continuing throughout adulthood. Such offenders view children as the main "target" for their sexual gratification. Eighty-one percent of offenders in this category were themselves sexually victimized as children.* Their psychosexual development appears to have been arrested at the point of onset of their own victimization. These offenders are most often male, and most frequently prey on male children. Emotionally, such offenders view themselves as a child and regard the child as a peer. They target victims of the same age that they were when their sexuality was fixated. As is true for regressed offenders, they also believe that they are offering love. Neglected children with an emotionally or physically absent parent are at high risk of being engaged by these fixated offenders.

Neither the regressed nor the fixated group perceive their behavior as exploitative. They "lovingly" describe their feelings of emotional intimacy and closeness with the children as if the youngsters were consenting partners. When coercion is used in a "gentle" context, the victims often become confused between "emotional love" and "physical love," and are unable to distinguish the exploitative aspects of this "loving" relationship. Although these children seem to gain

---

*A. N. Groth, personal communication, 1985.

some healthy emotional strengths from the more appropriate nurturing aspects of the relationship, their inability to separate the exploitative from the appropriate behavior often interferes with their ability to choose mutually satisfying friends or partners throughout the rest of their lives.

The most disturbed group are those fixated and regressed offenders who use violence to engage the child, in a way that is similar to that of the child rapist. Their family life is dysfunctional; usually it is characterized by hostility and ineffectual and destructive family relationships. Such offenders do not provide any nurturance for the child and are totally self-serving in the abusive relationship. Their major goal appears to be the attainment of power and control. In such cases the victims readily express their anger over the persistent, negative, abusive relationship and clearly identify the exploitative aspects. This type of offender tends to be involved in incestuous abuse where the child often appears to have weak ego strengths reflecting the lack of nurturance received from the abuser, the ineffectiveness of the nonoffending parent, and the disorganization of the entire family. Since so few family strengths are available to assist the child with the rehabilitative process, the prognosis is guarded.

In summary, the sexually abusive acts against children are extremely variable in their nature. The etiological underpinnings are complex and are similarly diverse. Children's reactions to having been abused are, in turn, nonspecific and fail to define a discrete syndrome. The symptoms often related to sexual abuse reflect an individual child's reaction to a stressor based on the child's developmental history and family supports. These symptoms are discussed in chapter 47.

Additional Concerns

Several family and individual characteristics that, although they do not describe a discrete syndrome, are often associated with child sexual abuse are discussed in the following text.

"Secret-keeping" is a common theme running through all child sexual abuse cases, whether overt or covert. Sometimes the secret-keeping is achieved at the behest of the offender; for example: "This is our little secret, so don't tell Mommy or she'll make me go away and I can't be your Daddy any more." Some offenders offer children rewards for not telling, such as money or material items. Others misrepresent moral standards by saying "This is sex education," or "All dads and daughters do this." The younger the child, the easier it is to gain his or her cooperation in the secret-keeping.

An identified game that "is just ours" (father and daughter) is sufficient to lure the young child into a secret abusive situation. In addition, because of their feelings of guilt and confusion, children may not tell about the acts that they have experienced. Lack of discussion of the sexual issues by other family members enhances the quality of secrecy and denies the child permission to talk about the abuse.

Some offenders are less adept at getting children to keep secrets through kindness and coercion and must rely on threats of violence. It has been alleged that animals have been mutilated or murdered in front of children, who were told if they did not cooperate the same would happen to them or to their families. Beatings and other sadistic acts of violence are sometimes used to intimidate the children into maintaining the secret.[6,16]

Secret-keeping causes two serious problems. It creates an imbalance of family structure by setting up alliances between the secret holders,[9] and it isolates the child from the resources that could offer physical and emotional protection. It forces the child to live a lie. When forced by coercion or threats to keep the incest secret, children will often develop a façade in order to cope with the many lies they must tell. Many adults who were molested as children have subsequently described the cheerful façade they always kept in place in an effort to counteract their negative self-depreciating feelings. Eventually it inhibited them from becoming assertive, to the extent that it became impossible for them to express dissatisfaction with any situation. Additionally, it blocked their ability to achieve close loving relationships because they could not disclose a recurrent, critical, abusive, and psychologically meaningful event that was occurring in their lives. They remember that as preteens and early adolescents they often felt out of place within their peer group: "How could I talk to other girls about kissing boyfriends for the first time when I'd been having sex with my dad for seven years?"

The offender and victim collude with one another to protect other family members from their dreadful secret. Unfortunately, this withdrawal also distances the victim from other possible sources of nurturance. This collusion also includes the nonoffending parent in the family. Of 178 cases in Montgomery County, Maryland, studied by one of the authors (LB), prior to disclosure to authorities, 25 percent of the nonoffending parents had already been told about the abuse by the victim. This parent often confronted the offender, who either denied what he had done or admitted it, promising never to do it again. Not realizing how difficult it is to control abusive behavior, the nonoffending spouse would accept this promise of restraint. Inevitably, when the abuse did recur, the victims felt the nonoffending parent could not or would not protect them. The *entire* family then often colluded to protect itself from "outsiders." This secrecy strongly impairs trust, healthy communication, and the expression of normal emotional responses; ultimately it alienates the child and family from the development of healthy relationships, both within the family and outside of it. In essence, it locks the child within a psychological prison.

Gelinas[5] describes a *traumatic neurosis* related to child sexual abuse. The first stage of this process is built around the need for the victim to repress the incestuous incidents they find abhorrent and unacceptable. At the very least, there appears to be a tendency to repress the emotions attendant on the sexual acts. The second stage of this process comes when the abuse is disclosed. At this point, the repressed issues and emotions are no longer contained, and the victim is forced to relive and reexperience these events. The ensuing emotional reaction is very much like a typical stress neurosis and needs to be taken into consideration at the time of the assessment.

In his studies of the relationship between incest and multiple personality, Putnam[13] describes the use of dissociative defense mechanisms by victims of sexual abuse. Similar to Gelinas's work, this theory is based on the emotional unacceptability of incest to the victim and the resulting strong need to blot the events and feelings out of consciousness. The assessment of abuse must take these dissociative tendencies into consideration, both in terms of understanding the victim's reaction and in terms of recognizing abuse when the victim either denies it or is inconsistent in reporting it.

Prior to the onset of the sexual relationship, the children's world is often relatively simple and carefree. When the abuse begins, children become confused by the sexual behavior directed toward them and requested of them by the adult. The strategies used to engage children in the abusive behavior communicate a quality of exclusivity to the relationship. As a result, not only does the adult (parental incest) behavior frighten the children, but, because of the special solicitude of the adult, it engenders a state of confusion as well. Children become conflicted between wanting the abusive parent's sole attention and not wanting the heavy burden of a powerful secret relationship that distances them from their nonoffending parent and siblings.

Initially children may experience guilt over the special attention they are receiving from the offender while such attention is withdrawn from or reduced to the siblings and the nonoffending parent. Additional guilt may also develop around the sexual arousal and physical pleasure that may be experienced as the result of the sexual contacts. This guilt is later augmented by an additional increment of self-blame for "participating in the abuse." The offender may further exploit children's egocentrism by implying that the child is to blame for starting the abuse. This is further complicated by the victim's preexisting oedipal feelings; the child has now become a realistic and apparently victorious rival of the nonoffending parent's position in the family. This guilt and fear of the newly attained power are made more disturbing by the child's inability to cope with the offender's ever-increasing emotional and sexual demands.

The secrecy pact thus causes a state of emotional isolation that worsens as the abuse continues; this, in turn, necessitates the development of a "public" façade with family, friends, school, and elsewhere in the community. The façade serves to divert attention away from the child; it is a survival technique selected unconsciously from the child's limited psychological options and controlled by the youngster's position of dependency. Although initially effective, the repression of negative feelings becomes internalized; these emotions are then experienced by the child as poor self-esteem, alienation, poor body image, and a variety of behavioral symptoms. Initially, these symptoms are often the only identifying clues that direct outsiders' attention to the child.

Long-term Sequelae

The sequelae of sexual abuse during childhood are as variable as the syndrome. Freud's description of the etiology of neurosis was linked in part to the repression of incestuous fantasies. While many workers in the field of child sexual abuse feel that the fantasies reported by Freud may well have been in actuality child sexual abuse experiences, the need to repress the reality or fantasy of incest is a major theme in the psychodynamic response to such incidents. This need uses a great deal of psychological energy and may well compromise the child's psychological development.

Lourie[12] has reported that the locus of emotional harm in incest is related to the positive and negative relationships within the family context in which the abuse takes place. He hypothesized that the greatest harm comes when a disturbed family, through specific dynamics, allows the incest to occur. The sexual nature of the abuse takes its toll with the appearance of secondary symptoms of a sexual nature. In nonincestuous child sexual abuse there have been no similar attempts to describe the parameters of harm. In addition, the feeling of betrayal, discussed earlier, disturbs the development of interpersonal relationships. When the most secure dependency relationships are disturbed, the child learns not to trust. Depression and borderline personality are diagnoses that often follow from such familial disturbances.

The sexual nature of the problem may lead to embarrassment and guilt, which in turn lead to self-denigra-tion. This is true even when the abuse is at the hands of a stranger and the child has played a purely victim role. Child victims may experience sexual dysfunction as adults, because they see these earliest sexual experiences as so unpleasant and destructive.

REFERENCES

1. BAIZERMAN, M., and THOMPSON, J., "Adolescent Female Prostitution Has Very Little to Do with Sex: Some Provocative Insights and Questions About Adolescent Female Prostitution," Paper presented at the Third National Conference on Sexual Victimization of Children, Washington, DC, 1984.

2. CAHILL, M. E. "Sexually Abused Children: Fact, Not Fiction," *Proceedings of the House of Representatives, Subcommittee on Crime, Serial #12, 95th Congress, 1st Session.* Washington, D.C.: U.S. Government Printing Office, 1977.

3. DE FRANCIS, V. *Protecting the Child Victim of Sex Crimes Committed by Adults,* Denver, Colo.: American Humane Association, 1969.

4. FINKELHOR, D. *Sexually Victimized Children.* New York: Free Press, 1979.

5. GELINAS, D. J. "The Persisting Negative Effects of Incest," *Psychiatry,* 46 (1983): 13.

6. GROTH, A. N. "Patterns of Sexual Assault Against Children and Adolescents," in A. W. Burgess, et al., eds., *Sexual Assault of Children and Adolescents,* Lexington, Mass.: Lexington Books, 1978, p. 15.

7. ———. *Men Who Rape: The Psychology of the Offender.* New York: Plenum Press, 1979.

8. ———. "The Incest Offender," in S. M. Sgroi, ed., *Handbook of Clinical Intervention in Child Sexual Abuse.* Lexington, Mass.: Lexington Books, 1982, pp. 215–240.

9. KARPEL, M. A. "Family Secrets: I. Conceptual and Ethical Issues in the Relational Concept; II. Ethical and Practical Considerations in Therapeutic Management," *Family Process,* 19 (1980): 295.

10. KEMPE, C. H., and HELFER, R. *Helping the Battered Child and His Family.* Philadelphia: J. B. Lippincott, 1972.

11. LOURIE, I. S. "Family Dynamics and the Abuse of Adolescents," *Child Abuse and Neglect,* 3 (1979): 967–974.

12. ———. "The Locus of Emotional Harm in Incest: The Study of Non-Victims of Incestuous Families," *Clinical Proceedings, Children's Hospital National Medical Center,* 40 (1984): 46–51.

13. PUTNAM, F. *The Diagnosis and Treatment of Multiple Personality Disorder.* New York: Guilford Press, forthcoming.

14. RUSSELL, D. "The Incidence and Prevalence of Intrafamilial and Extra-familial Sexual Abuse of Female Children," *Child Abuse and Neglect,* 7 (1983): 133–146.

15. SGROI, S. M. "An Approach to Case Management," in S. M. Sgroi, ed., *Handbook of Clinical Intervention in Child Sexual Abuse.* Lexington, Mass.: Lexington Books, 1982, pp. 81–109.

16. SUMMIT, R. "Sexual Child Abuse, the Psychotherapist, and the Team Concept," in *Dealing with Sexual Child Abuse,* vol. 2. Chicago: National Committee for the Prevention of Child Abuse, 1978,

31 / Childhood Depression: An Update

Leon Cytryn and Donald H. McKnew, Jr.

Introduction

Since the publication in 1979 of our chapter on childhood affective disorders in volume 2 of this *Handbook,* [11] there has been an ever-increasing interest in this subject, as evidenced by the proportion of presentations devoted to it by professional societies and by numerous publications in major psychiatric journals. Advances in this field have occurred in several areas: offspring studies and child development, genetics, classification, diagnosis, epidemiology, treatment, and biological correlates. This chapter is devoted to elucidating the progress made since the publication of chapter 16 in volume 2.

Clinical Picture (Nosology)

In our earlier chapter we proposed an operational classification of childhood depression that included three types of this illness—acute, chronic, and masked depression of childhood.

The first two categories have remained operationally valid and have proved useful in research and clinical work. However, masked depressive reaction has proved to be a difficult and controversial clinical entity. Fortunately, several investigators have wrestled with this issue and a consensus is emerging. Almost all who have studied depressed children find that severe depression is frequently associated with aggressive and somatic symptoms. If the acting-out behavior predominates and the depression seems secondary and of lesser magnitude in the clinical picture, then the child should properly be diagnosed as having a conduct disturbance of the appropriate type with depressive features. On the other hand, if the child fits the established criteria for a depressive disorder, that should be the primary diagnosis, with other diagnostic features stated as ancillary. In such a way, the acting-out symptoms would become an integral part of the depressive picture rather than a mask.[12] Pfeffer and Plutchik[38] have described a spectrum of children who present various combinations of assaultive and suicidal behaviors. Puig-Antich[41] found that as many as 40 percent of children with major depression had a concomitant conduct disorder. Interestingly, when the depression was successfully treated, the conduct disorder also remitted, thus suggesting the possibility of some link between these two disorders rather than merely a coincidence. Weissman and associates[64] found a large incidence of anxiety disorders in depressed children. A link between these two disorders is suggested by the finding that a joint clinical picture of depression and anxiety occurs more frequently in children of parents who had both of these disorders.[19] The authors of this last study found also that childhood depression frequently coexisted with both conduct and anxiety disorders.

In recent years we and other investigators have sought to bring the diagnostic classification of children in line with the recent reclassification of adult affective disorders.[12] While still taking into account age-specific differences, this would permit a diagnostic uniformity across age groups. In the field of adult affective disorders, the most generally accepted classification has been the Research Diagnostic Criteria (RDC) of Spitzer, Endicott, and Robins.[58,59] At about the same time, Weinberg developed his Criteria for Childhood Depression.[65] Recently the RDC was incorporated, with some modification, into the *Diagnostic and Statistical Manual of Mental Disorders* (DSM-III).[1] Kovacs and Beck[29] devised a self-rating children's diagnostic inventory (CDI), based on Beck's Diagnostic Inventory (BDI). A point-by-point comparison of the diagnostic criteria proposed by us with those of Weinberg, CDI, and DSM-III indicates a striking overlap, with only minor exceptions (which are mostly semantic in character). This comparison led us to conclude that: (1) childhood and adult diagnostic criteria for affective disorders are similar; (2) DSM-III is a valid instrument for diagnosing childhood depression; (3) our categories of acute and chronic depressive reactions can be subsumed under the headings of "Major Depressive Disorder," "Dysthymic Disorder," or "Atypical Depressive Disorder" (DSM-III). The acute depressive reaction would have the following "other features" (DSM-III): "single episode" and severe "psychosocial stressors." The chronic depressive reaction meets DSM-III criteria for "recurrent episodes," usually with a positive family history.

For diagnostic purposes, DSM-III provides a unifying framework in the diagnosis of affective disorders of children as well as adults. Further, it offers flexibility by allowing grading of severity as well as by including several features pertinent to children at various developmental levels. As DSM-III continues to be used, it will doubtless be modified to include more features unique to children. The diagnostic process has been aided by the development of several operational interview instruments that have lessened the reliance on the interviewer's intuition and clinical skill; at the same time they have increased the richness, scope, and reliability of the diagnostic interview. This increased reliability allows investigators or clinicians to compare, with confidence, the findings of their studies and the characteristics of their patients with those of other investigators who are using the same diagnostic instruments.

Some interview instruments used in child psychiatry represent a modification of existing instruments for adults. The Kiddie-SADS (K-SADS),[44] based on the Schedule for Affective Disorders and Schizophrenia (SADS),[58] and the CDI are examples of such modification of adult instruments. Another group of interview instruments has been developed exclusively for use in children. The Diagnostic Interview Schedule for Children (DICA)[22] and the Children's Assessment Scale (CAS)[24] are examples of this group. Currently, an interview instrument called the Diagnostic Interview Schedule for Children (DISC) is being developed by the National Institute of Mental Health[9]; historically, it is derived from three existing instruments: K-SADS, DICA, and the Interview Schedule for Children (ISC).

All these instruments are intended for use with children and adolescents ages six to eighteen. Some five-year-olds can be successfully interviewed using these instruments, provided they are bright and have a fairly good time sense. (The latter is needed to establish the duration of various symptoms and behavior.) However, it should be stressed that, regardless of the child's age and the instrument used, it is imperative to get a good history of the child's disorder from the parent. In a recently completed study[19] the children were administered the K-SADS while their mothers were interviewed, with the same instrument, *about* the child. The results of this study show that in one-quarter of the cases, mother and child agreed on a given diagnosis. However, one-half of the diagnoses would have been missed if the parents alone had been interviewed and another one-quarter if the children alone were interviewed. There is a possibility that, in a case where the parent and child agree on a diagnosis, the severity of the disorder is higher than in cases where they disagree. This hypothesis has yet to be systematically explored.

The K-SADS was originally designed for use with RDC. Recently the K-SADS has been modified for use with both RDC and DSM-III.[19] This instrument is probably the most thorough and exhaustive tool available, and is particularly suitable in a research setting. The CAS, on the other hand, is intended to be used only with DSM-III. It is easier to administer and particularly useful in clinical practice. The DISC is specifically intended for use by lay examiners in epidemiological studies.

Epidemiology of Childhood Depression

Relatively few investigators have studied the frequency with which childhood depression occurs within the general population. Just as is true in the adult epidemiological studies, the wide variance in reported prevalence is probably due to the different diagnostic instruments used. In the Isle of Wight study, Rutter and associates[56,57] reported that three out of 2,199 prepubertal children were depressed. This study was the first to report the existence of childhood depression in the general population. However, the study was not specifically designed to investigate depression, and the reported prevalence, therefore, might have been underestimated. Using DSM-III criteria, Kashani and Simonds[25] reported a frequency of depression of 1.9 percent in a sample of fifty-three children who were born at the University of Missouri-Columbia Hospital and whose parents were attending a family practice clinic for a medical condition. This study did distinguish between children who had a major depression and those who had only a dysphoric mood, but it did not address the issue of major and minor subtypes of depression.

A representative sample of 641 nine-year-old New Zealand children was studied by Kashani and co-workers.[26] The methods used to assess the prevalence of depression included a parent's questionnaire based on DSM-III criteria, teacher's report of school behavior based on Rutter's Child Scale B,[56] and the K-SADS-E (Epidemiology). The diagnoses of major and minor depression, present or past, were based on the child's meeting the appropriate levels of RDC. In addition to the child's K-SADS-E interview, information obtained from the parents and teachers was used both to corroborate the child's statements and, especially, to establish the timing of the past depressive episodes. The current prevalence of major and minor depression was estimated as 1.7 and 3.6 percent respectively. The past prevalence of major depression was estimated as 1.0 percent and of minor depression, 8.5 percent.

Family Studies

Family studies of affective disorders in childhood lag behind adult studies in many ways. The methodology of the child studies generate the following problems:

1. Childhood studies have involved small and not necessarily randomized samples.
2. Diagnostic criteria differ from study to study, and only in a minority of studies have well-defined operational criteria been used.
3. Use of normal controls and controls with other psychiatric or nonpsychiatric pathology is rare.
4. Even when proper diagnostic criteria have been used with the parents, the timing of parental illness in the life of the child, especially at the time of the child's psychiatric evaluation, is usually unreported.
5. The mental state of the spouse of the ill proband is similarly ignored.
6. Association of a depressive disorder in children with an antecedent undesirable life stress is even less clear than in adults. In both children and adults the findings in the life-events literature are hampered by the fact that life events may be the consequence of, the cause of, or confounded with a psychological disorder.[23]
7. There is a broad range of nonspecific psychopathology existing in infants and toddlers at risk for affective illness.[18,69] Yet a diagnosable depressive picture usually does not emerge until age six to seven.[14]

8. There is a paucity of well-conducted studies that follow children at risk for affective illness past adolescence; in particular there is a lack of continuity into adulthood until the subjects pass the age of morbid risk in adults.
9. Currently available genetic models have not yet been applied to affective disorders in childhood and adolescence.

OFFSPRING STUDIES

It is difficult to group the number of studies of children and adolescents born to affectively ill parents because of the widely divergent criteria used to characterize the parents and their offspring. Probably the earliest study of parents with depressive illness was Rutter's pioneering work, *Children of Sick Parents.* [54] Of the 137 children of 43 depressed parents, nearly 50 percent had a diagnosable psychiatric disorder. The disorders included conduct disturbances, neurotic behavior disturbances, mixed behavior disturbances, and neurotic illness. None of the children was diagnosed as depressed. Other studies, whose number approaches thirty, date since the early 1970s. Only nine of those* used affective diagnoses for the children. The incidence of depressive disorders ranged from 7 to 65 percent; however, most of these studies did not clearly distinguish between major and minor depressions. There was also a conspicuous absence of mania and depressive psychosis in those children, consistent with the findings of Anthony and Scott. [2] In a number of investigations, depressive symptoms were reported that did not satisfy precise diagnostic criteria.† Rutter [54] found no difference between the diagnostic pattern of children whose parents did suffer from affective illness and that of children whose parents were troubled with nonaffective psychiatric illness. In addition to an array of psychiatric symptoms that did not satisfy the diagnostic criteria for any given condition, a number of studies‡ reported disturbances, adjustment reactions, various personality disorders, minimal brain dysfunction, sociopathic behavior, and drug problems. More recently a number of investigators used children of normal controls.§ Although the rate of depression varied in these studies, it was significantly lower in the control group than in children of parents with affective disorders.

Use of Nonaffective Psychiatric Controls. Most of these studies have used groups of schizophrenic parents as controls and produced conflicting findings. Some investigators [51,52,53] have reported that children of depressed mothers have peer relationships and school behavior similar to those of normal controls and more appropriate than those of the children of schizo-

phrenic mothers. Other investigators [60,61] have reported that children of depressed mothers as well as the offspring of schizophrenic mothers were rated by teachers and peers as more disturbed than children of normal controls on such measures as impatience, defiance, disturbed behavior in the classroom, withdrawal, aggression, unhappiness, and a lessening of creativity, initiative, and comprehension.

NIMH STUDIES OF OFFSPRING

For many years the authors of this chapter have been involved in the study of the offspring of parents with a major affective illness. The children have been seen at various stages of development. We have chosen this strategy because illness tends to aggregate in families, and such children are, accordingly, at high risk for affective illness. Thus such families provide an opportunity to study affective disorders and other psychopathology at all stages of development and ultimately to discover the genetic and rearing practices that may be at the root of the illnesses that so many of these youngsters endure.

Our first offspring study [31] was exploratory, open, and without controls. We saw thirty children (ages six to fifteen) from fourteen families in which one parent was hospitalized at the National Institute of Mental Health (NIMH) for major depressive illness (twelve bipolar, two unipolar). Using two structured interviews done four months apart, sixteen of the thirty children were found to meet the Weinberg criteria [65] for depression on at least one of the interviews.

In our second offspring study [13] we saw nineteen children (ages five to fifteen) of thirteen hospitalized major depressive parents (seven bipolar, six unipolar) and twenty-one same-age children of thirteen normal parents. The control group was matched to the index group on age within two years, sex, and socioeconomic status (within one point on the Hollingshead-Redlich scale). Parents were assessed by the Life Schedule of Affective Disorder and Schizophrenia (L-SADS). [35,59] All children were interviewed and rated by a member of our team who was blind to parental diagnosis and the purpose of the study. The children were seen at four-month intervals using the previously mentioned structured interview, which elicits all types of psychopathology, and on each occasion they were interviewed by a different interviewer. The results were analyzed in two ways: using the individual children as a unit of analysis and using the families as units of analysis. Of the nineteen children of manic-depressive parents, twelve were depressed at one or both interviews, using the Weinberg criteria; only five of twenty-one control children were depressed at one or both interviews. The difference was statistically significant. When using the families as units of analysis, we employed both Wein-

*See references 4, 13, 16, 19, 33, 37, 63, 66, and 67.
†See references 20, 32, 36, 62, and 67.
‡See references 8, 17, 20, 41, and 62.
§See references 4, 13, 19, 37, 62, 63, 66, and 67.

berg and DSM-III criteria. Of the thirteen index families, as measured by Weinberg criteria, eleven had at least one child who was depressed; and of thirteen control families, three had a depressed child. The difference was statistically significant. When DSM-III criteria were used, a similar statistical difference was obtained. No child manifested manic or psychotic symptoms.

FOLLOW-UP STUDIES

Since there is some evidence that affective illness occurs at a higher rate in the children of families in which one or more parent is affectively ill, a question that then arises concerns the continuity or discontinuity of this phenomenon over time. Eighteen children of manic-depressive parents who had been seen in our earlier offspring studies[3] were followed up. The mean age of the children was ten years when first seen; at follow-up, it was fourteen years. The interviewers and diagnostician were blind as to the original diagnosis. Of the twelve originally diagnosed as depressed by Weinberg criteria, only two were asymptomatic four years later. Of the remaining ten, seven retained their diagnostic depressive label using DSM-III criteria (mostly dysthymic) and three had switched to other psychopathology. Of the six who were originally diagnosed as Weinberg negative, five remained asymptomatic at follow-up, while one had a major depressive disorder.

In a long-term follow-up of depressed children, Poznanski and associates[39] found that about 50 percent of them remained depressed as young adults and the remainder had other psychopathology.

Pearce, as discussed by Rutter,[55] reported that when both children and adults were diagnosed by his operational criteria for depressive syndromes, an impressive continuity was found: Of thirty-seven children diagnosed as depressed by Pearce's criteria, thirty-one were diagnosed as having a depressive syndrome in adulthood, using the same criteria. Rutter notes that such continuity is impressive and stands in contrast to the lack of continuity that results when traditional clinical diagnoses, rather than strict operational criteria, are employed. As he sees it, this contrast may be explained by the concomitant nondepressive disorders that overshadowed the presence of a depressive syndrome.

One group of investigators examined twelve adolescents whose mothers had been psychotic during the child's infancy.[21,27] They found significantly less competence in the children of depressed mothers than in those children whose mothers have nonaffective diagnoses. Another follow-up study of children[28] of depressed mothers indicated a general increase of emotional disturbance during adolescence as measured by the rate of school dropout and by overall adjustment.

All the findings suggest that depression or related psychological problems in childhood is not an evanescent phenomenon but is often a precursor of significant psychopathology in adolescence.

Recently Kovacs and associates[30] reported their findings in a carefully designed study. Surprisingly, children with dysthymic disorder were at greater risk for chronic mood disorder than children with a major depressive episode.

Trait and State Markers

Less research has focused on trait and state markers. Puig-Antich and associates* have concentrated on prepubertal major depression of endogenous type. They have reported hypersecretion of cortisol in 10 percent of this group and have found a positive dexamethasone suppression test (DST) in two-thirds of the cases. Similar DST results have been reported by Poznanski and coworkers.[40] However, both cortisol hypersecretion and positive DST return to normal upon recovery. Other important findings concern the secretion of growth hormone (GH). Hypersecretion of GH in sleep (especially during the delta stage of sleep) occurs in prepubertal children with major depression. Also, there is diminished GH secretion in response to an insulin tolerance test. Both findings are similar to those in adults but are more pronounced in prepubertal children. Although the GH data are quite suggestive of a trait, they do not yet fulfill all the criteria of a genetic marker as enumerated by Rieder and Gershon,[50] especially the state-independence and the relative absence of such a trait in non-ill relatives of prepubertal children with major depression.

In a study of children with a bipolar affective disorder, McKnew and associates[34] found the children to have a clear-cut response to lithium carbonate and a strongly augmented average evoked response (AER) to sensory stimuli; again, this paralleled findings in adults.[5,6,7] However, both the alteration in the 3-methoxy-4-hydroxy-phenylglycol urinary excretion (as reported in chapter 16 in volume 2 of this *Handbook*)[11] and that of the AER have to be considered state markers, since they return to normal once the child has recovered.

In addition to the just-mentioned studies that support the similarity between adult and childhood depression, two noteworthy findings stress the differences between depressive disorders at these two ages.[42] Imipramine hydrochloride was thought to be generally effective in major depressive disorders in children, but

---

*See references 42, 43, 45, 46, and 47.

in double-blind studies it was found to be no more effective than placebo unless plasma levels were greater than 155 ng per ml. Similarly, an early report[31] found sleep architecture in depressed children to be like the patterns in adult depressed patients; this too was not confirmed in subsequent studies. Two recent reviews discussed the issue of continuity and discontinuity of affective disorders, asking whether the disorders seen and diagnosed in childhood are identical with the same disorders seen in adults.[14,15]

Studies of Infants and Toddlers of Bipolar Parents

Cytryn, McKnew and associates[14] and Gaensbauer, Harmon, and coworkers[18] investigated attachment behavior, the nature of affiliative expression, and the quality of social relationships in infants of parents with bipolar illness (ages twelve to eighteen months).

The following results of this study are most relevant to a developmental perspective: (1) There was an increase over time, from twelve to eighteen months, of insecure, ambivalent attachment, in the proband infants. (2) These infants displayed a lesser capacity for self-regulation of their emotional equilibrium, especially in handling fear and anger. And (3) Only rarely did the infants show predominantly depressive mood. We found no neurological deficit in any of these infants nor any abnormalities in developmental milestones. When these infants reached age two, Zahn-Waxler, McKnew, and colleagues[69] studied problem behaviors. The psychological symptoms included: phobias, sleep disturbances, eating problems, excessive shyness, passivity, hyperactivity, poor impulse control, self-punitive behaviors (head banging), excessive dependency, social language problems, disturbances in regulation of affect, temper tantrums, echolalia, and resistance to physical contact. Children with a bipolar parent were rated as having both significantly more problems and more severe problems than children from control families.

Zahn-Waxler and associates[69] studied peer interactions in the same children and controls. During the period of reunion following separation from the mother, children of bipolar parents manifested a number of striking behavior patterns: They showed more inappropriately displayed aggression, hurting their friends with greater frequency than did controls; they showed substantially less altruism toward their peers, most noticeably reflected in less sharing; and they displayed heightened emotion during the argument between two adults and little emotion following a fight (controls showed the reverse pattern). Following exposure to a climate of anger, the high level of emotion shown by the proband children consisted primarily of distress, while for the controls, the high level of emotion following the anger consisted primarily of positive emotion.

Zahn-Waxler and associates[68] used the same children to investigate the development of object relations in infants and toddlers. Children from both bipolar and normal families showed normal developmental patterns of cognitive growth. However, children from the bipolar families failed to make the normal transition from self-oriented imitative play to inclusion of others in such play. In addition, at age twenty-six months, children from bipolar families were more frequently judged to be insecure in their attachment relationship to the mother. Early impairments in object relations were thus manifested in tasks that involved interactions with real or symbolic others.

Conclusion

The studies reviewed here indicate that there is continued growth and sustained interest in the field of affective disorders in children. Most findings support the concept of continuity of such disorders throughout the life cycle, extending from precursors in infants and toddlers up to adulthood. Some results, however, do not support this concept of continuity. It is hoped that this issue will be resolved by means of long-term follow-up, adoption, and twin studies and the development of stable genetic markers.

REFERENCES

1. AMERICAN PSYCHIATRIC ASSOCIATION. *Diagnostic and Statistical Manual of Mental Disorders,* 3rd ed. (DSM-III). Washington, D.C.: American Psychiatric Association, 1980.
2. ANTHONY, E. J., and SCOTT, P. "Manic-depressive Psy-chosis in Childhood," *Journal of Child Psychology,* 1 (1960):53–72.
3. APTER, A., et al. "A Four-year Follow-up of Depressed Children," *Journal of Preventive Psychiatry,* 1 (1982):331–335.

4. BEARDSLEY, W. R. "Disorder in Children at Risk," Paper presented at the annual meeting of the American Psychiatric Association, Los Angeles, 1984.

5. BUCHSBAUM, M. S. "The Average Evoked Response Technique in Differentiation of Bipolar, Unipolar and Schizophrenic Disorders," in H. Akiskal, ed., *Psychiatric Diagnosis: Exploration of Biological Criteria.* New York: Spectrum Publications, 1978.

6. ———. "Neuropsychiological Reactivity, Stimulus Intensity Modulation and the Depressive Disorders," in R. A. Depue, ed., *The Psychobiology of the Depressive Disorders: Implications for the Effects of Stress.* New York: Academic Press, 1979, pp. 221–242.

7. BUCHSBAUM, M. S., et al. "AER in Affective Disorders," *American Journal of Psychiatry,* 128 (1971):19–25.

8. CONNERS, C. K., et al. "Children of Parents with Affective Illness," *Journal of the American Academy of Child Psychiatry,* 18 (1979):600–607.

9. COSTELLO, A. "Structured Interview: The DISC," Paper presented at the research forum of the annual meeting of the American Academy of Child Psychiatry, San Francisco, 1983.

10. CYTRYN, L., and MCKNEW, D. H., JR. "Affective Disorders," in J. D. Noshpitz, ed., *Basic Handbook of Child Psychiatry,* vol. 2. New York: Basic Books, 1979, pp. 321–340.

11. CYTRYN, L., GERSHON, E. S., and MCKNEW, D. H. "Is Childhood Depression a Genetic Illness?" *Integrative Psychiatry,* 2 (1984):17–23.

12. CYTRYN, L., MCKNEW, D. H., and BUNNEY, W. E., JR. "Diagnosis of Depression in Children: Reassessment," *American Journal of Psychiatry,* 137 (1980):22–25.

13. CYTRYN, L. et al. "Offspring of Patients with Affective Disorders, II." *Journal of the American Academy of Child Psychiatry,* 21 (1982):389–391.

14. CYTRYN, L., et al. "A Developmental View of Affective Disturbances in the Children of Affectively Ill Parents," *American Journal of Psychiatry,* 141 (1984):219–223.

15. CYTRYN, L., et al. "Developmental Issues in Risk Research: The Offspring of Affectively Ill Parents," in M. Rutter, C. E. Izard, and P. B. Read, eds., *Depression in Young People.* New York: Guilford Press, 1985, pp. 163–188.

16. DECINA, P., et al. "Clinical and Psychological Assessment of Children of Bipolar Probands," *American Journal of Psychiatry,* 140 (1983):548–553.

17. EL-GUEBALY, N., et al. "Psychosocial Adjustment of the Offspring of Psychiatric Inpatients: The Effect of Alcoholic, Depressive and Schizophrenic Parentage," *Journal of the Canadian Psychiatric Association,* 23 (1978):281–289.

18. GAENSBAUER, T. J., et al. "Social and Affective Development in Infants with a Manic-depressive Parent," *American Journal of Psychiatry,* 141 (1984):223–230.

19. GERSHON, E. S., et al. "Diagnoses in School-age Children of Parents with a Bipolar Affective Disorder: Patients and Normal Controls," *Journal of Affective Disorders,* 8 (1985):283–291.

20. GREENHILL, L. L., and SHOPSIN, B. "Survey of Mental Disorders in the Children of Patients with Affective Disorders," in J. Mendlewicz and B. Shopsin, eds., *Genetic Aspects of Affective Illness.* New York: Spectrum Publications, 1979.

21. GRUNEBAUM, H., et al. "Children of Depressed and Schizophrenic Mothers," *Child Psychiatry and Human Development,* 8 (1978):219–228.

22. HERJANIC, B., and WELNER, Z. "Structured Interview: The Dica," Paper presented at the Research Forum, Annual Meeting of the American Academy of Child Psychiatry, San Francisco, 1983.

23. HIRSCHFELD, R.M.A., and CROSS, C. K. "Epidemiology of Affective Disorders," *Archives of General Psychiatry,* 39 (1982):35–46.

24. HODGES, K., et al. "The CAS Interview for Children: A Report on Reliability and Validity," *Journal of the American Academy of Child Psychiatry,* 21 (1982):468–473.

25. KASHANI, J. H., and SIMONDS, J. F. "The Incidence of Depression in Children," *American Journal of Psychiatry,* 136 (1979):1203–1205.

26. KASHANI, J. H., et al. "Depression in a Sample of Nine-year-old Children: Prevalence and Associated Characteristics," *Archives of General Psychiatry,* 40 (1983):1217–1227.

27. KAUFFMAN, C., et al. "Superkids: Competent Children of Psychotic Mothers," *American Journal of Psychiatry,* 11 (1979):1398–1402.

28. KOKES, R. F., et al. "Child Competence and Psychiatric Risk," *Journal of Nervous and Mental Disease,* 168 (1980):348–352.

29. KOVACS, M., and BECK, A. T. "An Empirical-clinical Approach Toward a Definition of Childhood Depression," in J. B. Schultenbrandt and A. Raskin, eds., *Depression in Childhood.* New York: Raven Press, 1977, pp. 1–26.

30. KOVACS, M., et al. "Depressive Disorders in Childhood," *Archives of General Psychiatry,* 41 (1984):229–237.

31. KUPFER, D. J., et al. "Imipramine and EEG Sleep in Children with Depressive Symptoms," *Psychopharmacology,* 60 (1979):117.

32. KUYLER, P. L., et al. "Psychopathology Among Children of Manic-depressive Patients," *Biological Psychiatry,* 15 (1980):589–597.

33. MCKNEW, D. H., et al. "Offspring of Manic-depressive Patients," *British Journal of Psychiatry,* 134 (1979):148–152.

34. MCKNEW, D. H., et al. "Lithium in Children of Lithium Responding Parents," *Psychiatric Research,* 4 (1981):171–180.

35. MAZURE, C., and GERSHON, E. S. "Blindness and Reliability in Lifetime Psychiatric Diagnosis," *Archives of General Psychiatry,* 36 (1979):521–525.

36. O'CONNELL, R. A., et al. "Children of Bipolar Manic-depressives," in J. Mendlewicz and B. Shopsin, eds., *Genetic Aspects of Affective Illness.* New York: Spectrum Publications, 1979.

37. ORVASCHEL, H., et al. "Assessing Psychopathology in Children of Psychiatrically Disturbed Parents: A Pilot Study," *Journal of the American Academy of Child Psychiatry,* 20 (1981):112–122.

38. PFEFFER, C. R., PLUTCHIK, R., and MIZRUCHI, M. S. "Suicidal and Assaultive Behavior in Children: Classification, Measurement and Interrelations," *American Journal of Psychiatry,* 140 (1983):154–157.

39. POZNANSKI, E. O., KRAHENBUHL, V., and ZRULL, J. P. "Childhood Depression: A Longitudinal Perspective," *Journal of the American Academy of Child Psychiatry,* 15 (1976): 491–501.

40. POZNANSKI, E. O., et al. "The Dexamethasone Suppression Test in Prepubertal Depressed Children," *American Journal of Psychiatry,* 139 (1982):321–324.

41. PUIG-ANTICH, J. "Major Depression and Conduct Disorder in Prepuberty," *Journal of the American Academy of Child Psychiatry,* 21 (1982):118–128.

42. PUIG-ANTICH, J. "Age and Sex Effects on Sleep/neuroendocrine State and Trait Markers of Major Depressive Disorder," in M. Rutter, C. E. Izard, and P. B. Read, eds., *Depression in Young People.* New York: Guilford Press, 1985, pp. 341–382.

43. PUIG-ANTICH, J., et al. "Cortisol Hypersecretion in

Prepubertal Depressive Illness: A Preliminary Report," *Psychoneuroendocrinology,* 4 (1979):191–197.

44. PUIG-ANTICH, J., et al. *Adaptation of Schedule for Affective Disorders and Schizophrenia for School Age Children, Epidemiologic Version, Kiddie-SADS-E with DSM-III,* 3rd ed., addenda. Monograph, Department of Child and Adolescent Psychiatry, New York State Psychiatric Institute.

45. PUIG-ANTICH, J., et al. "Prepubertal Endogenous Major Depressives Hyposecrete Growth Hormone in Response to Insulin-induced Hypoglycemia," *Biological Psychiatry,* 16 (1981):801–818.

46. PUIG-ANTICH, J., et al. "Growth Hormone Secretion in Prepubertal Major Depressive Children in Response to Insulin-induced Hypoglycemia," Paper presented at the annual meeting of the American Academy of Child Psychiatry, Washington, D.C., 1982.

47. PUIG-ANTICH, J., et al. "Growth Hormone Secretion in Prepubertal Children with Major Depression. Parts I–IV," *Archives of General Psychiatry,* 41 (1984):455–483.

48. PUIG-ANTICH, J., et al. "Imipramine in Prepubertal Major Depressive Disorders." *Archives of General Psychiatry,* in press.

49. RASKIN, A. "Depression in Children: Fact or Fallacy," in J. G. Schultenbrandt and A. Rankin, eds., *Depression in Childhood.* New York: Raven Press, 1977, pp. 141–146.

50. RIEDER, R., and GERSHON, E. S. "Genetic Strategies in Biological Psychiatry," *Archives of General Psychiatry,* 35 (1978):866–873.

51. ROLF, J. E. "The Social and Academic Competence of Children Vulnerable to Schizophrenia and Other Behavior Pathologies," *Journal of Abnormal Psychology,* 80 (1972):225–243.

52. ———. "Peer Status and the Directionality of Symptomatic Behavior: Social Competence Predictors of Outcome for Vulnerable Children," *American Journal of Orthopsychiatry,* 46 (1976):74–88.

53. ROLF, J. E., and GARMEZY, N. "The School Performance of Children Vulnerable to Behavior Pathology," in M. Roff, ed., *Life History Research in Psychopathology,* vol. 3. Minneapolis: University of Minnesota Press, 1974, pp. 87–107.

54. RUTTER, M. *Children of Sick Parents: Environmental and Psychiatric Study.* Institute of Psychiatry, Mandsley Monographs, No. 16, London: Oxford University Press, 1966.

55. RUTTER, M. "Developmental Psychopathology: Issues and Perspectives," in M. Rutter, C. E. Izard, and P. B. Read, eds., *Depression in Young People.* New York: Guilford Press, 1985, pp. 3–37.

56. RUTTER, M., TIZARD, J., and WHITMORE, K. *Education, Health and Behaviour.* Huntington, N.Y.: Krieger, 1981.

57. RUTTER, M., et al. "Isle of Wight Studies," *Psychological Medicine,* 6 (1976):313–332.

58. SPITZER, R. L., ENDICOTT, J., and ROBINS, E. *Research Diagnostic Criteria for Selected Group of Functional Disorders,* 2nd ed. New York: Biometrics Research Division, New York State Psychiatric Institute, 1975.

59. SPITZER, R. L., ENDICOTT, J., and ROBINS, E. "Research Diagnostic Criteria: Rationale and Reliability," *Archives of General Psychiatry,* 35 (1978):773–782.

60. WEINTRAUB, S., NEALE, J. M., and LIEBERT, D. E. "Teacher Ratings of Children Vulnerable to Psychopathology," *American Journal of Orthopsychiatry,* 45 (1975):839–845.

61. WEINTRAUB, S., PRINZ, R. J., and NEALE, G. M. "Peer Evaluations of the Competence of Children Vulnerable to Psychopathology," *Journal of Abnormal Child Psychology,* 6 (1978):461–473.

62. WEISSMAN, M. M., and SIEGEL, J. "The Depressed Woman and Her Rebellious Adolescent," *Social Casework,* 53 (1972):563–570.

63. WEISSMAN, M. M., et al. "Children of Affectively Ill Parents," paper presented at the annual meeting of the American Psychiatric Association, Los Angeles, 1984.

64. WEISSMAN, M. M. et al. "Depression and Anxiety Disorders in Parents and Children: Results from the Yale Family Study," *Archives of General Psychiatry,* 41 (1984):845–852.

65. WEINBERG, W. A., et al. "Depression in Children Referred to an Educational Diagnostic Center; Diagnosis and Treatment," *Journal of Pediatrics,* 83 (1973):1065–1972.

66. WELNER, Z., GARRISON, W., and RICE, J. "Blind High-Risk Study of Depressives' Offspring," paper presented at the annual meeting of the American Psychiatric Association, Los Angeles, 1984.

67. WELNER, J., et al. "Psychopathology in Children of Inpatients with Depression: A Controlled Study," *Journal of Nervous and Mental Disease,* 164 (1977):408–413.

68. ZAHN-WAXLER, C., et al. "Cognitive and Social Development in Infants and Toddlers with a Bipolar Parent," Paper presented at the annual meeting of the American Academy of Child Psychiatry, Washington, D.C., 1982.

69. ZAHN-WAXLER, C., et al. "Problem Behaviors and Peer Interactions of Young Children with a Manic-depressive Parent," *American Journal of Psychiatry,* 141 (1984):236–240.

70. ZAHN-WAXLER, C., et al. "Altruism, Aggression, and Social Interaction in Young Children with a Manic-depressive Parent," *Child Development,* 55 (1984):112–122.

32 / Narcissistic Disorders in Children: Clinical and Developmental Characteristics

Efrain Bleiberg

Introduction

Narcissus' ill-fated plunge in pursuit of his beautiful image turned him into a ready symbol of the perils of self-absorption. Nowadays, powerful cultural forces support the individual's plunge into a life-style of frantic pursuit of beauty, success, wealth, power, and admiration. The media's cult of celebrity gives substance, as Lasch[25] noted, to "narcissistic dreams of fame and glory" (p. 21), fostering the hunger for glamour and excitement, unlimited consumption, and uninhibited gratification.

The idea of individuals living for themselves and for the moment hinders people's sense of community and historical continuity. Calculated seductiveness, manipulation, and expedience are rewarded in the political, business, and social arenas. At a societal as well as a familial level, commitments are fragile, loyalty suspect, and relationships (as suggested by a divorce rate approaching 50 percent) less than enduring. Closeness, trust, and attachment often lead to pain and disappointment. Increasingly isolated from the support of community, tradition, or extended family, the American nuclear family has become prone to breakup. Narcissism, as Lasch[25] suggested, may be the prototypical character of contemporary America.

Not surprisingly, narcissism and narcissistic disorders have become the focus of enormous interest in the psychiatric and psychoanalytic literature. In clinical practice, some of the complaints clinicians hear most often bear the hallmarks of narcissistic disorders: pervasive feelings of unhappiness, inner emptiness and boredom, dependence on others' approval and admiration, fears of closeness and intimacy, exploitativeness and manipulation in interpersonal relationships, intense anxiety and efforts to deny death and aging, and inability to experience love or meaning in life.

In the child psychiatric literature, however, narcissistic disorders have received relatively little attention. Few attempts have been made to examine narcissistic traits as they emerge in children. Current theories of narcissism include developmental formulations that are supported primarily by retrospective data, collected in the treatment of adults.[19,20,24] This chapter describes the clinical and developmental features that characterize narcissistic children.

The Concept of Narcissism

Perhaps the one point regarding narcissism upon which everyone agrees is that it is one of the most confusing and controversial psychiatric and psychoanalytic concepts. The prevailing confusion is heir to the bewildering diversity of meanings that the term narcissism has received since Freud's seminal paper "On Narcissism: An Introduction"[11] was written almost seventy years ago. Freud fueled the conceptual disarray by using narcissism in various ways and in different contexts.[34] The various meanings Freud[11,12,13,14] gave to the term narcissism refer to it as: a sexual perversion; the earliest stage of normal development (primary narcissism); the investment of psychic energy in the ego; a type of object choice or a mode of relating to the environment; a regressive response to object loss; and a category of patients (those suffering from narcissistic neurosis) whose narcissism precluded the development of transference, thus rendering them inaccessible to the therapeutic efforts of psychoanalysis.

Over the last three decades, the trend in psychoanalysis has been for explanations of narcissism to focus less on drives and psychic energy distribution. Increasingly, narcissism is considered under the aegis of the self. The self has proven to be a fruitful construct that draws together notions about a person's conscious and unconscious self-images, the integration and cohesion of those images, and the individual's capacity for autonomous functioning and regulation of well-being and self-esteem. From this perspective, Stolorow[45] defined mental activity as narcissistic "to the degree that its function is to maintain the structural cohesion, temporal stability and positive affective coloring of the self-representation" (p. 179).

Jacobson[17] suggested that fluctuations in self-esteem are proportionate to the degree of congruence between the actual mental self-representation and the wishful concept of the self (the self as "I would like to be," i.e., the ego ideal). Extending Jacobson's concept, Joffe and Sandler[18] proposed that the central feature of narcissistic disorders is a state of pain, overt or latent, caused by "a substantial discrepancy between the mental representation of the actual self and an ideal shape of the self" (p. 65) that has to be dealt with by the ego. In response to the affective-cognitive state of pain, the ego mobilizes a number of defensive and adaptive maneuvers. These can assume pathological proportions. Thus a wide range of clinical and developmental problems connected with self-object relationships, self-regard, and identity have been subsumed under the term narcissistic disorder.

The theoretical models developed by Kohut[23,24] and Kernberg[19,20] have given rise to a surge of interest in narcissistic disorders and to lively controversy. Kohut anchored his theory on a supraordinate concept of the self, which he defined as the primary psychic constellation, the center of experience, initiative, and autonomy. The primordial self of the infant, however, is weak and unsteady and lacks enduring structure, cohesiveness, or continuity. It requires the participation of the parents for any sense of cohesiveness. Without parental involvement, the infant's proto-self is vulnerable to fragmentation. Kohut coined the term self-object to designate the parental involvement in supporting the child's self. The term highlights the fact that, from the child's standpoint, the parents, inasmuch as they supply functions that the child is not yet capable of performing with his or her own psychic structure, are not experienced as separate persons but as parts of the self. This concept of merger with the self-objects is the key to Kohut's conceptual scheme. The self-objects, through their empathic responsiveness to the infant's narcissistic needs, provide the necessary experiences, indeed the basic building blocks, for the gradual development of a cohesive self.

Two primary narcissistic structures are the organizing poles of Kohut's postulated primordial self. One is the "grandiose" self, which contains the child's needs to joyfully display his or her unique traits, talents, and evolving capabilities, and be admired for them. The second basic narcissistic structure is the "idealized parent imago," which comprises the child's need to merge with the strength and power of an idealized parent. These two narcissistic needs flower via interaction with two basic self-object (parental) functions: the "mirroring self-object" and the "idealized self-object."

The idealized self-object refers to the parents' capacity to convey to the infant that the parents are powerful, able to care for, set limits for, and prevent him or her from feeling fragmented. Mirroring refers to the child's need, in Miller's[30] words, "to be understood, taken seriously, and respected" (p. 32) by the parents according to the infant's unique sensitivities, qualities, attributes, and biological rhythms. As Winnicott[49] asserted, babies look at their mother's face and find themselves there. The parents function as a mirror that reflects not only an image of the infant as he or she really is, but they color the image with their pride and acceptance of the infant's uniqueness—the "gleam in mother's eyes."[21]

In response to developmentally adequate and empathic mirroring, the child's *grandiose self* is transformed gradually into ambitions and purposes. In the course of this process, the mirroring function of the parents is internalized slowly, allowing children to develop an internal conviction of their own real, vital identity, and self-worth. Similarly, when children's needs to merge with idealized parents are not interfered with, their functions are internalized, guaranteeing an internal sense of competence, self-direction, goals, and self-enforcement of limits. Thus parental empathy weaves the thread that binds the self in a cohesive whole. Children gradually become more capable of self-regulation and more able to guarantee their own sense of self-cohesiveness.

Kohut's concept of transmuting internalization describes the process whereby the parents' capacity to reduce physical and psychological tension is slowly taken over by the infant. A manageable, empathic withdrawal of the parents' ministrations, brought about by inevitable parental failure to mirror or permit idealization, leads to a "bit-by-bit" accretion of psychic structure"[46] (p. 318). Gradually children become capable of performing for themselves those functions previously performed by the parents, which gives rise to the development of permanent psychic structure.

The stability and cohesiveness of the self are regarded as the central criteria in assessing psychopathology. On this basis, Kohut and his followers[33] distinguish three broad categories of psychological disorders. At the psychoneurotic end of the spectrum, the self has attained stable cohesiveness, and other people are recognized and experienced as relatively separate and independent. At the psychotic and borderline end of the spectrum, the self has never attained any adequate degree of cohesiveness and remains fragmented. It is between these two that Kohut places the narcissistic or primary selfdisorders.

Narcissistic disorders represent discrete structural

deficits in the self. These deficits are related both to failures in the transformation of the infantile narcissistic structures into their more mature forms and to disruptions in the internalization of the parents' functions. Arrested in self-development, narcissistic individuals thus live a life of desperate search for the missing pieces of inner structure, the self-objects who would complement their thwarted self and allow them to experience cohesiveness and well-being.

For Kohut, the pathogenesis of narcissistic disorders is inadequate parenting ("empathic failure"), particularly parental inability to function as mirroring and/or idealized self-objects. According to Kohut, disruptions in parental empathy occur when the parent perceives and responds to the child in terms of the parents' own needs, wishes, or fears. In Miller's words, [30] "the child would not find himself in his mother's face but rather the mother's own predicament" (p. 32). Empathic failure also occurs when parents find parenting a burden and/or are themselves in need of nurturance and parenting.

Kernberg [19,20] distinguishes between normal and pathological narcissism differently. He believes that narcissistic disorders reflect a specific pathological self-structure (a pathological development instead of an arrest in development). Normal narcissism, on the other hand, manifests the libidinal investment of an integrated self. For Kernberg, an integrated self-representation results from the cohesion of early self-images. One set of images corresponds to the infant experiencing tension, distress, anxiety, or frustration. Another set corresponds to the self-images based on early experiences of safety, pleasure, and comfort. This process of integration is not a separate developmental line (as Kohut postulates) but is linked intimately with the integration of the object representation.

Integrating the libidinal self-representation (the self-experiencing safety, pleasure, and comfort) with the aggressive self-representation (the self in distress, anxiety, or frustration) leads to a far more realistic and stable self. The pristine image of the self—experiencing safety, pleasure, and gratification—remains, however, as the matrix of the *ideal* self-representation. The pristine image of the all-gratifying parent provides the basis of the *ideal* object representation (in contrast to the actual object representation that results from the integration of gratifying and frustrating images of the object).

According to Kernberg [20] and Jacobson, [17] during the course of normal development there is progressive differentiation between self and object representations as well as between the actual self-image and the ideal self and ideal object representations. Over time, the ideal object, ideal self, and superego precursors are gradually integrated into the direction-giving, limiting,

self-critical, and self-rewarding structure called the superego. According to Kernberg, in pathological narcissism the ideal object, ideal self, and actual self representation are fused, resulting in a grandiose self-representation. This pathological formation, the grandiose self, emerges as a defense against intense early conflicts, particularly conflicts involving envy, aggression, and dependency. The defended-against self-image is that of a "hungry, enraged, empty self, full of impotent anger at being frustrated, and fearful of a world which seems as hateful and revengeful as the patient himself" [20] (p. 233).

While a predominance of aggression plays a central role in Kernberg's formulation, he leaves open whether the pathological development is caused by a constitutionally determined strong aggression, a lack of tolerance in regard to aggressive impulses, or severe frustration in the first years of life. For Kernberg, the designation narcissistic personality betokens a specific instance of borderline personality organization rather than a broad range of disorders, as Kohut and his followers suggest. Expanding on this notion, Rinsley [39] and Adler [1] proposed the concept of a spectrum of disorders in which the narcissistic personality represents a "higher level" manifestation of the borderline personality.

The American Psychiatric Association's third edition of the *Diagnostic and Statistical Manual* (DSM-III) [2] includes narcissistic personality among the personality disorders. The definition set forth there bears considerable resemblance to Kernberg's description of the clinical manifestations of pathological narcissism. In DSM-III, narcissistic personality is characterized by:

1. Grandiose sense of self-importance or uniqueness.
2. Preoccupation with fantasies of unlimited success, power, brilliance, beauty, or ideal love.
3. Exhibitionism.
4. Cool indifference or marked feelings of rage, inferiority, shame, humiliation, or emptiness in response to criticism, indifference of others, or defeat.
5. At least two of the following:
   a. Entitlement.
   b. Interpersonal exploitativeness.
   c. Relationships that alternate between overidealization and devaluation.
   d. Lack of empathy.

The DSM-III diagnostic criteria for narcissistic personalities refer to the relatively finished product of an adult characterological organization. During childhood, of course, character, is in the process of being formed, and children's behavior, including symptomatic behavior, changes as needs change, as new equilibriums and disequilibriums are achieved by the forces of development, and as maturation and experience provide them with new ways to deal with stress and conflict. The following section addresses the clinical manifestations of narcissistic disorders as they unfold in the context of the child's developing personality.

Clinical Manifestations of Narcissism

The clinical descriptions offered in the literature on narcissistic disorders in children cover a wide range of psychopathological manifestations. For A. Ornstein,[33] narcissistic children may give evidence of self-pathology very early in life and certainly by latency and adolescence. According to Ornstein (representing Kohut's perspective), the manifestations of primary self-pathology are: "lack of vigor and aliveness, obvious depression, low self-esteem, lack of pleasure in the self and its activities, lack of enthusiasm and initiative, and lack of long-term investments in goals and ideals" (p. 438). Ornstein points out that because these frequently bright and gifted children cannot develop their gifts and talents, chronic feelings of emptiness and worthlessness ensue. Significant manifestations of self-pathology are related to the repression and/or disavowal of infantile exhibitionism. These children may be either shy and awkwardly self-conscious or exhibitionistic clowns, constantly demanding the limelight. Finally, Ornstein believes that lack of integration of infantile narcissistic structures results in defects in impulse control. These children may feel chronically overstimulated and appear "impulse-ridden" or hyperactive.

An important point emphasized by Kohut and his followers is that "chronic narcissistic rage"[23] represents the child's effort to deal with disappointments in parental empathy. Thus the rage so often encountered in both adult and child narcissistic patients has a specific psychological flavor: "the need for revenge, for righting a wrong, for undoing a hurt by whatever means" (p. 380). Ultimately, the diagnosis of narcissistic disorders rests on the patient's developing a specific type of narcissistic transference, one in which the therapist is experienced as an idealized or mirroring self-object.

Kernberg[20] believes that the clinical manifestations of pathological narcissism in adults can be masked by superficially smooth and effective social adaptation. Underlying the surface adjustment, however, are serious distortions in *internalized* object relations. According to Kernberg, narcissistic patients manifest various combinations of intense ambitiousness, grandiose fantasies, feelings of inferiority, and overdependence on external admiration and acclaim. They are haunted by chronic feelings of boredom and emptiness and constantly seek brilliance, wealth, power, and beauty. Specially important manifestations of pathological narcissism are a major inability to love, experience concern, and understand other people empathically. Other prominent features are patients' chronic uncertainty and dissatisfaction with their lives, conscious or unconscious exploitativeness toward others, extreme self-centeredness, and intense feelings of entitlement.

Egan and P. Kernberg[8] compared this clinical picture with the manifestations of normal infantile narcissism. Noting that small children normally "keep themselves in the center of attention" (p. 42) and fantasize acquiring great power, wealth and beauty; they emphasize that normal children do not require universal admiration as sole owners of everything enviable and valuable. Further, normal children's demands are related to realistic needs and incapabilities. The demands of children burdened with pathological narcissism, according to Egan and Kernberg, are "excessive, can never be fulfilled, and are in fact secondary to an ongoing angry denigration and even destruction of supplies." Small children can be warmly grateful when their demands are met. In contrast, narcissistic patients are cool, aloof, and disregard others, except for momentary idealizations as potential sources of narcissistic gratification.

Egan and Kernberg also compare the capacity of children older than two and one-half years for genuine attachments, trust, and interest in others with narcissistic patients' inability to depend on others beyond immediate need gratification. The hallmarks of pathological narcissism in childhood are age-inappropriate grandiose fantasies, excessive demands, intense self-absorption, severe disturbances in interpersonal relationships, and an often overweening grandiosity that defensively reverses overwhelming feelings of inadequacy and helplessness.

Thus narcissistic children are brought for treatment for a variety of symptoms, including: disturbances in interpersonal relationships, coldness, exploitiveness, meanness, incessant efforts to control and manipulate; impulsivity and poor tolerance for frustration; school difficulties; mood swings, irritability, and labile self-esteem; persistent lying and chronic violation of rules; exhibitionism, haughtiness, arrogance, and constant requirements of attention and admiration; and self-doubts and intense envy. Such symptoms, of course, are not specific to narcissistic children, whose interpersonal adjustment and surface behavior vary. The same features may characterize borderline children or affective disorders or conduct disorders in childhood.

Some narcissistic children are cool and canny far

beyond their tender years. They are well controlled and capable. People are impressed with their remarkable strengths and generous supply of intelligence, charm, and shrewd awareness of what to do to elicit specific responses from the environment. Others are shy, socially clumsy, and pained by fears of shame and humiliation. Eager to comply with other people's wishes and expectations, they readily sacrifice themselves for others' sake. They are haunted by the possibility of being exposed as inferior, ugly, or inadequate. Still other narcissistic children are so destructive, defiant, and apparently lacking in remorse, concern, or constraints that psychiatric hospitalization or placement in a correctional facility becomes necessary, if only to contain them and provide relief to schools and parents.

Yet, in the midst of this diversity, there are certain common developmental features present in all narcissistic children. Examining these children against the background of the normal developmental process may provide the basis for a definition of narcissistic disorders in childhood that lends itself more readily to objective assessment, facilitates the differential diagnosis, provides clues about the pathogenesis of these disorders, and serves as a guide for treatment.

Developmental and Dynamic Characteristics of Narcissism

IDENTITY FORMATION: REAL SELF, FALSE SELF, AND AS-IF PHENOMENA

A young child's sense of identity is anchored by external indications (i.e., "I belong to the X's family, attend Y's school, and live in Z's neighborhood"). By midlatency, however, most children have developed what Erikson[9] calls a sense of "me-ness," which has cohesiveness, continuity, and relative autonomy. That is, children have a sense of "I am me, the same that was yesterday and is likely to be tomorrow," which is relatively independent of the children's feelings of the moment, their affiliation to a group or family, or their awareness of their own developmental changes.

A central developmental feature of narcissistic children is difficulty in developing a sense of "me-ness." Their self-experience is pervaded by feelings of lack of genuineness. Often they feel they spend their lives acting a role. Under some conditions the role they select is that of an impressively self-sufficient, amazingly precocious miniature adult; under other conditions it may be an ever-changing role—a chameleonlike performance—where the children continually and carefully monitor their environment to adapt by means of the most convenient ad hoc identity. What these children experience themselves to be and the image they attempt to present to the world is not based on an internal core sense of identity. It is based, instead, on what they perceive is expected from them or is conducive to obtaining admiration or advantage. Their subjective experience is that they present a front to others. Often they have little conscious awareness of what the façade is covering other than an abiding feeling that in some way they are flawed. Balint's notion[3] of the "basic fault" captures the child's experience of defectiveness, damage, incompleteness, a haunting sense that something is wrong or missing or bad inside. The ensuing façade is akin to Winnicott's concept[48] of the "false self." Making realistic plans for the future, setting reasonable goals for themselves, even seeing themselves in the future, all are extremely difficult tasks for narcissistic children. Consider Pete.

Pete was adopted when he was six months old. His adoptive mother remembers that when she first met him, he smiled easily and seldom cried. He would not allow her to feed him, demanding even then to hold the bottle himself. As Pete grew, he insisted on being in charge of his own and everyone else's affairs. When efforts were made to set limits, he responded with terrible temper tantrums. When Pete was almost two years old, his adoptive father walked out on the family shortly after the adoptive mother gave birth to a baby girl. Pete's newborn sister suffered from a congenital heart malformation and her demands for attention left mother emotionally drained. Pete's behavior, on the other hand, improved and he was soon talking of being mother's boyfriend. Mother remarried when Pete was three years old, whereupon his behavior deteriorated once again. He insisted on being in charge, and when limits were set he would throw furious tantrums. He began to hurt his younger sister, devising schemes that became increasingly more cruel and harmful. His nursery-school teacher described him as a provocative and exhibitionistic youngster who acted like a miniature adult and talked in adultlike sentences. He had a remarkable skill at picking out others' vulnerabilities, which reflected his heightened awareness of interpersonal nuances. As his behavior continued to deteriorate, both school and parents agreed that their resources had been exhausted and requested hospitalization for the child.

The hospital team effectively blocked Pete's omnipotent, pseudo-adult behavior and supported his mother in formally "firing" him from his job as her boyfriend. For the first time, Pete became anxious. He then began to steal articles of clothing from other children, insisting on dressing like others. By frantically imitating other children, he attempted to "steal" their ideas, attributes, expressions, gestures, and interests, all in the service of desperately seeking an identity. Needless to say, his efforts were futile and led only to superficial "as-if" phenomena,[7] which failed to provide the sense of purpose, vitality, and authenticity that only a cohesive core sense of identity ensures.

It is not difficult to detect in Pete many of the features postulated by DSM-III—grandiosity, inflated sense of self-importance, exhibitionism, and marked feelings of rage when his pretentions to omnipotence were challenged by his being frustrated or criticized. At the same time, these traits were not yet crystallized into a fixed character organization. Pete was far more impulsive and maladapted than is typical of adult narcissistic personalities. Also, he was much more vulnerable to panic in response to environmental challenge and more prone to demonstrate the underlying confusion he experienced about his identity.

An important question pertains to the specificity of these manifestations of distortions in self-development. Indeed, an inability to develop a cohesive sense of self is encountered commonly in psychotic and borderline children. However, narcissistic children are much less vulnerable to psychotic thinking and experience and can usually maintain adequate (sometimes outstanding) reality contact even when faced with stress or conflict. Differences in the capacity to maintain contact with reality suggest significant differences in the overall development and ego functioning of narcissistic, borderline, and psychotic youngsters.

RELINQUISHMENT OF OMNIPOTENCE

When normal children are between eight to eighteen months, they typically respond to the awareness of separation from mother by creating a wishful, omnipotent image of themselves. This transient sense of "I can do and have what I want" counters their anxiety over loss. Later they can achieve sufficient intrapsychic autonomy to tolerate the awareness of separation, and they are then able to relinquish the omnipotence. Narcissistic children, however, are those who fail to relinquish omnipotence. For them, grandiosity, often coupled with devaluation and contempt for others, continues to play a crucial role.

From the moment of admission, Joe, an eleven-year-old boy, strutted into the hospital like a frontier gunfighter ambling into a saloon. He disparaged all attempts by staff and peers to get along with him. He wished to impose what he called "admirable" solutions to every problem. His fury knew no bounds when his marvelous ideas were subordinated to the "incompetent" decisions of adults. Unhesitantly he shared his certainty of becoming the President of the United States, as soon as he graduated in nuclear physics and brain surgery.

Even though they fall short of their own grandiose standards, narcissistic children often manage to impress people with their good surface adjustment. According to Tooley,[47] they are "self possessed, convincing and attractive, [and] demonstrate a capacity for cool reality testing and shrewd assessment of interpersonal situations" (p. 307). Exquisitely aware of other people's motives and weaknesses, these children often excel in manipulating the environment.

Their apparently precocious development often makes them seem to be miniature adults. They rarely experience real adults as protectors, soothers, limit-setters, or effective interpreters of reality. This is the rationale for narcissistic children's desperate efforts to hold on to an illusion of self-sufficiency.

Brutality, neglect, unattunement, loss, and deprivation are indeed glaring aspects of the upbringing of some of these children. As a result, their very survival seems to demand a precocious development of self-reliance and self-nurturing. For others, overindulgent rearing and absence of realistic limits fail to curb the infantile omnipotence. But even in the absence of those conditions, narcissistic children feel pushed into premature closure of dependency and premature pseudodevelopment. This omnipotence, however, coexists with intact reality testing. It is as if the children were saying "I know what the world is, but I want it to be like I want, and now," and they behave accordingly.

SELF-ESTEEM AND RELIANCE ON EXTERNAL APPROVAL

By midlatency most children are developing an internally validated sense of self-worth. While external confirmation continues to be important, in the face of momentary failures, rejections, or losses, most children continue to experience themselves as worthy and valuable with some degree of independence from other people's judgments. A relatively stable and autonomous self-esteem buffers them against violent oscillations in the affective coloring of their self-experience.

In narcissistic children, however, this developmental accomplishment is seriously compromised. No matter how haughty and self-assured they appear at one moment, they present a striking proclivity to plunge abruptly into feelings of ignominy, failure, and worthlessness. To achieve a semblance of self-worth, they require endless supplies of attention, approval, and admiration. They feel compelled to meet exorbitant demands for perfection. To them, the world is a vast courtroom where an implacable jury constantly judges whether they have passed or failed the test of "greatness."

By virtue of their beauty, cleverness, or talents, some narcissistic children are able to secure quite a lot of the vitally needed admiration. But it is never enough. In fact, success only perpetuates an impossible dilemma: To feel good, external approval is needed. Yet dependency on others threatens children whose grandiosity and fear of vulnerability necessitate that they avoid dependency. Furthermore, they feel admired for their ability to perform according to other people's standards and expectations rather than for being the person they really are. Ultimately, their very achievement intensifies their alienation from authenticity.

OBJECT RELATIONS AND DEFENSE MECHANISMS

A crucial developmental acquisition during latency is the ability to withstand stress and conflict without undue regression. To deal with painful, distressing, or dangerous feelings or experiences, latency-age children intellectualize, repress, displace, and symbolize.[42] Fantasy and play become effective mechanisms with which to master traumatic experiences; relieve tension; express feelings, concerns, and ideas; and find more adaptive solutions to life's dilemmas. It is a time when children's ability to make sense out of what is happening and to understand cause-and-effect relationships independent of personal feelings, needs, and wishes is enormously enhanced. Finally, latency-age children establish a system of peer relationships that provides an additional—or alternative—source of support and identification.

Thus, by midlatency, most children have typically evolved a variety of coping mechanisms that prevent regression and disorganization. These mechanisms may take the form of intellectual efforts to make sense, aggressive assertion of competence, or reaching out to others for help or thrusting themselves into activity.

Narcissistic children, on the other hand, are extraordinarily vulnerable to the threat of helplessness or loss of control that, as in Pete's case, may reveal their underlying emptiness. In extreme cases, there may be a controlled excursion into craziness, where playing "crazy"[6] becomes an atttempt to master the otherwise terrifying experiences of lack of interpersonal control and the danger of a precarious sense of identity. Playing crazy illustrates a typical defensive maneuver of narcissistic children: to provoke actively what they fear to experience passively. Turning passive into active is an effective maneuver to prevent helplessness, particularly when anticipating rejection or harm. Narcissistic children believe the environment is incapable of supporting, soothing, or protecting them. They do not expect people to notice them, understand them, take them seriously, respect them, or respond to them as persons in their own right. In turn, they experience other people as tools that they are entitled to manipulate in order to gratify their own needs.

In order to avoid the experience of hunger and depletion, need gratification is of paramount importance to such children. A common fantasy is that what is good is limited, hence to have the "goods" means to deprive someone else. Expecting only a ruthless competition for scarce supplies, narcissistic children feel compelled to sever any emotional connection with experiences of themselves as helpless, rejected, dependent, hungry, lonely, or frustrated. They recall the events of abuse, neglect, desertion, or lack of empathy in their lives in explicit detail, but the affects linked to these experiences are not accessible. Rinsley[37] described these processes of isolation of affect in narcissistic children as a precocious obsessional organization.

Omnipotence and grandiosity are, of course, most effective maneuvers to disown and deny dependency needs. Narcissistic children deny the valuable, nurturing, protective aspects of the environment while they project their own helplessness and vulnerability onto other people. Thus these children develop a particular defensive configuration characterized by turning passive into active; splitting off the weak and vulnerable aspects of themselves from their self-experience; isolating affect, grandiosity, and omnipotence; and devaluating others. By blocking the child's interpersonal relations and healthy identifications, this defensive constellation further distorts the child's subsequent development.

MORAL DEVELOPMENT, GOALS, AND IDEALS

Another crucial developmental task of the late oedipal–latency period is to construct an internal set of rules of what is right and what is wrong. Normal children experience guilt for transgressing internal rules with relatively little need for external pressures to make them comply with those rules. An internalized set of goals, standards, moral prohibitions, and demands constitute the direction-giving, enforcing, and self-critical functions of the superego.[16]

Even those narcissistic children who generally behave appropriately will readily lie, cheat, and exploit if they think they can get away with it. For them, moral rules are not internal injunctions but concrete concerns regarding reproachful and punishing adults. The youngsters often believe that they are entitled to use, manipulate, exploit, and do whatever they want to do, and they experience no constraints of guilt or morality.

Narcissistic children not only lack internal norms but expect ruthless exclusion, brutal humiliation, inflexible retaliation, and lack of compassion if their failures or inadequacies should be discovered. It matters little whether the "crime" is a murderous assault against a sibling or an inability to handle a ball at a friendly ball game. The expected consequence for failure is equally terrible.

INTEGRATION OF LANGUAGE AND COGNITIVE DEVELOPMENT

Narcissistic children may be quite impressive, but their real accomplishments and school performance often fail to meet the brilliant promise suggested by their superficial charm and apparent creativity. Their verbal cleverness typically entails empty intellectualizations and word play. "Hot air" and tall tales are advanced in an attempt to cover up a poor grasp of concepts, a limited capacity for sustained attention, a basic difficulty in solving problems in reality, and difficulty in communicating thoughts and feelings effectively.

In many narcissistic children language develops precociously. As charming and impressive as it may be, when it is not coordinated with other ego functions, language usage can become little more than a means for manipulation and exhibitionistic gratification, a weapon to avoid closeness, and a defense against envy, anxiety, or shame.

In sum, the characteristic dynamic and developmental picture presented by narcissistic children consists of: (1) preserved contact with reality; (2) age-inappropriate persistence of omnipotence and grandiosity; (3) failure to develop a relatively autonomous, stable sense of identity—that is, predominance of false-self and as-if phenomena; (4) failure to develop an image of other people as helpful and reliable protectors, limit-setters, interpreters of reality, soothers, sources of support, and models for identification; (5) failure to develop a relatively autonomous and stable sense of self-worth; (6) a maladaptive, development-distorting constellation of defensive operations, characterized by the pervasive use of splitting, isolation of affect, turning passive into active, omnipotence, grandiosity, and devaluation of others; (7) failure to develop relatively autonomous, stable, direction-giving, enforcing, and self-critical functions; and (8) precocious language development not coordinated with other ego skills necessary for effective communication, sustained attention, and solving problems in reality.

Narcissistic children consistently present this developmental profile. In spite of the commonality of features, individual narcissistic patients can be placed along a continuum ranging from better integrated, relatively well adjusted, and higher-functioning children, to more labile, impulsive, poorly adjusted children who shade into the borderline spectrum.[1,39]

Narcissistic disorders may coexist with other DSM-III diagnoses, particularly affective disorders, conduct disorders, avoidant disorders of childhood, oppositional disorders, or overanxious disorders of childhood. A useful point to remember is that narcissistic injuries are an inevitable aspect of normal *or* pathological development. All children encounter those hurts as they attempt to develop a sense of self, establish boundaries, struggle with the limits of omnipotence, face their vulnerabilities, and deal with the pain and frustration of reality. Not surprisingly, narcissistic *traits* are present, to some degree, in everyone's developing character organization. The children described in this chapter are those for whom pathological narcissism is a central feature in their lives and maladjustment.

Pathogenesis of Narcissistic Disorders

A point of convergence for a majority of investigators studying the pathogenesis of narcissistic disorders[41,44] is the relevance ascribed to the earliest phases of development, particularly Mahler's separation-individuation process.[26,27] The achievement of *separation* refers to children's growing capacity to experience themselves as separate and distinct from mother. *Individuation* defines the evolution of increasingly effective coping and adaptive skills, the capacities that guarantee intrapsychic autonomy.

Increasing awareness of separation and growing autonomy lead to what Mahler designated the practicing subphase. "During these precious six to eight months [from the age of ten or twelve months to sixteen or eighteen months], the world is the junior toddler's oyster ... the child seems intoxicated with his own faculties and with the greatness of his own world. Narcissism is at its peak"[27] (p. 71). The maturational spurt in cognition, language, and upright locomotion of the practicing subphase bolsters children's sense of competence and provides them with a powerful tool to handle the newly acquired sense of separateness and the loss of the symbiotic unit with mother. The children's narcissistic investment in their achievements, their body, and the objectives of their expanding reality counters their own sense of smallness and vulnerability.

In a series of papers, Ringsley* (initially in collaboration with Masterson[29]) advances the notion that in both narcissistic and borderline individuals there are specific patterns of mother-child interaction that can be correlated with the separation-individuation process. According to Rinsley, the mothers of future borderline individuals take pride in their infants' dependency and find gratification in experiencing it. In multiple ways, these mothers reward their infants' passive-dependent, clinging behavior. As the infants begin spontaneously to display more active, exploratory, autonomous strivings, however, these mothers withdraw emotionally or punish this behavior in subtle or overt ways. The central message they communicate is "to grow up is to face the calamitous loss or withdrawal of maternal supplies, coupled with the related injunction

*See references 36, 37, 38, 39, 40, and 41.

that to avoid that calamity the child must remain dependent, inadequate, and symbiotic"[41] (p. 5). The overall developmental consequence for the future borderline individual, says Rinsley, is an inhibition of *both* separation and individuation.

Future narcissistic individuals, on the other hand, face a modified maternal injunction. As delineated by Rinsley,[41] these infants receive the consistent message that it is safe to go through the motions of growing up, but only if everything accomplished remains in relation to the maternal object. The overall effect of this form of mother-child interaction is "to inhibit or preclude separation while allowing a significant degree of individuation to proceed, to desynchronize the two subprocesses, as it were" (p. 6).

Rinsley's formulation finds confirmation in the patterns of interaction to be found in the families of narcissistic patients.[4,8,28] In their account of the family dynamics of their patient Matt, Egan and P. Kernberg[8] describe a mother who idealized her son and considered him her possession. Her controlling behavior toward her child betrayed how much the child's growing autonomy and separation threatened her.

Clinical experience suggests that narcissistic children possess notable attributes that increase the likelihood of their selection to play a special role in their families. Unusual beauty, precocious development (particularly language development), and uncommon gifts increase narcissistic children's likelihood of being invested with parents' narcissistic aspirations. An uncanny ability to perceive interpersonal cues often is a striking feature in these children's early life. Such talents fuel parents' efforts to use the child as a receptive screen on which to project parental fantasies and ambitions.

Particular circumstances surrounding the child's birth (e.g., a death in the family, older parents longing for a child and doubtful of their ability to conceive, etc.) endow a child with a special meaning to the family. Those special gifts and meanings are glorified by the parents, who perceive their child as an enlargement of themselves, a source of pride and gratification, the provider of the appreciation to which the parents feel entitled but have been denied. Thus, while inflating the child's omnipotence, the parents simultaneously need to tightly control the child's "performance." While the apple of the parents' eyes, the child may not fail or disappoint them since parental self-esteem has become entwined with the child's magnificence. At the same time parents ignore, ridicule, or reject those aspects of the child that are "weak," frustrated, sad, and vulnerable. Troubled by their own dependency and vulnerability, the parents withdraw emotionally from the child when he or she is helpless or in pain.

This developmental scenario can be summarized as follows: Narcissistic children's sense of omnipotence is enormously enhanced; their sense of uniqueness is fostered, and the exhibitionistic display of competence is rewarded. At the same time, vulnerability, "weakness," pain, or frustration repel the parent or elicit humiliation. The children's emerging sense of self soon reflects the shaping power of those injunctions. They begin to experience as "me" those aspects of themselves that elicit the parents' delighted response. They cannot, on the other hand, integrate a full range of feelings, needs, and self-images into their sense of self, as so many of these self-aspects failed to be mirrored and instead were linked with parental withdrawal. Although the following vignette is an extreme example, it is vividly illustrative:

Adopted when he was four months old, Jimmy soon realized that his adoptive mother carefully scrutinized her adoptive charges by going over them with a fine-tooth comb, so to speak, that would capture any indication of defectiveness. Two children preceding Jimmy and three in the four years that followed his adoption were returned as unacceptable to the adoptive agencies by this mother-inspector. Her reasons for discarding children ranged from discovering that "colored" blood marred one child's bloodstream to suspecting that another infant was infected with syphilis. The message was clear: Failure to live up to her standards of physical, intellectual, and racial "perfection" would result in abandonment. Not surprisingly, the handsome, bright, and verbal Jimmy struggled mightily to perform brilliantly while proclaiming that he was a genius.

ENVIRONMENTAL FACTORS/DEFECTS IN THE HOLDING ENVIRONMENT

There are other possible routes that may lead to a similar deformation of the child's early sense of self. These include gross inadequacies in what has been designated the "holding environment"[31] and in what Winnicott called "good-enough mothering."[49] Examples of such inadequacies include the violence and inconsistency that may be associated with growing up in an urban ghetto, some of the many deprivations associated with extreme poverty, the possible emotional exhaustion and lack of supports of single parents, the unstable home environment and craving for nurturance so often an aspect of adolescent parenthood, violence in the neighborhood, inconsistent management at home, frequent moves, inadequate nutrition, and/or substance abuse in the caretakers.

For many bright and resourceful children, deficits in the holding environment provide a powerful push toward premature closure of dependency needs, precocious self-sufficiency, and reliance on self-nurturing capacities. The emotional price paid by the children is their inability to develop a cohesive sense of self that integrates neediness, dependency, and vulnerability. Perhaps it is in this group that we find the reservoir of narcissistic rage that Noshpitz[32] perceives at the root of much delinquent violence by noting the "callous, unthinking cruelty" that typifies many of these youths, their "gross disrespect for the victim's life," and their indifference to human warmth and caring signal the presence of a narcissistic personality. Noshpitz asserts the picture becomes clear when these youngsters are apprehended for they are so often "arrogant, rather than repentant; angry, not crestfallen; haughty and demanding instead of apologetic and guilt-striken" (p. 17).

Adopted children need to integrate the narcissistic injury of their adoption.[43] They can never completely ignore their biological parents and the fact of abandonment. Furthermore, as Brinich[5] points out, there are specific obstacles to the achievement of an early reciprocal relationship between adoptive mother and child. First, many adopted children encounter disruptions in their early experiences of reciprocity; these act as stresses that foster self-sufficiency and closure of dependency. Second, adoptions are rarely finalized during the first months of the child's life. Until the adoption is finalized, it is natural that both the parents and child feel "on probation," a state of affairs that hampers the formation of a trusting, smoothly reciprocal attachment. Third, as Reeves[35] suggests, the adoptive mother "has 'got' a baby, but has not 'had' a baby" (p. 167). The biological mother's investment in the baby, derived from the sense that the child is a part of her, has been hypothesized as crucial for the development of the symbiotic mother-infant relationship. This relationship may pose a problem for adoptive parents, as the presence of the adopted child can serve to underscore the narcissistic injury of infertility.

CONSTITUTIONAL FACTORS

For other children, constitutional factors may play a significant role in determining a distortion in their self-experience. As Kernberg[19] suggested, children with a constitutionally low tolerance for frustration may feel that their needs are not met even by "average expectable"[15] parents. If these children are sufficiently capable, they may feel inclined to discard their needy aspects and to consolidate their self-image around competence and self-sufficiency. Physically handicapped children seem particularly vulnerable to narcissistic disorders. Handicapped children's sense of self inevitably becomes entangled with their body defect and with the impact the handicap has on the caretakers. It may be as if the world owes handicapped children something, and the parents often behave accordingly, so that pain or a sneeze may trigger frantic responses. Thus overvaluation of the body and a sense of entitlement may come both from within and without.

Conclusion

In summary, multiple routes can be traversed to reach a distorted sense of self. The narcissistic injury children encounter is the feeling that an integral aspect of self —the weak, helpless, vulnerable, sad, dependent self— has to be obliterated. Further, their neediness, sadness, and dependency are dangerous because they drive the love object away or lead to still more pain. But, like the Cheshire cat, the rejected self-experiences do not disappear altogether. They leave behind the disembodied grin of a narcissistic wound, the inevitable feeling of a hole inside.

Schizoid children hold themselves emotionally aloof from the real world and rely extensively on odd fantasies to protect themselves from disorganizing anxiety. In schizoid children, isolation, oddness, hypersensitivity to criticism, and suspiciousness are the central traits. On the other hand, grandiosity, feelings of entitlement, exploitativeness, and devaluation of others are not typically present. In contrast to narcissistic youngsters, schizoid children are more prone to idiosyncratic fantasies, odd speech, bizarre thinking, and intrusions of primary process thinking.

As previously mentioned, affective disorders may coexist with narcissistic disorders. In some instances, pure affective disorders can be differentiated from narcissistic disorders only with difficulty. The presence of a precipitating narcissistic injury or triumph is important if it initiates the affective change in the child with a narcissistic disorder. Also, there is a far more fleeting and rapidly shifting quality to the affect in narcissistic children, which stands in contrast to the greater persistence of the depressed in affective disorders.

Borderline children are more prone to lapses in reality contact and are markedly vulnerable to regression and disorganization. The sense of self in narcissistic children is less shifting than it is in borderline children. For borderline children, experiences of separation can be extremely painful and disorganizing. They are inclined to resort to extreme measures to prevent abandonment or separation. In consequence, borderline children rapidly become overinvolved and overly dependent on others. Narcissistic children, on the other hand, tend to be enormously threatened by dependency and will go to great lengths to prevent intense or close involvements.

Socialized conduct disorders can be differentiated by

the children's capacity to extend themselves to others and to form affectionate bonds. These capacities contrast with the inability to love and the lack of concern and loyalty characteristic of narcissistic children. On the other hand, the descriptive diagnosis of undersocialized conduct disorder may represent a particularly severe and malfunctioning form of narcissistic disorder.

REFERENCES

1. ADLER, G. "The Borderline-Narcissistic Personality Disorder Continuum," *American Journal of Psychiatry,* 138 (1981): 46–50.

2. AMERICAN PSYCHIATRIC ASSOCIATION. *Diagnostic and Statistical Manual of Mental Disorders,* 3rd ed. (DSM-III). Washington, D.C.: American Psychiatric Association, 1980.

3. BALINT, M. *The Basic Fault: Therapeutic Aspects of Regression.* London: Tavistock Publications, 1968.

4. BERKOWITZ, D. A., et al. "Family Contributions to Narcissistic Disturbances in Adolescents," *International Review of Psycho-Analysis,* 1 (1974): 353–362.

5. BRINICH, R.M. "Some Potential Effects of Adoption on Self and Object Representations," *Psychoanalytic Study of the Child,* 35 (1980): 107–135.

6. CAIN, A. "On the Meaning of 'Playing Crazy' in Borderline Children," *Psychiatry,* 27 (1964): 278–289.

7. DEUTSCH, H. "Some Forms of Emotional Disturbance and Their Relationship to Schizophrenia," *Psychoanalytic Quarterly,* 11 (1942): 301–321.

8. EGAN, J., and KERNBERG, P. "Pathological Narcissism in Childhood," *Journal of the American Psychoanalytic Association,* 32 (1984): 39–62.

9. ERIKSON, E. H. "Identity and the Life Cycle," in G. S. Klein, ed., *Psychological Issues,* (1959): 1–171.

10. FENICHEL, O. *The Psychoanalytic Theory of Neurosis.* New York: W. W. Norton, 1945.

11. FREUD, S. "Civilization and Its Discontents," in J. Strachey, ed., *The Standard Edition of the Complete Psychological Works of Sigmund Freud* (hereafter *The Standard Edition*), vol. 21. London: Hogarth Press, 1957, pp. 64–145.

12. ———. "Mourning and Melancholia," in *The Standard Edition,* vol. 14. London: Hogarth Press, 1957, pp. 243–258.

13. ———. "On Narcissism: An Introduction," in *The Standard Edition,* vol. 14. London: Hogarth Press, 1957, pp. 73–102.

14. ———. "The Unconscious," in *The Standard Edition,* vol. 14. London: Hogarth Press, 1957, pp. 166–215.

15. HARTMANN, H. *Ego Psychology and the Problem of Adaptation.* New York: International Universities Press, 1958.

16. HARTMANN, H., and LOEWENSTEIN, R. M. "Notes on the Superego," *Psychoanalytic Study of the Child,* 17 (1962): 42–81.

17. JACOBSON, E. *The Self and the Object World.* New York: International Universities Press, 1964.

18. JOFFE, W. G., and SANDLER, J. "Some Conceptual Problems Involved in the Consideration of Disorders of Narcissism," *Journal of Child Psychotherapy,* 2 (1967): 56–66.

19. KERNBERG, O. "Factors in the Psychoanalytic Treatment of Narcissistic Personalities," *Journal of the American Psychoanalytic Association,* 18 (1970): 51–85.

20. ———. *Borderline Conditions and Pathological Narcissism.* New York: Jason Aronson, 1975.

21. KOHUT, H. "Forms and Transformations of Narcissism," *Journal of the American Psychoanalytic Association,* 14 (1966): 243–272.

22. ———. "The Psychoanalytic Treatment of Narcissistic Personality Disorders: Outline of a Systematic Approach," *Psychoanalytic Study of the Child,* 23, (1968): 86–113.

23. ———. "Thoughts on Narcissism and Narcissistic Rage," *Psychoanalytic Study of the Child,* 27 (1973): 360–400.

24. ———. *The Restoration of the Self.* New York: International Universities Press, 1977.

25. LASCH, C. *The Culture of Narcissism: American Life in an Age of Diminishing Expectations.* New York: W. W. Norton, 1978.

26. MAHLER, M., and McDEVITT, J. "Thoughts on the Emergence of the Sense of Self, with Particular Emphasis on the Body Self," *Journal of the American Psychoanalytic Association,* 30 (1982): 827–848.

27. MAHLER, M., PINE, F., and BERGMAN, A. *The Psychological Birth of the Human Infant: Symbiosis and Individuation.* New York: Basic Books, 1974.

28. MANDELBAUM, A. "The Family Treatment of the Borderline Patient," in P. Hartocollis, ed., *Borderline Personality Disorders: The Concept, the Syndrome, the Patients.* New York. International Universities Press, 1977, pp. 423–438.

29. MASTERSON, J., and RINSLEY, D. "The Borderline Syndrome: The Role of the Mother in the Genesis and Psychic Structure of the Borderline Personality," *International Journal of Psycho-Analysis,* 56 (1975): 163–177.

30. MILLER, A. *Prisoners of Childhood.* New York: Basic Books, 1981.

31. MODELL, A. " 'The Holding Environment' and the Therapeutic Action of Psychoanalysis," *Journal of the American Psychoanalytic Association,* 24 (1976): 285–307.

32. NOSHPITZ, J. "Narcissism and Aggression," *American Journal of Psychotherapy,* 38 (1984): 17–34.

33. ORNSTEIN, A. "Self-Pathology in Childhood: Developmental and Clinical Considerations," in K. Robson, ed., *The Psychiatric Clinics of North America: Development and Pathology of the Self,* vol. 4. Philadelphia: W. B. Saunders, 1981, pp. 435–453.

34. PULVER, S. E. "Narcissism: The Term and the Concept," *Journal of the American Psychoanalytic Association,* 18 (1970): 319–341.

35. REEVES, A. "Children with Surrogate Parents: Cases Seen in Analytic Therapy and an Aetiological Hypothesis," *British Journal of Medical Psychology,* 44 (1971): 155–171.

36. RINSLEY, D. "Borderline Psychopathology: A Review of Aetiology, Dynamics and Treatment," *International Review of Psycho-Analysis,* 5 (1978): 45–54.

37. ———. "The Developmental Etiology of Borderline and Narcissistic Disorders," *Bulletin of the Menninger Clinic,* 44 (1980): 127–134.

38. ———. "Diagnosis and Treatment of Borderline and

Narcissistic Children and Adolescents," *Bulletin of the Menninger Clinic,* 44, (1980): 147–170.

39. ———. "Dynamic and Developmental Issues in Borderline and Related 'Spectrum Disorders,' " in M. H. Stone, ed., *The Psychiatric Clinics of North America: Borderline Disorders,* vol. 4. Philadelphia: W. B. Saunders, 1981, pp. 117–132.

40. ———. *Borderline and Other Self Disorders: A Developmental and Object-Relations Perspective.* New York: Jason Aronson, 1982.

41. ———. "A Comparison of Borderline and Narcissistic Personality Disorders," *Bulletin of the Menninger Clinic,* 48 (1984): 1–9.

42. SARNOFF, C. *Latency.* New York: Jason Aronson, 1976.

43. SCHECTER, M. "Observations of Adopted Children," *Archives of General Psychiatry,* 3 (1960): 21–32.

44. SETTLAGE, C. "The Psychoanalytic Understanding of Narcissistic and Borderline Personality Disorders: Advances in Developmental Theory," in R. F. Lax, S. Bach, and J. Burland, eds., *Rapproachment: The Critical Subphase of Separation Individuation.* New York: Jason Aronson, 1980, pp. 77–100.

45. STOLOROW, R. D. "Toward a Functional Definition of Narcissism," *International Journal of Psycho-Analysis,* 56 (1975): 179–185.

46. TOLPIN, M. "On the Beginnings of a Cohesive Self: An Application of the Concept of Transmuting Internalization to the Study of the Transitional Object and Signal Anxiety," *Psychoanalytic Study of the Child,* 26 (1972): 316–352.

47. TOOLEY, K. "The Small Assassins: Clinical Notes on a Subgroup of Murderous Children," *Journal of the American Academy of Child Psychiatry,* 14 (1975): 306–318.

48. WINNICOTT, D. W. "Ego Distortion in Terms of True and False Self," in *The Maturational Processes and the Facilitating Environment. Studies in the Theory of Emotional Development.* New York: International Universities Press, 1965, pp. 140–152.

49. ———. *The Maturational Processes and the Facilitating Environment: Studies in the Theory of Emotional Development.* New York: International Universities Press, 1965.

33 / The Borderline Child

Jules R. Bemporad, Henry F. Smith, and Graeme Hanson

Introduction

In volume 2 of this *Handbook* Chethik[5] presented a historical review of the concept of the borderline child, beginning with its evolution from Bender's[2] description in the 1940s of childhood schizophrenia. Most of the first writers were psychoanalysts interested in the ego functions, object relations, and psychodynamics of the condition. While some child analysts, such as Kernberg,[16] continue to explore such issues today, they have been joined by other investigators attempting to establish descriptive clinical criteria for a borderline syndrome in children. These two approaches highlight not only the tension between differing diagnostic nosologies, as Shaprio[22] has recently discussed, but also several important controversies. First, is this one "syndrome" or several "conditions"? If it is the latter, do these conditions exist on the same spectrum from an etiological, developmental, psychodynamic, or neurophysiological point of view? Finally, does the borderline child bear any relation to the borderline adult? Historically, the concept of the borderline child developed separately from though simultaneously with that of the borderline adult. Only occasional bridges were built between the two concepts, mainly by theoreticians interested in the etiological implications of Mahler's work.[12,24] Many authors have felt that the use of the term borderline to refer to several different descriptive types of children and adults is confusing and leads to premature closure on the preceding questions.

We would add to the historical papers cited in volume 2 Anna Freud's[10] 1956 contribution, which emphasizes the variety of difficulties these children present and recommends a broad assessment of their intrapsychic functioning from a developmental point of view, and Engel's[9] 1963 description of the psychological testing of borderline children. Engel noted the intrusion of primary process thinking, particularly on less structured tests, and the panic the child experiences at the disintegration of more advanced ego functioning. Recently Leichtman and Shapiro[18] have published the most comprehensive description to date of these psychological test patterns.

Since the publication of volume 2, several authors

have attempted to clarify the diagnostic criteria. Morales[20] divided borderline children into five subgroups, each manifesting a different primary feature: (1) sudden and severe regression; (2) unpredictable, impulsive, and murderous rages; (3) extreme but nondiscriminating dependency; (4) extreme separation anxiety; and (5) intensely narcissistic features. Gilpin, Sexson, and Ward[13] suggested similar clinical criteria for children, designated "true fluid borderlines," who did not fit the Group for the Advancement of Psychiatry criteria for any stable personality disorder. Finally, noting the inappropriateness for children of the DSM-III criteria for "borderline personality disorder" in adults, Vela, Gottlieb, and Gottlieb[23] suggested six diagnostic symptom clusters: (1) disturbed interpersonal relationships; (2) disturbances in the sense of reality; (3) excessive intense anxiety; (4) severe impulsive behavior; (5) neuroticlike symptoms; and (6) uneven or distorted development.

In a further effort to clarify the picture, several authors have tried to examine these children in the light of other theoretical perspectives or clinical entities. Grubbs,[14] for example, studied one borderline adolescent's cognition in Piagetian terms and found marked similarities with the preoperational thinking of younger children. Cohen and associates[6] compared these children to those with attention deficit disorders, and Marcus, Ovsiew, and Hans[19] suggested a research method for studying the neurological dysfunctions noted in borderline children.

However, there have been few large-scale investigations of these children. Follow-up studies, for example, might clarify their natural history and thus settle whether this is one syndrome or many, and whether, as Kernberg[16] has suggested, these children grow up to be borderline adults. Kestenbaum[17] attempted to do this with a small sample of seven children, diagnosed according to the criteria of Vela, Gottlieb, and Gottlieb.[23] She reported heterogeneous outcomes with adult diagnoses ranging from anxiety neurosis to paranoid schizophrenia. Only one of the seven met adult borderline criteria.

Research efforts might also validate the etiological hypotheses that have taken root in Margaret Mahler's theories and observations. One such study was attempted by Bradley[4] in 1979, which showed that prior to five years of age, borderline children suffer a greater number of separations from their mothers than do control populations. The study, however, was hampered by the use of adult criteria for diagnosing the children.

One of the major problems in diagnosing borderline children is that the pathology may not be evident at all times but may become manifest only at times of emotional stress. It has been found also that the syndrome is difficult, if not impossible, to recognize with certainty before school age since much of the behaviors may be within the normal range for younger children. Finally, the term borderline may encompass a group of disorders, each showing a relative preponderance of some aspect of the multiplicity of difficulties.

These children differ from those with pervasive developmental disorder (PDD) by their ability to relate to others, their fuller range of affects, and their greater ability to withstand changes in the environment. Borderline children also do not demonstrate oddities of movement, abnormalities of speech, or peculiarities of sensation typical of children with PDDs. The greatest distinction between these two conditions is the fluctuation of functioning found in borderline children so that they, at times of emotional security, may appear neurotic or even normal.

Borderline children also differ in significant ways from those with narcissistic disorders, which are described in chapter 32 in this volume. While both diagnostic groups present a healthy façade masking more severe psychopathology, the types of symptoms exhibited are quite distinct. Narcissistic children are consciously manipulative, grandiose, and pseudo–self-reliant. Borderline children openly seek help from others, fear for their own sanity, and demonstrate regressive dependency. Also, narcissistic children do not show the lapses in reality testing and are not vulnerable to disorganization. The narcissitic child appears to use others for boosting self-esteem and obtaining gratification while the borderline child needs others for a basic sense of security against terrifying affects and fantasies and for continued contact with reality.

The description of the borderline syndrome presented here derives from an intensive study[1] of twenty-four children who had been diagnosed independently as borderline by three experienced clinicians on the basis of similarity of the clinical picture to descriptions in earlier published case reports. These children did not fit suitably in any official diagnostic category but exhibited difficulties in many crucial areas of functioning. It was found that, although a child may be more impaired in one area than another, all twenty-four children were affected in the five major areas: (1) fluctuation of functioning, (2) nature and extent of anxiety, (3) thought content and processes, (4) relationship to others, and (5) deficiency in control. Using these five areas of psychopathology as a diagnostic guide, other children were found who fit the proposed clinical picture so that the syndrome appeared to manifest coherence and consistency. These areas are to be taken as a rough guide in which the overall profile rather than any one area of difficulty should be considered in diagnosis.

Areas of Psychopathology

FLUCTUATION OF FUNCTIONING

The characteristic of fluctuation of functioning describes these children's oscillation between neurotic and psychoticlike states secondary to environmental reassurance or threat. These children often present initially with neuroticlike defenses and behaviors but under the stress of fear or anxiety they will exhibit psychotic preoccupations or behaviors.

One eleven-year-old boy, for example, climbed on a pile of rocks and then became afraid that he could not get down again. As his fear escalated, he started talking wildly about monsters and even sharks coming to eat him. Once he was down safely with his counselor, the boy became calm and appropriate again.

Often unstructured play will elicit fantasies that arouse anxiety, resulting in increasingly chaotic and bizarre preoccupations.

Carl, a ten-year-old boy who was capable of behaving at an age-appropriate level for considerable periods of time and could be quite engaging and charming, entered the playroom with his new, inexperienced therapist. The boy began to build an Eiffel Tower of blocks and engaged in a reasonable verbal dialogue with the therapist. As the tower grew taller and the therapist expressed interest and enthusiasm for the child's activity, the boy became increasingly excited. Carl had a male and female doll climb the tower and begin to kiss on top of the tower. He then proceeded to have the doll couple engage in intercourse and then pretended the male doll was being anally penetrated. At this point, the boy pretended to jab a pencil at his own anus. Then he said that both dolls were pregnant and that he himself was pregnant. The dolls fell from the tower and were then encased in clay to become one amorphous lump of merged figures, which he then proceeded to dump into the water-filled sink. Throughout this play, Carl became increasingly excited, agitated, and anxious, with his activity proceeding at a frenetic pace. At one point in the heat of excitement, he grabbed at his therapist's genital area and then ran out of the playroom and back to the children's inpatient ward where, in the presence of his counselor and other known figures, he quite quickly regained composure. He appeared calm and quite appropriate when the therapist arrived on the ward.

This clinical characteristic of rapid fluctuation in functioning has been described extensively by Ekstein and Wallerstein,[7,8] who have written that borderline children could not master anxiety resulting from a lack of empathic response from others with neurotic defenses but were forced to retreat into bizarre fantasies in order to diminish their painful affects while maintaining their contact with needed others. Reassurance from others will result in a removal of stress and a return to a level of neurotic or near-normal functioning.

This propensity for utilization of psychoticlike bizarreness of thought or a sense of overwhelming panic may result from a freeing up of fantasy material that rapidly escalates to threatening themes even without the occurrence of a chance unempathic comment from others. Engel,[9] for example, found that standard projective test materials were sufficient to cause a sense of panic and mental disorganization in such children. It has been found that unstructured play or certain emotionally stimulating situations may result in the intrusion of disordered thinking and behavior as a means of response to overwhelming anxiety. However, these children do not persist in a dereistic world as would a psychotic child but gradually regain a realistic grasp of their environment.

NATURE AND EXTENT OF ANXIETY

A second clinical characteristic of the borderline child is difficulty in managing anxiety, which often escalates to panic. Borderline children often present with neurotic symptoms such as phobias or obsessions, which cannot withstand environmental stresses or internal fantasies. The children communicate their mounting sense of terror and rely on others to help them allay their fears. At other times, the children express their anxiety though frenzied action that may be destructive to self or others.

A further difficulty in borderline children's management of anxiety is their inability to respond to signal anxiety as a warning and to alter their behavior accordingly. Instead, the children experience signal anxiety as a threat in itself, impairing their capacity to learn from experience or to behave appropriately in emotionally adverse circumstances. While the fragile defenses are all too readily overwhelmed, borderline children do not retreat into a dereistic world of detachment and delusions that might lessen their discomfort. Therefore, as Frijling-Shreuder[11] has observed, borderline children may be more tormented by their anxiety than neurotic children, who can remain in contact with an unpleasant reality and still master anxiety, or than psychotic children, who may also be relatively free of anxiety by grossly distorting their experiential world. Borderline children remain in relative contact with their world and ask others to help them deal with their anxiety but cannot decrease this threat by themselves. Engel[9] was particularly struck by borderline children's ability to communicate their terror in understandable terms when confronted by alarming stimuli of unstructured projective tests.

The sources of this overwhelming anxiety appear closer to those observed in psychosis than in neurosis despite the neuroticlike quality of defenses. For instance, borderline children may not express concern over having disobeyed an authority figure or the expectation of punishment following the breaking of a social rule; rather they describe a sense of self-annihilation, body mutilation, or world catastrophe. Concerns about their bodies disintegrating or their minds falling apart are frequently expressed. One boy feared his insides would fall out when he defecated. Another child feared that water demons would drown him. He also could not tolerate the sound of thunder. While he could not describe his resultant panic specifically, he seemed to indicate that a thunderclap somehow pierced his body. As such, these children somewhat resemble Hoch and Polatin's description [15] of adult "pseudoneurotic schizophrenics" who unsuccessfully try to cope with psychotic fears with neurotic defenses.

THOUGHT CONTENT AND PROCESSES

The aforementioned difficulties in managing anxiety are related to borderline children's excessive fluidity of thought. Because of their poor differentiation between fantasy and reality, threatening ideas intrude into the stream of consciousness. These intrusions refer repeatedly to themes of bodily destruction, death, or psychological dyscontrol, and appear prompted either by an external stress, such as rejection by a needed other, or by a neutral stimulus that has taken on a particular threatening significance, such as the sight of a knife or toy gun. These intrusions of frightening themes may be clearly observed in unstructured play situations when the children's inner life is activated by the play materials and they begin to introduce fantasy into their play. Soon the associations turn to frightening overt sexual or aggressive fantasies that are acted out in play with increasing anxiety and physical activity until the use of displacement dissipates and the children themselves become part of the "play" they are describing.

Some borderline children are aware of their vulnerability to the intrusion of frightening themes with accompanying anxiety and attempt to defend themselves as best they can by avoidance of threatening situations, minor distortion of reality, or restricting their cognitive activities to relatively "safe" areas. As a result of these inadequate defensive maneuvers, borderline children often show a marked restriction in thinking or play, resulting in lopsided learning and academic performance. Play is often repetitive and unimaginative and conversation may be equally restricted. Frequently there is disparity between an impressive expertise with relatively obscure subjects and an amazing ignorance of commonplace practical knowledge. One ten-year-old boy could talk intelligently and in great detail about metallurgy but did not know his address, could not go to stores by himself, and had difficulty making change. A nine-year-old girl was familiar with ancient Egyptian embalming and burial rites while unable to maintain a social conversation with peers.

Other children exhibit an occasional concreteness in understanding language, particularly in the usage of idioms. Rosenfeld and Sprince, [21] for example, described a child who believed the school buildings would be destroyed when he was told that school would "break up" for the holidays.

RELATIONSHIP TO OTHERS

The vulnerability to the external vicissitudes of stress and the particular difficulty in grasping the meaning of idioms or other linguistic conventions make relationships difficult for borderline children. We have observed a variety of disturbed modes of relating in our sample. Often children may form a close, need-fulfilling relationship with one adult who is sought out as a source of security and protection against anxiety while relationships with others are fraught with fear and hostility. Other children appear to be able to substitute one person for another with little regard beyond the meeting of personal needs. Whatever the quality or depth of attachment, borderline children get along better with adults than with peers, who will not take pains to gratify needs and who will not tolerate the peculiarities of behavior. Some elementary-school-age borderline children are referred by their school teachers for asking or trying to sit on their laps and be cuddled like infants. One ten-year-old boy would wrap himself around his counselor's legs and try to climb up his body.

In peer-group situations, borderline children will tend to withdraw and be jealous of adult attention. They may torment smaller children while being fearful of children their own age. Their odd interests, peculiar behavior, and concrete thinking may cause others to tease them, further threatening peer relationships.

DEFICIENCY OF CONTROL

The clinical parameter of deficiency of control refers to those areas borderline children find so difficult to master in an age-appropriate manner. These include maintaining anxiety, managing anger, delaying gratification, and repressing primary process material. These difficulties represent a failure on many levels to contain negative affects and thoughts that too readily spill over into hyperactivity, impulsive acts, panic, and temper tantrums. Borderline children are deficient in the ability to modulate and sublimate drives that are activated by experience from without and fantasy from within. A ten-year-old boy used puppets to play out a scene of a bad child being punished. As the play continued, the punishment became more and more severe with increasing agitation on the child's part. He appeared panic-stricken, had to stop suddenly, and ran from the room. Some of these children are particularly sensitive to environmental tension, becoming barometers of familial stress and responding with inappropriate hyperactivity or tantrums, which results in their being scapegoated by family members.

These five categories describe the basic clinical profile of a borderline child (see table 33–1). While all of these areas of psychological function are affected to some extent, each child, however, may show more impairment in one area than another. Particular extremes of the syndrome are those children who also manifest symptoms of attentional deficit disorder such as hyperactivity, distractibility, and impulsivity in contrast to more schizoidlike children who are hypoactive, quiet, and solitary. Some borderline children exhibit additional symptoms that do not fall easily within any of the major symptom categories just described. These

features include a general lack of age-appropriate social functioning, inattention to personal grooming, and a failure to learn from experience. Such children may repeatedly pick their nose in public or walk around with pants or shirts unbuttoned, oblivious to the effect their behavior or appearance has on others. Other children show various "soft" signs suggestive of neurological impairment, such as poor concentration, hyperactivity, and mixed laterality. Finally, these children demonstrate an unevenness in development, with retardation in some functions, age-appropriate abilities in others, and precocious capacities in still others. This simultaneous functioning on different age levels is almost pathognomonic of the syndrome, but the particular pattern may vary from child to child.

A recent empirical study[3] suggests the validity of the borderline syndrome as a clinical entity as the five major areas of symptomatology were shown to cluster together in seventy borderline children when com-

TABLE 33–1

Major Areas of Psychopathology in the Borderline Child

I. Fluctuation of functioning
   A. Rapid decompensation secondary to objectively minimal emotional stress with rapid reintegration after reassurance from environmental figures
   B. Brief shifts from neurotic to psychotic ideation
   C. Recurrent intrusions of bizarre preoccupations and fantasies
   D. Extreme dependence of level of functioning on environmental support
II. Nature and extent of anxiety
   A. Difficulty containing anxiety with rapid escalation of anxiety to panic unless helped by environmental figures
   B. Inability to utilize signal anxiety
   C. Basis of anxiety residing in fears of destruction, mutilation, and emotional annihilation
   D. Greater suffering from anxiety due to inadequacy of neurotic defenses and lack of psychotic reconstitutive symptoms
III. Thought content and processes
   A. Inadequate "synthetic ego functions" with some gross distortions and concretizations but without stable delusions, hallucinations, or prolonged or profound loss of reality contact
   B. Excessive fluidity of thought between fantasy and reality with inability to control potentially frightening avenues of association
   C. Short "reality span" with recurrent but transient intrusion of grotesque and bizarre fantasy themes
   D. Concern with survival manifested by poorly developed defenses (obsessions, phobias, extreme dependency, merging) to ward off possibility of catastrophic destruction
   E. Proficiency in obscure areas of knowledge with lack of awareness of practical, everyday matters
   F. Heterogeneous cognitive defects
IV. Relationships to others
   A. Immature attachments to need-fulfilling adults (merging, primitive identification, dependency)
   B. Excessive reliance on others to maintain inner security, able to function well with trusted adult
   C. Poor relationship with peers, inability to utilize intellectual talents in group situations
V. Deficiency of control
   A. Difficulty delaying gratification or tolerating frustration
   B. Syncretic expression of anxiety and tension by action and aggression
   C. Difficulty containing inner life so that anxiety leads to action
VI. Associated symptoms
   A. Social awkwardness, lack of adaptiveness
   B. Neurological "soft" signs
   C. General unevenness in development

---

pared by blind raters to seventy random control patients and twenty-four seriously disturbed control children. While the presence of all five symptom areas did significantly differentiate the borderline group, two symptoms, poor impulse control and poor peer relations, occurred with high frequency in both control groups.

Etiology, Clinical Course, and Prognosis

Current knowledge of the causes of borderline syndrome is rudimentary and based largely on isolated clinical observations that stress metapsychological or psychodynamic aspects. While these observations are certainly valuable and serve as crucial aids in the treatment of such children, they add little to questions regarding etiology.

In the authors' evaluation of borderline children, we have been struck by the frequent finding of organic impairment and of a history of being raised in a chaotic home environment that often includes physical and sexual abuse. Twenty-two of our original sample of twenty-four children exhibited some form of organic involvement such as abnormal but non-diagnostic electroencephalograms, hyperactivity, learning disabilities, poor coordination, and speech problems. Bentivegna, Ward, and Bentivegna[3] reported a significantly higher frequency of organic indicators in their sample of seventy borderline children than in their two clinical control groups. Kernberg[16] also has noticed an "extraordinary" high incidence of organicity in her sample of borderline children and believes that this syndrome often overlaps with minimal brain dysfunction.

Neuropsychological evaluations of borderline children suggest a deficit on attentional tasks; a fragmented, piece-by-piece approach to problem-solving tests; language disorders; and numerous neurological abnormalities in coordination and motor functions.

Familial disturbance has also been found uniformly in the authors' group of borderline children. Of our original sample of twenty-four children, ten presented frank evidence of physical abuse. However, much more pervasive than abuse was a history of inconsistent care and of the involvement of the child in bizarre parental activities. For example, one patient had his head shaved by his mother despite ridicule from peers, another mother regularly wiped the seven-year-old patient after each bowel movement, another was force fed until he vomited, another was told repeatedly that his penis would fall off, another

was given LSD by his father when he was eighteen months of age, and another was washed in the tub by her father into her teens and modeled underwear for him. One child's mother believed the patient was a witch and treated her as a strange being; on one occasion she tried to pull out the child's tongue. One boy was sent to school in his sister's clothes. Many children witnessed their parents' sexual activities as well as recurrent arguments and physical fights. Almost every family presented a home atmosphere of actual and potential violence, of constant turmoil and disorganization and lack of consistency. The presence of chaotic families was found also by Bentivegna, Ward, and Bentivegna,[3] as well as Kernberg,[16] in their samples of borderline children.

The parents of these children were considerably disturbed. The fathers manifested instability in relationships and in emotional control. Some "kidnapped" the child from their estranged wives or subjected their families to scenes of violence and aggression. Many of the mothers exhibited symptoms of adult borderline personality disorder with instability, lack of empathy in relationships, distortion of essential aspects of everyday life, and poor frustration tolerance.

Organic deficits could contribute to difficulties in motor control, to the inability to contain anxiety, and to problems with learning and social cognitive skills. However, these neurological factors do not account for the entire clinical picture. Rather, the syndrome can be conceptualized as the result of a vulnerable child raised in an environment that lacks structure, stability, and adequate reality testing. Borderline states may be conceptualized as resulting from a combination of different etiological factors, the preponderance of each being responsible for the variations seen in each child.

The eventual fate of borderline children as adults is as yet unknown beyond clinical reports on individual cases. Gerleerd[12] and Weil[24] found that the few that they followed to adolescence were described as "odd" and socially peculiar. We have observed a variable outcome in the handful of children available for follow-up evaluation. One child subsequently experienced episodes of schizophrenia. Another is doing relatively well as an adolescent, although he remains somewhat shy and withdrawn. Others show continuing impairment in social relationships and in vocational abilities. One nineteen-year-old formerly borderline girl is functioning adequately in a group home but cannot return home for fear of "becoming crazy." While obviously premature at this state of knowledge, it may be conjectured that those children who had the best outcome were the least neurologically impaired, had intensive treatment, and experienced an improved environment either as a result of placement outside the home or of an amelioration of parental psychopathology. These limited follow-up evaluations confirm the variety of adult outcomes of borderline children previously reported by Kestenbaum.[17]

Validity of the Borderline Concept in Childhood

The existence of borderline conditions in childhood has been questioned[22,23] on the basis that there is a lack of uniformity of diagnosis, that children so diagnosed do not resemble adults with borderline personality disorder, and that there is no evidence that these children grow up to be borderline adults. While no pathognomonic test or symptom exists for borderline diagnosis in childhood, there is an agreement in the literature on the constellation of clinical symptoms that are manifested by these children. The paucity of large-scale research diagnostic studies remains a problem that hopefully will be remedied in the future.

The relation of the childhood syndrome to adult borderline disorders is unclear, and it may be that the only element the two conditions share is the label borderline. The descriptions of both syndromes appeared simultaneously in the literature with little effect on each other. Since the early contributions, a great deal of interest has focused on adult borderline disorders, with a widening of the originally described clinical array of symptoms. In contrast, the term borderline, when applied to children, continues to imply a condition on the border between neurosis and psychosis, with alternating manifestations of each. It could be argued that another diagnostic term should be used for these children so as to avoid confusion with adult borderline conditions. However, much of the early clinical as well as the current literature on these children utilized the term borderline as a diagnostic modifier and so this label has stuck, possibly for lack of a better nosological term. It may be best for these conditions to be called something else, just as childhood schizophrenia is now called pervasive developmental disorder. This might help in establishing the syndrome, whatever its label, independently from any relationship to borderline adults.

REFERENCES

1. BEMPORAD, J. R., et al. "Borderline Syndromes in Children: Criteria for Diagnosis," *American Journal of Psychiatry,* 139 (1982): 596–602.

2. BENDER, L. "Childhood Schizophrenia," *Nervous Child,* 1 (1942): 138–140.

3. BENTIVEGNA, S. W., WARD, L.B., and BENTIVEGNA, B. S.: "Study of a Diagnostic Profile of the Borderline Syndrome in Children," *Child Psychiatry and Human Development,* 15 (1985): 198–205.

4. BRADLEY, S. J. "The Relationship of Early Maternal Separation to Borderline Personality in Children and Adolescents: A Pilot Study," *American Journal of Psychiatry,* 136 (1979): 424–426.

5. CHETHIK, M. "The Borderline Child," in J. D. Noshpitz, ed., *Basic Handbook of Child Psychiatry,* vol. 2. New York: Basic Books, 1979, pp. 304–321.

6. COHEN, D. J., et al. "Borderline Syndromes and Attention Deficit Disorders of Childhood: Clinical and Neurological Perspectives," in K. S. Robson, ed., *The Borderline Child.* New York: McGraw-Hill, 1983, pp. 197–221.

7. EKSTEIN, R., and WALLERSTEIN, J. "Observations on the Psychology of Borderline and Psychotic Children," *Psychoanalytic Study of the Child,* 9 (1954): 344–369.

8. ———. "Observations on the Psychotherapy of Borderline and Psychotic Children," *Psychoanalytic Study of the Child,* 11 (1956): 303–311.

9. ENGEL, M. "Psychological Testing of Borderline Psychotic Children," *Archives of General Psychiatry,* 8 (1963): 426–434.

10. FREUD, A. "The Assessment of Borderline Cases," in: *The Writings of Anna Freud,* vol. 5. New York: International Universities Press, (originally published 1956.): 1969, 301–314.

11. FRIJLING-SCHREUDER, E. "Borderline States in Children," *Psychoanalytic Study of the Child,* 24 (1969): 307–327.

12. GERLEERD, E. R. "Borderline States in Childhood and Adolescence," *Psychoanalytic Study of the Child,* 13 (1958): 279–295.

13. GILPIN, D. C., SEXSON, S., and WARD, C. "Research on the Concept of the 'Borderline' Psychotic Child," in E. J. Anthony and D. C. Gilpin, eds., *Three Further Clinical Faces of Childhood.* New York: Spectrum Publications, 1981, pp. 231–242.

14. GRUBBS, J. H. "A Borderline Case in the Light of Piaget's Theory," in E. J. Anthony and D. C. Gilpin, eds., *Three Further Clinical Faces of Childhood.* New York: Spectrum Publications, 1981, pp. 295–305.

15. HOCH, P., and POLATIN, P. "Pseudoneurotic Forms of Schizophrenia," *Psychiatric Quarterly,* 23 (1949): 248–276.

16. KERNBERG, P. F. "Borderline Conditions: Childhood and Adolescent Aspects," in K. S. Robson, ed., *The Borderline Child.* New York: McGraw-Hill, 1983, pp. 101–119.

17. KESTENBAUM, C. J. "The Borderline Child at Risk for Major Psychiatric Disorder in Adult Life," in K. S. Robson, ed., *The Borderline Child.* New York: McGraw-Hill, 1983, pp. 49–81.

18. LEICHTMAN, M., and SHAPIRO, S. "A Clinical Ap-

proach to the Psychological Testing of Borderline Children," in K. S. Robson, ed., *The Borderline Child*. New York: McGraw-Hill, 1983, pp. 121–170.

19. MARCUS, J., OVSIEW, F., and HANS, S. "Neurological Dysfunction in Borderline Children," in K. S. Robson, ed., *The Borderline Child*. New York: McGraw-Hill, 1983, pp. 171–195.

20. MORALES, J. "The Borderline Spectrum in Children," in E. J. Anthony and D. C. Gilpin, eds., *Three Further Clinical Faces of Childhood*. New York: Spectrum Publications, 1981, pp. 221–230.

21. ROSENFELD, S. K., and SPRINCE, M. P. "An Attempt

to Formulate the Meaning of the Concept 'Borderline,'" *Psychoanalytic Study of the Child*, 18 (1963): 603–635.

22. SHAPIRO, T. "The Borderline Syndrome in Childhood: A Critique," in K. S. Robson, ed., *The Borderline Child*. New York: McGraw-Hill, 1983, pp. 11–29.

23. VELA, R., GOTTLIEB, H., and GOTTLIEB, E. "Borderline Syndromes in Childhood: A Critical Review," in K. S. Robson, ed., *The Borderline Child*. New York: McGraw-Hill, 1983, pp. 31–48.

24. WEIL, A. P. "Certain Severe Disturbances of Ego Development in Childhood," *Psychoanalytic Study of the Child*, 8 (1953): 271–287.

34 / Anxiety-Related Disorders: Recent Advances

Alexander R. Lucas and Keith G. Kramlinger

In recent years a number of advances have stimulated us to reconsider the causes of anxiety-related disorders and consequently to reexamine their classification. These advances have come in the areas of neurochemistry and psychopharmacology and are leading us to rethink the ways in which we can best categorize certain emotional and mental disorders. Anxiety as an emotion is basic to the concept of the psychoneurotic disorders and a major component of many other emotional and mental conditions. However, its mechanisms and biological substrate are still not fully understood. Heretofore the focus has fallen either on its psychological and psychodynamic meanings or on its physiological concomitants. Current advances in neurochemistry have reached a point at which the biological concomitants of anxiety are beginning to be understood; inevitably they involve quantifiable parameters that seem far removed from mental phenomena. Nonetheless, the chasm between neuronal events and mental phenomena is beginning to be bridged.

The purpose of this chapter is to consider the research advances of recent years as they pertain to our understanding of anxiety and of the disorders in which anxiety is a prominent component. Most of this work has come from animal studies and work with adult patients and has potential applicability to the understanding of many emotional states. Just how relevant this work is to disorders of children will be explored in this chapter and in chapter 5.

Elucidation of chemical events accompanying emotions may lead to a better understanding of the relationship among disorders and may indeed provide the foundation for building a new theory of mental disorder. Such new scientific advances should be integrated with the rich network of older concepts in the quest for a comprehensive theory of neurobiology.

Historical Concepts of Anxiety

According to Kandel,[19] the idea that anxiety is inborn and that a neutral stimulus can be associated with it through learning has come from two sources. Beginning with Charles Darwin and George Romanes, work in comparative and evolutionary biology showed that most animals, like humans, have inborn defensive behaviors. William James proposed that in animals and in humans these built-in defensive behaviors are triggered by anxiety, an inborn tendency to react to danger situations with fear. Experimental support for the notion that anxiety can be learned came from Pavlov's discovery[26] that defensive reflexes can be modified by experience and elicited by a previously neutral stimulus.

Freud[12] independently came to similar conclusions. Because painful stimuli are often associated with neutral stimuli, symbolic or real, he postulated that the repeated pairing of a neutral with a noxious stimulus can cause the neutral stimulus to be perceived as dangerous and to elicit the anxiety response. Freud called the situation that contains the determinant for such expectation a "danger situation." He stated that in this situation the *signal* of anxiety is given. Freud considered this signal anxiety to be an attenuated version of an inborn primal anxiety.

Freud's understanding of anxiety evolved from his

early drive theory. Initially Freud regarded neurotic anxiety as transformed libido and distinguished between this kind of morbid distress and the realistic fear occasioned by external danger. His later theory viewed the problem from the standpoint of the ego.[12] Both "real" anxiety and neurotic anxiety were regarded as occurring in response to a danger to the organism. In "real" anxiety, the threat emanates from a known danger coming from outside the individual person, whereas neurotic anxiety is precipitated by an unknown danger, often arising from internal sources or from a mixture of internal and external precipitants.[23]

Both Pavlov and Freud appreciated that anxiety can be learned, and each achieved the important insight that the ability to manifest anticipatory defense responses to danger signals is biologically adaptive. If the danger is external, anxiety acts as a signal and prepares the person for fight or flight. For internal danger, Freud suggested that instead of fight or flight the individual resorts to the use of psychological defense mechanisms.

Freud distinguished two kinds of anxiety-provoking situations. In the first (birth was the prototype), anxiety occurs as a result of excessive instinctual stimulation that the organism does not have the capacity to bind or to handle. In this situation, arising because the individual feels totally helpless, a panicky state results that is the basis of trauma. These traumatic states are most likely to occur in infancy or childhood when the ego is immature; however, they may occur also in adult life, notably in psychotic turmoil or in panic states when the ego organization is overwhelmed.

Freud distinguished "actual" anxiety, an automatic inborn response to external or internal danger, from signal anxiety, an acquired fear response in anticipation of danger, either internal (unconscious) or external. Actual anxiety is synonymous with fear. Subsequent to Freud's work, newer research has shown that acquired anxiety can further be subdivided into three forms on the basis of distinct clinical characteristics

and differential response to psychopharmacological agents. These forms are panic attacks, anticipatory anxiety, and chronic anxiety.[19] In addition to the biological adaptive function of anxiety, Kandel[19] has suggested that there are inherited variations in the predisposition to learn certain stimulus relationships, that is, a genetic predisposition to anxiety (see figure 34–1).

Definitions

Panic attacks are brief, spontaneous episodes of terror without a manifest or clearly identifiable precipitating cause. The attacks are characterized by a subjective sense of impending disaster accompanied by evidences of sympathetic crisis.

Anticipatory (or signal) anxiety also is typically of brief duration. Unlike panic attacks, anticipatory anxiety is triggered by an identifiable signal, real or imagined, that has come to be associated with danger.

Chronic anxiety is a persistent feeling of tension that cannot be related to obvious external threats. Panic attacks occur suddenly and without an apparent trigger, and are thus not under obvious stimulus control. In contrast, anticipatory and chronic anxieties are to some degree under stimulus control. This feature suggests that both forms are at least partially learned.[19]

Classification and Nomenclature

Earlier versions of the diagnostic manual used in American psychiatry reflected the prevalent thinking about cause. This was typified by the "reactions" in DSM-I, which presumed psychodynamic causes, and the psychiatric illnesses of DSM-II, which presumed

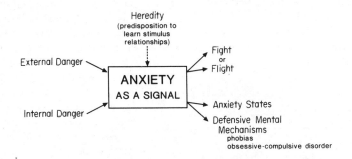

FIGURE 34–1

Integrated Scheme of Anxiety as a Mediator of Protective, Defensive, and Pathological Reactions to External and Internal Danger

biological causes. DSM-III[1] has attempted to be more objective by avoiding assumptions about etiology and by focusing on descriptions of behavior. This represents an advance in nosological rigor, if not in the understanding of causes. By serving as a phenomenological model, DSM-III has encouraged greater specificity in labeling and diagnosis. This is to be desired but, as Rapoport and Ismond[29] have pointed out, in many instances, seemingly clear, precise descriptions of behavior call for judgments that are difficult and subjective. Thus, while DSM-III has been touted as a boon to greater scientific rigor and clarity in psychiatric diagnosis, it can still reflect only the limited state of the art regarding the understanding of emotional disorder and psychiatric illness. Utilizing more specific clinical descriptions, DSM-III has encouraged a critical attitude toward clinical research in psychiatry. Rapoport and Ismond[29] have predicted that as our knowledge grows, DSM-IV may stipulate laboratory measures as validation of, or even as criteria for, certain diagnoses. The studies that may lead to knowledge requiring the revision of certain groupings of disorders will be reviewed in this chapter.

DSM-III includes sections on anxiety disorders of childhood or adolescence as well as on anxiety disorders that are not specifically related to children. However, the anxiety disorders category includes phobic disorders and anxiety states, which do occur regularly, although not frequently, in children.

The anxiety disorders considered to be *specific to childhood and adolescence* include separation anxiety disorder, avoidant disorder of childhood or adolescence, and overanxious disorder (see table 34–1). In separation anxiety disorder, excessive anxiety is aroused upon separation from familiar persons, usually the parents, or upon leaving home. It may occur during the preschool years, but the most extreme form is seen in children who refuse to go to school in order to avoid the trauma of separation. Avoidant disorder of childhood or adolescence is typified by fear of strangers, usually of such degree that social functioning is impaired. In contrast to the temporary social reticence shown by the shy, timid child, the withdrawing reaction persists in the individual with avoidant disorder. In the child with overanxious disorder, the characteris-

TABLE 34–1

DSM-III Classification of Anxiety Disorders of Childhood and Adolescence

309.21	Separation Anxiety Disorder
313.21	Avoidant Disorder of Childhood or Adolescence
313.00	Overanxious Disorder

TABLE 34–2

DSM-III Classification of Anxiety Disorders

	Phobic Disorders
300.21	Agoraphobia with Panic Attacks
300.22	Agoraphobia without Panic Attacks
300.23	Social Phobia
300.29	Simple Phobia
	Anxiety States
300.01	Panic Disorder
300.02	Generalized Anxiety Disorder
300.30	Obsessive Compulsive Disorder
308.30	Posttraumatic Stress Disorder, Acute
309.81	Posttraumatic Stress Disorder, Chronic or Delayed
300.00	Atypical Anxiety Disorder

tic finding is a state of excessive worrying and fearful behavior not focused on a specific situation or object. Anticipatory anxiety is typical of and tends to be generalized to include most events requiring someone to make a judgment or appraisal of the child's performance or appearance.

Subtypes grouped among the *anxiety disorders* (see table 34–2), more common in adults, are also to be found during the childhood and adolescent years. The *phobic disorders* include social phobia and simple phobia. Agoraphobia with or without panic attacks is presumed to be linked with childhood separation anxiety disorder, but the onset of the adult variety is usually not encountered until late adolescence or early adulthood. Phobic disorders involve a specific stimulus that, on encounter, initiates the anxiety response. The phobic object or situation is avoided thereafter in order to eliminate the flare-up of anxiety. In social phobia, the person is fearful of being observed and of possible humiliation. Simple phobia commonly involves an irrational fear of animals and fear of heights or closed spaces.

Among the anxiety disorders (or anxiety neuroses), the acute form, panic disorder, is seen both among children and adults; the chronic condition, generalized anxiety disorder, however, is applicable only to adults. Panic disorder involves recurrent episodes of intense terror, apprehension, and fear of impending doom. Like phobias, obsessive-compulsive disorder may be seen as a condition in which conspicuous or inappropriate behavior is used to ward off anxiety. Obsessive-compulsive disorder specifies the persistent presence of obsessions, compulsions, or both. Obsessions are ego-dystonic thoughts that are recurrent and persistent, and compulsions are repetitive activities or behaviors the patient feels driven to perform in order to ward off dire consequences. Posttraumatic stress disorder involves reactions to situations of extreme stress and psychological trauma. The category of atypical anxiety disorder is used for those instances of anxiety disorder that do not meet the criteria for the just-specified illnesses.

Psychosomatic Interrelationships

A model of anxiety with clinical implications for children will be presented here; it is based on the pathopsychological mechanisms of the hyperventilation syndrome (see figure 34–2). While these mechanisms can readily be understood within this scheme, the process can begin at any point. Thus the question of cause and effect remains a vexing one.

For decades, psychophysiological researchers have investigated the physiological accompaniments of emotions. The chemical changes underlying these physiological phenomena have been characterized in only the most rudimentary ways. Most of the work has been done in relation to depression and a lesser amount in relation to anxiety. The complexities and difficulties in defining the biochemistry of these disorders are illustrated by the sheer numbers of the many biochemical theories of depression that have been proposed.

It has been argued that in the study of anxiety, even highly complex animals like rats and monkeys may not be ideal substitutes for humans; at best, there are obvious differences in their cognitive and emotional makeup. It therefore seems even more farfetched and, at first, perhaps absurd to consider the problem of anxiety in the primitive marine snail *Aplysia.* Nonetheless, Kandel[19] has elegantly defended the rationale for studying the cellular basis for anxiety in this lowly mollusk. Along with his coworkers, and by means of a series of ingenious experiments, he has established models of anticipatory and chronic anxiety. Such models are beginning to elucidate the synaptic biochemical alterations that may underlie complex emotional reactions.

For many emotions that may be experienced acutely, there is also a chronic counterpart. The acute emotion often represents a biologically normal adaptive phenomenon, while the chronic emotion tends to represent a pathological reaction. Some examples of such pairings are fear and anxiety, grief and depression, and acute and chronic pain.[33] Table 34–3 suggests a few of the pathological emotions that can be conceptualized; there may indeed be many others.

In humans, there has been some interest directed toward tracing the developmental roots of anxiety by exploring situations that cause fear early in life.[6] In the early months of life, the situations that usually arouse fear involve various forms of physical stress. Later, during the first year of life, there is fear of

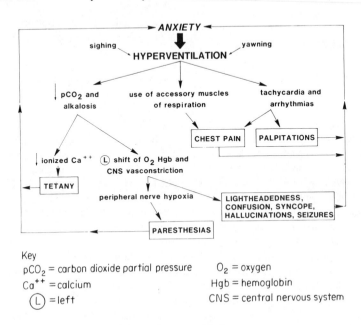

Key
pCO_2 = carbon dioxide partial pressure O_2 = oxygen
Ca^{++} = calcium   Hgb = hemoglobin
(L) = left   CNS = central nervous system

FIGURE 34–2

Pathophysiological Mechanisms of Hyperventilation

NOTE: Reprinted, by permission of the publisher, from S. P. Herman, G. B. Stickler, and A. R. Lucas, "Hyperventilation Syndrome in Children and Adolescents: Long-Term Follow-Up," *Pediatrics,* 67 (1981):186.

TABLE 34–3

Tentative Scheme of Human Emotions Related to Threats Against Fulfillment of Basic Needs

Basic need	Acute (adaptive emotion)	Chronic (pathological emotion)
Survival	Fear	Anxiety
Human tie	Grief	Depression
Body integrity	Acute pain	Chronic pain
Nourishment	Hunger	Dysorexia
Self-esteem	Anger	Hostility

strangers and of strange objects. Experimental situations have been created by the use of the "visual cliff" and an "approaching object," which elicit natural fear reactions in infants. In the visual cliff situation the infant is placed on a glass-covered table that appears to have a deep chasm between the child and its beckoning mother. The approaching object involves an expanding visual stimulus that appears to be rapidly approaching. At the end of the first year of life, infants begin to show fear of anticipated situations. Starting in the second year of life and continuing thereafter, noise, strangers, animals, and darkness all can precipitate fear. Bowlby[6] postulated that a more complex situation, and the prototype of anxiety in humans, is the fear of separation.

Recent Developments

The fact that certain subtypes of anxiety disorders (e.g., obsessive-compulsive disorder) frequently begin in childhood or adolescence and persist through adulthood suggests that parallels can be drawn between anxiety disorders of children and adolescents and anxiety disorders (and possibly other syndromes) of adults.[14,18] Clearer delineation of anxiety disorders in children and adolescents will necessarily await future direct studies on natural history, family history, biological markers, and treatment response. It is possible that illness and treatment paradigms of anxiety disorders of adults can be applied to the parallel conditions found among children and adolescents. Moreover, existing observations provide compelling motivation for doing so.

In recent years research on anxiety disorders has encompassed the search for improved nosology, methods of diagnosis, pharmacological treatment, and psychosocial intervention, as well as extensive study of the biological, behavioral, and social factors underlying the development of these disorders.

An appreciation of the epidemiology of these conditions is important to their understanding, but definitive data are sparse. Published prevalence rates for anxiety disorders vary widely, although consistency across studies is beginning to appear.[7,34]

Current knowledge of the familial nature and genetics of anxiety disorders, albeit suggestive, is still limited. Family studies[7] have shown that the frequency of anxiety disorders among first-degree relatives of persons so afflicted is consistently about 15 percent, with female relatives demonstrating a higher frequency than male relatives. The risk to a first-degree relative increases as a function of familial "loading": When neither parent is affected, the rate ranges from 8 to 15 percent; with only one affected parent, the rate increases to about 25 percent; and when both parents have anxiety disorder, the pooled rate becomes 40 percent. Unfortunately, no specific data are available that compare age at onset in childhood and adolescence with age at onset in adulthood.

In respect of separating genetic and environmental effects, studies of twins[7] provide a greater likelihood of drawing this distinction than studies of families. Such twin studies do in fact suggest a heritable variation for anxiety disorders: Among monozygotic twins concordance rates for anxiety disorders are significantly greater (17 to 30 percent) than for dizygotic twins (4 to 9 percent).

Thus evidence is accumulating suggesting that hereditary factors are important in the etiology of anxiety disorders. Studies are underway that are limited to specific diagnostic categories subsumed under the rubric anxiety disorders—for example, this has recently been done with panic disorders.[9] Such an approach should further our understanding of the role played by these hereditary factors.

The concern with genetic aspects in the etiology of anxiety disorders has led to considerable interest in the delineation and investigation of any associated phenomena that could serve as potential "markers" for their presence. Prominent among these has been the association between anxiety disorders (specifically, panic disorder) and the mitral valve prolapse syndrome.[3,10,20] There is an increased incidence of mitral valve prolapse in patients who present with panic disorder (30 to 50 percent), as compared to the prevalence of this condition in the general population (approximately 10 percent).[20] Conflicting data exist regarding both the degree of overlap of symptoms between these two disorders and their responses to pharmacological challenge with isoproterenol hydrochloride.[3,20] In order to account for these findings,[20] it has been proposed that an increased level of basal adrenergic activity is present that is mediated by or related to peripheral, and possibly central, catecholamine effects. As discussed later, similar pathophysiological mechanisms have been proposed for anxiety. Unfortunately, the nature and extent of the relationships between mitral valve prolapse and anxiety remain unclear. It is possible that the increased basal level of adrenergic activity observed in patients with mitral valve prolapse serves as only one of the many potential factors that together create a vulnerability to panic attacks.[20] Further delineation may provide useful insights into the mechanisms of anxiety.

In addition to the study of such associated phenomena, interest has been directed toward endocrine correlates of anxiety. Unfortunately, the absence of a reliable, reproducible, and specific model of human anxiety has made the clear elucidation of such factors a matter of considerable difficulty. Despite the lack of such a specific model, however, advances in understanding anxiety are being achieved through the use of pharmacological induction of anxiety. Sodium lactate,* isoproterenol,[28] and yohimbine hydrochloride[8] have each been used to produce episodes of anxiety and panic in humans. Such methods may be useful in differentiating anxious from nonanxious persons and in distinguishing between panic and generalized anxiety. It must be cautioned that (1) results thus far are preliminary, (2) the clinical relevance of this type of provocative testing remains to be demonstrated, and (3) anxiety attacks can indeed be induced with these agents, but the extent to which their symptoms and physiological correlates resemble the naturally occurring events is uncertain.

The endocrinological correlates[4,5,21] of spontaneous anxiety consist of elevations of plasma levels of catecholamines (epinephrine, norepinephrine), catecholamine metabolites (3-methoxy-4-hydroxy-phenylglycol, or MHPG), and cortisol. Such correlates suggest that the pituitary-adrenal axis is associated in an important way with anxiogenesis. Whether this is a cause-and-effect relationship, however, remains unclear.

It is evident that many of the somatic symptoms associated with anxiety are produced by a discharge of catecholamines. Thus, if peripheral catecholamine receptors are blocked by pharmacological means, behavioral responses to stress may be attenuated. A positive feedback process may exist in which catecholamines acting peripherally induce behaviors that augment the experience of anxiety. For example, anxiety-induced catecholamine-mediated tachycardia, a peripheral "behavior," contributes to the experience of palpitations and chest discomfort. This experience in a sensitized (anxious) person may exacerbate the preex-

isting anxious state via both indirect neuronal pathways operative through cognitive processes, such as the interpretation of the meaning of such an experience, and direct neuronal pathways from peripheral sensory afferents to central "anxiogenic" regions (e.g., the locus coeruleus).

The nucleus locus coeruleus of the pons has been advanced as being the central neuroanatomical site for the noradrenergic system; when overactive, it is this system that causes anxiety.[16,22] In animal studies, there are agents that increase noradrenergic activity in the locus coeruleus; the same substances have been reported to have anxiogenic properties in human beings.[8] It has accordingly been proposed that anxiolytic agents achieve their effects by inhibiting the locus coeruleus through various different neurochemical mechanisms (many of which remain unknown). The evolving understanding of the mechanism of action of one of these agents, the benzodiazepines, and of their effects on inhibitory control of noradrenergic function has improved the understanding of the neurobiology of anxiety.

Within the central nervous system, inhibitory neurotransmission is mediated predominantly by gamma-aminobutyric acid (GABA), which tends to be stored in synaptic vesicles.[25] Depolarization of GABAergic neurons results in the release of this previously stored GABA into the synapse. Here it interacts with one or more of the several subtypes of GABA receptors on the postsynaptic neuron. Such binding results in GABA-activated opening of chloride channels in the postsynaptic neuron; this, in turn, results in inhibition of these neurons.

Benzodiazepine receptors consist of glycoproteins located within neuronal cell membranes.[11] These glycoproteins bind benzodiazepines with high affinity and specificity. There are at least two subtypes of these receptor glycoproteins, which differ in their relative affinity for certain ligands. These receptors are closely associated with GABA receptors and chloride channels.

The binding of benzodiazepines to their specific receptor site potentiates the effect of GABA on the conductance of chloride.[25] Presumably, benzodiazepine-benzodiazepine receptor interaction changes the conformation of the benzodiazepine receptor molecule in such a way as to modify the coupling between the GABA receptor and the chloride channel. It has been suggested that the anxiolytic action of benzodiazepines may be due to two different but parallel brain mechanisms. One is the reduced excitation of noradrenergic neurons of the locus coeruleus. The other, however, may be the enhanced GABAergic stabilization of neurons within the limbic system.

Although less selectively anxiolytic in their actions

*See references 2, 15, 27, 28, and 31.

than the benzodiazepines, the group of barbiturates are the prototypic antianxiety drugs. The reason for the difference between these two classes of agents is not clear, but it may stem from different mechanisms of action. Barbiturates clearly do not occupy the same receptor sites as do benzodiazepines.[32] They may, however, bind to a separate site that is also adjacent to the chloride channels, where an effect on the coupling of the GABA receptor to the chloride channel may again be exerted. It is probably not irrelevant that barbiturates interact with a far larger number of GABA receptors than do the benzodiazepines, which interact with only a specific and limited receptor population.[11]

Possible mechanisms of action of alternative anxiolytic agents—such as beta-adrenergic blocking agents, alpha-adrenergic agonists, tricyclic antidepressants, monoamine oxidase inhibitors, and a newer agent, buspirone—have now been advanced. However, none has been as thoroughly investigated or has contributed as much to the understanding of the neurobiology of anxiety as has knowledge about the GABA-benzodiazepine receptor system.

Clonidine hydrochloride, an alpha-adrenergic agonist, is a potent inhibitor of locus coeruleus activity. It exerts its predominant effects presynaptically, resulting in reduced neuronal release of norepinephrine and, consequently, in reduced central sympathetic activity.[13]

The anxiolytic properties of beta-adrenergic blocking agents, on the other hand, may be attributed to the peripheral actions of these drugs.[24] Compounds such as propranolol hydrochloride may diminish somatic symptoms associated with anxiety-provoking situations by pharmacological blockade of peripheral beta-adrenergic neurons. In this way, catecholamine-related behavioral responses to stress could be attenuated. The peripheral manifestations of a centrally mediated anxiety state, which may in themselves contribute to anxiogenesis via a positive-feedback mechanism (described previously), are thus reduced. Central actions of these agents also may contribute to their antianxiety effects.

Buspirone is a uniquely structured compound having both dopamine agonist and antagonist properties; it appears to be anxiolytic without producing benzodiazepinelike side effects. It does not bind to benzodiazepine receptors and does not appear to influence GABA systems. It may be the first of many new antianxiety compounds that are not analogous of benzodiazepine structures and that accordingly possess a potentially different activity.[30]

The GABA system, the noradrenergic system, and other systems that are in the process of being delineated seem to be related in different ways to different syndromes. The notion that a single neurotransmitter or neurotransmitter system is specifically tied to a given clinical condition is being replaced by a perspective of biological systems interacting as mosaics. Within this framework, disturbances in one system precede or follow disturbances in others by variable amounts of time—in some cases, rather long periods of time.[35]

This effort at delineating the relationship of disturbances within various biological systems to psychosocial variables and to the major dimensions of symptomatology is one of the greatest challenges for psychiatric research today.

REFERENCES

1. AMERICAN PSYCHIATRIC ASSOCIATION. *Diagnostic and Statistical Manual of Mental Disorders,* 3rd ed. (DSM-III). Washington, D.C.: American Psychiatric Association, 1980.

2. APPLEBY, I. L., et al. "Biochemical Indices of Lactate-Induced Panic: A Preliminary Report," in D. F. Klein and J. G. Rabkin, eds., *Anxiety: New Research and Changing Concepts.* New York: Raven Press, 1981, pp. 411–423.

3. BOUDOULAS, H., KING, B. D., and WOOLEY, C. F. "Mitral Valve Prolapse: A Marker for Anxiety or Overlapping Phenomenon?" *Psychopathology,* 17 (Supplement 1) (1984): 98–106.

4. BOULENGER, J. P., and UHDE, T. W. "Biochemical Aspects of Anxiety," *Semaine des Hopitaux de Paris,* 58 (1982): 2573–2579.

5. ——. "Biological Peripheral Correlates of Anxiety," *Encephale,* 8 (1982): 119–130.

6. BOWLBY, J. *Attachment and Loss,* vol. 1. New York: Basic Books, 1969.

7. CAREY, G., and GOTTESMAN, I. I. "Twin and Family Studies of Anxiety, Phobic, and Obsessive Disorders," in D. F. Klein and J. G. Rabkin, eds., *Anxiety: New Research and Changing Concepts.* New York: Raven Press, 1981, pp. 117–135.

8. CHARNEY, D. S., HENINGER, G. R., and REDMOND, D. E., Jr. "Yohimbine Induced Anxiety and Increased Noradrenergic Function in Humans: Effects of Diazepam and Clonidine," *Life Sciences,* 33 (1983): 19–29.

9. CROWE, R. R. "The Role of Genetics in the Etiology of Panic Disorder," in L. Grinspoon, ed., *Psychiatric Update,* vol. 3. Washington, D.C.: American Psychiatric Press, 1984, pp. 402–410.

10. CROWE, R. R., et al. "Panic Disorder and Mitral Valve Prolapse," in D. F. Klein and J. G. Rabkin, eds., *Anxiety: New Research and Changing Concepts.* New York: Raven Press, 1981, pp. 103–114.

11. ENNA, S. J., "Role of γ-aminobutyric Acid in Anxiety," *Psychopathology,* 17 (Supplement 1) (1984): 15–24.

12. FREUD, S. "Inhibitions, Symptoms and Anxiety," in J.

Strachey, ed., *The Standard Edition of the Complete Psychological Works of Sigmund Freud,* vol. 20. London: Hogarth Press, 1959, pp. 87–156. (Originally published 1926.)

13. GILMAN, A. G., GOODMAN, L. S., and GILMAN, A., eds. *The Pharmacological Basis of Therapeutics,* 7th ed. New York: Macmillan, 1985.

14. GITTELMAN, R., and KLEIN, D. F. "Relationship Between Separation Anxiety and Panic and Agorophobic Disorders," *Psychopathology,* 17 (Supplement 1) (1984): 56–65.

15. GORMAN, J. M., et al. "Effect of Sodium Lactate on Patients with Panic Disorder and Mitral Valve Prolapse," *American Journal of Psychiatry,* 138 (1981): 247–249.

16. GRANT, S. J., and REDMOND, D. E., Jr., "The Neuroanatomy and Pharmacology of the Nucleus Locus Coeruleus," *Progress in Clinical and Biological Research,* 71 (1981): 5–27.

17. HERMAN, S. P., STICKLER, G. B., and LUCAS, A. R. "Hyperventilation Syndrome in Children and Adolescents: Long-Term Follow-Up," *Pediatrics,* 67 (1981): 183–187.

18. HOLLINGSWORTH, C. E., et al. "Long-Term Outcome of Obsessive-Compulsive Disorder in Childhood," *Journal of the American Academy of Child Psychiatry,* 19 (1980): 134–144.

19. KANDEL, E. R. "From Metapsychology to Molecular Biology: Explorations Into the Nature of Anxiety," *American Journal of Psychiatry,* 140 (1983): 1277–1293.

20. KLEIN, D. F., and GORMAN, J. M. "Panic Disorders and Mitral Valve Prolapse," *Journal of Clinical Psychiatry Monograph,* 2 (1984): 14–17.

21. KO, G. N., et al. "Panic-Induced Elevation of Plasma MHPG Levels in Phobic-Anxious Patients: Effects of Clonidine and Imipramine," *Archives of General Psychiatry,* 40 (1983): 425–430.

22. KOPIN, I. J. "Avenues of Investigation for the Role of Catecholamines in Anxiety," *Psychopathology,* 17 (Supplement 1) (1984): 83–97.

23. MACK, J. E., and SEMRAD, E. V. "Classical Psychoanalysis," in A. M. Freedman and H. I. Kaplan, eds., *Compre-* hensive Textbook of Psychiatry. Baltimore: Williams & Wilkins, 1967, pp. 269–319.

24. NOYES, R., Jr., et al. "Antianxiety Effects of Propranolol: A Review of Clinical Studies," in D. F. Klein and J. G. Rabkin, eds., *Anxiety: New Research and Changing Concepts.* New York: Raven Press, 1981, pp. 81–91.

25. PAUL, S. M., and SKOLNICK, P. "Benzodiazepine Receptors and Psychopathological States: Towards a Neurobiology of Anxiety," in D. F. Klein, and J. G. Rabkin, eds., *Anxiety: New Research and Changing Concepts.* New York: Raven Press, 1981, pp. 215–230.

26. PAVLOV, I. P. *Conditioned Reflexes: An Investigation of the Physiological Activity of the Cerebral Cortex,* G. V. Anrep, trans. and ed. London: Oxford University Press, 1927.

27. PITTS, F. N., and MCCLURE, J. N. "Lactate Metabolism in Anxiety Neurosis," *New England Journal of Medicine,* 277 (1967): 1329–1336.

28. RAINEY, J. M., Jr., et al. "A Comparison of Lactate and Isoproterenol Anxiety States," *Psychopathology,* 17 (Supplement 1) (1984): 74–82.

29. RAPOPORT, J. L., and ISMOND, D. R. *DSM-III Training Guide for Diagnosis of Childhood Disorders.* New York: Brunner/Mazel, 1984.

30. RIBLET, L. A., et al. "Pharmacology and Neurochemistry of Buspirone," *Journal of Clinical Psychiatry,* 43 (1982): 11–18.

31. RIFKIN, A., et al. "Blockade by Imipramine or Desipramine of Panic Induced by Sodium Lactate," *American Journal of Psychiatry,* 138 (1981): 676–677.

32. SNYDER, S. H. "Drug and Neurotransmitter Receptors in the Brain," *Science,* 224 (1984): 22–31.

33. SWANSON, D. W. "Chronic Pain as a Third Pathologic Emotion," *American Journal of Psychiatry,* 141 (1984): 210–214.

34. TORGERSEN, S. "Genetic Factors in Anxiety Disorders," *Archives of General Psychiatry,* 40 (1983): 1085–1089.

35. TUPIN, J., and WHYBROW, P. C. (Discussants). "Neurobiology of Anxiety II: Endocrine and Other Aspects," in *Perspectives on the VII World Congress of Psychiatry.* New York: Health Projects International, 1983, pp. 4–7.

35 / Tourette Syndrome: Clinical Features, Etiology, and Pathogenesis

Donald J. Cohen, Mark A. Riddle, and James F. Leckman

Introduction and Diagnostic Criteria

Tics are rapid, repetitive, purposeless, involuntary movements of functionally related muscle groups. Tourette syndrome (TS), the most debilitating of the tic disorders, is characterized by multiform, frequently changing motor and phonic tics and a range of behavioral symptoms. Prevailing diagnostic criteria include: (1) age of onset between two and fifteen years; (2) rapid, recurrent, repetitive, purposeless, involuntary motor movements affecting multiple muscle groups; (3) multiple vocal tics; (4) ability to suppress movements voluntarily for minutes to hours; (5) variations in the intensity of the symptoms over weeks or months; and (6) a duration of more than one year. "Emerging clinical research supports the need for refinements regarding age of onset, the "involuntary" character of the tics, and the full range of associated behavioral symptoms."

Many investigators consider TS to be a model for neuropsychiatric disorders with childhood onset—there appears to be a genetically determined biological vulnerability, an age-dependent expression of symptoms that may be related to central nervous system (CNS) ontogeny, sexual dimorphism, and environmental stress-dependent fluctuations in symptomatic severity.[31] Currently, multiple disciplines are studying TS in order to define the relationships between the behavioral, genetic, and neurochemical characteristics of the disorder.

Clinical Features of Tourette Syndrome

CLINICAL EXPRESSION

The motor and phonic tics of TS can be characterized by their frequency, complexity, and the degree to which they disrupt the patient's ongoing activities and daily life. *Simple motor tics* are fast, darting, repetitive, meaningless contractions of functionally related muscle groups. Examples include eye blinking, facial grimacing, nose twitching, shoulder shrugs, head or arm jerks, and finger movements. *Complex motor tics* are usually slower and more purposeful in appearance. They can involve any type of movement, including touching, kicking, hopping, throwing, or clapping, as well as gyrating, writhing movements or "dystonic" posturing. Often the patient will attempt to "camouflage" these movements. Repetitive grooming behaviors, such as brushing hair away from the face, are common examples of camouflaging. Complex motor tics may be organized, ritualistic, and "compulsive" in character—for example, the need to stand up repeatedly and move a piece of furniture into "just the right position" or to neatly arrange objects. Occasionally patients develop self-abusive behaviors, such as biting the inside of the mouth, head banging, or scratching scabs.

Linguistically meaningless noises and sounds, such as coughing, sniffling, spitting, barking, grunting, or hissing, typify *simple phonic tics.* *Complex phonic tics* involve the sudden ejaculation of inappropriate words or phrases, such as "Oops!" "Yup, you got it!" or "Why did I say that?" Patients may change the flow of speech by slurring a phrase, altering volume and/or pitch, or inappropriately accenting a word or phrase.

Coprolalia, the sudden utterance of obscenities, is the most socially distressing complex phonic symptom. Initially manifested by the abrupt utterance of first syllables (e.g., "fff, ffuu," or "sh, sh, shi") or single obscene words, this symptom may progress to more elaborate forms in which the swearing is embedded in longer statements and may take the form of sexual, hostile, or insulting statements (e.g., "Nice tits!" or "I love you, I hate you"). Coprolalia may lead to general argumentativeness and be consistent with a patient's emotional "short fuse." Most patients experience their coprolalic symptoms as ego dystonic or ego alien. Mental coprolalia—recurrent obscene thoughts—are difficult to evaluate but may be very distressing. The frequency of coprolalia differs dramatically in various studies, ranging from 15 percent to over 50 percent of patients. In the Orient, coprolalia is far less frequently observed, perhaps reflecting social constraint.

In a sizable proportion of TS patients, *specific learning disabilities* are present. These disabilities, in addition to difficulties in completing work, peer relationship problems, and graphomotor impairments, often interfere with optimal school and work performance.

Many TS patients manifest *mirroring or imitative phenomena,* such as echolalia, echopraxia, or pallilalia. These symptoms, also seen in other neuropsychiatric disorders of childhood, may be especially socially distressing.

Several behavioral symptoms commonly are seen in patients with TS, including diminished ability to concentrate, impulsiveness, frustration intolerance, hyperactivity, and obsessions and compulsions. As many as 50 to 60 percent of children with TS referred to clinical researchers in major medical centers satisfy the diagnostic criteria for *attention deficit disorder (ADD)* (inattentiveness and impulsivity) and hyperactivity. Since children with both TS and ADD present more complicated assessment and treatment issues than those with TS without ADD, they may be overrepresented in the referral populations seen by clinical researchers and subsequently described in the clinical literature. The onset of the ADD and hyperactivity often precede the onset of tics. Although most TS patients do not have primary learning disabilities, the ADD and hyperactivity can impair school performance substantially. Attentional problems persist during periods of tic remission and usually continue into adulthood.

The *obsessive-compulsive symptoms* seen in patients with TS usually appear late in the developmental course of the syndrome. Obsessive doubting or elaborate rituals may be severely disabling. Some patients need to "even out" actions or thoughts—for example, to touch first with the right and then the left hand; one patient had to swallow on the right side and then the left side of his throat.

PHENOMENOLOGY

A wide range of symptomatology and impairment is seen in patients with TS. In its most severe forms, patients may have almost constant, uncountable motor and phonic tics, paroxysms of full-body movements, shouting, and self-abusive behavior. Milder forms may present with only a few tics per minute or hour and are far less likely to come to diagnosis.

The frequency, severity, and mixture of symptoms may vary markedly over short and long periods of time and are place- and state-dependent. The bewildering waxing and waning of symptoms complicates diagnostic and therapeutic efforts—patients may "lose" their tics when they enter the doctor's office. Furthermore, tics may be inhibited in school but become nonstop as soon as the child arrives at home or be quiescent during focused activity but exacerbate while relaxing in front of the television. Although rigorous data are lacking, life events and stresses frequently seem to precede symptomatic exacerbations.

TS tics are currently described as "involuntary." This definition is consistent with the reported inner experience of many, especially younger, patients with TS. However, some children and many adult patients describe antecedent, fleeting sensory "signals" or "urges," suggesting the possible involvement of sensory systems, as well as motor pathways.[4] Patients may feel an increasing tension localized to a part of the body or throat; the tension will mount along with a sense of anxiety; finally patients will feel that they will explode unless they perform a tic or emit a sound. Following the discharge, a refractory period of reduced tension may be followed by a progressive increase in tension either at the same site or in some other part of the body. Some patients report "attending to" these inner signals in order to prevent or modify the occurrence of a tic. This ability to modify or inhibit tics calls into question the characterization of tics as "involuntary."

TS patients and their families usually are acutely aware of the emergence of a "new" tic. Patients describe some new tics as just appearing "out of the blue." Commonly, a nose sniffling or coughing tic may follow a cold or upper respiratory infection. Sometimes a new tic may follow a physical stimulus—a hair-straightening tic may have been preceded by hair repeatedly falling over the forehead. The observation of someone doing something (e.g., frowning) or saying something (e.g., an accented word or phrase) that the patient finds odd or distasteful may provide the template for a new tic. Some new tics (e.g., kissing or copropraxia) may be psychologically meaningful representations of specific wishes or desires. New tics usually last for about two months or longer.

NATURAL HISTORY

Attentional problems, impulsivity, and hyperactivity emerge during the late preschool years. These symptoms usually precede tics or develop concurrently with a few simple tics. Persistent motor and phonic tics occur later; the mean age of onset of motor tics is seven years, with a range from two to eighteen years, while the mean age of onset of phonic tics is eleven years. Often progressing in a rostral-caudal pattern, simple motor tics usually are followed by complex ones. Phonic symptoms develop after the motor symptoms. The most severe and disabling symptoms (e.g., rituals, compulsions, complex coprolalic descriptions of sexual or aggressive acts) tend to appear last, if at all. There are exceptions to this typical description; some patients experience the rapid emergence of symptoms over a brief interval of time or the onset of phonic tics prior to motor tics.

Clinical experience suggests that the most severely afflicted patients have the earliest age of onset and the most severe early behavior and ADD symptoms. These patients tend to have lifelong difficulties, in contrast to patients with fewer behavioral problems or no ADD, who may have long-term or even permanent remissions of major tics. In some cases, obsessive and compulsive symptoms may be the sole or major remaining symptom. Some adult TS patients will describe an "inner tension" or "constant struggle for inner peace" as their most distressful and disabling symptom. Typically, however, TS patients continue to have motor and phonic tics intermittently throughout life.

THE ORGANIZATION OF SYMPTOMS

The study of TS symptoms, particularly impulsivity, vocal tics, mirroring or imitative phenomena, and obsessions and compulsions, can enrich our understanding of the organization of mental life. Recent genetic and epidemiologic studies support the hypothesis that TS, chronic multiple tics, and obsessive-compulsive symptoms aggregate in families and are vertically transmitted (see the section entitled "Genetics"). Exactly what it is that is transmitted is not clear. What does seem clear is that TS symptoms reflect the release of constitutionally patterned and complexly organized behavioral systems. For example, imitation phenomena are commonly observed in humans and animals, and in certain circumstances are considered to be highly organized, adaptive, and "normal" behaviors —for example, a young child will imitate a repeatedly observed parental behavior, or an animal in a herd will follow (imitate) a leader that quickly leaves a feeding ground because of fear of an approaching predator. What is unique about imitative behavior in TS patients is that it usually involves aggressive, insulting, and socially inappropriate gestures. It is not imitative behavior per se that is unusual, but the social implications of the behavior.

Psychodynamic observers and theorists have noted that impulsivity (e.g., disinhibition) and obsessive-compulsive behavior (e.g., inhibition, which is sometimes understood as reaction formation in psychodynamic theories of psychological defense mechanisms) are frequently observed together and appear to be "connected" in some way. It is possible that in certain families with TS and obsessive-compulsive disorder (OCD), the same genotype may be expressed phenotypically as both impulsivity and obsessive-compulsive symptoms. In these individuals, the obsessive and compulsive behavior may not represent a defense against disinhibition but may be the behavioral expression of the biological endowment. The symptoms, although dynamically meaningful (e.g., why was a *particular* coprolalic or compulsive symptom expressed), would be biologically determined. In other words, a biological discharge would be "shaped" by complexly organized psychological desires and fantasies before it was expressed motorically. The discharge could be accompanied or followed by feelings of relief, guilt, shame, or confusion—the secondary psychological elaboration.

DIFFERENTIAL DIAGNOSIS

The differential diagnosis of tics includes choreiform, dystonic, athetoid, myoclonic, and hemiballismic movements and epilepsy, particularly temporal lobe seizures. In addition, spasms, synkinesia, and dyskinesias may be difficult to distinguish from tics.

Because of the increased recognition of TS in recent years, a patient with moderate-to-severe symptoms, including ADD and coprolalia, is unlikely to be misdiagnosed. However, it may be difficult to differentiate a child with severe ADD and hyperactivity from one with the early manifestations of TS. In addition, patients with amphetamine intoxication, cerebrovascular accident, Lesch-Nyhan syndrome, Wilson's disease, Sydenham's and Huntington's chorea, multiple sclerosis, schizophrenia, general paresis, and organic mental disorders may present with abnormal motor movements. However, these disorders can be distinguished from TS by clinical evaluation and appropriate laboratory tests. In practice, careful history and observation provide the diagnosis since no other disorder mimics the full TS.

PROGNOSIS

The long-term outcome for patients with TS ranges from complete remission of symptoms to severe debilitation that can require intermittent institutionalization. Ultimate social adaptation probably depends more on behavioral and attentional symptoms than on motor and phonic tics. Factors affecting outcome include intelligence, attentional problems, school achievement, the family's and patient's response to the illness, the severity of the motor and phonic symptoms, and the patient's response to medication and/or other therapeutic interventions.

Feeling unusual or different because of tics can lead to social isolation and dependence, which may interfere with optimal psychosocial development. Some TS patients experience intermittent episodes of depression that are frequently accompanied by feelings of social ostracism and isolation. Chronic dependence on medication, especially if accompanied by cognitive blunting or obtundation, may leave TS patients confused about what feelings are their own and what are due to the medication. Such confusion may exacerbate symptoms of depression and anxiety or reinforce feelings of social isolation.

Epidemiology of Tourette Syndrome

TS occurs in all major racial groups and appears to have a stable pattern of clinical expression across cultures. Boys are more commonly affected than girls. Estimates of the sex ratio (male: female) vary from three to one to nine to one. Until recently, TS was thought to be a rare disorder. However, with increasing medical recognition and public awareness, many more patients with TS are being diagnosed. As mentioned, patients with ADD in addition to TS may be more likely to come to diagnosis; milder forms may go unrecognized. Although definitive epidemiological studies are lacking, estimates of lifetime prevalence range from two to five per ten thousand. Epidemiological studies by Caine using full school populations suggest that there are many mild cases of TS that do not reach clinical diagnosis.*

*E. Caine, personal communication, 1985.

Etiology of Tourette Syndrome

Although both hereditary and environmental factors have been implicated, the etiology and pathogenesis of TS have not been established.

GENETICS

It is noteworthy that in his early writings, Gilles de la Tourette considered TS to be hereditary. Even so, there is only a modest literature on the familial nature of TS and chronic multiple tics (CMTs). Recent studies have demonstrated that TS and CMTs show a familial concentration,[24,33,36,37] and in families of TS patients, CMTs occur as a milder manifestation of the same etiologic factors.[35] Pauls and coworkers[35,37] give convincing evidence that susceptibility to TS and CMTs is transmitted vertically from one generation to the next. In addition, these studies suggest that the sex difference observed in the population is real and not an artifact of selection bias because more male relatives than female relatives are affected with either TS or CMTs. Furthermore, the sex difference seems to be related to the transmission since relatives of females are at greater risk for the disorder.

All of the evidence strongly supports the hypothesis of a major familial component being involved in the etiology of the disorder. The familial pattern can be explained by genetic models that incorporate both sex and severity differences.[23] Although no genetic model could be rejected statistically in these analyses, the solution that gave the best fit and the most reasonable estimate of population prevalence was one that closely resembled an autosomal dominant mode of transmission.

Anecdotal case reports of twins indicate a very high concordance rate for monozygotic twins for TS, in the range of 75 to 95 percent. In contrast, the results from a recent questionnaire study of thirty monozygotic twin pairs in which at least one twin had TS indicated only a 53 percent concordance for TS and a 76 percent concordance for TS or another tic disorder.[39] Concordant twin pairs also were frequently found to show differing levels in the severity of symptom expression. These more recent data provide support for the importance of environmental (nongenetic) factors in the expression of TS.

Recent family study data on first-degree relatives of TS patients suggest that TS and ADD are separate disorders and that they are independently transmitted in those families where the probands have both TS and ADD.[36] However, more data are needed before the relationship between TS and ADD can be completely understood, since the sample size for this study was small and since other investigators have suggested that the occurrence of ADD and TS may be due to the same underlying genetic factors.[12]

Approximately one-third of TS patients seen in our clinic also meet diagnostic criteria for OCD. The results of a preliminary family interview study indicate that the frequency of OCD among first-degree relatives was the same for relatives of TS-OCD probands as it was for TS-only probands, suggesting that the two disorders are not independent.[38]

While genetic factors appear to exert a powerful influence in the etiology of TS, they are not found in all patients. Even if the gene(s) underlying the disorder are identified, it will be necessary to explicate their molecular mode of action and to identify specific risk factors that may cause this vulnerability to be expressed.

ENVIRONMENTAL FACTORS

The onset of TS symptoms and the transitional periods that occur in its waxing and waning course often seem unrelated to environmental factors. However, clinical experience and pilot epidemiological studies indicate that periods of increased anxiety and emotional stress are regularly accompanied by an exacerbation of TS symptoms.[22]

A second environmental (nongenetic) factor known to exacerbate TS symptoms is exposure to stimulant medication. Recently investigators have reported several series of patients whose use of stimulants (e.g., methylphenidate hydrochloride, dextroamphetamine, or pemoline) correlated with the onset of motor and phonic tics. Stimulant medications can produce complex stereotypes in animals, which disappear when the stimulants are terminated; similarly, some children treated with stimulant medication develop simple motor tics (such as eye blinking or mouth puckering), which disappear with reduction or cessation of the medication. Whether stimulants actually can trigger or induce prolonged TS or CMTs that persist following the termination of medication remains controversial. However, cases have been reported in which this seems to have occurred.[18,32] The most convincing clinical evidence may come from tic-free children who received two courses of stimulant medication. During the first course, tics appeared after months of treatment and stopped with drug termination; during the second course of stimulants, tics appeared within days and persisted for months or continuously when stimulants were withdrawn. These children seem to have had TS "kindled" by repeated exposure to stimulants. A complication in this story is that some children—but, importantly, not all—who had TS emerge during the course of stimulant treatment had a family history of TS or tics and perhaps were genetically vulnerable. It is not possible to know whether a subgroup of ADD children who developed TS while taking stimulants were already on their way to developing TS.

Pathogenesis of Tourette Syndrome

NEUROCHEMISTRY

Several neurochemical systems have been implicated in the pathogenesis of TS. Pharmacological evidence supporting the role of dopaminergic systems includes: (1) the dramatic suppression of tics by dopaminergic receptor-blocking agents (e.g., haloperidol, pimozide), (2) the emergence of TS-like symptoms in psychiatric patients following withdrawal of neuroleptics (i.e., dopaminergic receptor blockers), (3) symptomatic exacerbations produced by stimulant medications, direct dopaminergic agonists, and (4) the amelioration of TS symptoms by dopaminergic autoreceptor stimulants (e.g., apomorphine, piribedil).[15] Neurochemical evidence of dopaminergic involvement includes lowered levels of cerebrospinal fluid (CSF) homovanillic acid (HVA, the principal metabolite of central dopamine) in many TS patients.[7,10] A "supersensitive dopamine receptor," with subsequent negative feedback to the presynaptic dopaminergic neuron, is one hypothesis that could explain these findings.[16]

The evidence for noradrenergic involvement in the pathogenesis of TS also comes primarily from clinical pharmacological studies. Clonidine hydrochloride, an imadozoline derivative that preferentially stimulates alpha$_2$-adrenergic presynaptic receptors, is effective in reducing the symptoms of TS in many receptors, is effective in reducing the symptoms of TS in many patients. Stimulation of these alpha$_2$-receptors results in a decreased release of norepinephrine (NE) at the synapse. Studies using microiontophoretic techniques have shown that clonidine inhibits the spontaneous firing of the locus coeruleus (LC, the primary site of noradrenergic cell bodies in brain) and reduces brain NE turnover. Clonidine also acutely lowers the concentration of plasma-free 3-methoxy-4-hydroxy-phenyl-glycol (MHPG, the principal central metabolite of NE).[27,28] However, there are several observations that raise questions about the role of NE in the pathogenesis of TS. First, clonidine is effective in ameliorating the symptoms of opiate withdrawal in addicted newborn infants[21]; yet studies in rat pups have shown that alpha$_2$-adrenergic receptors are not functional until twenty-one or more days of age, suggesting that clonidine may have other mechanisms of action. Second, our studies of CSF and urine MHPG and plasma NE in TS patients generally have not revealed differences from normal controls.

Finally, even after the LC is destroyed by neurotoxin, leading to almost complete reduction (less than 5 percent) of cortical NE, certain functions attributed to the LC and to clonidine remain intact. For example, LC-lesioned animals continue to show opiate withdrawal that is blocked by clonidine and clonidine-induced sedation. Although not as likely, alternate sites of action (e.g., peripheral) or systems (e.g., dopamine, serotonin, or histamine) may be involved in the therapeutic effect of clonidine in TS.

The mode of action of clonidine in TS also may involve indirect effects on the dopaminergic system.[30] The observation that a positive clinical response to haloperidol during a double-blind cross-over trial predicted a positive response to clonidine is consistent with this hypothesis.[5] In addition, results from animal studies indicate that noradrenergic activity can alter dopaminergic-mediated activity.[2] Serotonergic mechanisms have been suggested as the link between central noradrenergic and dopaminergic mechanisms.[6]

Currently there is insufficient evidence to support a hypothesis of direct serotonergic involvement in the pathogenesis of TS. Medications that act by increasing or decreasing serotonergic activity do not consistently affect TS symptoms. However, studies of CSF 5-hydroxyindoleacetic acid (5-HIAA, the principal central metabolite of serotonin) in TS patients have tended to reveal differences from normal controls, with TS patients showing lowered concentrations.

Although data are limited and contradictory, cholinergic systems also have been implicated in the pathogenesis of TS. Some clinical observations have suggested that cholinergic-enhancing agents (e.g., physostigmine, deanol acetamidobenzoate, choline, and lecithin) reduce TS symptoms, whereas anticholinergic agents (e.g., scopolamine) exacerbate the symptoms, supporting an acetylcholine-deficiency hypothesis.[41] These findings have not been replicated. In addition, elevated red-blood-cell choline was found in TS patients and their relatives; however, the relationship of this finding to brain cholinergic function is unclear.[19]

The expression of TS may involve several neurotransmitter systems operating in a cascading or reinforcing manner. Various aspects of the disorder may involve different neurotransmitters or a balance between them. For example, motor symptoms may express dopaminergic overactivity, while difficulties with inhibition (e.g., distractibility, coprolalia) may represent the engagement of noradrenergic or serotonergic mechanisms.

NEUROPHYSIOLOGY AND NEUROPSYCHOLOGY

The electroencephalogram (EEG), computed tomography (CT) scan, positron emission tomography (PET) scan, sensory and visual evoked response, premovement EEG potential, and neuropsychological test battery have been employed in the study of TS.

The high incidence of EEG abnormalities, observed in 35 to 65 percent of TS patients, has been interpreted as indicating neurophysiological dysfunction. Nonlocalized sharp waves and/or slowing are most frequently observed; epileptiform activity is uncommon. One study found that TS patients with abnormal EEGs were more likely to have other objective signs of neurological dysfunction or were taking haloperidol, a drug known to disturb the EEG.[3] We have found that TS patients with abnormal EEGs have a significantly earlier age of onset.[42] The EEG does not appear to be of either clinical or prognostic significance.

One study found six of sixteen (37 percent) subjects with TS had mildly to markedly abnormal CT scans using clinical criteria.[8] The most common abnormality was ventricular dilitation. Four of the six (67 percent) subjects with abnormal CT scans also had abnormal EEGs, while only one of the ten (10 percent) children with normal CT scan had an abnormal EEG. No localized CT findings have been reported in patients with TS. Our objective measurements of ventricular volume and cortical density are normal.

In a recent study, five patients with TS were compared with seven normal control subjects by PET scanning.[9] Overall cerebral glucose metabolism did not differ significantly between patients and control subjects. In the basal ganglia, however, glucose utilization in patients with TS averaged 16 percent above the control levels. This preliminary finding, although intriguing, leaves unanswered the question of whether altered basal ganglia function leads to TS movements or whether TS movements lead to altered basal ganglia function.

Preliminary studies of cortical somatosensory evoked potentials in patients with TS revealed no abnormalities,[34] while visually evoked responses showed wave IV amplitude changes.[14] Further studies are needed to clarify these observations; our preliminary findings suggest no abnormalities in event-related potentials.

A negative scalp recorded electrical potential (the readiness or premovement potential) during the half second or so preceding a willed, voluntary movement has been observed in normal human subjects[26] and patients with TS[34] following a request by the investigator to mimic a movement. These premovement potentials were not observed in TS patients preceding tics.[34] These results have been interpreted as indicating that simple tics are not generated through normal motor pathways utilized for willed movements. In addition, the absence of any observable potential change in the EEG prior to a tic suggests that tics originate in deep brain structures.

Neuropsychological testing of patients with TS has revealed mixed and sometimes conflicting results. Patients identified as showing evidence of "organicity" have abnormalities compatible with diffuse, nonlocalized, nonspecific CNS dysfunction. Frequently, using the age-appropriate Wechsler Intelligence Scale and/or a test of visual-motor integration (VMI) (e.g., the Bender-Gestalt), early case reports and surveys of unmedicated TS patients found average or above intelligence and VMI impairments. In the largest survey of 144 patients, a normal distribution of overall intelligence and subtest scores was found, except for a significantly increased Wechsler Intelligence Scale coding subtest.[13] More recent studies have involved some or all subjects on haloperidol and frequently have found normal IQ, VMI delays of two or more years, and a significant decrease on coding subtests.[17] A number of studies suggest that older patients (who have had their TS symptoms longer) have more impairments.

At least 50 percent of all school-age children with TS have school performance difficulties and may have specific areas of learning problems (math or reading). Difficulties often involve attention, self-monitoring, or motivation, all of which may be impaired further by medication and the need to inhibit symptoms. Careful neuropsychological assessment of these children revealed a normal distribution of IQ and no specific abnormalities, except in coding.[20]

NEUROPATHOLOGY

Only two detailed neuropathological descriptions of cases of TS have been reported in the literature.[40] One study found no evidence of a disease process; the other was interpreted as compatible with hypoplasia of the corpus striatum. Currently there is insufficient neuropathological evidence to suggest a pathological-anatomical correlate of TS.

ANIMAL MODELS

Several animal models, most of which involve the pharmacological induction of stereotypic behavior, have been studied for their relevance to TS.[17] One intriguing model involves stimulant-induced stereotypic behavior in the rat that is amplified by stress.[25,31] All proposed animal models for TS lack several features necessary to a complete model, which include the need to induce a disorder that is phenotypically similar to the human disorder, a symptomatic course that simulates the natural history of the human disorder, and a response to medications that is similar to that of the human disorder.

Future Developments

Basic and clinical researchers are currently attempting to elucidate the etiology, pathogenesis, and most effective treatment of TS. Recent developments in human behavioral genetics soon may be joined by those in molecular biology and result in the identification of the genetic defect(s) underlying the disorder. New imaging techniques, such as nuclear magnetic resonance and positron emission tomography, will allow for greater understanding of the anatomical structures and metabolic processes involved in the pathogenesis of TS. The use of medication challenges may add another dimension to our understanding of neurochemistry.[29] In addition, as our basic and clinical knowledge of TS increases, we can expect new medications to be developed that will treat more specifically the underlying defect(s) in TS.

ACKNOWLEDGMENTS

This research was supported by The Gateposts Foundation, Mental Health Clinical Research Center grant MH 30929, National Institute of Child Health and Human Development grant HD 03008, and the John Merck Fund.

REFERENCES

1. AMERICAN PSYCHIATRIC ASSOCIATION. *Diagnostic and Statistical Manual of Mental Disorders* (DSM-III). Washington, D.C.: American Psychiatric Association, 1980.

2. ANTELMAN, S. M., and CAGGIULA, A. R. "Norepinephrine-dopamine Interactions and Behavior," *Science,* 195 (1977): 646–653.

3. BERGEN, D., TANNER, C. M., and WILSON, R. "The Electroencephalogram in Tourette Syndrome," *Annals of Neurology,* 11 (1982): 382–385.

4. BLISS, J., COHEN, D. J., and FREEDMAN, D. X. "Sensory Experiences of Gilles de la Tourette Syndrome," *Archives of General Psychiatry,* 37 (1980): 1343–1347.

5. BORISON, R. L., et al. "New Pharmacological Approaches in the Treatment of Gilles de la Tourette Syndrome," in A. J. Friedhoff and T. N. Chase, eds., Gilles de la Tourette Syndrome, *Advances in Neurology,* vol. 35, New York: Raven Press, 1982, pp. 377–382.

6. BUNNEY, B. S., and DeRIEMER, S. A.; "Effects of Clonidine on Nigral Dopamine Cell Activity: Possible Mediation by Noradrenergic Regulation of Serotonergic Raphe System," in A. J. Friedhoff and T. N. Chase, eds., Gilles de la Tourette Syndrome, *Advances in Neurology,* vol. 35. New York: Raven Press, 1982, pp. 99–104.

7. BUTLER, I. J., et al. "Biogenic Amine Metabolism in Tourette Syndrome," *Annals of Neurology,* 6 (1979): 37–39.

8. CAPARULO, B. K., et al. "Computed Tomographic Brain Scanning in Children with Developmental Neuropsychiatric Disorders," *Journal of the American Academy of Child Psychiatry,* 20 (1981): 338–357.

9. CHASE, T. N., "Gilles de la Tourette Syndrome: Studies with the Fluorine-18-labeled Fluorodeoxyglucose Positron Emission Tomographic Method," *Annals of Neurology,* 15 (Supplement) (1984):S175.

10. COHEN, D. J., et al. "Central Biogenic Amine Metabolism in Children with the Syndrome of Chronic Multiple Tics of Gilles de la Tourette Syndrome: Norepinephrine, Serotonin, and Dopamine," *Journal of the American Academy of Child Psychiatry,* 18 (1979): 320–341.

11. COHEN, D. J., et al. "Interaction of Biological and Psychological Factors in the Natural History of Tourette's Syndrome: A Paradigm for Childhood Neuropsychiatric Disorders," in A. J. Friedhoff and T. N. Chase, eds., *Gilles de la Tourette Syndrome, Advances in Neurology,* vol. 35. New York: Raven Press, 1982, pp. 31–40.

12. COMMINGS, D. E., and COMMINGS, B. G. "Tourette's Syndrome and Attention Deficit Disorder with Hyperactivity —Are they Genetically Related? *Journal of the American Academy of Child Psychiatry,* 23 (1984): 138–146.

13. CORBETT, J. A., et al. "Tics and Gilles de la Tourette Syndrome: A Follow-up Study and Critical Review," *British Journal of Psychiatry,* 115 (1969)1229–1241.

14. DOMINO, E. F., et al. "Visually Evoked Responses in Tourette Syndrome," in A. J. Friedhoff and T. N. Chase, eds., Gilles de la Tourette Syndrome, *Advances in Neurology,* vol. 35. New York: Raven Press, 1982, pp. 115–120.

15. FEINBERG, M., and CARROLL, B. J. "Effects of Dopamine Agonists and Antagonists in Tourette's Disease," *Archives of General Psychiatry,* 36 (1979): 979–985.

16. FRIEDHOFF, A. J. "Receptor Maturation in Pathogenesis and Treatment of Tourette Syndrome," in A. J. Friedhoff and T. N. Chase, eds., Gilles de la Tourette Syndrome, *Advances in Neurology,* vol. 35. New York: Raven Press, 1982, pp. 133–140.

17. FRIEDHOFF, A. J., and CHASE, T. N., eds. *Gilles de la Tourette Syndrome, Advances in Neurology,* vol. 35. New York: Raven Press, 1982.

18. GOLDEN, G. S. "Gilles de la Tourette's Syndrome following Methylphenidate Administration," *Developmental Medicine and Child Neurology,* 16 (1974): 76–78.

19. HANIN, I., et al. "Red-cell Choline and Gilles de la Tourette Syndrome," *New England Journal of Medicine,* 301 (1979): 661–662.

20. HARCHERIK, D. F., et al. "Attentional and Perceptual Disturbances in Children with Tourette's Syndrome, Attention Deficit Disorder, and Epilepsy," *Schizophrenia Bulletin,* 8 (1982): 356–359.

21. HODER, E. L., et al. "Clonidine in Neonatal Narcotic Abstinence Syndrome," *New England Journal of Medicine*, 305 (1981): 1284.

22. JAGGER, J., et al. "The Epidemiology of Tourette's Syndrome: A Pilot Study," *Schizophrenia Bulletins*, 8 (1982): 267–278.

23. KIDD, K., and PAUL, D. L. "Genetic Hypotheses for Tourette Syndrome," in A. J. Friedhoff and T. N. Chase, eds., *Gilles de la Tourette Syndrome, Advances in Neurology*, vol. 35. New York: Raven Press, 1982, pp. 243–249.

24. KIDD, K. K., PRUSOFF, B. A., and COHEN, D. J. "Familial Pattern of Gilles de la Tourette Syndrome," *Archives of General Psychiatry*, 37 (1980): 1336–1339.

25. KNOTT, P. J., and HUTSON, P. H. "Stress-induced Stereotypy in the Rat: Neuropharmacological Similarities to Tourette Syndrome," in A. J. Friedhoff and T. N. Chase, eds., *Gilles de la Tourette Syndrome, Advances in Neurology*, vol. 35. New York: Raven Press, 1982, pp. 233–238.

26. KORNHUBER, H. H., and DEECKE, L. "Hirnpotentialanderungen bei Willkurbewegungen und passiven Bewwgungen des Menschen: Bereitschaftspotential und reafferente Potentiale," *Pfluegers Archiv*, 284 (1965): 1–17.

27. LECKMAN, J. F., MAAS, J. W., and HENINGER, G. R. "Covariance of Plasma-Free 3-methoxy-4-hydroxyphenethylene Glycol and Diastolic Blood Pressure," *European Journal of Pharmacology*, 70 (1981): 111–120.

28. LECKMAN, J. F., et al. "Effects of Oral Clonidine on Plasma 3-methoxy-4-hydroxyphenethylene Glycol (MHPG) in Man: Preliminary Report," *Life Sciences*, 26 (1980): 2179–2185.

29. LECKMAN, J. F., et al. "Clonidine in the Treatment of Gilles de la Tourette Syndrome: A Review," in A. J. Friedhoff and T. N. Chase, eds., *Gilles de la Tourette Syndrome, Advances in Neurology*, vol. 35. New York: Raven Press, 1982, pp. 391–402.

30. LECKMAN, J. F., et al. "Acute and Chronic Clonidine Treatment in Tourette's Syndrome: A Preliminary Report on Clinical Response and Effect on Plasma and Urinary Catecholamine Metabolites, Growth Hormone, and Blood Pressure," *Journal of the American Academy of Child Psychiatry*, 22 (1983): 433–440.

31. LECKMAN, J. F., et al. "The Pathogenesis of Gilles de la Tourette Syndrome: A review of Data and Hypotheses," in N. S. Shah, ed., *Movement Disorders*. New York: Plenum Press, forthcoming.

32. LOWE, T. L., et al. "Stimulant Medications Precipitate Tourette's Syndrome," *Journal of the American Medical Association*, 247 (1982): 1729–1731.

33. NEE, L. E., et al. "Gilles de la Tourette Syndrome: Clinical and Family Study of 50 cases," *Annals of Neurology*, 7 (1980): 41–49.

34. OBESCO, J. A., ROTHWELL, J. C., and MARSDEN, C. D. "The Neurophysiology of Tourette Syndrome," in A. J. Friedhoff and T. N. Chase, eds., *Gilles de la Tourette Syndrome, Advances in Neurology*, vol. 35. New York: Raven Press, 1982, pp. 105–114.

35. PAULS, D. L., et al. "Familial Patterns and Transmission of Gilles de la Tourette Syndrome and Multiple Tics," *Archives of General Psychiatry*, 38 (1981): 1085–1090.

36. PAULS, D. L., et al., "Evidence Against a Genetic Relationship Between Tourette Syndrome and Attention Deficit Disorders," *Archives of General Psychiatry*, in press.

37. PAULS, D. L., et al. "The Risk of Tourette's Syndrome and Chronic Multiple Tics Among Relatives of Tourette's Syndrome Patients Obtained by Direct Interview," *Journal of the American Academy of Child Psychiatry*, 23 (1984): 134–137.

38. PAULS, D. L., et al., "Evidence Supporting a Genetic Relationship Between Gilles de la Tourette's Syndrome and Obsessive Compulsive Disorder," submitted for review.

39. PRICE, R. A., et al. "A Twin Study of Tourette Syndrome," submitted for publication.

40. RICHARDSON, E. P., Jr., "Neuropathological Studies of Tourette Syndrome," in A. J. Friedhoff and T. N. Chase, eds., *Gilles de la Tourette Syndrome, Advances in Neurology*, vol. 35. New York: Raven Press, 1982, pp. 83–87.

41. STAHL, S. M., and BERGER, P. A. "Cholinergic and Dopaminergic Mechanisms in Tourette Syndrome," in A. J. Friedhoff and T. N. Chase, eds., *Gilles de la Tourette Syndrome, Advances in Neurology*, vol. 35. New York: Raven Press, 1982, pp. 141–150.

42. VOLKMAR, F. R., et al. "EEG Abnormalities in Tourette's Syndrome," *Journal of the American Academy of Child Psychiatry*, 23 (1984): 352–353.

36 / Sleep in Children: Recent Advances

Jovan G. Simeon

Introduction

It is estimated that about 50 million adults in the United States have "trouble with sleeping."[42] The incidence of sleep disorders is even greater if sufferers from excessive daytime somnolence and sleep-related problems are added. While relatively little is known about sleep and sleep disorders in children, recent research in this area has resulted in significant new knowledge. In daily practice, unfortunately, children's sleep problems are often unrecognized or minimized, and hence go untreated. Children and adolescents seldom complain of sleep difficulties, just as they seldom complain of any emotional, behavioral, or learning problems. The usual concerns and complaints commonly expressed by parents relate to irregular sleep habits, excessive or insufficient sleep, poor sleep, bedtime problems, night waking, nightmares, night terrors, sleepwalking, bedwetting, and daytime sleepiness. Sleep problems can, however, also cause serious and chronic disability (e.g., narcolepsy, sleep apnea–hypersomnia syndrome); at times they can even be fatal (e.g., sudden infant death syndrome (SIDS), accidental injuries during sleepwalking). Mild sleep problems may be symptomatic of serious but often misdiagnosed disorders, such as depression, sleep apnea, narcolepsy, and epilepsy.

To properly evaluate sleep events, the complete twenty-four-hour (circadian) sleep-wake cycle must be considered. To maintain the sleep-wake rhythm to the twenty-four-hour cycle, various indicators of time ("Zeitgebers") are necessary, such as clocks, mealtimes, and work and school schedules. In addition to the sleep-wake cycle, there are other circadian rhythms in humans, related to endocrine secretion, metabolism, temperature, and so forth. The secretion of some hormones is coupled with sleep. For example, human growth hormone is released soon after sleep onset (during stage 3–4 sleep), while peak values of prolactin occur between 5 and 7 A.M.; corticosteroid secretion, on the other hand, follows a secretory cycle independent of sleep. Unless the various circadian rhythms are synchronized daily, the different cycles may diverge, resulting in excessively variable and difficult sleep.[24] In such patients, a regular wake-up time may be a most effective Zeitgeber, as this is under voluntary control.

Most sleep problems can be evaluated and treated in the office. More complicated or difficult cases may require sleep laboratory evaluations. Such specialized clinical and research work is undertaken in sleep disorder centers. A decade ago the Association of Sleep Disorders Centers (ASDC) was formed; it currently has over forty centers operating in the United States and Canada. (For a list of these centers contact the Association of Sleep Disorders Centers, P. O. Box 2604, Del Mar, California, 92014.)

This chapter selectively reviews recent progress related to the development, methodology, prevalence, classification, diagnosis, findings in child psychiatric disorders, and the psychopharmacology of sleep and sleep disorders. Therapy is reviewed in chapter 53. A number of books and reviews of special interest to child psychiatrists deal with these topics in detail. Some are general texts,* while others deal with more specific topics, such as infancy,[3,4,6] adolescence,[16,17,18,19] parasomnias,[45,46,47] and research.[69] The journals *Sleep* and *Sleep Research* are also useful sources of information.

*See references 1, 5, 32, 38, and 51.

Sleep Development and Age Relationships

The ontogenetic development of sleep in childhood has been described elsewhere.* As the child grows older, there are decreases of total sleep time, rapid-eye-movement (REM) sleep, and stage 4 sleep; REM sleep cycles become longer, while sleep variability and disturbances increase. In infancy, sleep patterns develop according to a precise time schedule that allows for a determination of the conceptual age. Compared to full-term infants, premature infants reveal subtle but real differences of sleep-wake states, with more wakefulness and more irregular progression with age, suggesting unstable active sleep/wakefulness mechanisms.[6] The typical sleep problems of toddlers and young children are bedtime fears, sleep terrors, nightmares, and enuresis; while adolescents complain of difficulty falling asleep, nighttime arousals, difficulty getting up, overtiredness, and daytime sleepiness.[17,64] It appears that older children lose sleep during school days and recover the loss on nonschool nights.

Children of the same age show large individual differences in sleep requirements and patterns. Rigid sleep schedules may result in bedtime difficulties and insomnia, or in insufficient sleep with hyperactivity, irritability, and poor school performance. Nighttime sleep schedules are adequate if they are associated with optimal daytime alertness and energy.

To understand the mechanisms of normal and abnormal development of the sleep-wake cycle, it is essential to investigate the ontogenetic development of other circadian and ultradian rhythms, especially those of the endocrinological functions, and their relationship.

Methodology and Diagnosis

During the past two decades, remarkable progress in sleep research has resulted from advances in electronics, computers, and statistics. Polysomnographic evaluations have become the basic diagnostic and research method yielding objective data. They include the recording of sleep electroencephalogram (EEG), eye movements, electromyogram, air flow, respiratory effort, and electrocardiogram. Sleep in children has been investigated also by time-lapse video recordings in the home,[4,6] movies, twenty-four-hour polygraphic records,[27] quantitative computer EEG analyses,[69]

*See references 3, 5, 19, 38, and 62.

somatosensory evoked potentials,[25] and in-dwelling venous catheters for long-term plasma sampling of hormones. Sleep questionnaires have been specifically designed for use with children and adolescents.[5,16,70,71] (See table 36–1.)

Diagnostic evaluations of sleep complaints should include a pediatric examination and assessments of milestones, bedtime rituals, sleep habits, behavioral or learning problems, stress, and parental reactions. Sleep disorders may result from poor sleeping habits or stress, especially during rapid growth. Insomnia, hypersomnia, and parasomnias may be primary sleep disorders or may be due to medical or social factors. In adolescents with sleep problems affecting school performance or family life, the possibility of drug or alcohol abuse must be carefully explored. Most children with sleep disorders should be evaluated and treated in the office. Only a minority of patients require polygraphic investigations during sleep for diagnostic reasons or to monitor therapeutic efficacy. Such investigations have been useful also in the prediction of later outcome of brain-damaged or high-risk newborns as well as of those with hormonal and metabolic disorders[48]; these studies are essential as well for the differential diagnosis of nocturnal epilepsy and disorders of excessive daytime somnolence.

Prevalence of Sleep Problems

The few older prevalence studies on sleep in children are summarized in chapter 35 in volume 2 of this *Handbook*[1] as well as elsewhere.[1,48,69,71] More recent data have been obtained on normal preschool and school-age children, and on psychiatric patients. In normal toddlers the predominant problems are difficulty settling to sleep and night waking,[43] while older preschoolers show a prolongation of bedtime routines and delays in falling asleep; for example, 66 percent of normal five-year-olds required more than thirty minutes to fall asleep.[11] In normal grade-school children the most frequent sleep disorders were restless sleep and sleep talking[71]; more sleep problems were observed in children of lower socioeconomic class, with chronic medical problems, and with ear, nose, and throat allergies. Compared to either pediatric or normal controls, the rates of practically all sleep disorders in child psychiatric patients are significantly higher. In fact, the rates of parasomnias, nightmares, insomnia, and hypersomnia obtained from the child psychiatric samples are three to four times higher than those reported by pediatricians.[12] Similarly, compared to the findings with 1,300 normal children, the parents of 1,300 clinically referred, disturbed children reported

higher rates of nightmares, trouble sleeping, sleeping too little, overtiredness, and sleeping too much.[2] This author compared 962 normal schoolchildren to 103 child psychiatric patients; the latter's percent rates for sleep talking (33 percent), sleep-onset insomnia (31 percent), night waking (29 percent), enuresis (22 percent), and overtiredness (15 percent) were about three times higher than in the normal group. Poor or restless sleep (32 percent) was over six times more frequent. Nightmares (17 percent), early-morning waking (9 percent), daytime naps, and sleepwalking were also more frequent in the child psychiatric group. One or more moderate or marked sleep problems were reported in 17 percent of the normal schoolchildren. Another study was conducted of 120 unmedicated child psychiatric patients with more chronic and severe psychiatric disorders; in this instance even higher rates were reported for night and early-morning waking, sleep-onset insomnia, poor or restless sleep, and nightmares.[69,70] While there were no significant sex differences in the prevalence of sleep problems among the normal children, there were large differences between male and female psychiatric patients: more boys manifested sleep talking, enuresis, early-morning waking, and daytime naps, while more girls suffered from poor or restless sleep and night waking.

Due to differences in populations sampled, method of evaluation, age range, definition of symptoms, and severity criteria, it is difficult to compare the findings from these various studies. Nevertheless, the findings of different investigators show a remarkable degree of agreement. In summary, many normal and disturbed children suffer from a variety of sleep disorders; child psychiatric patients have more frequent and severe sleep problems than nonpsychiatric controls; there is a significant association between the frequency of sleep problems and psychopathology factors; many sleep problems occur in combinations; and for a number of sleep problems age is an important factor: for example, parental reports of nightmares and sleeping too little decrease as the child grows older, while overtiredness and sleeping too much increase. Longitudinal studies using more reliable methods are needed to clarify the clinical and prognostic value of sleep findings in children.

Sleep Disorders

The ASDC[8] has published a widely accepted classification of four types of sleep disorders: (1) disorders of initiating and maintaining sleep, where the chief complaint is poor sleep ("insomnia"); (2) disorders of excessive somnolence, which include a number of func-

SECTION IV / DEVIATIONS OF DEVELOPMENT

TABLE 36–1

Sleep Pattern Questionnaire

Record #: _____
Patient #: _____
Study #: _____

To Be Completed by Parents

Name of Child: _____ Date of Birth: _____ Sex: M ____ F ____

Date: _____

Numbers and Ages of
Brothers and Sisters: _____
_____
_____
_____

Please answer all questions as accurately as you can

	Never a Problem	Problem Only in Past	If a Problem: Mark How Many Days in the Past Week							Duration of Problem: Weeks, Months, Years
			1	2	3	4	5	6	7	
1. Poor or restless sleep										
2. Awakens at night										
3. More than 30 minutes to fall asleep										
4. Awakens before 6 a.m.										
5. Sleep walking										
6. Sleep talking										
7. Bedwetting										
8. Nightmares										
9. Excessive daytime sleepiness/tiredness										
10. Takes naps during the day										

11. During the past week (7 nights) what time has your child gone to bed on weekdays?
_____

12. Is the child fearful:
     of the dark? _____
     of sleeping alone? _____
     of going to bed? _____

13. Are there any other sleep habits, like snoring? _____
                              grinding the teeth? _____
     Others? (describe briefly) _____

14. Do any other members of the family have sleep problems?
     Mother _____ Father _____ Siblings _____
     Describe the problems briefly _____
     _____

15. Does the child share a bedroom?   Yes _____   No _____

16. Has there been medication given for:
     (a) Sleep problems?   Now ____ Past ____ Name of Medication _____
     (b) Medical problems?   Now ____ Past ____ Name of Medication _____

17. Describe briefly if your child has any:
     (a) Medical problems? _____
     (b) Behavioral problems? _____
     (c) Learning or school problems? _____
     (d) Emotional problems?   e.g. anxiety _____; depression _____
                              other _____

tional and organic conditions; (3) disorders of the sleep-wake schedule, where patients cannot sleep when they want, need, or expect to; and (4) dysfunctions associated with sleep, sleep stages, or partial arousals (parasomnias).

DISORDERS OF INITIATING AND MAINTAINING SLEEP

Night waking and bedtime difficulties, a common problem in older infants and toddlers,[67,68] made up about a third of the evaluations in a pediatric sleep disorders clinic.[28] Chronic childhood insomnia occurs much more frequently in emotionally disturbed children.[26] While insomnias are associated with a variety of psychiatric disorders in all age groups, in younger patients depression may be associated with hypersomnia.[40] In adults suffering from poor sleep, insomnia often starts in childhood. Childhood-onset insomniacs compared to adult-onset insomniacs take longer to fall asleep, sleep less, and have more ill-defined REM sleep, atypical EEG waves, soft neurological signs, and evidence of attention deficit and learning disorders[39]; many are sensitive to stimulants and noise. Adolescents often complain of difficulties in falling asleep or premature awakening; others suffer from the delayed sleep phase syndrome, where sleep-onset insomnia is associated with difficulty in morning awakening. If daytime sleepiness is excessive, a sleep apnea–hypersomnia syndrome and narcolepsy should be suspected. In otherwise normal eleventh- and twelfth-grade students, 12.6 percent reported chronic and severe sleep disturbance, whereas 37.6 percent reported occasional sleep disturbance. In contrast to adolescents with no sleep problems, those with poor sleep reported tension, worries, moodiness, a lesser ability in solving personal problems, and personality characteristics suggesting low self-esteem, mild depression, and daytime fatigue.[64]

DISORDERS OF EXCESSIVE SOMNOLENCE

Important progress has been made in the diagnosis and therapy of excessive daytime somnolence (EDS). Severe forms of EDS are usually associated with biological abnormalities. Children with EDS are often labeled lazy, inattentive, poor learners, hyperactive, mentally retarded, or having emotional problems.[57] Disrupted nighttime sleep and daytime somnolence are the typical presenting complaints of sleep apnea and narcolepsy, but the complaints are usually minimized by clinicians. If increasing the nighttime sleep results in no improvement, diagnostic evaluations for sleep apnea–hypersomnia and narcolepsy should be undertaken. These disorders often first appear during adoles-

cence. In contrast to preadolescent children, adolescents frequently complain of daytime sleepiness and tiredness; they do stay up later at night and this may lead to a chronic sleep deficit.[7] Cases with EDS require a thorough medical and sleep history and a physical examination. The objective measures of sleepiness are pupillography and multiple sleep latency testing (for an overview, see Orr[60]).

Sleep Apnea–Hypersomnia Syndrome. This disorder can occur in children of any age, but it increases markedly with age, affects mainly males, and can be acute or chronic. Predisposing factors include enlarged tonsils or adenoids, upper airway or maxillofacial abnormalities, hypothyroidism, and obesity.[22,35,61] The disorder is characterized by loud snoring followed by apneic pauses and brief arousals or restless movements. In addition to loud snoring, children with sleep apnea syndrome frequently manifest excessive daytime sleepiness, decreased school performance, reappearance of nocturnal enuresis, morning headaches, mood and personality changes, weight gain or loss, and hypertension.[33] Airway obstruction during sleep in children has been associated with behavioral, developmental, and academic problems.[74] The syndrome can affect intellectual functioning even more than in narcolepsy: Over one-third of children were misdiagnosed as borderline mentally retarded when first seen.[48] At first, cardiovascular and pulmonary abnormalities are found only during sleep or drowsiness, but after several years these complications become evident even during wakefulness.[48,74]

Sudden Infant Death Syndrome. SIDS occurs in two to three infants out of every thousand live births. Increased risk factors include prior intensive care, maternal addiction, short interpregnancy intervals, and male sex.[72] Compared with controls, "near miss for SIDS" infants are a heterogenous group with various unrelated respiratory, cardiac, or sleep-stage differences; the life-threatening events are more frequent during non-REM sleep.[34] Compared with normal infants, siblings of SIDS victims have a three- to fourfold higher risk for SIDS. Such siblings have longer intervals between active sleep epochs in the newborn period and a decreased tendency to enter short waking periods at two and three months of age, suggesting an increased tendency to remain asleep or a relative failure to arouse from sleep.[36]

Other Disorders of Excessive Somnolence. Of the variety of other disorders of excessive somnolence relevant to children and adolescents are those related to the use of drugs and alcohol; following the discontinuation of psychotropic drugs or alcohol; those associated with various psychiatric, metabolic (hypothyroidism, diabetes), and central nervous system disorders, and menstrual periods; an idiopathic form[73]; and rare conditions, such as the Kleine-Levin syndrome where hypersomnia episodes occurring typically in adolescent males are associated with excessive eating and frequently with weight gain or sexuality and mood disorders, representing some hypothalamic or diencephalic dysfunction.

Narcolepsy. This well-known syndrome has been described in detail in numerous texts (see Ablon and Mack[1]). Of particular relevance to child psychiatry is the fact that while about one-fifth of narcoleptics report problems with daytime sleepiness prior to age eleven, narcoleptic children are usually referred for medical evaluation only when their teachers complain about napping during class. Unrecognized microsleep episodes may precede the nap by several hours. Typically, such children are seen as lazy or poorly motivated, and an attention deficit and/or learning disorder may be the presenting complaint.[48] The child usually struggles against the excessive daytime sleepiness, sometimes with hyperactive behavior.[57] Hypnagogic auditory or visual hallucinations are vivid, often frightening, and not reported to the parents; such children may be reluctant to go to bed. In contrast to a seizure, when cataplexy occurs, the patient remains aware of the surroundings.

DISORDERS OF THE SLEEP-WAKE SCHEDULE

Sleep-wake rhythm difficulties usually result from a misalignment between the patient's circadian rhythms and environmental timetables (Zeitgebers). Computer techniques have enabled chronobiology to investigate the complex relations between various biological rhythms over prolonged periods of time. New therapeutic strategies can also be explored: Antidepressants, for example, appear to speed up the circadian cycle,[49] while lithium carbonate may lengthen it.[44] Many children and adolescents suffer from transient or persistent sleep-wake difficulties, but research data are practically nonexistent. The delayed sleep phase syndrome consists of delayed bedtimes and rising times. Such patients usually are younger than other insomniacs and show no psychiatric problems.[75] Their attempts to advance sleep onset results in insomnia, but sleep onset can be delayed.[77] In the non-twenty-four-hour sleep-wake syndrome, patients are unable to maintain a regular twenty-four-hour sleep-wake cycle. Such patients complain of periodic difficulties in getting to sleep and of extreme arousal problems. Some cases may be due to neurological malfunction, while others—such as blind or autistic children—do not perceive the usual environmental timetables. In the irregular sleep-wake pattern, a poor night's sleep and oversleeping lead to a self-reinforcing irregular pattern, where sleeping and waking are almost evenly spread over a twenty-four-hour day. Other circadian rhythms

(endocrine, temperature) also fluctuate erratically or flatten.[76]

DYSFUNCTIONS ASSOCIATED WITH SLEEP, SLEEP STAGES, OR PARTIAL AROUSALS (PARASOMNIAS)

Parasomnias are disorders that either occur during sleep or are exaggerated by sleep. About 5 percent of the U.S. population suffers from some clinically significant parasomnia. Some parasomnias are associated with specific sleep stages (e.g., somnambulism during arousal from delta sleep; painful erections during REM sleep); others occur almost any time during sleep (e.g., enuresis and bruxism) or occur predominantly during transitions from sleep to arousal (e.g., familial sleep paralysis). Arousal from delta sleep is difficult or almost impossible in some subjects, especially in children. In one study,[14] high-intensity auditory stimuli well above waking threshold values were given to both hyperactive and nonhyperactive children. These alarms failed to result in behavioral arousal for both groups during the first sleep cycle. When arousal from delta sleep is attempted, a state of confusion may result, characterized by a mixture of delta EEG waves (deep sleep) and waking EEG waves.

Somnambulism, sleep terrors, and some cases of enuresis may be due to an incomplete arousal from delta sleep. These disorders occur early in the night and most often in children who have more and deeper delta sleep than do adults. The children are difficult to arouse, and they can rarely recall the event in the morning. Different parasomnias often affect the same child.

Night terrors *(pavor nocturnus)* and somnambulism in childhood appear related primarily to genetic and developmental factors; their persistence is associated with psychological factors and with significant psychopathology in adulthood.[46,47] Attacks may be aggravated by stress, irregular sleep, and overtiredness. Somnambulism is also often associated with migraine.[9] In adults, somnambulism can be induced by various psychotropic drugs,[41] combined lithium-neuroleptic therapy,[20] sleep deprivation, or alcohol. The central issue in somnambulism, according to Broughton,[13] is why such subjects appear to have difficulty in fully waking up and why they manifest prolonged behavioral automatisms. The differential diagnosis of somnambulism includes nocturnal epilepsy and sleep drunkenness. Night terrors must be differentiated from nightmares (dream anxiety attacks)[10] and terrifying hypnagogic hallucinations; the latter may be due to narcolepsy, temporal lobe epilepsy, and depression.

Nightmares are more likely if REM sleep is increased, and may therefore be precipitated by fever and abrupt cessation of REM-suppressant drugs. It has been suggested that children who continue to have frequent nightmares at the age of ten or twelve could be considered at risk for developing schizophrenia.[37]

In the differential diagnosis of nocturnal epilepsy and pseudoseizures the standard polysomnogram is not sufficient, and full clinical EEG evaluations during sleep or after sleep deprivation are necessary. In some forms of epilepsy, often with temporal lobe EEG abnormalities, sleepwalking can occur more than twice a night, and behavior is complex and sometimes violent; these patients have no family history of parasomnias. Nocturnal epilepsy can present as a behavior problem in childhood. However, even when night terrors occur in epileptics, the mechanisms are nonepileptic and must be distinguished from nocturnal epileptic seizures with accompanying fear.[13] In a case of hypnogenic paroxysmal dystonia, the child displayed pseudoseizures characterized by nocturnal spasms during non-REM sleep.[54] Simultaneous EEG and videotaping (videosomnography) were used to establish the diagnosis and monitor the efficacy of carbamazepine therapy.[23]

Compared to normal subjects, children with sleep-related enuresis show multiple physiological changes throughout sleep, including bladders that are hyper-responsive to arousing stimuli[13]; during the enuretic episode, bladder pressures reached over 100 cm water, exceeding the levels that an awake child can inhibit. Recent data seem to have disproved the view that enuretic events are mainly associated with delta sleep, as they are not found to be associated with a particular sleep stage.[56] Also, with respect to the sleep-stage distribution of enuretic events, psychiatrically disturbed childen did not differ from the nondisturbed peers. According to Broughton,[13] the most important issue is not the sleep stage during which enuresis is most common, but why enuretic children show an insufficiently rapid or insufficiently complete awakening in response to vesicular stimuli.

Some of the other conditions classified as parasomnias are *jactatio capitis nocturna,* bruxism, familial sleep paralysis, impaired sleep-related penile tumescence, sleep-related cluster headaches, chronic paroxysmal hemicrania, and sleep-related asthma.

Sleep in Children with Various Psychiatric Disorders

As stated, survey and prevalence studies indicate clearly that child psychiatric populations suffer from more and greater sleep difficulties than do nonpsychiatric controls. Children with insomnia, hypersomnia,

and secondary enuresis are more likely to have other psychiatric disorders. While a number of psychological, medical, and environmental factors can cause sleep disturbances, pathological sleep can also lead to a variety of behavioral, learning, and medical problems.

Very little is known about any sleep patterns that may be characteristic for a child psychiatric diagnostic group or subgroup, or about any significant sleep changes during therapy and recovery. The identification of any sleep aspects typical of a child psychiatric disorder may have important implications in relation to the mechanisms, course, prognosis, and therapy of that disorder. Only in recent years have modern research techniques been used in the study of the sleep of children with depressive, attention deficit, conduct, and psychotic disorders.

DEPRESSION

In one study, sleep disturbances were a frequent complaint among depressed children.[50] In children with depressive symptomatology, preliminary sleep EEG findings compared to normative sleep data showed that the sleep continuity levels in the two groups were virtually identical.[52] Imipramine hydrochloride therapy of the depressed group resulted in decreased sleep efficiency, increased wakefulness, increased stage 2 sleep, decreased stage 4 sleep, and REM suppression—findings that contrast strikingly with those of tricyclic drug effects in adults (adults show increases of both total sleep time and delta sleep). Polysomnography evaluations of drug-free children with major depressive disorders, nondepressed children with emotional disorders, and normal children showed no differences among the three groups in respect to sleep stages.[65] In the course of structured interviews, the depressed and neurotic children reported a higher proportion of sleep disturbances. A number of fully recovered drug-free prepubertal patients with major depressive illness were compared to themselves while depressed and to nondepressed neurotic and normal children.[66] In each instance, in the recovered children there were significantly shorter REM period latencies and a higher number of REM periods.

ATTENTION DEFICIT DISORDER WITH HYPERACTIVITY

Parents report that restless sleep, very early rising, and difficulties in falling asleep are more frequent in children with attention deficit disorder with hyperactivity (ADDH) than in those with learning disabilities.[69] Compared to normal controls, sleep patterns in unmedicated hyperkinetic children showed longer REM onset latencies and greater amounts of movement time.[15] In the hyperkinetic group, spinal motoneuronal excitability was reduced during both sleep and wakefulness, but the spinal excitability was reduced only during sleep in the normal controls.[55,63] These findings indicate decreased reflex facilitation and central excitability in hyperkinetic children. A recent study of sleep architecture abnormalities reported that except for decreased REM activity, there were no differences between ADDH children and normal controls.[31] The findings of sleep EEG studies in hyperactive patients are still inconclusive, variable, and based on too few patients with large individual differences in their sleep patterns. ADDH children manifest varying severities of hypermotility, attentional deficits, impulsivity, excitability, emotional lability, "soft" neurological signs, and EEG abnormalities; any deviations of their sleep patterns from the norm may be related merely to some of these aspects of the disorder. Most sleep studies of the effects of stimulant medications or their withdrawal in ADDH children show several positive findings, but these are variable, difficult to interpret, and inconclusive.[69]

CHILDHOOD AUTISM AND PSYCHOSES

There have been very few all-night studies in autistic and psychotic children. In general, these studies have failed to show any major differences in sleep pattern between psychotic and normal children. In a series of studies of autistic children,[59] the findings suggested maturational defects, specifically related to REM sleep differentiation, and vestibular dysfunction. Computerized analyses were undertaken to explore the usefulness of automated techniques as applied to the sleep EEGs of seven psychotic children before and after drug therapy and of seven normal controls.[69] In addition, since sleep itself maximizes the manifestations of EEG seizure activity, such sleep investigations might have helped identify any patients who were also suffering from epilepsy. Visual evaluations of the EEG records showed various EEG abnormalities in four of the seven patients and in one of the controls. The automated quantitative sleep EEG analyses demonstrated that the patients had consistently higher percentages of stage 2 sleep and lower percentages of stage 4 sleep than did the controls. Significant drug-induced sleep EEG changes were also evident, illustrating the potential applicability of computerized sleep EEG methods in pediatric psychopharmacology.

Autistic and other psychotic children show great interindividual differences in the type and severity of their symptoms, organic pathology, intellectual and developmental levels, and so forth; these factors may be critical in relation to any sleep characteristics or problems.

MISCELLANEOUS CHILD PSYCHIATRIC DISORDERS

Using standard measurement techniques in a study of preadolescent boys with conduct disorders, the sleep EEG showed slight differences from that of normal boys. Automated measurements, however, revealed significantly higher delta wave counts among the conduct disorder group.[21] In Gilles de la Tourette patients, sleep was characterized by increases of stage 3 and stage 4 sleep, a greater number of awakenings, decreased percentage of REM sleep, paroxysmal events during stage 4 sleep, and motor tics during all sleep stages.[30] In patients with anorexia nervosa, insomnia and early-morning waking were associated with low body weight.[53] Compared to findings in healthy subjects, all-night sleep EEGs in anorexic patients showed decreases of REM activity and density; in those patients with normal EEGs, a decrease of delta sleep was seen.[58]

Pediatric Psychopharmacology and Sleep

The use of psychotropic drugs in the therapy of childhood sleep disorders is reviewed in chapter 53 of this volume. There has been little research on the effects of pharmacological compounds on the sleep of children. Drug therapy of psychiatric and nonpsychiatric disorders may result in sleep changes that are beneficial, adverse, or of yet unknown clinical significance. In adult patients, for example, single bedtime doses of tricyclics and neuroleptics, in contrast to multiple daily dosages, resulted in a significant increase in the number of frightening dreams.[29]

Daytime drowsiness and cognitive impairment are frequent complications of psychotropic medication. Any drugs that depress the respiratory center, such as hypnotics, are contraindicated in cases of sleep apnea. Withdrawal from any agent, including the stimulants, benzodiazepines, and alcohol, must be evaluated as a possible cause of sleep disorders. Even when drug effects on sleep are demonstrated in the clinic or the laboratory, the changes in the sleep patterns may be indirect, the result of drug-induced alterations of brain functions during wakefulness. Knowledge of the effects of drugs on sleep could help our understanding of the mechanisms underlying sleep as well as our grasp on the nature of various psychiatric disorders. The application of new recording techniques over prolonged periods of time, such as twenty-four-hour investigations and chronobiology, can demonstrate and possibly clarify the effects of various drugs on behavior, sleep, and other biological functions during growth and development.

Conclusions

Parents and professionals usually assume that childhood sleep difficulties are transient, developmental, and "outgrown sooner or later." While this may be true in most cases, data based on longitudinal studies are needed to determine the natural evolution of sleep events, their clinical significance, prognostic value, and possible causal associations with behavioral and medical problems. Chronically poor sleep has a significantly adverse effect on general well-being and daytime functioning. Even in the apparent absence of sleep difficulties, medical and psychological disorders may be due to a sleep disorder.

An assessment of the quality of sleep and of sleep habits should be an integral part of the routine diagnostic workup of a child. Child psychiatrists receive little training in the evaluation and treatment of sleep disorders. Parents and professionals alike need to be better educated. A better understanding of the biology of sleep should help the development of new therapeutic strategies dealing with sleep and other disorders as well as promote good health.

REFERENCES

1. ABLON, S. E., and MACK, J. E. "Sleep Disorders," in J. D. Noshpitz, ed., *Basic Handbook of Child Psychiatry,* vol. 2. New York: Basic Books, 1979, pp. 643–660.
2. ACHENBACH, T. M., and EDELBROCK, C. "Manual for the Child Behavior Checklist and Revised Child Behavior Profile," Monographs of the Society for Research, *Child Development,* 46 (1981):188.
3. ANDERS, T. F. "Biological Rhythms in Development," *Psychosomatic Medicine,* 44 (1982):61–72.
4. ANDERS, T. F., and SOSTEK, A. "The Use of Time Lapse Video Recording of Sleep-Wake Behavior in Human Infants," *Psychophysiology,* 13 (1976):155–158.
5. ANDERS, T. F., CARSKADON, M. A., and DEMENT, W. "Sleep and Sleepiness in Children and Adolescents," *Pediatric Clinics of North America,* 27 (1980):29–43.
6. ANDERS, T. F., KEENER, M., and HOLE, W. "Organization and Regulation of Sleep-wake States During the First Year of Life in Full-Term and Premature Infants," Paper presented at the 2nd Annual Stanford-San Francisco Psychoanalytic Institute Interdisciplinary Symposium on Development, Palo Alto, Calif., October, 1982.
7. ANDERS, T. F. et al "Sleep Habits of Children and the Identification of Pathologically Sleepy Children," *Child Psychiatry and Human Developments* 9 (1978):56–63.
8. ASSOCIATION OF SLEEP DISORDERS CENTERS. "Diagnostic Classification of Sleep and Arousal Disorders," 1st ed., Prepared by the Sleep Disorders Classification Committee, N. P. Roffwarg, Chairman, *Sleep,* 2 (1979):1–137.
9. BARABAS, G., FERRARI, M., and MATTHEWS, W. "Childhood Migraine and Somnambulism," *Neurology,* 33 (1983):948–949.
10. BEITMAN, B., and CARLIN, A. "Night Terrors Treated with Imipramine," *American Journal of Psychiatry,* 136 (1979):1087–1088.
11. BELTRAMINI, A. U., and HERTZIG, M. E. "Sleep and Bedtime Behavior in Preschool–Age Children," *Pediatrics,* 71 (1983):153–158.
12. BIXLER, E. O., et al. "Effectiveness of Temazepam with Short-, Intermediate-, and Long-term Use: Sleep Laboratory Evaluation," *Journal of Clinical Pharmacology,* 18 (1978): 110–118.

13. BROUGHTON, R. "Pathophysiology of Enuresis Nocturna, Sleep Terrors and Sleepwalking: Current Status and Marseilles Contribution. Henri Gastaut and the Marseilles School's Contribution to the Neurosciences," *Electroencephalography,* (Supplement 35) (1982):401–410.
14. BUSBY, K., and PIVIK, R. T. "Failure of High Intensity Auditory Stimuli to Affect Behavioral Arousal in Children During the First Sleep Cycle," *Pediatric Research,* 17 (1983): 802–805.
15. BUSBY, K., FIRESTONE, P., and PIVIK, R. T. "Sleep Patterns in Hyperkinetic and Normal Children," *Sleep,* 4 (1981):366–383.
16. CARSKADON, M. "Determinants of Daytime Sleepiness Adolescent Development, Extended and Restricted Nocturnal Sleep" (Ph.D. diss., Stanford University, 1979).
17. ———. "The Second Decade," in C. Guilleminault, ed., *Sleeping and Waking Disorders: Indications and Techniques.* Menlo Park, Calif.: Addison-Wesley, 1982, pp. 99–125.
18. CARSKADON, M. A., HARVEY, K., and DEMENT, W. "Sleep Loss in Young Adolescents," *Sleep,* 4 (1981):299–312.
19. CARSKADON, M. A., et al. "Pubertal Changes in Daytime Sleepiness," *Sleep* 2 (1980):453–460.
20. CHARNEY, D., et al. "Somnambulistic-like Episodes Secondary to Combined Lithium-Neuroleptic Treatment," *British Journal of Psychiatry,* 135 (1979):418–424.
21. COBLE, P. A., et al. "EEG Sleep 'Abnormalities' in Preadolescent Boys with a Diagnosis of Conduct Disorder," *Journal of the American Academy of Child Psychiatry,* 23 (1984):438–447.
22. COCCAGNA, G., et al. "Changes in Systemic and Pulmonary Arterial Pressures During Sleep in Normal and Some Pathological Disorders," in J. S. Meyer, H. Lechner, and M. Reineich, eds., *Cerebral Vascular Disease.* New York: Elsevier, 1977, pp. 193–195.
23. CROWELL, J. A., and ANDERS, T. F. "Hypnogenic Paroxismal Dystonia: A Case Report," Paper presented at the annual meeting of the American Academy of Child Psychiatry, San Francisco, October, 1983.
24. CZEISLER, C., et al. "Human Sleep: Its Duration and

Organization Depend on Its Circadian Phase," *Science,* 210 (1980):1264–1267.

25. DESMEDT, J. E., BRUNKO, E., and DEBECKER, J. "Maturation and Sleep Corrolates of the Somatosensory Evoked Potential," in J. E. Desmedt, ed., *Clinical Uses of Cerebral, Brainstem and Spinal Somatosensory Evoked Potentials,* vol. 7. Basel: S. Karger, 1980, pp. 146–151.

26. DIXON, K., MONROE, L., and JAKIM, S. "Insomniac Children," *Sleep,* 4 (1981):313–318.

27. FAGIOLI, I., and SALZARULO, P. "Sleep States Development in the First Year of Life, Through 24-h Recordings," *Early Human Development,* 6 (1982):215–228.

28. FERBER, R., BOYLE, P., and BELFER, M. "Insomnia in Toddlers Seen in a Pediatric Sleep Disorders Clinic," *Sleep Research,* 11 (1981):195.

29. FLEMENBAUM, A. "Pavor Nocturnus: A Complication of Single Daily Tricyclic or Neuroleptic Dosage," *American Journal of Psychiatry,* 133 (1976):570–572.

30. GLAZE, D. G., FROST, J. D., and JANKOVIC, J. "Sleep in Gilles de La Tourette's Syndrome: Disorder of Arousal," *Neurology,* 33 (1983):582–592.

31. GREENHILL, L., et al. "Sleep Architecture and REM Sleep Measures in Prepubertal Children with Attention Deficit Disorder with Hyperactivity," *Sleep,* 6 (1983):91–101.

32. GUILLEMINAULT, C., ed. *Sleeping and Waking Disorders: Indications and Techniques.* Menlo Park, Calif.: Addison-Wesley, 1982.

33. GUILLEMINAULT, C., and DEMENT, W. C. "Sleep Apnea Syndromes and Related Sleep Disorders," in R. L. Williams and I. Kararan, eds., *Sleep Disorders: Diagnosis and Treatment.* New York: John Wiley, 1978, pp. 9–28.

34. GUILLEMINAULT, C., and SOUQUET, M. "Sleep States and Related Pathology," *Advances in Perinatal Neurology,* 1 (1979):225–247.

35. GUILLEMINAULT, C., KOROBKIN, R., and WINKLE, R. "A Review of 50 Children with Obstructive Sleep Apnea Syndrome," *Lung,* 159 (1981):275–287.

36. HARPER, R., et al. "Periodicity of Sleep State Is Altered in Infants at Risk for Sudden Death Syndrome," *Science,* 213 (1981) 1030–1032.

37. HARTMANN, E., et al. "A Preliminary Study of the Personality of the Nightmare Sufferer: Relationship to Schizophrenia and Creativity?" *American Journal of Psychiatry,* 138 (1981):794–797.

38. HAURI, P. *Current Concepts: The Sleep Disorders.* Kalamazoo, Mich.: Upjohn, 1982.

39. HAURI, P., and OLMSTEAD, E. "Childhood-Onset Insomnia," *Sleep,* 3 (1980):59–65.

40. HAWKINS, D. R., et al. "Sleep Stage Patterns Associated with Depression in Young Adult Patients," in W. P. Koella and P. Levin, eds., *Sleep Nineteen Seventy-Six: Memory, Environment, Epilepsy, Sleep Staging: Proceedings.* Basel: S. Karger, 1977, pp. 424–427.

41. HUAPAYA, L. "Seven Cases of Somnambulism Induced by Drugs," *American Journal of Psychiatry,* 136 (1979): 985–986.

42. INSTITUTE OF MEDICINE. *Report of a Study: Sleeping Pills, Insomnia and Medical Practice.* Washington, D.C.: U.S. National Academy of Sciences, 1979.

43. JENKINS, S., BAX, M., and HART, H. "Behaviour Problems in Pre-School Children," *Journal of Child Psychology and Psychiatry,* 21 (1980):5–17.

44. JOHNSON, A., et al. "Influence of Lithium Ions on Human Circadian Rhythms," *Zeitschrift für Naturforschung* 35C (1980):503–507.

45. KALES, A., et al. "Hereditary Factors in Sleep-Walking and Night Terrors," *British Journal of Psychiatry,* 137 (1980):111–118.

46. KALES, A., et al. "Somnambulism: Clinical Characteristics and Personality Patterns," *Archives of General Psychiatry,* 37 (1980):1406–1410.

47. KALES, J., et al. "Night Terrors, Clinical Characteristics and Personality Patterns," *Archives of General Psychiatry,* 37 (1980):1413–1417.

48. KEENER, M. A., and ANDERS, T. F. "Sleep Disorders in Infants, Children and Adolescents," in J. O. Cavener, ed., *Psychiatry,* vol. 2. Philadelphia: J.P. Lippincott, 1985.

49. KRIPKE, D. F., et al. "Circadian Rhythm Phases in Affective Illnesses," *Chronobiologia,* 6 (1979):365–375.

50. KUPERMAN, S., and STEWARD, M.A. "The Diagnosis of Depression in Children," *Journal of Affective Disorders,* 1 (1979):213–217.

51. KUPFER, D., and REYNOLDS, C. "Sleep Disorders," *Hospital Practice,* 18 (1983):101ff.

52. KUPFER, D. J., et al. "Imipramine and EEG Sleep in Children with Depressive Symptoms," *Psychopharmacology,* 60 (1979):117–123.

53. LACEY, J. H., et al. "Weight Gain and the Sleeping Electroencephalogram: Study of Ten Patients with Anorexia Nervosa," *British Medical Journal,* 4 (1975):556–558.

54. LUGARESI, E., and CIRIGNOTTA, F. "Hypnogenic Paroxysmal Dystonia: Epileptic Seizure or a New Syndrome?" *Sleep,* 4 (1981):129–138.

55. MERCIER, L., and PIVIK, R. T. "Spinal Motoneuronal Excitability During Wakefulness and Non-REM Sleep in Hyperkinesis," *Journal of Clinical Neuropsychology,* 5 (1983): 321–336.

56. MIKKELSEN, I. J., et al. "Childhood Enuresis—Sleep Patterns and Psychopathology," *Archives of General Psychiatry,* 37 (1980):1139–1144.

57. NAVELET, Y., ANDERS, T., and GUILLEMINAULT, C. "Narcolepsy in Children," in C. Guilleminault, W. Dement, and P. Passouant, eds., *Narcolepsy.* New York: Spectrum Publications, 1976, pp. 171–177.

58. NELL, J. F., et al. "Waking and All-Night Sleep EEG's in Anorexia Nervosa," *Clinical Electroencephalography,* 11 (1980):9–15.

59. ORNITZ, E. M. "Neurophysiologic Studies," in M. Rutter and E. Schopler, eds., *Autism: A Re-appraisal of Concepts and Treatment.* New York: Plenum Press, 1978, pp. 117–139.

60. ORR, W. C. "Disorders of Excessive Somnolence (DOES)," in P. Hauri, ed., *Current Concepts: The Sleep Disorders,* Kalamazoo, Mich.: Upjohn 1982, pp. 52–62.

61. ORR, W. C., and MARTIN, R. J. "Obstructive Sleep Apnea Associated with Tonsillar Hypertrophy in Adults," *Archives of Internal Medicine,* 141 (1981):990–992.

62. PIVIK, R. T. "Order and Disorder During Sleep Ontogeny: A Selective Review," in P. Firestone, P. McGrath, and W. Feldman, eds., *Advances in Behavioral Medicine for Children and Adolescents.* Hillsdale, N.J.: Laurence Erlbaum, 1983.

63. PIVIK, R. T., and MERCIER, L. "Spinal Motoneuronal Excitability in Hyperkinesis, H-Reflex Recovery Function and Hymosynaptic Depression During Wakefulness," *Journal of Clinical Neuropsychology,* 3 (1981):215–236.

64. PRICE, V., et al. "Prevalence and Correlates of Poor Sleep Among Adolescents," *American Journal of Diseases of Children,* 132 (1978):583–586.

65. PUIG-ANTICH, J., et al. "Sleep Architecture and REM Sleep Measures in Prepubertal Children with Major Depression," *Archives of General Psychiatry,* 39 (1982):932–939.

66. PUIG-ANTICH, J., et al. "Sleep Architecture and REM Sleep Measures in Prepubertal Major Depressives. Studies

During Recovery from Depressive Episode in a Drug-Free State," *Archives of General Psychiatry,* 40 (1983):187–192.

67. RICHMAN, N. "Annotations—Sleep Problems in Young Children," *Archives of Diseases in Childhood,* 56 (1981):491–493.

68. ———. "A Community Survey of Characteristics of One- to Two-year-olds with Sleep Disruptions," *Journal of the American Academy of Child Psychiatry,* 20 (1981):281–291.

69. SIMEON, J. "Sleep Studies in Children with Psychiatric Disorders," in L. Greenhill and B. Shopsin, eds., *The Psychobiology of Childhood: A Profile of Current Issues.* New York: Spectrum Publications, 1984, pp. 85–114.

70. SIMEON, J. G., FERGUSON, H. B., and VARGO, B. "Sleep Problems in Child Psychiatry," Paper presented at the annual meeting of the American Academy of Child Psychiatry, San Francisco, October, 1983.

71. SIMONDS, J. F., and PARRAGA, H. "Prevalence of Sleep Disorders and Sleep Behaviors in Children and Adolescents," *Journal of the American Academy of Child Psychiatry,* 21 (1982):383–388.

72. VALDES-DAPENA, M. A. "Sudden Infant Death Syndrome: A Review of the Medical Literature 1974–1979," *Pediatrics,* 66 (1980):597–614.

73. VAN DEN HOED, J., et al. "Disorders of Excessive Daytime Somnolence Polygraphic and Clinical Data for 100 Patients," *Sleep,* 4 (1981):23–37.

74. WEISSBLUTH, M. "Modification of Sleep Schedule with Reduction of Night Waking: A Case Report," *Sleep,* 5 (1982):262–266.

75. WEITZMAN, E. D. "Disorders of Sleep and the Sleep/Wake Cycle," in K. J. Isselbacher, et al., eds., *Update One: Harrison's Principles of Internal Medicine.* New York: McGraw-Hill, 1981, pp. 245–263.

76. WEITZMAN, E. D., et al. "Relation of Cortisol, Growth Hormone, Body Temperature and Sleep in Man Living in an Enviornment Free of Time Cues," *Sleep Research,* 5 (1976): 219.

77. WEITZMAN, E. D., et al. "Chemobiological Disorders: Analytic and Therapeutic Techniques," in C. Guilleminault, ed., *Sleeping and Waking Disorders: Indications and Techniques.* Menlo Park, Calif.: Addison-Wesley, pp. 279–329.

37 / Attention Deficit Disorder: Diagnosis and Etiology

Robert D. Hunt, Richard W. Brunstetter, and Larry B. Silver

Attention deficit disorder with hyperactivity (ADDH) is a serious, frequently occurring disorder that disrupts the development of many children and frequently persists in a transmuted form into adulthood. Estimates indicate that ADDH with its characteristic symptoms of impulsivity, inattention, and hyperactivity affects over 200,000 children in the United States.[139,165] This significant disorder threatens academic learning, disrupts social and peer relations, and can greatly disturb functioning within the home and at school.[19,61,162,176]

The etiological roots of ADDH are both genetic and environmental. Its life course is highly affected by interpersonal relationships, life events, and treatment. The evidence of a genetic component to ADDH highlights the biological substrate of this common disturbance in attentional and behavioral modulation.[18,36,101] Biochemical factors may distinguish ADDH children from normal ones or be subtype-specific and eventually contribute to predicting medication response.

Follow-up studies have established the persistence of this disorder into adolescence[94,109] and adulthood.* ADDH children appear to be at increased risk of devel-

*See references 3, 32, 176, 180, and 188.

oping antisocial behavior,[145] alcoholism, and substance abuse.[42]

Recent developments in neurochemistry and cognitive psychology are beginning to clarify underlying mechanisms that affect the modulation of affect and information processing in this disorder. These methods may begin to define new dimensions of assessment and diagnosis that differentiate among possible educational and medical treatments.

Diagnostic Issues

The multiaxial, criterion-based classification of the third edition of the *Diagnostic and Statistical Manual of Mental Disorders* (DSM-III), established in 1978,[5] has had considerable impact on research and clinical work with the hyperactive or minimal brain dysfunctional child. DSM-III replaced the previous category of hyperkinetic reaction of childhood with that of attention deficit disorder and stated that attention deficit disorder (ADD) may occur either with or without hyperactivity and that a residual type may be diagnosed in older individuals where the initial symptoms have subsided but the core dysfunction persists. Underlying this shift in nomenclature was the suggestion that deficits in attention, and not in activity level, were the primary pathology of the disorder. Research in the past five years has sharpened issues of diagnosis and treatment.

The disorder is operationalized as follows:

Diagnostic criteria for Attention Deficit Disorder with Hyperactivity.

The child displays, for his or her mental and chronological age, signs of developmentally inappropriate inattention, impulsivity, and hyperactivity. The signs must be reported by adults in the child's environment, such as parents and teachers. Because the symptoms are clinically variable, they may not be observed directly by the clinician. When the reports of teachers and parents conflict, primary consideration should be given to the teacher reports because of greater familiarity with age-appropriate norms. Symptoms typically worsen in situations that require self-application, as in the classroom. Signs of the disorder may be absent when the child is in a new or a one-to-one situation.

The number of symptoms specified is for children between the ages of eight and ten, the peak age range for referral. In younger children, more severe forms of the symptoms and a greater number of symptoms are usually present. The opposite is true of older children.

A. *Inattention.* At least three of the following:
   (1) often fails to finish things he or she starts
   (2) often doesn't seem to listen
   (3) easily distracted
   (4) has difficulty concentrating on schoolwork or other tasks requiring sustained attention
   (5) has difficulty sticking to a play activity

B. *Impulsivity.* At least three of the following:
   (1) often acts before thinking
   (2) shifts excessively from one activity to another
   (3) has difficulty organizing work (this not being due to cognitive impairment)
   (4) needs a lot of supervision
   (5) frequently calls out in class
   (6) has difficulty awaiting turn in games or group situations

C. *Hyperactivity.* At least two of the following:
   (1) runs about or climbs on things excessively
   (2) has difficulty sitting still or fidgets excessively
   (3) has difficulty staying seated.
   (4) moves about excessively during sleep
   (5) is always "on the go" or acts as if "driven by a motor"

D. Onset before the age of seven.

E. Duration of at least six months.

F. Not due to Schizophrenia, Affective Disorder, or Severe or Profound Mental Retardation . . .

Diagnostic criteria for Attention Deficit Disorder without Hyperactivity.

The criteria for this disorder are the same as those for Attention Deficit Disorder with Hyperactivity except that the individual never had signs of hyperactivity (criterion C).

Diagnostic criteria for Attention Deficit Disorder, Residual Type.

A. The individual once met the criteria for Attention Deficit Disorder with Hyperactivity. This information may come from the individual or from others, such as family members.

B. Signs of hyperactivity are no longer present, but other signs of the illness have persisted to the present without periods of remission, as evidenced by signs of both attentional deficits and impulsivity (e.g., difficulty organizing work and completing tasks, difficulty concentrating, being easily distracted, making sudden decisions without thought of the consequences).

C. The symptoms of inattention and impulsivity result in some impairment in social or occupational functioning.

D. Not due to Schizophrenia, Affective Disorder, Severe or Profound Mental Retardation, or Schizotypal or Borderline Personality Disorders. (Pp. 43–45)[5]

Since the formulation of these clinical diagnostic concepts, researchers and clinicians have questioned both their validity for purposes of diagnosis and research and the actual existence of an authentic clinical syndrome.[21] At the time of their formulation, these criteria represented a theoretical effort to improve a nomenclature that had previously failed to distinguish among minimal brain dysfunction, learning disability, hyperactivity, and conduct disorder; they had not been empirically validated.[52] However, the focus on the attentional deficit as the underlying pathological process has generated its own set of difficulties. Attention is a broadbased and complex phenomenon that is more difficult to operationalize and to measure than activity or impulsivity. Questions persist as to whether the children who are diagnosed ADD without hyperactivity are related to ADD children with hyperactivity. Characteristics such as "doesn't seem to listen, easily distracted" may have different clinical significance when they are not associated with hyperactivity. Such behaviors may occur in a wide variety of dysfunctional states. Children who are being called ADD without hyperactivity may be inattentive for reasons quite separate from the presumed specific nervous system pathophysiology thought to underlie ADD.[52] While minimal brain dysfunction (MBD) may follow brain trauma or illness, evidence for a genetically determined disorder or syndrome is less conclusive.[135] A large number of attentional, perceptual, and motor deficits occur in normal seven-year-olds.[49] The extent to which ADDH is a valid syndrome with sufficient homogeneity to seek biological causes remains uncertain.[125]

There are many children whose difficulties with learning and behavior at home and in the school threaten their future adjustment and bring them to the attention of health and mental health professionals. Many of them are fidgety and cannot sustain academic effort in the classroom. Their primary difficulties occur in relation to the outside world, and these children can be distinguished from those whose suffering and uncertainty is turned inward. Efforts to aggregate this diverse group into one or several diagnostic categories have tended to be based on clincal experience rather than empirical research. Nosology has been influenced by controversy over etiology and the unstable requirements of existing systems for classification and disposition. The initial concept of "minimal brain damage" was forumulated to describe children with cognitive and behavioral problems similar to those seen in patients with known cerebral pathology. This concept finally gave way in the mid-1960s to one of "minimal brain dysfunction" because of the failure to demonstrate organic damage in the brains of the children. But the subsequent concept of brain dysfunction was not validated by studies such as those of Chen on the Collaborative Perinatal Data,[116] which failed to reveal a significant association between learning disabilities, hyperactivity, and soft neurological signs in affected children. Since children may have difficulties in any one or all of these areas, this may not often warrant the designation "syndrome."

Recent research has focused on the relationship between the symptoms of ADDH and levels of aggression or coexistence with conduct disorder. ADD with hyperactivity is at least twice as frequent as ADD without hyperactivity. Aggression, hyperactivity, and inattention can be reliably differentiated by teachers in the classroom.[128] Hyperactivity and aggression can be differentiated reliably in ADDH children during playroom observation.[111] While both hyperactive and nonhyperactive groups are rated by peers as socially "disliked," the hyperactive group is more likely to have conduct problems as well.[86] Children who most clearly fit the construct of ADDH are hyperactive across behavioral settings.[149] Loney, Kramer, and Milich[96] have demonstrated that the strongest predictor of difficulty in later life is not hyperactivity per se but the combination of hyperactivity and aggression. Satterfield, Hoppe, and Schell[145] reported a similar finding in demonstrating the ability to predict arrests for felonies in a group of hyperactive adolescent boys based on the appearance of an antisocial factor during initial evaluation eight years before.

Thus a large, heterogeneous group of behaviorally disturbed and dysfunctional children has not been successfully described by any theoretical approach that has yet been attempted. Research has been seriously impeded by these classificatory difficulties and idiosyncratic definitions, making it difficult to interpret. The importance of the problem is evident from follow-up studies, including, for example, the Kauai Studies[181, 182] and Robins's description of *Deviant Children Grown Up,*[129] which indicate that these are intransigent disorders associated with adult outcomes that are personally painful and costly to society.

The validity of any proposed disorder depends on demonstrated commonality of genetic background where applicable, clinical features, course and outcome, and response to treatment. Solid information about some of these dimensions in ADDH is just now beginning to become available. We still have very little data on the preschool development of children with these disorders and are only beginning to systematically monitor lifetime trajectories. Studies are needed that rigorously control for important clinical variables. The diagnosis of ADDH would likely be most valid in children with evidence of very early onset, absence of negative psychological effect from family, strong genetic loading, symptoms that are pervasive throughout all situations, prompt response to psychostimulants, and so forth. If relatively pure groups such as these can then be carefully followed into adulthood, we may define the essential features in order to compare them with children whose conditions are less classical. Greater diagnostic clarity would enhance meaningful etiological and treatment research.

Epidemiology of ADDH

ADDH has been variously estimated to affect 1 to 10 percent of elementary school–age boys in the United States.[141] A somewhat lower estimate, of about 2 to 3 percent, is derived from studies in England and China, suggesting that differences in cultures and in diagnostic criteria may contribute to this variability. Outcome studies of ADDH also suggest that cultural and familial variables alter the risk for subsequent development of antisocial behavior. A much greater frequency of antisocial behavior was noted in follow-up studies of ADDH children in Los Angeles[142] than in Canada.[174] ADD with hyperactivity is more prevalent in boys than girls, by a factor estimated at five- to nine-fold. The attentional disturbance may be more evenly distributed across genders, but the diminished hyperactivity and behavioral disruption of girls may decrease its recognition. In adults, symptoms of residual ADDH may be more apparent in women than men.[187]

Clinical Characteristics of ADDH

ADDH is a disorder of modulation that affects cognitive, motoric, social, and affective development. Although the behavioral manifestations are altered by life stages and events, the primary deficits may well pervade the modulation of attention, aggression, and activity during periods of stress and excitement throughout life. Monitoring of internal stimuli and feelings may be as impaired as difficulties in sustaining external attention. The problem of modulation usually affects attention to both internal and external events, and this affects development of the sense of self and the internal world of object relations.*

Important diagnostic and therapeutic distinctions can be made between children with learning or perceptual disabilities without the impulse disorder or hyperactivity of ADDH, who are described in chapter 38, and ADDH children. Children with primary learning disabilities (LD) may have more difficulty with information processing (peception, sequential organization or abstraction, memory storage and retrieval) and with motor integration and output but be less impulsive and distractible than those with ADDH. The LD child requires primarily special education and does not usually benefit from medication. Some, but not all, ADDH children are aggressive and have symptoms of conduct disorder. These distinctions are important for research and for clinical therapy. While the researcher often seeks children with maximum symptomatic homogeneity, the clinician must strive for a comprehensive evaluation of children with mixed symptomatology. Comprehensive treatment planning requires a complete survey of all related dimensions of cognition and behavior. The following clinical prototype reflects the heterogeneity of ADDH; children often do not fit neatly or exclusively into our diagnostic descriptions.

The untreated clinical expression of ADD changes with development. Since the development of attention is closely linked to the emergence of attachment, a close relationship exists between a child's early cognitive behavior and his or her interpersonal relationships. Careful history may disclose that ADD children were unusual infants. They cried a lot, were irritable, and slept less than most infants. They did not sustain play or exploration with one toy or object. They destroyed or lost even the most "childproof" toy. They wore out their clothes, toys, and mother's patience earlier than most toddlers. Many children with attentional deficits are identifiable during the first three years of life, even before the rigors of academic education demand the ability to sit still, master visual symbols, and sustain attention to immobile stimuli. By the time children are *age three* parents are usually able to accurately identify those who are overactive, inattentive, and difficult to discipline. These children are also more active, impulsive, and distractible during structured laboratory tasks. [17] ADDH alters parent/child interaction. Young hyperactive children are more irritable and noncompli-

ant toward their mothers. Their mothers are more directive, negative, and less interactive than mothers in control families. [108]

By elementary school, ADDH children frequently exhibit learning difficulties. Some appear to have primary *perceptual problems,* as evidenced by a tendency to reverse letters and numbers. Others have *reading difficulties (dyslexia),* perhaps secondary to the impulsivity of their visual scanning. Learning difficulties also may derive from impairment in other aspects of cognition. Attentional disturbance can impair discrimination of relevant versus distracting stimuli and disrupt processes of sustained vigilance or reflection. For example, the correct sequencing of information or the discrimination of a relevant pattern or concept often requires sustained focusing on subtle aspects of a stimulus, subject, or idea. The impulsive child may miss sequences and patterns through repeated distraction. Similarly, the abstract or idiomatic meaning of a word that is partially defined by its context may be lost to the child who processes information in rapidly shifting fragments.

In the classroom, the behavior of ADD children is characterized by restlessness, failure to finish subjects, impulsivity, short attention span, defiance of authority, and distractibility. If not treated, their schoolwork is often sloppy and disorganized. They may forget assignments, lose papers, and neglect handing in completed work. Since the symptoms of ADDH are usually most pronounced in a classroom where demands for sustained attention compete with many distractions, systematic teacher observations provide the best foundation for diagnosis. Behavior ratings from the teachers provide a standard referent for symptom quantification.

By middle childhood, attentionally impaired children are often enmeshed in conflict. Parents are unable to "make them mind"; teachers have difficulty helping them learn and behave in class; peers are annoyed by immature, attention-seeking behavior; neighbors may complain of their negligence, destruction of property, or "bad influence" on other children. Symptoms of depression and low self-esteem may complicate adaptation. Failure to channel efforts into a meaningful sequence of accomplishments often thwarts their achievement and gratification in relation to their apparent abilities and expectations. [35,71]

As ADD children become aware of their learning difficulties, their social isolation and poor self-control, depressive or sociopathic personality features may emerge. The low self-esteem frequently experienced by these children is, in part, a reflection of their lack of accomplishment, social rejection, and feelings of isolation and failure to sustain attachment. Their lack of sustained attention or interest leads to feelings of bore-

*See references 19, 26, 73, 92, and 176.

dom and diffusion of identity. Internal disorganization parallels the symptoms of behavioral chaos. They lack a sense of commitment, direction, and accomplishment. They fail to channel their efforts into a meaningful sequence of accomplishment. The development of emotional continuity—the internal linking of perception and understanding to feelings—may also be difficult for children with impaired attention and impulsivity.[47]

During adolescence, ADDH, when unmodified by appropriate intervention, is evident in continued learning difficulties and emotional-behavioral restlessness. Some ADDH teenagers have developed compensatory mechanisms through familial, educational, and psychotherapeutic intervention that enable them to exercise considerable behavioral control. Others persist in stimulus-seeking and risk-taking behavior. Some studies suggest a higher incidence of mixed-substance abuse in adolescents with residual ADDH—possibly as a means of diminishing motor restlessness and subjective anxiety. A few such teenagers may continue to self-administer "uppers" for their calming effect. However, prior treatment with stimulants does not increase the risk of substance abuse. Those ADDH adolescents with a history of childhood conduct disorder are at greater risk for subsequent antisocial and criminal behavior.[94,145]

Attentional deficit and impulsivity may persist into adulthood, although the motoric hyperactivity usually diminishes to manageable levels of restlessness. While some outgrow the effects of ADD, others continue to exhibit severe impulsivity and excitability as adults. These characteristics may emerge as excessive substance and alcohol abuse, risk taking, explosiveness, or antisocial activities. ADD may be a precursor to some later forms of major affective or interpersonal disorders.*

Fragmented attention and effort may lead to a life history of poor judgment and unfinished beginnings. Marriages may be disrupted, friendships brief, parenting inconsistent, and work records unproductive. ADDH adults may develop personality disorders or have substantial antisocial and legal difficulties as adults. Psychiatric inpatients, including those with psychosis and character disorder, reported a high incidence of symptoms of ADDH in childhood.[55] Studies of adult male alcoholics have shown that one-third had childhood ADDH and continued to have residual symptoms.[187] A substantial subset of adults carefully diagnosed as borderline personality have a history of learning disabilities and ADD in childhood. Symptoms of residual ADD coupled with complex partial seizures are frequent in adults with episodic uncontrollable rage

*See references 3, 19, 62, 65, 68, 71, 109, 124, 188, and 189.

attacks.[40] Adults with residual ADD who exhibit antisocial behavior are most likely to have had conduct disorder in childhood.

Follow-up and Outcome

Several recent follow-up studies attest to the persistence of ADDH into adolescence and adulthood and the vulnerability this creates for the development of conduct disorder and substance abuse. These studies range in method from true *prospective* studies, which longitudinally follow a cohort group,[53,65,70] and *follow-back* studies, which review a teenager's previous records,[180] to record-based *follow-up* studies in which children are identified from earlier records and assessed for current functioning.[129] Outcome may vary as a function of the clinical source of patients (whether referred from pediatric, school, psychiatric, or criminal services) and factors such as race, sex, social class, IQ, and the presence of coexisting diagnoses such as learning disorders or conduct disorder.

Prospective studies indicate that about 60 to 80 percent of adolescents continue to have difficulties in academic performance and self-image; about a quarter have identifiable problems with peer relationships and antisocial behavior.[170,175] Those children who had symptoms including more than one cluster of hyperactivity, inattention, and impulsivity were more likely to have later difficulty than those children who had previously exhibited only one area of symptoms. In a retrospective study of adults self-referred for residual ADDH, nearly half had no serious difficulties; the remaining had at least one major symptom area. This most frequently included dysphoria, labile mood, or anxiety disorder; and about half had alcohol or substance abuse.[178] In contrast, about 8 percent of normal adolescents gave a history of having had symptoms of ADDH as children.

Vulnerability of ADDH children for the development of subsequent conduct disorder is multidetermined as a function of social class, hyperactivity, and environmental influences. Conduct disorder (CD) is more likely to develop in those adolescents who continue to express the full symptom pattern of ADDH (inattention, impulsivity, and hyperactivity) even if they did not have CD as children. The ADDH children who no longer met criteria ADDH as adolescents did not have an increased incidence of CD as teenagers.[53] Social class effects are complex: Arrests for serious offenses were higher in upper- and lower-class children than for middle-class ADDH children; multiple arrests were overrepresented in lower-class ADDH children. The effect of ADDH on the vulnerability for CD was evident from the fact that non-ADDH brothers who were within one year of age of their ADDH probands (i.e., with similar family and socioeconomic status influence) had much lower arrest records than did their ADDH siblings.[13,142] The ADDH children who became delinquent were more hyperactive and had more normal electroencephalograms (EEGs) than ADDH children who did not become delinquent.

A longitudinal study of a ten- to fifteen-year follow-up of one hundred males diagnosed with ADDH in childhood and reassessed through standard interview of the proband and his parents showed the most common diagnoses were ADDH, conduct disorder, and substance abuse (31 percent, 20 percent, and 12 percent). The incidence of conduct disorder was higher in teenagers with persistent ADDH than in age-matched controls (45 percent in ADDH; 16 percent in controls), but there was no increase in the incidence of schizophrenia or affective disorder. Thus teenagers with continued ADDH were more likely to have antisocial behavior or to abuse substances.[54]

The ADDH syndrome may persist into late adolescence in over half of the children followed with the full cluster of impulsivity, inattention, and hyperactivity. Those young adults with only one symptom area are not significantly impaired. Those with the full syndrome of ADDH had a 50 percent chance of having CD; over half of those with CD had abused substances. High levels of aggression and delinquency in children predicted poorer outcome in adolescence and young adults.[96]

Conditions Associated with ADDH

Clinical studies increasingly differentiate subcategories of children with ADDH.[97,118] Potential clinical subtypes have been identified on the basis of (1) having a *family history* of attentional disorder, LD, alcoholism, or affective disorder[20]; (2) having a *medical history* of prenatal or birth trauma or illness[49]; (3) having *physical and neurological symptoms* including: minor physical anomalies,[126] presence of soft neurological signs such as delayed fine and gross motor coordination[150]; (4) *age of onset*; (5) having *behavioral symptoms* such as aggression,[111] conduct disorder,[64,146] and explosive dyscontrol[40]; (6) having *cognitive difficulties* such as specific learning disabilities;[9,90,95,117] and (7) having *affective symptoms,* including depression and separation anxiety.[33,56] Other factors that may affect clinical outcome and medication response include: (8) *family and cultural* structure and functioning[79]; and (9) *psy-*

chophysiological variables such as abnormalities in EEGs,[148] visual pursuit,[164] and electrocortical frequency response.[37] These subcategories may contribute to differential neurochemistry or response to medications.[183]

Many factors affect the processes of modulation, inhibition, association. and abstraction. It is important for therapeutic planning to recognize the varying patterns and associated symptoms frequently subsumed under ADD. Hyperactivity or attentional deficits may frequently coexist with or be independent from learning disorders, impaired motoric development, and affective disorder. Attentional disturbance is a frequent component of other more pervasive disorders such as autism, atypical development, and Tourette's syndrome.[27,82]

MINOR PHYSICAL ANOMALIES

The increased incidence of minor physical anomalies among attentionally impaired, hyperactive children may be evidence of a genetic disturbance or an *in utero* disruption of physical and cognitive-integrative integrity. Waldrop and Halverson[171] found an increased incidence of minor physical anomalies (stigmata) among those nursery-school children having higher levels of activity and aggression. Minor physical anomalies in newborns appear strongly predictive of preschool attention span, activity level, and aggressive-impulsive behavior.[11] Rapoport, Quinn, and Lamprecht[126] documented the presence of multiple minor physical anomalies in seventy-six severely hyperactive boys. High stigmata scores were associated with teachers' ratings of "hyperactivity" and conduct problems, fathers' history of childhood behavior disorders, and mothers' history of obstetrical difficulties. In addition, plasma dopamine beta-hydroxylase (DBH) showed a significant positive relationship with stigmata scores. These findings suggest the possibility of a genetic disorder that may be mimicked (phenocopied) by a traumatic event in early pregnancy.

MOTOR SKILLS

Frequently ADD children have a delay in development of fine and gross motor coordination, causing them to appear slow and awkward. Their handwriting is usually sloppy; gross motor coordination is often loose or clumsy. In spite of claims to the contrary, these children generally are poor athletes. Boys, probably because of their high activity level, are much more likely than girls to manifest the behavioral and motoric components of this disorder.[150,153] Some attentionally impaired children are fidgety and impulsive; others are slow but competent in information intake and visual motor performance, and appear grossly hypoactive. LD children may exhibit the impairment' of coordination but are less likely to be hyperactive and fidgety. Increased gross motor activity levels in ADDH children were documented using a solid-state monitoring device, regardless of time of day or setting. Treatment with d-amphetamine diminished activity levels in the classroom.[123] Gillberg and associates[51] report that about a third of seven-year-old Swedish children with behavioral and cognitive symptoms of ADD had hyperactivity.

Many children with coordination difficulties are intact cognitively or exhibit no other psychiatric diagnoses.[127,150] "Soft" neurological signs are developmentally or age-related[2] and are reliably elicited, persistent, but nonspecific; their clinical significance is not clear.[153] Some motoric symptoms occur in children with no behavioral or learning difficulties. The incidence of dysgraphia is 10 percent; dysdiadochokinesia occurs in 8 percent, and mirror movements in 14 percent, and choreiform movements were elicited in 11 percent of "normal" children.[150,169]

EEG ABNORMALITIES

Several investigators have reported that hyperactive children have a higher incidence of nonspecific EEG abnormalities that are not influenced by stimulant medications.[24,144,148] Computer-assisted spectrum analysis of the EEG has suggested some stimulant drug effects.[81] On a complex visual search task, the EEG spectrum of 16 to 20 Hertz appeared distinctive in children with hyperactivity or learning disability.[37] Methylphenidate appears to normalize the vigilance and evoked potential of ADDH children.[110] The effect of varying doses of methylphenidate on autonomic or behavioral responses in ADD appears linear.

PSYCHOPHYSIOLOGY

Psychophysiological studies in ADD have been pursued for at least two decades, and focused on peripheral or central measures. *Peripheral measures* of autonomic nervous system activity included skin conduction, blood pressure, pulse, and pupillary dilation. Collectively these measures suggest a decrease in the orienting response and relatively lower physiological reaction to laboratory-induced stress or anxiety.[193] *Central nervous system* measures include power spectrum analysis and evoked response to auditory or visual stimuli. The evoked potential (EP) is the summation of EEG activity after repeated presentation of a controlled sequence of stimuli. Following the presentation of the stimulus, a mathematical summation of the electrocortical response is performed at brief intervals

after the stimulus and is monitored for about 500 milliseconds. This technique produces a wave formation, the average evoked response, that follows a set of identical stimuli. Depending on the paradigm, the EP can be analyzed for the difference in clinical variables (age, sex, diagnosis), stimulus variables (intensity, frequency, duration, interstimulus interval), and task variables (attention to or away from the stimulus, presence of distractions).

Several earlier studies suggested that children with ADDH had increased variability of response. In response to increasingly intense stimuli, these children often demonstrate an enhanced or augmented response, similar to that of manic-depressed individuals.[15] Visual evoked potential (ERP) measures suggest that methylphenidate acts primarily on response-related processes rather than on stimulus evaluation. Methylphenidate effects were age dependent and affected the amplitude, but not the latency, of ERP.[60] An increase in EP latency seems related to a general effort at processing.[16,38]

AUTONOMIC DYSREGULATION

Differences in peripheral autonomic nervous system responses may also suggest a physiological basis for this disorder in some ADDH children. Investigators have reported lower levels of spontaneous skin conductance, increased variability and delay in reaction time, and decreased responsivity to an orienting stimulus in ADD.[121]

SOCIAL BEHAVIOR AND CONDUCT DISORDER

Untreated attentional dysfunction frequently includes an insensitivity to social cues. ADD children often ignore facial expressions, are unaware of danger, and fail to anticipate the effect their behavior will have on others. Social difficulties reflect the impetuousness with which they approach relationships. Attentionally impaired children may have difficulty integrating discrepant cues from different sensory modalities and hence miss subtle discrepancies between what is said and what is implied.[184] They often have little capacity for fairness, reciprocity, and taking turns. At school, recess provides too many opportunities for fights as the children bully or are bullied. ADD children may initially appear to be friendly, but they lose friends as quickly as they make them.

Children with ADDH have an increased risk for development of conduct disorder. Their impulsivity and propensity for action often precludes the exercise of good judgment. Their poor social skills place them at great risk of being used and scapegoated by other children to act deviantly. Family and social variables may strongly determine the likelihood of an ADDH child developing conduct disorder. Conduct disorder can be reliably differentiated from "pure" ADDH[111,128] and appears to be predictive of subsequent antisocial behavior. The arrest records of 110 adolescents who had childhood ADD, especially if associated with conduct disorder, demonstrated a higher incidence of serious delinquent offenses and penal institutionalization.[145]

FAMILY SETTING

Attention underlies the linkage of children's inner life to their external environment. In normal children, development of the capacity for sustained attention is enhanced by interaction with calm and predictable parents. An environment in which affection and rules are reliably provided allows safety for children to direct their attention to their "work" of practicing and exploration. A chaotic family, prone to explosiveness and disaster, creates an endless whirl of distraction requiring children's continued vigilance or worry. Children may not be able to focus energy toward the persistent pursuit of a goal. For ADDH children, with inherently dysfunctioning attentional capacities, the linkages are often impaired and familial inconsistencies may make for even greater distortion.

INTRAPSYCHIC AND AFFECTIVE DEVELOPMENT

The difficulties in learning and in social behavior frequently becomes evident to ADD children during elementary school. By this time, they may have been placed in special educational classes or programs, received medication and special therapy, and be known to teachers and fellow students as impaired. Depression or other disorders may occur as a subjective response to these life events or as a separate primary diathesis. The incidence of depression among ADDH children has been estimated to be 30 to 50 percent, depending on the clinical population and the methods and criteria utilized to determine the diagnoses.

The relationship between mood and behavior was examined in three diagnostic groups of children— those with depression, conduct disorder, and ADDH —by administration of standard psychiatric interviews and by ratings of the child's mood and behavior by parents, teachers and clinicians. Considerable symptom overlap occurred across diagnostic groups. About 40 percent of subjects with ADDH had significant symptoms of depression; about 50 percent had symptoms of conduct disorder. Similarly, about a third of the depressed children had evidence of motoric hyperactivity.[102] In another study of 178 children referred for psychiatric evaluation of school problems, 44

percent were motorically hyperactive; 75 percent of these also had coexisting depression as evidenced by sleep disturbance, somatic complaints, diminished social and academic interest, and self-deprecation.[167]

Differential Diagnosis

The occurrence of excessive motor activity and attentional inconsistancies is not limited to attention deficit disorder and hyperactivity. These are nonspecific responses of children to many kinds of stress and abnormality. What is unique to the concept of ADD is the absence of other possible causes and the presumption of a pattern of neurophysiological or neurochemical abnormalities that drives the motor and attentional disturbances.

For this reason it is important to distinguish ADD from a wide variety of conditions in which hyperactivity and attentional deficits occur as secondary, nonspecific manifestations. Among these conditions are such disorders as schizophrenia, affective disorder, mental retardation, and borderline personality disorder. It is also important in clinical assessment to determine whether additional diagnoses are indicated or whether other behavioral disturbances have arisen in association with the ADD. Among the possible additional diagnoses that need to be considered are affective disorders, anxiety disorders, antisocial personality disorder, conduct disorder in its various forms, and oppositional disorder. Hyperactivity may coexist with pervasive development disorder and be remediated by methylphenidate.[48] Attentional disturbance is a frequent component of more pervasive disorders such as autism, atypical development, and Tourette's syndrome.[28,82] These areas include disturbances in learning, motoric skills, and social behavior.

A child or adolescent can be overactive and have attentional problems for a number of reasons. The most common cause may be anxiety. Children, especially, frequently relieve their anxieties by increased muscle activity. Depression can also cause overactivity. Although depression often shows itself in quietness, withdrawal from people, and isolation, it may also appear as irritability, snapping at people, and bursts of temper. Children who express their depression in this way may appear to be hyperactive.

It should also be recognized that level of motor activity varies from individual to individual and that excess activity may be a normal variation rather than evidence of a disorder. Furthermore, many instances of attentional difficulty and hyperactivity can be directly traced to sociocultural factors including inconsistent, overstimulating child-rearing practices. Child abuse or excessive physical punishment may lead to ADDH symptoms—especially of episodic or situation-specific hyperactivity.

Many factors affect the processes of modulation, inhibition, association, and abstraction. Not all attentionally impaired children are motorically hyperactive; learning disabilities may occur without attentional problems. It is important for therapeutic purposes to recognize the varying patterns and associated symptoms frequently subsumed under ADD and to remember that hyperactivity or attentional deficits may frequently coexist with learning disorders, impaired motoric development, and affective disorder. Since many children have some, but not all, of the possible associated symptoms of ADDH, effective diagnosis and treatment planning requires consideration of the extent of the specific difficulties affecting these children.

LEARNING DISABILITIES

Since other chapters in this volume deal with the subject of learning disabilities at length, it will only be necessary here to remind the reader of their importance in considering the ADD child. A specific learning disability exists when cognitive functioning in one modality or area is impaired relative to other more general intellectual abilities. Many children with ADD may have specific reading or arithmetic disabilities.[54,62] Learning disabilities may reflect impairment in perception, cortical recognition, cross-modality integration, sequencing, abstraction, and memory storage and recall—functions that are linked by, but not exclusive to, attentional processes. In some cases, this attentional deficit may reflect a disturbance in attributing meaning to stimuli or, as shown by recent data, disturbances in physiological mechanisms that modulate arousal and intake of external stimuli in developmentally delayed children.[88] Psychiatric aspects of diagnosis and treatment of learning disabilities were recently reviewed by Hunt and Cohen.[74]

Etiology of ADDH

GENETIC CONTRIBUTIONS

Family studies of attentionally impaired children suggest a genetic contribution to the illness. It predominates in males (approximately five-to-one ratio) who may have a family history, usually paternal, of flight of attention, academic underachievement, reading difficulty, restlessness, and impulsivity.[20,178] Adoption studies suggest a strong contribution to this association.

Clinical observations suggest that parents of hyperactive children have an increased prevalence of mixed psychopathology (schizophrenia, affective disorders, and sociopathy) and a greater incidence of neurosis, antisocial behavior, "nervous breakdown," suicide, and alcoholism.[147] More than half of thirty-seven hyperactive children had a first- or second-degree relative with serious legal, psychiatric, or employment difficulties.[168] Heavy drinking was associated with behavioral difficulties in 22 percent of the fathers and 4 percent of the mothers. A history of learning difficulties was evident in nearly a fourth of fathers and 10 percent of mothers of hyperactive children.[109]

From a systematic psychiatric interview of the parents of fifty hyperactive children and fifty matched controls, Cantwell[18] found that nearly half of the parents of hyperactive children met clinical criteria for the diagnosis of a psychiatric disorder; this was in marked contrast to the virtual absence of psychiatric diagnoses in parents of controls. The main psychiatric diagnoses found in the parents of hyperactive children were alcoholism and sociopathy among fathers and hysteria among both parents. Sixteen percent of the fathers of hyperactive children gave a history of having been hyperactive themselves as children. Similar findings were reported by Morrison and Stewart[112] in their evaluation of parents of fifty-nine hyperactive and forty-one normal children. One-third of the parents of hyperactive children exhibited a psychiatric or behavioral disorder, usually consisting of alcoholism, sociopathy, or hysteria; over 10 percent of the hyperactive children had at least one parent with a history of childhood hyperactivity.

Adoption, sibling, and twin studies have also added further evidence of a genetic transmission of vulnerability to this disorder.[168] Using a systematic psychiatric examination, Morrison and Stewart[113] and Cantwell[18] compared the incidence of psychiatric disorder found in the nonbiological parents of adopted hyperactive children. (The biological parents of adopted hyperactive children were not available for examination.) These studies found no greater prevalence of a psychiatric disturbance or of childhood hyperactivity among the adoptive parents than existed in the parents of control children. A comparison of the incidence of "minimal brain dysfunction" in full and half siblings of seventeen MBD children found that 53 percent of their full siblings appeared to demonstrate MBD, while only 9 percent of the half siblings were symptomatic.[138] Comparisons of activity ratings by parents of ninety-three sets of monozygotic or dizygotic twins suggested a substantial genetic component to activity levels.[186] ADD children are overrepresented in studies of adoptees.[36]

While these studies do not define the extent of genetic and environmental influences in the transmission and expression of ADD, they do suggest a possible genetic component to the vulnerability for this disorder in children. The mechanism of inheritance is not clear since father-son transmission and variable penetrance appear likely. Familial studies have not yet clarified what is transmitted: an impaired ability to modulate impulses, an increased level of energy or aggression, or a more specific disruption of attentional or motoric integration.

There is substantial evidence for a genetic contribution to chronic multiple tics of Gilles de la Tourette syndrome (TS), in which motor and attentional disturbances frequently coexist.[85] Recent familial studies of TS suggest that in those probands with ADDH and TS, these dimensions segregate separately among relatives. Although the relatives of TS probands with ADDH had a higher incidence of ADD, this did not cosegregate with TS; the two factors, though separate, may be additive. Similarly, families of probands with TS alone (not associated with ADDH) did not exhibit an increased incidence of ADDH.[119] During the evaluation, the clinician may inquire about the following factors or events that may contribute to development of ADDH.

MEDICAL FACTORS IN ADDH

Transient variations in level of children's arousal, alertness, and motivation (their experience of the rewards and incentives for focusing on task) all may alter attentional functioning. Seizure disorders are frequently associated with ADDH.

Prenatal and Neonatal Contributions. Prenatal factors may contribute to the development of ADD. Prematurity, low birth weight, or maternal ingestion of substantial amounts of alcohol or barbiturates increases the infant's vulnerability to later attentional difficulties. Complications during labor and delivery resulting in fetal distress or anoxia may slightly increase risk of subsequent ADD—though most children who experience infantile anoxia do not develop ADD.

Natal and Perinatal History. Maternal consumption of excessive alcohol may be associated with mild fetal alcohollike syndrome predominantly characterized by nonaggressive attentional disturbance.[152] Behavioral and learning difficulties are often seen in children of normal intelligence born to alcoholic mothers.[152] When learning the medical history, the clinician should note the use of alcohol and other medications during pregnancy. While complications of pregnancy associated with bleeding, fetal anoxia or distress, or premature delivery may be associated with subsequent learning and behavioral disturbance, these factors do not account for a high percentage of children with ADDH.

Genetic-Metabolic Disorders. A number of genetic disorders may be present with early-onset learning difficulty: Wilson's disease (hepatolenticular degeneration) with characteristic Kayser-Fleisher rings; neuronal ceroid (Spielmeyer-Sjogren disease) with pigmentary retinal degeneration; juvenile-onset metachromatic leukodystrophy (MLM) may be evident by intellectual deterioration, emotional lability, and motor unsteadiness; juvenile Huntington's chorea is usually characterized by a jerky movement disorder and a family history; subacute sclerosine panencephalitis (SSPE) has a rapid deterioration; adrenoleukodystrophy is a sex-linked recessive disorder that causes behavioral and gait abnormalities in boys; Friedreich's ataxia is a spinocerebellar degenerative disease; and Neimann-Pick disease combines hepatosplenomegaly, motor disturbance, and intellectual deterioration.

Toxic or Traumatic Events in Children with ADDH. Cognitive and behavioral disturbance may follow toxic, metabolic, or traumatic damage to the brain. A childhood illness associated with high fever, encephalitis or meningitis, or seizure disorder may increase risk. Lead consumption through eating of old paint can impair cognition. Psychological trauma consisting of severe emotional neglect or abuse can be a source of behavioral and attentional disturbance. Children who are continuously disrupted from tasks, whose achievements are not praised and appreciated, may fail to develop effective task orientation.

Diet. Although frequent anecdotal reports suggest an etiological role for food additives, dyes, and high-carbohydrate or -sugar diets, controlled studies have usually failed to find a clear effect of challenge diets on expression of these symptoms. Although diet may affect the behavior and concentration of some children with ADD, it does not appear to greatly alter parent and teacher behavior ratings in controlled studies of groups of ADD children.[173]

ENVIRONMENTAL FACTORS IN ADDH

Children from chaotic homes may fail to develop the capacity to sustain the effortful focus of intellect and emotion that is derived from parents' reinforcing the pursuit of meaningful goals.[132,140] Attention may be diffused by a highly distracting environment or by anxiety about performance of a difficult academic task. Disturbances of attentional mechanisms may result from internal psychological conflicts that lead to preoccupation and an inward shift of attention.

Attentional disruption and hyperactivity may occur specific to a particular type of task or setting for some children.[10,41] Klein and Gittelman-Klein[87] found that of 155 subjects who were hyperactive in the classroom, only 25 percent were hyperactive at home. In more severe cases, the cognitive and behavioral disturbance occurs across settings, both at home and at school.

BIOCHEMICAL FACTORS IN ADDH

Given the clinical heterogeneity of ADDH and the difficulty of quantifying cognition and motoric function, it is not surprising that attempts to define a common neurochemistry remain rudimentary. The neurochemical effects of stimulants suggest a possible catecholaminergic substrate for ADDH. Dopaminergic and noradrenergic mechanisms may underlie discrete components of this disorder. The possible role of other neurotransmitters has not been well studied.

Enzyme Studies of ADDH.   Rapoport, Quinn, and Lamprecht[126] found that while hyperactive children with the highest scores for minor physical anomalies had increased levels of plasma DBH, no direct correlation existed between DBH levels and hyperactivity. The finding of normal DBH levels in a group of children with ADD was verified.[153] However, chronic treatment with methylphenidate decreased plasma DBH levels.[72] Rogeness and associates[131] reported diminished levels of DBH in undersocialized children with conduct disorder.

The low levels of platelet monoamine oxidase (MAO) found in many psychiatric diagnoses may be a source of nonspecific vulnerability to various major psychiatric illnesses.[114] Recent measures of MAO suggested that most children with ADD exhibit normal platelet concentration, although a subgroup with reduced activity may exist.[147] Shekim and coworkers[156] reported that ADDH children have lower levels of platelet MAO than controls. After two weeks of treatment with amphetamine the MAO returned to normal levels. ·

Amines in ADDH.   Shetty and Chase[160] measured cerebrospinal fluid (CSF) levels of the metabolites homovanillic acid (HVA) and 5-hydroxyindoleacetic acid (5-HIAA) in twenty-four hyperactive children without probenecid loading and compared these to six control subjects. They found no difference between patients and controls in baseline levels of either acid metabolite.

Shaywitz, Cohen, and Bowers[151] examined CSF levels of HVA and 5-HIAA in six children diagnosed as MBD compared to sixteen controls who had other neurological difficulties. After probenecid loading, a lumbar puncture was performed. While the average level of CSF HVA in MBD children was only slightly below that found in controls, the concentration of HVA/probenecid was found to be lower in MBD children than in controls.

Urinary Metabolite Measures in ADDH.   Wender and associates[180] found no differences between MBD and control groups in the twenty-four-hour excretion of 5-HIAA, HVA, or 3-methoxy-4-hydroxy-phenylglycol (MHPG), vanillylmandelic acid, metanephrine, and normethanephrine.

Recent studies of the noradrenergic system suggest an increased norepinephrine (NE) responsivity in ADDH, which may diminish following effective treatment. Studies of urinary MHPG excretion in children with ADDH have produced contradictory findings. Hunt and associates[77] and Shekim and coworkers[155,158] have reported bimodal twenty-four-hour urinary MHPG levels in untreated subjects with ADDH. Most ADDH children demonstrate diminished MHPG excretion compared to controls; a smaller percent excrete increased MHPG. Those ADDH children who had a favorable clinical response to d-amphetamine developed a further reduction in urinary MHPG excretion. The amphetamine responders had lower pretreatment levels of HVA.[157] Studies at the National Institute of Health also found decreased urinary MHPG excretion in amphetamine-responsive ADDH children.[14] Khan and Dekirmenjian[84] reported increased urinary levels in dietarily unrestricted outpatients as compared to their age-matched controls who may have had reduced levels of MHPG. Brown and colleagues[13] noted progressive decreases in twenty-four-hour urinary MHPG excretion measured on the third and eighth days of d-amphetamine treatment.

Serotonin Systems.   Coleman[29] reported a decreased concentration of serotonin (5HT) in whole blood of most of twenty-five hyperactive children. Rapoport, Quinn, and Lamprecht[126] found normal blood 5HT levels in hyperactive children. While treatment with either methylphenidate or imipramine hydrochloride improved behavior, only imipramine lowered blood 5HT levels.

Increased whole blood 5HT (hyperserotonemia) was associated with lower levels of plasma total protein-based tryptophan, with higher percent of free tryptophan.[80] But normal plasma free or total tryptophan was found in another study.[43]

Neuroendocrine Measures in ADDH.   A single dose of methylphenidate as a pharmacological probe produced increased human growth hormone (hGH) and decreased prolactin concentrations concurrent with the peak medication level; plasma catecholamines tended to decline following administration of this stimulant.[154]

Challenge Studies in ADDH.   Simultaneous indices of synthesis, release, catabolism, and receptor response along the pathway of a functional neurotransmitter system can now be obtained. By stimulating or inhibiting the system at a specific point and monitoring the response or impact at other moments, one can generate a map of neuronal sensitivity. The responsivity of these neurochemical systems may be assessed by sequential measures of amines and peptides following the administration of a single dose of a challenge agent such as the alpha-adrenergic agonist clonidine, which diminishes NE release and activity, or the alpha-2 antagonist yohimbine, which prompts NE release.

Studies with Clonidine in ADDH. Clonidine is an alpha-2 presynaptic noradrenergic agonist that decreases NE and MHPG release while prompting release of hGH. [4,25]

Clonidine was administered as a single-dose challenge agent to ADDH boys before, during, and after treatment with methylphenidate, in order to compare the responsivity of ADDH children with that of children with other diagnoses and to assess the effects of treatment. [77] The peak hGH level before treatment was greater than those observed following similar clonidine provocation in children with Tourette's syndrome or with short stature. After chronic treatment with methylphenidate, the release of hGH was reduced significantly. One day following the discontinuation of methylphenidate treatment, the hGH peak began to return toward pretreatment levels.

These results may indicate that a state of heightened noradrenergic receptor sensitivity occurs in untreated ADDH children, which subsequently decreases during treatment with methylphenidate. Other studies also suggest that chronic treatment with stimulant medication may diminish the activity and sensitivity of the noradrenergic system. A favorable response to d-amphetamine treatment was associated with a further reduction in twenty-four-hour urinary excretion of MHPG. [13,158] Chronic treatment of ADDH with methylphenidate appears to reduce plasma DBH levels. [72] Methylphenidate treatment reduces plasma NE release after exercise. [115] Thus response to long-term stimulant medication may be partially mediated by a down-regulation of NE system at several sites, including the presynaptic receptor and precursor enzymes, which may reduce net NE production and release.

The noradrenergic system has an important role in modulating neurobehavioral processes including affective state and level of activity and arousal. Recently Bloom and collaborators have shown that the NE–locus coeruleus neurons are activated during transitions in behavioral states and may regulate the level of cortical and behavioral arousal. [8,12,44,45] The pattern of behavioral and cognitive disturbance experienced by children with ADDH involves similar aspects of arousal, excitability, and distractibility, which appear to be partially mediated by the noradrenergic system.

Summary

Attention deficit disorder with hyperactivity is a serious, frequent, and long-lasting disorder. Its effects on children may persist into adulthood and create vulnerability for substance abuse, antisocial behavior, and impaired job and interpersonal performance. In childhood, ADDH is frequently associated with learning difficulties, delayed motoric development and control, disturbed interpersonal relationships at home and school, and depression and low self-esteem. Assessment requires behavioral quantification using parent and teacher rating scales, medical and neuromaturational examination, and psychiatric interview. Treatment is a collaborative endeavor requiring the coordinated skills of teachers, parents, therapist, and physician. Special education, behavioral shaping, psychotherapy, and medication all have a role in the optimal care of these children and collectively appear to improve learning, behavior, and outcome.

Advances in cognitive and neurochemical assessment increasingly illuminate underlying mechanisms of this disorder. ADDH children are impulsive, unreflective in their performance of cognitive tasks, and have great difficulty in organizing their work and sustaining their efforts. Research into the neurochemistry of ADDH is beginning to suggest underlying mechanisms of the disorder that may contribute to new pharmacological treatments.

ACKNOWLEDGMENTS

Dr. Hunt's research is supported by a grant from the MacArthur Foundation and the Mental Health Clinical Research Center. The authors gratefully acknowledge the assistance of Cathy Radmer, Research Assistant, with editing and preparation of this manuscript.

REFERENCES

1. AARSKOG, D., FEVANG, F. O., and KLOVE, H. "The Effect of Stimulants and Methylphenidate on Secretion of Growth Hormone in Hyperactive Children," *Journal of Pediatrics,* 90 (1977):136–169.

2. ADAMS, R. M., KOESIS, J. J., and ESTES, R. E. "Soft Neurological Signs in Learning Disabled Children and Controls," *Journal of Diseases in Childhood,* 12 (1974):614–618.

3. AMADO, H., and LUSTMAN, P. J. "Attention Deficit

Disorders Persisting in Adulthood: A Review," *Comprehensive Psychiatry,* 23 (1982):200–214.

4. AMARAL, D., and SINNAMON, H. "The Locus Coeruleus: Neurobiology of a Central Noradrenergic Nucleus," *Progress in Neurobiology,* 9 (1977):147–196.

5. AMERICAN PSYCHIATRIC ASSOCIATION. *Diagnostic and Statistical Manual of Mental Disorders,* 3rd ed., Washington, D.C.: American Psychiatric Association, 1980.

6. ANDRULONIS, P. A., et al. "Borderline Personality Subcategories," *Journal of Nervous and Mental Disease,* 170 (1982):670–690.

7. ANTON-TAY, F., and WURTMAN, R. J. "Brain Monoamines and Endocrine Function," in L. Martini and W. F. Ganong, eds., *Frontiers in Neuroendocrinology.* New York: Oxford University Press, 1971, pp. 45–66.

8. ASTON-JONES, G., and BLOOM, F. E., "Norepinephrine-containing Locus Coeruleus Neurons in Behaving Rats Exhibit Pronounced Responses to Non-Noxious Environmental Stimuli," *Journal of Neuroscience,* 1 (1981):887–900.

9. AUGUST, G. J., and STEWART, M. A. "Is There a Syndrome of Pure Hyperactivity?" *British Journal of Psychiatry,* 140 (1982):305–311.

10. BARKLEY, R. A., and JACKSON, T. I. "Hyperkinesis, Autonomic Nervous System Activity and Stimulant Drug Effects," *Journal of Child Psychology and Psychiatry,* 18 (1977):347–357.

11. BELL, R. Q., and WALDROP, M. F. "Temperament and Minor Physical Anomalies," *CIBA Foundation Symposium,* 89 (1982):206–220.

12. BLOOM, F. E., "Central Noradrenergic Systems: Physiology and Pharmacology," in M. E. Lipton, K. C. Killam, and A. DiMascio, eds., *Psychopharmacology: A 20 Year Progress Report.* New York: Raven Press, 1978, pp. 131–142.

13. BORLAND, B. L., and HECKMAN, H. K. "Hyperactive Boys and Their Brothers: A 25-year Follow-up Study," *Archives of General Psychiatry,* 33 (1976):669–675.

14. BROWN, G. L., et al. "Urinary 3-methoxy-4-hydroxyphenylglycol and Homovanillic Acid Response to d-amphetamine in Hyperactive Children," *Biological Psychiatry,* 16 (1981):779–787.

15. BUCHSBAUM, M. S., COURSAY, R. D., and MURPHY, D. L. "The Biochemical High Risk Paradigm: Behavioral and Familial Correlates of Low Monoamine Oxidase Activity," *Science,* 194 (1976):330–341.

16. CALLAWAY, E., and HALLIDAY, R. "The Effect of Attentional Effort on Visual Evoked Potential N1 Latency," *Psychiatry Research,* 7 (1982):299–308.

17. CAMPBELL, S. B., et al. "A Multidimensional Assessment of Parent-identified Behavior Problem Toddlers," *Journal of Abnormal Child Psychology,* 10 (1982):569–591.

18. CANTWELL, D. P. "Genetic Studies of Hyperactive Children: Psychiatric Illness in Biological and Adopting Parents," in R. Fieve, D. Rosenthal, and H. Brill, eds., *Genetic Research in Psychiatry.* Baltimore: Johns Hopkins University Press, 1975, pp. 273–280.

19. ———. *The Hyperactive Child: Diagnosis, Management, Current Research.* New York: Spectrum Publications, 1975.

20. ———. "Genetic Factors in the Hyperkinetic Syndrome," *Journal of the American Academy of Child Psychiatry,* 15 (1976):214–223.

21. ———. "A Clinician's Guide to the Use of Stimulant Medications for the Psychiatric Disorders of Children," *Journal of Developmental and Behavioral Pediatrics,* 1 (1980): 133–140.

22. CANTWELL, D. P. "Hyperactive Children Have Grown Up: What Have We Learned About What Happens to Them?" *Archives of General Psychiatry,* 42 (1985):1026–1028.

23. CAPARULO, B. K., et al. "Computed Tomographic Brain Scanning in Children with Developmental Neuropsychiatric Disorders," *Journal of the American Academy of Child Psychiatry,* 20 (1981):338–357.

24. CAPUTE, A. J., NIEDERMEYER, E. F., and RICHARDSON, F. "The Electroencephalogram in Children with Minimal Cerebral Dysfunction," *Pediatrics,* 41 (1968):1104–1114.

25. CEDARBAUM, J. M., and AGHAJANIAN, G. K. "Noradrenergic Neurons of the Locus Coeruleus: Inhibition by Epinephrine and Activation by the Alpha-antagonist Piperoxane," *Brain Research,* 112 (1976):412–419.

26. COHEN, D. J. "Minimal Brain Dysfunction: Diagnosis and Therapy," in J. Masserman, ed., *Current Psychiatric Therapies,* vol. 17. New York: Grune Stratton, 1977, pp. 57–70.

27. ———. "The Pathology of the Self in Primary Childhood Autism and Gilles de la Tourette Syndrome," *Psychiatric Clinics of North America,* 3 (1980):383–402.

28. COHEN, D. J., et al. "Clonidine Ameliorates Gilles de la Tourette Syndrome," *Archives of General Psychiatry,* 37 (1980):1350–1357.

29. COLEMAN, M. "Serotonin Levels in Whole Blood of Hyperactive Children," *Journal of Pediatrics,* 78 (1971):985–990.

30. CONNERS, C. K. "A Teacher Rating Scale for Use in Drug Studies with Children," *American Journal of Psychiatry,* 126 (1969):152–156.

31. COOPER, J. R., BLOOM, F. E., and ROTH, R. H., eds. "Catecholamines II: CNS Aspects," in *The Biochemical Basis of Neuropharmacology.* New York: Oxford University Press, 1978. pp. 161–196.

32. COWART, V. S. "ADD: Not Limited to Children," *Journal of the American Medical Association,* 16 (1982):286.

33. COX, W. H., JR., "An Indication for the Use of Imipramine in Attention Deficit Disorder," *American Journal of Psychiatry,* 139 (1982):1059–1060.

34. CRABTREE, L. H., JR., "Minimal Brain Dysfunction in Adolescents and Young Adults: Diagnostic and Therapeutic Perspectives," *Adolescent Psychiatry,* 9 (1981):307–320.

35. DAS, J. P., LEONG, C. K., and WILLIAMS, N. H. "The Relationship Between Learning Disability and Simultaneous-Successive Processing," *Journal of Learning Disabilities,* 19 (1978):618–625.

36. DEUTSCH, C. K., et al. "Overrepresentation of Adoptees in Children with Attention Deficit Disorder," *Behavior Genetics,* 12 (1982):231–238.

37. DYKMAN, R. A., et al. "Electrocortical Frequencies in Hyperactive, Learning Disabled, Mixed, and Normal Children," *Biological Psychiatry,* 17 (1982):675–685.

38. DYKMAN, R. A., et al. "Physiological Manifestations of Learning Disability," *Journal of Learning Disabilities,* 16 (1983):46–53.

39. EDDY, R. O., et al. "Human Growth Hormone Release: Comparison of Provocative Test Procedures," *American Journal of Medicine,* 56 (1974):179–185.

40. ELLIOTT, F. A. "Neurological Findings in Adult Minimal Brain Dysfunction and the Dyscontrol Syndrome," *Journal of Nervous Mental Disease,* 170 (1982):680–687.

41. ELLIS, M. J., et al. "Methylphenidate and the Activity of Hyperactives in the Informal Setting," *Child Development,* 45 (1974):217–220.

42. EYRE, S. L., ROUNSAVILLE, B. J., and KLEBER, H. D. "History of Childhood Hyperactivity in a Clinic Population of Opiate Addicts," *Journal of Nervous Mental Disease,* 170 (1982):5229.

43. FERGUSON, H. B., et al. "Plasma Free and Total Tryptophan, Blood Serotonin, and the Hyperactivity Syndrome: No Evidence for the Serotonin Deficiency Hypothesis," *Biological Psychiatry*, 16 (1981):231–238.

44. FOOTE, S., and BLOOM, F. E. "Activity of Norepinephrine-containing Locus Coeruleus Neurons in the Unanesthetized Squirrel Monkey," in E. Usdin, I. Kopin, and J. Barchas, eds., *Catecholamines: Basic and Clinical Frontiers.* New York: Pergamon Press, 1979, pp. 625–627.

45. FOOTE, S., ASTON-JONES, G., and BLOOM, F.E. "Impulse Activity of Locus Coeruleus Neurons in Awake Rats and Squirrel Monkeys is a Function of Sensory Stimulation and Arousal," *Proceedings of the National Academy of Science* (USA), 77 (1980):3033–3037.

46. FREEDMAN, L. S., et al. "Changes in Human Serum Dopamine Beta Hydroxylase Activity with Age," *Nature,* 236 (1972):310–311.

47. GARDNER, R. A. *The Objective Diagnosis of Minimal Brain Dysfunction.* Summit, N.J.: Creative Therapeutics, 1979.

48. GELLER, B., GUTTMACHER, L. B., and BLEEG, M. "Coexistence of Childhood Onset Pervasive Developmental Disorder and Attention Deficit Disorder with Hyperactivity," *American Journal of Psychiatry*, 38 (1981):388–389.

49. GILLBERG, C., and RASMUSSEN, P. "Perceptual, Motor and Attentional Deficits in Seven-year-old Children: Background Factors," *Developmental Medicine and Child Neurology*, 24 (1982):752–770.

50. GILLBERG, C., CARLSTROM, G., and RASMUSSEN, P. "Hyperkinetic Disorders in Seven-year-old Children with Perceptual, Motor and Attentional Deficits," *Journal of Abnormal Child Psychology and Psychiatry*, 24 (1983):233–246.

51. GILLBERG, C., et al. "Perceptual, Motor, and Attentional Deficits in Six-year-old Children. Epidemiological Aspects," *Journal of Child Psychology and Psychiatry*, 23 (1982):131–144.

52. GITTELMAN, R. "Hyperkinetic Syndrome: Outstanding Issues of Treatment and Prognosis," in M. Rutter, ed., *Behavioral Syndromes of Brain Dysfunction in Childhood.* New York: Guilford Press, 1984, pp. 201–223.

53. GITTELMAN, R., et al. "Hyperactive Boys Almost Grown Up: I. Psychiatric Status," *Archives of General Psychiatry*, 42 (1985):937–947.

54. GITTELMAN-KLEIN, R., and KLEIN, D. F. "Methylphenidate Effects in Learning Disabilities: Psychometric Changes," *Archives of General Psychiatry*, 33 (1976):655–664.

55. GOMEZ, R. L., et al. "Adult Psychiatric Diagnoses and Symptoms Compatible with the Hyperactive Child Syndrome: A Retrospective Study," *Journal of Clinical Psychiatry*, 42 (1981):389–394.

56. GORDON, M., and OSHMAN, H. "Rorschach Indices of Children Classified as Hyperactive," *Perceptual and Motor Skills*, 52 (1981):703–707.

57. GREENBERG, A., and COLEMAN, M. "Depressed 5-hydroxyindole Levels Associated with Hyperactive and Aggressive Behavior: Relationship to Drug Response," *Archives of General Psychiatry*, 33 (1976):331–338.

58. GREENHILL, L. L., et al. "Growth Hormone, Prolactin, and Growth Responses in Hyperkinetic Males Treated with d-amphetamine," *Journal of the American Academy of Child Psychiatry*, 20 (1981):135–147.

59. GUSTAVSON, K. H., et al. "Catechol-O-methyltransferase Activity in Erythrocytes and Plasma Dopamine-beta-hydroxylase Activity in Familial Minimal Brain Dysfunction," *Clinical Genetics*, 23 (1983):75–77.

60. HALLIDAY, R., CALLAWAY, E., and NAYLOR, H. "Visual Evoked Potential Changes Induced by Methylphenidate in Hyperactive Children: Dose/response Effects," *Electroencephalography and Clinical Neurophysiology*, 55 (1983): 258–267.

61. HALPERIN, J. M., and GITTELMAN, R. "Do Hyperactive Children and Their Siblings Differ in IQ Academic Achievement?" *Psychiatric Research*, 6 (1982):253–258.

62. HARRIS, L. P. "Attention and Learning Disordered Children: A Review of Theory and Remediation," *Journal of Learning Disabilities*, 9 (1976):100–110.

63. HECHTMAN, L., and WEISS, G. "Controlled Prospective 15-year Follow-up of Hyperactives as Adults: Non-medical Drug and Alcohol Use and Antisocial Behavior," *Journal of the American Academy of Child Psychiatry*, in press.

64. HECHTMAN, L., WEISS, G., and PERLMAN, T. "Hyperactives as Young Adults: Past and Current Antisocial Behavior (Stealing, Drug Abuse) and Moral Development," *Psychopharmacology Bulletin*, 17 (1981):107–110.

65. ———. "Hyperactives as Young Adults: Past and Current Substance Abuse and Antisocial Behavior," *American Journal of Orthopsychiatry*, 54 (1984):415–425.

66. HECHTMAN, L., et al. "Hyperactives as Young Adults: Various Clinical Outcomes," *Adolescent Psychiatry*, 9 (1985): 295–306.

67. HOPKINS, J., et al. "Cognitive Style in Adults Originally Diagnosed as Hyperactive," *Journal of Child Psychology and Psychiatry*, 20 (1979):209–216.

68. HOROWITZ, H. A. "Psychiatric Casualties of Minimal Brain Dysfunction in Adolescents," *Adolescent Psychiatry*, 9 (1981):275–294.

69. HOSHINO, Y., et al. "Plasma Cyclic AMP Level in Psychiatric Diseases of Childhood," *Folia Psychiatrica et Neurologica Japonica*, 34 (1980):9–16.

70. HOWELL, D. C., and HUESSY, H. R. "Hyperkinetic Behavior Followed from 7 to 21 Years of Age," in M. Gittelman, ed., *Strategic Interventions for Hyperactive Children.* Armonk, N.Y.: M.E. Sharpe, 1981, pp. 201–215.

71. HUESSY, J. H., METOYER, M., and TOWNSEND, J. "An 8–10 Year Follow-up of 84 Children Treated for Behavioral Disorder in Rural Vermont," *Acta Paedopsychiatrica*, 10 (1974):230–235.

72. HUNT, R. D. "Strategies for the Study of Neurochemical Aspects of Cognitive Dysfunction: Its Application in Attention Deficit Disorder."

73. HUNT, R. D., and COHEN, D. J. "Psychiatric Problems of Childhood," in H. Leigh, ed., *Psychiatry in the Practice of Medicine.* Menlo Park, Calif: Addison-Wesley, 1983, pp. 399–448.

74. ———. "Psychiatric Aspects of Learning Difficulties," *Pediatric Clinics of North America*, 31 (1984):471–497.

75. HUNT, R. D., MINDERAA, R. B., and COHEN, D. J. "Clonidine Benefits Children with Attention Deficit Disorder and Hyperactivity: Report of a Double-blind Placebo-Crossover Therapeutic Trial," *Journal of the American Academy of Child Psychiatry*, 24 (1985):617–629.

76. HUNT, R. D., et al. "Strategies for the Study of the Neurochemistry of Attention Deficit Disorder in Children," *Schizophrenia Bulletin*, 8 (1982):236–252.

77. HUNT, R. D., et al. "Possible Change in Noradrenergic Receptor Sensitivity Following Methylphenidate Treatment: Growth Hormone and MHPG Response to Clonidine Challenge in Children with Attention Deficit Disorder and Hyperactivity," *Life Sciences*, 35 (1984):885–897.

78. HUNT, R. D., et al. "Noradrenergic mechanisms in ADDH," in L. Bloomingdale, ed., *Attention Deficit Disorder and Hyperactivity*, vol. 3. New York: Plenum Press, forthcoming.

79. IDOL-MAESTAS, L. "Behavior Patterns in Families of

Boys with Learning and Behavior Problems," *Journal of Learning Disabilities*, 14 (1981):347–349.

80. IRWIN,, M., et al. "Tryptophan Metabolism in Children with Attentional Deficit Disorder," *American Journal of Psychiatry*, 138 (1981):1082–1085.

81. ITIL, T. M., and SIMEON, J. "Computerized EEG in the Prediction of Outcome in Drug Treatment in Hyperactive Childhood Behavior Disorders," *Psychopharmacology Bulletin* 10 (1974):36.

82. JAGGER, J., et al. "The Epidemiology of Tourette's Syndrome: A Pilot Study," *Schizophrenia Bulletin*, 8 (1982): 267–278.

83. JANSKY, J. J. *Developmental Reading Disorders (Alexia, Dyslexia)*. New York: Academic Press, 1980.

84. KHAN, A. U., and DEKIRMENJIAN, H. "Urinary Excretion of Catecholamine Metabolites in Hyperkinetic Child Syndrome," *American Journal of Psychiatry*, 138 (1981):108–109.

85. KIDD, K. K., PRUSOFF, B. A., and COHEN, D. J. "Familial Pattern of Gilles de la Tourette Syndrome," *Archives of General Psychiatry*, 37 (1980):1336–1342.

86. KING, C., and YOUNG, R. D. "Attentional Deficits With and Without Hyperactivity: Teacher and Peer Perceptions," *Journal of Abnormal Child Psychology*, 10 (1982): 483–495.

87. KLEIN, D. F., and GITTELMAN-KLEIN, R. "Problems in the Diagnosis of Minimal Brain Dysfunction and the Hyperkinetic Syndrome," *International Journal of Mental Health*, 4 (1975):45–60.

88. KOOTZ, J. P., and COHEN, D. J. "Modulation of Sensory Intake in Autistic Children: Cardiovascular and Behavioral Indices," *Journal of the American Academy of Child Psychiatry*, 20 (1981):692–701.

89. KOPIN, I. "Measurement of Neurotransmitter Turnover," in M. A. Lipton, A. DiMascio, and K. F. Killman, eds., *Psychopharmacology: Generation of Progress*, New York: Raven Press, 1978, pp. 933–942.

90. KUPIETZ, S. S., WINSBERG, B. G., and SVERD, J. "Learning Ability and Methylphenidate (Ritalin) Plasma Concentration in Hyperkinetic Children: A Preliminary Investigation," *Journal of the American Academy of Child Psychiatry*, 21 (1982):27–30.

91. LAL, S., et al. "Comparison of the Effect of Apomorphine and L-dopa on Serum Growth Hormone Levels in Man," *Clinical Endocrinology*, 4 (1975):277–278.

92. LAZOR, A., and CHANDLER, D. "Criteria for Early Diagnosis of Brain Dysfunction," *Canadian Psychiatric Association Journal*, 23 (1978):317–323.

93. LECKMAN, J. F., et al. "Acute and Chronic Treatment in Tourette's Syndrome: Clinical Response and Effects on Plasma and Urinary Catecholamine Metabolites, Growth Hormone, and Blood Pressure," *Journal of the American Academy of Child Psychiatry*, 22 (1984):433–440.

94. LERER, R. J., and LERER, M. P. "Response of Adolescents with Minimal Brain Dysfunction to Methylphenidate," *Journal of Learning Disabilities*, 10 (1977):223–228.

95. LEVINE, M. D., BUSCH, B., and AUFSEESER, C. "The Dimension of Inattention Among Children with School Problems," *Pediatrics*, 70 (1982):387–395.

96. LONEY, J., KRAMER, J., and MILICH, R. "The Hyperkinetic Child Grows Up: Predictors of Symptoms, Delinquency, and Achievement at Follow-up," in K. D. Gadow and J. Loney, eds., *Psychosocial Aspects of Drug Treatment for Hyperactivity*. Boulder, Colo: Westview Press, 1981, pp. 381–415.

97. LONEY, J., LANGBOURNE, J. E., and PATERNITE, C. E. "An Empirical Basis for Subgrouping the Hyper-kinetic/MBD Syndrome, *Journal of Abnormal Psychology*, 87 (1978):431–441.

98. LONEY, J., et al. "Hyperkinetic/aggressive Boys in Treatment: Predictors of Clinical Response to Methylphenidate," *American Journal of Psychiatry*, 135 (1978):1487–1491.

99. LOVINGER, R., et al. "The Role of Brain Amines in the Regulation of Growth Hormone Secretion in the Dog," *Endocrinology*, 96 (1975):178.

100. LYNN, R., GLUCKIN, N. D., and KRIPLE, B. *Learning Disabilities: The State of the Field*. New York: Social Research Council, 1978.

101. MCMAHON, R. C. "Biological Factors in Childhood Hyperkinesis: A Review of Genetic and Biochemical Hypotheses," *Journal of Clinical Psychology*, 37 (1981):12–21.

102. MADISON, R. "Overlap of Symptoms of Depression and Hyperactivity," Paper presented at the annual meeting of the American Academy of Child Psychiatry, Toronto, Ontario, October 1984.

103. MANHEIM, P., PAALZOW, L., and HOKFELT, B. "Plasma Clonidine in Relation to Blood Pressure, Catecholamines, and Renin Activity During Long-term Treatment of Hypertension," *Clinical Pharmacology and Therapeutics*, 31 (1982):445–451.

104. MARTIN, J. B. "Neural Regulation of Growth Hormone Secretion: Medical Progress Report," *New England Journal of Medicine*, 288 (1973):1384–1393.

105. ———. "Brain Regulation of Growth Hormone Secretions," in L. Martini and W. F. Ganong, eds., *Frontiers of Neuroendocrinology*. New York: Raven Press, 1976, pp. 129–168.

106. MARTIN, J. B., et al. "Inhibition by Apomorphine of Prolactin Secretion in Patients with Elevated Serum Prolactin," *Journal of Clinical Endocrinology and Metabolism*, 39 (1974):180–182.

107. MARTIN, J. B., et al. "Functions of the Central Nervous System in Regulation of Pituitary GH Secretion," in M. Motta, P. G. Crosignani, and L. Martini, eds., *Hypothalmic Hormones: Chemistry, Physiology, Pharmacology, and Clinical Uses*. New York: Academic Press, 1975, pp. 217–236.

108. MASH, E. J., and JOHNSTON, C. "A Comparison of the Mother-Child Interactions of Younger and Older Hyperactive and Normal Children," *Child Development*, 53 (1982): 1371–1381.

109. MENDELSON, W., JOHNSON, N., and STEWART, M. "Hyperactive Children as Teenagers: A Follow-up Study," *Journal of Nervous and Mental Diseases*, 153 (1971):273–279.

110. MICHAEL, R. L., et al. "Normalizing Effects of Methylphenidate on Hyperactive Children's Vigilance Performance and Evoked Potentials," *Psychophysiology*, 18 (1981): 665–677.

111. MILICH, R., LONEY, J., and LANDAU, S. "Independent Dimensions of Hyperactivity and Aggression: A Validation with Playroom Observation Data," *Journal of Abnormal Psychology*, 91 (1982):183–198.

112. MORRISON, J., and STEWART, M. "A Family Study of Hyperactive Child Syndrome," *Biological Psychiatry*, 3 (1971):189–195.

113. ———. "The Psychiatric Status of the Legal Families of Adopted Hyperactive Children," *Archives of General Psychiatry*, 28 (1973):888–891.

114. MURPHY, D. L., and DONNELLY, C. H. "Monoamine Oxidase in Man," in E. Usdin, ed., *Neuropsychopharmacology of Monoamines and Their Regulatory Enzymes*. New York: Raven Press, 1974, pp. 71–85.

115. NAGEL-HEIMKE, M., et al. "The Influence of Methylphenidate on the Sympathoadrenal Reactivity in Children

Diagnosed as Hyperactive," *Klinik Paediztrica,* 196 (1984): 78–82.

116. NICHOLS, P., and CHEN, T. C. *Minimal Brain Dysfunction: A Prospective Study.* Hillsdale, N.J.: Lawrence Erlbaum Associates, 1981.

117. O'BRIAN, J. "School Problems: School Phobia and Learning Disabilities," *Psychiatric Clinics of North America,* 5 (1982):297–307.

118. O'LEARY, S. G., and STEEN, P. L. "Subcategorizing Hyperactivity: The Stony Brook Scale," *Journal of Consulting and Clinical Psychology,* 50 (1982):426–432.

119. PAULS, D. L., et al. "Evidence Against a Genetic Relationship Between Tourette's Syndrome and Attention Deficit Disorder with Hyperactivity," *Archives of General Psychiatry,* in press.

120. PLOTKIN, D., HALARIS, A., and DEMET, E. "Biological Studies in Adult Attention Deficit Disorder: Case Report," *Journal of Clinical Psychiatry,* 43 (1982):501–502.

121. PORGES, S. W., et al. "The Influence of Methylphenidate on Spontaneous Autonomic Activity and Behavior in Children Diagnosed as Hyperactive," *Psychophysiology,* 18 (1981):42–48.

122. PORRINO, L. J., et al. "A Naturalistic Assessment of the Motor Activity of Hyperactive Boys, I: Comparison with Normal Controls," *Archives of General Psychiatry,* 40 (1983): 681–687.

123. PORRINO, L. J., et al. "A Naturalistic Assessment of the Motor Activity of Hyperactive Boys, II: Stimulant Drug Effects," *Archives of General Psychiatry,* 40 (1983):688–693.

124. QUINN, P. O., and RAPOPORT, J. L. "One Year Follow-up of Hyperactive Boys Treated with Imipramine and Methylphenidate," *American Journal of Psychiatry,* 132 (1975):241–245.

125. RAPOPORT, J. L., and FERGUSON, H. B. "Biological Validation of the Hyperkinetic Syndrome," *Developmental Medicine and Child Neurology,* 23 (1981):667–682.

126. RAPOPORT, J. L., QUINN, P. O., and LAMPRECHT, F. "Minor Physical Anomalies and Plasma Dopamine-beta-hydroxylase Activity in Hyperactive Boys," *American Journal of Psychiatry,* 121 (1974):386.

127. RIE, E. D., et al. "An Analysis of Neurological Soft Signs in Children with Learning Problems," *Brain and Language,* 6 (1978):32–46.

128. ROBERTS, M. A., et al. "A Multi-trait Multi-time Analysis of Teachers' Ratings of Aggression, Hyperactivity, and Inattention," *Journal of Abnormal Child Psychology,* 9 (1981):371–380.

129. ROBINS, L. N. *Deviant Children Grown Up: A Sociological and Psychiatric Study of Sociopathic Personality.* Baltimore: Williams & Wilkins, 1966.

130. ROBINSON, D. S., and NIES, A. "Demographic, Biologic, and Other Variables Affecting Monoamine Oxidase Activity," *Schizophrenia Bulletin,* 6 (1980):298–307.

131. ROGENESS, G. A., et al. "Biochemical Differences in Children with Conduct Disorder Socialized and Undersocialized," *American Journal of Psychiatry,* 139 (1982):307–311.

132. ROLLINS, B. C., and THOMAS, D. L. "Parental Support, Power and Control Techniques in the Socialization of Children," in W. Burr, ed., *Contemporary Theories About the Family,* vol. 1. New York: Free Press, 1979, pp. 317–364.

133. ROSE, J. C., and GANONG, W. F. "Neurotransmitter Regulation of Pituitary Secretion," in W. B. Essman and L. Valzelli, eds., *Current Developments in Psychopharmacology,* vol 3. New York: Spectrum Publications, 1976, pp. 87–117.

134. ROTH, J. A., YOUNG, J. G., and COHEN, D. J. "Platelet Monoamine Oxidase Activity in Children and Adolescents," *Life Sciences,* 18 (1976):919–924.

135. RUTTER, M. "Syndromes Attributed to 'Minimal Brain Dysfunction' in Childhood," *American Journal of Psychiatry,* 139 (1982):21–33.

136. RUTTER, M., and YULE, W. "Specific Reading Retardation," *Journal of Child Psychology and Psychiatry,* 16 (1975):181.

137. SACHAR, E. J. *Hormones, Behavior and Psychopathology.* New York: Raven Press, 1976.

138. SAFER, D. J. "A Familial Factor in Minimal Brain Dysfunction," *Behavioral Genetics,* 3 (1973):175–186.

139. SAFER, D. J., and ALLAN, R. P. *Hyperactive Children: Diagnosis and Management.* Baltimore: University Park Press, 1976.

140. SANDBERG, S. T., RUTTER, M., and TAYLOR, E. "Hyperkinetic Disorder in Psychiatric Clinic Attenders," *Developmental Medicine and Child Neurology,* 20 (1978):279–299.

141. SANDBERG, S. T., WIESELBERG, M., and SHAFFER, D. "Hyperkinetic and Conduct Problem Children in a Primary School Population: Some Epidemiological Considerations," *Journal of Child Psychology and Psychiatry,* 21 (1980):293–311.

142. SATTERFIELD, J. H., and SATTERFIELD, B. T. "A Ten-year Follow-up of Children with Attention Deficit Disorder and Hyperactivity—Preliminary Results," Paper presented at the sixth annual Research Conference on Attention Deficit Disorder with Hyperactivity, Austin, Texas, October 1985.

143. SATTERFIELD, J. H., and SCHELL, A. M. "Childhood Brain Function Differences in Delinquent and Non-delinquent Hyperactive Boys," *Electroencephalography and Clinical Neurophysiology,* 57 (1984):199–207.

144. SATTERFIELD, J. H., CANTWELL, D. P., and SATTERFIELD, B. T. "Pathophysiology of the Hyperactive Child Syndrome," *Archives of General Psychiatry,* 31 (1974):839–844.

145. SATTERFIELD, J. H., HOPPE, C. M., and SCHELL, A. M. "A Prospective Study of Delinquency in 110 Adolescent Boys with Attention Deficit Disorder and 88 Normal Boys," *American Journal of Psychiatry,* 139 (1982):795–798.

146. SATTERFIELD, J. H., SATTERFIELD, B.T., and CANTWELL, D. P. "Three-year Mulitmodality Treatment of 100 Hyperactive Boys," *Journal of Pediatrics,* 98 (1981):650–655.

147. SATTERFIELD, J. H., et al. "EEG Aspects in the Diagnosis and Treatment of Minimal Brain Dysfuncton," *Annals of the New York Academy of Science,* 205 (1973):274–282.

148. SATTERFIELD, J. H., et al. "Response to Stimulant Drug Treatment in Hyperactive Children: Prediction from EEG and Neurological Findings," *Journal of Autism and Childhood Schizophrenia,* 3 (1973):36–48.

149. SCHACHAR, R., RUTTER, M., and SMITH, A. "The Characteristics of Situationally and Pervasively Hyperactive Child Syndrome: A Retrospective Study," *Journal of Child Psychology and Psychiatry,* 22 (1981):375–392.

150. SHAFFER, D. "Longitudinal Research and the Minimal Brain Damage Syndrome," *Advances in Biological Psychiatry,* 1 (1978):18–34.

151. SHAYWITZ, B. A., COHEN, D. J., and BOWERS, M. B., JR. "CSF Monoamine Metabolites in Children with Minimal Brain Dysfunction: Evidence for Alteration of Brain Dopamine," *Journal of Pediatrics,* 90 (1977):67–71.

152. ———. "Cerebrospinal Fluid Monoamine Metabolites in Neurological Disorders of Childhood," in J. H. Wood, ed., *Neurobiology of Cerebrospinal Fluid,* vol. 1. New York: Plenum Press, 1980, pp. 219–236.

153. SHAYWITZ, S. E. "The Yale Neuropsychoeducational Assessment Scales," *Schizophrenia Bulletin,* 8 (1982):360.

154. SHAYWITZ, S. E., et al. "Psychopharmacology of Attention Deficit Disorder: Pharmacokinetic, Neuroendocrine and Behavioral Measures Following Acute and Chronic

Treatment with Methylphenidate," *Pediatrics,* 69 (1982): 688–694.

155. SHEKIM, W. O., DEKIRMENJIAN, H., and CHAPEL, J. L. "Urinary Catecholamine Metabolites in Hyperactive Children Treated with d-amphetamine," *American Journal of Psychiatry,* 134 (1979):1276–1279.

156. SHEKIM, W. O., et al. "Effects of d-amphetamine on Urinary Metabolites of Dopamine and Norepinephrine in Hyperactive Boys," *American Journal of Psychiatry,* 139 (1982): 485–488.

157. SHEKIM, W. O., et al. "Platelet MAO in Children with Attention Deficit Disorder and Hyperactivity: A Pilot Study," *American Journal of Psychiatry,* 139 (1982):936–938.

158. SHEKIM, W. O., et al. "Urinary MHPG and HVA Excretion in Boys with Attention Deficit Disorder and Hyperactivity Treated with d-amphetamine," *Biological Psychiatry,* 18 (1983):707–714.

159. SHEN, Y. C., and WANG, Y. F. "Urinary 3-methoxy-4-hydroxyphenylglycol Sulfate Excretion in 73 Schoolchildren with Minimal Brain Dysfunction Syndrome," *Biological Psychiatry,* 19 (1984):861–870.

160. SHETTY, T., and CHASE, T. N. "Central Monoamines and Hyperkinesis of Childhood," *Neurology,* 26 (1976):1000–1006.

161. SILVER, A., and HAGIN, R. *Search: A Scanning Instrument for the Identification of Potential Learning Disability: Experimental Edition.* New York: New York University Medical Center, 1975.

162. SILVER, L. B. "The Relationship Between Learning Disabilities, Hyperactivity, Distractibility, and Behavioral Problems: A Clinical Analysis," *Journal of the American Academy of Child Psychiatry,* 20 (1981):385–391.

163. SOLANTO, M. V., and CONNERS, C. K. "A Dose-response and Time-action Analysis of Autonomic and Behavioral Effects of Methylphenidate in Attention Deficit Disorder with Hyperactivity," *Psychophysiology,* 19 (1982):658–667.

164. SOSTEK, A. J., BUCHSBAUM, M. S., and RAPOPORT, J. L. "Effects of Amphetamine on Vigilance Performance in Normal and Hyperactive Children," *Journal of Abnormal Child Psychology,* 9 (1980):491–500.

165. SPRAGUE, R. L., and SLEATOR, E. K. "Methylphenidate in Hyperactive Children: Differences in Dose Effects on Learning and Social Behavior," *Science,* 198 (1977):1274–1276.

166. STARKE, K., and MONTEL, H. "Involvement of Alpha-receptors in Clonidine-induced Inhibition of Transmitter Release from Central Monoamine Neurons," *Neuropharmacology,* 12 (1973):1073–1080.

167. STATON, R. D., and BRUMBACK, R. A. "Non-specificity of Motor Hyperactivity as a Diagnostic Criterion," *Perceptual and Motor Skills,* 52 (1981):323–332.

168. STEWART, M. A., DEBLOIS, C. S., and CUMMINGS, C. "Psychiatric Disorder in the Parents of Hyperactive Boys and Those with Conduct Disorder," *Journal of Child Psychology and Psychiatry,* 21 (1980):293–311.

169. STINE, O. C., SARATSIOTER, J. M., and MOSSER, R. S. "Relationships Between Neurological Findings and Classroom Behavior," *American Journal of Diseases in Childhood,* 129 (1975):1036–1040.

170. THORLEY, G. "Review of Follow-up and Follow-back Studies of Childhood Hyperactivity," *Psychological Bulletin,* 96 (1984):116–132.

171. WALDROP, M., and HALVERSON, C. F. "Minor Physical Anomalies and Hyperactive Behavior in Young Children," in J. Hellmuth, ed., *Exceptional Infant,* vol. 2: *Studies of Abnormalities.* New York: Brunner/Mazel, 1971, pp. 343–389.

172. WEIL, A. P. "Learning Disturbances with Special Consideration of Dyslexia," *Issues in Child Mental Health,* 5 (1977):52.

173. WEISS, B., "Food Additives and Environmental Chemicals as Sources of Childhood Behavior Disorders," *Journal of the American Academy of Child Psychiatry,* 21 (1982):144–152.

174. WEISS, G. "Controversial Issues of the Pharmacotherapy of the Hyperactive Child," *Canadian Journal of Psychiatry,* 26 (1981):385–392.

175. ———. "Pharmacotherapy for ADDH Adolescents," Paper presented at the National Institute of Mental Health Workshop, Washington, D.C., September 1984.

176. WEISS, G., and HECHTMAN, L. "The Hyperactive Child Syndrome," *Science,* 205 (1979):1348–1353.

177. WENDER, P. H. *Minimal Brain Dysfunction in Children.* New York: Wiley-Interscience, 1971.

178. ———. "Psychiatric Genetics and the Primary Prevention of Psychiatric Disorders," *Biological Psychiatry,* 160 (1981):7–14.

179. WENDER, P. H., REIMHERR, F. W., and WOOD, D. R. "Attention Deficit Disorder ('Minimal Brain Dysfunction') in Adults," *Archives of General Psychiatry,* 38 (1981): 449–456.

180. WENDER, P. H., et al. "Urinary Monoamine Metabolites in Children with Minimal Brain Dysfunction," *American Journal of Psychiatry,* 127 (1971):1411–1415.

181. WERNER, E., and SMITH, R. *Kauai's Children Come of Age.* Honolulu: University of Hawaii Press, 1977.

182. WERNER, E., BERMAN, J., and FRENCH, F. *The Children of Kauai: A Longitudinal Study from the Prenatal Period to Age Ten.* Honolulu: University of Hawaii Press, 1971.

183. WERRY, J. S. "Drugs and Learning," *Journal of Child Psychology and Psychiatry,* 22 (1981):283–290.

184. WHALEN, C. K., et al. "A Social Ecology of Hyperactive Boys: Medication Effects in Structured Classroom Environments," *Journal of Applied Behavior Analysis,* 12 (1979):65–81.

185. WIIG, E. H., LAPOINTE, C., and SEMEL, E. M. "Relationships Among Language Processing and Production Abilities of Learning Disabled Adolescents," *Journal of Learning Disabilities,* 10 (1977):292–299.

186. WILLERMAN, L. "Activity Level and Hyperactivity in Twins," *Child Development,* 44 (1973)288–293.

187. WOOD, D. R., WENDER, P. H., and REIMHERR, F. W. "The Prevalance of Attention Deficit Disorder, Residual Type, or Minimal Brain Dysfunction, in a Population of Male Alcoholic Patients," *American Journal of Psychiatry,* 140 (1983):95–98.

188. WOOD, D. R., et al. "Diagnosis and Treatment of Minimal Brain Dysfunction in Adults," *Archives of General Psychiatry,* 33 (1976):1453–1460.

189. YELLIN, A. M., HOPWOOD, J. H., and GREENBERG, L. M. "Adults and Adolescents with Attention Deficit Disorder: Clinical and Behavioral Responses to Psychostimulants," *Journal of Clinical Psychopharmacology,* 2 (1982): 133–136.

190. YOUNG, J. G., and COHEN, D. J. "The Molecular Biology of Development," in J. D. Noshpitz, ed., *Basic Handbook of Child Psychiatry,* vol. 1. New York: Basic Books, 1979, pp. 22–62.

191. YOUNG, J. G., et al. "Platelet Monoamine Oxidase Activity in Children and Adolescents with Psychiatric Disorders," *Schizophrenia Bulletin,* 6 (1980):324–333.

192. YOUNG, J. G., et al. "Assessment of Brain Dysfunction in Clinical Pediatric Research: Behavioral and Biological Strategies," *Schizophrenia Bulletin,* 8 (1982):205–235.

193. ZAHAN, T. P., et al. "Minimal Brain Dysfunction Stimulant Drugs, and Autonomic Nervous System Activity," *Archives of General Psychiatry,* 32 (1975):381–387.

38 / Learning Disabilities: Recent Advances

Larry B. Silver and Richard W. Brunstetter

Introduction

This chapter reviews recent advances since the publication of the intial four volumes of the *Basic Handbook of Child Psychiatry.* [50,51]

"Learning disabilities" (LDs) is a generic term that refers to a heterogeneous group of disorders manifested by significant difficulties in the acquisition and use of listening, speaking, reading, writing, reasoning, or mathematical abilities. Although as yet there are no empirical findings to support the concept, these disorders are presumed to be due to central nervous system (CNS) dysfunction. [45] LD may occur concomitantly with environmental stresses (e.g., cultural deprivation, insufficient/inappropriate educational programs) or with other handicapping conditions (e.g., sensory impairment, mental retardation, emotional disorders); however, it is not considered to be the direct result of those factors.*

Special educators classify the disabilities either in general, descriptive terms or by identifying the specific areas of dysfunction. Generalists would label a difficulty with reading as dyslexia, a problem with writing as dysgraphia, and a disturbance with arithmetic as dyscalculia. On the other hand, a classification of specific LDs would include categories like perceptual, central processing, memory, motor, or language dysfunction (to be described later).

The *Diagnostic and Statistical Manual of Mental Disorders,* third edition (DSM-III) does not use the educators' terminology but refers to these disabilities as specific developmental disorders. [2] They are divided into subcategories, entitled developmental reading disorders, developmental arithmetic disorders, developmental language disorders, and developmental articulation disorders, or they may be designated as mixed specific developmental disorders.

Related clinical difficulties may be manifested by individuals with LDs. [50,52] Some may be hyperactive and/or distractible (attention deficit disorder in DSM-

III). Many show evidence of emotional, social, and family difficulties. The emotional problems may be independent or they may reflect the frustrations and failures experienced because of the presence of the LDs. They may also be another manifestation of a dysfunctional nervous system. For example, it is possible that an individual with an immature nervous system may have difficulty with impulsivity and impulse control; the consequence might be a behavior or conduct disorder. In general, in the course of evaluating a child or adolescent for LDs, it is important to assess the total individual and to note if other related difficulties are also present.

Learning is a complex function for which a cybernetics model is explanatory. This model describes learning in terms of input, central integration, storage, and output or expression. A fuller description of the specific learning disabilities can be found in chapter 20 of volume 2. [50]

Briefly, a child or adolescent might have difficulties with input, the process of receiving information into the brain. This comprises the group of perceptual problems and may involve any of the five senses. The two dysfunctions most commonly found are visual and auditory perceptual disabilities. Children with a visual perceptual disability may have difficulty organizing a percept in space; faced with a symbol, they may reverse it or transpose it. Or they may have difficulty with spatial relationships, confusing left and right or otherwise losing their bearings in space. Another variety of problems relates to difficulty in distinguishing the significant elements of a scene from the background, referred to as figure-ground discrimination. Depth perception may also be affected by visual perceptual deficits.

A child with auditory perceptual problems may find it hard to distinguish subtle differences in sound; he or she may misunderstand what is being said and perhaps respond incorrectly. Children may have difficulty with sound figure-ground or sound depth perception. Some children have difficulty processing sound as quickly as ordinary speech requires; this auditory lag causes them to miss part of what they hear.

*The views expressed in this chapter are those of the authors and may not reflect those of the National Institute of Mental Health.

In addition to input difficulties, a child may have problems relating to the integration of information after it has been perceived by the brain. He or she may assign symbols to an incorrect sequence or have difficulty inferring abstract meaning from the literal percepts. Again, these sequencing and/or abstraction problems may relate to visual or auditory inputs or both.

Once perceived and integrated, information must be stored for later retrieval. Some children have difficulty with memory. In certain cases, this disability involves only short-term memory, that is, memory which is retained only as long as one attends to the information. For others, the difficulty is with long-term memory—recalling information that has been permanently stored. Again, these disabilities can relate to visual, to auditory, or to both forms of input.

A final area of possible disabilities involves the process of getting information out of the brain. This output disability may include difficulty in expressing oneself in words, by means of language, or through muscle activity (motor output). Language disabilities usually involve difficulty with demand language. That is, children may have no limitation in their capacity to initiate a conversation, but when language is demanded, such as when asked a question, they find it hard to organize their thoughts or find the correct words.

A child with motor output disability may have a disturbance in either gross or fine motor performance. Gross motor difficulty might cause him or her to be clumsy or to have difficulty with skating or riding a bike; fine motor disabilities might cause the child to have a problem in organizing combinations of small muscles to work together. In school, the most commonly noted fine motor disability is in the area of written language. A parallel disability in coordinating the many muscles involved in speech production may be evidenced by poor articulation (dysarthria).

Etiology of Learning Disabilities

As noted earlier, it is presumed that LDs reflect a dysfunction of the CNS. Research on the brain functions underlying these disabilities has been hampered by the lack of an agreed-upon nosology. It is not always clear which disorder is being studied or what the character is of the different longitudinal patterns.

WHAT IS BEING STUDIED?

Researchers, whether within a given country or between countries, have found it difficult to achieve consensus on a definition of LDs. There is no agreed-upon standard test to establish their presence. Some researchers include subjects whose disability is defined by specific test scores; others accept subjects who are a certain number of years behind in particular academic skills. Still others employ criteria such as evidence of "soft signs of organicity." Efforts are now underway to establish basic definitions and procedures.

It is unusual also to find one site of dysfunction of the CNS (LDs) without finding other evidences of disturbance. Some children and adolescents are hyperactive and/or distractible; some show impulsivity or perseveration. If a researcher does not carefully define what is being studied, comparative analyses among studies is difficult.

A further complication takes form as the frequently found associated emotional problems. As noted earlier, these could contribute to the academic performance problems, they could be a consequence of the frustrations and failures experienced because of the academic problems, or they could be another reflection of a dysfunctional nervous system.

THE IMPORTANCE OF LONGITUDINAL PATTERNS

Once children or adolescents are identified as having LDs, it is important to classify them further according to the course of their disorder. There are individuals who seem to "mature" out of their disabilities by about the age of eight. Others show no further evidence of LDs by age twelve, reflecting only the residual missing skills or knowledge from previous grades. Still others will have their LDs for life. It is not known why this is true. There may be different etiological factors that can result in the same clinical or classroom picture; or a single etiological factor could result in different outcomes. Many studies focus on age group, thus mixing these different types. Longitudinal research is required to distinguish among these various groups of children; such differentiation is necessary for research to progress. Despite these difficulties, exciting research is underway.

Research on the Brain

Although research is proceeding in many areas, investigation of the CNS has as yet resulted in no firm findings. However, a number of basic themes are being studied.

As the necessary technology has taken time to develop, research on the brain and behavior has been slow in coming. One avenue of investigation led to the theory that some aspects of the problems with these children might be due to neurotransmitter deficiency.[49,58] We have just begun to learn the neurochemistry of the brain. Today we know of about fifty neurotransmitters, and it is estimated that there might be two hundred. With this knowledge, and aided by the ability to study neurotransmitter function through imaging techniques, such theories can be further developed.

Current research is focusing on chemical activities in the brain. This knowledge will lead to a better understanding of what controls brain behavior and interactions. Could this knowledge provide a breakthrough? Some animal research suggests a very promising lead. Research in molecular biology has begun to clarify how the genetic code results in brain development.[26] There appear to be specific expressed genes that code particular cells in the developing neural tube to be receptors for individual hormones. During each phase of fetal development, unique genetic messages result in chemicals that attach to specific receptor sites, stimulating growth of that particular area. In an apparently exact sequence, different sites are stimulated for specific periods of time, finally resulting in a fully developed CNS. This process continues throughout childhood. Having acquired hormonal sensitivity, a developing neuron may be subject to abnormal influences if hormonal agents are secreted at the wrong time or in excessive or insufficient amounts. Timing is of the essence in neuronal development, for the production of intricate neural circuitry requires the coordination of growth, differentiation, and circuit formation.

This process continues beyond birth into early childhood and perhaps beyond. What is the result of a different or defective genetic pattern? Would this result in a different or dysfunctional brain? If so, could this explain the familial patterns of learning and attentional problems?[31,48] On any particular day, could something interfere with the neurochemical messengers resulting in their not laying down the neuronal tracks scheduled for that phase of development? If so, what would this do to the functioning of the specific brain sites? What effect would this have on the later neuronal pathways that were to connect with these sites?

Animal studies during the prenatal and perinatal period show that phenobarbital inhibits or stops this vital neuroendocrine mediation of neuronal development.* Brain development is affected. This molecular genetic-neuroendocrine process is being actively researched. Such knowledge could clarify why some individuals develop brains that are "wired" differently. Knowledge of metabolites, toxins, or other chemicals

that impact on this development process might provide us with a major opportunity for prevention. Recently, for example, it has been noted with concern that during their pregnancy up to 80 percent of women take prescription or over-the-counter medication.[16,33] We do not know what these drugs do with respect to the developing brain. We do not know whether they could block or inhibit the just-described system, resulting in minimal or significant consequences depending on the time, amount, and length of time they circulate in the embryo. There is concern also that drugs taken during delivery or given to the child during the first year of life might interfere as well. The findings of this area of research could result in a major opportunity for preventive action.

Another aspect of brain development relates to lateralization of function. Many of the long-lasting influences of hormones on the brain are deduced from experiments in which, during different periods of development, fetal or newborn rodents are subjected to excesses or deficiencies of key hormones. Such studies have shown that imbalances of thyroid and adrenocortical hormones during different periods of development can have serious, long-lasting, and fairly obvious effects on adult brain function.

In contrast to these, the influence of the gonadal hormones is more subtle. In male mammals, during a brief period of pre- or postnatal development the testes secrete testosterone, a hormone that coincides with and, in fact, triggers sexual differentiation of the reproductive tract and brain. In rats, removal of the testes prior to this period of testosterone secretion prevents the masculine phenotype from developing; both the reproductive tract and the brain then develop in a feminine direction.[11,28] The role of the ovaries in early female development is less certain. Their removal early in life does not prevent the appearance of a feminine phenotype, though certain feminine behavioral traits may be altered.[26]

Lateralization of brain structure and function is linked to sexual differentiation. In our own species, the male brain is often cited as being more highly lateralized than the female brain. For example, males with left-hemisphere damage show deficits on verbal tests, and those with right-hemisphere damage show deficits on tests of nonverbal performance.[20,27] Brain-injured females, on the other hand, show deficits in test performance but do not show such marked laterality.

In general, LDs are more common in males than in females.[12,40] In addition, among normal subjects there is a sex difference in performance on verbal and spatial tasks. On the average, females score better than males on verbal tasks while males score better than females on spatial tasks.

It is suggested that both of these tendencies may be

*See references 3, 28, 29, 30, and 31.

related to the greater laterality of cerebral function in males, which in turn is the product of androgen exposure during early development. Evidence supporting this idea comes from studies of males and females with androgen abnormalities. For example, androgen-deficient males do less well than normal males on spatial tasks.[18] A condition called the adrenogenital syndrome leads to a state of androgen-insensitivity in girls and boys. Both groups in the study had been reared as girls. The girls with adrenogenital syndrome performed less well than normal girls on certain verbal tests. Unlike the average normal male, the androgen-insensitive males did better on verbal than nonverbal tests. These findings are consistent with the notion that the heightened presence of androgen increases nonverbal relative to verbal performance, whereas androgen absence (or insensitivity) has the opposite effect.

Several hypotheses seek to account for this interplay between androgens and cerebral lateralization in the development of cognitive abilities. One view suggests that the greater specialization in males of one hemisphere (usually the right) for the processing of spatial information may indeed produce higher ability in this regard. But it does so at the expense of verbal ability, which tends to be controlled by the opposite (usually left) hemisphere. According to this line of reasoning, "Strong left hemisphere specialization for verbal processing may put males at further risk for experiencing dyslexia by limiting their ability to compensate for either left hemisphere insults or unfavorable anatomic cerebral asymmetries[17] (p. 78). The unfavorable cerebral asymmetries refer to situations apparently present in a high percentage of dyslexic children in whom asymmetry of the cerebral hemispheres is reversed. In these children, the smaller and in some way less dominant temporal lobe is in control of verbal processing.[19,47]

Another line of investigation studied handedness. Investigators noted an elevated frequency of both autoimmune disease and developmental learning disorders in left-handed subjects.[5] Their study suggests that immune disorders may be linked to the development of left-handedness and of learning defects through the action of testosterone. In male fetuses, the right cerebral hemisphere usually develops earlier than the left. By thirty-one weeks of gestation, the left side has overtaken the right and become larger. That in males the left hemisphere matures later is further suggested by the observation that in boys, febrile convulsions during the first year of life may result in damage to the left temporal lobe.

Geschwind and Behan[15] suggest:

Delayed growth in the left hemisphere as a result of testosterone would account for the greater frequency of left-handedness in males. When testosterone effects are more marked and neuronal migration is interfered with to a greater extent, abnormalities in the formation of the left hemisphere will result —especially in males—such as those described by Galaburda and Kemper[14] in the left temporal speech area of a severe childhood dyslexic. This type of defect would account for the much greater incidence of learning disorders in boys. (P. 5099)

Geschwind and Behan have attempted to explain the mechanism underlying testosterone action on the development of the cerebral hemispheres. They note that neurons that will occupy the language area are formed and migrate to their ultimate locations before twenty weeks of gestation. Since twelve to twenty weeks of gestation is the period of maximum testosterone elevation in developing male fetuses, the hormone may affect some of these developing brain cells.[1] It could influence their division, their survival, their migration, or the formation of stable connections with other neurons. Why the result should be greater lateralization of function in one hemisphere rather than some sort of joint influence on both hemispheres is not known.

Indeed, explaining the possible linkage of androgens to brain lateralization is an especially intriguing problem that presents developmental neurobiologists with a major puzzle. How are they to make sense of the fact that a blood-borne substance, which presumably reaches both sides of the brain, can have selective effects on one side? Could it be that the hormone-receptive cells are not laid down in equal numbers on both sides of the developing brain, giving rise to an asymmetrical target for hormone action?

McEwen's view is that androgens per se do not cause dyslexia or the other developmental learning disorders that predominate in males.[26] He believes, rather, that these hormones alter, and perhaps restrict, cerebral development in such a way as to increase the chance that congenital defects or brain damage will have noticeable effects on cognitive ability. When more is known about the underlying mechanisms of prenatal brain development, ways of detecting and even preventing the abnormalities of brain development that give rise to learning disabilities may be discovered.

Current imaging techniques can picture brain function *in vivo*. Unlike previous technology, which showed brain structure, the position emission tomography (PET) scan and the newer nuclear magnetic resonance (NMR) scan can record brain function. These new methods are just beginning to be used with children and adolescents with LDs. It is hoped that such techniques will provide new information about brain dysfunction; from such knowledge might come better treatment or prevention efforts.

Although there is a relationship between nutrition and behavior, to date the research findings remain confusing. Data are available regarding the impact of toxins (lead,[5,33,34] mercury,[9] cadmium[20]) and on metabolites (glucose, specific amino acids) on brain function. The relationships of these substances to brain functioning and to LDs have yet to be clarified.

Major discoveries are yet to be made, such as finding new neurotransmitters or receptor sites. Research in the neurosciences is among the most rapidly advancing and most exciting of all scientific studies today. With these advances will come more knowledge about the basic brain dysfunctions that so evidently underlie LDs.

Research on Prenatal Factors

Several prenatal difficulties have been studied in relation to subsequent appearance of motor or cognitive disabilities: bleeding in pregnancy, maternal malnutrition and/or anemia, hypertension, feto-maternal blood incompatibility, prematurity (low birth weight or small size for gestational age), preeclampsia and eclampsia, placental difficulties, cord compression, and postmaturity.* Although some data are suggestive, no clear relationships to learning difficulties have emerged.

FETAL GROWTH

The nutritional status of the mother prior to and during her pregnancy is but one of the many factors that influence fetal growth and thus birth weight. Genetic factors, infections, placental abnormalities, toxins, and various metabolites are but some of the factors studied. Two new areas of research relate to maternal smoking and use of alcohol.

CIGARETTE USE BY PREGNANT WOMEN

There are no studies to date that address the relationship between cigarette smoking during pregnancy and LDs in the offspring. However, some studies address the long-term association between maternal smoking during pregnancy and other aspects of child behavior and development that may be related to LDs.†

In these studies the role of socioeconomic status was not fully clarified nor was whether the mother also used alcohol during pregnancy. These distinctions must be addressed in further research.

The British National Child Development Study collected data on almost 17,000 single births during 1958. Early analysis of the data led to the conclusion that

*See references 4, 22, 23, 24, 38, 39, and 57.
†See references 6, 7, 10, 37, 46, 53, 54, and 56.

maternal cigarette smoking was associated with a 28 percent increase in fetal and neonatal mortality rate, plus an average reduction of 170 grams in birth weight.[21]

A follow-up evaluation of these children at age seven and eleven revealed significant retardation in learning.[7,8] At age seven, maternal smoking was significantly related to decreased reading ability—the more the mother smoked, the greater the reading difficulty. At age eleven the same pattern persisted as did decreased performance in arithmetic and spelling.

Another large-scale prospective study was carried out in the United States. This Perinatal Collaborative Study[37] included 58,000 pregnant women. In a follow-up study when the children had reached age seven, Nichols and Chen[37] found a significant association between maternal smoking during pregnancy and learning difficulties, hyperactivity, impulsivity, and neurological soft signs.

ALCOHOL USE BY PREGNANT WOMEN

A recognized pattern of malformation called the fetal alcohol syndrome has been observed in children exposed to severe intrauterine alcohol levels.[55] This syndrome is characterized by a pattern of growth deficiency, characteristic dysmorphic facial features, CNS dysfunction as well as other evidence of system malformation.

Research is now underway on the effect of fetal alcohol exposure at the less severe end of a continuum of such effects. No results are yet available. One study,[45] however, suggests that this issue must be pursued; of eighty-seven children referred to the Yale Learning Disorders Unit, fifteen were born to mothers who had been alcoholic during the target pregnancy.

Research on Perinatal Factors

OBSTETRICAL TRAUMA

There have been investigations of the effects of asphyxia, dysfunction labor, abnormal presentations, or the use of forceps on the newborn.[36,38,39,57] The results do not confirm that LDs are a possible outcome of a specific form of trauma. However, before any clear relationships between such fetal difficulties and future cognitive, motor, or language development can be clarified, long-term follow-up studies are needed rather than clinical observations. These must employ specific measures of fetal stress—metabolic acidosis or fetal heart rate patterns.

OBSTETRICAL MEDICATION

With few exceptions, drugs used in obstetrical anesthesia and analgesia rapidly course the placenta and enter the fetal circulation. The ability of the neonate to metabolize many of these agents is poorly developed. As a result, after delivery, when elimination through the maternal circulation is no longer possible, the effects of drugs given during labor may persist for weeks.

It is known that narcotic analgesics may induce respiratory and CNS depression both in the mother and the neonate. In addition, nonnarcotic sedative-hypnotics, as well as general or inhalation anesthesia, may produce similar respiratory and CNS depression. Current research efforts are exploring the effects that reduce oxygen and secondary fetal acidosis have on fetal functioning in general and/or on the development of the CNS in particular.

MATERNAL POSITION

The suggestion has been advanced that maternal position during labor may contribute to possible fetal stress. Research is currently in progress on the influence of these factors. Some studies show that when the woman lies on her back while in labor, there is a resulting maternal hypotension with an attendant decrease in fetal oxygenation.[13] In many countries such a position is still preferred by most professionals.

Environmental and Genetic Research

ENVIRONMENTAL FACTORS

A recent prospective study by Nichols and Chen[37] highlights the importance of environmental factors in LDs. This study evaluated data from the massive Collaborative Perinatal Project of the National Institute of Neurological and Communicative Disorders and Stroke.[37] The cohort included a seven-year follow-up of 29,889 children and examined the role of three-hundred antecedent variables (by means of multivariate analysis). Among the results it was found that learning difficulties were strongly related to socioeconomic and demographic variables, in particular to large family size, low socioeconomic index scores, and frequent changes in residence. By way of contrast, most perinatal factors did not relate to LDs. An important finding was that LDs tended to run in families. In fact, the most powerful predictor of a child's own LD score was the

average LD score of his or her siblings. Taken by itself, of course, this finding does not permit any decision about the extent to which these correlations were determined either by environment or by genes. However, the importance of environmental factors is supported by the observation that estimated risks of learning disability were nearly identical for sibs and half sibs. More than that, the risks to other relatives did not vary systematically with the degree of relationship. This reemphasis of the importance of environmental factors must be considered with all studies.

GENETIC FACTORS

Most such studies have focused on one group of LDs, dyslexia. Omenn and Weber[40] studied twenty-one families in which there were multiple members with what the authors referred to as "specific dyslexia." They subdivided the dyslexia disability into three categories: visual predominant, auditory predominant, and mixed. Pedigree analysis revealed a pattern of inheritance compatible with an autosomal dominant mode of transmission. It is of interest that visual-predominant dyslexia clustered in families of probands with that subtype, whereas auditory-predominant dyslexia clustered in families of probands with the auditory-predominant subtype. Sociocultural deprivation did not appear to have been a significant factor in these families. This study lends support to the importance of genetic factors in at least some types of dyslexia. In addition, the results suggest that there are at least two types of dyslexia and that these are inherited separately. Possibly the two types reflect different groups of specific LDs that can result in a reading disability.

Finucci and associates[12] reported on the genetics of reading disability. In their study they included children whose reading skills lagged two or three years behind that of their classmates and whose reading disability could not be assigned to any known cause. Detailed studies were conducted of the family members of three children. Segregation analysis of the pedigrees suggested that the best hypothesis to fit these data was that of autosomal dominant transmission with sex limitation. The authors note that this hypothesis is the most attractive since it takes into account the well-recognized excess of males. Sex linkage was ruled out for most families since a common pattern involved father-to-son transmission.

LEARNING DISABILITIES AND OTHER GENETIC DISORDERS

In a large number of genetically determined disorders, LD may be one of the symptoms. Some of these disorders are summarized in a recent review by Moser.[32] Understanding of the mechanism by which a particular genetic pattern can lead to the phenotypic appearance of an LD may give some insight into the genetic mechanisms responsible for LDs in general. For example, the recent studies of Ratcliffe and his associates[42,43] have shown that persons with abnormal sex chromosomes show a high incidence of mild disturbances in reading and learning capacity. These findings relate to recent data on sex-related differences in normal development and to the observation that dyslexia is more common in boys. It is possible that in certain persons now classified among the group of learning disabled without cause there exists an underlying (although as yet unidentified) specific biochemical or chromosomal abnormality.

The Future

The major growth of research in the neurosciences will contribute significant knowledge concerning the causes and probable pathogenesis of learning disabilities. This new knowledge should result in better diagnosis and treatment as well as possible approaches to prevention.

REFERENCES

1. ABRAMOVICH, D. R., and ROWE, P. "Foetal Plasma Testosterone Levels at Mid-Pregnancy and at Term: Relationship to Foetal Sex," *Journal of Endocrinology,* 56 (1973): 621–622.

2. AMERICAN PSYCHIATRIC ASSOCIATION. *Diagnostic and Statistical Manual of Mental Disorders,* 3rd ed. Washington, D. C.: American Psychiatric Association, 1980.

3. AUROUX, M. "Behavioral Teratogenesis. A New Prospective of the Pathology of Prenatal Development," *Journal of Gynecology, Obstetrics, Biology and Reproduction,* 10 (1981):633–640.

4. BALOW, B., RUBIN, R., and ROSEN, M. "Perinatal Events as Precursors of Reading Disability," *Reading Research Quarterly,* 11 (1975):36–71.

5. BALOH, R., STURM, R., and GREEN, B. "Neuropsychological Effects of Chronic Asymptomatic Increased Lead Absorption," *Archives of Neurology,* 32 (1975):326–330.

6. BROMAN, S. H., NICHOLS, P. L., and KENNEDY, W. A. *Preschool IQ: Prenatal and Early Developmental Correlates.* Hillsdale, N. J.: Erlbaum, 1975.

7. BUTLER, N. R., and GOLDSTEIN, H. "Smoking in Pregnancy and Subsequent Child Development," *British Medical Journal,* 4 (1973):573–575.

8. BUTLER, N. R., GOLDSTEIN, H., and ROSS, E. M. "Cigarette Smoking in Pregnancy: Its Influence on Birth Weight and Perinatal Mortality," *British Medical Journal,* 2 (1972): 127–130.

9. CHANG, L. W. "Mercury," in P. S. Spencer and H. H. Schaumberg, eds., *Experimental and Clinical Neurotoxicology.* Baltimore: Williams & Wilkins, 1980, pp. 508–527.

10. DUNN, H. G., McBURNEY, A. K., INGRAM, S., and HUNTER, C. M. "Maternal Cigarette Smoking During Pregnancy and the Child's Subsequent Development: I. Physical Growth to the Age of 6½ Years," *Canadian Journal of Public Health,* 67 (1976):499–505.

11. FEDER, H. H. "Hormonal Actions on the Sexual Differentiation of the Genitalia and the Gonadotropin Regulating Systems," in N. J. Adler, ed., *Neuroendocrinology of Reproduction.* New York: Plenum Press, 1981.

12. FINUCCI, J. M., et al. "The Genetics of Reading Disability," *Annals of Human Genetics,* 40 (1976):1–23.

13. FLYNN, A. M., et al. "Ambulation in Labor," *British Medical Journal,* 2 (1978):591–593.

14. GALABURDA, A. M., and KEMPER, T. M. "Cytoarchitectonic Abnormalities in Developmental Dyslexia: A Case Study," *Annals of Neurology,* 6 (1979):94–100.

15. GESCHWIND, N., and BEHAN, P. "Left Handedness: Association with Immune Disease, Migraine and Developmental Learning Disorders," *Proceedings of the National Academy of Sciences (USA),* 79 (1982):5097–5100.

16. HEINONEN, D. P., SLONE, D., and SHAPIRO, S. *Birth Defects and Drugs in Pregnancy.* Littleton, Mass.: Publishing Sciences Group, 1977.

17. HIER, D. B. "Sex Differences in Hemispheric Specialization: Hypothesis for the Excess of Dyslexia in Boys," *Bulletin of the Orton Society,* 29 (1979):74–83.

18. HIER, D. B., and CROWLEY, W. F. "Spatial Ability in Androgen-Deficient Men," *New England Journal of Medicine,* 206 (1982):1202–1205.

19. HIER, D. B., et al. "Developmental Dyslexia," *Archives of Neurology,* 35 (1978):90–92.

20. INGLIS, J., and LAWSON, J. S. "Sex Differences in the Effects of Unilateral Brain Damage on Intelligence," *Science,* 212 (1981):693–695.

21. JOHNSTON, C. "Cigarette Smoking and the Outcome of Human Pregnancies: A Status Report on the Consequences," *Clinical Toxicology,* 18 (1981):189–209.

22. KAFFMAN, M., SIVAN-SHER, A., and CAREL, C. "Obstetrical History of Kibbutz Children with Minimal Brain Dysfunction," *Israeli Journal of Psychiatry and Related Sciences,* 18 (1981):69–84.

23. KAWI, A. A., and PASAMANICK, B. "Association of Factors of Pregnancy with Learning Disorders in Childhood," *Journal of the American Medical Association,* 166 (1958):1420–1423.

24. LILIENFELD, A. M., and PARKHURST, E. "A Study of the Association of Factors of Pregnancy and Parturition with the Development of Cerebral Palsy: Preliminary Report," *American Journal of Hygiene,* 53 (1951):262–282.

25. LUCIS, O., LUCIS, R., and SHAIKH, Z. A. "Cadmium in Pregnancy and Lactation," *Archives of Environmental Health,* 25 (1972):14–22.

26. McEWEN, B. S. "Gonadol Steroids Influences on Brain Development and Sexual Differentiation," in R. O. Greep, ed., *Reproductive Physiology,* vol. 4. Baltimore: University Park Press, 1983.

27. McGLONE, J. "Sex Differences in Human Brain Asymmetry: A Critical Survey," *Behavioral and Brain Sciences,* 3 (1980):215–263.

28. MANNING, D. E., STOUT, A. G., and ZEMP, J. W. "Effects of Maternal Phenobarbital Administration in Some Aspects of Neonatal Brain Development," *Federal Procedure,* 30 (1971):239.

29. MARTIN, J. C., et al. "Effects of Maternal Absorption of Phenobarbital Upon Rat Offspring Development and Function," *Neurobehavioral Toxicology,* 1 (1979):49–55.

30. MIDDAUGH, L. D., et al. "Effects of Prenatal Maternal Injections of Phenobarbital on Brain Neurotransmitters and Behavior in Young CST Mice," *Neurobehavioral Toxicology and Teratology,* 3 (1981):271–275.

31. MORRISON, J. R., and STEWART, M. A. "A Family Study of the Hyperactive Child Syndrome," *Biological Psychiatry,* 3 (1971):189–195.

32. MOSER, H. W. "Mental Retardation Due to Genetically Determined Metabolic and Endocrine Disorders," in I. Jacob, ed., *Mental Retardation.* Basel: Karger, 1982, pp. 2–26.

33. NATIONAL ACADEMY OF SCIENCES. "Non-prescription Drug Use and Pregnancy Outcomes," *The Blue Sheet,* 12 January 1983.

34. NEEDLEMAN, H. L., GUNNOE, C. G., and LEVITON, A. "Deficits in Psychological and Classroom Performance of Children with Elevated Dentine Lead Levels," *New England Journal of Medicine,* 300 (1979):689–695.

35. NEEDLEMAN, H. L., LEVITON, A., and BELLINGER, D. "Lead-associated Intellectual Deficit," *New England Journal of Medicine,* 306 (1979):367.

36. NELSON, K. B., and BROMAN, S. H. "Perinatal Risk Factors in Children with Serious Motor and Mental Handicaps," *Annals of Neurology.*

37. NICHOLS, P. L., and CHEN, T. C. *Minimal Brain Dysfunction: A Prospective Study.* Hillsdale, N. J.: Lawrence Erlbaum Associates, 1981.

38. NISWANDER, K. R. "The Obstetrician, Fetal Asphyxia, and Cerebral Palsy," *American Journal of Obstetrics and Gynecology,* 133 (1979):358–361.

39. NISWANDER, K. R., GORDON, M., and DRAGE, J. S. "The Effect of Intrauterine Hypoxia on the Surviving to 4 Years," *American Journal of Obstetrics and Gynecology,* 121 (1975):892–899.

40. OMENN, G. S., and WEBER, B. A. "Dyslexia: Search for Phenotypic and Genetic Heterogenecity," *Journal of Learning Disabilities,* 6 (1973):26–34.

41. PERLMAN, S. M. "Cognitive Abilities of Children with Hormone Abnormalities: Screening by Psychoeducational Tests," *Journal of Learning Disabilities,* 6 (1973):26–34.

42. RATCLIFFE, S. G. "Speech and Learning Disorders in Children with Sex Chromosome Abnormalities," *Developmental Medicine and Child Neurology,* 24 (1982):80–84.

43. RATCLIFFE, S. G., et al. "Kleinfelters Syndrome in Adolescence," *Archives of Diseases of Childhood,* 57 (1982): 6–12.

44. ROSENBERGER, P. B., and HIER, D. B. "Cerebral Asymmetry and Verbal Intellectual Deficits," *Annals of Neurology,* 8 (1980):300–304.

45. RUTTER, M. "Syndromes Attributed to 'Minimal Brain Dysfunction' in Childhood," *American Journal of Psychiatry,* 139 (1982):21–33.

46. SAXTON, D. W. "The Behavior of Infants Whose Mothers Smoke in Pregnancy," *Early Human Development,* 2 (1978):363–369.

47. SHAYWITZ, S. E., COHEN, D. J., and SHAYWITZ, B. A. "Behavior and Learning Difficulties in Children of Normal Intelligence Born to Alcoholic Mothers," *Journal of Pediatrics,* 96 (1980):978–982.

48. SILVER, L. B. "Familial Patterns in Children with Neurologically-Based Learning Disabilities," *Journal of Learning Disabilities,* 4 (1971):349–358.

49. ———. "A Proposed View on the Etiology of the Neurological Learning Disability Syndrome," *Journal of Learning Disabilities,* 4 (1971):123–133.

50. ———. "Minimal Brain Dysfunction," in J. D. Noshpitz, ed., *Basic Handbook of Child Psychiatry,* vol. 2. New York: Basic Books, 1979, pp. 416–439.

51. ———. "Therapeutic Interventions with Children Who Have Perceptual and Other Learning Problems," in J. D. Noshpitz, ed., *Basic Handbook of Child Psychiatry,* vol. 3. New York: Basic Books, 1979, pp. 605–614.

52. ———. "The Relationship Between Learning Disabilities, Hyperactivity, Distractibility, and Behavioral Problems: A Clinical Analysis," *Journal of the American Academy of Child Psychiatry,* 20 (1981):385–397.

53. STREISSGUTH, A. P., BARR, H. M., and MARTIN, D. C. "Offspring Effects and Pregnancy Complications Related to Self-Reported Maternal Use," *Developmental Pharmacology and Therapeutics,* 5 (1982):21–32.

54. STREISSGUTH, A. P., et al. "Effects of Maternal Alcohol, Nicotine and Caffeine Use During Pregnancy on Infant Development at 8 Months," *Alcoholism: Clinical and Experimental Research,* 4 (1980):152–164.

55. STREISSGUTH, A. P., et al. "Teratogenic Effects of Alcohol in Humans and Laboratory Animals," *Science,* 209 (1980):353–361.

56. STREISSGUTH, A. P., et al. The Seattle Longitudinal Prospective Study on Alcohol and Pregnancy," *Neurobehavioral Toxicology and Teratology,* 3 (1981):223–233.

57. THOMPSON, A. J., SEARLE, M., and RUSSELL, G. "Quality of Survival After Severe Birth Asphyxia," *Archives of Disease in Childhood,* 52 (1977):620–626.

58. WENDER, P. H. *Minimal Brain Dysfunction in Children.* New York: Wiley-Interscience, 1971.

59. YANAI, J., and BERGMAN, A. "Neuronal Deficits After Neonatal Exposure to Phenobarbital," *Exploratory Neurology,* 73 (1981):199–208.

39 / The Psychoses of Childhood

Marian K. DeMyer

Introduction

The goal of this chapter is to describe the main advances since the publication of volume 2 of this *Handbook* in the clinical description, etiology, biology, psychodynamics, and family dynamics of child psychoses. According to DSM-III,[1] psychotic disorders include pervasive developmental disorders, schizophrenia, some organic mental disorders, paranoid disorders, and some affective disorders. While some children undoubtedly fall into the latter three categories, most psychotic children meet the criteria for pervasive developmental disorders (PDD) and schizophrenia in childhood (SchCh). Of the three types of PDD, infantile autism (IA) is the most common. In fact, no papers have yet appeared concerning PDD, childhood type (ChTy), or PDD, Atypical Type (AtTy). It is rather mysterious that, during the 1970s, both of the terms childhood schizophrenia and child psychoses were infrequently used in the literature.[21]

What is the reason for the relatively infrequent use of the term childhood schizophrenia? Rutter[78] suggested that there may be no such entity. In chapter 14 in volume 2 of this *Handbook* Fish and Ritvo[28] argued that the insistence on the presence of delusions and hallucinations (D/H) as necessary criteria may have prevented many children from receiving the diagnosis. These authors believed that use of Bender's criteria[4] (which do not require D/H) would have resulted in more schizophrenic children being identified. Whether any of these statements are valid is moot, but the fact is that most of the recent literature on childhood psychoses deals with IA; this chapter will therefore be devoted largely to that entity. Perhaps in the next decade we shall see some studies of PDD AtTy, which may be nearly what Bender[4] called SchCh without D/H. In any event, with or without D/H, such cases are rare in children under thirteen years[55] of age and probably represent less than 1 percent of the cases referred to child psychiatry services.

Why is the term childhood psychoses so infrequently used now? For one thing, it is a generic term, and since only one type, IA, has received much recent attention, there is little need for a generic term. Although PDD is listed on page 367 of DSM-III as a type of psychosis, DSM-III omits any reference to "childhood psychoses" as such. The DSM-III definition of "psychosis" is "gross impairment in reality testing . . ." (p. 367) as evidenced by presence of D/H without insight. For SchCh, DSM-III clearly indicates that adult criteria are applicable and thus impairment of reality testing would be important. (See table 39–1 for DSM-III terms and diagnostic criteria.) Research from the 1970s suggests that perhaps the essence of the psychotic process in IA is a serious degree of social distance coupled with language[20] and symbolizing disabilities.[98]

Because it is difficult to separate progress in the first half of the 1970s from that of the second half, this chapter reports on the whole decade, which the author has reviewed elsewhere.[21] The emphasis here is on the later years of that decade and into the 1980s.

Diagnosis

Two thorny problems have been diagnostic reliability and validity. Kanner's criteria[49]—namely, absence of affective contact, desire for preservation of sameness, and failure to use communicative language—have been used by many investigators. On the surface these criteria appear simple but in actuality they have been difficult to apply. "Absence of affective contact" is a high-level construct whose definition depends on the presence of several behaviors in the child such as lack of eye contact, ignoring of humans, and lack of affectionate gestures. Each of these behaviors must be precisely defined if various observers are to agree as to

TABLE 39–1

Axis I[a]: DSM-III Terms and Diagnostic Criteria for Psychoses of Childhood[b]

Generic Term: Pervasive Developmental Disorders[c]	
Subclass	Diagnostic criteria

1. Infantile autism
   Full syndrome 299.00
   Residual 299.01
	All of the following:
	a. Onset before age 30 months
	b. Serious lack of social response
	c. Language deficit—gross
	d. Speech peculiar, if present
	e. Unusual responses to environment
	f. No delusions or hallucinations

2. Childhood-onset pervasive developmental disorder
   Full syndrome 299.90
   Residual 299.91
	a. Severe disturbance of emotional responses and social relationships
	b. Three or more of: excess anxiety; affect disturbance; resistance to change; peculiar motility; dysprody; abnormal sensation; self-mutilation
	c. onset between ages 2½ and 12 years
	d. No delusions or hallucinations

3. Atypical pervasive developmental disorder 299.8x	a. Distortion of social and language skills that cannot be classified as either 1 or 2 above b. No delusions or hallucinations

Generic Term: Schizophrenic Disorders[d]	
Subclass	Diagnostic criteria
Schizophrenic disorders in childhood (5 subtypes as for adults) Full syndrome 295.1x through 295.6x Residual 295.6x	As for adult schizophrenia, all of the following: a. At least one of six delusional, hallucinatory, or associational symptoms b. Impairment in two or more routine functions of living c. Continuous illness for at least six months

[a] If an individual has mental retardation in addition to a mental illness, this diagnosis is coded also on Axis I and is described in DSM-III beginning on p. 36. Borderline mental retardation is described on p. 322.
[b] This term appears nowhere in DSM-III.
[c] Described in DSM-III, pp. 86–92, under "Disorders Usually First Evident in Infancy, Childhood or Adolescence."
[d] Described in DSM-III, pp. 181–193, under "Schizophrenic Disorders."

whether it is present or absent. As with most human behaviors, Kanner's symptoms exist on a continuum of severity. It is difficult to locate reliably the point on that continuum where such a trait as social distance, for example, should be labeled as "absence of affective contact."

To circumvent these difficulties, a series of diagnostic checklists have appeared that have stipulated that a particular array of scores is needed for a diagnosis of IA. The older checklists seem gradually to have been replaced by the newer ones. Several authors have determined at least partially the reliability and validity of their rating instruments. Parks[70] reviewed five rating scales* (see table 39–2) and found that while "each of these instruments has contributed to the greater specification and quantification of the autistic syndrome," further reliability and validity studies are needed to make them more useful (p. 265). In this author's opin-

ion, all the existing checklists must be supplemented by histories and clinical judgment.

Other points of diagnostic disagreement concern the child's intelligence and whether signs of organic dysfunction may or may not be present. Kanner[49] himself set the critical diagnostic biases by observing that IA bore little resemblance to any known organic condition or to mental retardation. His views persisted from the 1940s through the 1960s. These statements, plus his observation that the parents of autistic children were cold and obsessive, lessened the impact of his statement that autistic infants were born "with innate inability to form the usual, biologically provided affective contact with people" (p. 250). Unfortunately, the professional community emphasized the supposedly obsessive, cold parents who were then "blamed" nearly universally for the creation of autism. Likewise, most of the professional community accepted Kanner's assertation that autistic children were of normal intelligence—especially if they possessed a splinter skill—and that a diag-

*See references 32, 54, 74, 76, 77, and 80.

TABLE 39-2

Diagnostic Instruments for Infantile Autism for Which Partial Reliability and Validity Have Been Determined

| Title | Format | Reliability[a] | | Validity[b] | | |
		Rater	Internal	Content	Concurrent	Discriminant
1. Diagnostic Checklist for Behavior Disturbed Children (E2)[74]	76 multiple-choice questions answered by parent	0	0	0	0	Psychotic vs. nonpsychotic
2. Behavior Rating Instrument for Autistic & Atypical Children (BRIAAC)[76,77]	8 empirically derived scales—e.g. adult relations, communication, drive, speech	+	+	+	A few scales	Mentally retarded?
3. Behavior Observation Scale for Autism (BOS)[32]	67 objectively defined items	+	0	0	0	Normal; mentally retarded
4. Childhood Autism Rating Scale (CARS)[80]	15 scales from Kanner and British Working Party	+	+	0	Not well described	0
5. Autism Behavior Checklist (ABC)[54]	57 items selected from 7 sources	+	+	0	Partial	Normal; mentally retarded

[a]No instrument tested for test-retest reliability.
[b]No instrument has been demonstrated to have construct validity.

nosis of autism could not be accepted if there were overt signs of brain pathology. For example, a cerebral-palsied child would not be called autistic in Kanner's sense even if the child possessed all of his cardinal symptoms.

The major problem with such thinking is that in many cases damage to brain substance is difficult to detect, especially if it does not affect the motor system. Each child must be thoroughly studied neurologically to detect subtle signs; and in those early years few children were given such careful scrutiny. In addition, even if no overt neurological signs are present, the central nervous system (CNS) may have been subjected to a variety of insults such as anoxia, trauma, or maldevelopment with resulting organic malfunction. Such "silent" insults may leave many brain areas free from defect but seriously undermine some crucial areas, such as the language centers or the limbic areas. These malfunctions may be undetectable in young children by current examination methods other than by direct study of their behavior.

In sum, the diagnosis of autism has heretofore been based on a number of uncertain measures. These included: (1) behavioral features that are difficult to define precisely, (2) rough estimates of basic biological intelligence, and (3) crude measures of the intactness of the CNS. The most recent effort to overcome these problems has been in DSM-III, where a behavioral diagnosis can be made separately from an intellectual diagnosis. Thus if a child meets the criteria for PDD, IA type, and also tests below IQ 70, then the diagnosis "mental retardation" would be coded also, both on Axis I. (See table 39–1.)

If the diagnostician locates a putative neurological cause such as congenital rubella, that diagnosis can be coded on Axis III. Thus we now can separate the important factors of behavior, intelligence, and neurological status. This allows for a study of their relationships not only to each other but to other important variables of child psychosis as well, and thus offers a major advance over making assumptions without prior study.

Presumably the "organic psychoses" as listed in DSM-III refer to both children and adults. While the "disintegrative psychoses" are not common and are poorly understood, they do occur. Properly speaking, they should be described in the section entitled "Disorders Usually First Evident in Childhood" and listed in the differential diagnosis of PDD. Rett's syndrome,[40] consisting of loss of speech, affective contact, and diminution of motor skills, can mimic PDD exactly. Age of onset has become important in diagnosis. In DSM-III, onset before thirty months is one of the chief criteria separating IA from the other two types of PDD. (See table 39–1.) (A clinical diagnostic strategy is outlined in chapter 57.)

Etiological Theories Past and Present

Initially, there was ready professional acceptance of the idea that IA represented a parentally caused condition in a biologically normal child. Despite this, however, two other hypotheses were advanced: (1) that parents were only partially responsible for autism (nature-nurture theory), and (2) that parents contributed little or nothing to the production of autism and that all autistic children were biologically defective (nature theory).[46]

While each theory had several variations, the sum of which would have been impossible to test in any one investigator's lifetime, some consistencies made possible a reasonable program of research. The various "nature" and "nature-nurture" theories, whatever their differences, emphasized the failure of parents to stimulate their autistic children as infants in a warm and adequate way. This parental lack was implied by some authors who emphasized the greater degrees of parental psychopathology or extremes of parental rage. The rationale was that inadequate parental practices would make infants so uncomfortable that they would withdraw from a bewildering set of circumstances and thereby fail to form social bonds or learn to speak. The alternative idea was that the infants mimicked in exaggerated form the sick personalities of the parents.[17]

Many varieties of biological defect were proposed. In general, they all appeared to involve the CNS, although the locus of the defect was theorized to be in any of a wide array of sites ranging from the general substance of the brain to such specific areas as the vestibular system, the reticular formation, or the cortex.[17]

In 1961 this author[17] began a program of research to test these three theories. It was clear that the psychopathology of the parents, their child-rearing practices, and the neurological state of the children must be described. Moreover, two control groups were essential: (1) parents whose children were normal and one of their normal children and (2) parents who had at least one nonpsychotic child with a developmental deficiency such as dysphasia or mental retardation. After twelve years of research, the resultant findings strongly supported the theory that autistic children were abnormal neurobiologically and that the parents were basically no different from any other group of people drawn from their socioeconomic class.[22] During this same period, other investigators were reporting results of similar import.[14]

By the end of the 1970s a series of family studies by several investigators[58] that had compared the parents of autistic children to other parent groups revealed that the "autistic" parents possessed no special parenting defects. They were as warm and relating to their autistic children as they were to their other offspring, and they displayed no more signs of psychopathology or of extreme character traits such as coldness, obsessiveness, social anxiety, or rage than did the control parents. These results have been so persuasive that no studies of parental personality, child-rearing techniques, or psychopathology have appeared from 1980 through 1983. In contrast, rearing the autistic child was a stressful situation, especially for the mothers. Indeed one-third of these women developed mild depressions during the period when autistic symptoms were at their height (two to four years of age)[18] and when community supportive services were not available in adolescence and adulthood.[19] The long-held idea that autistic children came from relatively higher socioeconomic classes was refuted by several studies in several countries.[33,36,91,94]

Studies of Neurobiological Import

At the same time that investigators were finding little to suggest the presence of unusual parental psychopathology, they were uncovering evidence of neurobiological dysfunction in psychotic children.[21] While the brain was usually thought to be the site of the lesion, the specific loci responsible for the characteristic autistic symptoms are still unknown. The major evidence for these conclusions came from comparisons of autistic children with normal children and with other impaired populations with respect to cognition, perception, neurological signs, electrophysiology, brain images, sex differences, genetics, biochemistry, and immunology.

NEUROLOGICAL EVALUATIONS

My group[17] performed thorough neurological evaluations of 150 autistic children and compared the findings with data from 48 nonpsychotic subnormal children and 43 normal children.[17] The results revealed significantly more signs of neurobiological dysfunction in the autistic and the subnormal children than in the normal groups. However, in this respect the autistic and subnormal children were nearly equal. These signs included observations made during neurological physical examination, a history of pre-, peri-, neo- and postnatal stresses, and abnormal tracings on the electroencephalogram (EEG). Only 14.2 percent of the autistic brain damage index scores fell within one standard deviation of the normal scores. This difference is remarkable because prescreening had eliminated from the study those autistic children with obvious neurological signs. Throughout the 1970s other investigators* studying smaller groups of autistic children reported results of similar character. They described multiple types of neurological findings, including "hard" and "soft" signs. This led to the inference that the ultimate causes of autism are multiple and can be due to nearly any type of brain insult. Within a total Swedish population the birth data for autistic infants showed reduced scores on optimum pregnancy and perinatal factors as compared with matched normals.[34]

Such neurological findings were often thought to be spurious; the investigators were criticized for contaminating their groups of autistic children with those who were "really retarded."[28] However, low brain damage indices and low prenatal optimality scores were frequently found in the low-IQ autistic children and high indices in higher-functioning children.[17,34] More than that, measures of family adequacy and amount of parental psychopathology were unrelated to the neurological diagnoses of the children.[17] That still leaves open the possibility that the low-functioning retarded and mute autistic child is a basically different entity than the higher-functioning autistic child with some speech and a higher IQ. That question is discussed in the section devoted to the relation of autism to mental retardation.

Coleman[13] reported 129 neurological conditions in which the autistic picture is found. It is especially apt to be associated with infantile spasms (about 37 percent)[73]; phenylketonuria, congenital rubella, postencephalitis (about 5 percent of cases)[97]; and fragile X syndrome[7,65] but is much less common in other chromosomal abnormalities such as Down's syndrome.

ELECTROPHYSIOLOGICAL STUDIES

After reviewing all EEG studies appearing in the 1960s and 1970s, Small[85] concluded that autistic subjects had significantly more abnormalities than did the normal controls. This led her to suggest that infantile autism is a CNS disorder. In evaluating the fact that there is so much disagreement among various investigators about the kinds of EEG abnormalities and the clinical correlations they make, Small attributed these differences to the technical difficulties that arise when one seeks to obtain adequate records from uncooperative children. Such differences might also be explained as evidence of differing amounts, types, and sites of brain pathology in the spectrum of autistic children.

*See references 24, 50, 51, 52, and 56.

OTHER ELECTROPHYSIOLOGICAL AND
PSYCHOPHYSIOLOGICAL STUDIES

Rapid eye movement sleep has been reported abnormal in IA.[89] Evidence of abnormal auditory brainstem responses (ABR) has been found in 23 to 33 percent of cases. This disturbance may be associated with symptoms of muscular hypotonia and inattentional symptoms.[25,38] Relatively similar findings by several investigators make the brain stem an area of special interest.[68,84,86] However, as Maurer and Damasio[63] pointed out, the brain-stem pathology may be "neither primary nor specific for IA." On the other hand, Tanguay and Edwards[88] have speculated that the brain-stem abnormalities may be primary and have an effect on the forebrain while the brain is developing.

In other psychophysiological research,[53] high-functioning autistic children who learned a research task had peripheral blood flow (PBF) measurements "consistent with sensory intake." Lower-functioning children who failed the task showed "PBF consistent with sensory rejection." Thus autistic children may avoid sensory experiences when they cannot make sense of them. A study of event-related electrical potentials[67] revealed an aberrant wave form that signified to the authors that autistic children "cannot evaluate stimuli." James and Barry[48] showed that autistic children had more disability in acquiring right ear dominance than did matched retarded children, a finding they interpreted to support the notion that autistic children had difficulty in establishing cerebral dominance.

BRAIN IMAGING

Based on findings from pneumoencephalograms (PEG)[42] and computerized tomography (CT),[37,45,75] a variety of brain abnormalities have been discerned in from 20 to 88 percent of autistic subjects. The heterogeneity of abnormalities suggested to Damasio and coworkers[15] that autism could be "consequent to a variety of CNS diseases." A number of anatomical abnormalities, such as unilateral and bilateral ventricular enlargement and reversed patterns of brain asymmetry, resemble those reported in major mental disease of adults. Among others, these have been noted in both adult and adolescent schizophrenic subjects.[81]

IMMUNOLOGICAL STUDIES

Weizman and associates[93] reported that 76 percent of autistic children may have an autoimmune reaction. Deykin and MacMahon[23] found an increased incidence of maternal viral infection and exposure during pregnancy of autistic children. Markowitz[61] discussed the importance of exploring viruses as a source of brain pathology in autism.

BIOCHEMICAL STUDIES

The search for biochemical markers during the 1970s covered many possibilities, but the serotonergic system was the most widely investigated. The first studies reported higher levels of serotonin (5HT) in IA. Later, however, it was found that low-IQ groups of all kinds had higher 5HT than did high-IQ groups. Also it turned out that it was the low-IQ autistic children who had elevated 5HT levels and that the higher-IQ autistic children had 5HT levels that were generally in the normal range.[21] Such evidence makes it mandatory to control for IQ in all 5HT studies. There was an earlier report that high 5HT efflux from red blood cells was a marker for IA; this was not confirmed by later studies.[6]

In order for biochemical research to be meaningful, multiple biological controls must be imposed. This is well illustrated by the research history of dopamine beta-hydroxylase (DBH). There had been early reports of differences in the DBH activity of autistic children. These lost significance when it was discovered that DBH activity increases with age and that the earlier studies had not been adequately age-controlled.[21]

Cohen and coworkers[11] reported cerebral spinal fluid (CSF) elevations of homovanillic acid (HVA) and 5-hydroxyindoleacetic acid (5-HIAA) in autistic patients as compared to epileptic patients. On the other hand, when the CSF 5-HIAA levels of autistic children were compared with those of nonautistic psychotic children, lower values were found. Gillberg, Svennerholm, and Hamilton-Hellberg[39] showed increases of only HVA and not 5-HIAA in autistic patients as against mentally retarded patients.

It is difficult to compare biochemical studies with one another because of differences in the diagnostic groups studied, in methods of experiment, in the small size of the populations sampled, and because of the numerous factors that affect the levels of these chemicals and their metabolites in the body. Nevertheless, the search for evidence of disordered biochemistry should continue, preferably with several centers participating in carefully planned, stepwise studies to eliminate the problems of too-small patient samples and diverse experimental methods.

STUDY OF SEX DIFFERENCES

The well-known difference in sex ratios of IA (2 to 4 boys to 1 girl) has stimulated studies of fairly large populations. The most consistent finding is that to a small but significant extent, autistic boys have higher cognition skills than do girls.[90,96] In the study by Schopler's group with the largest population ($N = 384$) and the most detailed testing, the boys also "showed more

unusual visual responses and more stereotypic play"
than the girls did[57] (p. 317). The authors interpreted
these results as providing some support for the mul-
tifactorial genetic transmission of autism. They speculated that males may have a lower threshold for brain
dysfunction than girls do and would therefore require
less "genetic liability" than girls to produce autism.

GENETIC STUDIES

Folstein and Rutter[30] have gathered evidence from
twin studies that indicate there may be a genetic component to autism. Sibling studies show not only a
higher rate of autism (2 percent versus 0.02 to 0.04
percent of the general population) but also an increased
incidence of language/cognitive disability in the
nonautistic siblings of autistic children.[3,66] The case
for a genetic component is somewhat weakened, however, by the finding that language functioning of the
involved parents is not measurably less adequate than
that of other parent groups.[99]

The Relationship of Infantile Autism to Other Related Conditions

Table 39–3 lists the chief differential DSM-III criteria
that distinguish among PDD and the four most closely
related disorders. Of these conditions, the relationship
between IA and mental retardation has been the most
widely studied. The disintegrative psychoses should be
listed in DSM-III. Also, the caveat that few mentally
retarded autistic children have the full autistic syndrome should be eliminated from the next diagnostic
manual.

MENTAL RETARDATION

When Kanner[49] implied that autistic children were
not retarded in the usual biological sense, the professional community generally agreed. From the 1940s
through the 1960s autistic children were widely regarded as pseudoretarded. As a rule their IQs were
estimated to be at the level of any splinter skill they
might possess and were thus usually overestimated.
The low IQs revealed after formal testing of certain
psychotic children were widely dismissed as spurious;
after all, everyone assumed that autistic children were
too negativistic to perform when tested. Indeed, because of the well-known scatter in the autistic child's
abilities, IQs were regarded as useless.

However, during the 1960s and 1970s several well-

TABLE 39–3

DSM-III Differential Diagnosis of Pervasive Developmental Disorders: Major Differential Features

Axis I

Infantile autism versus childhood-onset pervasive
developmental disorder.
> The chief differential criterion is that the former
> have onset before thirty months of age and the
> latter appear after thirty months of age.

Pervasive Developmental Disorder vs.:

1. Mental retardation
   a. Full-syndrome PDD rarely present.
   b. When both disorders present, both diagnoses should be made.
2. Schizophrenia in childhood
   a. Hallucinations, delusions, incoherence present.
3. Hearing impairment
   a. History of responding only to loud noises.
   b. Audiogram indicates deafness or hearing impairment.
4. Developmental language disorder, receptive type
   a. Eye or social contact made.
   b. Appropriate gestures used.

done studies using large populations of children disproved the foregoing assumptions. The results of these
studies included[21]:

1. All autistic children are testable if items within the
   child's mental age are used.
2. Most psychotic children score in the mentally retarded
   ranges.
3. While performance IQs are higher than verbal IQs,
   nevertheless, about 75 percent of autistic children have
   performance IQs of 68 or below.
4. IQs of autistic children are as stable over time as those
   of normal children—only about 10 percent show
   marked and sustained acceleration in mental development, and a similar percentage show a marked and
   sustained drop.
5. Splinter skills do not reduce the validity of IQ scores.
6. The most common splinter skills involve fitting and
   assembly tasks and the rote repetition of words or sentences.
7. The most common splinter disabilities are on verbal
   items requiring abstract thinking skills or symbolization.
8. IQ scores obtained in the preschool years are predictive
   of outcome.

9. Negativism is not an important factor in reducing IQ scores.
10. Those children with an initial evaluation of IQ 40 or below have a poor outcome. While not all children with IQs of 60 or above have a good outcome, those who have a fair or good status on follow-up do, in fact, come from this range.

As a group, autistic children are similar to mentally retarded children in that both are late in acquiring milestones such as hand dominance, right-left awareness, imitative acts,[18] gross and fine motor skills, the ability to draw geometric figures, and music performance.[18] In fact, Ornitz, Guthrie, and Farley[69] reported that in a group of seventy-four autistic children, in addition to the profound and well-known delays in language, nearly all aspects of development were delayed.

If so many autistic children are truly mentally retarded, then what is the difference between mentally retarded nonautistic children and their retarded autistic counterparts? In 1973 DeMyer, Bryson, and Churchill[20] reported that only two behavioral symptoms separated a psychotic group from a subnormal nonpsychotic group—the psychotic children displayed serious social withdrawal and noncommunicative behavior. In the last ten years one of the big advances has been the proliferation of studies that have attempted to locate critical differences between the two populations matched for mental age. (See table 39–4.) This matching is crucial because several important behaviors previously thought to be diagnostic of autism are strongly related to mental age and are found in other conditions, including normality. Such phenomena as echolalia, pronominal reversal, and lack of self-awareness[27] are three important examples.

Thumbnail results of studies (see table 39–4) conducted in the 1980s* tend largely to extend and support those of earlier workers such as Hermelin and O'Connor[43] and Wing and associates.[98] Some preliminary conceptions of the critical differences between mentally retarded and autistic subjects have been decided on. These concern the splinter disability of autistic children in their capacity to abstract and to symbolize. This may have its roots in deficiencies in manipulating images in a purposeful manner; that is to say, in whatever internal mental images autistic children may be able to form. Also, a severe deficiency in memory for events exists side by side with a reasonably good capacity to learn by rote and paired associate learning. According to Boucher,[5] autistic children do poorly in such memory tasks as recent event memory and free recall in which distinctive retrieval cues must be encoded at input. She speculated that their disability in verbal conversation may be partly due to an "inability to voluntarily bring to mind appropriate things to say" (p. 293). The foregoing literature should be studied in detail by those researchers interested in the critical differences between mental retardation and autism.

A common criticism of the early intelligence investigations was that the autistic groups were "contaminated" with retarded children and that the retarded autistic child was "rediscovered."[28] The implication of such a statement is that if a child has low enough cognitive skills, that child will not be able to relate positively to other humans or to communicate nonverbally on the basis of low general cognitive skills alone. Wing[95] tested this assumption in an epidemiological study and found it to be unverified. She located all the children ($N = 172$) in a London borough with an IQ below 50. Of these children, including some whose IQs were below 20, eighty-two were rated as sociable and "enjoyed and sought out social interaction."

Of the socially impaired, seventeen children demonstrated elaborate rituals or stereotypes needing "reasonably good fitting and assembly skills" in combination with aloofness. This pattern is what Wing termed "classic" autism in the "Kannerian sense," and it occurred in children with an IQ of 20 to 49. Those with IQs below 20 engaged in simple repetitive routines. It is apparent that the children in Wing's sample with "Kanner's" syndrome tested in the severely to moderately mentally retarded range, while those with less elaborate rituals were profoundly retarded. While a triad of social disability, communication failure, and stereotypes occurred with increasing frequency as IQ went down, the low IQs could not by themselves explain the presence of the triad.

Wing[95] speculated that the "problems in the socially impaired children are of a different order from those in the sociable group" (p. 40) and that, in addition to whatever other brain defects they and the sociable child may share in common, the socially aloof are afflicted with a specific brain defect of their own. Wing is not alone in speculating about specific brain locations that might be compromised in autism. A whole literature is developing on the subject, which will be reviewed only briefly here. Some putative locations such as the brain stem have been mentioned. However, the most frequent location cited is the left hemisphere.[16,59] Autistic children have been described as "right-hemisphere processors" while mentally retarded children use both hemispheres.[12,27] Bilateral temporal lobe involvement[44] and the mesial surface of the frontal and temporal lobes[64] have also been implicated. Ciaranello, Vanden Berg, and Anders[10] speculated that the damage probably occurs in the latter stages of neuronal development. Much more basic knowledge of normal and abnormal brain function is needed to localize the brain defects of autism.

*See references 5, 31, 41, 60, 62, 72, and 82.

TABLE 39–4

Differences Reported for Autistic Children Versus Normals and Mental Retardates When Mental Age Was Controlled

Authors	Date	Findings Concerning IA
Boucher[5]	1981	Poor memory for recent events.
Hammes and Langdell[41,a]	1981	Could form visual images but could not manipulate them purposefully and meaningfully.
Maltz[60]	1981	Performed better on concrete discrimination and worse on formal (abstract) discrimination tasks.
Riguet et al.[72]	1981	Impaired symbolic and imitative functions.
Masterton and Biederman[62]	1983	Preference for proximal rather than visual sensory input is probably an alternate strategy compensating for inability to use visual control of reaching.
Shah and Frith[82]	1983	Perform better on embedded figure task, showing good visual spatial orienting ability, but lack ability to manipulate visually presented stimulus objects or pictures mentally or to refer to stimulus meaning.
Frankel et al.[31, a]	1984	Probably show "stimulus overselectivity"—tend to respond to a restricted subset of multiple cues in a discrimination task.

[a]Only mentally retarded children used as controls. All other investigators used both normal and mentally retarded children.

We now come to the question of whether the retarded autistic child is basically a different entity from the autistic child who tests (least in performance scores) within the borderline-to-normal IQ range. Rutter[79] argued for the difference, pointing to the better outcome in higher-functioning autistic children. Higher-IQ children generally have better speech in the preschool years, and a few develop completely adequate language by adulthood. However, the majority continue to have difficulties in relating to people and controlling their emotions. It can be surmised also that higher-functioning autistic children may have less extensive damage to their brains while still suffering some damage to the centers that mediate social and abstraction skills. More definite knowledge will come only from comparative neurobiological studies of lower and higher cognitive skill IA groups.

DEVELOPMENTAL DYSPHASIAS

After conducting a series of language disability studies, Churchill[9] came to the conclusion that severe dysphasia is a necessary and sufficient condition to explain the symptoms of autism. Others argue that autism is basically a form of cognitive dysfunction.[79] A problem with pursuing either of these lines of reasoning too forcibly is that satisfactory definitions have not been formulated for either cognition or language. If there is a social intelligence dimension, as Wing's studies suggest, we will have to relate that factor to the language and cognition deficits of autistic people. However, language, cognition, and social intelligence are so closely intertwined that it may not be possible to define them

separately although we may learn much from the effort to do so.

Some autistic children with speech manifest dysphasic speech patterns. For example, many fluent autistic individuals have the semantic-pragmatic type of aphasia that has the following features: (1) the patients cannot understand wh— questions yet can obey simple commands; (2) they demonstrate good phonology and syntax; (3) their spontaneous speech is better than their elicited speech; (4) they demonstrate good verbal memory; (5) their conversation does not convey much information.

Tager-Flushberg[87] pointed out that pragmatic and semantic speech functions may be specially deficient in autism. In fact, however, most autistic patients (over 50 percent) are mute and remain so throughout their lives. Most of those who do have language tend to engage in word repetition—that is, echolalia—which may at times be used communicatively. Or they learn to communicate immediate needs by one word or a simple phrase. These children remain poor at discourse, at creating language on their own, or in the use or understanding of language abstractions.

By definition, aphasic children with typical autistic social and affective symptoms are called autistic, and there is verbal symptomatic overlap between fluent autistic subjects and those with developmental aphasia. Perhaps in addition to dysfunctional speech centers (which are not themselves clearly located),[2] there is in autism damage to those unknown parts of the brain that mediate social skills and nonverbal communication.

Because so many therapeutic efforts have been directed toward increasing the language skills of autistic children, additional language descriptions will be found in chapter 57.

SCHIZOPHRENIA

There are two schools of thought in regard to the relationship of infantile autism and schizophrenia. As noted in chapter 14 in volume 2 of this *Handbook,* Bender, Goldfarb, Ornitz, Fish, and Ritvo[28] support the idea that the two syndromes lie on a continuum of severity (e.g., IA children have lower IQs than SchCh). Rutter and Kolvin[28] on the other hand, believe they are separate entities. Before DSM-III, it was difficult to separate children called "autistic" from those called "schizophrenic." Some of the earlier criteria for childhood schizophrenia were excessively broad, and in any case there was a great deal of symptom overlap. However, in respect to any comparison of IA with SchCh, the literature remains sparse. Twenty years after an initial evaluation, Howells and Guirguis[47] reevaluated twenty child schizophrenic subjects. They found that while the patients were "quieter in adulthood, in other respects they were almost unchanged and retained most of the cardinal points (i.e., British Working Party criteria) of childhood schizophrenia" (p. 123). The only difference between those with onset before thirty months of age and the later-onset cases was that the latter "reported more hallucinatory experiences." When the authors used the criteria of Feighner and coworkers, all patients turned out to be adult schizophrenics. However, if Schneider's first-rank symptoms were applied, none were diagnosed as adult schizophrenics. Other follow-up studies[83] likewise have emphasized how little psychotic children change in adolescence and adulthood. However, Gillberg and Schaumann[35] estimated that about one-third deteriorate at the onset of puberty, with no environmental causes to explain the setbacks.

Petty and associates[71] documented three cases of IA (diagnosed according to DSM-III criteria) that by adolescence developed schizophrenia (also diagnosed according to DSM-III). The authors linked the two conditions principally on the basis of the presence of perceptual disturbances in both time periods; they feel that their view is buttressed by the results of neurobiological studies.

Even though schizophrenia commonly first becomes manifest during adolescence,[29] only a handful of papers have appeared in the last decade concerning the condition in adolescence. Likewise, only a few have appeared concerning SchCh. A small number of SchCh subjects demonstrated greater difficulties than normal children in recognizing emotion in facial expressions.[92] In comparison to nonschizophrenic psychiatrically disturbed children, SchCh patients were similar in verbal IQ but inferior in performance IQ, and also had more difficulties in paired associate learning.[8]

Summary

During the last decade the literature on childhood psychoses was dominated by studies of infantile autism. This entity is now considered to be a pervasive developmental disorder that can be caused by any one of the many conditions which can injure the brain in its pre-, peri-, or postnatal state. In occasional individual cases, a putative cause can be identified; often, however, no brain insult is apparent. Some research evidence suggests that genetics, autoimmune or virus diseases, or disordered biochemistry may play roles. It is now well established that the larger proportion of IA cases have mental retardation that is severe and long lasting. In addition, however, autistic persons suffer from social and symbolization disabilities that differentiate them from retarded individuals. Speculation abounds concerning the exact brain site(s) that may be responsible for the absence of affective contact and for autistic individuals' communication and symbolization splinter disabilities.

REFERENCES

1. AMERICAN PSYCHIATRIC ASSOCIATION. *Diagnostic and Statistical Manual of Mental Disorders,* 3rd ed. (DSM-III). Washington, D. C.: American Psychiatric Association, 1980.

2. ARNOLD, G., and SCHWARTZ, S. "Hemispheric Lateralization of Language in Autistic and Aphasic Children," *Journal of Autism and Developmental Disorders,* 13 (1983):129–139.

3. AUGUST, G. J., STEWART, M. A., and TSAI, L. "The Incidence of Cognitive Disabilities in the Siblings of Autistic Children," *British Journal of Psychiatry,* 138 (1981):416–422.

4. BENDER, L. "Schizophrenia in Childhood—Its Recognition, Description and Treatment," *American Journal of Orthopsychiatry,* 26 (1956):499–506.

5. BOUCHER, J. "Memory for Recent Events in Autistic Children," *Journal of Autism and Developmental Disorders,* 11 (1981):293–301.

6. BOULLIN, D., et al. "Towards the Resolution of Conflicting Findings," *Journal of Autism and Developmental Disorders,* 12 (1982):97–98.

7. BROWN, W. T., et al. "Autism Is Associated with the Fragile-X Syndrome," *Journal of Autism and Developmental Disorders,* 12 (1982):303–308.

8. CARTER, L., ALPERT, M., and STEWART, S. M. "Schizophrenic Children's Utilization of Images and Words in Performance of Cognitive Tasks," *Journal of Autism and Developmental Disorders,* 12 (1982):279–293.

9. CHURCHILL, D. W. *Language of Autistic Children.* New York: John Wiley & Sons, 1978.

10. CIARANELLO, R. D., VANDENBERG, S. R., and ANDERS, T. F. "Intrinsic and Extrinsic Determinants of Neuronal Development: Relation to Infantile Autism," *Journal of Autism and Developmental Disorders,* 12 (1982):115–145.

11. COHEN, D. J., et al. "Dopamine and Serotonin Metabolism in Neuropsychiatrically Disturbed Children: CSF Homovanillic Acid and 5-Hydroxyindoleacetic Acid," *Archives of General Psychiatry,* 34 (1977):545–550.

12. COLBY, K. M., and PARKINSON, C. "Handedness in Autistic Children," *Journal of Autism and Childhood Schizophrenia,* 7 (1977):3–9.

13. COLEMAN, M. "Studies of the Autistic Syndromes," in R. Katzman, ed., *Congenital and Acquired Cognitive Disorders,* vol. 57. New York: Association for Research in Nervous and Mental Disease, 1979, pp. 265–275.

14. COX, A., et al. "A Comparative Study of Infantile Autism and Specific Developmental Receptive Language Disorder: II. Parental Characteristics," *British Journal of Psychiatry,* 126 (1975):146–159.

15. DAMASIO, H., et al. "Computerized Tomographic Scan Findings in Patients with Autistic Behavior," *Archives of Neurology,* 37 (1980):504–510.

16. DAWSON, G. "Lateralized Brain Dysfunction in Autism: Evidence from the Halstead-Reitan Neuropsychological Battery," *Journal of Autism and Developmental Disorders,* 13 (1983):269–286.

17. DEMYER, M. K. "Research in Infantile Autism; A Strategy and Its Results," *Biological Psychiatry,* 10 (1975): 433–452.

18. ———. *Parents and Children in Autism.* Washington, D. C.: Victor H. Winston & Sons, 1979.

19. DEMYER, M. K., and GOLDBERG, P. "Family Needs of the Autistic Adolescent," in Schopler and Mesibov, eds., *Autism in Adolescents and Adults.* New York: Plenum Press, 1983, pp. 225–250.

20. DEMYER, M. K., BRYSON, C. Q., and CHURCHILL, D. W. "The Earliest Indicators of Pathological Development: Comparison of Symptoms During Infancy and Early Childhood in Normal, Subnormal, Schizophrenic and Autistic Children," in J. I. Nurnberger, ed., *Biological and Environmental Determinants of Early Development,* vol. 51. Bethesda, Md.: Williams & Wilkins, 1973, pp. 298–332.

21. DEMYER, M. K., HINGTGEN, J. N., and JACKSON, R. K. "Infantile Autism Reviewed: A Decade of Research," *Schizophrenia Bulletin,* 7 (1981):388–451.

22. DEMYER, M. K., et al. "Parental Practices and Innate Activity in Normal, Autistic and Brain-Damaged Infants," *Journal of Autism and Childhood Schizophrenia,* 2 (1972): 49–66.

23. DEYKIN, E. Y., and MACMAHON, B. "Viral Exposure and Autism," *American Journal of Epidemiology,* 109 (1979):826–836.

24. ———. "Pregnancy, Delivery and Neonatal Complications Among Autistic Children," *American Journal of Diseases of Children,* 134 (1980):860–864.

25. FEIN, D., SKOFF, B., and MIRSKY, A. F. "Clinical Correlates of Brainstem Dysfunction in Autistic Children," *Journal of Autism and Developmental Disorders,* 11 (1981): 303–315.

26. FERRARI, M. "Childhood Autism: Deficits of Communication and Symbolic Development: I. Distinctions from Language Disorders," *Journal of Communication Disorders,* 15 (1982):191–208.

27. FERRARI, M., and MATTHEWS, W. S. "Self-recognition Deficits in Autism: Syndrome-Specific or General Developmental Delay?" *Journal of Autism and Developmental Disorders,* 13 (1983):317–324.

28. FISH, B., and RITVO, E. R. "Psychoses of Childhood," in J. D. Noshpitz, ed., *Basic Handbook of Child Psychiatry,* vol. 2. New York: Basic Books, 1979, pp. 249–304.

29. FLAHERTY, L., and SARLES, R. M. "Psychosis During Adolescence: A Review," *Journal of Adolescent Health Care,* 1 (1981):301–307.

30. FOLSTEIN, S., and RUTTER, M. "Genetic Influences in Infantile Autism," *Nature,* 265 (1977):726–728.

31. FRANKEL, F., et al. "Stimulus Overselectivity in Autistic and Mentally Retarded Children—A Research Note," *Journal of Child Psychology and Psychiatry,* 25 (1984):147–155.

32. FREEMAN, B. J., et al. "Behavior Observation Scale for Autism: Initial Methodology, Data Analysis, and Preliminary Findings in 89 Children," *Journal of the Academy of Child Psychiatry,* 17 (1978):576–588.

33. GILLBERG, C. "Infantile Autism and Other Childhood Psychoses in a Swedish Urban Region: Epidemiological Aspects," *Journal of Child Psychology and Psychiatry,* 25 (1984):35–43.

34. GILLBERG, C., and GILLBERG, I. C. "Infantile Autism: A Total Population Study of Reduced Optimality in the Pre-, Peri-, and Neonatal Period," *Journal of Autism and Developmental Disorders,* 13 (1983):153–166.

35. GILLBERG, C., and SCHAUMANN, H. "Infantile Autism and Puberty," *Journal of Autism and Developmental Disorders,* 11 (1981):365–371.

36. ———. "Social Class and Infantile Autism," *Journal of Autism and Developmental Disorders,* 12 (1982):223–228.

37. GILLBERG, C., and SVENDSEN, P. "Childhood Psychosis and Computed Tomographic Brain Scan Findings," *Journal of Autism and Developmental Disorders,* 13 (1983):19–32.

38. GILLBERG, C., ROSENHALL, U., and JOHANSSON, E. "Auditory Brainstem Responses in Childhood Psychosis," *Journal of Autism and Developmental Disorders,* 13 (1983): 181–195.

39. GILLBERG, C., SVENNERHOLM, L., and HAMILTON-HELLBERG, C. "Childhood Psychosis and Monoamine Metabolites in Spinal Fluid," *Journal of Autism and Developmental Disorders,* 13 (1983):383–396.

40. HAGBERG, B., et al. "A Progressive Syndrome of Autism, Dementia, Ataxia, and Loss of Purposeful Hand Use in Girls: Rett's Syndrome: Report of 35 Cases," *Annals of Neurology,* 14 (1983):471–479.

41. HAMMES, J. G. W., and LANGDELL, T. "Precursors of Symbol Formation and Childhood Autism," *Journal of Autism and Developmental Disorders,* 11 (1981):331–346.

42. HAUSER, S. L., DELONG, G. R., and ROSMAN, N. P. "Pneumoencephalographic Findings in the Infantile Autism Syndrome. A Correlation with Temporal Lobe Disease," *Brain,* 98 (1975):667–688.

43. HERMELIN, B., and O'CONNOR, N. *Psychological Experiments with Autistic Children.* Oxford: Pergamon Press, 1970.

44. HETZLER, B. E., and GRIFFIN, J. L. "Infantile Autism

and the Temporal Lobe of the Brain," *Journal of Autism and Developmental Disorders,* 11 (1981):317–330.

45. HIER, D. E., LeMAY, M., and ROSENBERGER, P. B. "Autism: Association with Reversed Cerebral Asymmetry," *Neurology,* 28 (1978):348–349.

46. HINGTGEN, J. N., and BRYSON, C. Q. "Recent Developments in the Study of Early Childhood Psychoses: Infantile Autism, Childhood Schizophrenia, and Related Disorders," *Schizophrenia Bulletin,* 5 (1972):8–54.

47. HOWELLS, J. G., and GUIRGUIS, W. R. "Childhood Schizophrenia 20 Years Later," *Archives of General Psychiatry,* 41 (1984):123–128.

48. JAMES, A. L., and BARRY, R. J. "Developmental Effects in the Cerebral Lateralization of Autistic, Retarded and Normal Children," *Journal of Autism and Developmental Disorders,* 13 (1983):43–56.

49. KANNER, L. "Autistic Disturbances of Affective Contact," *Nervous Child,* 2 (1943):217–250.

50. KINEGAN, J.-A., and QUARRINGTON, B. "Pre-, Peri-, and Neonatal Factors in Infantile Autism," *Journal of Child Psychology and Psychiatry,* 20 (1979):119–128.

51. KNOBLOCH, H., and PASAMANICK, B. "Some Etiologic and Prognostic Factors in Early Infantile Autism and Psychosis," *Pediatrics,* 55 (1975):182–191.

52. KOLVIN, I., OUNSTED, C., and ROTH, M. "Studies in the Childhood Psychoses: V. Cerebral Dysfunction and Childhood Psychoses," *British Journal of Psychiatry,* 118 (1971):407–414.

53. KOOTZ, J. P., MARINELLI, B., and COHEN, D. J. "Modulation of Response to Environmental Stimulation in Autistic Children," *Journal of Autism and Developmental Disorders,* 12 (1982):185–193.

54. KRUG, D. A., ARICK, J. R., and ALMOND, P. J. "Autism Screening Instrument for Educational Planning: Background and Development," in J. Gilliam, ed., *Autism: Diagnosis, Instruction, Management, and Research.* Austin: University of Texas at Austin Press, 1979, pp. 64–78.

55. KYDD, R. R., and WERRY, J. S. "Schizophrenia in Children Under 16 Years," *Journal of Autism and Developmental Disorders,* 12 (1982):343–357.

56. LOBASCHER, M. E., KINGERLEE, P. E., and GUBBAY, S. S. "Childhood Autism: An Investigation of Aetiological Factors in Twenty-Five Cases," *British Journal of Psychiatry,* 117 (1970):525–529.

57. LORD, C., SCHOPLER, E., and REVICKI, D. "Sex Differences in Autism," *Journal of Autism and Developmental Disorders,* 12 (1982):317–330.

58. McADOO, W. G., and DeMEYER, M. K. "Research Related to Family Factors in Autism," *Journal of Pediatric Psychology,* 2 (1978):162–166.

59. McCANN, B. S. "Hemispheric Asymmetries and Early Infantile Autism," *Journal of Autism and Developmental Disorders,* 11 (1981):401–411.

60. MALTZ, A. "Comparison of Cognitive Deficits Among Autistic and Retarded Children on the Arthur Adaptation of the Leiter International Performance Scales," *Journal of Autism and Developmental Disorders,* 11 (1981):413–426.

61. MARKOWITZ, P. I. "Autism in a Child with Congenital Cytomegalovirus Infection," *Journal of Autism and Developmental Disorders,* 13 (1983):249–253.

62. MASTERTON, B. A., and BIEDERMAN, G. B. "Proprioceptive Versus Visual Control in Autistic Children," *Journal of Autism and Developmental Disorders,* 13 (1983):141–152.

63. MAURER, R. G., and DAMASIO, A. R. "Vestibular Dysfunction in Autistic Children," *Developmental Medicine and Child Neurology,* 21 (1979):656–659.

64. ———. "Childhood Autism from the Point of View of

Behavioral Neurology," *Journal of Autism and Developmental Disorders,* 12 (1982):195–205.

65. MERYASH, D. L., SZYMANSKI, L. S., and GERALD, P. S. "Infantile Autism Associated with the Fragile-X Syndrome," *Journal of Autism and Developmental Disorders,* 12 (1982):295–301.

66. MINTON, J., et al. "Cognitive Assessment of Siblings of Autistic Children," *Journal of the American Academy of Child Psychiatry,* 21 (1982):256–261.

67. NIWA, S.-I., and OHTA, M. "P300 and Stimulus Evaluation Process in Autistic Subjects," *Journal of Autism and Developmental Disorders,* 13 (1983):33–42.

68. NOVICK, B., et al. "An Electrophysiologic Indication of Auditory Processing Defects in Autism," *Psychiatry Research,* 3 (1980):107–114.

69. ORNITZ, E. M., GUTHRIE, D., and FARLEY, A. H. "The Early Development of Autistic Children," *Journal of Autism and Childhood Schizophrenia,* 7 (1977):207–229.

70. PARKS, S. L. "The Assessment of Autistic Children: A Selective Review of Available Instruments," *Journal of Autism and Developmental Disorders,* 13 (1983):255–267.

71. PETTY, L. K., et al. "Autistic Children Who Become Schizophrenic," *Archives of General Psychiatry,* 41 (1984): 129–135.

72. RIGUET, C. B., et al. "Symbolic Play in Autistic, Down's, and Normal Children of Equivalent Mental Age," *Journal of Autism and Developmental Disorders,* 11 (1981): 439–448.

73. RIIKONEN, R., and AMNELL, G. "Psychiatric Disorders in Children with Earlier Infantile Spasms," *Developmental Medicine and Child Neurology,* 23 (1981):747–760.

74. RIMLAND, B. *Infantile Autism: The Syndrome and Its Implications for a Neural Theory of Behavior.* New York: Appleton-Centry-Crofts, 1964.

75. ROSENBLOOM, S., et al. "High Resolution CT Scanning in Infantile Autism: A Quantitative Approach," *Journal of the American Academy of Child Psychiatry,* 23 (1984):72–77.

76. RUTTENBERG, B. A., et al. "An Instrument for Evaluating Autistic Children," *Journal of the American Academy of Child Psychiatry,* 5 (1966):453–478.

77. RUTTENBERG, B. A., et al. *Behavior Rating Instrument for Autistic and Other Atypical Children,* rev. ed. Philadelphia: Developmental Center for Autistic Children, 1977.

78. RUTTER, M. "Childhood Schizophrenia Reconsidered," *Journal of Autism and Childhood Schizophrenia,* 2 (1972):315–337.

79. ———. "Cognitive Deficits in the Pathogenesis of Autism," *Journal of Child Psychology and Psychiatry,* 24 (1983): 513–531.

80. SCHOPLER, E., et al. "Toward Objective Classification of Childhood Autism: Childhood Autism Rating Scale (CARS)," *Journal of Autism and Developmental Disorders,* 10 (1980):91–103.

81. SCHULZ, S. C., et al. "Ventricular Enlargement in Teenage Patients with Schizophrenia Spectrum Disorder," *American Journal of Psychiatry,* 140 (1983):1592–1595.

82. SHAH, A., and FRITH, U. "An Islet of Ability in Autistic Children: A Research Note," *Journal of Child Psychology and Psychiatry,* 24 (1983):613–620.

83. SHAPIRO, T., and SHERMAN, M. "Long-term Follow-up of Children with Psychiatric Disorders," *Hospital and Community Psychiatry,* 34 (1983):522–527.

84. SKOFF, B. F., MIRSKY, A., and TURNER, D. "Prolonged Brainstem Transmission Time in Autism," *Psychiatric Research,* 2 (1980):157–166.

85. SMALL, J. G. "Psychiatric Disorders and EEG," in E. Niedermeyer and L. da Silva, eds., *Electroencephalography,*

Basic Principles, Clinical Applications and Related Fields. Baltimore: Urban and Schwarzenberg, 1982, pp. 439–459.

86. SOHMER, H., and STUDENT, M. "Evidence from Auditory Nerve and Brainstem Evoked Responses for an Organic Brain Lesion in Children with Autistic Traits," *Journal of Autism and Childhood Schizophrenia,* 8 (1978):13–20.

87. TAGER-FLUSBERG, H. "On the Nature of Linguistic Functioning in Early Infantile Autism," *Journal of Autism and Developmental Disorders,* 11 (1981):45–56.

88. TANGUAY, P. E., and EDWARDS, R. M. "Electrophysiological Studies of Autism: The Whisper of the Bang," *Journal of Autism and Developmental Disorders,* 12 (1982):177–184.

89. TANGUAY, P. E., et al. "Rapid Eye Movement (REM) Activity in Normal and Autistic Children During REM Sleep," *Journal of Autism and Childhood Schizophrenia,* 6 (1976):275–288.

90. TSAI, L., STEWART, M. A., and AUGUST, G. "Implication of Sex Differences in the Familial Transmission of Infantile Autism," *Journal of Autism and Developmental Disorders,* 11 (1981):165–173.

91. TSAI, L., et al. "Social Class Distribution of Fathers of Children Enrolled in the Iowa Autism Program," *Journal of Autism and Developmental Disorders,* 12 (1982):211–221.

92. WALKER, E. "Emotion Recognition in Disturbed and Normal Children: A Research Note," *Journal of Child Psychology and Psychiatry,* 22 (1981):263–268.

93. WEIZMAN, A., et al. "Abnormal Immune Response to Brain Tissue Antigen in the Syndrome of Autism," *American Journal of Psychiatry,* 139 (1982):1462–1465.

94. WING, L. "Childhood Autism and Social Class: A Question of Selection?" *British Journal of Psychiatry,* 137 (1980):410–417.

95. ———. "Language, Social, and Cognitive Impairments in Autism and Severe Mental Retardation," *Journal of Autism and Developmental Disorders,* 11 (1981):31–44.

96. ———. "Sex Ratios in Early Childhood Autism and Related Conditions," *Psychiatry Research,* 5 (1981):129–137.

97. WING, L., and GOULD, J. "Severe Impairments of Social Interaction and Associated Abnormalities in Children: Epidemiology and Classification," *Journal of Autism and Child Developmental Disorders,* 9 (1979):11–29.

98. WING, L., et al. "Symbolic Play in Severely Mentally Retarded and in Autistic Children," *Journal of Child Psychology and Psychiatry,* 18 (1977):167–178.

99. WOLCHIK, S. A. "Language Patterns of Parents of Young Autistic and Normal Children," *Journal of Autism and Developmental Disorders,* 13 (1983):167–180.

40 / An Overview of the Eating Disorders

L. K. George Hsu

It is safe to say that the eating disorders—anorexia nervosa and bulimia nervosa—are diseases of our times. This is an epoch in which improved health care and overall affluence have all but eliminated malnutrition and starvation in the developed countries; it is ironic that just at this time these disorders have emerged as public health hazards. Both are serious disorders and may lead to death; yet for the affected patients, who are usually young, attractive, and intelligent, at least in the early stages, they are ego syntonic. These intriguing conditions have stimulated a deluge of publications. This chapter reviews the recent developments in diagnosis, epidemiology, clinical features, and theories of etiology.

Diagnoses of Anorexia Nervosa and Bulimia Nervosa

The emergence of the eating disorders as diagnostic entities has been hampered by a lack of agreement or understanding among researchers as to their etiology, cardinal features, course, and outcome. Thus, for instance, many clinicians still regard anorexia nervosa as an appetite disorder, when in fact the anorectic patient's refusal to eat is certainly not related to a loss of appetite. Among other things it is due to a fear of weight gain and a need to maintain control and be slim. Many diagnostic issues remain unresolved and great gaps in our knowledge of the two disorders persist, but recent attempts, such as that by the American Psychiatric Association,[2] have produced succinct and useful definitions of the disorders, which are contrasted in table 40–1.

DIAGNOSIS OF ANOREXIA NERVOSA

Table 40–2 is a list of diagnostic criteria for anorexia nervosa that retains most of what is present in the DSM-III.[2]

The cardinal feature of anorexia nervosa is the relentless pursuit of thinness,[11] most commonly expressed by willful starvation and excessive exercising, less often by vomiting and laxative/diuretic abuse. Strictly speaking, anorexia nervosa is not really an eating disorder, because most patients will agree to eat

TABLE 40–1

Comparison of Anorexia Nervosa and Bulimia Nervosa

	Anorexia Nervosa		Bulimia Nervosa
	Restrictor Subgroup (60%)	Bulimic Subgroup (40%)	
Cardinal Features	Emaciation Drive for thinness Behavior directed to weight loss		Binge eating/ Vomiting/ Laxative abuse Fear of fatness
Weight	Low		Normal or overweight
Amenorrhea (Female)	Present		Variable
Binge eating	Absent	Present	Present
Vomiting/purging	Usually Absent	Present	Present

provided that eating is not accompanied by weight gain. For operational purposes the degree of weight loss necessary to qualify for a diagnosis of anorexia nervosa should be specified. Furthermore, simply relying on weight loss as a criterion may inadvertently define normal or overweight subjects as suffering from the syndrome (e.g., a premorbidly obese subject of 100 kg may have lost weight to 60 kg and thus qualify for the diagnosis even though she* is not emaciated) and thus destroy the classical image of the illness. A low body weight is thus proposed as an additional criterion. Less severe cases should not be excluded; to that end a staging of body weight is suggested. Disturbance of body image is an accepted diagnostic feature, but the concept is difficult to define.[74] Indeed, all the recent studies suggest that overestimation of body width is *not* a characteristic feature of the illness and should therefore be deleted from the symptom list.[43,74,148] Amenorrhea in females is a recognized feature of the disorder[129] and should be included. The distinction between the restrictor (or abstainer) and the bulimic (or vomiting) subgroups has been the subject of much recent research† and should therefore be drawn. Finally, concurrent or previous Axis I or II diagnoses should be specified if present.

DIAGNOSIS OF BULIMIA NERVOSA

The cardinal feature of bulimia (Greek for "ox appetite") is the presence of recurrent episodes of binge eating. When they occur, the episodes are of varying duration (from minutes to hours) and frequency (up to ten times a day). Initially the binge eating is almost always described as pleasurable and soothing, but there soon follow depression, guilt, and a fear of loss of control. A relatively normal body weight is maintained

*Females outnumber males by a ratio of 10 to 1 for the eating disorders. Hence, the feminine pronoun is used throughout this chapter.

†See references 5, 19, 44, 65, and 144.

by self-induced vomiting, laxative/diuretic abuse, prolonged fasting, or excessive exercising. A fear of fatness is always present particularly after a binge, but bulimic patients do not seem to be striving for an unrealistically low weight. No clear demarcation exists between bulimia as defined in DSM-III and eating binges[126] or great variations in dietary intake.[95] Binge eating[145] occurs in nearly half of all anorexia nervosa patients[19,77,125] and in 30 percent of obese subjects who seek treatment.[55] Binges also occur sporadically in many normal-weight subjects, particularly in those dieting to control weight.[68,101,154] Thus, in order to define bulimia as a syndrome, it is necessary to distinguish it from anorexia nervosa with bulimic features on the one hand and from milder forms of binge eating on the other. The term bulimia nervosa has therefore been proposed for a diagnosable, severe form of the disorder and will be so used in this chapter. (See table 40–3.)[131]

Debate continues on whether the two eating disorders are separate, dichotomous syndromes.[1,6,118,131] Existing evidence suggests that the consistency of asso-

TABLE 40–2

Diagnostic Criteria for Anorexia Nervosa

A. Intense fear of becoming obese, which does not diminish as weight loss progresses.
B. Emaciation as a result of weight loss of at least 15 percent of original body weight.
   1. Grade 1: Body weight less than 85 percent of average weight for height.
   2. Grade 2: Body weight less than 75 percent of average weight for height.
C. Behavior directed toward weight loss.
D. Amenorrhea in the female.
E. Subgroup:
   1. Bulimic: Presence of bulimic episodes.
   2. Restrictor: Absence of bulimic episodes.
F. No known physical illness that could account for the weight loss and emaciation.

TABLE 40–3

Diagnostic Criteria for Bulimia Nervosa

A. Recurrent episodes of binge eating (rapid consumption of a large amount of food in a discrete period of time, usually less than two hours), frequency of at least once a week over the previous four weeks.

B. Awareness that the eating pattern is abnormal and fear of not being able to stop eating voluntarily once the binge eating begins.

C. Intense fear of fatness, depressed mood, and self-deprecatory thoughts following eating binges.

D. Termination of binge eating episodes by self-induced vomiting or use of cathartics.

E. Repeated attempts to lose weight by severe dieting, self-induced vomiting, or use of cathartics or diuretics.

F. The bulimic episodes are not related to a concurrent anorexia nervosa or any known physical disorder.

ciation of the cardinal features and the course and outcome of the two disorders form relatively distinct aggregates. Thus, from an operational and treatment point of view, it is best at this stage to regard them as separate conditions.

These classifications and criteria use body weight as the feature that distinguishes between the two eating disorders. More recently, researchers have suggested that bulimic behavior may be of greater diagnostic, prognostic, and etiological significance than low body weight. For example, the bulimic patients, whether of normal or low body weight, more often are emotionally labile and impulsive and more likely to be premorbidly obese.* They are more likely also to have a family history of obesity, alcoholism, and depression.[81,125,144] However, at this stage it seems premature to abandon the previous classification as so many issues remain unresolved.[50]

Epidemiology of the Eating Disorders

How common is anorexia nervosa? The answer to the question depends on how the condition is defined and what population is being studied. According to the best estimate, in the 1970s in southern England one in one hundred private school girls age sixteen and over[28] and one in two hundred college women were affected.[16] There is no reason to suppose that the prevalence in the

*See references 5, 19, 24, 44, 50, 85, 125, and 144.

United States is any lower.[123] In general, females outnumber males by about ten to one.[24,42,87] The syndrome is more common in the middle and upper classes[28,87,92,147] and in those who must strive to maintain a thin body shape[31,41,48,161] such as athletes, ballerinas, and models. It appears to be uncommon among the blacks in this country,[87,92] and the disorder is rare in developing countries.[15]

Bulimia nervosa appears to be more common than anorexia nervosa. According to two questionnaire surveys, between 4.5 and 19 percent of college females and 0.4 and 5 percent of college males in this country met criteria for bulimia.[66,126] Pope, Hudson, and Yurgelun-Todd[123] surveyed three hundred women by questionnaire at a suburban shopping mall and found that 10.3 percent reported a lifetime history of bulimia diagnosable by DSM-III criteria; at the time of the survey half of them reported that they were still actively bulimic. Three percent of women attending a family planning clinic in England[22] and 4 percent of students attending a university psychiatric clinic in this country[140] fulfilled the criteria for bulimia. It seems safe to assume, therefore, that bulimia is probably four to five times more common than is anorexia nervosa. Like anorexia nervosa, it also affects more females than males.[65,126]

The incidence of eating disorders appears to be increasing. Case register and hospital record studies in the United States and in Switzerland have reported a two- to three-fold increase in the incidence of anorexia nervosa between the early 1960s and the mid-1970s.[87,158] This confirmed a continuing trend reported by other earlier studies.[92,147] Crisp, Palmer, and Kalucy[28] surveyed nine school populations in southwest London. Relying on teacher's reports, medical records, and personal interviews, they also reported an increase in the incidence of anorexia nervosa.

Direct evidence to support the increase in incidence of bulimia nervosa is lacking. However, Pope, Hudson, and Yurgelun-Todd[123] estimated that 2.2 million American women probably have a lifetime history of bulimia (narrowly defined as binge eating weekly and vomiting or purging). Such evidence as does exist supports their estimate and suggests that bulimia is a major public health problem.

Clinical Features of the Eating Disorders

A description of the clinical features of anorexia nervosa can be found in volume 2 of the *Basic Handbook of Child Psychiatry*[136] and in several review articles[29,64,108]and monographs.[13,24,42] This section therefore is devoted to an account of the clinical features of bulimia nervosa.

All patients with bulimia nervosa report that they feel too fat and that they are dieting. In about 40 percent of bulimic persons, the dieting led at first to anorexia nervosa, which then gave way to the full range of bulimic symptoms. [34,94,131] Following the prolonged dieting, an experience of intense hunger ensues along with a craving for high-carbohydrate ("junk") food. Presently the temptation to eat becomes overwhelming. After the first bite is taken, a feeling of abandon, even liberation, follows, and the patient gives herself over to the binge. This in turn may last from several minutes to two hours and may recur several times a day; ultimately it is terminated by a sense of intolerable fullness and guilt. Several thousand calories may be consumed in one single binge. The fear of fatness and the guilt over the loss of control thereupon usually leads to self-induced vomiting, or the patient may take large amounts of laxatives and diuretics to dispose of the calories. A new resolve to "start over" usually follows, and a state of rigid dieting (sometimes with the aid of diet pills) returns until the next binge.

Many bulimic individuals will admit that before the fullness and the guilt set in, a binge is pleasurable, soothing, and comforting. The sense of oblivion, abandon, and liberation may reinforce it. Bulimic patients are thus caught between two opposing desires, a drive for thinness and rigid control versus an urge to eat as much as they want and to be free from constraints. For a while, the rigid dieting during the day fulfills their desire to be slim and to gain control, while the evening binge satisfies the craving for forbidden foods and bestows a sense of liberation. The vomiting or laxative or diuretic abuse is an inconvenience, but it is experienced as necessary if the price of weight gain is to be avoided. In time, the binge eating and vomiting become coping mechanisms, ways of adapting to life situations. The bulimic behavior may serve as an escape when the patients are depressed, angry, tense, anxious, frustrated, or under stress, or as a means of celebration when they are happy. It may even become a punishment they visit on significant others or a way they use to manipulate them. When the bulimia cycle becomes entrenched, life for the bulimic is the cycle.

Many bulimic patients are able to function well in their daily life, particularly in the realm of work. [85] However, when asked specifically about such symptoms as anxiety or depression in conjunction with their eating disturbance, they usually report significant dysphoria, emotional lability, intolerance to stress, and undue sensitivity in interpersonal situations. [36,85,86,125] Two questionnaire surveys [36,85] found many bulimic individuals to experience suicide ideation frequently. On direct interview, Hudson, Laffer, and Pope [80] found almost half of their patients to fulfill DSM-III criteria for major depression. Poor impulse control, as expressed by alcohol/substance abuse and kleptomania, has been documented also by many researchers.* In my experience, some 10 percent of bulimic patients fulfilled DSM-III criteria for borderline personality disorder. The relationship of bulimia nervosa to affective disorder and borderline personality disorder is currently the subject of investigation.

Relationship Between Eating Disorders and Other Psychiatric Disturbances

In particular, the relationship between affective illness and eating disorders has begun to receive considerable attention. Various authors have stated that the eating disorders perhaps are variants of affective disorders. [18,70,80] The evidence for this contention from a family history perspective is discussed later.

Both anorectic and bulimic patients sometimes are quite depressed, and suicide and attempted suicide occur commonly. However, both clinical impression and standardized interviews suggest that the depression associated with the eating disorders is usually not as severe or as persistent as it is in major depression.† In fact, eating-disorder patients usually complain of mood changes that parallel changes in the acceptance of their weight and shape or in their control over their eating behavior. Psychometric testings confirm such clinical findings. [76,144]

Biological marker studies have yielded inconclusive findings. High plasma cortisol level, dexamethasone nonsuppression, and low urinary 3-methoxy-4-hydroxy-phenylglycol (MHPG) occur in both anorectic and affective disorder patients, [152] but in anorectic patients these changes are reversible with weight gain. The characteristic sleep electroencephalogram (EEG) changes in anorexia nervosa [109] resemble those that occur in patients with chronic medical illnesses more so than those in patients with primary affective disorder.

Long-term follow-up studies of anorexia nervosa suggest that the disorder tends to "breed true"; in those who fail to recover, the core symptoms seem to remain stable over time. [73] While depression is common at follow-up, it is usually overshadowed by the more prominent anorectic features. No long-term outcome studies for bulimia nervosa are available, and it is not clear whether or not bulimia nervosa may change over time into major depression. The usefulness of anti-

*See references 19, 29, 42, 85, 125, and 144.
†See references 4, 33, 42, 85, and 131.

depressants in anorexia nervosa is controversial[42]; in bulimia, however, the evidence for the efficacy of antidepressants is stronger. [124] However, it would be fallacious to argue that bulimia is related to major depression on the basis of its response to medications that have been designated as antidepressants. [22]

In sum, the existing evidence does not support the view that the eating disorders are variants of affective illness, but it does seems to suggest that a family history of depression and a state of depression may predispose an individual to develop an eating disorder. [22,42,79]

Atypical psychosis with prominent affective features sometimes develops in eating-disorder patients and seems to run an independent course. [61,78] Certain borderline personality symptoms such as affective instability, impulsivity, physical self-damaging acts, chronic feelings of emptiness and boredom, and identity disturbance are seen in some bulimic patients; others manifest symptoms of other impulse control disorders such as alcoholism, substance abuse, and kleptomania. [42,143] Social phobia is common in bulimic patients whereas obsessive-compulsive features are more common in the abstaining anorectic patients. As a rule, however, these features are overshadowed by the more prominent anorectic and bulimic behaviors.

Endocrine Disturbances in the Eating Disorders

A number of detailed reviews of endocrine disturbances in anorexia nervosa have appeared recently.* The endocrine findings most often have been compared to those of subjects with starvation due to other causes and to data arising from patients with major depression. It must be stated at the outset that the endocrine changes in anorexia nervosa are largely (but not entirely) a product of the starvation state and low body weight of the patient. Discrepancies in findings sometimes occur, but they are probably related to differences in subject selection in respect to such factors as duration of illness, severity of weight loss, and whether or not the patients are bingeing and vomiting. The following sections summarize the endocrine changes in anorexia nervosa and what little is known about the changes in bulimia.

THE HYPOTHALAMIC-PITUITARY-ADRENAL AXIS

Plasma cortisol levels are increased in anorexia nervosa, and the normal diurnal excursions in the pattern

*See references 42, 63, 83, 152, and 155.

of cortisol levels is flattened. Dexamethasone nonsuppression occurs both in anorexia nervosa and bulimia nervosa. These changes are due in part to an increased half-life of cortisol, which occurs also in starvation from other causes, and in part to increased activation of the hypothalamic-pituitary-adrenal (HPA) axis which occurs also in major depression (although not in other starvation states). The increased half-life of cortisol can be corrected by administration of triiodothyronine (T_3), which is low in both anorexia nervosa and in starvation from other causes. With even a small amount of weight gain, the HPA activation in anorexia nervosa usually reverts to normal. In sum, it seems that the HPA disturbances in anorexia nervosa resemble those found in starvation as well as those found in major depressive illness.

THE HYPOTHALAMIC-PITUITARY-THYROID AXIS

Normal or low normal thyroxine (T_4) levels and low T_3 levels occur in anorexia nervosa. The decrease in T_3 is associated with an increase in the inactive, reverse form of T_3. Thyrotropin levels and thyrotropin response to thyrotropin-releasing hormone (TRH) appear to be normal and different from those that occur in major depression. These findings are similar to those that occur in euthymic patients with a variety of chronic illnesses; in anorexia nervosa they are likely to represent an adaptation to starvation.

HYPOTHALAMIC-PITUITARY-OVARIAN AXIS

Low plasma estradiol and serum gonadotropins and prepubertal circadian patterns of luteinizing hormone (LH) and follicle-stimulating hormone (FSH) occur in anorexia nervosa. These changes may be ascribed to a reversion of hypothalamic-pituitary-ovarian (HPO) activity to prepubertal or pubertal functioning. The mechanism of the initiation of this reversion is unknown. Loss of body weight and fat, malnutrition, and increased physical activity do not fully explain the changes as some of them also occur in normal-weight bulimic patients. In states of malnutrition, estradiol is metabolized more to 2-hydroxy estrone (at the expense of estriol), a substance with antiestrogen properties. This may explain how changes in HPO activity are sustained once the weight loss has begun. Recovery of body weight alone does not always normalize HPO activity, and it is generally agreed that symptom remission (e.g., overcoming the fatness phobia and chaotic eating) is necessary also for functional recovery of the HPO.

Release of LH and FSH from the anterior pituitary by luteinizing hormone-releasing hormone (LHRH) usually is impaired in anorexia nervosa if the LHRH is injected as a bolus of 50 or 100 mcg. However, if the LHRH is pulsed rather than injected as a bolus, no defect in LH or FSH release occurs even at low body weight. In any case, both LH and FSH release tend to normalize with weight gain.

GROWTH HORMONE AND PROLACTIN

Resting growth hormone (GH) levels are elevated in anorexia nervosa. This seems to be secondary to the starvation state, and even before any substantial weight gain occurs, normal levels appear with increased caloric intake. GH responses to provocative tests such as the use of glucose loading, bromocriptine mesylate, and TRH have been reported as impaired. This suggests a disturbance in the control mechanisms, but such disturbances are usually reversible with weight gain. The normal rise in GH during sleep is apparently retained in anorexia nervosa.

Hyperprolactinemia is associated with amenorrhoea; in anorexia nervosa, however, prolactin levels are usually normal. Nocturnal prolactin levels are low and prolactin response to TRH is impaired in anorexia nervosa, but again these changes are usually reversible with weight gain.

ARGININE VASOPRESSIN AND CEREBRAL SPINAL FLUID OPIOID ACTIVITY

Defects in urinary concentration or dilution suggestive of abnormal secretion of the antidiuretic hormone arginine vasopressin have repeatedly been demonstrated in anorexia nervosa. Such defects are related either to a simple deficiency of vasopressin secretion or, more commonly, to erratic fluctuations in plasma levels of the hormone that bear no apparent relation to changes in plasma levels of sodium.[53] Furthermore, the average concentration of arginine vasopressin in the cerebral spinal fluid (CSF) of anorectic patients varies much more from the mean than it does in normal subjects; indeed, the normal CSF/plasma ratio of arginine vasopressin is reversed. This abnormal osmoregulation of arginine vasopressin is not immediately corrected by improvement of weight and nutritional status, but, after a few months with normal weight maintenance, it does revert to normal. The significance of these changes is unclear. They may reflect alterations in catecholamine metabolism or they may be due to the fact that the patients are inducing vomiting.[42]

Higher levels of CSF opioid activity have been reported to occur in severely underweight anorectic patients.[91] In animal studies opioid agonists seem to stimulate eating and the opioid system seems to play an important role in stress response. At present these findings must be regarded as preliminary.

Metabolic Disturbances in the Eating Disorders

Most of the metabolic changes in anorexia nervosa are due to the starvation; in bulimia nervosa, they tend to occur as a result of the vomiting/purging/diuretic abuse.[42,63] Leukopenia, relative lymphocytosis, mild subclinical iron and folic acid deficiency, and bone marrow abnormalities in the form of hypocellularity with the presence of large amounts of gelatinous acid mucopolysaccharide are all found to occur, but they are reversible with improved nutritional status and weight gain. Similarly, in anorexia nervosa low erythrocyte sedimentation rates and plasma fibrinogen levels return to normal with clinical improvement. Hypercarotenemia and hypercholesterolemia are sometimes found; they too may be related to the starvation state and excessive intake of vegetables and cheese. Abnormal glucose tolerance involving insulin resistance may ensue as a result of the starvation state; such an abnormality, however, may persist after full recovery of weight.[28,42,150] The reduced basal temperature and abnormal thermoregulation in anorexia nervosa apparently are reversible with weight gain.

Defective antidiuretic hormone (ADH) regulation occurs in anorexia nervosa,[50] and such abnormalities in water conservation are closely linked with those in thermoregulation. Such changes occur also in individuals with simple weight loss without anorexia nervosa.[149]

Etiology of the Eating Disorders

There are currently six main theories organized within different conceptual frameworks that attempt to explain the etiology of anorexia nervosa. Some aspects of these theories apply also to bulimia nervosa. Logically, they are not mutually exclusive, and to some degree they do overlap.

THE SOCIAL-CULTURAL THEORY

As already mentioned in the section on epidemiology, social-cultural factors appear to be involved in the development of the eating disorders. Evidence will be summarized according to the current emphasis on slimness, the contradictory role of women in modern society, and the vulnerability of the adolescent female.

The importance of physical attractiveness in western society is undeniable. In the female this attractiveness involves a dimension of slimness. Several surveys indicate that the majority of young women are unhappy about their weight and want to be slimmer.[17,82,114] In contrast, men prefer to be bigger and heavier.[17,82,114] Garner and Garfinkel,[48] reviewing data from *Playboy* centerfolds and Miss America Pageant contestants in the last twenty years, found a significant trend towards slimness. Except for height and waist, all measurements of *Playboy* centerfold girls decreased significantly. Thus, for instance, the average Playmate in 1959 weighed 91 percent of average, while in 1978 she weighed only 83.5 percent of average. Since 1970, the winners of the Miss America Pageant had a mean weight of only 82.5 percent of average and weighed significantly less than the average contestant. Meanwhile, over the last twenty years the number of diet articles in six women's magazines has increased substantially. However, this emphasis on thinness and dieting is occurring in a population that is becoming heavier.[48] Over the last twenty years weight statistics from the Society of Actuaries indicate an increase in average weight for all women below the age of thirty years. It is possible that such pressure on women to diet and appear slim, particularly in those of the upper social class,[54,67] may precipitate the development of anorexia nervosa. This is supported by the finding that the condition is much more common in women such as ballerinas, modeling students, and athletes, who must control their size and shape rigorously.[31,41,48] Under such circumstances it is perhaps not surprising that Branch and Eurman[8] found that the anorectic patient's friends and relatives actually admire her slimness, specialness, and control.

Boskind-Lodahl and White[6] regarded the "cultural heritage of sexual inequality" to be directly responsible for the development of eating disorders in women. However, since such inequality presumably exists also in developing countries, it is difficult to see why the disorder is so rare there.[15] Selvini Palazzoli[116,117] emphasized the complex and contradictory roles women have to play in modern society. Self-definition and achieving a feminine identity may be particularly problematic for the modern female.[102,115] High-achieving women may experience lower self-esteem[102] and a heightened fear of success that revolve around fear of loss of femininity and of interpersonal rejection.[71,115] Many college women have reported difficulty in integrating "masculine" ideals such as independence and assertiveness with traditional concepts of feminin-

ity.[32] Such role diffusion and insecurity presumably intensify the striving for perfection and control.

The dilemma confronting the modern female may explain why adolescence tends to be a particularly difficult phase for the white girl who is likely to have a poor self-image, great self-consciousness, low self-esteem, and a high level of instability.[134] The Ten State Nutrition Survey,[45,46] which in 1968 to 1970 studied over 40,000 individuals from all age groups with respect to their nutritional status, has provided also a good deal of insight into why the current cultural emphasis on slimness has hit the middle- and upper-class white adolescent females the hardest. The survey findings may be summarized as follows:

1. There is a tendency at all ages for the female to be fatter (as measured by triceps fatfold) than the male.
2. A prepubertal fat gain occurs in both sexes, but during adolescence proper, the female gains fat while the male loses fat.
3. Higher income is associated with greater fatness for males at all ages and for females through early adolescence. In the female, however, there is an income-related reversal of relative fatness during adolescence—that is, during adolescence females in lower-income families started out being leaner but ended up being fatter than those in higher-income families. Garn and Clark[45,46] speculated that this reversal occurs as a result of conscious dieting on the part of the higher-income females.
4. White males tend to be fatter than black males at all ages. White females are also fatter than black females through early adolescence, but thereafter a reversal of relative fatness occurs similar to that for higher- and lower-income females. This differential fatness pattern between the two races remains even after controlling for family income. Garn and Clark[45,46] again speculated that this reversal occurred as a result of conscious dieting on the part of the white female.

These findings suggest that fatness is related to being female, white, and from a high-income family. It is obvious that the cultural emphasis on thinness has its most powerful impact on the white teenage girl from a higher-income family.

That such social-cultural pressure generates a greater likelihood for the development of anorexia nervosa and bulimia in women is probably not in dispute. It is obvious, however, that not all women exposed to such pressure develop an eating disorder. Other factors must occur also to precipitate the final development of the illness.

FAMILY PATHOLOGY THEORY

Early investigators all emphasized the role of family pathology in anorexia nervosa.[20,62,96] Charcot[20] advocated separation of the patient from the family as part of treatment. Gull[62] found relatives to be the worst attendants to the patient. Laseque[96] described the striking degree of family enmeshment, and he urged clinicians not to overlook the family pathology. Other early investigators likewise have described the adverse influence of the family on the patient.[30,162]

Attempts to identify a typical anorectic mother[21,90,93,110] or a typical anorectic father[58,93,110,137] have produced no consistent findings.[27,88] This may be related, at least in part, to methodological shortcomings such as inadequately defined terms and non-standardized observational methods. More recently, Bruch[13,14] emphasized the façade of happiness and stability that hid deep disillusionment and secret competition of the parents. Also, she found the parents to be enormously preoccupied with outward appearance and success. Palazzoli[116] found certain characteristics to be present in anorectic families: rejection of communicated messages, poor conflict resolution, covert alliance of family members, blame shifting, and rigidity. Both Palazzoli and Bruch found the parents to be overprotective but also to involve the sick child in their covert competition and conflict. They seemed to use the child to discharge some of their own unfulfilled longings. Minuchin and his coworkers[105,106,107] advocated an open systems model for psychosomatic illness, including anorexia nervosa. This system included such elements as extrafamilial stress, family organization and functioning, the vulnerable child, physiological and biochemical mediating mechanisms, and the symptomatic child. The system could be activated at any point and the parts could affect each other, but these authors have emphasized the family pathology element almost exclusively. They hypothesized that certain family characteristics were related to the development and maintenance of psychosomatic symptoms in children and that the child's psychosomatic symptoms played a major role in maintaining family homeostasis. The family characteristics identified by Minuchin and his colleagues were enmeshment, overprotectiveness, rigidity, and lack of conflict resolution. Meanwhile, the child was used to maintain stability and avoid open conflict, and thus was often caught (triangulated) in the parents' covert conflict. The illness enabled the parents to submerge their conflicts in favor of protecting or blaming the sick child, who was then defined as the sole family problem.

However, few studies exist to confirm that such family interaction pathology occurs in anorexia nervosa, or that such pathology is causally related to the development of the disorder. Crisp, Harding, and McGuinness[26] found that the psychoneurotic status of the parents worsened significantly as the patient's weight increased with treatment. This was particularly so if the marital relationship was poor. Increased parental psychoneurotic morbidity was associated with a poor six-month outcome for the illness. However, several important factors, including case selection, family therapy effects, and parental anxiety over the patient's impending discharge, were uncontrolled. Foster and Kupfer[38] telemetrically recorded the nocturnal motility of a patient with anorexia nervosa; they found that her nocturnal "arousal" was correlated with visits by specific family members, such as her twin sister and her mother, during the previous day. The extent to which such findings can be generalized, however, is questionable. Strober[143] found higher marital discord among the parents of the bulimic anorectic patients when compared with restrictor anorectics, but Yager[162] found great diversity in the family interaction pattern of the eating-disordered patients.

One issue that is related to family environment is the role of *genetic factors* in the pathogenesis of anorexia nervosa. Several large-scale studies have found an increased incidence of the condition in the family members of the patients.[27,67,108,147] Twin studies[3,42,79] have yielded a concordance of about 50 percent for monozygotic and 10 percent for dizygotic twins. Adoptive studies, however, are needed to tease out environmental from genetic factors. In this connection, Crisp and Toms[25] described a remarkable case of a male chronic anorectic whose adoptive son as well as the girl who stayed with the family as a war evacuee both developed anorexia nervosa.

Crisp and his coworkers have suggested that family weight pathology may be specifically related to the pathogenesis of the illness.[23,88] In a well-controlled study of the parents of anorectic patients, Halmi, Struss, and Goldberg[67] failed to confirm this.

Several detailed studies of psychiatric disorders in the families of eating-disordered patients have been published recently. Strober and coworkers[144] compared the relatives of bulimic patients with those of restrictor anorectics; they found that the fathers of bulimic patients were more impulsive, less tolerant of frustration, and more dissatisfied with family relations, while the mothers of bulimic patients were more depressed and hostile. The presence of more severe paternal and maternal depression and paternal impulsivity was predictive of greater severity in the patients' bulimic states. On psychiatric interview, affective disorders, alcoholism, and substance abuse disorders were more prevalent among the first- and second-degree relatives of bulimic patients. In a study of 420 first-degree relatives of 89 eating-disordered patients, Hudson and associates[81] found an increased risk of affective disorder among the first-degree relatives of both anorectic and bulimic patients. In fact, the risk achieved a level similar to that of the families of bipolar disordered patients. Winokur, March, and Mendels[160] found that in comparison with a control group, there was a doubling of affective illness in the parents of anorectic patients. Thus familial prevalence of affective illness and perhaps of alcoholism as well appears to be increased in the eating-disordered patients.

In sum, it remains to be substantiated that specific abnormal family interaction patterns occur in anorexia nervosa and that they are causally related to the development of the condition. Most of the studies quoted ignored the effect of this exasperating illness on family interaction and thus failed to distinguish between family pathology occurring as stress reactions as opposed to preexisting patterns.[162] The need for well-controlled direct observation studies of family interaction and anorexia nervosa is obvious. The role of family interaction in the pathogenesis of bulimia nervosa has not been clearly formulated. Familial affective disorder and perhaps alcoholism and other impulse control disorders may predispose an individual to develop an eating disorder.[22,79,144]

INDIVIDUAL PSYCHODYNAMIC THEORY

Earlier psychoanalytic interpretation of anorexia nervosa considered it to be related to a rejection of female genital sexuality and oral impregnation fantasies by means of starvation. This was accompanied by a regression to pregenital defense mechanisms in the face of conflict around primitive sadistic and cannibalistic oral fantasies.[37,84,139,151] Object-relation theorists considered it to be related to the introjection (and repression) of a bad object consequent upon the early ambivalent relationship with an aggressively overprotective and unresponsive,[116] or an aggressive and castrating,[146] or a domineering and controlling[136] mother. On a more superficial level, it is generally recognized that starvation serves as an expression of hostility, control, and aggression toward the family.[146,151] Psychoanalytic explanations of bulimia nervosa consist mainly of comments within the interpretations for anorexia nervosa.[72,104,112] Among other possibilities, bulimia is considered to be related to a less rigid character structure,[104] a desperate acting out after failure to remain in control,[112] or else a desire for pregnancy.[98] The lack of specificity in such interpretations limits their usefulness. Both Bruch[12] and Palazzoli[116] have found the psychoanalytic approach to be relatively ineffective.

In 1931 Langdon Brown[10] observed that anorexia nervosa was a pathological manifestation of the detachment of the growing individual from parental authority. Bruch[11,12,13,14] repeatedly has stated that anorexia nervosa is a struggle for a self-respecting identity. That such a struggle took the form of willful starvation suggested serious psychological developmental defects. Central to such defects was the failure of the parents

to regard the patients as individuals in their own right; they failed to transmit a sense of competence and self-value to their children. The youngsters were treated instead as something to complement the parents' needs and their sense of worth, and value was to be derived from being needed by each parent. In short, the children were made to feel that they were their parents' property. The illness in turn represented the children's effort to escape from this role and to establish a modicum of control. Their disturbed perception of bodily sensation is related to their lack of autonomy along with a paralyzing sense of ineffectiveness. As a result, such patients misinterpreted their biological functioning and social role, and came to regard thinness and starvation as evidence of specialness and self-control in an exaggerated and concrete way. Palazzoli[116] and Boskind-Lodahl and White[6] echoed such views. Neither Bruch nor Palazzoli offered any detailed explanation for the dynamics of bulimia nervosa.

The individual psychodynamic theory is plausible except that it has never been empirically tested; its emphasis on early parent-child interaction does not lend itself easily to such testing. A recent single case study[127] provided some evidence of abnormal mothering in a case of male anorexia nervosa.

THE DEVELOPMENTAL PSYCHOBIOLOGICAL THEORY

Brown[10] stated that a fear of growing up and assuming adult responsibility was highly characteristic of anorectic patients. Crisp[23,24,26] repeatedly has commented that anorexia nervosa was rooted in the biological and consequently experiential aspects of normal adult weight. Starvation in anorectic patients represented a phobic avoidance of adolescent/adult weight. Anorexia nervosa was thus a disorder of weight pivoting around the specific maturational changes of puberty, both biological and psychological. The psychobiological regression reflected the patients' need to avoid adolescent and related family turmoil. The severe dieting was reinforced by the relief that arose from the sense of control and the low weight; this was further intensified as biological and related psychological childhood was reexperienced and postpubertal experience was concurrently eliminated. Meanwhile, the children's advance into adolescence threatened the rigid and experience-denying parents. Thus the illness could sometimes serve to avert a rekindling of buried and denied but unresolved parental conflicts and psychopathology. Needless to say, the illness brought its own problems in its train, but they were deemed to be the price that patients and their families had to pay in order to avoid deeper and more fundamental discord. Crisp has emphasized repeatedly that the maturational demands of adolescence and the presence of family pathology were not specific to the condition. Indirect and partial support for this view has come from several sources. For one thing, the immature pattern of gonadotropin release in anorectic patients, which reverts to normal after weight gain,[7,89] may be construed as evidence for the biological regression in anorexia nervosa. Second, Frisch[39,40] has found that puberty hinges on the individual attaining a critical amount of fatness. And third, clinical experience suggests that anorectic patients will often agree to eat provided that weight gain does not occur, thereby indicating that weight rather than eating is involved in the issue of control. Nevertheless, this theory of "weight phobia" has never been empirically tested. One study found anorexia nervosa patients to be different from other phobic patients in terms of skin conductance changes.[132]

COGNITIVE-BEHAVIORAL THEORY

The cognitive-behavioral theory of the etiology of anorexia nervosa emphasizes cognitions and behaviors rather than early childhood experience, family interaction, or biological processes.[42,47] However, it does draw on individual psychodynamic and psychobiological concepts. Garner and Bemis[47] and Garfinkel and Garner[42] have set out their views systematically on this point. As they see it, anorexia nervosa is the final common pathway of a multiply determined pathogenetic sequence. The starting point, however, occurs with introverted, sensitive, and isolated adolescents arriving at the idea that weight loss will somehow alleviate their distress and dysphoria. The dieting that ensues is a means to achieve slimness as well as an expression of ascetic control. It is soon reinforced by a gratifying sense of success, approval, and concern from others. The negative reinforcement of avoiding food and weight gain gradually becomes more prominent, and the increasing isolation, which occurs as a result of starvation, decreases the patients' responsiveness to other issues and considerations. Progressive weight loss secures a "safety margin,"[24] and the complex of anorectic cognitions and behaviors become autonomous. This theory is intuitively familiar and consistent with the patients' own reports. However, the more crucial questions may be why more dieters do not move toward this final common pathway and what distinguishes between a "normal dieter" and a committed anorectic. Garner, Garfinkel, and O'Shaughnessy[49] recently provided some evidence to suggest that anorectic individuals, compared to "normal dieters," may be interpersonally less effective, more distrustful, and more lacking in interoceptive awareness.

Cognitive-behavioral explanations for bulimia nervosa have been set forth systematically by several researchers.[34,100,135] They have incorporated a functional analysis of cognitions and behaviors involved in the binge-purge process. Antecedents for a binge include prolonged dieting leading to feelings of hunger and deprivation, and negative feeling states such as depression, a sense of failure, self-critical thoughts, anxiety, or frustration in relation to outside stress for which the subject has limited coping skills. Other investigators have emphasized the importance of "restraint" as an antecedent. Restrained eaters are found to increase their intake when made to feel anxious,[69] when distressed,[120] when consuming alcohol,[121] or after they believe that they have broken their diet and failed.[100,119,138] Boskind-Lodahl and White[6,157] hypothesized that the bingeing provides the bulimic individual with a release from tensions and dilemmas, and that such tensions and dilemmas are directly related to strivings to achieve an exaggerated ideal of femininity and acceptance from men. Food represents the only area of their life where they can indulge excessively without fear of disapproval or reprisal, at least for the moment.

Again, such explanations make intuitive sense and are consistent with the patients' own description of the process. But again, not all dieters or anorectics become bulimics. The cognitive-behavioral theory may explain how the bulimic process perpetuates itself, but it does not really convey why some dieters or anorectics develop it and others do not.

BIOLOGICAL THEORIES

Russell[128,129,130] has suggested repeatedly that a primary hypothalamic dysfunction of unknown etiology occurs in anorexia nervosa, one that is only partially dependent on weight loss and psychopathology. Early onset of amenorrhea, the incomplete recovery of hypothalamic function, and the persistence of amenorrhea despite weight gain have been cited as evidence for a primary hypothalamic disorder.[89,130] Furthermore, several reports of hypothalamic tumor presenting as anorexia nervosa have appeared.[42,103] Finally, in animals the role of the ventromedial hypothalamic nucleus in the regulation of feeding and satiety appears to be well established.[97]

However, the significance of all these findings remains controversial. An accurate dietary history is difficult to obtain in most eating-disordered patients, and amenorrhea preceding the onset of eating disturbance probably occurs in only a small proportion of patients. Emotional disturbance, not specifically related to anorexia nervosa, may cause amenorrhea. The incomplete recovery of hypothalamic function may be related to inadequate weight gain,[149] abnormal eating habits, or the simple fact that recovery may take time. The eating disorder that occurs in association with a hypothalamic tumor often has atypical features. Since the vast majority of anorectic patients have no demonstrable anatomical hypothalamic pathology, in those cases where typical "anorectic" features occur in association with demonstrable hypothalamic pathology it remains possible that this infrequent association is entirely due to chance. Thus the evidence for a primary hypothalamic disturbance in anorexia nervosa is far from compelling.

The noradrenergic system in the medial hypothalamus in rats seems to regulate intake and body weight directly.[97] Thus, for instance, norepinephrine (NE) injected into the medial hypothalamus of the satiated rat in physiological doses elicits an eating response, increases its preference for carbohydrates, and increases its meal size, meal duration, and rate of eating; while chronic infusion of NE into the medial hypothalamus stimulates food intake and body weight gain. Medial hypothalamic injection of the alpha-adrenegeric agonist clonidine hydrochloride and certain tricyclic antidepressants such as desipramine hydrochloride also induce an eating response in the satiated rat. Conversely, a decrese of noradrenergic innervation to the paraventricular hypothalamus leads to a decrease of daily intake and body weight and a selective decline in carbohydrate ingestion. Food deprivation, which stimulates intake and carbohydrate preference in the animal, increases the turnover rate of endogenous NE in the medial hypothalamus. Extrapolating animal data to human psychopathology is hazardous, but such findings, if replicated in humans, are clearly of significance in the treatment of these distressing disorders.

However, no direct evidence exists for medial hypothalamic noradrenergic system dysfunction in anorexia nervosa. MHPG, an important end product of NE, is reduced in anorexia nervosa,[52,59,67] but it normalizes on weight gain.[59] Reduced plasma levels of dopamine and NE in anorexia nervosa are also weight related.[42]

Hypothalamic functions in normal-weight bulimic patients have so far not been studied extensively. At this stage, the role of the hypothalamus in the pathogenesis of this disorder is therefore entirely speculative.

Finally, Green and Rau[56,57] found 14- and 6-per-second positive spiking in the temporal and occipital region in the EEGs of some of their bulimic patients and hypothesized that such neurological dysfunction is related to the compulsive overeating. Certainly not all bulimic individuals show such EEG abnormality,[156] and the significance of the 14- and 6-per-second positive spikes is unclear.[111]

Conclusion

The two eating disorders, anorexia nervosa and bulimia nervosa, have apparently become major public health hazards in this country. Some progress has been made in the classification and description of these disorders, and a clearer picture of the endocrine and metabolic disturbances has emerged. Social-cultural factors bearing on the development of the disorders and the final common pathway of the pathogenesis of the disorders seem to be better understood. Several testable etiological theories are available. The challenge is now to identify the vulnerable individual and to prevent the onset of the disorders.

REFERENCES

1. ABRAHAM, S. F., and BEUMONT, P. J. "How Patients Describe Bulimia or Binge-eating," *Psychological Medicine,* 12 (1982):625–635.

2. AMERICAN PSYCHIATRIC ASSOCIATION. *Diagnostic and Statistical Manual of Mental Disorders,* 3rd ed. (DSM-III). Washington, D.C.: American Psychiatric Association, 1980.

3. ASKEVOLD, F., and HEIBERG, A. "Anorexia Nervosa: Two Cases in Discordant MZ Twins," *Psychotherapy and Psychosomatics,* 32 (1979):223–228.

4. BENTOVIM, D. I., MARILOV, V., and CRISP, A. H. "Personality and Mental State (P.S.E.) with Anorexia Nervosa," *Journal of Psychosomatic Research,* 23 (1979):321–325.

5. BEUMONT, P.J.V., GEORGE, G.C.W., and SMART, D. E. "Dieters and Vomiters and Purgers in Anorexia Nervosa," *Psychological Medicine,* 6 (1976):617–622.

6. BOSKIND-LODAHL, M., and WHITE, W. C. "The Definition and Treatment of Bulimarexia in College Women—A Pilot Study," *Journal of the American College Health Association,* 27 (1978):84–97.

7. BOYAR, R. N., et al. "Anorexia Nervosa: Immaturity of the 24-hour Luteinizing Hormone Secretory Pattern," *New England Journal of Medicine,* 291 (1974):861–865.

8. BRANCH, C.H.H., and EURMAN, L. K. "Social Attitudes Toward Patients with Anorexia Nervosa," *American Journal of Psychiatry,* 137 (1980):632–633.

9. BROTMAN, A. W., HERZOG, D. B., and WOODS, S. W. "Antidepressant Treatment of Bulimia," *Journal of Clinical Psychiatry,* 45 (1984):7–9.

10. BROWN, W. L. "Anorexia Nervosa," in L. Brown, ed., *Anorexia Nervosa.* London: C. W. Daniels, 1931, pp. 11–17.

11. BRUCH, H. "Perceptual and Conceptual Disturbances

in Anorexia Nervosa," *Psychosomatic Medicine,* 24 (1962): 187–194.

12. ———. "Psychotherapy in Primary Anorexia Nervosa," *Journal of Nervous and Mental Disease,* 150 (1970): 51–67.

13. ———. *Eating Disorders.* New York: Basic Books, 1973.

14. ———. "Psychological Antecedents of Anorexia Nervosa," in R. A. Vigersky, ed., *Anorexia Nervosa.* New York: Raven Press, 1977, pp. 1–10.

15. BUHRICH, N. "Frequency of Presentation of Anorexia in Malaysia," *Australia–New Zealand Journal of Psychiatry,* 15 (1981):153–155.

16. BUTTON, E. J., and WHITEHOUSE, A. "Subclinical Anorexia Nervosa," *Psychological Medicine,* 11 (1981):509–516.

17. CALDEN, G., LUNDY, R. M., and SCHLAFER, R. J. "Sex Differences in Body Concepts," *Journal of Consulting Psychiatry,* 23 (1959):378.

18. CANTWELL, D. P., et al. "Anorexia Nervosa—an Affective Disorder?" *Archives of General Psychiatry,* 34 (1977):1087–1093.

19. CASPER, R. C., et al. "Bulimia," *Archives of General Psychiatry,* 37 (1980):1030–1035.

20. CHARCOT, J. M. *Disorders of the Nervous System.* London: New Sydenham Society, 1889.

21. COBB, S. *Emotions and Clinical Medicine.* New York: W. W. Norton, 1950.

22. COOPER, P. J., and FAIRBURN, C. G. "Are Eating Disorders Forms of Affective Disorders?" *British Journal of Psychiatry,* 148 (1983):96–97.

23. CRISP, A. H. "Diagnosis and Outcome of Anorexia Nervosa," *Proceedings of the Royal Society of Medicine,* 70 (1977):464–470.

24. ———. *Anorexia Nervosa—Let Me Be.* London: Plenum Press, 1980.

25. CRISP, A. H., and TOMS, D. A. "Primary Anorexia Nervosa or Weight Phobia in the Male," *British Medical Journal,* 1 (1972):334–338.

26. CRISP, A. H., HARDING, B., and McGUINNESS, B. "Anorexia Nervosa: Psychoneurotic Characteristics of Parents: Relationship to Prognosis," *Journal of Psychosomatic Research,* 18 (1974):167–173.

27. CRISP, A. H., HSU, L.K.G., and HARDING, B. "The Starving Hoarder and Voracious Spender—Stealing in Anorexia Nervosa," *Journal of Psychosomatic Research,* 24 (1980):225–231.

28. CRISP, A. H., PALMER, R. L., and KALUCY, R. S. "How Common Is Anorexia Nervosa? A Prevalence Study," *British Journal of Psychiatry,* 128 (1976):549–554.

29. CRISP, A. H., et al. "Clinical Features of Anorexia Nervosa," *Journal of Psychosomatic Research,* 24 (1980): 179–191.

30. CROOKSHANK, F. G. "Anorexia Nervosa," in L. Brown, ed., *Anorexia Nervosa.* London: C. W. Daniel, 1931, pp. 19–40.

31. DRUSS, R. G., and SILVERMAN, J. A. "Body Image and Perfectionism of Ballerinas," *General Hospital Psychiatry,* 2 (1979):115–121.

32. DUNN, P. K., and ONDERCIN, P. "Personality Variables Related to Compulsive Eating in College Women," *Journal of Clinical Psychology,* 37 (1981):43–49.

33. ECKERT, E. D., et al. "Depression in Anorexia Nervosa," *Psychological Medicine,* 12 (1982):115–122.

34. FAIRBURN, C. G. "A Cognitive Behavioral Approach to the Management of Bulimia," *Psychological Medicine,* 11 (1981):707–711.

35. ———. "Binge Eating and Its Management," *British Journal of Psychiatry,* 141 (1982):631–633.

36. FAIRBURN, C. G., and COOPER, P. J. "Self-induced Vomiting and Bulimia Nervosa: An Undetected Problem," *British Medical Journal,* 1 (1982):1153–1155.

37. FENICHEL, O. "Anorexia," in *The Collected Papers of Otto Fenichel,* vol. 2. New York: W. W. Norton, 1954, pp. 288–295.

38. FOSTER, F. G., and KUPFER, D. J. "Anorexia Nervosa: Telemetric Assessment of Family Interactions and Hospital Events," *Journal of Psychosomatic Research,* 12 (1975):19–35.

39. FRISCH, R. E. "Weight in Menarche," *Pediatrics,* 50 (1972):445–450.

40. ———. "Food Intake, Fatness and Reproductive Ability," in R. A. Vigersky, ed., *Anorexia Nervosa.* New York: Raven Press, 1977, pp. 149–162.

41. FRISCH, R. E., WYSHAK, G., and VINCENT, L. "Delayed Menarche and Amenorrhea in Ballet Dancers," *New England Journal of Medicine,* 303 (1980):17–19.

42. GARFINKEL, P. E., and GARNER, D. M. *Anorexia Nervosa: A Multidimensional Perspective.* New York: Brunner/Mazel, 1982.

43. GARFINKEL, P. E., MOLDOFSKY, H., and GARNER, D. M. "The Stability of Perceptual Disturbances in Anorexia Nervosa," *Psychological Medicine,* 9 (1979):703–708.

44. ———. "The Heterogeneity of Anorexia Nervosa," *Archives of General Psychiatry,* 37 (1980):1036–1040.

45. GARN, S. M., and CLARK, D. C. "Nutrition, Growth, Development, and Maturation—Findings from the Ten State Nutrition Survey of 1968–1970," *Pediatrics,* 56 (1975):306–319.

46. ———. "Trends in Fatness and the Origins of Obesity," *Pediatrics,* 57 (1976):443–456.

47. GARNER, D. M., and BEMIS, K. "A Cognitive Behavioral Approach to Anorexia Nervosa," *Cognitive Therapy and Research,* 6 (1982):1–27.

48. GARNER, D. M., and GARFINKEL, P. E. "Social Cultural Factors in the Development of Anorexia Nervosa," *Psychological Medicine,* 10 (1980):647–656.

49. GARNER, D. M., GARFINKEL, P. E., and O'SHAUGHNESSY, M. "Clinical and Psychometric Comparison Between Bulimia in Anorexia Nervosa and Bulimia in Normal Weight Women," in D. E. Redfern, ed., *Understanding Anorexia Nervosa and Bulimia.* Columbus, Ohio: Ross Laboratories, 1983, pp. 6–13.

50. GARNER, D. M., OLMSTED, M. P., and GARFINKEL, P. E. "Does Anorexia Nervosa Occur on a Continuum?" *International Journal of Eating Disorders,* 2 (1983):11–20.

51. GARNER, D. M., et al. "Cultural Expectations of Thinness in Women," *Psychological Medicine,* 38 (1976):327–336.

52. GERNER, R. H., and GWIRSTMAN, H. E. "Abnormalities of Dexamethasone Suppression Test and Urinary MHPG in Anorexia Nervosa," *American Journal of Psychiatry,* 138 (1981):650–653.

53. GOLD, P. W., et al. "Abnormalities in Plasma and Cerebral Spinal Fluid Arginine Vasopressin in Patients with Anorexia Nervosa," *New England Journal of Medicine,* 308 (1983):1117–1123.

54. GOLDBLATT, P. B., MOORE, M. E., and STUNKARD, A. J. "Social Factors in Obesity," *Journal of the American Medical Association,* 192 (1965):1039.

55. GORMALLY, J., et al. "The Assessment of Binge Eating Severity Among Obese Persons," *Addictive Behaviors,* 7 (1982):47–55.

56. GREEN, R. S., and RAU, J. H. "Treatment of Compul-

sive Eating Disturbances with Anticonvulsant Medication," *American Journal of Psychiatry,* 131 (1974):428–432.

57. ———. "The Use of Diphenylhydantoin in Compulsive Eating Disorders: Further Studies," in R. A. Vigersky, ed., *Anorexia Nervosa.* New York: Raven Press, 1977, pp. 377–382.

58. GROEN, J. J., and FELDMAN-TOLEDANO, Z. "Educative Treatment of Patients and Parents in Anorexia Nervosa," *British Journal of Psychiatry,* 112 (1966):671–681.

59. GROSS, H. A., LAKE, C. R., and EBERT, M. H. "Catecholamine Metabolism in Primary Anorexia Nervosa," *Journal of Clinical Endocrinology and Metabolism,* 49 (1979): 805–809.

60. GROSS, H. A., et al. "A Double-blind Controlled Trial of Lithium Carbonate in Primary Anorexia Nervosa," *Journal of Clinical Psychopharmacology,* 1 (1981):376–381.

61. GROUNDS, A. "Transient Psychosis in Anorexia Nervosa," *Psychological Medicine,* 12 (1982):107–113.

62. GULL, W. W. "Anorexia Nervosa (Apepsia Hysterica, Anorexia Hysterica)," *Transactions of Clinical Endocrinological Metabolism,* 49 (1874):805–809.

63. HALMI, K. A. "Anorexia Nervosa: Recent Investigations," *Annual Review of Medicine,* 29 (1978):137–148.

64. ———. "Anorexia Nervosa," in H. I. Kaplan, A. M. Freedman, and B. J. Sadock, eds., *Comprehensive Textbook of Psychiatry,* vol. 2, 3rd ed. Baltimore: Williams & Wilkins, 1980, pp. 1882–1890.

65. HALMI, K. A., and FALK, J. R. "Anorexia Nervosa: A Study of Outcome Discriminators in Exclusive Dieters and Bulimics," *Journal of the American Academy of Psychiatry,* 21 (1982):369–375.

66. HALMI, K. A., FALK, J. R., and SCHWARTZ, E. "Binge Eating and Vomiting: A Survey of a College Population," *Psychological Medicine,* 11 (1981):697–706.

67. HALMI, K. A., STRUSS, A., and GOLDBERG, S. C. "An Investigation of Weights in Parents of Anorexia Nervosa Patients," *Journal of Nervous and Mental Disease,* 166 (1978): 358.

68. HAWKINS, R. C., II, and CLEMENT, P. F. "Development and Construct Validation of a Self-Report Measure of Binge-Eating Tendencies," *Addictive Behaviors,* 5 (1980): 219–226.

69. HERMAN, C. P., and POLIVY, J. "Anxiety, Restraint, and Eating Behavior," *Journal of Abnormal Psychiatry,* 84 (1975):666–672.

70. HERZOG, D. B. "Bulimia: The Secretive Syndrome," *Psychosomatics,* 23 (1982):481–485.

71. HOFFMAN, L. W. "Fear of Success in Males and Females," *Journal of Consulting and Clinical Psychology,* 42 (1974):353–358.

72. HOGAN, C. C. "Psychodynamics," in C. P. Wilson, ed., *Fear of Being Fat.* New York: Jason Aronson, 1983, pp. 115–128.

73. HSU, L.K.G. "Outcome of Anorexia Nervosa—A Review of the Literature (1954–1978)," *Archives of General Psychiatry,* 37 (1980):1041–1046.

74. ———. "Is There a Disturbance of Body Image in Anorexia Nervosa?" *Journal of Nervous and Mental Disease,* 170 (1982):305–307.

75. ———. "Editorial: Etiology of Anorexia Nervosa," *Psychological Medicine,* 13 (1983):231–238.

76. HSU, L.K.G., and CRISP, A. H. "The Crown-Crisp Experiential Index Profile in Anorexia Nervosa," *British Journal of Psychiatry,* 136 (1980):567–573.

77. HSU, L.K.G., CRISP, A. H., and HARDING, B. "Outcome of Anorexia Nervosa," *Lancet,* 1 (1979):61–65.

78. HSU, L.K.G., MELTZER, E. S., and CRISP, A. H.

"Schizophrenia and Anorexia Nervosa," *Journal of Nervous and Mental Disease,* 169 (1981):273–276.

79. HSU, L.K.G., et al. "Bipolar Illness Preceded by Anorexia Nervosa in Identical Twins," *Journal of Clinical Psychiatry,* 45 (1984):262–266.

80. HUDSON, J. I., LAFFER, P. S., and POPE, H. G. "Bulimia Related to Affective Disorder by Family History and Response to the Dexamethasone Suppression Test," *American Journal of Psychiatry,* 139 (1982):685–687.

81. HUDSON, J. I., et al. "Family History Study of Anorexia Nervosa and Bulimia," *British Journal of Psychiatry,* 142 (1983):133–138.

82. HUENEMANN, R. L., et al. "A Longitudinal Study of Gross Body Composition and Body Conformation and Then Association with Food and Activity in a Teenage Population," *American Journal of Clinical Nutrition,* 18 (1966): 325–338.

83. ISAACS, A. J. "Endocrinology in Anorexia Nervosa," in P. Dally, and J. Gomez, eds., *Anorexia Nervosa.* Heineman, London, 1979, pp. 159–209.

84. JESSNER, L., and ABSE, D. W. "Regressive Forces in Anorexia Nervosa," *British Journal of Medical Psychology,* 33 (1960):301–312.

85. JOHNSON, C. L., and LARSON, R. "Bulimia: An Analysis of Moods and Behavior," *Psychosomatic Medicine,* 44 (1982):341–351.

86. JOHNSON, C. L., et al. "Bulimia: A Survey of 500 Patients," in P. L. Darby et al., eds., *Anorexia Nervosa: Recent Developments.* New York: Alan R. Liss, 1982, pp. 159–172.

87. JONES, D. J., et al. "Epidemiology of Anorexia Nervosa in Monroe County, New York: 1960–1976," *Psychosomatic Medicine,* 42 (1980):551–558.

88. KALUCY, R., CRISP, A. H., and HARDING, B. "A Study of 56 Females with Anorexia Nervosa," *British Journal of Medical Psychology,* 50 (1977):381.

89. KATY, J. L., et al. "Weight and Circadian Luteinizing Hormone Secretory Pattern in Anorexia Nervosa," *Psychosomatic Medicine,* 40 (1978):549–567.

90. KAY, D.W.K., and LEIGH, D. "The Natural History, Treatment and Prognosis of Anorexia Nervosa, Based on a Study of 38 Patients," *Journal of Mental Science,* 100 (1954): 411–431.

91. KAYE, W. H., et al. "Cerebral Spinal Fluid Opioid Activity in Anorexia Nervosa," *American Journal of Psychiatry,* 139 (1982):643–645.

92. KENDELL, R. E., et al. "The Epidemiology of Anorexia Nervosa," *Psychological Medicine,* 3 (1973):200–203.

93. KING, A. "Primary and Secondary Anorexia Nervosa," *British Journal of Psychiatry,* 109 (1963):470–479.

94. LACEY, J. H. "Bulimia Nervosa, Binge Eating, and Psychogenic Vomiting: A Controlled Treatment Study and Long-Term Outcome," *British Medical Journal,* 1 (1983): 1609–1613.

95. LACEY, J. H., et al. "Variations in Energy Intake of Adolescent Schoolgirls," *Journal of Human Nutrition,* 32 (1978):419–426.

96. LASEQUE, C. "On Hysterical Anorexia," *Medical Times Gazette,* 2 (1873):265.

97. LIEBOWITZ, S. F. "Hypothalamic Noradrenergic System: Role in Control of Appetite and Relation to Anorexia Nervosa," in D. E. Redfern, ed., *Understanding Anorexia Nervosa and Bulimia.* Columbus, Ohio: Ross Laboratories, 1983, pp. 54–59.

98. LINDNER, R. "Solitaire: The Story of Laura," in *The Fifty-Five Minute Hour: A Collection of True Psychoanalytic Tales.* New York: Holt, Rinehart & Winston, 1955, pp. 115–168.

99. LONG, C. G., and CORDLE, C. J. "Psychological Treatment of Binge Eating and Self-Induced Vomiting," *British Journal of Medical Psychology,* 55 (1982):139–145.

100. LORO, A. D., and ORLEANS, C. S. "Binge-eating in Obesity," *Addictive Behavior,* 6 (1981):155–166.

101. LUCAS, A. R. "Pigging Out," *Journal of the American Medical Association,* 247 (1982):82.

102. MARCIA, J. E., and FRIEDMAN, M. L. "Ego Identity Status in College Women," *Journal of Personality,* 38 (1970): 249–263.

103. MAWSON, A. R. "Anorexia Nervosa and the Regulation of Intake: A Review," *Psychological Medicine,* 4 (1974): 289–380.

104. MINTZ, I. L. "Psychoanalytic Description: The Clinical Picture of Anorexia Nervosa and Bulimia," in C. P. Wilson, ed., *Fear of Being Fat.* New York: Jason Aronson, 1983, pp. 83–113.

105. MINUCHIN, S. *Families and Family Therapy.* Cambridge, Mass.: Harvard University Press, 1974.

106. MINUCHIN, S., et al. "A Conceptual Model of Psychosomatic Illness in Children," *Archives of General Psychiatry,* 32 (1975):1031–1038.

107. MINUCHIN, S., et al. *Psychosomatic Families: Anorexia Nervosa in Context.* Cambridge, Mass.: Harvard University Press, 1978.

108. MORGAN, H. G., and RUSSELL, G.F.M. "Value of Family Background and Clinical Features as Predictors of Long-term Outcome in Anorexia Nervosa," *Psychological Medicine,* 5 (1975):355–371.

109. NEIL, J. F., MERIKANGAS, J. R., and FOSTER, F. G. "Waking and All-Night EEG in Anorexia Nervosa," *Clinical Electroencephalography,* 11 (1980):9–15.

110. NEMIAH, J. C. "Anorexia Nervosa," *Medicine,* 29 (1950):225–268.

111. NIEDERMEYER, E. "Abnormal EEG Patterns (Epileptic and Paroxysmal)," in E. Niedermeyer and F. L. daSilva, eds., *Electroencephalography, Basic Principles, Clinical Applications and Related Fields.* Baltimore: Urban & Schwarzenberg, 1982, pp. 155–177.

112. NOGAMI, Y., and YABANA, F. "On Kibarashi-gui," *Folia Psychiatrica et Neurologica Japonica,* 31 (1977):159–166.

113. NURNBERGER, J. H., and GERSHON, E. S. "Genetics," in E. S. Paykel, ed., *Handbook of Affective Disorders.* New York: Guilford Press, 1982, pp. 126–145.

114. NYLANDER, I. "The Feeling of Being Fat and Dieting in a School Population," *Acta Sociomedica Scandinavica,* 3 (1971):17–26.

115. ORLOFSKY, J. L. "Identify Formation, Achievement, and Fear of Success in College Men and Women," *Journal of Youth and Adolescence,* 7 (1978):49–62.

116. PALAZZOLI, M. S. *Self-Starvation.* New York: Jason Aronson, 1974.

117. PALAZZOLI, M. S., et al. "Family Rituals: A Powerful Tool in Family Therapy," *Family Process,* 16 (1977):445–453.

118. PALMER, R. L. "The Dietary Chaos Syndrome: A Useful New Term?" *British Journal of Medical Psychology,* 52 (1979):187–190.

119. POLIVY, J. "Perception of Calories and the Regulation of Intake in Restrained and Unrestrained Subjects," *Addictive Behaviors,* 85 (1976):338–340.

120. POLIVY, J., and HERMAN, C. P. "Clinical Depression and Weight Change: A Complex Relation," *Journal of Abnormal Psychology,* 85 (1976):338–340.

121. ———. "The Effects of Alcohol on Eating Behavior," *Addictive Behaviors,* 1 (1976):121–125.

122. POPE, H. G., and HUDSON, J. I. "Treatment of Bulimia with Antidepressants," *Psychopharmacology,* 78 (1982):176–179.

123. POPE, H. G., HUDSON, J. I., and YURGELUN-TODD, D. "Anorexia Nervosa and Bulimia Among 300 Suburban Women Shoppers," *American Journal of Psychiatry,* 141 (1984):292–294.

124. POPE, H. G., et al. "Bulimia Treated with Imipramine: A Placebo-controlled, Double-blind Study," *American Journal of Psychiatry,* 140 (1983):554–558.

125. PYLE, R. L., MITCHELL, J. E., and ECKERT, E. D. "Bulimia: A Report of 34 Cases," *Journal of Clinical Psychiatry,* 42 (1981):60–64.

126. PYLE, R. L., et al. "The Incidence of Bulimia in Freshman College Students," *International Journal of Eating Disorders,* 2 (1983):61–74.

127. RAMPLING, D. "Abnormal Mothering in the Genesis of Anorexia Nervosa," *Journal of Nervous and Mental Disease,* 168 (1980):501–504.

128. RUSSELL, G.F.M. "Metabolic Aspects of Anorexia Nervosa," *Proceedings of the Royal Society of Medicine,* 58 (1965):811–814.

129. ———. "Anorexia Nervosa—Its Identity as an Illness and Its Treatment," in J. H. Price, ed., *Modern Trends in Psychological Medicine,* vol. 2. London: Butterworths, 1970, pp. 131–164.

130. ———. "The Present Status of Anorexia Nervosa," *Psychological Medicine,* 7 (1977):353–367.

131. ———. "Bulimia Nervosa: An Ominous Variant of Anorexia Nervosa," *Psychological Medicine,* 9 (1979):429–448.

132. SALKIND, M. R., FINCHAM, J., and SILVERSTON, T. "Is Anorexia Nervosa a Phobic Disorder?" *Biological Psychiatry,* 15 (1980):803–808.

133. SECORD, P., and JOURARD, S. "The Appraisal of Body-cathexis and the Self," *Journal of Consulting Psychology,* 17 (1953):343–347.

134. SIMMONS, R. G., and ROSENBERG, F. "Sex, Sex Roles, and Self-Image," *Journal of Youth and Adolescence,* 4 (1975):229–258.

135. SLADE, P. D. "Towards a Functional Analysis of Anorexia Nervosa and Bulimia Nervosa," *British Journal of Clinical Psychology,* 21 (1982):167–179.

136. SOURS, J. A. "The Primary Anorexia Nervosa Syndrome," in J. D. Noshpitz, ed., *Basic Handbook of Child Psychiatry,* vol. 2. New York: Basic Books, 1979, pp. 568–580.

137. ———. "Depression and the Anorexia Nervosa Syndrome," *Pediatric Clinics of North America,* 4 (1981):145–158.

138. SPENCER, J. A., and FREMOUW, N. J. "Binge-eating as a Function of Restraint and Weight Classification," *Journal of Abnormal Psychology,* 28 (1979):262–267.

139. SPERLING, M. "A Re-evaluation of Classification, Concepts, and Treatment," in C. Wilson, ed., *The Fear of Being Fat: The Treatment of Anorexia Nervosa and Bulimia.* New York: Jason Aronson, 1983, pp. 51–82.

140. STANGLER, R. S., and PRINZ, A. M. "DSM-III: Psychiatric Diagnosis in a University Population," *American Journal of Psychiatry,* 137 (1980):937–940.

141. STRICKER, E. M. "The Central Control of Food Intake: A Role for Insulin," in B. G. Hoebel and D. Novin, eds., *The Neural Basis of Feeding and Reward.* Brunswick, Maine: Haer Institute for Electrophysiological Research, 1982, pp. 227–239.

142. STROBER, M. "An Empirically Derived Typology of

Anorexia Nervosa," in J. L. Darby, ed., *Anorexia Nervosa.* New York: Alan R. Liss, 1980, pp. 185–196.

143. ———. "The Significance of Bulimia in Juvenile Anorexia Nervosa," *International Journal of Eating Disorders,* 1 (1981):28–43.

144. STROBER, M., et al. "Validity of the Bulimia-restricter Distinction in Anorexia Nervosa," *Journal of Nervous and Mental Disease,* 170 (1982):345–351.

145. STUNKARD, A. J. "Eating Patterns and Obesity," *Psychiatric Quarterly,* 33 (1959):284–292.

146. SZYRYNSKI, V. "Anorexia Nervosa and Psychotherapy," *American Journal of Psychotherapy,* 27 (1973):492–505.

147. THEANDER, S. "Anorexia Nervosa: A Psychiatric Investigation of 94 Female Patients," *Acta Psychiatrica Scandinavica,* Supplement 214 (1970).

148. TOUYZ, S. W., et al. "Body Shape Perception and Its Disturbance in Anorexia Nervosa," *British Journal of Psychiatry,* 144 (1984):167–171.

149. VIGERSKY, R. A., ANDERSON, A. E., and THOMPSON, R. H. "Hypothalamic Dysfunction in Secondary Amenorrhea Associated with Simple Weight Loss," *New England Journal of Medicine,* 21 (1977):1141–1145.

150. WACHSLICHT-RODBARD, H., et al. "Increased Insulin Binding for Erythrocytes in Anorexia Nervosa," *New England Journal of Medicine,* 300 (1979):882–887.

151. WALLER, J., KAUFMAN, M. R., and DEUTSCH, F. "Anorexia Nervosa: A Psychosomatic Study," *Psychosomatic Medicine,* 2 (1940):3–16.

152. WALSH, B. T. "Endocrine Disturbances in Anorexia Nervosa and Depression," *Psychosomatic Medicine,* 44 (1982):85–91.

153. WALSH, B. T., et al. "Treatment of Bulimia with Monoamine Oxidase Inhibitors," *American Journal of Psychiatry,* 139 (1982):1629–1630.

154. WARDLE, J., and BEINHART, H. "Binge Eating: A Theoretical Review," *British Journal of Clinical Psychology,* 20 (1981):97–109.

155. WEINER, H. "Abiding Problems in the Psychoendocrinology of Anorexia Nervosa," in D. E. Redfern, ed., *Understanding Anorexia Nervosa and Bulimia.* Columbus, Ohio: Ross Laboratories, 1983, pp. 47–53.

156. WERMUTH, B. M., et al. "Phenytoin Treatment of the Binge-Eating Syndrome," *American Journal of Psychiatry,* 134 (1977):1249–1253.

157. WHITE, W. C., and BOSKIND-WHITE, M. "An Experiential-Behavioral Approach to the Treatment of Bulimarexia," *Psychotherapy: Theory, Research and Practice,* 18 (1981):501–507.

158. WILLI, J., and GROSSMANN, S. "Epidemiology of Anorexia Nervosa in a Defined Region of Switzerland," *American Journal of Psychiatry,* 140 (1983):564–567.

159. WILLIAMS, J. G., BARLOW, D. H., and AGRAS, W. S. "Behavioral Measurement of Severe Depression," *Archives of General Psychiatry,* 27 (1972):330–333.

160. WINOKUR, A., MARCH, V., and MENDELS, J. "Primary Affective Disorder in Relatives of Patients with Anorexia Nervosa," *American Journal of Psychiatry,* 137 (1980): 695–697.

161. YATES, A., LEEHEY, K., and SHISSLAK, C. M. "Running—An Analogue of Anorexia?" *New England Journal of Medicine,* 308 (1983):251–255.

162. YAGER, J. "Family Issues in the Pathogenesis of Anorexia Nervosa," *Psychosomatic Medicine,* 44 (1982):43–60.

163. YOUNG, J. C. "Anorexia Nervosa," in L. Brown, ed., *Anorexia Nervosa.* London: C. W. Daniel, 1931, pp. 41–49.

41 / Adolescent Substance Abuse: Etiology and Dynamics

John E. Meeks

History of Psychiatrists' Attitudes Toward Substance Abuse

In recent years the massive increase in the use of psychoactive drugs has attracted the growing attention of psychiatrists. Because of the large numbers of their patients who use drugs, child and adolescent specialists have been particularly involved. Although the problem is widespread, it is by no means universal; nor is it always clinically serious. Many of these youngsters use drugs only once or twice and thereafter show no sustained interest. Others use them more regularly but drop them easily when the drug use poses any threat to family relationships, personal productivity, or their

psychotherapy. However, there is a significant number of patients whose regular use of drugs causes real clinical concern. This has led to considerable professional discussion and a reawakening of interest in the topic of drug dependency and addiction. Despite this, however, some professionals are reluctant to treat individuals whose difficulties result primarily from extensive drug ingestion. Other psychiatrists are willing to treat these patients, but they do so because they consider drug use to be merely another symptom of anxiety and depression. That is, they treat the drug-dependent patient from the theoretical standpoint that resolving underlying conflicts and promoting psychological growth will remove the patients' need for drug use and stop the addictive behavior.

Much of the early theoretical literature was founded

on this conceptual base. To some extent, this misunderstanding of the nature of the process of chemical dependency resulted from inexperience; it was a relatively infrequent state of affairs for the addict to come to treatment. Even though some of his ideas on etiology have not stood the test of time, Knight[11] actually struggled with these patients and was accordingly more realistic. Traditional psychotherapy maintains an expectation for introspection and for persistent efforts to understand and resolve painful internal conflicts. In addictions, however, denial is a prominent symptom; most such patients are poorly motivated for traditional psychotherapy. Since very few addicts were successfully treated through analytic psychotherapy, much of the theorizing about their difficulties stemmed from "armchair" speculations. In brief, these did not achieve an in-depth understanding of the nuances of addictive behavior.

The history of psychiatry's involvement with addiction, then, is one of both neglect and misunderstanding. This has contributed to an unfortunate estrangement between psychiatry and drug counselors; in some areas this, in turn, has resulted in virtually excluding psychiatrists from the drug treatment process. Some degree of polarization has occurred since psychiatrists often minimize the importance of the actual drug use and emphasize instead the psychopathology of the individual drug user. On the other extreme, many drug counselors and spokespersons for self-help recovery groups deny the presence of any psychological preconditions for addiction and insist that it is a biological illness. This dichotomizing has had an unfortunate impact on many patients who are in dire need of the insights available from both perspectives.

Concepts of the Illness: Etiology

HEREDITARY INFLUENCES IN THE DEVELOPMENT OF SUBSTANCE ABUSE BEHAVIORS

It has long been recognized that substance abuse is transmitted from one generation to another. The evidence is particularly well documented in the case of alcoholism,[3,4,5] but clinical experience suggests that the same situation holds for drug dependency in general. Severe alcoholism in particular appears to be genetically transmitted,[10] a finding that is supported by twin studies and the study of adopted youngsters with genetic loading from substance-abusing biological parents.[8]

In the case of less severe drug abuse, considerable debate continues regarding the relative roles of genetic as opposed to learned behavior transmission. Parents who drink heavily or who regularly utilize other drugs in the presence of their children do provide a model of stress management, adaptation, and recreation that acts as a powerful influence. Some studies suggest that these influences are particularly strong if the drug use disrupts crucial family traditions.[23]

There is also some evidence to suggest that alcoholism shares a common genetic base with illnesses in the depressive spectrum.[4,22] However, recent studies have challenged the assumption of a genetic link between the two syndromes,[5] and this issue remains somewhat controversial. The assumption has always been an attractive one because of the obvious dysphoria that tends to accompany and perhaps to underlie substance abuse.

Social, economic, and life-style background variables are surprisingly unimportant[2] factors in determining patterns of drug use in adolescents. The only real exception is religious involvement, which has a clear negative correlation with drug use. Political conservatism and positive college plans are also correlated, but less strongly. Obviously, all three of these factors are at least partially influenced by personality structure as well as cultural factors. Other factors such as economic level, urbanicity, and parents' educational level seem to have minor correlation with drug use.

BIOLOGICAL ASPECTS

The Alcoholics Anonymous (AA) community has strongly supported the "disease concept" of alcoholism,[1] a view of the disorder that has also been broadened to include patterns of abuse of other substances. This widely utilized model is a *treatment* concept. It evolved out of widespread personal and clinical experience that suggests that some individuals react very positively to the experience of intoxication the very first time they are exposed to it. It has also been suggested that these individuals progress in their substance abuse according to a predictable and tragic schedule that is life-threatening. A corollary of this view holds strongly that even after the cessation of drinking or other drug use the person continues to remain alcoholic—that is, vulnerable to recurrence. In other words, the illness remains and awaits only the contact with the agent to reappear in full flower. Thus AA members refer to themselves as "recovering" alcoholics and not as recovered alcoholics.

This concept does not confront etiological issues. No definite statements are made regarding the biological roots of the disease, its biochemistry, or its hereditary origin. Although there is a strong implication that alcoholics are born and not made, the concept addresses treatment issues rather than offering a theoretical view.

A second group of important biological issues relates

to the complications of prolonged and heavy substance abuse. These include some clearly defined sequelae of alcoholism such as liver damage, delerium tremens, Korsakov syndrome, and others. Many physical complications of drug use are related to withdrawal states, including the psychosis associated with amphetamine use and the convulsive disorders that may follow withdrawal of barbiturates from addicted individuals. Among many adolescents who use drugs heavily, withdrawal of any psychoactive agent may produce more subtle organic effects. These are important mainly because they complicate the initial treatment period and interfere with the therapeutic alliance. (This is discussed more fully in chapter 59).

Long-term drug use, particularly polydrug use, also produces subtle changes in intellectual and cognitive functioning that appear to be organic. Many drug-using adolescents display changes in electroencephalographic patterns as well as evidence of reversible neurological-based abnormalities on psychological testing.

Psychodynamics of Substance Abuse

Many theories seek to explain the dynamics of substance abuse, but at this time there does not appear to be any universally accepted psychological formulation that fully accounts for this behavior. The concepts that have been advanced range from simple paradigms to highly complex and sophisticated theories. Many of these conceptual models appear to have resulted from "armchair" theorizing or were derived from experience with only a limited number of individuals with substance abuse problems. There is a tendency also to confuse limited or brief drug use with more sustained and serious patterns of dependency. In any case, this chapter discusses the range of concepts that have been proposed with comments regarding their applicability, areas of usefulness, and deficiencies.

Early discussions of drug abuse tended to focus on the drugs' obvious relationship to impulse satisfaction.[7] The "oral" orientation of the drug user, particularly the alcoholic, was noted, with considerable discussion of the "bottle equals breast" equation. Addiction was thus viewed as virtually synonymous with fixation at the earliest need satisfaction level of personality development. Addicted individuals were regarded as dependent, needy, and desirous of primitive comfort and the bliss of satiation.

The surface attractiveness of this theory was reinforced by its clinical applicability to some alcoholics, to many heroin addicts, and to other substance abusers who indeed manifested passivity, excessive dependency, and strong tendencies to escape from the demands of maturity. However, the model was unable to explain the occurrence of substance abuse in many individuals who did not show these personality patterns, or to account for the abuse of substances that did not lead to physiological satiation.

A second line of psychological theorizing in regard to substance abuse has focused on the use of psychoactive chemicals not only in the service of impulse gratification but as an artificial way of dealing with psychological discomfort. This distress could arise from structural deficiencies and/or from internal conflict. In this set of theories, the drugs were seen as agents of self-medication utilized to calm anxiety, lift depression, or provide "self-soothing"[13]; this made it possible to account for individual preference and specific drug choice. These formulations range from the commonsense suggestion that depressed people choose stimulants while those who were anxious might use calming drugs all the way to more sophisticated proposals, such as that of Wieder and Kaplan's[21] "ego prostheses." This concept suggested that adolescents chose particular drugs in an effort to self-completion; they sought to reinforce structural personality defects by means of pharmacologically mediated "psychic Band-Aids."

Both lines of thought regarding the basic causes of vulnerability to substance abuse led to efforts to recognize, describe, and demonstrate the presence of an "addictive personality." Initial findings in this area were promising; however, they did not differentiate adequately between the causes of substance abuse and the eventual results of that activity.[6,12,20] In other words, there appears to be a teleologic trap in that many of the observed characteristics of the so-called addictive personality may be more the result of continued and excessive drug use than expressions of its etiological origin. However, as will be noted later, there are certain personality characteristics, common defenses, and life experiences that appear to increase the likelihood that an individual—at least an adolescent—will possess an increased vulnerability to substance abuse.

The concept of an addictive personality might well be an overstatement of the degree to which personality structure explained addiction. However, it is balanced by an opposing view at the opposite end of the spectrum. As espoused by Pattison and others,[17] this viewpoint regards most alcohol addiction as a bad habit. That is, the authors assert that in normal individuals a variety of external circumstances may lead to drug use. In response to a feedback loop, using the drugs gradually leads to learned addictive behavior. This viewpoint is espoused also by Newton[16] who described a sequence of stages of drug involvement, each of which draws the adolescent further into the next portion of the downward spiral. Newton proposes that adolescents first use drugs to enjoy the high, but then, as tolerance develops, negative social effects appear and destructive developmental events occur. The drugs are then clung to desperately merely to maintain an approximation of normal mood and a sense of well-being. This model resembles the viewpoints of AA and Narcotics Anonymous (NA); in its every variation the strong implication is that aside from the substance abuse itself, no pathology necessarily exists. There is some recognition that developmental tasks have been neglected and/or delayed during the period of substance abuse so that removal of the offending substance will not immediately place an adolescent back in the mainstream. Training and relearning are recognized as necessary in order to correct the defects that have resulted from the drug use.

Recent psychoanalytic formulations have emphasized viewing the drug as a psychological object rather than merely as a chemical that is knowingly used either to meet needs or to diminish emotional discomfort. Addictive behavior is recognized to be similar to emotional dependencies on human beings; the addict, however, tends to withdraw from human contact as the drug use proceeds. Within the framework of this formulation, adolescents are seen as ambivalently attached to the drug. They view the drug as a controllable source of emotional gratification and a means of regulating feeling states or affects.[15,19,24] (It is interesting to note that many of these recent psychoanalytic ideas were foreshadowed over fifty years ago by Rado.[18]) When adolescents begin to recognize that the need for the drug is no longer under their volitional control, this becomes a source of concern and conflict. The resulting stress can stimulate a denial response in which adolescents insist that they can "take or leave" the drug even though objective evidence points overwhelmingly to a blind dependency on the substance. Alternatively, their response to the evidence of mounting dependency might be to stop the drug for a period of time in order to prove that they can "give it up," only to return to drug use later.

From this perspective, the addictive behavior is viewed as an omnipotent avoidance of human relationships that are perceived as dangerous, undependable, and potentially humiliating or painful. The magic substance at once alleviates internal conflicts and softens the impact of external frustration.[25] This model has a number of things to recommend it. First, it accounts for a wider range of the behaviors typically observed in drug-dependent individuals than do most of the other formulations. It has the additional advantage of explaining the success of AA and NA in interrupting the pattern of substance abuse. These treatment approaches emphasize the necessity for abstinence. They stress the need to forswear omnipotent self-sufficiency and to embrace instead satisfying substitutions of supportive and acceptable affiliation with a group.

Work with large populations of adolescent substance abusers reinforces the relevance of this general model; it also suggests the need to expand and understand it within a developmental framework. Chapter 25 in volume 2 of this *Handbook* explores the psychodynamics and personality structure of behaviorally disordered adolescents, a category to which a significant percentage of adolescent substance abusers belong.[14] A review of the patients admitted to an inpatient unit specializing in the treatment of psychiatrically disturbed youngsters whose illness was complicated by heavy drug use highlights the frequency with which there was a prior impairment of adaptive skills.[26] This was often evidenced by a history of attention deficit disorder or learning disability. One is impressed also with the patterns of childhood neglect and abuse reported by the adolescents; this includes a strikingly high percentage of physical or sexual abuse at the hands of parenting figures.[25] Both the deficiencies in the ego apparatus and the interference with safe dependency act to diminish the development of internal trust; adolescents are left with no faith either in their capacity to master their own feelings or in the dependability of the surrounding environment. The resulting overwhelming anxiety and despair encourage the development of a "pseudo-competency"; this encompasses distortions of reality ("Who wants a stupid nine-to-five job anyway? That's for suckers") and the artificial maintenance of a sense of well-being ("Who cares what happens tomorrow? Let's party tonight"). Because of the need for secrecy and the expectation of censure, drug use inevitably leads to a further alienation from constructive adults. Obviously the recurrent state of intoxication also disrupts both the motivation for learning and the capacity to grasp and implement new social, academic, and vocational skills. Gradually the adolescents become even less competent in the skills for mastery of the world as well as in the ability to gain and maintain emotionally satisfying human relationships. As a direct result of drug use, psychological and physical deterioration will take a toll as well, so that with the passage of time, the individuals need to move further into the illusory sense of pseudocompetence.

The concepts just described do explain the observed tendency toward deterioration in the substance-abusing adolescents. There is a predictable downhill course to the illness that tends to accelerate until it reaches a point of crisis. It is this crisis that often brings youngsters to the attention of legal authorities or medical centers. Occasionally, however, there are spontaneous remissions, even when the youngsters are seriously dependent on psychoactive chemicals. As mentioned earlier, most dependent individuals periodically try to "kick the habit." Because of the inherent flexibility and buoyancy of adolescence, during these abstinent periods the teenagers may fortuitously come into positive contacts with people. These encounters may, in turn, provide the necessary ingredients for significant human attachment and genuine emotional growth. The contacts may be with important adults such as coaches or charismatic teachers; more often, however, they entail satisfying acceptance by friends. Most "spontaneous cures" follow attachments where genuine tender affection is present as a major component.

The ideas and formulations just described apply to youngsters with serious problems in substance abuse. They are not intended as explanations for the widespread recreational use of illegal substances among adolescents. The general social acceptance of intoxication and the widespread rebellion against social rules are entirely different topics that go beyond the scope of this chapter.[9] They relate to serious substance abuse only in that they provide a much greater opportunity for the exposure of vulnerable youngsters to potentially

crippling agents. If drugs were not so commonly available, some vulnerable youngsters might simply never encounter the precipitating cause of their substance abuse problem. Even if this were not true, a more unequivocal definition of drug use as a deviant rather than a normative and expected form of adolescent behavior might draw therapeutic attention more rapidly to abusing youngsters and also undercut a major element in denial. It is difficult to convince youngsters that they have a drug problem when they see the majority of their classmates engaging regularly in the self-administration of illegal substances. In any case, as mentioned earlier, teenagers who are not drug dependent may use drugs with some regularity but still be able to give up that use in response to relatively minor external intervention such as decreased availability, parental detection and disapproval, minor scrapes with legal authorities, or even the recognition that a regular pattern of drug use is incompatible with their own long-range plans.

Unfortunately, not all abusing youngsters so readily escape from the escalating syndrome of dependency on chemical agents.

REFERENCES

1. ALCOHOLICS ANONYMOUS. New York: Alcoholic Anonymous World Services, 1976.

2. BACHMAN, J. G., JOHNSTON, L. D., and O'MALLEY, P. M. "Smoking, Drinking and Drug Use Among American High School Students: Correlates and Trends, 1975–1979," *American Journal of Public Health,* 71 (1981):59.

3. CLONINGER, C. R., et al. "Alcoholism and Affective Disorders: Familial Associations and Genetic Models," in D. W. Goodwin and C. K. Erickson, eds., *Alcoholism and Affective Disorders.* New York: SP Medical and Scientific Books, 1979, pp. 3–14.

4. CLONINGER, C. R., et al. "Inheritance of Alcohol Abuse: Cross Fostering Analysis of Adopted Men," *Archives of General Psychiatry,* 38 (1981):861.

5. EGELAND, J., and HOSTETTER, A. M. "Amish Study I: Affective Disorders Among the Amish, 1976–1980," *American Journal of Psychiatry,* 140 (1983):56.

6. GENDREAU, P., and GENDREAU, L. P. "The 'Addiction-Prone' Personality: A Study of Canadian Heroin Addicts," in H. Shaffer and M. E. Burgless, eds., *Classic Contributions in the Addictions.* New York: Brunner/Mazel, 1981, pp. 191–202.

7. GLOVER, E. "On the Etiology of Drug Addiction," in E. Glover, ed., *On the Early Development of Mind.* New York: International Universities Press, 1956.

8. GOODWIN, D. W., et al. "Alcohol Problems in Adoptees Raised Apart from Alcoholic Biologic Parents," *Archives of General Psychiatry,* 28 (1973):238.

9. GRUNSPOON, A. "Marijuana," *Scientific American,* 221 (1969):17.

10. HRUBEC, A., and OMENN, G. S. "Evidence of Genetic Predisposition to Alcoholic Cirrhosis and Psychosis: Twin Condordances for Alcoholism and Its Biological End Points by Zygosity Among Male Veterans," *Alcoholism: Clinical and Experimental Research,* 5 (1981):207.

11. KNIGHT, R. P. "The Psychodynamics of Chronic Alcoholism," *Journal of Nervous and Mental Disease,* 86 (1937): 538.

12. MacANDREW, C., and GEERTSMA, R. N. "A Critique of Alcoholism Scales Derived from the MMPI," *Quarterly Journal for the Study of Alcohol,* 25 (1981):58.

13. MAROHN, R. C. "Adolescent Substance Abuse: A Problem of Self Soothing," *Clinical Update in Adolescent Psychiatry,* 1 (1983).

14. MEEKS, J. E. "Behavioral and Antisocial Disorders," in J. D. Noshpitz, ed., *Basic Handbook of Child Psychiatry,* vol. 2. New York: Basic Books, 1979, pp. 482–530.

15. MEISSNER, W. W. "Addiction and Paranoid Process: Psychoanalytic Perspectives," *International Journal of Psychoanalytic Psychotherapy,* 8 (1980):273.

16. NEWTON, M. *Gone Way Down: Teenage Drug-Use Is a Disease.* Tampa, Fla.: American Studies Press, 1981.

17. PATTISON, E. M. "Types of Alcoholism Reflective of Character Disorders," in M. R. Zales, ed., *Character Pathology: Theory and Treatment.* New York: Brunner/Mazel, 1984, pp. 84–116.

18. RADO, S. "The Psychoanalysis of Pharmaeothemia," *Psychoanalytic Quarterly,* 2 (1933):1.

19. SUGARMAN, A., and KURASH, C. "Marijuana Abuse, Transitional Experience, and the Borderline Adolescent," in

J. Lichtenberg and S. Smith, eds., *Adolescent Addiction: Varieties and Vicissitudes, Psychoanalytic Inquiry* #2. Hillsdale, N. J.: The Analytic Press, 1982, pp. 519–538.

20. VALLIANT, G. E. "Natural History of Male Psychological Health: VIII. Antecedents of Alcoholism and Orality," *American Journal of Psychiatry,* 137 (1980):181.

21. WIEDER, H., and KAPLAN, E. H. "Drug Use in Adolescents: Psychodynamic Meaning and Pharmacogenic Effect," *Psychoanalytic Study of the Child,* 24 (1969):399.

22. WINOKUR, G. "Alcoholism and Depression in the Same Family," in D. W. Goodwin and C. K. Erickson, eds., *Alcoholism and Affective Disorders.* New York: SP Medical and Scientific Books, 1979.

23. WOLIN, S. J., et al. "Disrupted Family Rituals; A Factor in the Intergenerational Transmission of Alcoholism," *Journal of Studies on Alcohol,* 41 (1980):199.

24. WURMSER, L. "Psychoanalytic Considerations of the Etiology of Compulsive Drug Use," *Journal of the American Psychoanalytic Association,* 22 (1974):820.

25. WURMSER, L., and ZIENTS, A. "The Return of the Denied Superego," in J. Lichtenberg and S. Smith, eds., *Adolescent Addiction: Varieties and Vicissitudes, Psychoanalytic Inquiry* #2. Hillsdale, N. J.: The Analytic Press, 1982, pp. 539–580.

26. YENDALL, L. T., FROMM-AUCH, D., and DAVIES, P. "Neurological Impairment of Persistant Delinquency," *Journal of Nervous and Mental Disease,* 170 (1982):257.

SECTION V

Therapeutics

Saul I. Harrison / Editor

Introduction / Therapeutic Interventions in Child and Adolescent Psychiatry: Status and Prospects

Saul I. Harrison

In the late 1970s, aspects of my introductory chapter to volume 3 of this *Handbook* resembled a sermon. Clinicians were exhorted to acknowledge the existence of treatment methods derived from conceptual frameworks at variance with their preferred theoretical orientation. Following acknowledgment of those alien treatments, the next step urged was familiarity with the other therapeutic approaches and their indications so that they might be considered during clinical assessments and recommended when indicated.

It is gratifying to report that our status now appears to be one of progress. Today it is doubtful that there are many therapists encumbered by the lack of cognizance that existed only a few years ago. There is also a marked diminution in the type of deprecating nonacknowledgment that so often appeared as a defensive replacement for the earlier lack of awareness. Increasingly, the détente of quiet recognition includes constructive engagement. The most encouraging growth, however, appears to be in the area of mutual enrichment, as will be evident by the frequency with which multimodal therapeutic approaches are described in the chapters that follow.

It will be noted in those chapters, however, that substantial opportunities remain to enhance specificity and refinement in prescriptive efforts to mix the various therapeutic approaches. With increasing specificity of diagnostic assessment, child psychiatric treatment increasingly finds itself on the threshold of targeted therapeutic interventions. It is likely that the future will encompass technologically assisted procedures as well. Accompanying the requirements posed by those kinds of advances, clinicians will find themselves faced increasingly with the challenge of assuring that we not retreat from our field's traditional sensitivity to the child's and family's human features.

Despite the often surprising instances, cited in chapter 1 of volume 3 of this *Handbook,* in which treatment innovations with children pioneered subsequent therapeutic advances in adult psychiatry, child psychiatric treatment methods appear to lag behind those of adult psychiatry. Clearly, these analogies leave much to be desired, and there are disadvantages inherent in this kind of derivative thinking. Nevertheless, it is worth noting that the ésprit of adult psychiatric treatment today calls to mind the medical zeitgeist in relation to infectious diseases that was taking place when I became part of the profession four decades ago. Another less than perfect analogy links our knowledge base today with the status of molecular biology two decades ago.

In summary, the view from the interior is positive. The direction in which we are moving, however, is not affected only by internal factors. Child psychiatric treatment is being buffeted by external fiscal pressures that create artificial shortages (and that always seem so unfair when compared to the profusion and cost of weapons systems). This does not refer to utilization review; as unpleasant as it sometimes feels to be reviewed, the major potential contribution of peer review is in minimizing inappropriate treatments and keeping a youngster in the "sick role" longer than necessary. The truly noxious external factors that create artificial shortages are the cost-containing time limits imposed by third-party payers; these factors in particular result in the application of incomplete treatments. It is pathetic but true that it is not uncommon for eating disorders, for instance, to be treated with behavioral modification techniques alone or with tricyclics alone or with individual psychodynamic therapies alone or with family therapy alone primarily because that is all the economic constraints will permit. Elements of that scenario border on a form of prostitution; the analogy breaks down, however, because prostitution sometimes is characterized as a victimless crime; there is no question as to who is victimized by such cost-containment efforts.

The child psychiatric therapeutic professions are caught in a Catch-22, so to speak. If we go along with these restrictions, the communication perceived by third-party payers is that the restrictions are acceptable. If we do not go along, we have to turn away patients in need while negatively affecting our institutional and/or personal exchequer. As a consequence of the field's failure thus far to reverse those limiting trends, the general tendency is to go along. This generates a most unwelcome reminder of the surgeon who operates on a known polysurgical addict with the rationalization that it is better that the unnecessary surgery be performed with skill rather than by someone else who might not be as skillful.

It will have to be left to future volumes of this *Hand-*

book to record progress in dealing with these vexing "external" problems. In any case, the chapters that follow report encouraging "internal" advances in child and adolescent psychiatric therapeutic interventions.

42 / Advances in the Psychopharmacology of Childhood and Adolescence

Wayne H. Green and Magda Campbell

Introduction

The goal of this chapter is to summarize the progress made in psychopharmacology since the publication of chapter 23 in volume 3 of this *Handbook.* Since DSM-III was published in 1980,[1] DSM-III nomenclature was used in the majority of studies that are reviewed in this chapter. The newer developments since the 1979 *Handbook* were in the following areas: (1) diagnosis, (2) methodology, (3) efficacy of psychoactive drugs in depression, (4) efficacy of psychoactive drugs in aggressiveness and conduct disorder, aggressive type, (5) search for newer psychoactive agents, (6) long-term efficacy of psychoactive drugs, (7) effects of psychoactive drugs on cognition and learning, (8) relationship of clinical response and blood levels of psychoactive drugs, and (9) short- and long-term safety of psychoactive drugs.

Developments in diagnosis[32,59] and methodology[8,10,25] have been reviewed elsewhere and will not be included here.

Efficacy of Psychoactive Drugs in Major Depression

In the course of the past few years, the existence of major depression in prepubertal children and adolescents has been confirmed.* However, in spite of great progress in the area of diagnosis, in the development of appropriate rating instruments, and in measuring the bioavailability of drugs, the therapeutic efficacy of antidepressants has not been firmly established in this age group. In thirteen prepubertal children, ages six to twelve years, imipramine hydrochloride was studied: in six, in an open fashion, and in seven, under double-blind and placebo-controlled conditions. At five weeks of treatment, only plasma levels of imipramine differentiated responders from nonresponders; in the first group the mean level was 231 ng per ml, whereas in the nonresponders it was 128 ng per ml ($p < 0.05$).[57] Of twenty hospitalized children, ages seven to twelve

*See references 19, 20, 43, 44, and 55.

years, after three weeks of imipramine administration (75 mg/day), four had remitted; all had plasma concentrations between 125 and 225 ng per ml.[68] At six weeks, twelve of sixteen children had remitted; eleven of the twelve responders had a total plasma tricyclic concentration between 125 and 225 ng per ml. In an open study involving twelve children, ages five to eleven years, Geller and associates[30] found nortriptyline hydrochloride to be effective in reducing symptoms of depression, with the onset of response ranging from two to eight weeks. In another open trial, twenty-one children, whose ages ranged from six to thirteen years, were treated with imipramine in daily doses of 75 to 225 mg (3.8 to 5.0 mg/kg).[23] Fourteen showed improvement in one or more areas of functioning, while the remaining seven showed either no change or a worsening of their behavior. In a sample of thirty prepubertal children, plasma levels of imipramine and desmethylimipramine were significantly higher in the twenty responders (mean 283.85 ng/ml) than in those who failed to respond (mean 144.7 ng/ml).[58] Those who suffered from psychotic depression were less likely to show improvement than those who were not psychotic. Thus it can be concluded that antidepressants are effective in alleviating symptoms of depression in prepubertal children.

It appears that the maintenance plasma level of antidepressant in prepubertal children predicts the clinical response: Higher plasma levels are associated with alleviation of symptoms, while at least some of the nonresponders have low plasma levels.

However, in a sample of thirty-two adolescents, irrespective of daily dose or plasma level (249 mg/d, 301 ng/ml in nonresponders and 249 mg/d, 378 ng/ml in responders),[56] imipramine was not effective.

Efficacy of Psychoactive Drugs in Aggressiveness and in Conduct Disorder, Aggressive Type

There has been a recent literature review on pharmacotherapy in the management of severe aggressive behavior in children. It was found that, in well-designed studies, the efficacy of anticonvulsants and psychomotor stimulants was not demonstrated; among the neuroleptics, haloperidol appeared to be the most promising drug.[9] Critical reviews of the literature[11,12] and a well-designed study involving a relatively large sample of carefully diagnosed aggressive children[3,18,48,52] (referred to in the section entitled "Effects of Psychoactive Drugs on Cognition and Learning"), strongly suggest that lithium carbonate is an effective therapeutic agent for this group and that its long-term safety should be further studied under careful clinical and laboratory monitoring.

A current project involves the administration of molindone hydrochloride (18–155 mg/d, mean, 40.5 mg/d) to children, ages six to eleven years, who have been diagnosed as undersocialized conduct disorder with aggressivity. Preliminary results suggest that this agent will also bring about a lessening of the target symptoms.[36] No definitive statement can be made at the present time. However, because to date molindone appears to be infrequently associated with tardive dyskinesia, it merits further study.

Results of a pilot study suggest that chlordiazepoxide may be contraindicated in children with severe impulsivity and aggressiveness, while in children with symptoms of mild depression, anxiety, and withdrawal, it merits further study.[50]

Search for Newer Psychoactive Agents

The therapeutic effectiveness of magnesium pemoline in hyperactive children has now been demonstrated in well-designed studies. In a major double-blind and placebo-controlled study, Conners and Taylor[24] compared pemoline to methylphenidate hydrochloride. The subjects were sixty children, six to eleven years of age; multiple assessments were carried out by multiple raters. Pemoline (mean daily dose 60.4 mg or 2.25 mg/kg) had slower onset and longer duration of action than methylphenidate; it was, however, almost equally effective in reducing behavioral symptoms and improving cognitive functions. The most common untoward effects were insomnia, anorexia, headache, stomachache, irritability, and crying. The advantage of this drug over methylphenidate or dextroamphetamine is that it requires only a single morning dose. While sustained-release tablets of methylphenidate are now available, they are produced only in 20 mg tablets. Thus they may be useful when a child requires at least a 20 mg daily dose of methylphenidate or a multiple thereof.

In Tourette's disorder, haloperidol is, at the present time perhaps the most effective drug[5]: In conservative doses (0.5–8.0 mg/day) it yields decreases of target symptoms.[5,6,65] Even at these levels, however, but particularly at higher doses, sedation, depression, and deterioration of cognitive functions and school performance were observed. Pimozide, a neuroleptic, has recently been approved by the Food and Drug Administration for the treatment of Tourette's disorder. In daily doses of 1.0 to 2.0 mg it appears to be effective in reducing both vocal and motor tics. [6,65] Even with very conservative doses careful monitoring, including electrocardiogram, is recommended. Little is known about the safety of pimozide in children and adolescents. It is contraindicated in treating simple tics or tics not associated with Tourette's disorder. [51]

Clonidine hydrochloride is reported to be effective in reducing the symptoms in Tourette's disorder, without major untoward effects. [7,45,65] However, its use is still investigational.

Preliminary studies indicate that fenfluramine hydrochloride, an antiserotonergic agent, is a medication that offers some promise in the treatment of autistic children. [31,61] Fourteen autistic subjects, ages two and one-half to eighteen years, received fenfluramine in doses of 1.5 mg per kg over a period of four months. Ritvo and collaborators [61] reported a decrease of motility disturbances, a lessening of withdrawal, an increase in socialization, and improvement in the spontaneous use of language. The only untoward effects noted were decrease of appetite and weight and transient lethargy. It appears, however, that the responders were high-functioning autistic children and that baseline serotonin levels were not related to clinical response. Further studies are needed to establish the efficacy and safety of fenfluramine in this group of children.

No strong association of behavioral and learning problems with food additives has been demonstrated in carefully designed studies: Less than 5 percent of these children are sensitive to additives. [22,27]

The alleged positive effects of carbamazepine in aggressive children diagnosed as conduct disorder have yet to be demonstrated.

Long-term Efficacy of Psychoactive Drugs

The long-term therapeutic efficacy of psychoactive drugs was investigated in a few studies; all but one [14,15] are retrospective. In a prospective study, haloperidol was shown to be effective in decreasing symptoms of stereotypies, fidgetiness, hyperactivity, withdrawal, and abnormal object relations in autistic children, when given over a period of six months and up to two and one-half years. [14,15] This effect was achieved in thirty-six patients, ages two years and four months to seven years and ten months; daily doses of haloperidol ranged from 0.5 to 3.0 mg. Medication was discontinued every six months. One week after the drug discontinuation, worsening of behavioral symptoms was rated in most children, requiring resumption of drug administration at the end of the four-week placebo period. Thus behavioral deterioration was not only statistically but also clinically significant. There was no diminution of therapeutic efficacy over time, which is important in daily practice. Compliance was excellent. Withdrawal and tardive dyskinesia were the only untoward effects observed under careful clinical monitoring; they will be discussed in the section entitled "Short- and Long-term Safety of Psychoactive Drugs."

All children who participated in this ongoing study were enrolled in special educational programs. A number of children did not require continuation of haloperidol administration after the six-month treatment periods, because even after the drug was withheld, they maintained their gains.

Seventy-five hyperactive children were reexamined ten to twelve years after their initial evaluation. [67] During the first five years of treatment six of these children received amphetamine for six to forty-eight months; twenty-seven received chlorpromazine for six to forty-eight months; nine had a mixed drug history; and thirty-five of the children had received no drug longer than six months. When at ten-year follow-up a comparison was made to forty-four controls, who were matched for age, sex, socioeconomic status (SES), and IQ, the hyperactive subjects (now mean age 19.5 years) had significantly more car accidents, more moves of domicile over ten years, and completed less schooling. In the same sample, there was no difference between a subgroup of twenty-one hyperactive subjects who had been treated with 25 to 200 mg chlorpromazine daily for eighteen to forty-eight months and a subgroup of seventeen hyperactive subjects matched for SES, sex, IQ, and age who had received chlorpromazine for less than six months. The comparison included a variety of variables, such as psychiatric assessment, school and work histories, drug abuse, and court referrals. Thus pharmacotherapy, type of drug, or duration of drug administration do not seem to have significantly altered the clinical course of these children in affecting final outcome. It should be noted that a definitive statement cannot be made because of methodological inadequacies.

Effects of Psychoactive Drugs on Cognition and Learning

Werry and Aman [69] conducted a study of aggressive and hyperactive children of normal intelligence. They found that the adverse effect of neuroleptics on cognition may be a function of dose rather than of the drugs per se. Further research has shown that the same drug may have different effects on children in different diagnostic categories. [2,13,52]

A study was designed to make an objective assessment of the effects of haloperidol on discrimination learning and on behavioral symptoms in autistic children. The study was conducted under placebo-controlled and double-blind conditions, and employed multiple raters using a variety of rating scales. The research format involved a combination of intensive and extensive design [66]; the duration of the study was fourteen weeks. It involved a laboratory-based, computer-controlled, operant conditioning apparatus that performed several functions: It presented visual and auditory stimuli, recorded responses, offered reinforcers according to a specified schedule, and noted the duration of stereotypies and motor activity. Forty children, ages 2.33 to 6.92 years, completed this clinical trial. [2] Where compared to placebo, doses of haloperidol ranging from 0.5 to 3.0 mg per day (mean 1.11) or 0.019 to 0.217 mg per kg per day (mean 0.058) were followed by significant facilitation and retention of discrimination learning. At the same doses, no side effects were observed, while symptoms of stereotypies, withdrawal, hyperactivity, abnormal object relationships, fidgetiness, negativism, and labile and angry affect decreased. Whereas the decrease of these symptoms under haloperidol, and not under placebo, was significant outside of the laboratory, within the laboratory haloperidol failed to affect stereotypies and motor activity. Untoward effects were observed only above optimal doses (dosage was individually regulated); excessive sedation and acute dystonic reaction were those most frequently seen.

In young autistic children, most of whom function on a retarded level, haloperidol when given over a period of four weeks had a positive effect on learning in the laboratory. At similar doses, however, it had some negative effects on cognition in children of normal intelligence. [52] These children participated in a double-blind, placebo-controlled study designed to make a critical assessment of the efficacy of haloperidol and lithium. They were treatment-resistant and diagnosed as conduct disorder, undersocialized, aggressive. [18] The entire sample consisted of sixty-one hospitalized children, ages 5.2 to 12.9 years. Twenty of these children received haloperidol; optimal doses ranged from 1.0 to 6.0 mg per day (mean 2.95), or 0.04 to 0.21 mg per kg per day (mean 0.096). A cognitive battery was administered in the laboratory to each child, on baseline and at the end of a four-week drug period. Though drug effects on cognition were mild, haloperidol did yield significant decreases in Porteus Maze test quotient scores and a slowing of reaction time on a simple reaction time task. [52] Lithium administration

had an adverse effect on qualitative scores on the Porteus Mazes. Neither drug significantly affected the Stroop Test, the Matching Familiar Figures Test, short-term recognition, memory, and concept attainment tasks. With respect to decreasing the target symptoms, [18] both lithium (given to twenty-one children) and haloperidol were significantly and clinically superior to placebo. However, haloperidol yielded significantly more untoward effects than did lithium at therapeutic doses. The most common untoward effects with haloperidol were excessive sedation and acute dystonic reaction; with lithium, the prominent side effects were stomachache, headache, and tremor of the hands. Optimal doses of lithium ranged from 500 to 2,000 mg per day (mean 1,166); serum level of 0.32 to 1.51 mEq per 1 (mean 0.993) and saliva level of 0.81 to 5.05 mEq per 1 (mean 2.515). Saliva and serum lithium levels were highly correlated ($r = 0.83$); the saliva-to-serum ratio was 2.53 across patients. [48] Most untoward effects occurred during high doses of lithium; the few children who had untoward effects on low doses had relatively high lithium levels in saliva. [48] It should be noted that these children did not suffer from affective disorders. However, the families of those children who were receiving lithium had a greater incidence of affective disorders in the form of depression, psychiatric hospitalization for depression, and suicide attempts than the families of children receiving haloperidol or placebo, even though the assignment of patients to treatment was random. The presence or absence of such family history did not affect the magnitude of response to lithium in the child. [18]

For review of the literature on the effect of psychoactive drugs on cognition in children, a chapter by Campbell and associates is recommended. [17]

Relationship of Clinical Response and Blood Levels of Psychoactive Drugs

The relationship between clinical improvement and blood levels of antidepressants was discussed earlier.

The relationship between behavioral response to haloperidol and its serum levels was investigated in infantile autism. In twenty-eight autistic children, ages two years and ten months to six years and eleven months, a significant relationship was found between a reduction of stereotypies and lessening of withdrawal and of the levels of haloperidol in serum (mean 3.025 ng/ml). [53] Serum level and dosage (haloperidol, mean dosage 1.0 mg/day) revealed no association. By way of contrast, in the case of methylphenidate, plasma levels are significantly associated with dosage[70] but fail to differentiate responders from nonresponders.[38]

At the present time, the only two clinical situations for which routine monitoring of drug levels in blood is recommended are (1) the measuring of plasma levels of antidepressant in children with major depression and (2) the careful monitoring of serum lithium levels, which was discussed earlier.

For a comprehensive review of this topic, an article by Gualtieri and associates is recommended.[39]

Short- and Long-term Safety of Psychoactive Drugs

There are recently published studies and review articles addressing the issues of safety with psychoactive drugs (haloperidol*; lithium[11,18,48,60]; pemoline[24]) and chapters summarizing the literature.[17,34,42] Of particular concern are the adverse effects associated with long-term administration of psychoactive drugs. This can be evaluated in terms of the impact of these agents on growth and on the development of abnormal movements. There has been a controversy over the effects of psychomotor stimulants on height and weight[63] (for a critical review of evidence, see Roche and associates[62]). Mattes and Gittelman[47] conducted a longitudinal study of eighty-six hyperactive children, who received methylphenidate (average daily dose 40 mg) for up to four years. After one year, the children's height percentiles based on the National Center for Health Statistics (NCHS) Growth Charts[41] showed a 1.4 percentile decrease (nonsignificant). After four years there was an 18.1 percentile decrease in height ($p < 0.001$). There was also a significant decrease in weight percentile ($p < 0.001$) during these four years. In a subgroup of thirty-four children, the addition of thioridazine hydrochloride did not influence the adverse effect of methylphenidate on growth. Thus stimulants given in moderate to high doses may have an adverse effect on growth.[62]

There are reports on both short- and long-term effects of neuroleptics on growth. In two well-designed studies, involving a total of seventy-six preschool-age autistic children, haloperidol (in daily doses of 0.5 to 3.0 mg/day) had no significant effect on linear growth or weight when administered over four to eight weeks cumulatively, and when compared to placebo.[33]

In a prospective study involving forty-two autistic children, haloperidol administration over a period of

six months resulted in a significant increase in weight (8.2 percentile, $p < 0.05$).[33] There was no significant change in height percentile, as measured by NCHS Growth Charts.[41] The subjects, whose ages ranged from 2.0 to 7.6 years, received haloperidol in daily doses ranging from 0.5 to 3.0 mg. Further studies are required in order to make a definitive statement on the effect of prolonged neuroleptic administration on these parameters. There are two reports based on small patient samples, ranging from eight[35] to twenty[28] children. They indicate that this class of drugs does not affect adversely height and weight when given over a period of one and up to six years.

The appearance of tics was reported to be associated with administration of stimulants to children with attention deficit disorder (ADD). In a sample of 1,520 such children, treated with methylphenidate, fourteen (0.92 percent) developed tics de novo, and in six (0.39 percent) there was worsening of preexisting tics.[26] Of one hundred children who were evaluated for Tourette's syndrome, in fifteen the symptoms of this disorder were associated with stimulant (methylphenidate, dextroamphetamine, and/or pemoline) treatment for ADD.[46] Others suggest children who develop tics while receiving stimulants probably have a genetic predisposition and would have developed tics with no medication,[21] and that stimulants probably do not significantly accelerate the onset of Tourette's disorder.[64]

The reported prevalence of neuroleptic-induced tardive and withdrawal dyskinesias ranges from 0.5 to 67.6 percent in adult psychiatric patients (for review, see Berger and Rexroth[4] and Gardos and Cole[29]). In children, retrospective studies suggest the prevalence ranges from 8 to 51 percent (for review, see Campbell et al.[15]). In a carefully conducted prospective study involving fifty-eight autistic children, the prevalence rate was 22 percent.[16,49] The latter study underscores the need to attempt to differentiate (1) stereotypies from tardive dyskinesias, (2) stereotypies that were suppressed by neuroleptic administration and that reemerge after neuroleptic withdrawal from withdrawal dyskinesias, and (3) neuroleptic-related dyskinesias from "abnormal" movements seen in normal children.[16,49] The topography of neuroleptic-related dyskinesias is the same in children as in adults: the buccolingual area is most frequently involved[16,37,40,49] (though not all reports are in agreement[54]). The duration of movements varies: In a sample of thirteen children, the movements ceased in as few as sixteen days and, in all cases,[49] by nine months. In ten of the thirteen children, the movements remitted spontaneously, and in the remaining three children, the movements ceased upon the reinstitution of haloperidol. The children who developed movements were receiving haloperidol over a period of time extending from 3.5

*See references 2, 12, 15, 17, and 30.

months to 42.5 months, cumulatively. At the time the movements developed, their daily doses ranged from 0.5 mg to 7.5 mg (0.02–0.16 mg/kg).

It is recommended that neuroleptics be prescribed judiciously, and only when benefits outweigh the risks of developing neuroleptic-induced dyskinesias. Once a child develops dyskinesias, neuroleptic administration should be withheld, if clinically possible.

ACKNOWLEDGMENT

Dr. Campbell's work was supported in part by NIMH Grants MH–32212 and MH–40177; by a grant from Stallone Fund for Autism Research; and aided by Social and Behavioral Sciences Research Grant No. 12–108 from the March of Dimes Birth Defects Foundation.

REFERENCES

1. AMERICAN PSYCHIATRIC ASSOCIATION. *Diagnostic and Statistical Manual of Mental Disorders,* 3rd ed. (DSM-III). Washington, D.C.: American Psychiatric Association, 1980.

2. ANDERSON, L. T., et al. "Haloperidol in the Treatment of Infantile Autism: Effects on Learning and Behavioral Symptoms," *American Journal of Psychiatry,* 141 (1984): 1195–1202.

3. BENNETT, W. G., et al. "EEG and Treatment of Hospitalized Aggressive Children with Haloperidol or Lithium," *Biological Psychiatry,* 18 (1983):1427–1440.

4. BERGER, P. A., and REXROTH, K. "Tardive Dyskinesia: Clinical, Biological, and Pharmacological Perspectives," *Schizophrenia Bulletin,* 6 (1980):102–116.

5. BOGOMOLNY, A., ERENBERG, G., and ROTHNER, A. D. "Behavioral Effects of Haloperidol in Young Tourette Syndrome Patients," in A. J. Friedhoff and T. N. Chase, eds., *Advances in Neurology,* vol. 35, *Gilles de la Tourette Syndrome.* New York: Raven Press, 1982, pp. 427–432.

6. BORISON, R. L., et al. "New Pharmacological Approaches in the Treatment of Tourette Syndrome," in A. J. Friedhoff and T. N. Chase, eds., *Advances in Neurology,* vol. 35, *Gilles de la Tourette Syndrome.* New York: Raven Press, 1982, pp. 377–382.

7. BRUUN, R. D. "Clonidine Treatment of Tourette Syndrome," in A. J. Friedhoff and T. N. Chase, eds., *Advances in Neurology,* vol. 35, *Gilles de la Tourette Syndrome.* New York: Raven Press, 1982, pp. 403–405.

8. CAMPBELL, M., COHEN, I. L., and PERRY, R. "Psychopharmacological Treatment," in T. H. Ollendick and M. Hersen, eds., *Handbook of Child Psychopathology.* New York: Plenum Press, 1983, pp. 461–484.

9. CAMPBELL, M., COHEN, I. L., and SMALL, A. M. "Drugs in Aggressive Behavior," *Journal of the American Academy of Child Psychiatry,* 21 (1982):107–117.

10. CAMPBELL, M., GREEN, W. H., and DEUTSCH, S. I. *Child and Adolescent Psychopharmacology.* Beverly Hills, Calif.: Sage Publications, 1985.

11. CAMPBELL, M., PERRY, R., and GREEN, W. H. "Use of Lithium in Children and Adolescents," *Psychosomatics,* 25 (1984):95–106.

12. CAMPBELL, M., SCHULMAN, D., and RAPOPORT, J. L. "The Current Status of Lithium Therapy in Child and Adolescent Psychiatry," *Journal of the American Academy of Child Psychiatry,* 17 (1978):717.

13. CAMPBELL, M., et al. "The Effects of Haloperidol on Learning and Behavior in Autistic Children," *Journal of Autism and Developmental Disorders,* 12 (1982):167–175.

14. CAMPBELL, M., et al. "Haloperidol in Autistic Children: Effects on Learning, Behavior, and Abnormal Involuntary Movements," *Psychopharmacology Bulletin,* 18 (1982): 110–112.

15. CAMPBELL, M., et al. "Long-term Therapeutic Efficacy and Drug-Related Abnormal Movements: A Prospective Study of Haloperidol in Autistic Children," *Psychopharmacology Bulletin,* 19 (1983):80–83.

16. CAMPBELL, M., et al. "Neuroleptic-Induced Dyskinesias in Children," *Clinical Neuropharmacology,* 6 (1983): 207–222.

17. CAMPBELL, M., et al. "Pharmacotherapy," in C. E. Walker and M. C. Roberts, eds., *Handbook on Clinical Child Psychology.* New York: John Wiley & Sons, 1983, pp. 1109–1130.

18. CAMPBELL, M., et al. "Behavioral Efficacy of Haloperidol and Lithium Carbonate," *Archives of General Psychiatry,* 41 (1984):650–656.

19. CARLSON, G. A., and CANTWELL, D. P. "Diagnosis of Childhood Depression: A Comparison of the Weinberg and DSM-III Criteria," *Journal of the American Academy of Child Psychiatry,* 21 (1982):247–250.

20. CHAMBERS, W. J., et al. "Psychotic Symptoms in Prepubertal Major Depressive Disorder," *Archives of General Psychiatry,* 39 (1982):921–927.

21. COMINGS, D. E., and COMINGS, B. G. "Tourette's Syndrome and Attention Deficit Disorder with Hyperactivity: Are They Genetically Related?" *Journal of the American Academy of Child Psychiatry,* 23 (1984):138–146.

22. CONNERS, C. K. *Food Additives and Hyperactive Children.* New York: Plenum Press, 1980.

23. CONNERS, C. K. and PETTI, T. "Imipramine Therapy of Depressed Children: Methodologic Considerations," *Psychopharmacology Bulletin,* 19 (1983):65–69.

24. CONNERS, C. K., and TAYLOR, F. "Pemoline, Methylphenidate and Placebo in Children with Minimal Brain Dysfunction," *Archives of General Psychiatry,* 37 (1980):922–930.

25. CONNERS, C. K., and WERRY, J. S. "Pharmacotherapy," in H. C. Quay and J. S. Werry, eds., *Psychopathological Disorders of Childhood,* 2nd ed. New York: John Wiley & Sons, 1979, pp. 336–386.

26. DENCKLA, M. B., BEMPORAD, J. R., and MACKAY, M. C. "Tics Following Methylphenidate Administration," *Journal of the American Medical Association,* 235 (1976):1349–1351.

27. DENNY, F. W., et al. "Defined Diets and Childhood Hyperactivity, Consensus Conference," *Journal of the American Medical Association,* 248 (1982):290–292.

28. ENGELHARDT, D. M., and POLIZOS, P. "Adverse Effects of Pharmacotherapy in Childhood Psychosis," in M. A. Lipton, A. DiMascio, and K. F. Killam, eds., *Psycho-*

pharmacology: A Generation of Progress. New York: Raven Press, 1978, pp. 1463–1469.

29. GARDOS, G., and COLE, J. O. "Overview: Public Health Issues in Tardive Dyskinesia," *American Journal of Psychiatry,* 137 (1980):776–781.

30. GELLER, B., et al. "Nortriptyline in Major Depressive Disorder in Children: Response, Steady-State Plasma Levels, Predictive Kinetics and Pharmacokinetics," *Psychopharmacology Bulletin,* 19 (1983):62–65.

31. GELLER, E., et al. "Preliminary Observations on the Effect of Fenfluramine on Blood Serotonin and Symptoms in Three Autistic Boys," *New England Journal of Medicine,* 307 (1982):165–169.

32. GITTELMAN-KLEIN, R., SPITZER, R. L., and CANTWELL, D. P. "Diagnostic Classification and Psychopharmacological Indications," in J. S. Werry, ed., *Pediatric Psychopharmacology.* New York: Brunner/Mazel, 1978, pp. 136–167.

33. GREEN, W. H., et al. "Effects of Short- and Long-term Haloperidol Administration on Growth in Young Autistic Children," Paper presented at the 31st annual meeting of the American Academy of Child Psychiatry, Toronto, October 10–14, 1984.

34. GREEN, W. H., et al. "Neuropsychopharmacology of the Childhood Psychoses: A Critical Review," in D. W. Morgan, ed., *Psychopharmacology: Impact on Clinical Psychiatry.* St. Louis: Ishiyaku EuroAmerica, 1985, pp. 139–173.

35. GREENHILL, L. L., et al. "Growth Hormone, Prolactin, and Growth Responses in Hyperkinetic Males Treated with D-Amphetamine," *Journal of the American Academy of Child Psychiatry,* 20 (1981):84–103.

36. GREENHILL, L. L., et al. "Molindone Hydrochloride in the Treatment of Aggressive, Hospitalized Children," *Psychopharmacology Bulletin,* 17 (1981):125–127.

37. GUALTIERI, C. T., ct al. "Tardivc Dyskincsia and Other Movement Disorders in Children Treated with Psychotropic Drugs," *Journal of the American Academy of Child Psychiatry,* 19 (1980):491–510.

38. GUALTIERI, C. T., et al. "Clinical Studies of the Methylphenidate Serum Levels in Children and Adults," *Journal of the American Academy of Child Psychiatry,* 21 (1982): 19–26.

39. GUALTIERI, C. T., et al. "Blood Level Measurement of Psychoactive Drugs in Pediatric Psychiatry," *Therapeutic Drug Monitoring,* 6 (1984):127–141.

40. GUALTIERI, C. T., et al. "Tardive Dyskinesia and Other Clinical Consequences of Neuroleptic Treatment in Children and Adolescents," *American Journal of Psychiatry,* 141 (1984):20–23.

41. HAMILL, P. V. V., et al. *N.C.H.S. Growth Charts, 1976.* Monthly Vital Statistics Report, Health Examination Survey Data, National Center for Health Statistics Publication (HRA) 76–1120, vol. 25, Suppl. 3, 1976, pp. 1–22.

42. KLEIN, D. F., et al. *Diagnosis and Drug Treatment of Psychiatric Disorders: Adults and Children,* 2nd ed. Baltimore: Williams & Wilkins, 1980.

43. KOVACS, M., et al. "Depressive Disorders in Childhood: I. A Longitudinal Prospective Study of Characteristics and Recovery," *Archives of General Psychiatry,* 41 (1984): 229–237.

44. KOVACS, M., et al. "Depressive Disorders in Childhood: II. A Longitudinal Study of the Risk for a Subsequent Major Depression," *Archives of General Psychiatry,* 41 (1984):643–649.

45. LECKMAN, J. F., et al. "Clonidine in the Treatment of Tourette Syndrome: A Review of Data," in A. J. Friedhoff and T. N. Chase, eds., *Advances in Neurology,* vol. 35, *Gilles*

de la Tourette Syndrome. New York: Raven Press, 1982, pp. 391–401.

46. LOWE, T. L., et al. "Stimulant Medications Precipitate Tourette's Syndrome," *Journal of the American Medical Association,* 247 (1982):1729–1731.

47. MATTES, J. A., and GITTELMAN, R. "Growth of Hyperactive Children on Maintenance Regimen of Methylphenidate," *Archives of General Psychiatry,* 40 (1983):317–321.

48. PERRY, R., et al. "Saliva Lithium Levels in Children: Their Use in Monitoring Serum Lithium Levels and Lithium Side Effects," *Journal of Clinical Psychopharmacology,* 4 (1984):199–202.

49. PERRY, R., et al. "Neuroleptic-Related Dyskinesias in Autistic Children: A Prospective Study," *Psychopharmacology Bulletin,* 21 (1985):140–143.

50. PETTI, T. A., et al. "Effects of Chlordiazepoxide in Disturbed Children: A Pilot Study," *Journal of Clinical Psychopharmacology,* 2 (1982):270–273.

51. "Pimozide Approved for Tourette's Syndrome," *FDA Drug Bulletin,* 14 (1984):24–25.

52. PLATT, J. E., et al. "Cognitive Effects of Lithium Carbonate and Haloperidol in Treatment-Resistant Aggressive Children," *Archives of General Psychiatry,* 41 (1984):657–662.

53. POLAND, R. E., et al. "Relationship of Serum Haloperidol Levels and Clinical Response in Autistic Children," *Abstracts of the 13th CINP Congress* (Jerusalem, Israel), vol. 2, June 20–25, 1982, p. 591.

54. POLIZOS, P., and ENGELHARDT, D. M. "Dyskinetic and Neurological Complications in Children Treated with Psychotropic Medication," in W. E. Fann, et al., eds., *Tardive Dyskinesia. Research and Treatment.* Jamaica, N.Y.: Spectrum Publicatons, 1980, pp. 193–199.

55. PUIG-ANTICH, J. "Affective Disorders in Childhood: A Review and Perspective," *Psychiatric Clinics of North America,* 3 (1980):403–424.

56. ———. "Childhood Affective Disorders," Paper presented at the Psychopharmacology Update in Childhood Disorders, Course 32, American Psychiatric Association, 136th annual meeting, New York, April 30–May 6, 1983.

57. PUIG-ANTICH, J., et al. "Plasma Levels of Imipramine (IMI) and Desmethylimipramine (DMI) and Clinical Response in Prepubertal Major Depressive Disorder: A Preliminary Report," *Journal of the American Academy of Child Psychiatry,* 18 (1979):616–627.

58. PUIG-ANTICH, J., et al. "Imipramine Effectiveness in Prepubertal Major Depressive Disorders I. Relationship of Plasma Levels to Clinical Response of the Depressive Syndrome," *Archives of General Psychiatry,* in press.

59. RAPOPORT, J. L., and ISMOND, D. R. *DSM-III Training Guide for Diagnosis of Childhood Disorders.* New York: Brunner/Mazel, 1984.

60. REISBERG, B., and GERSHON, S. "Side Effects Associated with Lithium Therapy," *Archives of General Psychiatry,* 36 (1979):879–887.

61. RITVO, Æ. R., et al. "Effects of Fenfluramine on 14 Outpatients with the Syndrome of Autism," *Journal of the American Academy of Child Psychiatry,* 22 (1983):549–558.

62. ROCHE, A. F., et al. "The Effects of Stimulant Medication on the Growth of Hyperkinetic Children," *Pediatrics,* 63 (1979):847–850.

63. SATTERFIELD, J. H., et al. "Growth of Hyperactive Children Treated with Methylphenidate," *Archives of General Psychiatry,* 36 (1979):212–217.

64. SHAPIRO, A. K., and SHAPIRO, E. "Do Stimulants Provoke, Cause or Exacerbate Tics and Tourette's Syndrome?" *Comprehensive Psychiatry,* 22 (1981):265–273.

65. ———. "Clinical Efficacy of Haloperidol, Pimozide,

Penfluridol, and Clonidine in the Treatment of Tourette Syndrome," in A. J. Friedhoff and T. N. Chase, eds., *Advances in Neurology,* vol. 35, *Gilles de la Tourette Syndrome.* New York: Raven Press, 1982, pp. 383–390.

66. TURNER, D. A., et al. "Intensive Design in Evaluating Anxiolytic Agents," in F. G. McMahon, ed., *Principles and Techniques of Human Research and Therapeutics,* vol. 7, *Psychopharmacological Agents,* ed. J. Levine, B. C. Schiele, and W. J. R. Taylor. Mt. Kisco, N.Y.: Futura Publishing Company, 1975, pp. 105–118.

67. WEISS, G., et al. "Hyperactives as Young Adults. A Controlled Prospective Ten-Year Follow-up of 75 Children," *Archives of General Psychiatry,* 36 (1979):675–681.

68. WELLER, E. B., et al. "Childhood Depression: Imipramine Levels and Response," *Psychopharmacology Bulletin,* 19 (1983):59–62.

69. WERRY, J. S., and AMAN, M. G. "Methylphenidate and Haloperidol in Children," *Archives of General Psychiatry,* 32 (1975):790–795.

70. WINSBERG, B. G., et al. "Methylphenidate Oral Dose Plasma Concentrations and Behavioral Response in Children," *Psychopharmacology,* 76 (1982):329–332.

43 / Advances in Child Behavior Therapy

Alan E. Kazdin

During the last several years there has been a tremendous amount of activity within the field of child behavior therapy. Numerous intervention techniques, clinical problems, and settings have been investigated.[18,20] Controlled outcome research is currently available for many clinical problems, including hyperactivity, anxiety disorders, social skills deficits, antisocial behavior and delinquency, habit disorders, autism, mental retardation, and a variety of physical illnesses and health-related problems.[5,14] The literature is vast in part because individual clinical problems may respond to different treatment techniques, each of which has its own literature. Treatments are based on variations of reinforcement, punishment, modeling, systematic desensitization, rehearsal, cognitive therapies, self-control strategies, and others. Moreover, these treatments have been applied in many different settings, including the home, school, group living arrangements, institutions, and the community at large. The diversity of child behavior therapy, the breadth of applications, and the scope of outcome research preclude covering the field in depth in anything less than a separate handbook.[5]

Although child behavior therapy encompasses a number of clinical techniques, these techniques do not define the field. Child behavior therapy is an *approach* toward treatment and an *evaluation* of therapeutic change. The central characteristic is an empirical approach toward the investigation of clinical problems and therapy techniques. There is no single substantive position, etiological view, narrow set of techniques, or codified series of propositions that encapsulates the field.[11] Consequently, the scope of the field is extraordinarily broad and includes many different, and often competing, conceptual views and treatment techniques; these in turn are applied to the full gamut of problems seen in clinical settings. The purpose of this chapter is to identify the characteristics of child behavior therapy, to illustrate the range of conceptual views and treatment approaches, and to discuss recent advances in identifying which treatments are effective. Along with describing advances in outcome research, the chapter discusses issues and limitations raised by current research.

Characteristics of Child Behavior Therapy

Few characteristics can be identified that uniformly encompass all of the conceptual views, clinical techniques, or treatment foci of child behavior therapy.[16] Nevertheless, as a whole, several features convey why child behavior therapy can be delineated meaningfully as a unique approach toward the treatment of childhood disorders.

CONCEPTUAL VIEWS

Child behavior therapy draws heavily from diverse conceptual models regarding the bases for behavior and therapeutic change. At the most general level, abnormal child behavior is assumed to be on a continuum with normal behavior. Thus the task for behavior therapy is to understand behavior per se and the factors that account for its emergence, maintenance, and alteration. Within the context of behavior therapy, of course, knowledge of these factors is ultimately applied toward therapeutic ends.

For expository purposes, current views of behavior can be cast generally as *mediational* and *nonmediational*. Nonmediational views focus on the direct connections between environmental or situational events and behaviors. Operant conditioning, which views behavior as a function of its consequences, represents a nonmediational view. Child behavior problems can be viewed as deficits or excesses in performance that can be altered directly through the application of antecedent and consequent (e.g., rewarding and punishing) events. In contrast, mediational views emphasize the cognitive underpinnings of behavior. Environmental events influence behavior according to mediational views, but these events are processed by the child whose perceptions, plans, goals, beliefs, expectations, self-statements, and attributions influence how given events produce their effects. Indeed, it is largely the cognitive processes that imbue an event with meaning and determine its impact.

The dominant view within child behavior therapy can be referred to as a *social learning theory* of behavior. Social learning theory reflects a broad orientation that recognizes the importance of both cognitive and environmental influences and their reciprocal interaction.[2] Primacy has been given to cognitive processes as the underlying basis for the acquisition and persistence of behavior. But within the field, the primacy of cognitive mechanisms is by no means universally endorsed.

PRIMACY OF BEHAVIOR

Within child behavior therapy, overt behavior plays a major part in the assessment and treatment of clinical dysfunction. Whenever possible, clinical problems are operationalized in terms of overt behavioral referents. Children's symptoms, syndromes, and disorders, such as childhood fear and avoidance, enuresis, autism, depression, and others, are conceptualized primarily as problems in behavior. This does not mean that problems are viewed solely in terms of overt actions. Many clinical problems encompass subjective experience and psychophysiological concomitants, as, for example, in anxiety or affective disorders. However, the main basis for seeking treatment, identifying the treatment focus, and evaluating treatment outcomes is considered to be overt behavior.

Typically, evaluation of child behavior therapy relies on multiple assessment methods. Self-report, observed

behavior, psychophysiological responses, and other modalities are all regarded relevant to the problem.[17] Overt behavior is usually emphasized, especially samples of performance that reflect the child's functioning in everyday situations. For example, it may be important to show that after treatment, children with attention deficit disorder have become less impulsive on laboratory measures. However, the major criterion to evaluate the impact of treatment is the effect on performance in the situations (e.g., at school and at home) in which behavior was initially identified as problematic.

USE OF PARAPROFESSIONALS

Some types of behavioral treatment involve meeting with children in individual therapy sessions, in a fashion similar to that of traditional models of treatment. More commonly, however, therapy involves working directly with and training those persons who are responsible for the care, management, and education of children. Within child behavior therapy, parents and teachers in particular frequently serve as the agents of change.[14]

Several different factors have pointed to the need to train those who are in contact with children. First, parents, teachers, institutional staff, and peers unwittingly encourage and support many of the problem behaviors identified as worthy of intervention (e.g., obstinancy, tantrums, antisocial behavior).[19] Hence, changing the behaviors of those in contact with the child is often a prerequisite for effective treatment. Second, treatment effects often can be more readily accomplished in the naturalistic setting than in the therapist's office. Parents and teachers have immediate access to the problems as they occur; if suitably trained, they can bring to bear potent events (e.g., their own attention and affection) to promote prosocial behavior. Third, behavioral problems are often situation specific. For example, a child who is disruptive at home may not be so at school or vice versa. Consequently, it is advantageous when treatments are designed for and implemented in those situations in which behavior is problematic. When treatment is conducted in a special setting (e.g., day treatment or inpatient service), the attempt is made to encourage extension of the treatment outside of settings where the behaviors ultimately need to be performed.

DIRECTIVE AND ACTIVE TREATMENT PRESCRIPTIONS

A common feature among child behavior therapy techniques is the use of directive and active treatment prescriptions. Treatments provide prescriptions about what children and/or their caretakers need to do to produce therapeutic change. Behavioral techniques do not rely heavily on such therapeutic processes as catharsis, insight, the therapeutic relationship, and attributional processes. To be sure, during the course of therapy any of these processes might be important and contribute specific beneficial effects. Yet such processes are not viewed as carrying the major burden of producing change in the problem behaviors. Rather, explicit training experiences are prescribed in treatment. Therapy sessions are frequently used as the context in which actions for change are planned and often rehearsed.

The treatment model for many child behavior therapy techniques is that the child or persons who are responsible for his or her care must do something (behave) differently to develop the desired behaviors. Characteristically, extensive opportunities for rehearsal and practice are included as part of treatment. Alternatively, or additionally, opportunities to provide consequences for performance of the desired responses are arranged in everyday situations. Therapeutic change is conceptualized as learning new behaviors that are to be performed in the natural environment.

SCOPE OF TREATMENT APPLICATIONS

As noted, the range of childhood problems and intervention techniques encompassed by child behavior therapy is vast. In addition to the usual clinical problems seen by mental health professionals, child behavior techniques have been extended widely to education and special education, rehabilitation of mentally retarded and disabled populations, and pediatrics. To sample the range of techniques, diverse conceptual positions, and the empirical approach of the field, two major techniques for the treatment of conduct problems will be illustrated.

Treatment of Conduct Problems: Selected Techniques

The term conduct problems generally refers to children who act out and evince aggressive or oppositional behaviors, tantrums, excessive whining, teasing, arguing, and so on. Such behaviors obviously can vary in severity from mild forms, which try the patience of parents and teachers in the average home or classroom, to those severely aggressive behaviors that can lead to serious injury. In the *Diagnostic and Statistical Manual of Mental Disorders* (DSM-III), these conduct problems usually encompass the symptoms delineated

by oppositional (313.81) and conduct disorders (312.00).[1] Many different behavior therapy techniques have been developed to treat oppositional and aggressive behavior, including parent management training, cognitively based treatment, operant conditioning, social skills training, and others.[15] Two of these are discussed in the next sections to convey the general approach, conceptual diversity, and recent advances within the field.

PARENT MANAGEMENT TRAINING

Background and Underlying Rationale. Parent management training refers to procedures that train parents to alter their child's behavior in the home. The parents meet with a therapist or trainer who teaches them to use specific procedures to alter their interactions with their child, to promote prosocial behavior, and to decrease deviant behavior. Training is based on the general view that conduct problem behavior is inadvertently developed and sustained in the home by maladaptive child-parent interactions. By altering these interaction patterns, antisocial child behavior can be decreased.

Patterson[19] has developed a theoretical framework, referred to as *coercion theory,* and has provided supporting research to explain specific interaction patterns that lead to the development of antisocial behavior in the home. Coercion is defined as a type of interpersonal interaction in which deviant behavior of one person (e.g., the child) is supported or directly reinforced by the other person (e.g., the parent). The notion of coercion is designed to explain a particular type of interaction pattern often referred to as a reinforcement trap. Deviant behavior performed by a child directed toward a parent—usually the mother—may be reinforced (rewarded) when the parent gives in or complies. The "trap" is that while parents may yield in an effort to stop the child's aversive behavior at that time (e.g., tantrum), in doing so, they inadvertently increase the likelihood that the behavior will recur in the future.

From the child's perspective, *positive reinforcement* —that is, compliance on the part of the parent—has been provided for aversive behavior. Thus the aversive behavior is likely to increase in the future. From the standpoint of the parent, *negative reinforcement* is operative. The aversive behavior of the child terminated when the parent complied with the request. Termination of the aversive event increases the likelihood that the parent will comply in the future. The fact that aversive child behavior will increase in the long run does not decrease the parent's compliance with the child's demands because compliance is successful in terminating the child's aversive behavior in the short run.

The critical feature of coercion theory and its supporting research, which are detailed in Patterson's book,[19] is that the findings have served as the basis for developing an effective treatment, namely, parent management training. The general purpose of this training is to alter the pattern of interchanges between parent and child so that prosocial rather than coercive behavior is directly reinforced and supported within the family. Because parents of aggressive children are less effective in their parenting skills than parents of normal children, family interaction can serve as the vehicle for altering child behavior.

Characteristics of Treatment. The most obvious characteristic of parent management training is that treatment is achieved primarily through the parents, who directly implement several procedures they learn in therapy. The child may be seen as part of an initial interview or observed while interacting with the parents at the clinic or in the home. However, as a rule, the therapist does not intervene directly with the child. A second feature is that training usually includes didactic instruction in social learning principles. These principles include concepts from operant conditioning such as reinforcement, punishment, and extinction as they apply to social interaction in the home and everyday situations. Third, parents are trained to identify, define, and observe problem behavior in new ways. The identification and definition of problem behavior are based on precise descriptions of behavioral problems in terms that are as objective as possible. The careful specification of the problem is essential for the delivery of reinforcing or punishing consequences for concrete behaviors and for evaluating if the program is working. Fourth, the treatment sessions cover the concepts and procedures of several content areas. Considerable time is devoted to positive reinforcement in which the use of social praise, attention, and tokens or points following prosocial behavior are incorporated in the program. Punishment is covered also, especially the use of time out from reinforcement, loss of privileges, and loss of tokens. The emphasis is on training parents how to apply procedures consistently in the home. Fifth, the sessions provide opportunities for parents to see how the techniques are implemented and to practice using the techniques. To develop parental skills, the therapist uses instructions, modeling, role playing, and rehearsal. Also, treatment sessions usually review the behavior-change program that has been implemented in the home over the course of the previous week.

The immediate goal of the program is to develop specific skills in the parents. This is usually achieved by having parents apply their skills initially to relatively simple behaviors that can be observed easily and that are not enmeshed with more provoking interactions (e.g., punishment, battles of the will, coercive inter-

changes). Another initial purpose is to help parents reestablish control over child behavior in the home. As the parents become more proficient, the focus of the program can address the child's more severely problematic behaviors and encompass other problem areas such as school behavior.

Efficacy of Treatment. Parent management training has been evaluated in hundreds of outcome studies with behavior-problem children varying in age and severity of dysfunction. The work of Patterson and his colleagues, which has spanned almost two decades, exemplifies the outcome research on parent training. Over two hundred families have been seen; their children are primarily aggressive, ages three to twelve years, referred for outpatient treatment.[19] The effectiveness of treatment has been evaluated by parental and teacher reports of deviant behavior as well as by direct observation of child behavior at home and at school. Several studies have demonstrated marked changes over the course of treatment and have shown that the changes surpass those achieved with variations of family-based psychotherapy, control conditions designed to rule out patient expectancies and contact with the therapist, and changes without intervening treatment.[15] Follow-up assessment has shown that the gains are often maintained one year after treatment, a finding that has been replicated several times.

The effects of parent management training apparently extend beyond the child referred for treatment. Deviant behaviors of siblings, who are at risk for conduct disorder, improve as well, even though siblings are not a direct focus of treatment. In addition, maternal psychopathology, particularly depression, has been shown to decrease systematically following parent management training. These changes suggest that a behavioral focus on family interaction patterns can affect multiple aspects of dysfunctional families.

COGNITIVE (PROBLEM-SOLVING) THERAPY

Background and Underlying Rationale. Cognitive therapy focuses on the cognitive processes that are presumed to underlie the child's maladaptive behavior. The child's cognitive processes that serve as the focus of change may include perceptions, self-statements, attributions, expectations, strategies, and problem-solving skills. The assumption of cognitive therapy is that children with deviant behavior suffer a deficiency in particular processes or an inability to use or apply cognitive skills. The relationship between cognitive processes and behavioral adjustment has been evaluated extensively by Spivack, Platt, and Shure.[23] These investigators have identified cognitive processes or interpersonal cognitive problem-solving skills that underlie social behavior. These processes, presented in table 43–1, are assessed by presenting the child with hypothetical interpersonal problems (e.g., getting one's toy back from a sibling, entering a game that one's peers are already playing) and asking the child how many different ways the goal could be achieved, the consequences of particular actions, and so on.

Ability to engage in these problem-solving steps is related to behavioral adjustment, as measured in teacher ratings of acting-out behavior and social withdrawal in children. Disturbed children tend to generate fewer alternative solutions to interpersonal problems, to focus on ends or goals rather than on the intermediate steps to obtain them, to see fewer consequences associated with their behavior, to fail to recognize the causes of other people's behavior, and to be less sensitive to interpersonal conflict arising in the behaviors of others.[23] Several studies have shown that deficits in problem-solving skills and the relation of these deficits to maladaptive behavior cannot be accounted for by other variables such as socioeconomic class, child intel-ligence, gender, or ability to comprehend social situations.[23]

Characteristics of Treatment. Cognitive therapy for conduct-problem children has several characteristics. First, the emphasis is on *how* the child approaches situations. Although it is obviously important that the child ultimately select appropriate means of behaving in everyday life, the primary focus is on the thought *processes* rather than on the *outcome* or behavioral acts that result. For example, the approach may be conveyed by presenting the child with a task involving confrontation of another individual, say, procuring the return of a toy from a sibling or peer. The focus of the training is to help the child develop the cognitive processes that will generate alternative solutions to the problem rather than merely engaging in concrete behaviors to obtain the toy. Of course, process and outcome are quite related. Indeed, the focus of treatment is precisely on the underlying cognitive processes so that socially acceptable and effective solutions to interpersonal problems can be identified. If the child masters the process of problem solving, he or she is likely to be equipped to handle diverse situations that arise.

Second, the treatment attempts to teach the child to engage in a step-by-step approach to solve problems. The method is usually achieved by having the child make statements to himself or herself (self-instructions) that direct attention to certain aspects of the problem or tasks that lead to effective solutions. The statements may include: (1) What is my problem? (2) What am I supposed to do? (3) What is my plan? and (4) How do I do it? After each question, the child states the answer to himself or herself and thus approaches the particular task or problem in a systematic, step-by-step fashion. The steps help the child generate solutions, identify consequences if different courses of action were selected, sense the feelings of others, and so on.

Third, treatment utilizes structured tasks involving games, academic activities, stories, or, for young children, even puppets. The tasks provide the child with an opportunity to apply the particular processes or steps. Over the course of treatment, specific tasks continue to be used, but they are more likely to consist of vignettes involving real-life interpersonal situations.

Fourth, the therapist usually plays an active role in treatment. He or she models the cognitive processes by making verbal self-statements, applies the series of statements noted earlier to particular problems, provides cues to the child to prompt the use of the skills, and delivers feedback and praise to develop correct use of the skills. Finally, treatment usually involves the combination of several different procedures. These include modeling the use of problem-solving skills, prac-

TABLE 43–1

Interpersonal Cognitive Problem-Solving Skills That Underlie Social Behavior

Process	Definition
1. Alternative Solution Thinking	The ability to generate different options (solutions) that can solve problems in interpersonal situations.
2. Means-ends Thinking	Awareness of the intermediate steps required to achieve a particular goal.
3. Consequential Thinking	The ability to identify what might happen as a direct result of acting out in a particular way or choosing a particular solution.
4. Causal Thinking	The ability to relate one event to another over time and to understand why one event led to a particular action of other persons.
5. Sensitivity to Interpersonal Problems	The ability to perceive a problem when it exists and to identify the interpersonal aspects of the confrontation that may emerge.

tice and role playing, the application of reinforcement and mild punishment (loss of points or tokens), and others. The various techniques that are used in treatment are all directed toward the goal of developing use of the problem-solving and self-instructional steps rather than altering the deviant behaviors directly.

Efficacy of Treatment. Several outcome studies have examined variations of cognitively based therapies with children.[24] For example, research with different age groups has shown that developing interpersonal problem-solving skills improves behavioral adjustment in the classroom and interpersonal attributes such as popularity and likeability.[23] Importantly, they demonstrated a relationship between deficits in specific problem-solving skills and behavioral adjustment at different ages along with a correlation between change in these skills and improvement in adjustment. Few studies have elaborated the factors that contribute to treatment outcome. Different problem-solving skills and the impact of particular skills on behavior are known to vary as a function of age.[23] Both laboratory and treatment studies have suggested that the child's age and stage of cognitive development influence both the extent to which behavior is mediated by self-statements and the content of the statements.[7]

ADVANTAGES OF PARENT TRAINING AND COGNITIVE THERAPY

Parent training and cognitive therapy have been highlighted because they represent promising treatment approaches within child behavior therapy. Moreover, each technique illustrates the general approach of behavior therapy in developing and evaluating treatments. Specifically both treatments: (1) are based on underlying conceptual models about the nature and emergence of deviant child behavior, (2) have provided direct evidence that specific (family or cognitive) processes are in fact related to child adjustment, (3) have specified concrete procedures (in treatment manual form)[6] that can be applied clinically, and (4) have been subjected to rather extensive empirical research. These features are essential for the identification of effective and empirically based treatment techniques.

LIMITATIONS OF PARENT TRAINING AND COGNITIVE THERAPY

At the present time, neither treatment can be said to have demonstrated unequivocally that gains are invariably produced and furthermore that these gains controvert the poor prognosis of antisocial children. The evidence of beneficial effects is greater for parent management training than for cognitive therapy at present, but major questions remain about child and family factors that interact with outcome.

An important issue is the optimal focus of treatment. This is germane to treatment of conduct-disordered children in general and is reflected as well in the two specific treatments just highlighted. Parent management training focuses on family interaction, and cognitive therapy focuses on the child. Yet the child's presenting problem often does not convey the range of problems that may need to be addressed in treatment. Many of the risk factors for antisocial behavior (e.g., parent psychopathology, marital discord) often reflect current dimensions that impact directly on clinical management and the implementation and feasibility of treatment. Thus even if parent management training is an effective treatment for conduct disorders, it might not be applicable in a large proportion of cases because of the chaotic family conditions in which the child is enmeshed. Often families are not interested in or in a position to engage in the sort of treatment regimen required by parent management training. Analogously, the value of cognitive therapy may be limited for many children by their severe cognitive deficits and/or by maladaptive cognitive problem-solving skills of their parents that render the treatment difficult to apply or simply ineffective. Work is currently underway to identify those factors that interfere with the feasibility of implementing these procedures.

Recent Advances

PARENT AND FAMILY VARIABLES IN CHILD TREATMENT

While it is not surprising to child mental health professionals that parent and family variables have important impact on child treatment, the unique contribution of child behavior therapy has been to explore many influences empirically and to show how these variables contribute to outcome.

For example, research has examined factors that contribute to parent perception of child deviance. As might be expected, the evidence suggests that perception of child deviance depends heavily on factors other than the child's actual behavior. Parental psychopathology, particulary maternal depression and anxiety, is a strong predictor of how the child's behaviors will be perceived, somewhat independently of what these behaviors actually are.[8]

Once parents are in treatment, family variables have been shown to be important to outcome. For example, investigators have shown that the success of parent management training depends on the social interactions that mothers have outside of the home with relatives and social agencies.[27] An inverse relationship has been found between the number of extrafamilial interactions of mothers and parent-child problems in the home. Moreover, parents with negative interactions outside of the home are less likely to show therapeutic change in parent training or to maintain the gains that have been achieved. Thus in cases where maternal social networks are deficient, parent training alone may not be effective.

RESPONSE COVARIATION

The assessment of childhood problems in behavior therapy has revealed important information about the organization of behavior. Treatment research has demonstrated that the alteration of a given area of performance may have an impact on several other areas of child functioning as well. For example, changing social behavior at home or at school may alter a variety of other behaviors that are seemingly unrelated (e.g., self-stimulation, studying, and others). Moreover, over the course of treatment both increases and decreases occur in concomitant behaviors, some of which would be regarded as desirable and others which would be regarded as undesirable. [14]

For example, in one study ruminative vomiting was eliminated in a three-year-old girl. [4] The behavior was eliminated by suppressing another behavior (lip smacking) that always preceded regurgitation. When rumination decreased, crying decreased and smiling and spontaneous social interaction increased. Stereotypic play with objects and head slapping, however, also increased. Several other studies have carefully shown complex relations between changes in one or more behaviors and other behaviors as well. [12]

Research in child behavior therapy has begun to explore how behaviors are organized by measuring multiple behaviors in children over time and across situations. The work has revealed that behaviors are organized into clusters, or sets of responses that covary. The clusters may vary over time and across situations. For example, in one study children referred for treatment because of highly disruptive behavior were observed over an extended period (approximately three years). [25] Observations were made of several behaviors at home and at school to determine correlations among different classes of behavior. As an illustration, working on assignments at school for one child was positively correlated with engaging in self-stimulatory behaviors and negatively correlated with fiddling with objects, staring into space, and not interacting with others. For this same child, several other behaviors were intercorrelated at home. Specifically, sustained play with toys was inversely associated with compliance with adult instructions, social interactions with adults, and self-stimulation.

Interestingly, altering one behavior in the cluster

leads to systematic changes in other behaviors. For example, in the previous study, changing a specific problem behavior at school affected other behaviors with which that behavior was correlated. Also, changes at school were associated with changes in behaviors at home. Again, the concomitant changes of treatment were neither necessarily desirable nor undesirable from the standpoint of how these changes might be evaluated by parents or mental health professionals. In one case, for example, improvements at school were associated with increases in peer interactions at home and oppositional behavior at school. Thus both desirable and undesirable changes were evident.

In general, behaviors that tend to be negatively correlated with a particular behavior that is increased in frequency tend to decrease; behaviors that tend to be positively correlated with the behavior that is increased tend to increase as well. Thus the direction of change in concomitant behaviors can be predicted by understanding the organization of behavior (i.e., the intercorrelations among different behaviors) before treatment begins.

Research on the covariation of responses has raised both theoretical and practical issues. On the theoretical plane, research has suggested that the clusters of behaviors cannot be explained adequately by existing models of personality and behavior, whether psychoanalytic, trait, or learning theories. [12] Further, those more specific notions that often are proposed to account for broad changes following treatment, such as symptom substitution or generalization, do not explain these data on response covariation. Clinically, response covariation may have important implications. Once the cluster of behaviors is known, impact on a particular behavior can be achieved indirectly. For example, engaging in solitary play is inversely correlated with aggressive behavior in conduct-problem children. Therefore, increasing the frequency of solitary play during one part of the day markedly decreases aggressive behavior at other times. [26] The therapeutic implications of response covariation are only now beginning to be explored.

ASSESSMENT OF TREATMENT OUTCOME

Research in child behavior therapy has become increasingly concerned with evaluating the clinical significance of treatment effects. Clinical significance refers to evidence that changes produced in treatment are not merely statistically significant but also have clear impact on the child's functioning in everyday life. [10] The clinical significance of treatment effects has been evaluated primarily by comparing treated children with peers who are functioning well in everyday life. If behavior of referred children departs from a normative group before treatment and falls within the range of the normative group after treatment, the magnitude of change is often considered to be clinically significant. Essentially, on the dimensions assessed, treatment has moved the patient group to within the realm of acceptable behavior, which is "normal" in more than the statistical sense.

The use of normative data as a basis for judging treatment effects is an extremely important advance in treatment evaluation. The advance is critical in child treatment because normative levels of behavior may vary greatly as a function of the child's developmental stage and chronological age. Normative data provide the necessary baseline to judge initial deviance of the target problem and to measure the impact of treatment in returning children to adaptive levels of functioning.

Current Limitations

DIAGNOSIS OF CHILDHOOD DISORDERS

A major difficulty in child behavior therapy is to evaluate the population to whom treatments are to be addressed. The primary focus of treatment is on relatively isolated presenting problems and circumscribed target behaviors. These behaviors are often assessed with extreme care and methodological sophistication that has little precedence in the child treatment literature. Yet there have been no uniform methods of assessing the whole child in a comprehensive fashion that permit a standard means of communicating their characteristics.

Proponents of behavior modification have eschewed psychiatric diagnosis because of the model of behavior upon which such systems as DSM-I and DSM-II have been based. DSM-III, however, emphasizes descriptive features, and its focus falls on the patient's presenting symptoms rather than on presumed etiologies as the basis for reaching a diagnosis. These features make psychiatric taxonomy more compatible with the orientation of behavior therapists. Nevertheless, DSM-III has yet to be incorporated into descriptions of the children to whom behavioral treatments are applied.[13]

On the other hand, the failure of the behavioral literature to adopt a standard method of defining child populations and assessing the range of their dysfunction (e.g., across multiple axes) introduces ambiguity in evaluating that literature. In most studies, it is impossible to discern important characteristics of the children who have been treated. Until further research begins to adopt standardized methods of describing the populations and the range, severity, and duration of their clinical impairment, there will be difficulty in unambiguously evaluating the impact of treatment and disseminating these treatments to practitioners outside of behavior therapy.

THE FOCUS OF TREATMENT

Child behavior therapy generally focuses on discrete behaviors that define the child's clinical dysfunction. Translation of symptoms into observable behaviors has facilitated the design and implementation of treatment and the assessment of therapeutic change. Yet the primary (and occasionally exclusive) focus on overt behaviors raises potential problems in developing effective treatments.

To begin with, children may present similar overt symptoms but differ considerably in other characteristics that may be quite relevant to the efficacy of alternative treatment procedures. For example, considerable research has been devoted to developing interpersonal skills among socially withdrawn children and adolescents. One of the problems is the failure to examine the bases for social withdrawal before treatment. Children may fail to interact with peers and adults for a variety of reasons, which include lack of interest in social interaction, severe anxiety in interpersonal situations, depression, or genuine deficits in the requisite social skills. It is important to assess these distinctions preparatory to applying social skills training. Training children how to interact with others and directly reinforcing the interaction may vary their beneficial effects as a function of the reasons for the child's social skills deficits. Focusing on concrete target behaviors by itself may yield effective therapeutic techniques; however, long-term treatment effects may be limited by not making diagnostic distinctions among children whose presenting problems may be similar from the standpoint of current behavior.

Similarly, the focus of behavioral treatment is on current child behavior. Here, too, the focus itself cannot be faulted. Yet behavior therapy tends to eschew the relevance of the child's past history, including the duration, severity, and breadth of the presenting problem. Presumably children with longer histories of dysfunction, a larger number of symptoms contributing to the disorder, and more severely dysfunctional behavior will respond less well. An important issue within behavior therapy is the absence of information on these dimensions of dysfunction.[13]

Conclusions

Too often, child behavior therapy is viewed as a singular approach toward treatment or a specific set of treatment intervention techniques. Given the diversity of interpretations of clinical problems and an ever-expanding range of treatments, homogeneity of approaches within child behavior therapy is illusory. Heterogeneity of conceptual views and treatments is not problematic within the field because of the unifying commitment to empirical research. The hallmark of behavior therapy is the commitment to careful assessment of therapeutic change along with an empirical evaluation of treatment outcomes. This characteristic is not to be taken lightly because most of the alternative treatments for children and adults have not been subjected to controlled outcome research,[9,21,22] and progress on empirical research on child psychotherapy continues to be slow.[3]

Many of the techniques currently under investigation in child behavior therapy may not ameliorate a large number of the disorders that children present clinically. At this early stage of development, an important contribution of child behavior therapy is to place the questions of treatment efficacy for childhood disorders firmly in the arena of empirical research. Conceptual approaches and treatment techniques have broadened within behavior therapy. There is increased recognition that narrow views of clinical problems delimit the range of effective techniques that are explored. There is no need to be parochial about the techniques that warrant application as long as there is recognition that the ultimate criterion for advocating a technique needs to be based on demonstrable effectiveness.

ACKNOWLEDGMENT

Completion of this chapter was facilitated by a Research Scientist Development Award (MH00353) from the National Institute of Mental Health.

REFERENCES

1. AMERICAN PSYCHIATRIC ASSOCIATION. *Diagnostic and Statistical Manual of Mental Disorders,* 3rd ed. (DSM-III). Washington, D.C.: American Psychiatric Association, 1980.
2. BANDURA, A. *Social Learning Theory.* Englewood Cliffs, N.J.: Prentice-Hall, 1977.
3. BARRETT, C. L., HAMPE, E., and MILLER, L. "Research on Psychotherapy with Children," in S. L. Garfield and A. E. Bergin, eds., *Handbook of Psychotherapy and Behavior Change: An Empirical Analysis,* 2nd ed. New York: John Wiley & Sons, 1978, pp. 411–435.
4. BECKER, J. V., TURNER, S. M., and SAJWAJ, T. E. "Multiple Behavioral Effects of the Use of Lemon Juice with a Ruminating Toddler-age Child," *Behavior Modification,* 2 (1978):267–278.
5. BORNSTEIN, P. C., and KAZDIN, A. E., eds. *Handbook of Clinical Behavior Therapy with Children.* Homewood, Ill.: Dorsey Press, 1985.
6. CAMP, B. W., and BASH, M. S. *Think Aloud Program: Group Manual.* Champaign, Ill.: Research Press, 1980.
7. COLE, P. M., and KAZDIN, A. E. "Critical Issues in Self-instruction Training with Children," *Child Behavior Therapy,* 2 (1980):1–23.
8. GRIEST, D. L., and WELLS, K. C. "Behavioral Family Therapy with Conduct Disorders in Children," *Behavior Therapy,* 14 (1983):37–53.
9. HERINK, R., ed. *The Psychotherapy Handbook.* New York: New American Library, 1980.
10. KAZDIN, A. E. "Assessing the Clinical or Applied Significance of Behavior Change Through Social Validation," *Behavior Modification,* 1 (1977):427–452.
11. ———. *History of Behavior Modification: Experimental Foundations of Contemporary Research.* Baltimore: University Park Press, 1978.
12. ———. "Symptom Substitution, Generalization, and Response Covariation: Implications for Psychotherapy Outcome," *Psychological Bulletin,* 91 (1982):349–365.
13. ———. "Psychiatric Diagnosis, Dimensions of Dysfunction and Child Behavior Therapy," *Behavior Therapy,* 14 (1983):73–99.
14. ———. *Behavior Modification in Applied Settings,* 3rd ed. Homewood, Ill.: Dorsey Press, 1984.
15. KAZDIN, A. E., and FRAME, C. "Treatment of Aggressive Behavior and Conduct Disorder," in R. J. Morris and T. R. Kratochwill, eds., *The Practice of Child Therapy.* New York: Pergamon Press, 1983, pp. 167–192.
16. KAZDIN, A. E., and WILSON, G. T. *Evaluation of Behavior Therapy: Issues, Evidence, and Research Strategies.* Cambridge, Mass.: Ballinger, 1978.
17. MASH, E. J., and TERDAL, L. G., eds. *Behavioral Assessment of Childhood Disorders.* New York: Guilford Press, 1981.
18. OLLENDICK, T. H., and CERNY, J. A. *Clinical Behavior Therapy with Children.* New York: Plenum Press, 1981.
19. PATTERSON, G. R. *Coercive Family Process.* Eugene, Oreg.: Castalia, 1982.
20. ROSS, A. O. *Child Behavior Therapy.* New York: John Wiley & Sons, 1981.
21. SCHAEFER, C. E., and MILLMAN, H. L. *Therapies for Children.* San Francisco: Jossey-Bass, 1977.
22. SCHAEFER, C. E., JOHNSON, L., and WHERRY, J. N. *Group Therapies for Children and Youth.* San Francisco: Jossey-Bass, 1982.
23. SPIVACK, G., PLATT, J. J., and SHURE, M. B. *The Problem-Solving Approach to Adjustment.* San Francisco: Jossey-Bass, 1976.
24. URBAIN, E. S., and KENDALL, P. C. "Review of Social-cognitive Problem-solving Interventions with Children," *Psychological Bulletin,* 88 (1980):108–143.
25. WAHLER, R. G. "Some Structural Aspects of Deviant Child Behavior," *Journal of Applied Behavior Analysis,* 8 (1975):27–42.
26. WAHLER, R. G., and FOX, J., III. "Solitary Toy Play and Time Out: A Family Treatment Package for Children with Aggressive and Oppositional Behavior," *Journal of Applied Behavior Analysis,* 13 (1980):23–39.
27. WAHLER, R. G., and GRAVES, M. G. "Setting Events in Social Networks: Ally or Enemy in Child Behavior Therapy?" *Behavior Therapy,* 14 (1983):19–36.

44 / Treatment of Psychic Trauma in Children

Lenore Cagen Terr

Introduction

When any field is new and when the spectrum of signs, symptoms, and psychodynamics is first being delineated, strategies for treatment will lag far behind; this holds true in the case of psychic trauma in childhood. Some techniques did evolve from 1940s wartime work with traumatized adults[20,33] and from individual psychotherapy[25] or psychoanalysis[15] with neurotic or frightened child patients. But many more therapeutic possibilities are currently under investigation and others, obviously, have not even been thought of or "invented" yet. Hence this chapter can only be a preliminary one at best and cannot be considered a complete outline of the treatment possibilities for childhood trauma. The chapter covers principles of prevention and explores techniques of group intervention, family treatment, play therapy, conditioning therapy, treatment with medication, and individual psychodynamic psychotherapy.

Prevention of Psychic Trauma

There is no way entirely to prevent the occurrence of psychic trauma. However, the risk of being emotionally overwhelmed under circumstances of expected disaster is certainly less if one can avoid conditions of intense surprise. Hence children who live in areas at high risk for natural disasters such as earthquakes, tornados, cyclones, and floods should be offered preparatory exercises in their homes, day-care centers, and schools for such *expected* disasters. The extent to which preparation in one area would help the child cope in other areas is unknown. What happens when children well trained in earthquake safety techniques find themselves in a life-threatening terrorist attack? This is the seemingly unsolvable problem for the preventionist.

Psychoanalyst Rangell[34] and sociologist Luchterhand[27] have separately made the point that man-made disasters create more severe and more lingering posttraumatic effects than do natural catastrophes. These authors' reasoning makes some sense; one probably cannot become as angry at indiscriminate nature or at God as one might feel at man. Theoretically we should be able to prevent man-made disasters. Such approaches as worldwide political actions (especially to limit nuclear weapons and to establish international population control); statewide vigilance concerning the licensing of child care operations and the overseeing of schools; neighborhood watchfulness on behalf of any youngster, either a recognizable one or a stranger; local enforcement of animal leashing laws; public concern about industrial methods (such as slag heaping or sloppy enforcement of building and fire safety codes); and careful personal adherence to established safety rules probably could prevent many instances of childhood psychic trauma.

Even with very careful public and private actions regarding the protection of youngsters, however, children will nonetheless fall prey to terrorist attacks, accidents, acts of human or animal violence, epidemics, and natural catastrophes. The medical community, therefore, must remain alert to an age-old, continuing, and future problem for young people—that of the traumatic event and its emotional aftermath.

CHILD SNATCHING

"Child snatching" is one precipitant of childhood psychic trauma against which preventive techniques eventually may prove particularly effective. When one divorcing parent steals and hides children from the other parent, some of these stolen youngsters will become psychically traumatized either by the stealing parent or, ironically, by the "rescuing" one.[42] Although we cannot entirely stop child snatching, federal law,[31] uniform custody acts,[8,36] and international accords among nations[21,47] should serve to avert many such cases. Furthermore, if primary physicians were to record the parents' social security numbers, car registration numbers, drivers' licenses, and/or union memberships whenever a new child "enrolls" in their practices, retrieval of parentally stolen children would be easier and faster than it is now.[42] If school systems were to insist that full records from transferring schools be made available in all instances of new student registrations,[42] another mechanism of child-stealing prevention would come into operation. Eventually such preventive techniques would probably make child snatching so difficult that it would become considerably less prevalent. But man-made misuses and abuses of youngsters will never fully disappear. Regardless of the possible consequences and despite any "deterrent" examples from others, some individuals—for their own pressing emotional reasons—will do horrible things to children.

PUBLIC INFORMATION AND PREVENTION

In the case of some traumatic events, one terrifying concomitant is the lack of immediately available information. Without on-the-spot cognitive understanding, a major coping technique is lost to the victim. Because most "leaders" who endure an intense, unexpected event are themselves psychically overwhelmed, they become quite unable to help the rest of their fellow victims and cannot deliver meaningful instructions or direction. The author of this chapter interviewed five survivors of two commercial airline crashes; in each instance, no pilot or flight attendant was reported to have made a public announcement. During the chaos, each victim was on his own. This, of course, would be particularly difficult for children—especially if their parents are absent, dead, immobilized, or unable to help them. Disasters connected with the military can be of somewhat different character because army personnel are trained to convey instructions and to assert leadership—as are Federal Bureau of Investigation and Special Weapons and Tactics (SWAT) teams, which specialize in rescuing hostages.[10] We already know that trauma victims suffer a kind of inertia based upon the "fear of further fear," an emotion that strikes them from the first moments of their paralyzing terror.[40] Unless such "paralyzed" victims are given firm orders to move, they may stay put rather than enter into any new and, as far as they are concerned, potentially more dangerous space.

Public health methods of reaching child victims during moments of acute panic—especially at the time of natural disasters such as tornados and hurricanes—might include the child-oriented use of the radio and television. Simply worded statements that those over three would understand could be inserted into the public announcements and disaster advisories directed toward adults. (When at age five I heard the radio announcements regarding the Japanese attack on Hawaii and the Philippines, I construed that "they" were stealing our "pearls" and our "vanilla." An explanation of these momentous events aimed directly at children might have averted what turned out to be a longstanding misunderstanding.)

On the afternoon of the devastating Southern California, San Fernando Valley, earthquake in 1971,[6] one social agency near Los Angeles developed the unique idea of using a radio talk show to answer call-in questions from bystanders and victims of all ages. The "show" was enthusiastically received and may have had some preventive value. After its very worthwhile early intervention, however, the agency did not provide much follow-up counseling, thereby incompletely fulfilling its own mandate to offer treatment in addition to striving to prevent.

Early Intervention

The Beverly Hills Nightclub disaster of 1977 did not affect youngsters as direct victims. At the time that it happened Lindy, Grace, and Green, a research group from the University of Cincinnati, set up an informal storefront drop-in clinic for victims and the families of victims.[26] They discovered that even though treatment was offered at no cost, the vast majority of directly or indirectly involved persons did not voluntarily seek help. It is clear that psychically traumatized individuals—both adults and children—do not like to think of themselves as "sick," "changed," or "neurotic." (This is only one of the reasons that the old term traumatic neurosis is not a particularly effective designation.)

In order to provide services, mental health professionals must go directly to the frightened children and parents. The clinicians cannot expect psychic trauma victims to come to them asking for help. A recent study of the community of Othello, Washington, confirmed this point.[1] After the Mt. St. Helens eruption of May 18, 1980, the number of hospital emergency room visits, episodes of domestic violence, and diagnoses of stress-aggravated illness, psychosomatic illness, and mental disorder increased significantly. Adams and Adams demonstrated that these stressful effects lasted for at least seven months (the length of their study period). Despite the insistence of some individuals that the eruption had not affected the community, this was a statistically significant change.

After the Vicksburg, Mississippi, tornado of 1953, Bloch, Silber, and Perry[7] made the point that one could not reach the child victims without seeing their parents first. This approach was employed in the 1976–1981 Chowchilla kidnapping studies. But some recent researchers have dealt directly with the traumatized youngsters without necessarily interviewing their parents at all. Aylon[3] worked directly with some terrorized Israeli children who had been segregated from the caretaking adults on their *kibbutzim* at the time of attack. As part of their work with the Los Angeles Police Department, Pynoos and Eth[32] have interviewed a number of child witnesses to violence without necessarily interviewing the children's parents. Depending on the point of contact chosen by the therapist, children can be interviewed alone or in child groups at their singular institutions (schools especially), or they may be treated as part of their family group.

One cannot overemphasize the importance of community and medical preplanning for early interventions in the face of possible disaster.[4,9,30,46] By mobilizing teams of mental health workers right from the beginning of a catastrophe, some serious emotional casualties may be averted. The National Institute of Mental Health has published a disaster manual aimed at assisting those mental health professionals dealing with children.[14]

As a result of the battlefield experiences of World War II, we have been made aware that prompt intervention and rapid return to ordinary routine can be ameliorative for battle-shocked soldiers (although the follow-ups in these reports were nonexistent or very short term).[20,33] Prompt intervention, unfortunately, does not seem to stop the progression of posttraumatic symptoms in children. For example, I began treating one parentally kidnapped child (Wanda, age five) within twenty-four hours of the time her father and a detective forcibly brought her back home from a two-year illegal stay on an island with her mother.[41,45] During the months following this traumatic but legal kidnapping, Wanda developed debilitating new symptoms. Despite the preventive and treatment approaches that were being actively employed during this interval, the symptoms and signs kept adding up. A similar inexorable progression of posttraumatic effects was observed in other cases. In one instance, a four-and-one-half-year-old boy was first seen in psychiatric treatment about forty-eight hours after his release from a terrifying day-long confinement in a broken-down elevator. In another, a nine-year-old girl was interviewed for the first time seven days after her grandmother, with whom she had been staying, was murdered.[45] Thus far, at least, no adequate proof has been brought forward to demonstrate convincingly that early intervention in childhood psychic trauma will abort the steady progression of subsequent posttraumatic symptomatologies.

The field awaits new techniques for early intervention that would eventually offer more effective means for preventing the advance of progressive posttraumatic symptoms in overwhelmed youngsters.

Group Therapies in Psychic Trauma

Psychic trauma sufferers cannot vent all their rage directly on their tormenters. As a result child victims and their families may become extremely angry[12] at covictims, community leaders, fellow townsfolk, and/or professional helpers (rescue workers, medical teams, and, of course, psychiatrists[43]). This phenomenon represents displacement of trauma-induced rage from the unavailable "villains" to innocent but accessible targets. Some of the victims' anger also may be expressed in the form of posttraumatic reenactments.[40]

In order to establish strong therapeutic relationships that will weather the angry storms which are at times inevitable, mental health workers should, if possible, organize family groups before the results of a catastrophe become apparent.[40] Lasting and valuable therapeutic relationships can be set up prior to the relief or despair, which will come once the results of a disaster are known. Such preformed groups may outlive the community fragmentation[13] that often follows a peacetime disaster.

Children may be included—perhaps to their benefit—in professionally organized multifamily or multiage therapeutic groupings; alternatively, they might be segregated in groups consisting solely of children. The latter type of child grouping can be organized in classrooms or even at nursery schools, especially when an unexpected shock or a sudden misfortune strikes a classmate. This type of group approach has worked quite well on the college level for the prevention of contagion and for treatment (for instance when one student in a dormitory commits suicide or is raped)[5,35]; it is currently under investigation for much younger age groups. Such techniques should be considered by those professionals consulting to schools and to other natural child groupings, such as juvenile halls, residential treatment centers, and pediatric wards. Any limitation on the spread of highly communicable posttraumatic fears and symptoms[43] is a worthwhile public health child psychiatric goal.

Isaiah Zimmerman, a clinical psychologist who is consulted by the U.S. State Department, has sought to formulate contingency plans for U.S. citizens taken hostage by terrorists in foreign countries. He suggested that groups of recovered hostages be kept together and away from home for several days in order to form small and informal groupings in a spontaneous fashion. After a day or two, these rescued or released citizens could attend a large professionally run "mini-marathon" session lasting three to four hours to which any affected children would also be invited. Buffered for a while from contact with nonaffected family members and protected, though not restricted, from the press, such victims might have time and space enough to ally voluntarily with some fellow victims, to be completely evaluated physically and psychiatrically, and to settle down a bit from the massively stressful experience they had endured.[49] Zimmerman's "plan" has not been evaluated scientifically, but some of his ideas may apply to community catastrophes as well as to the foreign kidnappings for which they were originally designed.

One type of early grouping that may create more problems than it resolves is the large survivor- or victim-organized community meeting. Bringing everybody together under nonprofessional direction may further community fragmentation rather than prevent it.[40]

Among social workers and court personnel who work with sexually abused youngsters, the use of rape groups and incest groups has recently achieved popularity. Systematic study of this method, however, has yet to establish its cost-effectiveness or therapeutic worth. In a group, a youngster obtains reassurance from the knowledge that other children, too, have undergone sexual horrors, and a child may be able to vent considerable rage, but there could be some spread of symptoms within this small therapeutic community. A therapeutic group may actually introduce some fears by exposing a stranger-raped little girl to the potentially shocking new information that men can have sexual relations with boys or that children may pose for pornographic photos. The professional must constantly balance the contagious effects of childhood trauma with the benefits of grouping victim strangers, one with the other.

Interventions with the Family

In evaluating the effects of psychic trauma upon a given child, a fuller understanding of the process will emerge if the entire family is evaluated. Siblings *are* quite prone to "catch" contagious posttraumatic symptoms,[41] and this might well be prevented by appropriate psychiatric interpretation to the brothers and sisters of a traumatized youngster. Parents, also, may themselves be traumatized by the event(s) or they may "catch" symptoms transmitted by their overwhelmed child.[40] They will need help for this. Parents may provide the psychiatrist with the traumatized child's full developmental history. A previously vulnerable child will manifest more severe posttraumatic symptoms than will an essentially "normal" youngster.[40] In the course of the evaluation parents may reveal their connectedness or the lack of connectedness to their communities (an important factor in assessing the long-term prognosis for symptom severity),[43] and they may tell the psychiatrist about earlier or intervening family disruptions or serious illnesses (again, important in determining long-term symptom severity in a traumatized youngster).[43] Thus, whenever possible, the immediate families of traumatized children should be evaluated, both for data gathering and prognostication and, hopefully, for prevention and treatment.

An overwhelmed child may be treated in conjunction with the family or parents. This is especially appropriate when the entire family has been subjected to the same catastrophic event. The problem in using this approach is that even if the external experience was the same for each family member, the child victim's interpretation of the dangers, the meanings, and the personal turning points relating to the disaster is unique; it is a function of his or her own history, cognitive and perceptual capacities, vulnerabilities, and stage of development. These individual impressions of and meanings given to the traumatic event must be interpreted just as vigorously as are the more general posttraumatic effects shared throughout the family. Thus, even if the family is usually seen together as a group, each traumatized member will probably benefit from some individual psychotherapeutic sessions.

Child psychoanalyst Erna Furman has developed one particular treatment technique called parent guidance[16] or filial therapy (see chapter 9 in volume 3 of this *Handbook*),[17] which may be helpful in cases of childhood trauma. Furman suggests that parents may function as auxiliary therapists. The parent learns from the professional therapist what would be helpful to say to the child, and then works steadily along these lines at home. Because posttraumatic symptoms are so repetitive, the parent would have more opportunity than would a professional to explain or to interpret play behaviors, reenactments, and dreams to the overwhelmed youngster. "Parent guidance" may help traumatized children to: (1) feel that their parents understand them, (2) see that their "weird" current behaviors may be connected to their past ordeal, and (3) know that their parent has enough emotional stamina to focus directly on them after a catastrophe. This style of parent education and indirect psychotherapy of children may help also to limit the contagious spread of posttraumatic symptoms among nontraumatized siblings and the victims' friends.

Individual Treatments of Psychic Trauma

EXPERIMENTAL THERAPIES

In this section, a few types of treatment will be presented about which thus far little is known. They therefore cannot be considered standard and should not be employed except under rigorous research conditions. Hypnotism and amytal interviews have been successfully employed for soldiers during and after the battles of World War II,[20] but they have not been carefully studied in severely stressed children. There is something about "borrowing" or "bypassing" voluntary ego controls and coping mechanisms even temporarily from an already traumatized youngster that gives me pause. It is not clear whether such techniques will take a future position in the therapeutic armamentarium for childhood psychic trauma, but we will not know without definitive investigation and full reporting in the literature.

A number of drugs are being used currently for adult panic attacks and phobias (benzodiazepines such as alprazolam [Xanax], beta-blocking agents, the tricyclics, and the monoamine oxidase inhibitors[36,38]); these eventually may have some ameliorative effects when used in conjunction with psychotherapy for posttraumatically stressed youngsters. At this point these drugs have not entered the standard pharmacopeia for childhood trauma, and we must await more information before using them. Posttraumatic stress disorders are far more complex than ordinary phobias or panic disorders, for which there already is some data on pharmacotherapy with children.[19] In most likelihood, the entire spectrum of posttraumatic effects in childhood will eventually require a combined therapeutic approach including drugs, if proven effective, along with psychotherapy.

DESENSITIZATION THERAPIES

In both adult and children's phobias, considerable success has been reported following the use of relaxation techniques along with prescribed tasks requiring increasing contacts with a feared item. The psychodynamics of psychic trauma are probably different form those of phobia. Many phobias are the displacement of an internal anxiety to an external object, whereas posttraumatic fears develop as overgeneralizations of external objects reminiscent of the actual event.[40] However, there *are* many symptomatic similarities between the two conditions, particularly the panic attacks, the avoidances, and the quickly increasing number of feared items in the early stages.

Silverman and Geer,[39] using the standard deconditioning techniques for phobia, treated an adult female patient who had been severely frightened years earlier when her brother had threatened that a bridge on which she was standing at the time would collapse. The investigators claimed that by means of desensitization, their patient overcame longstanding repetitive nightmares and bridge phobias. If fears are the only symptoms or signs apparent after a traumatic incident, such conditioning therapies should work well both for adults[22] and for school-age children. In most psychic trauma, however, while the fears may be the most obvious findings, there are far more serious underlying changes present as well that affect the entire personality and the life attitudes of the victim.[43] In such instances removing the fears would only be nicking the top of the iceberg.

With the passage of time, some psychically traumatized children spontaneously decondition some of their trauma-related fears; they do this simply by forcing themselves or by being forced to face the trauma-connected stressors.[43] Those children who do manage to accomplish this spontaneous deconditioning feel some relief. Any therapy that can bring about this same result faster is to be encouraged—with the important reminder that desensitization treatment may have to take an ancillary position to psychodynamic psychotherapy in many instances of psychic trauma. Those techniques that stand the greatest chance of effecting a "cure" or that at least offer the most benefit to the traumatized young person are likely to be the methods that aim at combatting the child's trauma-inspired sense of extreme helplessness.

PLAY THERAPY

Like other approaches to childhood trauma, play techniques are not fully worked out; however, considerable work has already been done in this field.[44] In 1938 David Levy developed a nondirective, noninterpretive abreactive play technique that he called release therapy.[23] Levy intended this sometimes wild and messy play treatment to mirror the abreactions by means of which battle-traumatized soldiers under hypnosis or sodium amytal infusion subsequently gained significant relief. A problem with Levy's technique was the chaos it might create in the office or the playroom. Furthermore, the technique came to be used in the late 1940s and 1950s for far more kinds of emotional disturbances in youngsters than just psychic trauma. "Abreactive therapy" was attended by some rather uncomfortable countertransference stirrings in child psychiatrists who followed Levy. For all these reasons, release therapy never gained popularity. Levy did show, however, that frightened children could gain relief by massive physical expression without the therapist making any accompanying psychiatric interpretation or clarification.

"Preset play" has useful applications in childhood trauma. Here therapists purposely stack their toy shelves with objects directly reminiscent of the child's own trauma. David Levy[24] originally suggested this approach, and others including Shapiro[37] and Mac-Lean[28] have refined it considerably. The therapist "happens to have" something on hand that promotes trauma-related play in the child patient. Sometimes the psychiatrist can suggest that the child bring to the office a particular toy which the psychiatrist knows— usually from ancillary information—the child has been using in posttraumatic play. Once I purchased two toy planes—a Pan Am jet and an American Airlines 747 —just before a three-year-old who had recently crashed on a Pan Am plane in Central America was scheduled for evaluation. The youngster repeatedly ignored, looked past, and "accidentally" tried to mutilate the miniature Pan Am jet. He would not "voluntarily" play with it. Instead, he played at crashing with the little American Airlines aircraft. The intensity of feelings and the accompanying memories elicited with this "preset play" were quite striking.

Gardner has applied his mutual storytelling technique to the treatment of childhood trauma.[18] A frightened child is encouraged to tell a story, and the therapist imposes a new ending to the child's traumatically derived "story." Over fifty years ago Waelder suggested that schoolteachers use such new endings in storytelling with emotionally upset youngsters.[48] Gardner offered a single case to demonstrate the efficacy of his type of play treatment for psychic trauma, and he reported that the child patient he described was cured.

In some cases of psychic trauma, especially those in which the child exhibits extreme guilt, the "corrective dénouement" technique of play therapy may be successfully employed. Here the therapist seeks to dramatize with the child a different way in which the whole traumatic event might have been handled—if indeed there *was* a different way.[44] In one of my cases, the grandmother of a nine-year-old girl opened her apartment door to a murderer after admonishing the child first to call the police. The child had not known how to do this. In therapy the psychiatrist showed the child how to phone the police. The child and the therapist also practiced ways the grandmother might have avoided opening the door. Using this series of different outcomes, the child realized that she had had no real basis for control of the actual events and, thus, no guilty responsibility for her grandmother's violent death.

For the carefully selected patient, a therapeutic message may come to the child through "corrective dén-

ouement" play. It conveys a sense that the child could *never* have known how to handle the horrible events, and that he or she therefore could not have done anything other than what was done. Where the child feels responsible for injuries or deaths to others during a traumatic event, this adjunctive technique can be particularly effective. If a child has inadvertently taken on adult responsibilities without adult "know-how," this play technique may provide profound relief, though it is unlikely that it would effect a cure.

The utilization of real posttraumatic play as part of office or hospital play therapy is extremely difficult to arrange.[44] Posttraumatic play is so secret, so specific (employing only certain toys and special places), and so personal that it may only be observed by professionals under a few special circumstances. These include situations in which the therapist is connected with an institution where the traumatized child already lives[15]; a trauma involving an extremely underprivileged child who owns few, if any, of his or her own toys; treatment conducted by a talented therapist who somehow inspires a wish in a child to sacrifice privacy (see Erikson[11]); or therapy in which the psychiatrist *asks* the child to bring toys from home in order to show what he or she has been usually playing there. It is very useful to the child, however, for the psychiatrist to observe posttraumatic play whenever possible and to interpret it successfully.[41] This play can be debilitating, and any mechanism for relieving the child of the need to play out the trauma repeatedly is worthy of the therapist's efforts.

Psychotherapy in Cases of Psychic Trauma

In working with the traumatized child in individual psychotherapy, the available treatment options include abreaction, suggestion, clarification, and interpretation. An extreme sense of helplessness, awareness of the evanescence of life and of the fragility of connections with loved ones, profound distrust of the future, and ongoing cognitive-perceptual distortions are four of the major areas that will require vigorous verbal interventions by the therapist. Metaphoric interpretations (deep interpretations couched in the language of humor, "stories," or acted-out "scenarios") may be employed successfully with traumatized children. Direct, straight-out talk to the traumatized youngster him- or herself can also be helpful. As opposed to youngsters with more subtle in-dwelling fantasies and neurotic conflicts, traumatized children require little to no psychiatric "probing." They *know* their experience —unless it happened when they were infants or young toddlers—and they are quite aware of what they play, what they think, and what they do. With the traumatized child, therapy is not a matter of a long unraveling process—rather it is the treatment process itself, the interpretations and the clarifications, that create the technical problems. The child may not respond quickly, if at all. Guilt—sometimes quicker to yield in the neurotic youngster—does not surrender to standard interpretation in the case of a traumatized child. In trauma the guilt hides a sense of helplessness so profound that the guilty torment is needed, clung to by the patient, in order to reestablish some sense of personal control. The same is true in regard to the omens and the perceptual distortions that follow externally precipitated childhood terrors. They come so immediately and are so closely related to the ordeal that even though the omens and distortions are interpreted and /or clarified repeatedly by the psychiatrist, the child may nonetheless cling to them.

It is rapidly becoming apparent just how longlasting, how extensive, and how progressive are the effects of psychic trauma in youngsters.[43] The problem is, now that we know that the effects of an actual disaster are extremely invasive and longlasting, how can we offer treatment for these posttraumatic difficulties in the most effective and efficient way?

REFERENCES

1. ADAMS, P., and ADAMS, G. "Mount Saint Helens's Ashfall: Evidence for a Disaster Stress Reaction," *American Psychologist,* 39 (1984):252–260.

2. ANTON, A. "The Hague Convention on International Child Abduction," *International and Comparative Law Quarterly,* 30 (1981):537.

3. AYLON, O. "Children as Hostages," *The Practitioner,* 226 (1982):1773–1781.

4. BARTON, A. *Communities in Disaster.* Garden City, N.Y.: Doubleday, 1969.

5. BINNS, W. A., KERKMAN, D., and SCHROEDER, S. O. "Destructive Group Dynamics: An Account of Some Peculiar Interrelated Incidents of Suicide and Suicidal Attempts in a University Dormitory," *Journal of the American College Health Association,* 14 (1966):250–256.

6. BLAUFARB, H., and LEVINE, J. "Crisis Intervention in an Earthquake," *Social Work,* 17 (1972):16–19.

7. BLOCK, D., SILBER, E., and PERRY, S. "Some Factors in the Emotional Reaction of Children to Disaster," *American Journal of Psychiatry,* 113 (1956):416–422.

8. BODENHEIMER, B. "Interstate Custody," *Family Law Quarterly,* 14 (1981):203.

9. COHEN, R., and AHEARN, F. L., JR., eds., *Handbook for Mental Health Care of Disaster Victims.* Baltimore: Johns Hopkins University Press, 1980.

10. EICHELMAN, B., SOSKIS, D. A., and REID, W. H., eds. *Terrorism: Interdisciplinary Perspectives.* Washington, D.C.: American Psychiatric Press, 1983.

11. ERIKSON, E. *Childhood and Society.* New York: W. W. Norton, 1950.

12. ERIKSON, K. *Everything in Its Path.* New York: Simon & Schuster, 1976.

13. ———. "Loss of Communality at Buffalo Creek," *American Journal of Psychiatry,* 133 (1976):302–305.

14. FARBEROW, N., and GORDON, N. *Manual for Child Health Workers in Major Disasters.* Rockville, Md.: National Institute of Mental Health, 1981.

15. FREUD, A., and BURLINGHAM, D. *War and Children.* New York: Medical War Books, 1943.

16. FURMAN, E. "Treatment of Under-fives by Way of Parents," *Psychoanalytic Study of the Child,* 12 (1957):250–262.

17. ———. "Filial Therapy," in J. D. Noshpitz, ed., *Basic Handbook of Child Psychiatry,* vol. 3, ed. S. I. Harrison. New York: Basic Books, 1979, pp. 149–158.

18. GARDNER, R. *Therapeutic Communication with Children: The Mutual Storytelling Technique.* New York: Science House, 1971.

19. GITTELMAN, R., and KLEIN, D. "Controlled Imipramine Treatment for School Phobia," *Archives of General Psychiatry,* 25 (1971):204–207.

20. GRINKER, R., and SPIEGEL, J. *Men Under Stress.* Philadelphia: Blakiston, 1945.

21. HAGUE CONFERENCE ON PRIVATE INTERNATIONAL LAW, FOURTEENTH SESSION (1980). *International and Comparative Law Quarterly,* 30 (1981):556.

22. KIPPER, D. A. "The Desensitization of War-induced Fears," *Current Psychiatric Therapies,* 16 (1976):41–47.

23. LEVY, D. "Release Therapy in Young Children," *Psychiatry,* 1 (1938):387–390.

24. ———. "Release Therapy," *American Journal of Orthopsychiatry,* 9 (1939):713–736.

25. ———. "Psychic Trauma of Operations in Children," *American Journal of the Diseases of Children,* 69 (1945):7–25.

26. LINDY, J., GRACE, M., and GREEN, B. "Survivors: Outreach to a Reluctant Population," *American Journal of Orthopsychiatry,* 51 (1981):468–478.

27. LUCHTERHAND, E. "Sociological Approaches to Massive Stress in Natural and Man-Made Disasters," *International Psychiatric Clinics,* 8 (1971):29–53.

28. MacLEAN, G. "Psychic Trauma and Traumatic Neurosis: Play Therapy with a Four-Year-Old-Boy," *Canadian Psychiatric Association Journal,* 22 (1977):71–76.

29. NOYES, R., et al. "Diazepam and Propranolol in Panic Disorder and Agoraphobia," *Archives of General Psychiatry,* 41 (1984):287–292.

30. PARAD, H., RESNIK, H., and PARAD, L., eds. *Emergency and Disaster Management.* Bowie, Md.: Charles Press Publishers, 1976.

31. PARENTAL KIDNAPPING PREVENTION ACT, Public Law No. 96–6111, §§6–10, Stat. 3568, 1980.

32. PYNOOS, R., and ETH, S. "Witness to Violence: The Child Interview," *Journal of the American Academy of Child Psychiatry,* in press.

33. RADO, S. "Pathodynamics and Treatment of Traumatic War Neurosis," *Psychosomatic Medicine,* 4 (1942): 362–368.

34. RANGELL, L. "Discussion of the Buffalo Creek Disaster: The Course of Psychic Trauma," *American Journal of Psychiatry,* 133 (1976):313–316.

35. SEIDEN, R. H. "Suicidal Behavior Contagion on a College Campus," in N. L. Farberow, ed., *Proceedings: Fourth International Conference for Suicide Prevention.* Los Angeles: Suicide Prevention Center, 1968, pp. 360–367.

36. SHADER, R. I., GOODMAN, M., and GEVER, J. "Panic Disorders: Current Perspectives," *Journal of Clinical Psychopharmacology,* 2 (1982):25–105.

37. SHAPIRO, S. "Preventive Analysis Following a Trauma: A 4½ Year Old Girl Witnesses a Stillbirth," *Psychoanalytic Study of the Child,* 28 (1973):249–285.

38. SHEEHAN, D. V. "Panic Attacks and Phobias," *New England Journal of Medicine,* 307 (1982):156–158.

39. SILVERMAN, I., and GEER, J. "The Elimination of a Recurrent Nightmare by Desensitization of a Related Phobia," *Behavioral Research and Therapy,* 6 (1968):109–111.

40. TERR, L. "Children of Chowchilla: A Study of Psychic Trauma," *Psychoanalytic Study of the Child,* 34 (1979):547–623.

41. ———. " 'Forbidden Games': Post-Traumatic Child's Play," *Journal of the American Academy of Child Psychiatry,* 20 (1981):741–760.

42. ———. "Child Snatching: A New Epidemic of an Ancient Malady," *Journal of Pediatrics,* 103 (1983):151–156.

43. ———. "Chowchilla Revisited: The Effects of Psychic Trauma Four Years After a Schoolbus Kidnapping," *American Journal of Psychiatry,* 140 (1983):1543–1550.

44. ———. "Play Therapy and Psychic Trauma: A Preliminary Report," in C. Schaefer, and K. O'Connor, eds., *Handbook of Play Therapy.* New York: Wiley-Interscience, 1983, pp. 308–319.

45. ———. "Time Sense Following Psychic Trauma: A Clinical Study of Ten Adults and Twenty Children," *American Journal of Orthopsychiatry,* 53 (1983):244–261.

46. TIERNEY, K. *Crisis Intervention Programs for Disaster Victims: A Source Manual for Smaller Communities.* Rockville, Md.: U.S. Department of Health, Education, and Welfare (ADM), 1979.

47. UNIFORM CHILD CUSTODY JURISDICTION ACT, 1973 California Statute, Chapter 693.

48. WAELDER, R. "The Psychoanalytic Theory of Play," *Psychoanalytic Quarterly,* 2 (1933):208–224.

49. ZIMMERMAN, I. "Adaptation to Terrorism and Political Violence," Paper presented at the annual meeting of the Los Angeles Group Psychotherapy Society, Los Angeles, June 1983.

45 / Treatment of Failure to Thrive and Growth Disorders in Infants and Children

Irene Chatoor and James Egan

Treatment of any condition or disorder is more effective when it specifically addresses the individual factors that generate the disturbance. One important advantage of a developmental classification of eating and growth disorders in infants and children (see chapter 29) is that it delineates specific difficulties that characterize certain growth disorders in a number of areas: in children's physical and emotional development, in their interactions with their caretakers, and in their family and social environment. Chatoor and associates[3] have defined three types of growth disorders that are associated with three specific developmental stages: (1) disorders of homeostasis, (2) disorders of attachment, and (3) disorders of separation and individuation. Each of these disorders will be described and appropriate therapy and intervention will be reviewed.

Disorders of Homeostasis

In the first two months of life, the major developmental tasks are stabilization of the autonomic and motor systems and establishment of a regular feeding pattern. For some infants, prematurity or organic illness interferes with the development of these basic skills. When rapid respirations or intubation prohibit oral feedings, infants are prevented from learning to associate sucking with filling of the stomach and relief of hunger tension. Consequently, when these infants recover medically and should be physically able to feed, they are often unable to suck, swallow, and regulate their milk intake by signals of hunger and satiation. Bernbaum and associates[1] showed that regular offering of a pacifier during gavage feedings facilitated infants' learning to suck and swallow. Later these infants learned to feed more quickly and gained weight faster than did a control group (infants with similar difficulties who were not given a pacifier). Furthermore, although both groups were taking in the same amount of milk through gavage feedings, the infants who were stimulated to suck a pacifier seemed to absorb their feedings more effectively.

Additional support for the use of a pacifier during gavage feedings or for the establishment of sham feedings comes from Dowling.[5] In a study of infants with esophageal atresia who had had only gastrostomy feedings for the first months of life, Dowling observed that these children had severe difficulties learning how to suck, chew, and swallow. After surgical repair they were expected to feed orally; when approached with food, however, they whimpered and whined. They not only lacked oral skills in handling the feedings, but they also appeared completely unaware of feelings of hunger or satiation. In addition, these children showed marked delays in gross motor and speech development. They lacked motivation and vitality and showed general affective and intellectual dullness. With a second group of infants born with esophageal atresia, Dowling introduced oral sham feedings. The mothers were instructed to hold their infants and to have them suck from a bottle whose milk was then collected from the esophageal fistula at the neck. At the same time the mothers were to feed the infants through the gastrostomy tube. Children who had been fed this way quickly learned to signal their hunger and satiety. The mothers could read these cues and feed the infants accordingly. Once surgically corrected, the infants learned to feed orally without much difficulty. Following the children's affective, motor, and speech development, Dowling concluded that all the developmental deficits of the first group of infants with gastrostomy feedings could be avoided by the introduction of sham feedings.

Other infants at risk during the development of homeostasis are those with delays in the coordination of the oral musculature. These infants frequently choke during feedings. For an inexperienced mother, infant distress of this kind creates severe anxiety. A person trained in motor development, such as an occupational or physical therapist, can teach the mother specific feeding techniques that will facilitate motor development and better feeding. Such an early intervention can prevent a vicious cycle of infant distress and parental anxiety that so frequently leads to further complications during subsequent stages of the infant's development.

A related problem during the infant's early establishment of feedings is the inability to coordinate sucking and breathing. As demonstrated by Murray, Fink, and Gaiter,[12] some infants who present with abnormal

sucking and breathing patterns tire quickly. They fall asleep after having taken in only small amounts of milk and presently fail to thrive because their milk intake is inadequate. Once again, the mothers experience great anxiety; more than that, they are frequently exhausted because of prolonged feeding periods during both the day and the night. Effective intervention should consider the mother's need for rest along with the infant's difficulty in feeding. In order to get mother and infant through this developmental crisis until the infant establishes a more mature sucking and breathing pattern, a "mother's helper" might have to be introduced. Infants with severe feeding problems of this nature might need supplemental feedings through a nasogastric tube until they are able to suck and breathe without difficulty.

Some problems may occur because the mother has difficulties in reading her infant's cues. She might under- or overstimulate and under- or overfeed the baby. Such mothers need to be helped to establish a communication pattern with their infants. This would help at once to facilitate regulation of the infant's motor and autonomic systems, to establish a feeding pattern in accord with the infant's cues, and to prepare the mothers for the next developmental stage. The therapist serves as an interpreter between mother and infant by reinforcing mutual cueing and helping the mother read her infant's signals more effectively. Videotaping of mother and infant during feeding and play is not only useful for diagnostic purposes[4] but can serve also as a powerful therapeutic tool. The therapist can watch the tape replay together with the mother, share observations with her, and help her to become a better self-observer.[13] Through this technique as well as through interventions during direct observations of mother and infant, the mother can be made more aware of her infant's cues and of contingent responses on her part. It is important for the therapist to focus on positive and contingent interactions and to ignore maladaptive responses as much as possible so that the mother does not feel criticized and suffer a further fall in self-esteem. The therapist should strive rather to strengthen the mother's confidence and to help her fulfill her wish to become an effective caretaker.

Attachment Disorders

The most common cause of growth failure by far is a disturbance in the mother-infant attachment. This is generally due to the emotional unavailability of mother, her physical absence, or both. The most frequent bases for emotional unavailability are maternal depression or a lack of adequate parenting in the mother's own childhood combined with a variety of psychosocial privations. Frequently a multiplicity of factors can be discovered. Proper treatment entails directing therapeutic measures at each of the component parts contributing to the dysfunction of parenting.

Because of the complexity of the issues involved, a multidisciplinary team comprised of child psychiatrists, nurses, pediatricians, nutritionists, and occupational therapists is generally required for effective treatment. Best results are obtained when the same team members have been working together over a period of time with a unified approach. In order to maintain a cohesiveness of purpose, these teams should meet on at least a weekly basis to review the patients currently under their charge. Because of the large number of personnel involved, the seriousness of the disorder and the frequency of inanition, hospitalization is frequently necessary both to accomplish a thorough assessment and to undertake nutritional rehabilitation. In severe cases, nasogastric tube feedings during the night are necessary in order to augment the oral feedings.

An initial hospitalization provides an opportunity for continued observations and for mobilizing the infant's innate capacities. The improvement in the infant's feeding and affect can be used to activate the mother and to engage her in the treatment process. Hospitalization can help forge an alliance between the mother and the mental health team; this will offer a greater likelihood that treatment of the mother-infant dyad will continue after nutritional rehabilitation is completed and the baby has been discharged from the hospital.

Frequently these infants are developmentally delayed in many areas and a thorough developmental assessment is necessary. This is generally the province of child psychiatrists and psychologists, but may well include an occupational therapist. The occupational therapist often assesses the gross and fine motor development as well as certain aspects of perceptual and social functioning. A plan can then be developed for specific techniques of infant stimulation to be undertaken by the nursing and occupational therapy staff. During the hospitalization, it is very important to assign a primary care nurse and to keep the number of caretakers as low as possible in order to facilitate a special relationship between infant and caretakers. With this type of multidisciplinary intervention in the hospital, infants frequently gain weight and progress developmentally. But, as Harris[10] accurately emphasizes, "changes in growth and cognition are frequently rapid; changes in personality and behavior are much slower. Recovery from growth failure does not indicate that the parent-child relationship is adequate, it is only a first step" (p. 241).

Because the mothers generally present with a variety of social, developmental, and psychological disturbances, they too require a careful assessment of their developmental history, their current psychosocial functioning, and caretaker/infant interactions. If specific areas of disturbance are discovered, efforts at remediation can be undertaken. For example, if the mother is suffering from clinical depression, tricyclic antidepressants might well be indicated. If, on the other hand, there is a reactive depression to serious psychosocial stresses and privations, efforts at psychological intervention can be undertaken by a psychiatrist, psychologist, or social worker. These efforts are aimed at elucidating inhibitions and obstacles to effective parenting. These interventions are generally done in a supportive and nurturing fashion. When this is accomplished, one generally discovers that the mother's capacities to nurture the child more effectively can be mobilized.

Many of these mothers have tangible difficulties in their lives that contribute to the dysfunction in their parenting. Accordingly, a skilled social worker is needed, not just to provide direct psychological treatment for the parent but also to assist in mobilizing psychosocial services in support of the entire family. These may range from finding day care, a homemaker or visiting nurse, to arranging financial assistance in the form of welfare, food stamps, and so forth.

As the feeding disorder improves and the infant becomes more engageable, the sense of progress frequently has a positive stimulating effect on the mother. Her improved affective involvement in turn tends to reinforce the infant's feeding and development. These mothers often need to be nurtured themselves before they can nurture their infants. Only then are they able to benefit from developmental guidance to help them in understanding their infants' needs. As this therapeutic alliance develops, the clinician may be able to help the mother psychotherapeutically to see how the "ghosts" from her own childhood may be interfering in her new relationship with her infant.[8]

Those mothers with severe character pathology need intensive support by a team of professionals. The infant's growth and development must be closely supervised. In some cases, infant day care is utilized to meet the baby's needs for appropriate attention and stimulation while the mother is being helped to work on her own difficulties.

Drotar, Malone, and Negray[6] point also to the influence of the family as a stress-buffering or stress-producing system. They emphasize a bidirectional-transactional model of development: "The infant affects and is affected by the marital, or parental partner, relationship which in turn influences and is influenced by parenting" (p. 931). They suggest a family-centered outreach program in the home to: (1) engage relevant family members in treatment, (2) identify environmental stressors, (3) assess family resources, (4) establish a context for communication among various family subsystems critical to the infant's nurturing, and (5) identify and remediate the dysfunctional patterns and focal conflicts that affect the care and nurturing of the child.

In some situations the pathology of the mother or the disruptions within the family are so severe that the infant needs to be placed in alternate full-time care.[11] These are difficult decisions to make. A therapeutic trial with the mother should always be attempted before this intervention is suggested.

Disorders of Separation

Based on the work of Egan, Chatoor, and Rosen[7] and these authors,[2] it can be stated that oppositional food refusal on the part of infants, toddlers, and children can lead not only to failure to thrive but also to linear growth retardation (dwarfism). It is of more than academic interest to distinguish growth failure secondary to attachment disorders from growth failure secondary to disorders of separation. The treatments involved are quite distinct and, indeed, many aspects of the treatment of attachment disorders would not only be unhelpful but would be pathogenic in the treatment of separation disorders. Thus efforts at coaxing and encouraging eating will only exacerbate a disorder of separation, and developmental stimulation is usually unnecessary because these children have frequently received too much attention. By the time they are seen, their cognitive development is usually age appropriate if not precocious.

The central symptom of disorders of separation is the child's refusal to eat as part of the battle for autonomy with the parent, who is usually overanxious about the child's food intake. Mother and child become trapped in a pattern of maladaptive interactions around food. The parent coaxes, distracts, or forces the child to eat, while the child refuses the food, plays with it, or throws it around. The child seems unaware of physiological feelings of hunger; instead, emotional needs for attention or anger toward mother dictate eating behavior. These children have failed to develop somatopsychological differentiation.[9]

Therapeutically, the first intervention for a separation disorder focuses on helping the parents become aware of the importance of the developmental task of somatopsychological differentiation. They must begin to learn about their role in helping the infant attain this

ability and that this is accomplished by separating mealtime from playtime. The parents are instructed to feed the child at regular mealtimes and, if the interval between meals is too long, to schedule regular snacks. They are asked to assume a neutral stand about the child's food intake, not to praise if the child eats well and not to coax or force the child if he or she does not want to eat. In this way the child's attention can be refocused on the inner state of hunger or fullness instead of being drawn into constant interactions with the parents. If the child does not want to eat, the parents are encouraged to set firm limits by terminating the meal, and to make up for the loss of attention during feedings by playing with the child before or after meals. The parents often need much support in learning to trust the infant's ability for nutritional self-regulation, to read the infant's cues, and to respond in a contingent manner.

Some parents can use this developmental guidance to alter their own and their child's behavior around feeding. Because of their own conflicts around parenthood or eating, however, other parents have greater difficulty with change. Psychotherapy may be useful in helping them overcome these conflicts. Because these mothers often have a rather elaborate defensive organization with frequent use of reaction formation, as well as a generally neurotic level of character pathology, they may benefit from exploratory psychodynamic psychotherapy as well as from straightforward behavioral counseling. Since many more children with separation disorders come from intact families than do those with attachment disorders, the fathers frequently need to be involved in order to foster a strong alliance between the parents and to have the father participate appropriately in parenting. The involvement of the father frequently diminishes the mother's pathological tie to the infant. With these multiple therapeutic interventions, one can begin to see significant improvement occur fairly quickly.

In some situations hospitalization is indicated either for assessment or to provide a "parentectomy." This requires limiting parent access to the children at feeding times. Frequently one must impose strict rules prohibiting parental involvement during feeding. The primary care nurse assumes total responsibility for the eating situation, preferably in the parent's absence. The mother's involvement is limited to nonnutritive issues. With this intervention, the infant usually begins to eat more and to gain weight. This progress often is received ambivalently by the mothers. They are relieved to see their child's weight gain and their anxiety about the child starving to death is reduced; nonetheless, they are frequently hurt by the notion that someone else is better equipped to feed their child. In order to maintain therapeutic alliance with the mother, empathic work regarding these issues is essential.

After the child has established a healthy eating pattern, the mother and father are helped to resume feeding their child. The children are frequently testy with their parents and try to reestablish the old patterns of interaction. The parents will then need much reinforcement to maintain a neutral stand about the child's food intake and to set firm limits to the child's provocative feeding behaviors. Once the child realizes that the old games do not work any more, he or she usually gives them up. The parents feel strengthened in their ability to set limits appropriately and are better prepared to deal with the other developmental aspects of separation and individuation.

Summary

While there are relatively distinct differences in the treatment of feeding disturbances due to disorders of homeostasis, attachment, and separation, it should be borne in mind that many infants present a picture of compromised eating and that growth retardation is due to a combination of organic factors, disturbances of attachment, and aspects of separation disorder. Although relatively common, such disorders require the most distinct efforts at precise treatment interventions because the effects of some of the interventions are mutually exclusive.

REFERENCES

1. BERNBAUM, J., et al. "Nonnutritive Sucking During Gavage Feeding Enhances Growth and Maturation in Premature Infants," *Pediatrics,* 71 (1983):41–45.

2. CHATOOR, I., and EGAN, J. "Nonorganic Failure to Thrive and Dwarfism Due to Food Refusal: A Separation Disorder," *Journal of the American Academy of Child Psychiatry,* 22 (1983):294–301.

3. CHATOOR, I., et al. "Non-organic Failure to Thrive: A Developmental Perspective," *Pediatric Annals,* 13 (1984): 829–843.

4. CHATOOR, I., et al. "Pediatric Assessment of Nonorganic Failure to Thrive," *Pediatric Annals,* 13 (1984):844–850.

5. DOWLING, S. "Seven Infants with Esophageal Atresia: A Developmental Study," *Psychoanalytic Study of the Child,* 32 (1977):215–256.

6. DROTAR, D., MALONE, C., and NEGRAY, J. "Psychosocial Intervention with Families of Children Who Fail to Thrive," *Child Abuse and Neglect,* 3 (1979):927–935.

7. EGAN, J., CHATOOR, I., and ROSEN, J. "Failure to Thrive: Pathogenesis and Classification," *Clinical Proceedings, Children's Hospital National Medical Center,* 36 (1980):173–180.

8. FRAIBERG, S., ADELSON, E., and SHAPIRO, V. "Ghosts in the Nursery," *Journal of Child Psychiatry,* 14 (1975): 387–421.

9. GREENSPAN, S. I., and LIEBERMAN, A. F. "Infants, Mothers and Their Interaction: A Quantitative Clinical Approach to Developmental Assessment," in S. I. Greenspan and G. H. Pollock, eds., *The Course of Life,* vol. 1, *Infancy and Early Childhood.* Bethesda, Md.: National Institute of Mental Health, 1980, pp. 271–312.

10. HARRIS, J. C. "Nonorganic Failure to Thrive Syndromes," in P. Y. Accardo, ed., *Failure to Thrive in Infancy and Early Childhood.* Baltimore: University Park Press, 1982, pp. 240–241.

11. MALONE, C., and DROTAR, D. "A Prospective Study of Failure to Thrive: Outcome Data for the Children up to the Age of Two," Paper presented at the 30th annual meeting of the American Academy of Child Psychiatry, San Francisco, 1983.

12. MURRAY, S. L., FINK, R., and GAITER, J. "Nutritive Sucking Patterns in Infants at Risk for Sudden Infant Death," Paper presented at the International Conference on Infant Studies, New York, March 1984.

13. STERN, D. *The First Relationship: Infant and Mother.* Cambridge, Mass.: Harvard University Press, 1977.

46 / Treatment of Victims of Physical Abuse and Neglect

Richard Galdston

Introduction

The past years have brought increased recognition of child abuse and neglect as a problem worthy of public concern. Most state legislatures have followed the example set by the federal Congress in declaring child abuse and neglect to be reportable conditions, thereby affirming the seriousness with which these bodies regard the problem.[4]

The communication media have devoted considerable time to detailing instances of child abuse as part of the competition for the public's attention. The portrayal of violence, especially that associated with sexual acts, continues to be a highly marketable item.

The response of the public and of their elected leaders has brought a significant increase in the perception of child abuse as one manifestation of the domestic dimensions of violence. The inclination to place child abuse, rape, and marital assaults within a category of related problems bespeaks an acknowledgment of the undercurrent of violence that can erupt from disturbances of domestic life.

This chapter considers recent developments concerning physical abuse and neglect in four sections: detection, reporting, treatment, and prevention.

Detection of Abuse and Neglect

The detection of instances of suspected child abuse or neglect has been facilitated by the establishment of family services and child care clinics designed to serve the lower socioeconomic segments of society within urban ghettos.

Availability of personnel familiar with the clinical stigmata of child abuse and neglect has increased the likelihood of earlier detection of cases among the populations seeking pediatric services. Identification of the child considered to be "at risk" for abuse or neglect

makes it possible for others to monitor the child's developmental course. The problem of the "false positive," of a child erroneously suspected of having been abused, is a hazard that cannot be completely avoided. It is the price of public alertness in the screening process.[3]

The suburban and rural areas present different problems that call for greater initiative in reaching out to families whose children are less likely to gain notice through public services.[12] The skewing of the relative prevalence of child abuse and neglect toward the urban lower class may be a consequence of the greater likelihood of detection within an urban setting. It is more difficult to establish reliable figures of case incidence in the suburban and rural communities.

The derivation of data remains approximate because of the variation in services throughout the country. The Task Force on Psychiatry and Child Abuse of the American Psychiatric Association recently estimated that there are 1.5 million cases of child abuse and neglect reported yearly. The American Academy of Child Psychiatry estimates that at least 4,000 of these children die.[1]

The question of whether the incidence is increasing is of theoretical interest. The fact that child abuse exists warrants attention, not only to the welfare of the children involved but because of the significance of the problem as a symptom of an underlying sociocultural affliction.[7]

Reporting Abuse and Neglect

In 1963 the Deputy Chief of the Children's Bureau of the Department of Health, Education and Welfare, Katherine Bain, M.D., warned, "No one believes that requiring doctors or hospitals to report cases of suspected physical abuse will end, or even, lessen such abuse."[21] Despite the seemingly official unanimity that led to mandating the reporting of suspected cases, the response remains diffuse and frequently ineffective. Child abuse can be considered to be a psychiatric, a social, an economic, a medical, or a legal problem. It can be viewed as a moral or religious issue. Responsibility for converting case detection into a responsive intervention remains a point of weakness in the chain of events needed to attain effective treatment.

Although the law protects against legal action stemming from the reporting of unproven cases, the vicissitudes of administrative retaliation make it difficult for those charged with such reporting to know exactly when to do so and when not to.[17] Legal action has been initiated against agencies for failing to report child abuse. When cases are reported appropriately, the responsibility is passed on. Usually it falls to social agencies charged with the welfare of children or to the police. Typically, these personnel are overworked and undertrained for the task. Professional ambiguities about the particulars of child abuse and neglect become compounded by administrative deficiencies that reflect an underlying societal ambivalence regarding the welfare of children. The reporting process is rendered an endeavor of uncertain outcome, with consequences that can vary from benign neglect to militant prosecution depending on factors that have little to do with the clinical details of the case in question.

Treatment of Those Who Abuse or Neglect Children

There is a medical aphorism that the length of text devoted to therapeutics varies inversely with the understanding of the etiology of the problem. The wide variety of therapeutic interventions for child abuse and neglect developed in recent years suggests limits in the level of understanding of the problem's etiology. This is complicated further by the prevailing concern about the cost of social welfare. The public desire for cost containment has interfered with the ability to individualize treatment.

The various treatment approaches developed can be grouped into four main categories.

SELF-HELP MOVEMENTS

Patterned on the model of Alcoholics Anonymous, the Parents Anonymous movement has experienced considerable success. Under the aegis of leaders chosen from the group members, groups are formed to offer peer support in dealing with shared issues. The group offers its members aid and comfort and the opportunity

to explore experiences with the avowed goal of helping each other become better parents.[6,16]

Participation in these groups depends on the parents' ability to sustain their own motivation for change. Unless assigned under legal duress, the parents must be capable of initiative sufficient to sustain them. This requirement limits the utility of the self-help route to those who are capable of helping themselves. There are many parents whose abuse of their children reflects their inability to help themselves. For them some other course of treatment is needed.

THE "HOT LINE"

The use of the telephone to share personal concern about problems has been developed to contend with child abuse (comparable to the Hot Line approach to drug problems and possible suicide). The underlying principle rests on the belief that two heads are better than one; that it is helpful for the sufferer to share the burden of anxiety with another through ventilation, catharsis, and reasoning over the telephone. The use of the telephone to register reality, to seek sympathy and possible clarification about an immediate crisis offers the abusing parent relief from the lonely subjective sense of distress.

Hot Line programs for child abuse seldom offer other services. Opportunities to implement referrals for further treatment are limited. The solutions implicit in the approach are ad hoc and can be justified by its immediacy and the assumption that something is better than nothing.

THE TEAM APPROACH

Many agencies and hospitals have assigned professionals to groups organized for the purpose of offering a team approach for the treatment of cases suspected of child abuse or neglect.[18] This arrangement encourages the pooling of skills and collaboration in sharing responsibility for the treatment of detected cases. The involvement of the team members reduces the likelihood of cases becoming lost to follow-up, a great hazard in dealing with psychological problems of a chronic nature.

The effectiveness of the team is enhanced greatly by the support of the sponsoring institution, which is important in protecting individual participants from the ravages of "burn-out," the loss of morale than can befall a professional contending with the treatment of cases of child abuse. The advantages of group support can be transmitted to the patients, most of whom feel themselves to be isolated and beset with a multitude of problems both social and psychiatric in nature.

Yet the advantage of enhanced group morale inherent in the team approach is accompanied by the potential hazard of diffusion of personal responsibility. To cope with this risk, the team should have a leader responsible for the specific implementation of planned interventions. Maintenance of planning tends to be a persistent problem because the therapeutic potential of clinics, agencies, and public hospitals remains vulnerable to the vicissitudes of funding coupled with the ad hoc mentality of so much administration of social intervention. [19]

THERAPEUTIC TECHNIQUES

Among specific therapeutic techniques that have been applied are parent effectiveness training (PET), surrogate mothering, behavior modification, intervention by family agents, and methods that draw on psychoanalytic principles.

Parent Effectiveness Training. PET rests on the premise that maltreatment of children is due in part to cognitive deficits in the parents that can be remedied by direct instruction. The treatment is based on education and has the advantage of a simple pedagogic approach. Those parents who are capable of identifying with the instructor enough to sustain learning will likely profit from the information provided. The approach depends on the capacity of the instructor to reach the parents and the parents' ability to learn alternative child-rearing techniques.

Behavior Modification. Behavior Modification is a related approach discussed in chapters 5 and 11 in volume 3 [14,24] and in chapter 43 in this volume. The principles are applied to child-rearing practices and carry with them the hazards of negative reinforcement merging into concealed sadism.

Surrogate Mothering. In surrogate mothering, the services of a paraprofessional homemaker are provided; she participates in the household by helping the mother and child to relate to each other in a more constructive fashion. [20] This technique appears particularly suited to patients in rural areas, where physical isolation makes difficult their inclusion in groups of agency programs. The model of the visiting nurse offers a prototype of the merits of this relationship.

Psychoanalytic Principles. Psychoanalytic principles have been utilized in the training of family intervention agents to work in a housing project with high-risk families. The approach was developed to employ inhabitants of a housing project to help neighbors burdened with child abuse and neglect. [22] Similar programs have been developed to offer the principles of psychoanalytic understanding to parents and children who can participate in a therapeutic day care center as a basis for a long-term relationship. [8,11]

PRINCIPLES FOR TREATMENT

The following principles for the treatment of victims of physical abuse and neglect have been derived from my fifteen-year experience in the treatment of 150 children between the ages of six months and four years in the Parents' Center Project for the Study in Prevention of Child Abuse in Boston.

Having been subjected to abuse and neglect appears to readily result in disordered ego development. Most notably, the child's competence in the purposeful direction of aggression in the service of the self remains undeveloped. The capacity to employ aggression either remains liable to discharge through impulsive or compulsive repetition or undergoes atrophy from disuse.

Treatment rests on the establishment of a relationship within an interpersonal environment designed to promote mastery of the tasks of ego development. This requires an emotional climate designed to help the child gain the freedom to enact rather than merely to be acted upon. Such initiative can be restored only through the adjustment of relationships in response to children's needs and according to their abilities at the moment.

The individualized attention required to accomplish this requires a ratio of at least one adult for the care of three children. The staff should possess great energy, patience, and willingness to learn from personal experience.

The course of treatment typically encompasses three phases: *recovery, engagement* and *growth.* These are determined by the state of the children's aggression in relation to their surroundings.

The *recovery* phase is ushered in with intervention that protects the child from parental aggression. The phase is marked by apathy that serves as sensory retreat from stimuli too threatening for the child to bear. Inactivity allows flight and withdrawal affords the child a haven.

During this phase the child's need to preserve a sense of safety through retreat should be respected. When caretakers introduce stimuli, they should do it with meticulous attention to the child's relative intolerance. Interactions easily accepted by normal children often prove to be more than the abused child can tolerate at this time. Ingenuity combined with respectful sensitivity will gradually enable the child to come out of hiding, as it were, into a world of objects while simultaneously allowing the child to claim some initiative for the process.

The phase of recovery can consume considerable time. Children must be allowed to recover according to their own needs rather than in response to an externally imposed schedule. The staff's therapeutic efforts will be enhanced if they are enriched with the support of informed understanding. Without such an appreciation of the process, it will be difficult for child care staff to preserve the fortitude required to expend effort without immediate results.

The onset of the *engagement* phase is marked by eruptions of aggression that are often abrupt, unpleasant, unpredictable, and disturbing. These temper outbursts signal progress and provide a force for growth. Usually they take the form of physical or verbal attacks on other children or adults who formerly were the attacker's favorites. Often the only apparent provocation is attention to the child. At that point, the child typically bursts into emotional activity that is best described as a tantrum. The attack continues until a response of restraint is forthcoming. Closure is effected by an attentive adult's physical constraints containing the tantrum within an emotional response. The adult must neither go away nor give in. The adult must endure, remain with, and partake of the child's experience in a sustained relationship. By doing so the child is allowed to feel a sense of self within that of another, so to speak.

During the early part of the engagement phase, these attacks occur frequently. They are followed by a marked increase in the child's basal level of vitality in verbal and facial expression. The episodes appear to function as a sort of existential affirmation. They serve as what could be designated as an entity crisis. It is as if children define themselves as being, feeling, and doing in relation to the presence of another person, whose mutual response is measured to establish the separate existence of each party in the pair.

Within the entity crisis, the child makes a specific demand upon the adult to participate emotionally and physically through the provision of compassion and comforting. Usually this exchange is demanded by the child without acknowledging gratitude. Acknowledgment is implied by the rapid increase in signs of orientation to persons, places, and relationships that follow. There ensues a rapid increase in the children's engagement with their world.

It is out of the entity crisis that the child becomes enabled to define a self in relation to others via the respectful exercise of aggression. Mutuality as a way of being becomes possible. The child starts to acquire the wherewithal to benefit from the social experience of engagement with others and develops skill at recognizing those with whom he or she can and cannot engage. Usually the parents remain intolerant of the child's newly found aggression. The child learns to respect these parental limitations and confines efforts to engage to those who have demonstrated their ability to participate.

The outpouring of aggression in these engagements confront children with a bewildering array of inclinations that leave them buffeted by ambivalence. The children's ambivalence requires protracted patience

from the adult coupled with explicit instructions about how they can proceed to make up their mind in effecting choices. This process helps the children learn that it is possible to sort out personal experience so as to lend some order to their experience of others who are involved with the objects of the children's desire.

During the latter part of the engagement phase, a great deal of time and energy has to be devoted to the ordering of options. This enables the children to acquire a sense of self in conjunction with each of their desires and associated feelings. The adult should maintain a level of attention that is responsive without being intrusive. This helps the children to sort out sensations and to elaborate motor responses that are personally satisfying and socially appropriate. Through the repetition of this experience, the children establish that they are and that they can do something with who they are. Once they know this, they are able to grow.

For children who have been abused and neglected, *growth* is limited by past experience. Even when the past has been overcome, it remains a fact of personal history. It is as if the inconstancy of objects past is embedded within the children. The poverty of protection that marked abused children's early experience appears as memory encoded in habitual apprehension and vulnerability to regress in response to perceived danger. The long-term limitations of ego growth defy discrete delineation because of the multiplicity of variables involved. It can be assumed only that the provision of early and sustained comforting and protection will afford abused children an enhanced opportunity to realize their potential for utilizing aggression in the service of growth and development.

No single treatment technique has a claim to universal effectiveness.[5] The complexity of factors that contribute to the maltreatment of children make it necessary that each case receive individual diagnostic evaluation. Treatment should be designed according to the particulars of the case, and planning requires a realistic assessment of the alternatives available within the community. Whatever else it may represent, child abuse and neglect result from a disordered relationship between parents and child. Relief can be obtained only through the addition of another relationship that is helpful.

Prevention of Abuse or Neglect

Child abuse and neglect are disorders of behavior with serious social consequences that are both acute and far-reaching. Psychiatry as a specialty and medicine as a profession have been relatively ineffective in achieving primary prevention of these conditions. Alcoholism, addictions, acts of criminal intent, and related sociopathic behavior share in this resistence to prophylaxis. [23]

Attempts at primary prevention have rested largely on advocacy programs. Dissemination of information has produced a more widely informed public with a more responsive judicial system. [15] Many communities require that domestic court procedures include a person selected specifically as advocate for the child's interests as distinct from the interests of the community or the parents. Paradoxically, advocacy as a movement carries with it the potential for increased polarization of parent versus child, male versus female, and society versus family. The tendency for fragmentation is the price paid for the benefits derived from greater militancy in advocating action.

The emergence of the advocacy movement reflects an underlying crisis mentality indicative of the belated recognition of a longstanding problem for which social action has long been insufficient. It has been said that violence is "as American as apple pie"! That it makes its way into the home to emerge as child abuse and neglect, spousal attacks, or just plain assault and battery indicates the depth of ambivalence with which domestic partners live with one another and their issue. [13]

Secondary prevention by reducing the recurrence rate among families determined to be liable to abuse and neglect represents a more feasible goal. The various techniques reported to have achieved success in preventing recurrence share one factor in common—an increase in the amount of personal attention devoted to the members of the family. Two features characterize all these forms of attention: the expressly declared disapproval of violence as a means of treating children and a strongly avowed concern for the welfare of children. It is important to realize that affirmation of these two values is a clear instance of social interference with individual freedom to set personal standards. Indeed, effective secondary prevention requires some infringement upon personal liberty to do as one would with one's children. Society imposes standards and enforces their priority, often against the inclination of abusing or neglectful parents.

Focusing on the discrepancy between social and individual priorities highlights the relationship between the process of superego formation and the role of culture in offering values to support the function of the family. The term culture encompasses dual meanings. On one hand, culture comprises an accumulation of values cherished by society; on the other hand, it represents an activity devoted to the raising of subsequent generations—for example, agriculture. When society fails in the function of supporting the raising of children, its culture becomes less competent. Several observers have described abusing and neglectful parents as immature and suffering from deficits in superego structure. [10,21] It is among the disenculturated that child abuse and neglect occur, among those whose values fail to hold to the primacy of the health and welfare of their children. [9]

Culture affords a context in which the individual can identify with prevailing social values to form the body of personal persuasions that make up the superego. Child abuse and neglect can be viewed as a manifestation of cultural failure to induce and/or sustain in individuals the priority of regenerative functions.

Secondary preventive efforts in child abuse and neglect lead to the conjunction between culture and the process of individual superego formation. How we learn to value what we want and why we do so strongly influences how we raise our children. More effective means are needed to enhance the cultural valuation assigned to the welfare of the individual in order to support the function of the family as an agency for the reproduction of adults through the raising of their children.

Studying the clinical particulars of individual superego development in concert with object relations offers an opportunity to learn about the determinants of parental values and the efficacy of the cultural context to promote child raising.

REFERENCES

1. AMERICAN ACADEMY OF CHILD PSYCHIATRY. "Child Abuse—the Hidden Bruises," *Facts for Families,* 1.

2. AMERICAN PSYCHIATRIC ASSOCIATION, Task Force on Psychiatry and Child Abuse. *Report to the Council on Children, Adolescents and Their Families.* 29 June, 1984.

3. BESHAROV, D. J. "Overreach of the Guardian State," *Wall Street Journal,* 2 April 1984.

4. CHILD ABUSE PREVENTION ACT. Hearings before the Subcommittee on Children and Youth of the Committee on Labor and Public Welfare. S.1191, March 26, 27, 31, and April 24, 1973.

5. COHN, A. H. *Evaluation of Child Abuse and Neglect Demonstration Projects: 1874–1977,* vols. 1 and 2. Washington, D.C.: National Center for Health Services Research,

(PHS) 79–3217–1, U.S. Department of Health, Education and Welfare, 1978.

6. COLLINS, M. C. *Child Abuser: a Study of Child Abusers in Self-help Group Therapy.* Littleton, Mass.: PSG Publishing Company, 1978.

7. FISCHOFF, J. "Abused Children: A Psychiatrist Examines Violence in the Family," *The American Family Unit II Report No. 1.* Philadelphia: Smith, Kline and French Laboratories, 1975.

8. GALDSTON, R. "Violence Begins at Home: The Parent's Center Project for the Study and Prevention of Child Abuse," *Journal of the American Academy of Child Psychiatry,* 10 (1971):336–350.

9 ———, "The Domestic Dimensions of Child Abuse," *Psychoanalytic Study of the Child,* 36 (1981):391–414.

10. GREEN, A. H. "Psychiatric Treatment of Abused Children," *Journal of the American Academy of Child Psychiatry,* 17 (1978):356–371.

11. ———. "Expanding Psychiatry's Role in Child Abuse Treatment," *Hospital and Community Psychiatry,* 30 (1979): 702–705.

12. HELFER, R. E., and SCHMITT, B. D. "The Community Based Child Abuse and Neglect Program," in R. E. Helfer and C. H. Kempe, eds., *Child Abuse and Neglect: The Family and The Community.* Cambridge, Mass.: Ballinger Publishing Co., 1976.

13. LANGLEY, R., and LEVY, R. *Wife Beating: The Silent Crisis.* New York: Simon & Schuster, 1977.

14. McGEE, J. P., and SAIDEL, D. H. "Individual Behavior Therapy," in J. D. Noshpitz, ed., *Basic Handbook of Child Psychiatry,* vol. 3, ed. S. I. Harrison. New York: Basic Books, 1979, pp. 72–107.

15. NEWBERGER, E. H., and BOURNE, R. "The Medicalization and Legalization of Child Abuse," *American Journal of Orthopsychiatry,* 46 (1976):593–607.

16. PARENTS ANONYMOUS. "Frontiers" (Spring 1984).

17. SCHETKY, D. H., and BENEDEK, E. P. *Child Psychiatry and the Law.* New York: Brunner/Mazel, 1980.

18. SCHMIDT, B. D. *The Child Protection Team Handbook.* New York: Garland Press, 1978.

19. SHAY, S. W. "Community Council for Child Abuse Prevention," in C. H. Kempe and R. E. Helfer, eds., *The Battered Child,* 3rd ed. Chicago: University of Chicago Press, 1980, pp. 330–346.

20. STEELE, B. F. "Psychodynamic Factors in Child Abuse," in C. H. Kempe and R. E. Helfer, eds., *The Battered Child,* 3rd ed. Chicago: University of Chicago Press, 1980, pp. 49–85.

21. U.S. DEPARTMENT OF HEALTH, EDUCATION, AND WELFARE. Welfare Administration, Children's Bureau, cited in *Pediatrics,* 31 (1963):895–898.

22. U.S. DEPARTMENT OF HEALTH, EDUCATION, AND WELFARE. *Intervention at Early Age in High Risk Families,* Final Report, Grant No. MH 12168, Principal Investigator, E. Pavenstedt. Washington, D.C.: National Institute of Mental Health, September 1970–August 1973.

23. U.S. DEPARTMENT OF HEALTH, EDUCATION, AND WELFARE. *Child Abuse and Neglect: The Problem and Its Management,* OHD #75-30073. Washington, D.C.: U.S. Government Printing Office, 1975.

24. WETZEL, R. J., BALCH, P., and KRATOCHWILL, T. R. "Behavioral Counseling: The Environment," in J. D. Noshpitz, ed., *Basic Handbook of Child Psychiatry,* vol. 3, ed. S. I. Harrison. New York: Basic Books, 1979, pp. 181–192.

47 / Intervention in Cases of Child Sexual Abuse

Ira S. Lourie and Linda Canfield Blick

Introduction

Child sexual abuse does not describe a mental health syndrome so much as it defines a type of behavior to which a child has been exposed. Intervention and related treatment, therefore, require that each case be understood in terms of both its own unique etiology and its emotional consequences. Cases come to light in a number of ways: They are disclosed by the child's verbal report, through inferences made by an adult observer of the child's symptoms, by the discovery of a physical injury that requires medical attention, or by someone observing the sexual act directly. Once recognized, the situation must be assessed, including a process of validation. As a consequence of factors unique to child sexual abuse, intervention inevitably is a dual process in which the acute effects of the sexual incident(s) and the disclosure of the abuse must be dealt with simultaneously at the outset. Longer-term therapeutic goals can then focus on the more complex sequelae of the abuse and the dynamics that lead up to it.

Disclosure of Sexual Abuse

In all cases of child sexual abuse, before one can intervene the case must first be disclosed. Disclosure occurs in three ways: (1) intentionally—when the child consciously plans to tell someone and proceeds with a self-report of the abuse to a parent, teacher, friend, sibling, or trusted adult; (2) unintentionally—when a third party notices a consistent change in the child's affect or behavior and questions the child; and (3) accidentally—when someone walks in on the abuse in progress, the child contracts a sexually transmitted disease, a sexually related physical injury is discovered, or through discovery of a pregnancy. All such disclosures should be assessed and investigated as described in the following sections. When children are abused by strangers, there is usually a vigorous response to the disclosure by the parents, and the treatment process begins easily. When the abuse is within the family, however, or at the hands of a close family friend or relative, there is often reluctance on the part of family to believe and respond to the report. In fact, there is often a complete denial of the possibility of any such occurrence. In those cases where the child's report has not been responded to, the child feels a sense of intense helplessness and may withhold further attempts to communicate while the abuse continues.

SYMPTOMS

When children have been unsuccessful in reporting abuse or have not been able to do it at all, the only hope of disclosure is through knowledgeable observation of the child's behavior. Table 47–1 highlights some of the behavioral symptoms likely to be present in sexually victimized children, which could indicate the presence of abuse. Many of these behaviors are nonspecific to abuse and occur as well when children suffer from other kinds of psychological trauma. In order to diagnose sexual victimization as the basis of a child's problem, the therapist must, therefore, rely on validation of the case by a trained investigator, a statement from the child, corroborative medical evidence consistent with sexual abuse (which is present in only 10 to 15 percent of the instances), a confession from the abuser, or an eyewitness account of the victimization.

Assessment of Sexual Abuse

Assessment of child sexual abuse requires an investigation that goes beyond the usual child mental health evaluation. Symptoms are usually assessed in terms of their origin within multiple contexts: the individual (developmental), the family, and the environment. Child sexual abuse differs in that regardless of the presence of symptoms, the investigation first focuses on an action taken toward a child and only then proceeds with the traditional assessment of the emotional effects

of the abuse on that child. Finally, both the symptoms and the underlying dynamics (pathological or healthy) of all family members are explored. The added step of first investigating the nature of the abuse before exploring any resultant symptoms is most important in determining the need for child protection.

These major issues related to the abuse must be assessed initially:

1. By whom was the child victimized? What was their relationship, if any?
2. What type of victimization did the child suffer?
3. At what age did the victimization begin? At what age did it stop?
4. How was the child engaged: coercion, deception, intimidation?
5. Were violence or threats of violence used in the commission of the victimization?
6. What is the nonoffending parent(s) attitude? What is the perpetrator's attitude?
7. Is the child presenting behavioral symptoms? If so, what are they?
8. How was the victimization disclosed: intentional, unintentional, accidental?
9. Is the child able to discuss the abuse?

The assessment period should include: four to eight individual sessions with the child, an individual session with the nonoffending caretaker(s) and siblings, a review of the child's social and academic performance at school, a complete medical examination by a physician experienced with sexually victimized children, and the caretaker's written observations of the child's behavioral and social performance. If the offender is admitting the abuse and is cooperative, a meeting should be arranged to discuss his abusive activity. This will include engagement of the child, types of sexual behavior performed on the child, and strategies used to inhibit the child's disclosure of the abuse. The clinician should review records from child protective services, law enforcement, medical examinations, any previous psychological or psychiatric evaluations, and schools. It is important to interview the parents/caretakers for information about behavioral changes or symptoms present in their children. If the child is old enough, he or she can be asked to fill out a behavioral questionnaire to assist in this process.

VALIDATION

Validation of a report of child sexual abuse is extremely important and has both legal and therapeutic ramifications. Without validation, neither criminal justice nor community child protective service involvement are available to the child and family. Some unvalidated incidents, especially those that are incest related, may go untreated and uncontrolled. In order to ensure that the need for protection of abused and

TABLE 47–1

Symptom Chart for Sexually Victimized Children

Preschool	School Age	Adolescents
Regressive behaviors—thumb sucking, bed wetting, baby talk Nightmares	Sleep disturbances Running away School problems—academic	Sleep disturbances Running away School problems—academic or social
Sleeping with a previously discarded toy (sign of regression) Child clings to nonoffending parent(s)—excessively fearful of separation	Overly compliant *or* aggressively acting out Poor body image	Overly compliant *or* pseudomature Aggressively acting or fighting with peers
Child initiates sexual behavior with peers, younger children, older people, toys, animals Child draws pictures of sexual activity or talks about it Child masturbates *excessively* Child acts adultlike	Difficulty with peer relation Discomfort in taking gym (disrobing in front of others) Child has advanced knowledge of sex Enuresis Depression Child has difficulty trusting	Difficulty with peer relationships Pervasive sense of mistrust Substance abuse Poor body image Confusion over sexual identity or fear of opposite sex Pregnancy one or more times at an early age
	Fugue state	Clinical depression Suicide ideation Somatic compliants Depersonalization or dissociation

neglected children is met (see section entitled "Protection of the Child Victim"), the verification of the true nature of the incident affords community agencies the necessary preconditions for mandatory intervention.

From the legal perspective, sexual abuse is particularly difficult to validate; it is a behavior that occurs in secrecy and there are, therefore, no witnesses. Of further importance is the fact that very little corroborating physical evidence is ever present; medical evidence is only available in 10 to 15 percent of the cases. There is also a strong judicial prejudice against a child's ability to remember and to tell the truth when reporting a crime committed by an adult, especially a parent. At present, child developmental specialists know that even very young children can accurately describe significant life events and do not have the information necessary to develop complex fantasies that detail the kinds of sexual behavior they report; nevertheless, their testimony is often disallowed.[10] The ability of a child to testify should be based on an evaluation of that child's capacity to do so rather than on any preconceived notion or prejudice about the ability of child witnesses in general. In 1985 the state of Maryland enacted a law that prohibits discrimination of child witnesses solely on the basis of age.* While this is a

movement in the right direction, the efficacy of such legislation is not yet tested.

There have also been recent attempts to develop more appropriate methodologies to obtain testimony from children. The use of video equipment is primary in these efforts. California and Texas have experimented with the use of videotaped interviews of the child. The purpose is to question the child in a more humane, less stressful situation and thereby obtain more objective and valid testimony. Using this technique requires a neutral interviewer specially skilled in interviewing abused children. The disadvantage of this procedure comes when children must tell the story to a new person who may make them uncomfortable and resistant; however, it bypasses the problem of so-called prejudiced interviews by involved therapists. A similar technique is the use of closed circuit television during the testimony of the child witness. Using this procedure children would not have to face an abuser who had made threats against them or face a courtroom full of adults. Both of these video techniques raise serious, unanswered constitutional questions related to the right of the accused to face the accuser and the right of cross-examination. However, videotaped interviews have been used effectively to confront alleged offenders and precipitate confessions.

Several important factors make disclosure and sub-

*Section 9–103, Courts and Judicial Proceedings Article, *Annotated Code of Maryland,* 1984 replacement volume, 1985 cumulative supplement (1985).

sequent validation of child sexual abuse particularly troublesome. Two of these are the shame and guilt associated with the abuse. These feelings naturally make victims of all ages reluctant to report the abuse, let alone describe it in detail and/or testify concerning it. Also, one must combat the aspects of secret keeping and collusion that most often accompany sexual abuse and that interfere with the intervention process (this is discussed in chapter 30). Added to these are the feelings of embarrassment associated with discussing sexual matters in general, and all the more so in a public setting. Issues of love and dependency also impede the validation process. The family and/or the victim may care for and/or rely on the perpetrator; this often leads them to protect the abuser: "I don't want Daddy to go to jail." Some victims are reluctant to discuss the abuse for fear of retribution by the perpetrator (especially in cases involving violence or those in which there have been threats).

The interview techniques for validating child sexual abuse are based on the same principles as any child mental health assessment. However, because of the collusive nature of incest families and the guilt, love, and fear factors mentioned earlier, clinicians must be extremely adept at those techniques that assure the highest degree of disclosure by the child and family. The interviewer must also be one who believes that child sexual abuse can occur. Most important, the victim must be made to feel safe and supported. The child must be interviewed by that person mandated by law (in some jurisdictions this person is in child protection; in others the interviewer is in law enforcement). The person should be a skilled interviewer who understands the unique resistances in these cases and who can control the environment so as to make the child most at ease. The interviewer must know the type of questions that can help victims feel more comfortable about the abuse and that are likely to elicit information about abuse from reluctant victims. The use of sexually correct dolls, freestyle investigative drawings, or Groth's anatomical drawings[12] is an essential addition to age-appropriate interview materials. Clinicians must not be hesitant to ask nonleading questions about sexual matters. If we cannot talk about it, why should we expect others to be able to?

Sgroi, Blick, and Porter[16] have developed a five-phase validation procedure to assist professionals of all disciplines in properly assessing a child sexual abuse report. The five phases include:

1. Engagement of the Child
   a. Who is the offender?
   b. How did the offender gain access to the child?
   c. How did the offender gain the child's cooperation?
   d. What was the duration and frequency of the abuse (look for patterns)?

2. Progressive Sexual Behaviors
   a. Child sexual abuse occurs over time, progressing from less intimate forms of abuse (exposure, voyeurism, fondling) to more intimate forms of abuse (masturbation, oral-genital acts) and sometimes to intercourse. This progression is not seen with child rapists.
3. Strategies Used to Maintain the Secret
   a. Methods include fear of abandonment, death threats, other physical threats, or the secret can be maintained by the child out of a sense of duty or fear of the consequences of the disclosure on the family.
4. Disclosure: Accidental or Planned (Intentional)
   a. Accidental disclosure varies from discovery of a pregnancy (x-rays of a ten-year-old revealing a pregnancy), to a witness walking in on an abusive act, to discovery of a sexually transmitted infection or an abuse-related injury requiring medical attention.
   b. Planned disclosure is a conscious choice of the victim to report the abuse.
5. Suppression Phase
   a. This occurs when pressure is placed on the child victim by one or more family members to retract allegations of abuse.

Through interviewing the child victim, then the siblings and other nonoffending family member(s), this information is obtained. It is then analyzed in conjunction with a review of the aforementioned behavioral symptoms displayed by the child and a medical examination. The report can then be validated.

NATURE OF THE ABUSIVE SITUATION

The nature of the abusive situation is another part of the initial assessment. In terms of the child's reactions, the fact that a stranger abused a child on one occasion has different ramifications than the occurrence of multiple episodes with close relatives or friends. Other factors relate to the acts or progression of acts involved. Being flashed by a stranger or having one's pants pulled down for exploration by a teenager will have a lesser (although not necessarily less traumatic) effect than being raped by an acquaintance or abused by one's father over a period of weeks, months, or years. Similarly, the use of violence and/or threats as the means for initiating the abuse will have different effects than when seduction, coercion, or deception is employed.

As stated in chapter 30, any incident of child sexual abuse falls between the extremes of both the stranger /incest and the interpersonal/sexual victimization continua. Exploration of these two areas gives valuable insight into the etiology of the abuse and the expected reactions of both the involved adult(s) and child. Without this basic information describing the abusive situation, no rational decisions can be made about how best to intervene. Exploration of these data will also include a basic understanding of the developmental history of the child, the involved adult(s), and the family in which the child lives.

DEGREE OF VICTIMIZATION

Along with this information, the degree to which the child has been "victimized" needs to be determined. While most people agree that child sexual abuse is harmful to the child, as previously discussed, it is evident that each child will react differently. There are several factors that appear to determine the degree of harm in incest: the age of the child; the amount of violence versus caring attendant on the abuse; the degree of disorganization in the family; the innate psychological strength of the child; and the response of the family and community to the child. While no generalizations should be made about the effects of these factors, they do offer a framework with which to approach the concept of degree of victimization.

PROTECTION OF THE CHILD VICTIM

Protection of the child victim is a vital concern. Once it has been determined that child sexual abuse has occurred, the primary issue becomes protecting the child from further abuse. In the case of abuse at the hands of a stranger, protection is easily arranged; the closer the relationship between the perpetrator and the child, however, the more complicated it becomes. In cases of incest, protecting a child from his or her own parent or parents is in fact most difficult. The disclosure of sexual abuse is often so painful, however, and the abuse is so often accompanied by threats concerning disclosure, that affected children must be placed in a position where they can be protected from further abuse as well as from their own ambivalence.

As part of this protection, the use of public agencies is mandatory. In all states the reporting of suspected child abuse is required by law.[5] Abuse outside the family should always be reported to law enforcement agencies, while incest or abuse by a caretaker must be reported to the appropriate community agency (child protective services and/or law enforcement). These resources alone have the capacity to protect children. Mental health practitioners can help rehabilitate families and individuals but cannot protect children.

The therapeutic value of police and court intervention in child sexual abuse is controversial, especially in cases of incest. Most investigators* feel that such official sanction of the abuser is necessary for child protection and in order to help relieve the child of guilt. Experience teaches that there are some instances in

*See references 4, 7, 9, 11, and 15.

which arrest and/or incarceration of a parent or relative can increase guilt and emotional harm to a child victim. This can be minimized by an appropriate professional approach helping the child place the responsibility for the abuse and all the ramifications of reporting on the offending parent. "He knew it was wrong when he did it, even if he didn't know it was against the law, because he told you to keep it secret. It was his *choice* to abuse you." The need to protect any particular child must take all these factors into consideration, and professional expertise must be called upon to prevent mishandling of the investigation and subsequent intervention.

In cases of incest, current thinking holds that effective treatment is more likely when the involved adult is removed (at least temporarily) from the home.[4] This allows the child to feel protected and to understand that the adult was the person who was in the wrong. The responsibility for the abuse is clearly removed from the child and the burden of the consequences is placed with the offending adult. This also allows the adult to escape from a situation within which he has not been able to maintain control and to begin to understand the impact of his actions. When an adult refuses to acknowledge the abuse, his removal from the home and, if necessary, incarceration are mandatory. It is important to note that removal of the child from the home is destructive in that it validates the victim's sense of personal wickedness while dislodging the child from whatever support the family or the community can offer. The removal of the child is an alternative of last resort, to be resorted to only when the family is so destructive that it is the only means of protecting the youngster from a dangerous situation. Even in these cases, once treatment has begun and improvements made, the perpetrator should be removed from the home in order to facilitate the return of the child.

Removal of the offender from the home is a very effective therapeutic tool in that it precipitates change in each family member's role. A nonoffending parent who has previously taken a passive role must take a more active position in the family. This parent must overcome doubts about the ability to run a household or to be a giving, effective parent. The child victim may feel angry about having felt abandoned by this parent and by the lack of protection from abuse; there is also skepticism on the part of the child about the remaining parent's parenting skills. In helping the nonoffending parent deal with these feelings, a stronger parent/child relationship is formed, which reconstructs the balance within the family structure and creates an atmosphere in which abuse is much less likely to recur.

The children in the family must also make some major adjustments. The victim(s) must give up the special alliance held with the abuser. This brings with it a loss of power and often a loss of a sense of love. Unfortunately, the victim(s) must also face the impact that the disclosure has on the rest of the family. Without intervention parents and nonvictimized sibs have a tendency to blame the victim for the changes in the family structure and may lead to retraction of the allegations of abuse. At a minimum, abused children will turn this blame toward themselves and feel that they are the cause of the family distress and, sometimes, even the abuse itself.

An important part of the intervention related to removal of the abuser from the home is education that will help the family understand the reasons for the removal. All family members need to be informed that removal of the offender is neither a punishment nor a recommendation that the family be dissolved. It is designed first as a protection for the child. Second, it protects the offender from the compulsive urges to abuse the child and thus from the further emotional or legal consequences of reabuse. Third, it serves as a time-out period in which to reduce familial stress.

This educational process allows the family to understand why the offender was removed. It helps decrease the anxieties caused by speculation that the removal is a form of punishment which will lead to permanent separation. A final important conclusion that must be made is that the family has the ultimate decision-making power concerning reunification or divorce.

The experience of child sexual victimization undermines the foundations of the child's basic sense of love, security, and trust. Since this violation impedes the establishment of a trusting relationship, the therapists' first formidable task is to establish trust. This often requires months to accomplish. The therapist plays a significant role in this process by gently encouraging the child to talk about the victimization and by providing educational information about this phenomenon, saying, for example, "It wasn't your fault" or "Many children have experienced a touching problem [sexual abuse] in their own homes . . . by people they know . . . or strangers."

Children whose victimization was violent or involved bizarre or ritualistic behavior will be much more difficult to engage. The more severe the abusive situations, the stronger the defensive structure the child needs to erect in order to survive emotionally. Feelings are hidden through repression and dissociation. These victims can often create a pseudomature façade that may all to easily convince professionals they have escaped trauma.

The single most significant factor in the rehabilitation of the child victim is the attitude of the nonoffending caretaker.[2] The parent or caretaker who blames the child for the abuse and/or views the youngster as permanently damaged is inflicting additional psycho-logical injury on that child. Such a stance creates an atmosphere that perpetuates the dynamics leading to the abuse. Conversely, the parent who believes the child, is supportive, and takes whatever measures might be necessary to protect the child creates a positive atmosphere in which both sexual victimization and interpersonal issues can be addressed and expedites the treatment process. Because of this, it is critical that the child's caretaker(s) receive: (1) psychotherapy to help deal with their own feelings about the victimization, (2) education to understand the phenomenon and the effect it has had on their child, and (3) guidance in assisting that part of the therapeutic process which is aimed at the child.

Most child victims of sexual abuse experience feelings of guilt and shame over what has happened; these arise both from the nature of the abuse and the effects of its disclosure.[13] In addition, the children are caught between both positive and negative feelings toward the perpetrator, nonoffending parent(s), and siblings. They must further face and assimilate society's negative attitudes about sexual abuse. The abusive acts themselves create confusion for the child over both the etiology of the victimization and the difference between emotional love and physical love. Eventually, the emotional consequences of this trauma may range in severity from symptoms of psychosis or multiple personality through various less serious behavioral reactions to cases in which the child appears symptom-free. Gelinas[8] has described a traumatic neurosis as accompanying both the sexual abuse and its disclosure. Putnam[14] has described the dissociative aspects of a child's reaction to child sexual abuse, which sometimes lead to the development of multiple personalities. Both of these phenomena are described in chapter 30.

Treatment Process

Following an assessment that addresses the issues discussed earlier, a treatment plan for the child, adult, and family can be developed. Treatment of child sexual abuse has two distinct phases. The first is the management of the abusive incident(s) and the issues related to disclosure. The second is the exploration of the individual and family problems that underlie the abuse. Both phases begin with the assessment and proceed concurrently. This section addresses those underlying treatment issues that are unique to child sexual abuse or that require special emphasis. It should be understood that these issues take place within the context of the customary practice of child mental health intervention.

The therapist must play a dual role: both as a child advocate and as a psychotherapist. As an advocate, the therapist will be responsible for reporting to related courts on happenings with the victim and the offender. Concerning the victim, the therapist may be called on to make recommendations about placement and family separation and reunification. Concerning the offender, the therapist may be called on to report violations in the legal agreements made in the case, which include reabuse, returning home, or having unsupervised visits before they are court ordered, or poor attendance in therapy. The therapist must be willing to take an authoritarian role and to advocate legally for the child and/or the offender.

Treating a sexually abused child can be a complex and lengthy process. However, children with few and mild symptoms, who have supportive caretakers, and who have suffered abuse of short duration that did not involve violence may need less extensive treatment. Sexual abuse damages the child's development from both psychological and physical perspectives. Children introduced to adult life experiences prematurely have not yet developed the sophisticated ego apparatuses that are necessary to assimilate the experience or to resolve such powerful value conflicts in a healthy fashion. In general, the younger the victim and the lengthier and more extensive the abuse, the greater is the degree of resulting psychological trauma.

Effective treatment of a sexually victimized child first requires a proper evaluation of the complaint. Validation of such a report is a complex, time-consuming but necessary process. It is rendered more difficult because in these cases traditional legal standards of evidence are minimal. Once a complaint has been validated by mandated child protection and law enforcement authorities and the child's protection has been assured, treatment can begin.[15]

Treatment is indicated for children when they have observable symptoms (see table 47–1) or when they are not able to talk about the abuse even if no symptoms are present. If the child appears to be symptom-free, is able to talk about the abuse freely and appropriately, and has the support of at least one parent, continuing treatment need not be recommended at that time. However, it is important to leave the child victim and caretakers with information that helps them understand that:

1. The victimization was not the child's fault.
2. The child did the right thing by telling.
3. There may be a time either in the near future or much later on when the child may want therapeutic assistance in working with the memories of the victimization—this is normal.
4. If problematic behavioral symptoms develop, a new evaluation should be performed.

5. Child sexual victimization is a pervasive problem. The child could be approached again sexually by the same or other perpetrators, and several sessions on prevention are, therefore, imperative in order to assist the child in appropriate prevention/avoidance techniques.

Effective treatment of child victims can begin only after the child is in a safe environment. In incest cases, the offender should be ordered to leave the home during the initial treatment phases. Removal of the offender provides a safe environment for the child(ren), symbolizes the seriousness of the sexually victimizing behavior, and allows the nonoffending parent/child relationship to develop gradually to a healthy level. The offender should be placed in a situation where, over time, he can become less defensive and more amenable to intervention. Unfortunately, this is not always possible. In such cases the child will need to be removed to assure his or her safety.

Various combinations of individual, group, and dyad sessions involving the child victim, nonoffending caretakers, offender, and possibly siblings can be of value. Individual psychotherapy gives the child an unpressured opportunity to sort out and define the many feelings that result from the impact of the abuse. Since control was taken from the child during the abusive situation, it is important to reestablish it by giving the school-age child or adolescent an opportunity to establish age-appropriate goals. For both offending and nonoffending parents, individual psychotherapy can help resolve the conflicts that led to that person's role in the abuse as well as offering needed support. Another important use of individual psychotherapy is the development of a more definite sense of self, which can lead to clearer boundary structures between family members. Nonoffending mothers should be helped to find ways to become less dependent on an abusive husband and to become more effective in communicating with and supporting their abused children.

Intermittent sessions involving various groupings of family members are useful both in investigating the problems and in breaking down barriers to communication and treatment. At first, such sessions between the child and the nonoffending caretaker(s) are helpful in discussing each other's feelings, developing open channels of communication, establishing a better relationship for the child's protection, redefining appropriate parent/child roles, and resolving existing problems. At later stages of treatment, offender/child meetings can be extremely useful in restructuring, renegotiating, and, if desired, rebuilding family relationships. Such meetings should take place only at a time when both the offender and victim are ready.

Group therapy is extremely helpful both for the victimized children and for the offending and nonoffending parents. Most children believe themselves to be unique, isolated cases and do not realize the prevalence of the problem. Immediately after group therapy sessions, children report relief from such feelings of being an isolated exception. Within the context of offender groups, offenders too are often able to share feelings about their abusive behavior as well as their own prior victimization as children. Nonoffending parents can often use groups of other parents for support and understanding of the problem and its solutions.

The use of self-help and other types of support groups is increasingly becoming an integral part of treatment of child sexual abuse. Parents United International is the leader among such groups. Incorporated in 1975, its purpose is to provide a structured program to protect incest victims, support the emotional growth and monitor the behavior of offenders, and offer a supportive atmosphere where all willing family members can discuss their feelings about this otherwise taboo subject. The ultimate goals are the rebuilding of the individual and the establishment of a better-functioning family structure. While family reunification is not a requirement of the Parents United program, nor is it a stated goal for each family, the program works toward that goal with families that desire it.

Parents United provides two kinds of service: support and therapy. Support services include a "buddy" system where older members help new members deal with the stresses and emotions related to disclosure of child sexual abuse. With offenders, this support helps them admit what they have done and accept the legal constraints that will prevent them from further abusive behavior. Peer involvement in the administration of the program and the development of the therapeutic milieu are also seen as part of the supportive aspects of the program. Therapeutic services include a variety of group modalities, including groups for offenders, nonoffending parents, victims of different ages, and adults molested as children, along with various combinations of these groups. Therapeutic issues addressed are the impact of the abuse, individual problems, family problems, living skills and vocational concerns, sex education, assertiveness training, communication, and parenting skills.

In addition to psychotherapeutic modalities just discussed, treatment of the offender can be approached socially and medically. Social issues include role clarification and parenting education, and may include assertiveness training and the development of job and independent living skills. New medical techniques for treating offenders are being developed based on hormonal and physiological aspects of sexual behavior.[5] Berlin[3] has introduced the use of weekly medrooxyprogesterone acetate (Depo-Provera) injections to decrease the production of testosterone and, therefore, the sexual urges of repeat sexual offenders. Abel[1] has developed a behavioral technique in which a penile transducer, or plethysmography, is used to help control arousal.

REFERENCES

1. ABEL, G. G. "The Outcome of Assessment and Treatment at the Sexual Behavior Clinic and its Relevance to the Need for Treatment Programs for Adolescent Sex Offenders in New York State," Paper presented at the Prison Research Education/Action Project Press Briefing, Albany, New York, 1984.

2. ANDERSON, L., and SHAFER, G. "The Character Disordered Family: A Community Treatment Model for Family Sexual Abuse," *American Journal of Orthopsychiatry*, 10 (1979):436–445.

3. BERLIN, F. S., and MEINECKE, C. F. "Treatment of Sex Offenders with Antiandrogenic Medication: Conceptualization, Review of Treatment Modalities and Preliminary Findings," *American Journal of Psychiatry*, 138 (1981):601–607.

4. BERLINER, L., and STEVENS, D. "Clinical Issues in Child Sexual Abuse," in J. Contee and D. Shore, eds., *Social Work and Child Sexual Abuse*. New York: Haworth Press, 1982, pp. 93–108.

5. BRADFORD, J. M. "Organic Treatments for the Male Sexual Offender," *Behavioral Sciences and the Law*, 3 (1985): 355–375.

6. BULKLEY, J. *Child Sexual Abuse and the Law*. Washington, D.C.: American Bar Association, 1981.

7. BURGESS, A. W., HOLMSTROM, L., and McCAUSLAND, M. "Counseling Young Victims and Their Families," in A. W. Burgess et al., eds., *Sexual Assault of Children and Adolescents*. Lexington, Mass.: Heath and Co., 1978, pp. 181–204.

8. GELINAS, D. J. "The Persisting Negative Effects of Incest," *Psychiatry*, 46 (1983):13.

9. GIARRETTO, H., GIARRETTO, A., and SGROI, S. M. "Coordinated Community Treatment of Incest," in A. W. Burgess et al., eds., *Sexual Assault of Children and Adolescents*. Lexington, Mass.: Heath and Co., 1978, pp. 231–240.

10. GOODMAN, G. S. "The Child Witness: Conclusions and Future Directions for Research and Legal Practice," *Journal of Social Issues*, 40 (1984):157.

11. GROTH, A. N. *Men Who Rape: The Psychology of the Offender*. New York: Plenum Press, 1979.

12. ———. *Anatomical Drawings: For Use in the Investigation and Intervention of Child Sexual Abuse*. Newton Center, Mass.: Forensic Mental Health Associates, 1984.

13. PORTER, F. S., BLICK, L. C., and SGROI, S. M. "Treatment of the Sexually Abused Child," in S. M. Sgroi, ed., *Handbook of Clinical Intervention in Child Sexual Abuse*. Lexington, Mass.: Lexington Books, 1982, p. 115.

14. PUTNAM, F. *The Diagnosis and Treatment of Multiple Personality Disorder*. New York: Guilford Press, in press.

15. SGROI, S. M. "Introduction: The State of the Art in Child Sexual-Abuse Intervention," in S. M. Sgroi, ed., *Handbook of Clinical Intervention in Child Sexual Abuse.* Lexington, Mass.: Lexington Books, 1982, p. 3.

16. SGROI, S. M., BLICK, L. C., and PORTER, F. S. "A Conceptual Framework for Child Sexual Abuse," in S. M. Sgroi, ed., *Handbook of Clinical Intervention in Child Sexual Abuse.* Lexington, Mass.: Lexington Books, 1982, pp. 9–37.

48 / Treatment of Childhood Depression

Leon Cytryn and Donald McKnew, Jr.

Introduction

The all-encompassing goal of therapeutic intervention with depressed children is to help patients reach the highest level of functioning of which they are capable. For any therapeutic intervention, however, the ultimate goal will vary from case to case, depending on many factors. Some therapists and patients seek to relieve the present symptoms without attempting to alter patients' basic personality characteristics. Others may be more ambitious and strive toward the realization of patients' full potential. Such strivings are limited by the nature of patients' past and present life circumstances, their motivation, and the strength of their determination to seek change. Sometimes even the most motivated patients and their families are frustrated by the most mundane circumstances, such as the availability of treatment and monetary and time considerations.

Family Intervention

The child psychiatrist or other child therapist can choose from or combine a number of types of treatment that are usually most effective in the earlier stages of childhood depression. The most important of these is some kind of family intervention. This can include intensive family psychotherapy, in which all family members are encouraged to discuss what they know about the problem and the circumstances that precipitate it and are guided to see how changes in their own behavior may alleviate it.[9] It can also include periodic counseling of the parents, with or without direct contact with the child.[11] All work with families contains

a certain amount of insight therapy and a certain amount of guidance, and children and parents may benefit from both. The choice of method will depend on the severity and length of the illness, the age of the child, and the intelligence, motivation, and insightfulness of the parents. The younger the child, the more responsive he or she will be to environmental changes alone.

Parent Counseling

Some of the families that mental health professionals see are not aware of the potential harm their child-rearing methods can wreak on children. For instance, consider the family that farmed out their son all week to a grandmother and brought him home for the weekend. Coming herself from an emotionally deprived background, the mother experienced difficulty understanding the potentially traumatic impact of this situation. In such cases, it is often not feasible to help the parents by interpreting the child's feelings of rejection; rather the therapist has to be directive and point out to the parents the relationship between the child's life situation and his depression. Unless it is specifically contraindicated, all activities that will bring the parents closer to or more in touch with their children are encouraged. The therapist may suggest also to the parents that they help the children cope more effectively with any specific depressive issues that may have arisen in the children's life. If there has been a recent death, the family will be advised to talk about it with the children openly and to answer frankly any questions they may have. Grief may be lightened by being brought out in the open. If children are depressed about not having friends, parents may be advised as to how to go about teaching and helping the children to make more friends.

When children are older, in grade school, or when depression is of long duration or great intensity, work with families should include the affected child and often other family members as well. In such cases, it must often be supplemented by the therapist's individual work with the depressed child and with the parents —particularly if, as so often happens, one or both parents are depressed. Whenever it can be used, a form of therapy that interprets what is going on but does not direct the family in so many words as to what to do generally is most efficacious in producing long-term benefits.

When the therapist tells the family to spend more time with their children or to stop sending them away during the week, this is a form of direct guidance. But when the therapist tries to get the family to understand the process of scapegoating, in an effort to decrease depreciation and rejection of a child, this entails valuable insight. In the course of scapegoating, a child is blamed for virtually every untoward event that occurs. Naturally the child's self-esteem is forced lower than ever. Therapists can help some families undo this process. Therapists can get families to see that scapegoating pulls children down, takes away their natural desire to accomplish things, makes them wonder whether life is worth living. When the members of the family come to realize this, apparently all by themselves, they are likely to abandon the scapegoating habit much faster than if they are simply given direct counseling or guidance.

The same process can work in cases in which children are depressed because they have suffered a major loss or bereavement. The therapist can help the family understand that such an occurrence may affect a child more deeply than an adolescent or an adult, because more mature individuals have a wider array of interests and a greater number of understanding friends to buoy them up. The therapist may also explain that because of children's developmental needs, their more fragile sense of self, and their greater emotional dependency, they may feel that the loss of a favorite friend or relative or even a pet means the loss of their world. Given these insights into the situation, many families can come to their own conclusions about what to do.

Parent Therapy

If the parent of a patient suffers from a depressive illness, it is important to provide appropriate treatment for him or her, in order to improve the patient's functioning and to furnish a more available source of care

as well as a nondepressed model for the child to follow and with whom to identify.

Individual Therapy with the Child

In some cases of childhood depression, family therapy and parental counselling or treatment may not suffice and individual psychotherapy for the child will be indicated. In such a circumstance, the specific goals of treatment differ only slightly from those with adult patients. A crucial element is the attempt to develop a close empathic and trusting relationship with the therapist. In addition to their professional qualifications, therapists have to be sensitive persons who can respond intuitively to the child's needs. Many distinguished therapists, such as David Levy[8] and Frederick Allen,[2] have gone so far as to say that the therapeutic relationship itself accounts for most of the successes achieved in psychotherapy with children. All would agree that that kind of relationship is the cornerstone of such therapeutic work.

Second in importance is what Franz Alexander[1] called a corrective emotional experience: Children come to experience a different and a more healthy response from their therapist than they had experienced before in their outside life. The therapist accepts the children in their totality without criticism and judgment. Where appropriate, the therapist expresses approval of the children, which often stands in contrast to so much previously experienced disapproval. Since low self-esteem and hopelessness are the hallmarks of childhood depression, therapists have to make special efforts to convey to the children that they are valued as a person irrespective of the their shortcomings and that, as therapists, they have firm hopes about each child's ability to overcome difficulties in becoming a self-respecting person.

A third important element is encouraging children to ventilate all their feelings and thoughts, such as fears, worries, sadness, hopelessness, conflicts with important people, anger, and distortions about self and others. Although Anna Freud[5] stressed that ventilation is not sufficient, nevertheless it is important that children feel free to get things off their chest with appropriate affect in a nonthreatening and supportive situation.

The final goal is the interpretation by the therapist of the basis for children's feelings and conflicts. With the help of the therapist, the children must become aware of their feelings. They have to learn to understand their unrealistic perceptions of themselves and others, to begin to unravel their neurotic conflicts, and to try out the alternative ways available to them to cope with their life circumstance in a more effective and adaptive manner.

Probably the most commonly used form of psychological therapy is *analytically oriented psychotherapy,* with sessions scheduled once or twice a week. [12] This technique is based on the premise that people's emotional difficulties arise from largely unconscious conflicts, accompanied by painful feelings, which lead to distorted views of oneself and others. Whether used with an individual, a family, or a group, this form of therapy has a common base of operations. If patients are intellectually and emotionally ready, this therapy strives to give them insight into their personal difficulties. Perhaps more important still, it makes use of what English child analyst David Winnicott [18] called "the holding situation." This refers to the therapist-patient environment. Therapists who employ this type of treatment use what James Strachey [17] called the *mutative interpretation.* Such interpretation encourages patients to express in therapy all the bad things they feel about themselves. They project these feelings by attributing these negative characteristics to the therapist; or if they are being treated in a group, they may also project them onto some of the group members. The therapist, group members, or both interpret to patients the largely unconscious maneuver; by doing so they give patients back a corrected, realistic version of their often distorted ideas and feelings. If this process is repeated often enough, patients can gradually acquire a new idea or picture of themselves and of the people in the world around them, and thus begin to change.

Another method of psychological treatment is *behavior modification.* [4,19] (See chapter 43) This method is based on various learning and behavior theories that hold that human behavior is governed not by unconscious forces but rather by specific environmental factors. Behaviorists stress environmental responses that influence behavior and pay little attention to insight or to any of the other intrapsychic factors discussed previously. The emphasis is on manipulating environmental conditions in order to alter certain behaviors. Such behavioral alteration is often achieved by reward and punishment systems. The so-called *positive reinforcement* involves a system of rewards that may be tangible, such as food, money, or candy, or intangible, such as privileges or praise. *Negative reinforcement* seeks the extinction of undesirable behavior. The most common techniques used toward this goal include either purposeful ignoring of a specific behavior or some form of punishment.

A variant of behavioral therapy is developed and modified for use in children by Aaron Beck and Maria Kovacs [7] at the University of Pennsylvania. Their basic assumption is that emotional disturbances, including depression, are caused by distortion in thinking on a conscious level. According to this theory, the disturbed

thinking of a depressed person includes three major elements: (1) negative self-esteem (2) negative view of the past and present, and (3) hopeless outlook for the future. Cognitive therapy attempts to correct this disturbed thinking by direct examination of patients' views, with the goal of helping them gradually to adopt a realistic view of themselves, their environment, and their destiny.

Sometimes all the preceding techniques fail because of the truly hopeless nature of the child's situation. In such a case, it is crucial that the therapist acknowledge this reality.

Although the goals of therapy are basically the same for all children, regardless of age, the technique employed obviously has to be tailored to children's chronological age and the degree of their cognitive or emotional readiness. Clearly young children require play therapy that employs dolls and other play materials and games. Through these media, children can express in their own way all the problems that older children verbalize more directly. However, children as young as five or six can talk about and discuss their difficulties in a reasonable manner; indeed, they may require only a minimum of nonverbal activities such as play or games. In any case, the level of interpretation has to be adjusted to the age of the child.

Community Collaboration

There are many cases, of course, where family conditions make traditional psychiatric intervention unfeasible. In such cases, therapists may have to collaborate or work with community resources such as schools, juvenile courts, halfway houses, foster homes, and the police. On behalf of their depressed patients, therapists may have to get involved with community agencies and keep in touch until the particular problems of interest to the agencies are solved. In the course of treatment of depressed children, it is often necessary to go to schools for meetings with teachers, arrange for halfway houses or foster homes, talk to the police, and testify in court.

Pharmacotherapy

In the past twenty-five years there has been a great increase in the use of drugs for the treatment of depression in adults. More recently, drugs have been employed also in the management of depression in children. At this point only tentative answers are available as to their usefulness; however, it looks as though they are going to be as helpful with children as they are with adults.

We feel strongly that if drugs seem necessary for a depressed child, they should always be used in conjunction with psychotherapy and never as the only method of treatment. Our stand is based on observations made by a number of therapists that in many adult depressed patients drugs alone may not be sufficient to bring about adequate improvement. Almost all adult patients respond to the combined use of drugs and psychotherapy, and there is increasing reason to believe that the same is true of children. If children are sufficiently disturbed as to require drugs, they need psychotherapy too, in order to help them understand and work through the disturbing and sometimes even terrifying experiences they have been through while ill.

TRICYCLIC ANTIDEPRESSANTS

As mentioned in chapter 16 in volume 2 of this *Handbook,*[3] there have been a number of inconclusive studies about the use of tricyclic antidepressants in depressed children. Most of these studies reported approximately a 75 percent improvement rate; nonetheless, it has been very difficult to assess the true worth of such medication in children as opposed to possible placebo effect.

Two groups of investigators have conducted well-designed double-blind studies with tricyclics in children. Puig-Antich and associates[16] first conducted an open study of thirteen children with major depressive disorder. Eight children who failed to respond to ward therapy received imipramine hydrochloride for one month, and six of the eight showed demonstrable improvement. A subsequent study[15] suggested that in such children the degree of improvement correlated well with their plasma levels of imipramine and desimipramine hydrochloride. In his most recent study, Puig-Antich[14] studied thirty-eight prepubertal children who satisfied the unmodified Research Design Criteria for a major depressive disorder in a double-blind, placebo-controlled design. This time there was no statistical difference in the degree of improvement between the drug and placebo groups. Subsequently, the investigators split the imipramine-treated group into two subgroups: one with a high plasma level of imipramine and desimipramine (greater than 155 ng/ml) and one with a low plasma level of the drugs (less than 155 ng/ml). All patients with the high plasma level showed clinical improvement, while only 22 percent of the low-plasma-level group showed such a response. However, this was significantly lower than the placebo group, which showed a 68 percent improvement.

Preskorn, Weller, and Weller[13] treated with imipramine twenty hospitalized children diagnosed by DSM-III criteria as major depressive disorder. When the plasma level of imipramine and desimipramine was in the range of 125 to 225 ng per ml, 92 percent of the children showed clinical improvement as opposed to 25 percent improvement in those children with plasma levels above and below this range. The authors point out that despite some evidence of the efficacy of imipramine in childhood depression, no study has convincingly demonstrated a drug/placebo difference. In view of the fact that the drug has a potentially serious cardiotoxic effect, such a finding should make everyone prudent in prescribing imipramine to children. Side effects may include dry mouth, nausea, constipation, somnolence, tachycardia, and anorexia. Given these considerations, careful monitoring of the cardiovascular system (blood pressure and electrocardiogram) is indicated.

LITHIUM CARBONATE

Much of the criticism that has been leveled at antidepressant drug studies applies as well to lithium studies in children—open design, heterogeneous diagnostic grouping, and no defined length of study or follow-up. A number of different child psychiatric conditions have been reported to be responsive to lithium; they include hyperactivity, cyclic mood changes, aggressive behavior, and explosive outbursts. A previous lithium study conducted by McKnew and coworkers[10] yielded a good response for bipolar conditions.

In connection with the use of lithium, a number of factors should be noted.

Time Response. It takes approximately four to seven days before a significant therapeutic effect is apparent.

Dose. In contrast to some European reports, which stress the frequent need for the use of adult doses in children (usually 1500–1800 mg/day), our experience indicates that in most children (ages six to twelve) 900 mg per day is the maximum dose needed to maintain a therapeutic plasma level of 0.5 mEq per l to 1.5 mEq per l.

Side Effects. Although adult side effects include diarrhea, nausea, weakness, tremor, hypo- and hyperthyroidism, blurred vision, drowsiness, polyuria, and polidypsia, our findings to date confirm earlier reports about the relative rarity of side effects in children. Recently there have been some reports of permanent kidney damage in adults after prolonged lithium administration. The renal changes included interstitial nephritis and tubular necrosis. So far, no such complications have been reported in children. However, prudence would dictate: (1) the contraindication of lithium in children with renal, cardiovascular, or thyroid disease; (2) periodic screening of thyroid (thyroid-stimulating hormone, triiod othyronine, and thyroxine) and renal function (urine concentration test and

creatinine clearance); and (3) caution in determining the length of lithium therapy in children. The need, safety, and maintenance dosage of lithium in children has yet to be determined.

REFERENCES

1. ALEXANDER, F., and FRENCH, T. *Psychoanalytic Therapy. Principles and Applications.* New York: Ronald Press, 1946.
2. ALLEN, F. H. *Psychotherapy with Children.* New York: W. W. Norton, 1942.
3. CYTRYN, L., and McKNEW, D. H., JR. "Affective Disorders," in J. D. Noshpitz, ed., *Basic Handbook of Child Psychiatry,* vol. 2. New York: Basic Books, 1979, pp. 321–340.
4. ENGEL, M. "Developmental Deviations," in J. D. Noshpitz, ed., *Basic Handbook of Child Psychiatry,* vol. 2. New York: Basic Books, 1979, pp. 184–194.
5. FREUD, A. "Introduction to the Technique of Child Analysis," *Nervous and Mental Disease Monograph,* no. 48. New York: Nervous and Mental Disease Publishing Co., 1928.
6. GREENSPAN, S. I., LOURIE, R. S., and NOVER, R. A. "A Developmental Approach to the Classification of Psychopathology in Infancy and Early Childhood," in J. D. Noshpitz, ed., *Basic Handbook of Child Psychiatry,* vol. 2. New York: Basic Books, 1979, pp. 157–164.
7. KOVACS, M., and BECK, A. T. "An Empirical-Clinical Approach Toward a Definition of Childhood Depression," in J. G. Schultenbrandt and A. Raskin, eds., *Depression in Childhood.* New York: Raven Press, 1977, pp. 1–26.
8. LEVY, D. "Release Therapy," *American Journal of Orthopsychiatry,* 9 (1939):713–737.
9. LEWIS, M. "Differential Diagnosis," in J. D. Noshpitz, ed., *Basic Handbook of Child Psychiatry,* vol. 2. New York: Basic Books, 1979, pp. 144–156.
10. McKNEW, D. H., et al. "Lithium in Children of Lithium Responding Parents," *Psychiatric Research,* 4 (1981):171–180.

11. NAGERA, H., and BENSON, R. M. "Normality as a Syndrome," in J. D. Noshpitz, ed., *Basic Handbook of Child Psychiatry,* vol. 2. New York: Basic Books, 1979, pp. 165–172.
12. POZNANSKI, E. O. "The Hospitalized Child," in J. D. Noshpitz, ed., *Basic Handbook of Child Psychiatry,* vol. 3, ed. S. I. Harrison. New York: Basic Books, 1979, pp. 567–578.
13. PRESKORN, S., WELLER, E., and WELLER, R. "Depression in Children: Relationship Between Plasma Imipramine Levels and Response," *Journal of Clinical Psychiatry,* 43 (1982):450–453.
14. PUIG-ANTICH, J. "Psychobiological Correlates of Major Depressive Disorder in Children and Adolescence," in L. Grinspoon, ed., *Psychiatry 1982 Annual Review.* Washington, D.C.: American Psychiatric Press, 1982, pp. 288–295.
15. PUIG-ANTICH, J., PEREL, J. M., and LUPATKIN, W. "Plasma Levels of Imipramine (IMI) and Clinical Response in Prepubertal Major Depressive Disorder," *Journal of the American Academy of Child Psychiatry,* 18 (1979):606–627.
16. PUIG-ANTICH, J., et al. "Pre-pubertal Major Depressive Disorder," *Journal of the American Academy of Child Psychiatry,* 17 (1978):695–707.
17. STRACHEY, J. "The Nature of the Therapeutic Action of Psychoanalysis" *International Journal of Psycho-Analysis* 15 (1934):127–159.
18. WINNICOTT, D. W. "Hate in the Countertransference," *International Journal of Psychoanalysis,* 30 (1949):69–74.
19. WERRY, J. S. "Behavioral/Learning Theory Formulations," in J. D. Noshpitz, ed., *Basic Handbook of Child Psychiatry,* vol. 2. New York: Basic Books, 1979, pp. 100–110.

49 / Treatment of Narcissistic Disorders in Children

Efrain Bleiberg

Fundamental to consideration of treatment of narcissistic disorders in children and adolescents is an appreciation of the developmental, clinical and pathogenetic underpinnings of the problem, which are addressed in chapter 32 in this volume.

According to Rinsley,[19,21] the treatment of children

with borderline or narcissistic conditions should seek, as goals, to:

1. Establish and maintain a stable, predictable (average expectable) environment within which individualized understanding and resolution of psychopathology may

be developed and carried out, and provide appropriate opportunities for otherwise healthy growth and development.

2. Control untoward symptomatic behavior.
3. Unravel the complex strands of communication and interaction from which the patient's psychopathology has emerged and become manifest by working with the patient's family.
4. Reestablish the patient's blighted processes of separation-individuation and identity formation.

Outpatient Treatment

The majority of children with narcissistic disorders can be treated as outpatients, providing that: their behavior or symptomatology is dangerous to neither self nor others and does not cause social ostracism; they have a reasonable capacity to make use of the growth-enhancing agencies, persons, and mechanisms of the community (most significant is the ability to engage in age-appropriate behavior and academic achievement in school); and their family is able, in spite of pathological features, to support growth and change. In particular, this includes parental appreciation of the child's need for treatment.

Residential or Inpatient Treatment

For a minority of youngsters with narcissistic disorders, developmentally appropriate goals can be pursued only in an inpatient or residential setting. Hospital and residential treatment is required when: the youngster's behavior is seriously disruptive, bizarre, dangerous to self or others, or elicits destructive responses from the environment; or when the child gives evidence of progressive psychosocial deterioration and/or escalation of distress despite adequate outpatient efforts. [2,18,19,25]

In addition, group home or foster placement may be indicated when: the child's ability to utilize home, school, church, and other growth-enhancing persons or agencies in the community is severely limited or compromised; or when parental-familial psychopathology is so severe that the child's removal from a clearly dysfunctional, destructive family environment is necessary.

There is a growing consensus in the field that those youngsters requiring inpatient or residential treatment require a therapeutic setting with the following features:

1. A consistent "holding" environment, [15,19,20] which sets firm limits, confronts the child's omnipotence, controls

manipulative and provocative behavior, is not destroyed by the child's rage, and clearly conveys to the child that he or she will be cared for and protected.

2. A sensitive and empathic "mirroring" environment [26] that carefully perceives and responds to the child as a unique being in his or her own right. The environment needs to take the child seriously; nurture the development of the child's real competence, autonomy, and individuality; and clearly convey to the child that vulnerability, pain, sadness, or dependency needs will *not* drive the caretakers away.
3. A thorough integration of every aspect of the child's life —school, family, individual therapy, leisure, peer interactions, and so forth—so that efforts in every one of these areas are mutually supportive. [13,19] As a specialized aspect of the milieu, the school needs to be empathically attuned to narcissistic children's fears of failure and humiliation and to their difficulties in acknowledging ignorance or asking for help. At the same time, the school must maintain expectations for adequate (as opposed to exceptional) performance and needs to set limits on provocative, exhibitionistic, or manipulative behavior. Often individualized tutoring is necessary to remediate the gaps in knowledge and learning skills that the children have attempted to conceal with bravado and exhibitionism. Personal projects should be designed to foster the children's capacity for sustained attention, realistic ambitions, and sense of purpose.

Marohn and associates [13] proposed a sophisticated model for the inpatient treatment of delinquent adolescents, a subgroup of which they classified as narcissistic-delinquents. Such youngsters, as is typical of narcissistic children requiring hospitalization or residential treatment, see themselves as well adjusted, deny problems, go through the motions of engagement in treatment, and are skillful at using others for their own needs, particularly for self-esteem regulation.

In Marohn's model [13] the milieu is conceptualized on three levels. The first level consists of sameness, consistency, and permanence, a dependable environment with a basic structure. Included in this basic structure are a safe space with no drugs or weapons available, a predictable schedule, and a consistent set of rules with clear consequences for breaking rules. The second level includes the development of the essential tasks of adolescence—school, peer relations, increased capacity for verbal expression of needs and feelings and for planning and anticipating. Participation in these activities is both a goal and an expectation. The third level involves developing individual treatment approaches based on an understanding of the youngster's specific needs, defenses, and deficits. The essence of this treatment model is, according to Marohn and coworkers, [13] that

staff members serve as external egos or self-objects, providing externally those psychological functions which the delinquent lacks internally, and helping to set limits on his behavior, to delay, to plan, to anticipate, to soothe himself, to modulate the intensity of his experiences, to look inside himself, to identify affect, to assuage hurt feelings, to organize fragments, and to clear up confusion. (P. 279)

CASE EXAMPLE

Jay, a bright and resourceful twelve-year-old boy, was admitted to the hospital after a long history of defiance, provocativeness, manipulative behavior, and inordinate need to be in control. The first two months in the hospital, Jay behaved like a perfect little gentleman, a most ingratiating and charming boy, in accordance with his plan to convince his father that all would go well if only he would take him home in a few months, in time to celebrate his thirteenth birthday. Staff members consistently communicated to Jay their awareness that trusting and expressing his worries and concerns would probably be hard for him, and that they knew he had more confidence in his ability to "trick" people than in his ability to share thoughts and feelings. Nevertheless, their agreement with his parents was that he would stay in the hospital until his underlying difficulties (the "things that really bothered him") were resolved.

Confronted with this message, the honeymoon was soon over. Jay became increasingly more provocative and manipulative. He excelled at identifying other children's weak spots and ruthlessly poured salt on their wounds. They were soon responding to his subtle messages. Like a puppeteer pulling the strings, he smugly sat back and grinned while other children decompensated, became anxious, silly, or aggressive. Staff intervened by restricting Jay to his room when *other* children were acting up. As expected, his response upon being sent to his room was "I don't care." At the same time, staff members made a concerted effort to identify, recognize, and respond to the slightest expression of Jay's genuine feelings, interests, or ideas. Along those lines, staff attempted to empathize with how difficult it was for Jay to stop acting or manipulating, as if he were condemned to the lonely role of actor on a stage or puppeteer. Repeatedly staff members shared their appreciation that he could not just relax and be himself. This approach seemed to help decrease the child's frantic pushiness and enabled him to take the first cautious steps toward developing a relationship with several staff members. Only then, after four months in the hospital, did Jay begin individual psychotherapy.

Specific Therapeutic Interventions with Narcissistic Children

INDIVIDUAL PSYCHOTHERAPY OR PSYCHOANALYSIS

Many agree that individual psychodynamic psychotherapy or psychoanalysis is an essential ingredient in the treatment of narcissistic youngsters, whether as a part of a comprehensive inpatient treatment or in an outpatient setting. There are widely divergent views, however, regarding the optimal therapeutic approach. Masterson[14] and Rinsley[19] identify three stages that the psychotherapy process should transverse before

therapy can be considered successful: (1) a resistance (testing) stage; (2) a definitive (working through) stage; and (3) a resolution (separation) stage. Exemplifying the application of O. Kernberg's[6,7,8] viewpoint to the psychotherapy of narcissistic children, Egan and P. Kernberg[3] emphasized as the central therapeutic tool the systematic clarification, confrontation, and interpretation of the typical narcissistic defenses of omnipotent control, devaluation, splitting, and projective identification. An essential element in this treatment approach is the thorough exploration and resolution of the child's underlying rage and envy, and related fears of retaliation and deprivation.

Kohutian therapists[4,16,17,24] believe that the treatability of narcissistic patients is predicated on the therapist's ability to adopt an empathic point of view. This literally entails the capacity of therapists to put themselves in the patient's shoes. Only from that perspective can therapists appreciate and understand the enormous pain and associated rage the patient experiences in reaction to seemingly trivial events. In the Kohutian model, therapists' pivotal function is to facilitate, via empathic understanding and acceptance, the development of the characteristic narcissistic transferences, namely the idealizing and the mirror transference. Both positions are reactivations of the child's original (and unmet) narcissistic needs: the need to share in the omnipotence of an idealized parent and the need for reflection of the child's displays of grandiosity and exhibitionism. In idealizing transferences, therapists are experienced by children as omnipotent and God-like.[24] In mirror transferences, the children see therapists only in terms of their responsiveness, similarity, or actual convergence with the patients' warded-off grandiosity.

The central feature of these transference positions is that patients rely upon therapists to regulate their self-esteem and stabilize their narcissistic equilibrium. The ultimate challenge to therapists' empathy is their acceptance of the fact that patients experience and treat them as an extension, a substitute for each patient's own psychological structure, rather than as an independent and separate person. In the soil of an empathic therapeutic relationship, patients' narcissistic transferences come to flower. Transmutative internalizations can then take place and patients' arrested narcissism is transformed into more mature forms.[9,11,23]

Naturally, the therapeutic approaches of Kernberg and Kohut differ. Kernberg[6] expects patients to be so consumed with envy that they cannot tolerate dependency or accept anything good coming from therapists: "All the patient's efforts seem to go into defeating the analyst, into making analysis a meaningless game, into systematically destroying whatever they experience as good and valuable in the analyst" (p. 70). Patients may *appear* dependent and may *seem* to idealize therapists, but in fact they are maneuvering to further exploit and devalue. Therapists must consistently address a patient's envy, greed, aggression, and devaluation while gradually helping the patient accept the unbearable feelings of smallness, hunger, and humiliation. For Kohutian therapists, on the other hand, a patient's coldness, arrogance, rage, and efforts to devalue the therapist are all attempts to ward off underlying, unmet narcissistic needs for idealized and mirroring self-objects. [10,11,16,17]

No matter what theoretical orientation or technical approach therapists take, they still must face the puzzling challenges of narcissistic youngsters. Typically, protracted and nonrelatedness marks the opening phase of the therapy. Youngsters may appear aloof and indifferent, suspicious and provocative, demanding to control the sessions or bent on reducing the therapist to the role of captive audience of an elaborate show. Consider Sam.

Sam, an impish-looking boy of six, insisted on the therapist's silent admiration of the elaborate fortified castles and walled cities that he built with his Lego set. His constructions were indeed meticulous and rather impressive. Whenever the therapist attempted to shift his role from that of "admiring spectator" to an active participant, Sam would immediately pretend to be a skunk, whose fetid odor would keep people away.

These initial gambits provide a window on the child's conflicting wishes and contrasting experiences: He feels both wonderful and smelly, entitled to admiration and simultaneously flawed and undeserving. Older latency-age and adolescent narcissistic patients often present themselves as "hot shots" filled with bravado and pretensions of self-sufficiency. The "hot shot" presentation typically signals the conflicting wishes to hide behind an omnipotent façade, thus protecting a precarious sense of autonomy, versus the wish that the therapist, in contrast to other people, would not be fooled and would call the bluff. The empathic dilemma for the therapist is when to respect patients' need to "hide" and when to respond to their need to be found out. At times, it is empathic *not* to be empathic. "Excessive" empathy only stirs up the child's fears of loss of autonomy and personal boundaries as well as anxieties that hidden vulnerabilities will be revealed by the "too-clever" therapist. At the same time, the therapist's attunement, respect, and acceptance of the child are necessary to assuage the child's fears of the consequences of genuine communication. With careful handling of children's vulnerability, therapists counter the children's conviction that their self-esteem will be deflated and their sense of self shattered at the hands of an unempathic partner.

A consistent and systematic exploration of the de- fensive function of children's omnipotence—the need to cover up their basic narcissistic vulnerability—paves the way for the possibility of the children inviting the therapist to share in their activities and their life. Jimmy, a ten-year-old boy, hospitalized while in therapy, initially subjected the therapist to ruthless tyranny and depreciation. The therapist interpreted the child's difficulties in getting what he felt he needed. These interpretations were followed with a play theme consisting of Jimmy pretending that his father was the president of the United States who needed Jimmy's guidance in order to run the country. Jimmy instructed the therapist to play the role of the father-president and delighted in barking orders that he expected the therapist to translate into directives for the country. This play theme provided the therapist with the opportunity to interpret the child's fantasy: If he could share in the omnipotence of the father-president, he would not have to feel little, helpless, lonely, or envious.

Perhaps the greatest obstacles therapists contend with during the initial phase of treatment stem from countertransference. Typical countertransference reactions described in the literature [3,8,24] include: dread of the sessions and irritation; feelings of being fooled by patients with related wishes to show them who is "really in charge"; feelings of worthlessness, helplessness, and defeat; verbal or nonverbal rejection of patients; boredom or indifference. For Kohutian therapists rejection of patients' idealizations or early interpretation of aggressive tendencies (instead of seeing the aggression as a defense against idealization) is an indication of countertransference. [24] On the other hand, followers of Kernberg would consider uncritical acceptance of the idealization, *without* addressing the patient's aggression, to be a blatant form of countertransference.

The middle stage of therapy (Masterson [14] and Rinsley's [19] definitive stage) begins when children are able to consider, in their relationships with the therapist, that there is a major section of their life that has been unlived, which until now they have denied and set aside. The children turn to face their own vulnerability, pain, helplessness, and wishes for dependency, and are filled with stark panic. Jimmy became quite anxious as the therapist invited him to explore feelings of vulnerability. Cautiously, however, he shared a long-held (and previously secret) fantasy: He had an imaginary twin who, in contrast to Jimmy, was a frightened, needy child. Jimmy could invoke the presence of this twin at will and just as readily make him disappear.

Not surprisingly, intense resistances and intensified reliance on old defensive mechanisms accompany every move in this phase of the treatment; these resistances include renewed efforts to devalue the therapist, to provoke abandonment and rejection, or to gain control of the sessions. The therapist offers empathic acknowledgment of the utter terror the children must feel as they enter this unexplored portion of their own self-experiences and gives recognition to the degree of courage required to venture much further; these responses often are helpful in supporting the children's progress.

Quite commonly, somatic complaints appear at this juncture, reflecting both children's reconnection with their own feelings of pain and vulnerability as well as their shift to a safer (and more primitive) way of requesting care and attention. This turn of children's attention to their own body also conveys underlying feelings of inadequacy and defectiveness. Strong compensatory mechanisms are called into play as the children suddenly begin to experience a host of feelings they had not allowed themselves to feel before.

If the therapist can "survive" the combined onslaught of the children's neediness and demandingness on the one hand and their provocative efforts to deny that very same neediness on the other hand, the definitive (middle) stage of treatment is underway. Themes of dependency, nurturance, safety, autonomy, and separation become available for exploration, often mixed with oedipal themes of competition, fears of body integrity, and guilt over oedipal fantasies. The children's internalization of the therapist, as an accepting object who can perceive them and respect them for what they are, plays an important role in their therapeutic progress. Identification with this accepting object is a critical factor in helping the children arrive at a more integrated and realistic self-image. Ultimately, these processes of identification and internalization[22] will give rise to more benign, realistic, and autonomous ideals and limit-setting capacities as well as to more stable regulation of self-regard.

In the final stage of individual psychotherapy, the children have an opportunity to test their readiness to relinquish pathological defenses, particularly omnipotence. The involvement with the psychotherapist is perhaps the first relationship in which the children have experienced trust and dependency. How they handle termination is a sensitive indicator of their internal changes. Some reactivation of old symptoms can be expected. While still in the hospital, Jimmy had progressed to the point of attending public school. There he quickly alienated his classmates with his petulance, tall tales about extraordinary accomplishments, magnificent accounts of his unique family, and efforts to be the center of attention. As a peer described him, he was generally regarded as "full of hot air." Despite this regression to old patterns, Jimmy presented to his therapist a rosy picture of his social life in school. As he described it, he was liked by his peers, was eagerly sought out as a playmate, and had already developed close ties with two or three boys who could not wait to have him spend the night at their homes.

Once the true picture was revealed by a teacher's report, Jimmy sheepishly acknowledged that he had lied as he was afraid to disappoint his therapist. He was so anxious to succeed that he felt compelled to be "marvelous." There was a painful gap between the ideal he felt he should meet and his actual performance. As he realized the impact of his grandiosity on his schoolmates, the gap widened.

This incident stimulated a host of important issues: Jimmy's fears that his success was contingent upon the support provided by the hospital and therapist; his ideal expectations, projected onto the therapist; his fantasy that the therapist could love him only if he was "marvelous"; his fears of not being ready to terminate; and last, but certainly not least, his difficulties in dealing with the sadness and loss associated with termination.

Family Therapy

Kohutian therapists have long advocated treating parents of narcissistic children. The goal of this effort is both to consolidate their own cohesive selves and to enable them to be empathically responsive to their children's narcissistic needs. As A. Ornstein[16] stated: "since parental empathy is the sine qua non for the execution of parental self-object functions, the remobilization of these functions will depend on the parents' ability to become empathic toward the now symptomatic child. This may require the treatment of one or both parents, since this capacity cannot be grafted onto the parents' personalities" (p. 452).

Berkowitz and associates[1] agree that in families with a narcissistically disturbed child or adolescent, the youngster has been used for the maintenance of parental self-esteem. The youngster's separation attempts severely threaten his or her narcissistically vulnerable parents. They in turn defensively project onto the child their devalued estimations of themselves and threaten to extrude the youngster prematurely from the family. These authors attempt to deal with the parents' narcissistic vulnerability in family therapy sessions. Within this context, the narcissistic child or adolescent is helped to negotiate a healthier, more phase-appropriate, and less family-destabilizing separation.

Rinsley[19] makes a strong case for the necessity of family therapy in the treatment of children or adolescents with borderline or narcissistic disorders. He believes that narcissistic psychopathology in children and adolescents is the consequence of their systematic experience of depersonification throughout childhood—that is, the child was perceived by the parents as a parent, a sibling, a spouse, and so forth. According to Rinsley, only an alteration of that nexus of depersonifying communications and interactions will allow children to resume their arrested development.

From the perspective of family systems theory, the child's symptomatology is seen as playing an essential role in maintaining the family's precarious structure. As Haley[5] stated: "Symptoms are contracts between people that serve many functions, including protective ones. Not only will parents resist improvement in a disturbed adolescent [or] child, but the child will resist improvement if something is not done about the family" (p. 282). In studying resistances to change in hospitalized young patients, Mandelbaum[12] identified, at the core of their resistances, "grave anxiety and panic that autonomy and independence will shatter the family unit and cause the parents to hurt one another, divorce, or abandon the patient forever" (p. 430). In fact, common precipitants of symptoms in narcissistic youngsters are failed efforts to help one or both parents or the family as a whole. The "rescuer" fantasy underlies some of the most tenacious resistances to treatment in narcissistic patients.

The overall principles proposed by Mandelbaum for the family treatment of the borderline patient apply as well to the family treatment of the narcissistic child. According to Mandelbaum, treatment should be directed at the family matrix rather than at the identified patient. Therapists establish their control early, setting the rules and boundaries for carrying out the treatment. Their active intervention encourages preservation of boundaries, avoids the perpetuation of myths, blocks disruptions of family interactions, and prevents helplessness over establishing controls. Furthermore, the therapists' interventions prevent irrational projections, particularly those that would assign to the child an omnipotent role endowed with precocious power and authority. Therapists select issues for the family to examine that "lead to a systematic unfolding of those dysfunctional elements weakening and destroying the parental executive function"[12] (p. 434). Basic objectives in the treatment are to:

1. *Establish the parents in an executive position.* The therapist encourages negotiations between parents regarding setting and carrying out rules and regulations, and praises them when they succeed in coming to an agreement about how to run the family.
2. *Disentangle the child from his or her "special" role in the family and institute clear boundaries within the family.* Sexual or marital conflicts between parents are the parents' business and theirs alone to solve. The child has to be freed from the role of partner in a powerful coalition with one parent against the other or as mediator between parents, alternately allied with one or the other. The child is blocked from solving adult difficulties while the parents are stopped from becoming involved in

those developmental issues that children can work out on their own, with peers, or with the appropriate parent, at the appropriate time and place.
3. *Assist the parents in developing realistic perceptions, expectations, and responses to the child.* The therapist encourages the parents to demand from the child consistent adherence to realistic constraints and limits. Parental expectations of the child are brought into line with the child's genuine strengths and weaknesses. The child's dependency needs and vulnerabilities are legitimized while the therapist coaches the parents to respond appropriately to such needs. While children are often relieved *not* to be permitted to be omnipotent and in charge, they can relinquish omnipotence only if they are reassured consistently that there will be a place for them in the family even if they are not "wonderful" or special, indeed even if they are vulnerable and in pain.

As Mandelbaum[12] observed, the therapist emphasizes that the family members

should become clear and real to each other, consistent and dependable individuals who could be counted on to protect personal space, to give empathy, to express affect, to balance all good with some bad and all bad with some good. . . . [The child is] consistently advised that as he changes he will no longer be held accountable for the difficulties his parents have in their marital relationship, in their relationships with their families of origin, in their conflicts with their other children. This reassurance is experientially observed and tested. (P. 437–438)

Clinical experience suggests that best results are obtained when individual psychotherapy is carefully coordinated with family treatment. At home, in school, and in the therapy sessions, the child slowly deals with the unresolved dilemmas of both the past and the present, but in new ways.

Prognosis of Children with Narcissistic Disorders

The literature devoted to the prognosis of youngsters with narcissistic disorders is strikingly meager. The unsettled nature of the diagnostic nosology of narcissistic disorders in children contributes to this state of affairs. Many such children are labeled as suffering from conduct disorders, affective disorders, attention-deficit disorders, schizoid or oppositional disorders, or borderline conditions. Lack of systematic longitudinal studies accounts for a paucity of empirical data regarding the later outcomes of the narcissistic disorders of childhood. Hence statements about prognosis are risky, to say the least. Kernberg[6,8] suggested that the following point to a better prognosis in adults with narcissistic personality disorders: (1) a capacity to experience depression, mourning, and guilt; (2) the patient can accrue some secondary gain or advantage from being involved in treatment; (3) transference reactions in which guilt feelings predominate versus those with predominantly paranoid feelings; (4) the presence of a capacity to sublimate and achieve real creativity in some area of their lives; (5) a higher degree and quality of superego integration, as manifested by evidence of reasonable honesty and a capacity to keep promises versus consistent lying or involvement in antisocial behavior; (6) the absence of life circumstances that grant unusual degrees of narcissistic gratification and that reinforce the patient's need for power and admiration; and (7) reasonably good impulse control and anxiety tolerance.

Careful clinical and longitudinal studies of children and adolescents are necessary to ascertain the validity and prognostic power of these criteria. Many questions remain unanswered to explain the predicament of often gifted children who plunge into a life of empty, angry, envious alienation. Much clinical refinement is needed if we are to help these children break the grip that narcissism has fastened on their loneliness.

REFERENCES

1. BERKOWITZ, D. A., et al. "Family Contributions to Narcissistic Disturbances in Adolescents," *International Review of Psycho-Analysis,* 1 (1974):353–362.

2. EASSON, W. *The Severely Disturbed Adolescent: Inpatient, Residential, and Hospital Treatment.* New York: International Universities Press, 1969.

3. EGAN, J., and KERNBERG, P. "Pathological Narcissism in Childhood," *Journal of the American Psychoanalytic Association,* 32 (1984):39–62.

4. GOLDBERG, A. "On the Prognosis and Treatment of Narcissism," *Journal of the American Psychoanalytic Association,* 22 (1974):243–254.

5. HALEY, J. *Uncommon Therapy: The Psychiatric Techniques of Milton H. Erickson, M.D.* New York: W. W. Norton, 1973.

6. KERNBERG, O. "Factors in the Psychoanalytic Treatment of Narcissistic Personalities," *Journal of the American Psychoanalytic Association,* 18 (1970):51–85.

7. ———. "Contrasting Viewpoints Regarding the Nature and Psychoanalytic Treatment of Narcissistic Personalities: A Preliminary Communication," *Journal of the American Psychoanalytic Association,* 22 (1974):255–267.

8. ———. *Borderline Conditions and Pathological Narcissism.* New York: Jason Aronson, 1975.

9. KOHUT, H. *The Analysis of the Self: A Systematic Approach to the Psychoanalytic Treatment of Narcissistic Personality Disorders.* New York: International Universities Press, 1971.

10. ———. "Thoughts on Narcissism and Narcissistic Rage," *Psychoanalytic Study of the Child* 27 (1973):360–400.

11. ———. *The Restoration of the Self.* New York: International Universities Press, 1977.

12. MANDELBAUM, A. "The Family Treatment of the Borderline Patient," in P. Hartocollis, ed., *Borderline Personality Disorders: The Concept, the Syndrome, the Patients.* New York: International Universities Press, 1977, pp. 423–438.

13. MAROHN, R., et al. *Juvenile Delinquents: Psychodynamic Assessment and Hospital Treatment.* New York: Brunner/Mazel, 1980.

14. MASTERSON, J. *Treatment of the Borderline Adolescent: A Developmental Approach.* New York: Wiley-Interscience, 1972.

15. MODELL, A. " 'The Holding Environment' and the Therapeutic Action of Psychoanalysis," *Journal of the American Psychoanalytic Association,* 24 (1976):285–307.

16. ORNSTEIN, A. "Self-Pathology in Childhood: Developmental and Clinical Considerations," in K. Robson, ed., *The Psychiatric Clinics of North America: Development and Pathology of the Self,* vol. 4. Philadelphia: W. B. Saunders, 1981, pp. 435–453.

17. ORNSTEIN, P. "On Narcissism: Beyond the Introduction, Highlights of Heinz Kohut's Contributions to the Psychoanalytic Treatment of Narcissistic Personality Disorders," in J. E. Gedo et al., eds., *The Annual of Psychoanalysis,* vol. 2. New York: International Universities Press, 1975, pp. 127–149.

18. POTTER, H. "A Service for Children in a Psychiatric Hospital," *Psychiatric Quarterly,* 8 (1934):16–33.

19. RINSLEY, D. *Treatment of the Severely Disturbed Adolescent.* New York: Jason Aronson, 1980.

20. ———. *Borderline and Other Self Disorders: A Developmental and Object-Relations Perspective.* New York: Jason Aronson, 1982.

21. ———. "A Comparison of Borderline and Narcissistic Personality Disorders," *Bulletin of the Menninger Clinic,* 48 (1984):1–9.

22. SANDLER, J., and ROSENBLATT, B. "The Concept of the Representational World," *Psychoanalytic Study of the Child,* 17 (1962):128–145.

23. TOLPIN, M. "On the Beginnings of a Cohesive Self: An Application of the Concept of Transmuting Internalization to the Study of the Transitional Object and Signal Anxiety," *Psychoanalytic Study of the Child,* 26 (1972):316–352.

24. TYLIM, I. "Narcissistic Transference and Countertransference in Adolescent Treatment," in A. J. Solnit et al., eds., *The Psychoanalytic Study of the Self,* vol. 33. New Haven: Yale University Press, 1978, pp. 279–292.

25. WARDLE, C. "Residential Care of Children with Conduct Disorders," in P. Barker, ed., *The Residential Psychiatric Treatment of Children.* New York: John Wiley & Sons, 1974, pp. 48–84.

26. WINNICOTT, D. *Playing and Reality.* New York: Basic Books, 1971.

50 / Treatment of the Borderline Child

Jules R. Bemporad, Henry F. Smith, and Graeme Hanson

The borderline child typically presents with so varied and extensive a multiplicity of deficits that effective treatment generally involves more than one modality and one provider. While individual psychotherapy may be considered the mainstay of treatment efforts, pharmacotherapy, family counseling, academic remediation, and, not infrequently, day hospitalization or residential placement are required. Each of these treatment modalities plays a singular role in the overall therapeutic goal that strives beyond symptom reduction to promote appropriate developmental skills, compensate for possible organic deficits, maximize potential for learning, ameliorate the child's everyday living situation, and eventually alter the child's estimation of self and others. These various treatment modalities are presented separately for convenience of exposition but, in reality, they tend to be used simultaneously, necessitating a primary clinician to coordinate various involved professionals and agencies.

Individual Psychotherapy

Much of the literature on the treatment of borderline children emphasizes individual psychotherapy and specifically the patient-therapist relationship. Chethick's chapter[3] in volume 2 of this *Handbook* focused primarily on the borderline child's narcissistic fantasy world, the nature of the transference tie, and the problem of structuralization.

There has been much debate over the relative value of ego-supportive as opposed to interpretive techniques in the psychotherapy of these children. While the controversy may be fueled in part by the fact that different authors seem to be talking about children at opposite ends of the borderline diagnostic spectrum, it nonetheless remains a lively and useful clinical issue.

In the mid-1950s Ekstein and Wallerstein[4,5] observed sudden regressions within the therapy hour, which seemed to occur in response to inadvertent rebukes, failures in comprehension, inappropriate interpretations, or lapses in empathic contact on the part of the therapist. Finding that direct interpretation of fantasied play material often led to panic and loss of contact or to superficial compliance, they warned of the danger of mistimed and misphrased interpretation. They recommended instead that the therapist maintain the displacement with these children, join them in their own mode of thought and level of ego functioning to "interpret within the metaphor," and reserve direct interpretation until they show a capacity for fuller understanding.

In 1963 Rosenfeld and Sprince[12] noted that borderline children, in contrast to neurotic children, used interpretation as an invitation to produce more fantasy and to act out impulsively. They later cautioned that interpretation of regression led to panic and loss of control and recommended the use of ego-supportive techniques to facilitate repression, encourage displacement, and discourage the emergence of unconscious material until the child's ego could cope with it.[13]

Anna Freud[6] also noted the negative reaction of the breakthrough of unconscious material in response to interpretation. She therefore recommended clarification of frightening affects and of those internal and external dangers that the child's weakened ego cannot master satisfactorily.

Gilpin[7] described the psychotherapy of "true fluid borderline." She advocated an active approach to let these children know the therapist can help organize their primary process world and to clarify both the nature of their difficulties and the therapeutic relationship as it develops. Paulina Kernberg,[8] too, emphasized clarification and confrontation in the areas of transference, external reality, and the communicative process between the therapist and the patient, stressing especially the here and now. Pine[11] discussed his borderline subtypes in terms of the specific focus of psychotherapy in each case, recommending a variety of interpretive and supportive maneuvers, depending on the particular subtype, the particular child, and the particular moment in the course of the psychotherapy. When asked, "Shall we interpret?" he answers, "It all depends," a point of view consistent with the thrust of this chapter.

In response to the need for a comprehensive and synthetic approach to the psychotherapy of these children, this chapter spells out various aspects of their treatment within the context of psychodynamic psychotherapy, the course of which is divided into three phases with specific tasks to be addressed in each phase: (1) allaying anxiety and forming an alliance, (2) promoting ego development, and (3) internalization.

FIRST PHASE: ALLAYING ANXIETY AND FORMING AN ALLIANCE

The two major tasks of the first phase are closely related. The degree of anxiety experienced by borderline children in the face of a new and threatening relationship inhibits the formation of a therapeutic alliance in the beginning. Rosenfeld and Sprince[12,13] described this dilemma clearly. These children are frightened by dangers they imagine to be coming from outside and from inside themselves. The therapist must bear this anxiety with them, often without the benefit of knowing its source. If the therapist tries, in fact, to identify the source of the anxiety with common psychotherapeutic approaches such as the elaboration of fantasy, clarification, or interpretation, the anxiety may escalate to panic. In an attempt to deal with mounting anxiety, such children may then become aggressive and attack either the therapist or themselves. The therapist may be forced to restrain them physically, despite knowing that physical contact may increase their panic.

The problem of closeness may manifest itself in another way. These children initially may treat the therapist as if he or she were not there, or were an inanimate object, or, via projection, they may regard the therapist as "crazy" and insist on distance. At the same time, they may make clear their longing for physical closeness and touching, even insisting on it. From a psychological perspective, such children demand a kind of merger or symbiotic attachment. In this regard, the therapist is asked to function as an empathic parent in the most demanding of circumstances.

The patients' dilemma of setting a comfortable distance between themselves and another person is similar to that ascribed to borderline adults by Modell.[9] He recalled Schopenhauer's simile of the freezing porcupines, cited by Freud in his "Group Psychology," for whom the problem is to be close enough not to freeze in the cold but not so close as to prick one another with their quills.

As participants in this dilemma, therapists, especially at the start of therapy, must be ready constantly to adjust their own physical and emotional distance from their patients, while seeking to gain their trust. Respecting the child's wishes, the therapist allows the child to make use of him or her at whatever developmental level the patient can best manage. There may be very little mutual interaction in the beginning.

It is useful for therapists, at the start of therapy, to present themselves in as nonthreatening a way as possible. In this endeavor they will usually refrain from direct interpretation and may even interrupt the free associative play of the child if it threatens to provoke too much anxiety. For example, when David, a slight ten-year-old, after several sessions involving the exploration through drawings and puppet play of his perverse sexual and aggressive fantasies, became increasingly excited and anxiously spoke about stabbing women in the "tits" and cutting off the doctor's penis, the therapist had to curtail the elaboration of this material and shifted to more structured activities.

It is also useful to adopt a reality-based, ego-supportive approach in the beginning, avoiding dynamic exploration. This may include acknowledgment of the child's anxiety and clear statements about the purpose of therapy and the therapist's intentions. Activities may include the use of concrete simple shared tasks, such as model building, and the limited gratification of wishes, such as a dish of candy on the office table. As it is for less disturbed children, it is particularly helpful for borderline children to have a safe private place in the office in which to keep their drawings and other productions, such as a shoe box or special folder. These considerations not only aid in allaying the child's anxiety but also help to build a relationship of trust and an alliance.

The task of allaying anxiety and forming an alliance in the first phase of individual psychotherapy must include work with the family and the school. These modalities will be discussed in detail later. There is room for debate as to whether all of these tasks should be performed by one or several therapists. Weger, Gilpin, and Morales[15] have described a case in which collaborative therapy was used successfully to treat a borderline child and his mother. They noted the inordinate strain such families can impose on one therapist. Unquestionably, this is true; however, when the primary focus is the individual work with the child, the therapist can avoid fragmentation and act as a particularly effective family therapist and case manager if it is feasible for one clinician to undertake most of the work. In either event, it is vital that someone must take overall responsibility for the management of the comprehensive treatment program.[14]

SECOND PHASE: PROMOTING EGO DEVELOPMENT

The goal of promoting ego development in the second phase of therapy is to encourage the borderline child's entry into latency-age functioning and to aid progress with the developmental tasks of latency.

Therapists, therefore, work to encourage defensive structure, interpretation of reality, channeling of aggression, impulse control, peer relatedness, school performance, and the pursuit of gratifying age-appropriate activities. With this last endeavor, they hope to bring these children recognition from the environment and the sense of social usefulness so important to the latency-age child's self-esteem. Indeed, the growth of self-esteem is a useful monitor of any given child's progress.

There are differences of opinion as to how these ambitious goals can best be achieved in therapy. Ekstein and Wallerstein[5] described beautifully the process of joining the child in play at the patient's own level of communication, avoiding direct interpretation of the material. In this way the therapist's ego serves as a bridge between the patient's primary process thinking and the outside world and as a facilitator of further ego development. Chethik[3] has outlined in detail this aspect of the work, which he sees as providing a bridge to the patient's "narcissistic fantasy world."

As noted earlier, however, the play and fantasy material of the borderline child is fraught with pitfalls for the patient so that the therapist must remain alert, as in the beginning of therapy, to the dangers of regression, panic, and loss of control. Also, there are quieter dangers; borderline children can be masterful in isolating the therapist. These patients may retreat autistically into a secure world of ritualized play and thereby avoid the fearful challenge of the therapist and the outside world. Here the danger is one of stalemate, boredom, and, ultimately, treatment failure.

When this stalemate occurs in therapy, it should be considered a sign that these children are successfully avoiding the frightening realities of their everyday lives, and it is incumbent on the therapist to find ways of talking with them about the real events of their lives, the pain of their sense of failure, and the distortions they adopt to explain and avoid this pain. When the alliance with borderline children is relatively secure, they will often begin to reveal how different they feel from other children. One ten-year-old boy began, in displacement, to talk about himself as Pinocchio, who wanted so much to be a "real boy." Such statements can serve as cues that their anxiety has so diminished that they can begin to look at the problems they face in real life, at their image of themselves and their sense of defect. Many borderline children feel an intense pressure to perform and succeed in social situations at the same time as they are acutely aware that they find this much more difficult than do less disturbed children. The combination of this pressure and the sense of being different is a painful subjective experience and often drives these children to withdraw even further.

At this stage in therapy, children may begin to talk frankly about the difficulties they are having at school with peers and at home with parents and other family members. Therapists then can lend, so to speak, their own egos to the examination of what the child's world is really like as well as to the examination of the child's fears and distortions of that world.

Such discussions can further strengthen the alliance, encourage identification with the therapist, and promote the child's own observational skills. In this setting, with a more secure alliance and a firm support for the child's ego functioning, the exploration of dynamic material can then be encouraged.

The sequence of steps need not be as outlined. In practice, all phases include a mixture of play, accompanied by clarification and interpretation of the issues that emerge in displacement, and a focus on the here and now with an attempt to clarify the child's perception of the world. What should be emphasized is the necessity for adjusting one's techniques flexibly to avoid the twin dangers of panic and stagnation and the necessity for monitoring, moment by moment, the state of the child's ego functioning. The constant empathic readjustment required of the therapist is a challenging and sometimes exhausting process.

Family meetings at this stage may be useful in several ways. They can help to clarify pathological family interaction and to help the parents understand the nature of the child's difficulties. If therapists choose to conduct such meetings themselves, it affords the additional advantage of giving the child a chance to see the therapist grappling with some of the problems the child faces every day. They may discuss such meetings afterward, comparing notes, so to speak.

On the more practical side, meetings with the family and the school help the therapist to find the child's areas of potential strength in order to encourage further ego growth and self-esteem. With the parents and the school assisting, the therapist can guide the child toward age-appropriate, peer-related activities, hobbies, and socially useful achievements. Some of these children have unusual talents or interests that they have allowed to hypertrophy in isolation from their peers, such as map making, electronics, antique radio collecting, photography, or botany. While such activities are isolating and herald the need for encouraging peer group interaction, they can also be capitalized on as potential sources of gratification and self-esteem. This potential can be enhanced if the talent or interest can be channeled into situations where they may achieve some peer group and social recognition, such as a science or nature club, a school newspaper, or, as they get older, academic and vocational pursuits. More than one therapist has hoped to find a place for a borderline adolescent patient as a computer programmer, botanist, or forest warden.

Activities such as sports, clubs, scouting, church groups, and camping, which are useful for social and physical development, involve risk for borderline children. Only in the setting of a trusting relationship with the therapist and with the therapist's encouragement can they begin to take such risks in group situations.

This second phase of individual psychotherapy constitutes the core of the therapeutic experience. It is a lengthy phase, during which the child and therapist "face the world" together. They face not only the external world, which the child finds so confusing, but also the child's own inner world, which has its special dangers as well as comforts. Ultimately, the examination of inner and outer reality proceed simultaneously, and in this context the child may gain sufficient confidence to progress into latency and, perhaps, beyond it.

FINAL PHASE: INTERNALIZATION

The final stage of individual psychotherapy for borderline children is a matter of considerable debate. Rosenfeld and Sprince[13] wondered how the ego-supportive methods they recommended might adversely affect the course of the child's therapy, perhaps preventing affective and libidinal growth. They referred, nonetheless, to a "later period of treatment when the borderline picture gradually changes and internalized conflict can become the center of treatment" (p. 515). Ekstein and Wallerstein[5] also noted that "as regressive trends lessen and as the neurotic aspects of the child's ego become stabilized, interpretations aim at giving insight and thus eventually approximate those used with the neurotic child" (p. 311).

Chethik[3] disputed the findings of Ekstein and Wallerstein[5] and of Rosenfeld and Sprince,[13] asserting that the quality of change from borderline to neurotic personality organization during the course of psychotherapy was contrary to his experience: "Essentially it has been our experience through therapy that improvement in functioning may be profound, but borderline children nonetheless remain borderline children" (p. 318). By the end of therapy he reported improvement in adaptation to reality, control of regression, defensive structure, and ego functioning but did not observe "the marked changes in synthetic function, in the ability to neutralize energy, in the capacity for repression as a major defense, and in libidinal object relations that are necessary for the development of a neurotic personality structure" (p. 318).

Anthony[1] put it clearly:

It is not possible to terminate with a borderline child; one can bring proceedings to a halt; one can make other arrangements; one can create a progressive program; and one can monitor development over time. But we need to follow our borderline child into borderline adolescence and into the borderline adult, and watch not only what therapy does for him but what fate does for him, and also what he is eventually able to do for himself. (Pp. 307–308)

Though we would disagree with Anthony's assumption that the borderline child necessarily becomes the borderline adult (see chapter 33), our experience with termination is similar. Frequently there is no final stage to the treatment of borderline children.

With increased mastery, self-esteem, security, and control, these children begin to make real progress toward age-appropriate levels of functioning, but with each internal advance, they simultaneously grow older, so that the environment makes increasing demands on them. Each developmental task in latency becomes a new opportunity to reopen and review therapeutic work, but soon adolescence brings another set of particularly troublesome internal and external demands. It has been found that if psychotherapy can continue into young adulthood, these patients may do relatively well. The frequency of appointments can be markedly reduced or eliminated altogether during temporary periods of calm and then increased again at times of stress. In this manner, some patients have been able to achieve success in college, choose careers, master separation from parents, and make great strides toward heterosexual intimacy, free from disabling anxiety. But therapy has never been fully terminated.

The therapist, then, becomes like the transitional object the borderline child may never before have enjoyed, discarded but not forgotten, lying in the attic, taken out and reexamined at intervals, waiting to be passed on to the next child or grandchild. So patients will on occasion contact their therapists again for a brief visit or series of visits, especially at times of developmental crisis, even into adulthood. As therapy remains open-ended, so do the boundaries between patients and their therapists, patients never fully separating, never fully internalizing their therapists to make the process their own. Rather, the experience more often is reflected in the words of one adult borderline patient who told her therapist after the therapy had ended: "When I am confronted with a difficult decision, I try to think how you would handle it, what questions you would ask me, what advice you would have." And so patients continue in this way to check in with their therapists long after the meetings in fact have ended.

Day or Residential Treatment

Borderline children have serious and chronic failures and distortions in a wide range of ego functions, along with incomplete mastery of the most important developmental tasks. The more severe cases require a treatment approach that can address the myriad areas of pathology. As Chethik[3] indicated, an intensive day or residential treatment program with a multidisciplinary approach is often the treatment of choice.

Frequently, borderline children are entangled in mutually regressive relationships with their families and are in serious difficulty with their outside environments. These children fail in almost all important aspects of latency-phase functioning, such as the development of stable and meaningful peer relationships, academic accomplishment, the development of successful sublimatory channels, the increasing control of impulses with stabilization of an internalized superego, relative independence from parental figures, and confident mastery of the body with gratification from motoric play activities.

A good milieu treatment program with personnel skilled to deal with these various areas of functioning can provide therapeutic components to help borderline children in ways that an outpatient individual or family therapy program alone cannot provide. In addition, many consider it important for children to have intensive individual psychotherapy as one component of the multidisciplinary team approach of the residential or day treatment program.

As mentioned, these children often are enmeshed in destructive and regressive relationships with their parents. There are difficulties in separation and individuation with pathological identification and projections on the part of both parents and children.

Separating borderline children by placing them in residential settings can help them and their families clarify and confront these issues. For example, a ten-year-old boy with a two-year history of severe school phobia was assigned a powerful role in the family functioning by virtue of threatening to kill himself or his parents if forced to go to school. On the day of admission to a residential program, when his mother was to say good-bye, she became tearful, ashen, and looked terrified. In a nonverbal way, she communicated palpably an overwhelming feeling of catastrophe. The staff observing this parting scene was greatly impressed with how panic-stricken the mother was at leaving her son. Thus a powerful component of the boy's psychological difficulties became much clearer.

Separating borderline children from their families can interrupt the vicious cycle of the remarkable intertwining of the psychopathologies of children and parents, which results not only in keeping children from progressing and mastering appropriate developmental tasks but frequently leads to periods of mutual regression in both parents and children.

A structured, consistent, and reliable therapeutic unit can offer a safe and supportive environment for such children as well as act as an auxiliary ego in their various areas of ego impairment. For instance, borderline children frequently have weakness in the area of reality testing; the therapeutic milieu can be especially helpful in strengthening this function by being sensitive to the child's vulnerability in this area and by making special efforts to be clear and concise about the operations and activities in the therapeutic milieu, as well as to clarify and correct distortions in the child's perception of the milieu. This strengthening of reality testing by the staff complements the work being done in the individual psychotherapy. In regard to this aspect of the milieu function, it is imperative that the staff meet regularly in team meetings to share experiences and observations of the children and their peers since it is typical of these children to form different and shifting levels of relationships with different people. They tend also to split their perceptions and experiences of people, which can result in conflicting approaches by the staff. This split perpetuates the child's lack of ego integration, which is often a reflection of what happened in the child's experience at home before coming to treatment. Related to this is the importance of having a variety of staff sharing responsibility for the care of the child, with no one person being totally responsible. This helps minimize the reestablishment of the regressive, destructive relationships such children have with their parents, although they will often tend to re-create these relationships with staff and therapists, a typical transference phenomenon.

Borderline children have a major difficulty with the capacity for signal anxiety and with the observing function of the ego. Personnel in the therapeutic milieu can help children with both of these limitations. Experienced staff can learn to recognize when children are approaching an area of intrapsychic conflict that will lead to overwhelming anxiety and panic. The staff's recognition of this danger and immediate intervention, either through verbal clarification or, more commonly, through distraction or displacement, can help these children develop their own ability to use anxiety as a cue to institute extensive and protective maneuvers. This recognition of the child's state by a staff member, who can offer a sympathetic comment about it, can be a prototype for the observing ego function, which may be strengthened in a consistent, observant, and concerned milieu.

Often the borderline child's progress in strengthening various ego functions comes through the processes of internalization and identification with beloved counselors in the therapeutic setting. Establishing a trusting and emotionally stable relationship with borderline children is notoriously difficult. A trained and experienced counselor, however, sensitive to the special characteristics of such children, may succeed where an individual psychotherapist fails to establish a powerful and meaningful relationship. Counselors are involved in a real way in much of the child's everyday life. In the rituals of waking, getting dressed, feeding, and punishments, they function much like parents. Since actions speak louder than words, it is not uncommon for borderline children to internalize the prohibitions and warnings as well as the praise and positive comments of their counselors. A vivid example is what happened with a child who initially became wildly out of control and had to be removed bodily to the quiet room. After a year of intensive inpatient treatment, that child was able to say when getting out of control "I have to go to the quiet room now" and go there on his own. This is a remarkable example of the internalization of the counselor's role in helping the child maintain control.

The role of the school is crucial in the overall treatment of borderline children. Many of these children have a variety of cognitive and perceptual motor integration deficits. Special education teachers, with the help of good neuropsychological testing, can help elucidate the specific nature of each child's learning difficulties and identify the most effective approach to learning. All too often, the child's academic difficulties have been attributed to behavioral and psychological factors. Strong emphasis should be placed on the importance of paying particular attention to evaluating the borderline child's neuro-cognitive functions.[2,8] As mentioned earlier, these children fail in many areas of latency-phase functioning. School and academic mastery occupy a major role in their lives. Through appropriate individually designed special education, these children can increase their mastery of school situations and thereby gain significantly in self-confidence. Also, it has been found that when children with learning difficulties based on central nervous system dysfunction can be given an explanation of their difficulties, there is often a sense of relief, a decrease in self-devaluation, and an increase in self-esteem.

Since a high proportion of borderline children have associated neuropsychological handicaps, specific educational strategies must be developed to meet their individual needs. Children with concomitant attentional disorders, for example, will need help with impulsivity and inattention. Such modifications as smaller group and tutorial meetings, extra emphasis on organization, seating arrangements that maximize teacher-student interaction, specific time goals, and shorter tasks with frequent alternation of active and quiet projects have proven useful. Children with problems in auditory or visual perceptual tasks, sequencing, or short-term memory functions require careful, repeated instructions, the teaching of strategies that utilize their talents, and remedial training where indicated for handicaps. Separate cognitive training programs may be built into the overall treatment plan.

Similarly, the special problems posed by borderline children with language disorders need to be considered. Such children may have great difficulty not only in reading and writing but in understanding the more abstract components of a therapeutic dialogue or of everyday speech. If a child has no concept of time, or does not understand sentences with prepositional phrases, or cannot match words such as "sad" or "angry" with the feelings they denote, appropriate modifications in the usual therapeutic and educational program will be indicated.

Ideally, the borderline child's educational experience will be integrated within the entire treatment program either by having the schooling on site with the day or residential treatment program or at least by having a close collaboration between the extramural educational staff and the mental health staff. The mental health staff can help teachers understand the special psychological characteristics of these children (such as their frequent fluctuation in functioning, their impulse control problems, their need for adult auxiliary egos, etc.). The educational staff can help the mental health staff understand the special characteristics of a particular child's cognitive style and limitations so that they can then tailor their interventions accordingly.

In summary, an intensive day or residential treatment program may be the treatment of choice for the more severely handicapped borderline child and can provide a wide variety of support in the areas of defective ego functioning that these children typically manifest.

Pharmacotherapy

Pharmacological treatment of borderline children aims at reduction of specific target symptoms, which vary from child to child. Petti[10] has reviewed the major classes of psychotropic agents in relation to the treatment of borderline children, indicating the applicability of each, while also stressing that medication should be used in conjunction with psychotherapy and not as a definitive treatment in itself. Appropriate use of psychotropic agents may prove essential in preventing decompensation in crisis situations or in reducing certain symptoms that interfere markedly with a child's environmental adjustment and mastery of developmental tasks. The creation of a more tranquil inner state or the reduction of distractibility and aimless activity will foster more effective functioning and greater receptivity to positive experiences with others.

A significant number of borderline children also present symptoms of attention deficit disorder (ADD),[2,8] and this aspect of the clinical picture is ameliorated by psychomotor stimulants such as methylphenidate hydrochloride or dextroamphetamine. As with children with ADD only, these drugs decrease distractibility, hyperactivity, and impulsivity.

The panic attacks and crippling anxiety of borderline children may respond to major tranquilizers. However, maintenance on these drugs is not advised and their use is limited to acute crisis situations. Usually thioridazine hydrochloride is the preferred medication from this group because of its presumed reduced likelihood of extrapyramidal side effects.

Other pharmacological agents that have been used with borderline children are antidepressants and lithium carbonate. Petti[10] has found antidepressants, particularly imipramine hydrochloride, to be highly effective when there is a definite depressive component in the clinical manifestations. Antidepressants have been credited with increasing the control of aggression, hostility, and hyperactivity, and improving school performance. To minimize the possibility of undesirable cardiovascular or central nervous system side effects, maintenance therapy is not recommended with these drugs. Gradual discontinuation is recommended to avoid withdrawal reactions once the depressive symptoms have abated.

Careful study of the use of lithium in the treatment of borderline children has not been reported. Nevertheless, lithium's effect on symptoms such as mood swings, aggressive behavior, and extreme emotionality suggest that further consideration should be given to the use of this drug in the treatment of selected children.[10]

Coffee* has treated thirty-five borderline children with medication as part of an overall therapeutic effort. She bases the choice of psychotropic agents on the child's symptom picture, family history of illness, and results of projective tests. Bizarre behavior, family history of schizophrenia, and evidence of dereistic thinking on testing would favor the use of a neuroleptic. The presence of mood disorder, family history of bipolar affective disorder, and themes of depression on testing prompt the use of an antidepressant or lithium. Symptoms of ADD and a family history of alcoholism are indications for the use of stimulants. Coffee stresses that each child's profile is somewhat unique and a medication regimen has to be tailor made to fit the varying clinical manifestations. In agreement with Petti,[10] she views medication as only a part of a total treatment plan and does not advocate long-term or maintenance use of medication.

*B. Coffee, personal communication, 1985.

Summary

Our knowledge of borderline syndromes of childhood is still rudimentary regarding etiology, outcome, and treatment. The clinical manifestations are gradually coalescing into a reliable diagnostic profile with a group of key symptom areas, the preponderance of which may vary from child to child. Most borderline children show some evidence of organic impairment, combined with long-term exposure to a chaotic home environment and a deprivation of crucial socialization experiences resulting in a multiplicity of symptoms, developmental arrests, and distorted views of themselves and others. Treatment of so complex a syndrome (or group of syndromes) has to be equally complex and comprehensive. The key to treatment is flexibility, with the utilization of multiple modalities that aim at remediating the defects of the child and restoring a path toward more normal developmental progress. An intensive day or residential treatment program may be the treatment of choice for the more severely handicapped borderline child and can provide a wide variety of support in the areas of defective ego functioning that these children typically manifest.

REFERENCES

1. ANTHONY, E. J. "Summing up the Borderline Child," in E. J. Anthony and D. C. Gilpin, eds., *Three Further Clinical Faces of Childhood.* New York: Spectrum Publications, 1981, pp. 307–313.

2. BEMPORAD, J. R., et al. "Borderline Syndromes in Childhood: Criteria for Diagnosis," *American Journal of Psychiatry,* 139 (1982):596–602.

3. CHETHIK, M. "The Borderline Child," in J. D. Noshpitz, ed., *Basic Handbook of Child Psychiatry,* vol 2. New York: Basic Books, 1979, pp. 304–321.

4. EKSTEIN, R., and WALLERSTEIN, J. "Observations on the Psychology of Borderline and Psychotic Children," *Psychoanalytic Study of the Child,* 9 (1954):344–369.

5. ———. "Observations on the Psychotherapy of Borderline and Psychotic Children," *Psychoanalytic Study of the Child,* 11 (1956):303–311.

6. FREUD, A. "The Assessment of Borderline Cases," in *The Writings of Anna Freud,* vol. 5. New York: International Universities Press, 1969, pp. 301–314. (Originally published 1956.)

7. GILPIN, D. C. "The True Fluid Borderline in Psychotherapy," in E. J. Anthony and D. C. Gilpin, eds., *Three*

Further Clinical Faces of Childhood. New York: Spectrum Publications, 1981, pp. 257–268.

8. KERNBERG, P. F. "Borderline Conditions: Childhood and Adolescent Aspects," in K. S. Robson, ed., *The Borderline Child.* New York: McGraw-Hill, 1983, pp. 101–119.

9. MODELL, A. "Primitive Object Relationships and the Predisposition to Schizophrenia," *International Journal of Psycho-Analysis,* 44 (1963):282–292.

10. PETTI, T. A. "Psychopharmacologic Treatment of Borderline Children," in K. S. Robson, ed., *The Borderline Child.* New York: McGraw-Hill, 1983, pp. 235–256.

11. PINE, F. "A Working Nosology of Borderline Syndromes in Children," in K. S. Robson, ed., *The Borderline Child.* New York: McGraw-Hill, 1983, pp. 83–100.

12. ROSENFELD, S. K., and SPRINCE, M. P. "An Attempt to Formulate the Meaning of the Concept 'Borderline,' " *Psychoanalytic Study of the Child,* 18 (1963):603–635.

13. ———. "Some Thoughts on the Technical Handling of Borderline Children," *Psychoanalytic Study of the Child,* 20 (1965):495–517.

14. SMITH, H. F., BEMPORAD, J. R., and HANSON, G. "Aspects of the Treatment of Borderline Children," *American Journal of Psychotherapy,* 36 (1982):181–197.

15. WEGER, L., GILPIN, D. C., and MORALES, J. "The Borderline Child in the Jones Family: Collaborative Therapy with a Borderline Child," in E. J. Anthony and D. C. Gilpin, eds., *Three Further Clinical Faces of Childhood.* New York: Spectrum Publications, 1981, pp. 243–255.

51 / Advances in the Treatment of Anxiety-Related Disorders

Keith G. Kramlinger and Alexander R. Lucas

Recently there has been much interest and a great many advances in the area of anxiety-related disorders. In view of this, one would expect there to be much research activity directed toward the treatment of such disorders in children. Surprisingly, this is not the case. On the contrary, there is a paucity of both new data and new findings regarding the treatment of anxiety disorders in children. During the entire five-year period, 1979 through 1983, no articles in the major child psychiatric journal *(Journal of the American Academy of Child Psychiatry)* dealt with the treatment of anxiety disorders. Moreover, in the journal's 1983 index, there was not a single reference to "anxiety." In 1982, there was only one article.

Anxiety continues to be a ubiquitous presence in the emotional disturbances of children, but until recently little has changed in the treatments used for its alleviation. During the past fifty years, psychotherapeutic approaches and largely ineffective psychopharmacological interventions have been the primary treatment modalities. The growing knowledge gained from the studies reviewed in chapter 34 in this volume makes this an unusually fertile area for potential investigations with children. Some intriguing work is beginning in the area of separation anxiety disorders. Until more data becomes available, however, we must content ourselves with possibilities and speculation about future advances.

Heretofore, treatment approaches have been primarily psychotherapeutic with the child and family, aiming either to induce internal changes in the child or to alter his or her environment. The verbal/play therapy approach involves psychotherapeutic techniques aimed at enabling the child to become aware of the sources of his or her anxiety and at strengthening the child's ability to cope with these feelings. The environmental manipulations aim either at reducing or eliminating the presumed sources of anxiety in the child's environment. In contrast to these approaches, behavioral treatments attempt to decrease the child's overt reactions or to make him or her more able to confront the anxiety-provoking situations, and they try to do so without addressing the inner life of the child. Psychopharmacological approaches aim at reducing symptoms associated with anxiety and seek to make the child more comfortable in anxiety-provoking situations.

Medications have frequently been used in the treatment of children's anxiety disorders. They have included sedatives and minor tranquilizers (antianxiety drugs), as well as drugs having antihistaminic properties. While some favorable results have been achieved in reducing relatively mild anxiety in some children, on the whole the results have been discouraging. The classic antianxiety drugs, particularly of the benzodiazepine group, tend not to reduce anxiety in children. On the contrary, through their disinhibiting effects they may in fact aggravate the symptoms. Barbiturates have an unpredictable effect. While they may calm some anxious children, they stimulate others. It is of interest that the antihistaminic drugs, notably diphenhydramine hydrochloride and related agents, most reliably diminish anxiety in children.

Data from Studies in Adults

Various effective therapeutic interventions—pharmacological, psychotherapeutic, and behavioral—are now available for adults suffering with anxiety disorders.[1,17] There is some controversy about which interventions to employ and in what combination to employ them for each of the anxiety disorders. Currently there is an expanding knowledge base founded on clinical experience and research findings that is becoming increasingly useful in guiding therapeutic interventions.

Of the pharmacological agents currently used to treat anxiety, the benzodiazepines are the most widely known and prescribed. Other drugs of potential use in specific types of anxiety disorders are the tricyclic antidepressants, monoamine oxidase inhibitors (MAOIs), beta-adrenergic blocking agents, clonidine hydrochloride, and a newer agent, buspirone.

Psychotherapy seeks to help by bringing conflicts into consciousness with the aim of resolving them and thus diminishing anxiety. Cognitive therapy involves teaching anxious patients to control anxiety by developing mastery of those situations in which anxiety has occurred in the past.

Behavioral therapy attempts to induce anxiety either by exposing the patient to an anxiety-provoking situation (*in vivo* exposure) or by having the patient fantasize the context in which he or she typically becomes anxious (systematic desensitization). However it is achieved, control of the patient's responses at that moment appears to provide a crucial corrective emotional experience. This in turn leads to the critical feeling of mastery that the patient must acquire in order to be able to cope with future anxiety-provoking situations.[16]

Current nosological schemata separate the anxiety disorders into four discrete entities: panic disorder, obsessive-compulsive disorder, phobic disorders, and generalized anxiety disorder. Despite significant clinical and phenomenological differences among these four conditions, it is clear that they all share overlapping symptomatology. Occasionally, this serves as a complicating factor and leads to difficulties in reaching a specific diagnosis. This is particularly likely when treating patients who either are experiencing less than the full complement of symptoms required for diagnosis (*"forme fruste"*) or are having two or more clearly definable syndromes simultaneously (e.g., panic dis-

order complicated secondarily by phobic disorder—simple phobia, social phobia, and/or agoraphobia). Children, particularly those who have psychoneurotic disorders, tend to have mixed symptomatology.

These difficulties in attaining specific and precise diagnoses understandably complicate therapeutic approaches. It is evident that various aspects of anxiety respond differentially to the various treatment modalities—for some aspects, pharmacological intervention is best; for others, psychotherapy; and for still others, a behavioral approach. Treatment programs thus cannot be determined only by symptom constellations (diagnosis) and need to be tailored to the individual patient.

PANIC DISORDER

In panic disorder, drugs are effective at blocking the panic attacks, but the chronic anticipatory anxiety and phobic/avoidant behavior are not so effectively treated.[1,17]

Panic attacks perhaps reflect an inadequacy of some neurobiological regulatory system, which leads to paroxysmal episodes of great intensity but without any apparent psychological content. These panic episodes are blocked by antidepressant medication,[21] but the mechanism by which this occurs is not clear and may be unrelated to the antidepressant effect.

Panic attacks seem to respond dramatically to the tricyclic antidepressant imipramine hydrochloride.[1,17] Unlike the delayed effect seen in depression, in panic disorders, once the appropriate dose is reached, the response to imipramine is rapid. For treatment of adults with this condition, current dosage recommendations for tricyclics are often in the range of 150 to 225 mg per day (it is important to recognize the sensitivity of some patients to these drugs). Many patients experience significant improvement while taking smaller doses. When imipramine therapy is discontinued, panic attacks tend to recur.

MAOIs are also effective in reducing panic attacks.[1,17] Studies that compared tricyclics and MAOIs found both to be effective.[21] Given the need for dietary restrictions with MAOIs, for most patients the treatment of choice is one of the tricyclic antidepressants.

Some patients may require the addition of a benzodiazepine on a time-limited basis. Alprazolam, a structurally unique benzodiazepine with possible mild antidepressant properties, has been reported to be effective in blocking panic attacks.[1] However, doses (6 mg/day) higher than those normally recommended may be required in order to obtain a clinical response. Sedation may be a problem, and it is not yet established whether tolerance to the drug's antipanic effects may occur. Other benzodiazepines do not appear to have specific antipanic or antidepressant effects. They may be of use in treating any coexisting anticipatory or chronic anxiety that has developed secondary to panic attacks. However, it is not clear how often the addition of benzodiazepines is actually of any lasting benefit, and their prolonged use should be avoided in panic disorders.

The secondary phobic and avoidant symptoms that so frequently develop do not respond well to drug treatment,[13,16] and some form of psychosocial intervention is usually required for these. Both dynamically oriented supportive psychotherapy and behavioral therapy have proved fairly effective in addressing these anxious avoidant phenomena that develop in the interim between panic attacks.[13] Support in the form of encouragement and sympathy, persuasion, and *in vivo* exposure—all within the context of a patient-therapist relationship—have been associated with good success in treatment.

OBSESSIVE-COMPULSIVE DISORDER

Obsessive-compulsive disorder is one of the most treatment-resistant conditions seen by psychiatrists. Pharmacological intervention, including the use of neuroleptics, tricyclic antidepressants, MAOIs, lithium carbonate, and benzodiazepines, has not given consistent benefit. Other somatic therapies—electroconvulsive treatment and even leukotomy—have had only limited success. Psychosocial interventions emphasizing behavioral treatment have provided only partial response.[1,7,17]

Recently an investigational drug of the tricyclic antidepressant class, clomipramine hydrochloride, has emerged as consistently effective in the treatment of obsessive-compulsive disorder in children, adolescents, and adults.[2,7,12] It seems effective for both the primarily obsessional and the primarily ritualizing patients. However, its effects are often partial. Obsessional thinking persists but interferes less with patients' activities, and intrusive thoughts are resisted more easily. Obsessional symptoms disappear entirely in only about 15 percent of patients. Dosages of 75 to 300 mg per day are needed, and effective response may not occur for four to six weeks. Among all the drugs, clomipramine (not yet available in the United States) is the most promising agent for the treatment of obsessive-compulsive disorder.

Obsessive-compulsive disorder is chronic. It often starts in childhood and continues throughout adulthood.[11] Hence patients need long-term support and directive interventions. Pharmacological treatment is just one dimension of a multifaceted approach.[12] In psychotherapy with these patients, it helps to encourage them to take risks and to push themselves into work, school, or other activities that can enhance their self-esteem and distract them from obsessional thoughts. A supportive family is a distinct advantage and may be a critical influence in the patient's ultimate outcome.[12]

PHOBIC DISORDERS

In the treatment of patients with specific phobias and avoidant behaviors, psychotherapy and behavioral training are more effective than the use of anxiolytic drugs. In some patients, behavioral training may be more effective than psychotherapy.[14] Behavioral treatment of these dysfunctional states with regimens that emphasize the patient's prolonged confrontation with or "exposure" to the feared stimulus has produced consistent improvement.[16] From 65 to 75 percent of phobic patients who complete behavioral treatment show substantial, clinically significant improvement. These positive effects appear to endure at follow-up of four to nine years.

Controversy exists regarding the use of anxiolytic drugs as adjunctive treatment during behavioral training. It is reasoned by some that such adjunctive treatment would reduce avoidant behavior and hence optimize the critical factor in the treatment of patients with phobias—namely, the gradual exposure to situations in which the phobic reactions occur. Patient selection for this type of adjunctive therapy requires careful attention.[15] An ideal candidate would be a person who is motivated to try to understand the symptoms and to work to gain mastery over them. Patients who can achieve this sense of mastery often become less desperate and more able to explore a variety of nondrug means of coping with the anxiety, thus avoiding the risk of long-term drug dependency.

In conditions such as stage fright, test anxiety, experimental stress, and acute anxiety, studies examining single doses of beta-adrenergic blocking agents indicate that these agents can be effective in some instances without causing impairment or interfering with alertness and concentration.[5]

GENERALIZED ANXIETY

There is a paucity of research comparing the effectiveness of various forms of treatment in patients with generalized anxiety. In clinical psychiatric practice, most patients with significant symptoms of generalized anxiety will be treated with psychotherapy, with or without the addition of pharmacological agents. Studies comparing behavioral approaches with medication tend to suggest that some combination may be best.[1,16,17]

There have been attempts to predict which patients are most likely to respond to benzodiazepines; these studies suggest that higher levels of anxiety predict a better response. Other reliable predictors related to a good outcome of pharmacological intervention include (1) lack of chronic difficulties, (2) absence of overexposure to drugs, (3) anxiety occurring in the context of stress, and (4) the physician's degree of comfort with the patient and with prescribing drugs, as well as positive expectations about their use.[1] The largest drug-placebo differences occur in respect to subjective and somatic symptoms of anxiety.[19] However, it seems that even those patients who experience significant benefits on benzodiazepine therapy have more symptoms than do nonanxious patients seen in general medical practice.

Beta-adrenergic blocking agents offer the clinician an alternative to benzodiazepines in the treatment of anxiety disorders. Despite the fact that these agents have not been dramatically successful in widespread clinical practice, the potential benefit of beta-blockers in generalized anxiety states has been demonstrated in several investigations.[6,18] Although the antianxiety effects were variable in studies comparing beta-adrenergic blockers with placebo, doses of 40 to 240 mg per day of propranolol hydrochloride or its equivalent were generally superior to placebo. However, in other studies comparing beta-adrenergic blockers with benzodiazepines, the benzodiazepines were consistently (if not always statistically) more effective. The hypothesis that these agents are more effective for somatic symptoms of anxiety than for the subjective experience of anxiety has not always been upheld. In fact, studies using the highest doses of beta-adrenergic blockers yielded the greatest reduction in the subjective experience of anxiety.

DIFFERENTIAL THERAPEUTICS

The actual study of anxiety disorders—their etiology, biology, and treatment—is still in its early stages. Available research does not yet provide conclusive evidence to permit more specific treatment recommendations, particularly in generalized anxiety disorder. It is, however, important to integrate pharmacological and psychosocial interventions effectively in the treatment of these conditions. Consideration of these two aspects separately in a two-stage differential assessment of symptomatology may prove useful in achieving such an integration.

The diagnostic entity that most closely approximates the individual patient's experience, such as panic disorder, obsessive-compulsive disorder, phobic disorder, or generalized anxiety disorder, is most useful as a guide toward the development of a comprehensive treatment program. This is achieved after the formulation of an orderly, stepwise, and hierarchical differential diagnosis. Such a formulation is facilitated by attention to the descriptive features of the patient's symptoms.

Pharmacological interventions should be considered in the presence of features or syndromes such as panic attacks, obsessions, compulsion, circumscribed identifiable stressors, or generalized anxiety, as discussed in the previous section. Unfortunately, more specific data to assist rational selection of pharmacological agents are not currently available. Indeed, the most difficult question in the pharmacological approach to anxiety may be not so much which agent to employ but rather whether one should institute pharmacological treatment at all.

Subsequent to this determination, since any form of anxiety may be complicated secondarily by phobic/avoidant behaviors, an assessment of these factors, with a goal toward the selection of the most appropriate psychosocial intervention, needs to be undertaken. Additionally, since many of these disorders are chronic or only partially remediable despite optimal management with currently available means, it is of paramount importance not to overlook the psychological effects such distressing and disabling conditions have on patients and their families. Under such circumstances the need for appropriate long-term supportive psychosocial intervention seems self-evident.

Application to Children

The work of Gittelman-Klein and Klein[9] demonstrates that knowledge obtained from the treatment of adult patients with anxiety disorders can have relevance to work with children and adolescents. These investigators noted that a large proportion of adult agoraphobic patients had a childhood history of severe separation anxiety and that their response to initial panic had been clinging, dependent behavior. Gittelman-Klein and Klein postulated that the agoraphobic patients were suffering from a disruption in the biological process that regulates the anxiety triggered by separation. They assumed that panic anxiety was a pathological variant of developmentally normal separation anxiety, which suggested that imipramine, which relieved panic anxiety, would be useful in disorders involving separation anxiety. The medication was accordingly tried in agoraphobic adults and in school-phobic children.

A placebo-controlled, double-blind study of imipramine in forty-five school-phobic children, ages seven to fifteen years, was carried out.[9] During the six-week study the patients and family also received weekly psychotherapeutic management. It turned out that imipramine was significantly more effective than placebo in relieving the primary symptom of anxiety and causing the treated children to feel better after their return to school. The drug also had a beneficial effect on secondary symptoms of stomachache, nausea, dizziness, headache, and vague aches and pains.

Significant dosages were required in the range of 100 to 200 mg per day. No child responded to less than 75 mg per day. Gittelman[8] cautioned that a daily dose of 5.0 mg per kg of body weight should not be exceeded because of possible serious cardiovascular side effects. That this warning cannot be taken lightly is illustrated by the sudden death of a six-year-old girl who was receiving 300 mg (14.7 mg/kg) of imipramine.[20] Saraf and associates[20] pointed out that children receiving doses of 3.5 mg or more of imipramine per kilogram are likely to show an increase in P-R interval on the electrocardiogram.

Gittelman-Klein and Klein[10] found that imipramine modified the child's level of anxiety in response to separation, enabling return to the classroom. They emphasized that psychotherapy and counseling for the family were used also and that drug therapy should not be viewed as the sole treatment for school phobia.

In another study, Berney and coworkers[3] reported a twelve-week trial of 40 to 75 mg of clomipramine per day in school-phobic children. Little change in anxiety resulted with either placebo or clomipramine. At the end of the trial, 40 percent of the children were still not attending school and 75 percent still experienced significant separation anxiety. Undoubtedly, however, the dosage levels employed were too low to dismiss clomipramine as ineffective in the treatment of school phobia. As noted earlier, in daily doses ranging from 100 to 200 mg, clomipramine has been shown to be significantly more effective than placebo in controlling the symptoms of obsessive-compulsive children and adolescents.[7]

Conclusion

In many of its manifestations, anxiety has defensive and adaptive value and should not necessarily be eliminated simply because it is there. However, when warranted by the clinical condition, treatment is necessary. Treatment approaches need to be individually tailored. Psychosocial approaches, including psychotherapeutic, behavioral, and environmental techniques, still have an important place in the treatment of most anxiety-related disorders in children. The availability of effective medications for use in these disorders is most welcome. When clinically indicated, medications that have proven effective with adults may be tried in appropriate doses. However, the evaluation of the efficacy of such approaches in children awaits further study. Given the potential toxicity of psychotropic medications and their unknown short-term and long-term risks when used in children, cautious use is advised.[4,22] It should be noted that when these drugs are used by physicians unfamiliar with their effects, the relative risk is increased. Again, when such medications are used, appropriate attention must be paid to side effects in order to prevent serious complications. Research is needed to clarify further the clinical varieties of anxiety, to improve psychosocial interventions, and to develop more effective pharmacological treatments.

REFERENCES

1. ALTESMAN, R. I., and COLE, J. O. "Psychopharmacologic Treatment of Anxiety," *Journal of Clinical Psychiatry,* 44 (1983):12–18.
2. ANANTH, J. "Clomipramine in Obsessive-Compulsive Disorder: A Review," *Psychosomatics,* 24 (1983):723–727.
3. BERNEY, T., et al. "School Phobia: A Therapeutic Trial with Clomipramine and Short-Term Outcome," *British Journal of Psychiatry,* 138 (1981):110–118.
4. BIEDERMAN, J., and JELLINEK, M. S. "Psychopharmacology in Children," *New England Journal of Medicine,* 310 (1984):968–972.
5. BRANTIGAN, C. O., BRANTIGAN, T. A., and JOSEPH, N. "Effect of Beta Blockade and Beta Stimulation on Stage Fright," *American Journal of Medicine,* 72 (1982):88–92.
6. COLE, J. O., ALTESMAN, R. I., and WEINGARTEN, C. H. "Beta-blocking Drugs in Psychiatry," in J. O. Cole, ed.,

Psychopharmacology Update. Lexington, Mass.: Collamore Press, 1980, pp. 43–68.
7. FLAMENT, M. F., et al. "Clomipramine Treatment of Childhood Obsessive-Compulsive Disorder: A Double-Blind Controlled Study," *Archives of General Psychiatry,* 42 (1985): 977–983.
8. GITTELMAN, R. "Anxiety Disorders in Children," in *Psychiatry Update,* vol. 3. Washington, D.C.: American Psychiatric Press, 1984, p. 415.
9. GITTELMAN-KLEIN, R., and KLEIN, D. F. "Controlled Imipramine Treatment of School Phobia," *Archives of General Psychiatry,* 25 (1971):204–207.
10. ———. "School Phobia: Diagnostic Considerations in the Light of Imipramine Effects," *Journal of Nervous and Mental Disease,* 156 (1973):199–215.
11. HOLLINGSWORTH, C. E., et al. "Long-Term Outcome

of Obsessive-Compulsive Disorder in Childhood," *Journal of the American Academy of Child Psychiatry,* 19 (1980):134–144.

12. INSEL, T. R. "An Update on Obsessive-Compulsive Disorder," *Currents,* 3 (1984):5–7.

13. KLEIN, D. F., et al. *Diagnosis and Drug Treatment of Psychiatric Disorders: Adults and Children,* 2nd ed. Baltimore: Williams & Wilkins, 1980.

14. KLEIN, D. F., et al. "Treatment of Phobias. II. Behavior Therapy and Supportive Psychotherapy: Are There Any Specific Ingredients?" *Archives of General Psychiatry,* 40 (1983):139–145.

15. MCCURDY, L. M. (Discussant). "Current Therapies in Anxiety," in *Perspectives on the VII World Congress of Psychiatry.* New York: Health Projects International, 1983, pp. 13–17.

16. MARKS, I. "Behavioral Treatment Plus Drugs in Anxiety Syndromes," in D. F. Klein and J. Rabkin, eds., *Anxiety: New Research and Changing Concepts.* New York: Raven Press, 1981, pp. 265–289.

17. MAVISSAKALIAN, M. "Pharmacologic Treatment of Anxiety Disorders," *Journal of Clinical Psychiatry,* 43 (1982):487–491.

18. NOYES, R., JR., et al. "Antianxiety Effects of Propranolol: A Review of Clinical Studies," in D. F. Klein and J. Rabkin, eds., *Anxiety: New Research and Changing Concepts.* New York: Raven Press, 1981, pp. 81–93.

19. RICKELS, K. "Use of Antianxiety Agents in Anxious Outpatients," *Psychopharmacology,* 58 (1978):1–17.

20. SARAF, K. R., et al. "EKG Effects of Imipramine Treatment in Children," *Journal of the American Academy of Child Psychiatry,* 17 (1978):60–69.

21. SHEEHAN, D. V., BALLENGER, J., and JACOBSON, G. "Relative Efficacy of Monoamine Oxidase Inhibitors and Tricyclic Antidepressants in the Treatment of Endogenous Anxiety," in D. F. Klein and J. Rabkin, eds., *Anxiety: New Research and Changing Concepts.* New York: Raven Press, 1981, pp. 47–67.

22. "Use of Approved Drugs for Unlabeled Indications," *FDA Drug Bulletin,* 12 (1982):4–5.

52 / Tourette Syndrome: Assessment and Management

Donald J. Cohen, Mark A. Riddle, and James F. Leckman

Introduction

Clinical management of children and adults with Tourette syndrome (TS) depends on a thorough understanding of pathogenesis, natural history, and associated features of the disorder. (See chapter 35.) While TS is a biologically based, neurobiological dysfunction, assessment and treatment must approach the patient from a developmental point of view in which difficulties are understood as reflecting various types of interactions between the underlying diathesis and experiential factors. The goal of assessment is to specifically define these difficulties and their roots, while treatment aims at facilitating the patient's overall development and not just the suppression of motor and phonic symptoms.

Assessment of Children with Tourette Syndrome

The assessment of a child with TS usually requires several hours of interviewing and observation with the child and family, as well as information obtained from parents using standardized clinical assessment instruments (e.g., a list of tic symptoms and a behavioral checklist), over a period of several weeks. A thorough evaluation includes information regarding motor and phonic tics, psychosocial functioning, cognition and school achievement, previous medications, and a behavioral pedigree of the extended family. Although the diagnosis of TS is essentially based on the history and observation, a neurological examination and appropriate laboratory tests may provide additional diagnostic data.

TICS

The nature, frequency, severity, and extent of impairment produced by the motor and phonic tics needs to be assessed from the onset of their expression until the present. It is important to review with the child and family the waxing and waning course as well as factors (e.g., particular stresses or states of excitement) associated with the onset, worsening, or amelioration of various symptoms. The degree to which relationships with family members and peers, school performance, and the child's sense of well-being and self-worth have been affected by the tics requires careful exploration.

The great variability in symptomatic expression seen in TS patients—the waxing and waning course, the exacerbation produced by stress or anxiety, and the ability of many to control their symptoms for brief periods of time—can lead to a bewildering clinical picture that the patient, parents, teacher, and clinician each "see" differently. Information obtained from multiple sources over the longest possible period of time is essential for clarifying the clinical picture so that a consensus can emerge regarding the patient's strengths, problems, and the nature of the symptomatic fluctuations. The use of standardized clinical assessment instruments, which are usually developed and employed for research purposes, can help in clarifying many clinical issues.

The Tourette's Syndrome Global Scale (TSGS)[5] is a rating instrument specifically designed to permit across-subject comparisons among patients with TS. Using the TSGS, motor and phonic tics are rated according to their frequency and disruptiveness using defined anchor points. Other domains contributing to the TSGS are ratings of motor restlessness, behavioral difficulties, and school and learning problems. This scale can be used by clinicians to quantify their clinical impressions on a weekly basis.

The Tourette Syndrome Symptom List (TSSL) is an instrument designed for parents to use to record observations of their children.[2] The TSSL, which contains twenty-nine items divided into three domains (overall motor tics, overall phonic tics, and overall behavioral problems), can be filled out daily. The Conners Parent Questionnaire is a forty-eight-item checklist that assesses general behavioral disruptiveness on a weekly basis.[3] Both rating forms are simple and straightforward and can be filled out reliably by most parents. Teachers also may be asked to complete a symptom checklist.

As the evaluation proceeds and the child becomes more comfortable, he or she will reveal symptoms with less suppression or inhibition. Only when there is confidence in the doctor is a child or adult likely to acknowledge the most frightening and bizarre symptoms (e.g., "disgusting" habits, obsessive thoughts, or rituals). A well-conducted assessment allows the family to feel that their full story has been heard—sometimes for the first time after having seen many physicians. This assessment process can be therapeutically important and lead to an easing of the immediate crisis. In addition, nothing is more useful for developing confidence than the family and child's belief that the clinician has "heard" what they have been through and understands how they are coping with the tragedy they have experienced.

PSYCHOSOCIAL FUNCTIONING

Prior to receiving a diagnosis and explanation of TS, the family (and child) may think the child is going "crazy." By the time of the evaluation, children may be distressed and confused by their own experiences. Teasing by peers and criticism from parents who may have scolded, bribed, threatened, and perhaps beaten children to get them to stop their "weird" and embarrassing behavior may have threatened children's sense of well-being and self-esteem. Time spent alone with children in an unstructured setting can facilitate evaluation of the extent to which they have internalized feelings of worthlessness, hopelessness, or anger toward parents. Family issues, including parental guilt, need to be addressed throughout the evaluation. Relevant factors elicited during a sensitive evaluation can be approached through clarification, education, and therapeutic discussion with the child and family.

COGNITION AND SCHOOL ACHIEVEMENT

The child with TS who has school problems requires assessment of cognitive functioning and school achievement. Since children with TS with cognitive difficulties rarely have clearly delineated learning disorders, the evaluation of their difficulties can be similar to that for other children with school performance problems (e.g., school reports, psychoeducational testing, discussion with teachers). The average IQ of TS patients is normal; their problems often include distractibility, reduced perseverance, and difficulty keeping themselves and their work organized. Many have impairments in penmanship (graphomotor skills) and compulsions that interfere with writing. Determining specific problem areas can help in the recommendation of alternatives (e.g., the use of a typewriter or more emphasis on oral reports). It is also important to establish the degree to which the child's feelings (e.g., anger, depression) and attempts to inhibit symptoms affect school performance.

PREVIOUS MEDICATIONS

Previous medications need to be reviewed in detail. If a child has received stimulant medications, it is important to determine why the medication was prescribed, whether there were any preexisting tics or compulsions, and the temporal relation between the stimulants and new symptoms. Catecholaminergic agonists are contained in other drugs, such as in antihistamine combinations used in treating allergies and in medications used for asthma. If such drugs were used in the past, it is important to know their effects. Children who developed tics on stimulants may have shown improved attention and learning with the use of these medications.

Frequently children have been tried on other medications before being assessed by the current clinician. The child's response to these medications, the dosages used, the initial positive and negative responses, and the rationale for their discontinuation need to be assessed. A family may report that haloperidol was not useful with a child or that he or she had unacceptable side effects. A careful history may reveal that the child improved on haloperidol but then developed akathisia, which was not recognized, or that the side effects were dose-related and probably controllable. Was the medication used at the correct dosage, with adequate monitoring, for a long enough time? Patients and families may not recognize important side effects, such as fearfulness or school phobia, that may be related to haloperidol and not primarily to psychological issues.

BEHAVIORAL PEDIGREE OF THE EXTENDED FAMILY

A detailed behavioral pedigree of the extended family, including tics, attentional problems, learning disorders, and compulsions, can clarify many family issues. A grandfather's TS may have been diagnosed as Sydenham's chorea; an uncle may have been thought simply to be odd or weird. Parents may be embarrassed about acknowledging their own symptoms—if a father is asked about his obvious eye-blinking and throat-clearing tics, initially he may deny that he ever had tics or that he ever noticed them. Only when the mother comments on noticing them "when he's nervous" will he be able to "remember" his childhood and current symptoms.

Patients with TS have family histories that are strongly positive for tics, TS, and obsessive-compulsive disorder. The presence of these disorders in parents or siblings may alter the family's perception of an individual child's difficulties, exacerbate tension, or strengthen identification between the child and parent.

NEUROLOGICAL EXAMINATION

Neurological examination should include documentation of neuromaturational difficulties as well as other neurological findings. Approximately half of TS patients have nonlocalizing, so-called soft neurological findings suggesting disturbances in the body schema and integration of motor control. While these findings have no specific therapeutic implications, they probably strengthen the diagnosis of TS and may define a clinical subgroup. Neurological findings also are important as "baseline" data, since the use of medications may cloud the neurological picture.

Children with paroxysmally abnormal electroencephalogram (EEG) tracings sometimes have been treated as epileptics, but anticonvulsants are of no consistent value in TS. Computed tomography (CT) of the brain generally produces normal results, and the EEG and CT scans are not necessary for the diagnosis or treatment of TS. Yet concerned clinicians are likely to feel comforted by a normal EEG and CT scan; at the least, other disorders affecting movement (such as seizures or basal ganglia disorders) are more or less ruled out.

LABORATORY TESTS

No diagnostic laboratory tests are specific for TS. Chemical studies may include electrolytes, calcium, phosphorous, ceruloplasmin, and liver function tests—all related to movement difficulties of various types. These tests are useful as baseline measurements, particularly if medication is to be prescribed.

ASSESSMENT PROBLEMS

Although prevailing diagnostic criteria require that all children with a one-year history of suppressible multiple motor and phonic tics, however minimal, should be diagnosed as having TS, in practice clinicians may deviate from this rigorous research approach. In talking with families, we tend to consider severity and associated features (particularly complex motor and phonic symptoms as well as attention problems and general disinhibition) in the diagnosis of TS. For example, we might use the term nervous habits, rather than TS, to describe the throat clearing, facial grimacing, and occasional shrugging of an otherwise normal, competent youngster. However, since there are genetic implications, and some families and patients want to have full disclosure of the physician's thoughts, the clinician may want to raise the possible relationship between the patient's symptoms and TS. The problem is, while not everyone who twitches has TS, in the absence of diagnostic tests, it may be hard to draw the line. For research purposes, it is necessary to maintain clear diagnostic criteria.

Patients with the most severe symptoms of TS and past treatment with medication may present problems in differential diagnosis. For example, Sam, a fourteen-year-old boy, presented for evaluation two months after abrupt withdrawal from haloperidol. In addition to nonspecific learning and speech articulation problems and a longstanding history of social isolation, Sam developed "motor tics" at age eleven during a trial on methylphenidate hydrochloride. Although the movements improved with haloperidol, problems with sedation and cognitive blunting led to the referring physician's decision to discontinue it. Two months later Sam was confused, disorganized, aggressive toward his caretakers, and intermittently appeared psychotic. Whether Sam's involuntary movements were motor tics, manifestations of TS, or stereotypies in a boy with pervasive developmental disorder or schizophrenia was difficult to ascertain. Short-term hospitalization for observation, evaluation, and institution of medication was necessary to clarify Sam's diagnosis.

When a child is currently on a medication but still is having serious tic or behavioral difficulties, hard clinical judgment is called for. Today TS patients frequently will be on haloperidol, clonidine hydrochloride, a phenothiazine, or some combination at the time of evaluation. The clinician will have to decide whether to increase the medication(s) and see if the child improves or discontinue the medication(s) and observe the child's response. Discontinuation from haloperidol may lead to severe withdrawal-emergent exacerbation for up to two to three months. Thus if haloperidol is withdrawn, it cannot be expected that the child's "real" status will be visible for quite a while. Some children may improve for a few weeks after haloperidol discontinuation and then exacerbate after another week or so, remain worse for a while, and then gradually improve. With discontinuation of haloperidol, cognitive blunting, feeling dull, decreased motivation, social phobias, excessive appetite, and sedation may lift rather quickly, over days to several weeks, while emergent tic symptoms remain or become worse. Thus the decision to discontinue haloperidol must be planned so as to disrupt the child's life as little as possible.

If a child on clonidine is not benefiting, tapering the medication over one or two weeks may be followed by increased anxiety lasting for a few days. Exacerbation of TS symptoms usually is milder than with haloperidol, and children do not get worse during withdrawal than they were before the initiation of treatment. Less is known about withdrawal from phenothiazines, but withdrawal-emergent dyskinesias and exacerbations can occur.

When symptoms are poorly controlled, a clinician will have to decide whether to attempt to "clean out" a child's system by discontinuation of all medication or to change dosage. The presence of serious side effects probably would lead to attempted detoxification, but careful assessment of the child and family's coping and response to intervention can guide such decisions.

Another complication in the assessment of a child with TS is that parents may themselves have TS or an associated disorder, such as obsessive-compulsive disorder. There are several implications of this multigenerational sharing of symptoms. Clinicians may feel inhibited in sharing fully their impressions of the child's social and personality problems if they observe similar difficulties in the parents, for fear that they may hurt their feelings. Also, parents may feel an additional burden of guilt if they recognize that they have contributed genetically to their child's disorder. On the other side, parents with TS or tics may have more sympathy for their child's dilemmas and greater capacity to appreciate how life can proceed in spite of them. In addition, they may be interested in receiving treatment for themselves, or other family members, if there is success in the treatment of the child.

Families frequently ask if TS is a "medical" or "emotional" disorder. These terms carry with them ideological and psychological weight. A well-conducted assessment, in which all aspects of the child's development and current functioning are discussed, is an important step in undoing the epistemologically mischievous disjunction between body and mind. While TS arises on the basis of neurophysiological dysfunction and thus is "biological," it is apparent that its manifestations affect the child in many areas of life and are exacerbated by emotional and social tensions. Thus the treatment of TS must address the child as a whole person and not just as a collection of physical symptoms. This orientation to TS and its treatment can be conveyed implicitly during the assessment—as the clinician analyzes medical, psychosocial, and psychological issues—and usually requires explicit discussion at the end of the evaluation.

Management of Children with Tourette Syndrome

Effective treatment is now available for many patients with TS. There are several approaches to treatment.

MONITORING

Initially, unless there is a state of emergency, the clinician can follow the patient for several months before deciding with the family on a specific treatment plan. The goals of this first stage of treatment are to establish a baseline of symptoms; define associated difficulties in school, family, and peer relations; obtain necessary medical tests; monitor, through checklists and interviews, the range and fluctuations in symptoms and the specific areas of greatest difficulty; and establish a relationship. If there is ongoing exposure to stimulants, they should be discontinued if medically feasible.

EDUCATION AND REASSURANCE

Families vary in their understanding of TS and their ideas about prognosis. In addition to their personal experience, what patients and parents have read or been told may greatly influence their perception of TS.

Patients and families deserve a frank discussion of available treatments, prognosis, and emerging knowledge of genetic factors. Given the availability of effective treatments, we are generally optimistic when discussing prognosis. Literature from the Tourette Syndrome Association and professional journals also may be helpful.

MEDICATION

Available pharmacological agents are effective in suppressing the symptoms of TS in the majority of patients. However, drugs are not curative, and patients may need to remain on them for extended periods of time.

Haloperidol. Since the early 1960s, haloperidol (Haldol) has been the drug of choice in treating TS. This agent has been found effective in numerous clinical studies, and its use for the control of TS symptoms has been approved by the Food and Drug Administration (FDA)[9]; surprisingly, no rigorous, double-blind study of haloperidol efficacy has been published. Haloperidol is most effective at low doses. It is not unusual for patients to experience improvement in their symptoms with as little as 0.5 mg p.o. per day. The effectiveness of haloperidol in controlling symptoms usually can be determined after several days at a given dosage level. The dose usually is not increased more rapidly than 0.5 mg every three to seven days. At doses above 1 mg per day, a twice-daily divided dosage regimen usually is best. The higher the dose, the more likely are unwanted physical and psychological effects. Patients, of whatever age, rarely show a fully favorable response above 7 mg per day. Even if the medication has been effective in controlling the tics, the side effects of the medication are judged by many patients and their families to be worse than the disorder. Indeed, only about a third of patients who have shown a favorable response choose to remain on this medication long term (for more than one year).[11] Although some patients, particularly those on low doses, do not experience any side effects on haloperidol, many do. These include dysphoria (feeling like a "zombie"), depression, phobias, sedation, cognitive dulling, excessive weight gain, acute dystonic reaction, parkinsonian symptoms, and akathisia. The extrapyramidal side effects may be effectively treated with antiparkinsonian medications, such as benztropine maleate (Cogentin).

Clonidine. The first report in 1979 of the value of clonidine (Catapres) in treating TS has been followed by other case reports and open and closed trials, suggesting that from 40 to 70 percent of TS patients benefit from its use.[1,2,6] Clonidine has been approved by the FDA for use only in hypertension, but clinicians prescribe it without special government approval for TS if they understand its indications and share the basis for their decision with the family and patient. Many clinicians use clonidine as the drug of first choice because of its relative safety and the low occurrence of side effects. Although many patients with TS show a favorable response to the drug, this favorable outcome often takes two to three months to develop. The reasons for this latency of response are not clear. In general, clonidine is started at low doses of 0.05 mg per day and slowly titrated over several weeks to 0.15 to 0.30 mg per day. Doses above 0.5 mg per day may be beneficial but often lead to undesirable side effects. As with haloperidol, the best responses are in those patients who respond at the lower dosages.

In a twenty-week, single-blind, placebo-controlled trial of clonidine in thirteen patients with TS, six patients were judged to be unequivocal responders to clonidine, based on a greater than 25 percent reduction in symptoms after eight weeks of treatment, a greater than 25 percent worsening of symptoms following placebo substitution, and a greater than 25 percent reduction in symptoms after a second eight-week period of clonidine treatment.[7] Six other patients were judged to have an equivocal response by satisfying at least one of the three operational criteria. All patients were followed for one year in an open design; all experienced an overall reduction in their symptoms during the one-year period (mean = 50 percent reduction, range = 12–90 percent reduction). Significant improvements in motor and phonic tics as well as in associated behavioral problems were observed. Double-blind, placebo-controlled studies are needed to establish definitively the efficacy of clonidine. Comparative studies, using haloperidol, clonidine, pimozide, and other medications effective in TS, are needed to establish their differential efficacy with respect to specific symptoms, both short and long term.

At low doses, the side effects of clonidine include fatigue that usually "wears off" after several weeks and dry mouth. At higher doses, orthostatic hypotension can occur. Electrocardiogram (EKG) changes (prolongation of the PR interval) also have been reported. Untoward psychological effects, including increased irritability, also have been reported at higher doses. In addition to the usual workup described earlier, a baseline EKG should be obtained prior to the initiation of clonidine.

Haloperidol and Clonidine. Haloperidol and clonidine have been used in combination, but there is only anecdotal information about this approach. The combination has been used in two clinical situations: (1) for patients whose symptoms are not fully controlled on haloperidol, or who are having serious side effects when medication is increased, yet who cannot have their haloperidol fully discontinued because of the severity of symptoms or the emergence of an exacerbation with tapering; and (2) for patients who are on clonidine but still having motor and phonic symptoms. It has appeared that patients can be managed with smaller doses of haloperidol if clonidine is added to the regimen and, on the other hand, that haloperidol may improve the tic control for some patients on clonidine. In general, quite small doses of both medications have been used when the drugs are combined, and no serious side effects have been reported in addition to what is seen with the drugs used individually.

Pimozide. Pimozide (Orap) is a potent neuroleptic used widely in Europe in the treatment of psychosis; several open and blind clinical studies have shown pimozide to be at least as effective as haloperidol in the treatment of TS.[8,10,12] Pimozide is a diphenylbutylpiperidine derivative, chemically distinct from haloperidol, clonidine, or the phenothiazines. Its mode of action appears to be preferential inhibition of postsynaptic dopamine receptors.

Treatment with pimozide is initiated at 1 mg per day, and dosage is gradually increased, on clinical indications, to a maximum of 6 to 10 mg per day (0.2 mg/kg) for children and 20 mg per day for adults. The long half-life (fifty-five hours) of pimozide makes once-daily dosage possible. Major side effects are similar to those described for haloperidol. Pimozide also causes EKG changes in up to 25 percent of patients, including T-wave inversion, U waves, QT prolongation, and bradycardia. EKG changes are observable within one week and at doses as low as 3 mg per day. The manufacturer recommends discontinuation of pimozide with the occurrence of T-wave inversion or U waves, seen in up to 20 percent of patients; dosage should not be increased if there is prolongation of the QT interval (corrected). A series of cardiac deaths have occurred in healthy patients. As with haloperidol, tardive dyskinesia must be considered a long-term possibility. In addition to the usual clinical and laboratory monitoring, patients receiving pimozide should receive regular EKG monitoring.

Other Medications. A variety of other medications, particularly neuroleptics, have been used to treat patients with TS.[4] Some phenothiazines may be as effective as haloperidol. Agents that primarily affect serotonergic or cholinergic systems, although interesting from a research perspective, have not found a place in the treatment of TS.

Choice of Medication. The clinician's choice of a first drug is a difficult decision. Haloperidol has the longest "track record," and its therapeutic benefits and side effects are well defined; the only other major contender as a first drug today is clonidine, which is less well defined and less likely to be dramatically effective. Those clinicians who favor clonidine as a first drug do

so because of its limited side effects and positive effect on attention; however, when a rapid response is needed, haloperidol may be more effective. Until more evidence accumulates, it will be difficult to decide if a patient should have a several-month course of clonidine before starting haloperidol or the other way around. When a patient is started on haloperidol, it may be more difficult to discontinue the drug; withdrawal symptoms are usually less severe at usual doses of clonidine. Some clinicians have added low-dose clonidine to low-dose haloperidol with good results, but no controlled studies have been reported. Whether pimozide will become an alternative to haloperidol may depend on the seriousness and frequency of observed side effects, especially cardiac toxicity. Until further evidence is available, pimozide might be reserved for patients who do not benefit from the other drugs.

ACADEMIC INTERVENTION

Children with attentional and learning problems require educational intervention similar to the approaches used in the management of other forms of attention deficit disorder and learning disabilities. TS patients may require special tutoring, a learning laboratory, a self-contained classroom, a special school, or residential school, depending on the severity of academic and associated behavioral problems. It may be difficult to convince a school district of the need for special school provisions for a bright TS patient who does not have specific learning disabilities but whose attentional problems limit optimal functioning. Since TS is an uncommon disorder, schools need to be informed about the nature of the syndrome and the way it affects attention and learning. A homebound program, which deprives children of their legal right to the least restrictive educational environment and an adequate education, should be avoided. At home, children with TS may regress academically and behaviorally; they require the structure provided by well-designed school programs.

GENETIC COUNSELING

Since the precise mode of inheritance of TS is still not known, only generalizations about genetic counseling are possible. It is known that: (1) TS and multiple tics aggregate in families and are on the same spectrum; (2) boys are more commonly affected than girls (estimates of the male to female sex ratio vary from three to one to nine to one); (3) obsessive-compulsive disorder is found in more than 10 percent of TS patients and is on the same spectrum; and (4) attention deficit disorder occurs in more than 20 percent of patients with TS. Parents considering having another child should be told that having a first-degree relative (parent or sib) with TS increases the risk of having the disorder from one in many hundreds or thousands to one in four or five. The risk is much higher for male offspring. For a young adult with TS who is thinking about having a child, genetic counseling must be done cautiously and with sensitivity regarding the meaning of the information. The offspring of a mother with TS are at quite high risk. At present, there is no method for prenatal diagnosis. In providing genetic counseling, it is important to emphasize the uncertainties as well as the increasing knowledge about treatment.

PSYCHOTHERAPY

Psychotherapy probably is not effective in reducing tics. However, psychotherapy and other counseling techniques can help the patient and his or her family adjust more adaptively to life with TS. If the child has internalized, self-deprecating thoughts in response to teasing or scolding by peers or parents, psychotherapy is indicated. Family therapy may be recommended for families preoccupied with concerns about blame or guilt. Individual and/or family psychotherapy can facilitate the adolescent patient's separation and emancipation from parents. Parent support groups, which have been organized by various chapters of the Tourette Syndrome Association, provide parents the opportunity to share their experiences and concern.

HOSPITALIZATION

Short-term hospitalization may be useful during crises. However, because phonic symptoms and bizarre behaviors may be difficult to tolerate in the hospital, TS patients often are unwelcome on an inpatient neurology or psychiatry service. When patients are hospitalized, there is a tendency to use medication for sedation, not only because of the patient's needs but because of the anxiety of the clinical staff and other patients. Yet the availability of an inpatient service willing to accept a TS patient in crisis can be reassuring for both the patient and the physician.

MULTIPLY HANDICAPPED TS PATIENTS

Most patients with TS can be treated effectively using techniques described earlier. The most difficult treatment problems arise for the adolescent or adult with chronic, severe TS and multiple associated social, occupational, and interpersonal difficulties. It is not uncommon for severely afflicted patients to have limited social and personal resources and to be rigidly enmeshed in ambivalent and hostile relations with their exhausted families. Disentangling what is "Tourette's" and what are the associated problems is a major, long-term therapeutic task. Some of these problems include the manifestations of chronic treatment with medication, confusion about longstanding status as a "patient," and internalized feelings of worthlessness, hopelessness, and helplessness. Patients may no longer know what is under their control and what is primarily a manifestation of TS. Allowing patients to recount their experience and helping them in their attempt to comprehend what they are doing are initial goals of the therapeutic work. Those patients who have become chronically dependent and unable to function on their own require assistance in establishing a social support network. Patients also may need vocational guidance, a halfway house program, individual psychotherapy and/or family counseling, and advocacy, in addition to judicious use of medication. Even in desperate situations, therapeutic commitment combined with the patient's determination and courage can lead to satisfying therapeutic results.

NONCONVENTIONAL TREATMENT

As with many other chronic disorders of unknown etiology, a range of therapeutic modalities have been used with TS that are not specific for the disorder but that have generated enthusiastic endorsements. Nutritional therapies, involving the elimination of certain foods and additives plus the utilization of large doses of vitamins and minerals, have been used with TS as well as other serious disorders. While no adequate scientific basis for this approach has been defined in TS, and while there is no body of rigorous data determining efficacy, there are many advocates and anecdotal reports of the benefits of nutritional treatments. Because of waxing and waning, suggestibility, and other factors, anecdotal reports are hard to evaluate; however, as in other areas, further studies of the effects of nutrition on brain function are indicated. Similarly, there are clinicians engaged in testing TS patients for specific environmental and food allergies, using standard skin-testing procedures. Desensitization and elimination diets have been used with TS patients; again, anecdotal reports support the usefulness of this approach for some patients, but there is no body of scientific evidence to support it. Biofeedback and hypnosis also have been used in the treatment of TS but have not been shown to be effective. The structure, optimism, and sense of doing something active for oneself provided by these "nonconventional" treatments may account, in part, for their acceptance by patients and families. Further, rigorous studies would be required to determine their long-term efficacy.

Overview: The Developmental Perspective

Throughout the assessment and treatment of TS, the clinician maintains a developmental perspective, considering each intervention in light of the child's overall needs and with an eye to the future. Thus the institution of medication may seem appropriate for reducing symptoms at present; the clinician, however, must consider whether medication is in the child's long-term interests. It is far easier to start haloperidol than to discontinue it; for most medications, the long-term side effects remain poorly defined. On the other hand, there are serious and long-lasting consequences of social ostracism, self-depreciation, school maladjustment, and familial distress. Amelioration of symptoms and specific treatment interventions in these areas may be critical to long-term social adjustment and competence.

There are also developmental factors in the patient-therapist relationship. Since TS is a chronic and often lifelong disorder, families and patients need to establish a long-term relationship with a clinician or clinic with expertise in TS and in general aspects of child development/child psychiatry. As with other chronic disord-ers, there are expectable, "normative" tensions in the physician-patient relationship that relate to periods of exacerbation, "doctor shopping," and experimental and fad treatments. Families and patients will naturally feel anger toward the physician for not having the complete cure or knowledge they desire, and the therapist must deal with his or her own feelings of anger and inadequacy in the face of exacerbations. There is a natural tendency for families to search for new treatments; the clinician must be prepared to help guide them in this search and counsel them about potentially useful and also apparently dangerous or useless "remedies." While common to other chronic disorders, these therapeutic issues may be compounded in TS because of the multigenerational nature of the disorder in some families. However, the rapid expansion in biological, genetic, and pharmacological knowledge in TS offers considerably more promise for therapeutic efficacy during the coming years.

ACKNOWLEDGMENTS

This research was supported by The Gateposts Foundation, Mental Health Clinical Research Center grant MH 30929, National Institute of Child Health and Human Development grant HD 03008, and the John Merck Fund.

REFERENCES

1. BRUUN, R. D. "Gilles de la Tourette Syndrome: An Overview of Clinical Experience," *Journal of the American Academy of Child Psychiatry,* 231 (1984):126–133.

2. COHEN, D. J., et al. "Clonidine Ameliorates Gilles de la Tourette Syndrome," *Archives of General Psychiatry,* 37 (1980):1350–1357.

3. CONNERS, C. K. "Symptom Patterns in Hyperkinetic, Neurotic, and Normal Children," *Child Development,* 41 (1970):667–682.

4. FRIEDHOFF, A. J., and CHASE, T. N., eds. *Gilles de la Tourette Syndrome, Advances in Neurology,* vol. 35. New York: Raven Press, 1982.

5. HARCHERIK, D. F., et al. "A New Instrument for Clinical Studies of Tourette Syndrome," *Journal of the American Academy of Child Psychiatry,* 23 (1984):153–160.

6. LECKMAN, J. F., et al. "Clonidine in the Treatment of Gilles de la Tourette Syndrome: A Review," in A. J. Friedhoff and T. N. Chase, eds., *Gilles de la Tourette Syndrome, Advances in Neurology,* vol 35. New York: Raven Press, 1982, pp. 391–402.

7. LECKMAN, J. F., et al. "Short- and Long-term Treat-ment of Tourette's Syndrome with Clonidine: A Clinical Perspective," *Neurology,* 35 (1985):343–351.

8. ROSS, M. S., and MOLDOFSKY, H. "Comparison of Pimozide with Haloperidol in Gilles de la Tourette Syndrome," *Lancet,* 1 (1977):103.

9. SHAPIRO, A. K. and SHAPIRO, E. "Clinical Efficacy of Haloperidol, Pimozide, Penfluridol, and Clonidine in the Treatment of Tourette Syndrome," in A. J. Friedhoff and T. N. Chase, eds., *Gilles de la Tourette Syndrome, Advances in Neurology,* vol. 35. New York: Raven Press, 1982, pp. 383–386.

10. ———. "Controlled Study of Pimozide vs. Placebo in Tourette Syndrome," *Journal of the American Academy of Child Psychiatry,* 231 (1984):161–173.

11. SHAPIRO, A. K., SHAPIRO, E., and EISENKRAFT, G. J. "Treatment of Gilles de la Tourette's Syndrome with Clonidine and Neuroleptics," *Archives of General Psychiatry,* 40 (1983):1235–1240.

12. ———. "Treatment of Gilles de la Tourette Syndrome with Pimozide," *American Journal of Psychiatry,* 140 (1983): 1183–1186.

53 / Treatment of Sleep Disturbances in Children— Recent Advances

Jovan G. Simeon and H. Bruce Ferguson

Introduction

This chapter reviews recent advances in the management of sleep disorders and problems in children and adolescents. Like so many other difficulties children experience, sleep disturbances may seem to be a greater problem for their parents than for the children themselves. Usually children have very little control over their environment and little awareness of its effects on sleep. It is important, therefore, to assess the role of environmental factors, including the attitudes and reaction of family members to the perceived disturbances. Parents may know very little about their children's sleep patterns or complaints; even chronic and serious sleep problems in children may be minimized or ignored by both parents and professionals. Professionals vary in their attitudes and management of such problems. Some feel that sleep problems are transient, developmental phenomena, while others believe that these problems are usually related to psychopathology. The association between sleep disorders and other childhood psychiatric disorders and symptoms has not been explored systematically. What is known is summarized in chapter 36 in this volume. It is evident that children do suffer from sleep disturbances previously attributed only to adults, such as insomnia. Sleep problems, like other symptoms, must be managed in the context of the overall medical, personal, and family problems of each individual child.

In general, the therapy of sleep disorders takes the form of environmental manipulation, behavior modification, and/or pharmacotherapy. This overview of treatment advances relates primarily to new techniques in behavioral management and recent data on the use of medication. Extremely few psychopharmacology research reports focusing on sleep and sleep-related disorders in children have been published. By far the largest number of drug studies have focused on enuresis. New findings about drug effects on sleep and sleep-related problems have emerged. Usually they are the products of studies with adults or have arisen in the course of research and drug trials in other child psychiatric disorders, such as attention deficit disorder, depression, anxiety, and psychosis. While treatment of the primary condition and environmental modifications comprise the main therapeutic approaches, various medications can offer rapid symptomatic relief. Nevertheless, there has been a general reluctance to prescribe psychotropic drugs for sleep problems in children.[29] While it may be prudent to err on the side of caution, the short-term use of medication does appear safe and can greatly facilitate the effects of behavioral interventions. In specific sleep disorders such as narcolepsy, drugs may be needed on a long-term basis. Long-term pharmacotherapy also can benefit sleep disorders accompanying other medical and psychiatric conditions such as allergies, nocturnal asthma, epilepsy, or chronic psychoses.

Evaluation of Sleep

In general, child psychiatric patients have a high incidence of sleep problems. Any routine diagnostic evaluation in child psychiatry must include a systematic inquiry of sleep patterns and behavior. Parent/child sleep questionnaires can facilitate the evaluation, demonstrate therapeutic effects, and assist in the management of individual patients. If there are concerns about the child's sleep, the following areas must be reviewed[24]:

1. The presence and manifestations of any sleep disturbances.
2. A history of the pregnancy, delivery, and neonatal period.
3. Developmental history.
4. Current sleep pattern, including daytime naps, presleep routine, bedtime, sleep latency, frequency and times of night waking, parents' understanding and reactions, and sleep latency after night waking.

5. The sleeping arrangements for the child.
6. The child's behavior during the day.
7. Any problems in other developmental areas, such as feeding or toilet training.
8. Any significant, identifiable life event preceding the onset of the sleep disturbance, such as hospitalization, birth of a sibling, death in the family, or move to a new dwelling.

Sleep Hygiene

Good sleep hygiene may improve or cure many sleep problems. Before any intervention is initiated, individual differences in sleep needs and habits must be considered. Many environmental factors disturb healthy sleep but often go unrecognized for long periods. Noise interferes with sleep onset, although once the first sleep cycle has gotten underway it is very difficult to arouse sleeping children with noise stimuli.[10] Sensitivity to noise during sleep increases with age, but there are wide individual variations. Occasional loud noises are more bothersome than constant noise. Some adaptation to noise occurs, but it may never be complete. Moderate bedroom temperatures (55° to 75° F) are optimal for good sleep, while extremes of barometric pressure are associated with increased sleepiness.

Food and drink may also affect sleep. Milk seems to improve sleep while caffeine and other stimulants are powerful disturbers of sleep.[7] Insomniacs can be very sensitive to stimulants, even to a single cola drink or cup of chocolate. Drinking alcohol typically results in poor sleep. Various behavioral factors also affect sleep. Habitual afternoon or early-evening exercise deepens sleep more than morning or late-evening exercise. Marked increases in exercise load produce unpredictable changes in sleep. Anxiety and stress typically cause poor sleep and, if present, should be taken into account before any environmental changes are made. Since many people sleep poorly in novel conditions, if environmental changes are attempted, they must be tried for more than one night.

Disorders of Initiating and Maintaining Sleep

Various types of insomnia can afflict children and adolescents.* These include the settling and waking problems of young children and the insomnias characteristic of older children and adolescents.

*See references 2, 17, 24, 26, 29, and 40.

TREATMENT OF BEDTIME SETTLING AND NIGHT WAKING PROBLEMS

A substantial proportion of young children have difficulty settling at bedtime or after night waking. While many parents are tolerant,[67] persistent problems often lead to requests for professional help. Circumscribed sleep difficulties that are not symptomatic of more pervasive behavioral or family dysfunction can often be managed very effectively by a behavioral approach.[28,70] This requires the therapist to undertake a careful analysis of the individual problem, obtaining records of child and parent behaviors and a history of the development of the difficulty. Bedtime problems must be resolved first and rituals, transitional objects, and nightlights may be used to minimize difficulties. The key element of behavioral approaches involves making parents aware that returning repeatedly to the child's bedside can maintain waking behavior. With the therapist's support and guidance, parents must stop such secondary reinforcement. To accomplish this, the goals and systematic steps of the treatment program must be set out along with clear rules for their attainment. Although there are few systematic data, general clinical experience attests to the efficacy of such approaches.

Toddlers frequently have fears that prevent them from falling asleep. Such distress at bedtime is often related to separation anxieties and requires consistent limit setting throughout the day. If one initiates setting firm limits only at bedtime, it may serve merely to intensify the panic. Such problems need to be worked out through counseling and psychotherapy, reassuring the child and allowing better sleep habits to develop. Children also learn a set of sleep-onset associations. In older infants and toddlers, fear and stress at bedtime may lead to maladaptive learning of poor sleep habits. Children can become conditioned against relaxation in their beds, particularly when crying results in being picked up or rocked. New associations may be learned gradually, and during this relearning period crying must not be rewarded.

Parental pressure for help with these distressing problems often leads to drug treatment. In one study,[37] a quarter of 159 firstborn children had sedatives prescribed by the time they were eighteen months old. Two-thirds of the parents of toddlers suffering from severe night waking reported improvement with the phenothiazine derivative trimeprazine tartrate, but the gains were modest. Following drug discontinuation, the frequency of night waking returned to predrug levels, indicating that the common practice of a trial of hypnotics does not break the pattern of waking.[46] The long-term use of hypnotics is not recommended.[29,46] In general, medications are recommended mostly for emergency short-term use; diphenhydramine hydrochloride[49] or chloral hydrate are probably the agents most frequently used.[24] Clinical experience indicates that diphenhydramine is effective and safe for children who are not anxious. For children presenting with anxiety or extreme fear reactions, a short-acting benzodiazepine (e.g., oxazepam, triazolam) may be most useful.

Surveys reveal that waking problems in young children are common.[45,67] Parents appear frequently to allow the child into their bed. This occurs in apparently healthy families, a finding that runs counter to the traditional notion that this practice is at the root of much childhood psychopathology.[47]

TREATMENT OF CHILDHOOD AND ADOLESCENT INSOMNIAS

Insomnia in children and adolescents can be primary or it can be symptomatic of other disorders, such as depression, anxiety, attention deficit disorder, somatic complaints, neurotic symptoms, or acute psychotic decompensation. The successful therapy of the primary disorder may in itself result in a normalization of sleep patterns. In cases of transient and situational insomnia persisting for more than a few nights, hypnotic medications may be indicated to allow the patient to rest and to avoid conditioning, which may lead to persistence of the sleep difficulty. Chronic insomnias may require extended direct treatment with behavioral techniques or medication.

A group of persistent insomnias result from conditioning of maladaptive sleep-onset associations; these may best be treated with behavioral techniques such as relaxation training and "stimulus-control" therapy. Most of the information about such techniques is derived from work with adult patients, but these methods could be as effective with adolescents. Biofeedback and relaxation training may help insomnias associated with tension and anxiety.[8,25] Conditioned insomnia can also be treated by "stimulus-control" behavior therapy.[64] The following rules are recommended for adolescents[8]:

1. Go to bed only when sleepy.
2. Use the bed only for sleeping.
3. If unable to sleep, get up and move to another room; stay up until you are really sleepy, then return to bed.
4. Repeat step 3 as often as necessary throughout the night.
5. Set the alarm and get up at the same time every morning regardless of how much you slept during the night.
6. Do not nap. Milder insomnias can be relieved by reading in bed, watching TV, and so forth, but the insomniac must rise at a predetermined hour, no matter how poor the night's sleep. Otherwise a day-night reversal of sleep and wakefulness may result. These rules can be modified appropriately for use with younger children.

While the treatment of insomnias has been studied extensively only in adults, the experience thus gleaned can be used tentatively to guide the treatment of children and adolescents. The NIH Consensus Development Conference (1983) on drugs and insomnia in adults recommended that treatment of insomnia should start with the assessment and necessary correction of sleep habits and hygiene and that psychotherapy, behavioral therapy, and pharmacotherapy should be considered. When pharmacotherapy is indicated, the benzodiazepines are the drugs of choice for adults.[14] Detailed knowledge about the efficacy and side effects of psychotropic drugs in childhood and adolescent insomnia, however, awaits further controlled studies.

When benzodiazepine hypnotics are prescribed as part of the short-term management of insomnia (and in their rare long-term use), it is important to keep in mind that hypnotics may mask an insomniac's medical, behavioral, and psychological problems and thus delay appropriate treatment. Flurazepam hydrochloride and temazepam are marketed as hypnotics. Temazepam has a shorter half-life (eight to twelve hours), but new benzodiazepines with even shorter half-lives (two to six hours) have been developed (e.g., oxazepam, triazolam). While currently available hypnotics show development of tolerance and cross-tolerance, the dependence liability of the new rapidly eliminated benzodiazepines in adults and children is not known. However, physical addiction is not usually a problem, and flurazepam (the most frequently prescribed hypnotic) has been demonstrated to remain effective after even one month of continuous use.[30] Adverse psychomotor effects have been demonstrated the day following flurazepam ingestion[27,48]; thus cognitive or psychomotor impairment may well be a problem when slowly eliminated benzodiazepines are given over longer periods.

Benzodiazepines are generally safer than other hypnotics. The barbiturates are an older class of drugs; relative to the benzodiazepines, they have many disadvantages: acute overdose toxicity, depression of respiratory centers, physical dependence, stimulation of hepatic drug metabolizing enzymes, and withdrawal symptoms. Thioridazine is not recommended for insomnia as it is a poor hypnotic and has adverse and toxic side effects.

Although adult patients withdrawn from hypnotics are reported to develop "rebound insomnia," the existence of this phenomenon remains controversial. Precipitous withdrawal from certain hypnotics can result in anxiety, agitation, and dizziness. Withdrawal delirium and seizures have been reported following abrupt cessation of barbiturates or high chronic doses of benzodiazepines.[13] Procedures for drug withdrawal of central nervous system (CNS) depressants require first stabilizing the patient on a steady dose and then a gradual tapering the dose to avoid seizures and other adverse effects.

Other hypnotics include chloral hydrate, which promotes relatively normal sleep. However, its severe toxic effects at dosages only five to ten times greater than the clinically effective dose make it a poor risk for outpatient therapy. If benzodiazepines are not helpful, sedative antidepressants could be used, although tricyclic antidepressants have the potential for adverse and toxic side effects. In insomniac adults who were hyperactive as children, low doses of amitriptyline hydrochloride (10 to 50 mg) have proven effective; this medication seems to retain efficacy over years without habituation. Recent studies with a variety of child psychiatric patients show that both benzodiazepines[58] and new-generation antidepressants—for example, maprotiline hydrochloride and bupropion[54,59]—have resulted in symptomatic improvement of a range of different sleep problems.

Disorders of Excessive Somnolence

SLEEP APNEA

The sleep apnea syndrome can occur in infants, children, and adolescents as well as in adults, although often it is not diagnosed until adolescence. Daytime sleepiness results from the brief arousals caused by the many apneic episodes. Sleep apnea patients may occasionally complain of poor sleep; the use of hypnotics, however, is strictly contraindicated as the ensuing depression of respiratory functions will aggravate the apnea. Apneas can be due to respiratory obstruction, CNS dysfunction, or a mixture of these. The mechanisms underlying apneas are not well understood.[36,62] The treatment of the sleep apnea–hypersomnia syndromes is limited; most of the information available relates to the treatment of obstructive apneas. Any causes contributing to airway obstruction must be corrected, such as swollen adenoids, respiratory allergies, nocturnal asthma, and obesity. Guilleminault, Korobkin, and Winkle[23] reported on the management of fifty children with obstructive apneas. Eight of their patients had a tracheostomy; thirty had tonsillectomy/adenoidectomy (three subsequently required tracheostomy); and twelve were managed by diet and administration of steroids, oral medroxyprogesterone acetate, acetazolamide, or protriptyline hydrochloride. Some adolescents suffer from severe nighttime apnea

and impaired daytime functioning but have no obvious obstruction. In such cases, a small tracheostomy that functions at night but is closed during the day results in marked improvements of sleep and behavior. Some children have disturbed sleep, a history of snoring, and chronic respiratory or ear infections, but no obvious obstruction during wakefulness; such youngsters should have polygraphic monitoring with ear oximetry to rule out sleep apnea. Home monitoring with an apnea monitor may be useful in individuals at high risk for sudden infant death syndrome and for those treated with theophylline or atropine.

NARCOLEPSY

Narcolepsy is a rare disorder of unknown etiology. It can be extremely incapacitating, and intellectual, social, and emotional development can all be affected. Parent and teacher counseling is important in order to manage problems related to academic performance and social adjustment. Amphetamine, methylphenidate hydrochloride, or pemoline can control the sleep attacks,[11,51] while imipramine hydrochloride and chlorimipramine hydrochloride can reduce cataplectic and sleep paralysis attacks. Protriptyline, an antidepressant with stimulant properties, is also useful in treating cataplexy attacks in adults, while reducing the stimulant dosage needed to control sleepiness.[50] In a seven-year-old narcoleptic boy, a single morning dose (2.5 mg) of protriptyline relieved both sleepiness and cataplexy.[69] Drug discontinuation resulted in relapse, with further improvement following protriptyline reinstatement. In children, when symptoms clearly interfere with academic and social functions, medication may be necessary. While patients can experience considerable relief from multiple short naps, most will require CNS stimulants. Initially, very small dosages of stimulants should be used to minimize the development of drug tolerance. Tolerance development can be delayed by instituting drug "holidays."

Disorders of the Sleep–Wake Schedule

Children and adolescents can show various disorders of sleep-wake schedules, but the predominant problems are likely to be irregular sleep-wake patterns and the delayed-sleep-phase insomnia syndrome. Disruptions of the sleep-wake rhythm are corrected by regular sleep-wake schedules, a basic precondition for good sleep. Behavioral techniques have been evaluated more systematically in adult patients but can be adjusted for children, depending on their age. Such techniques have included reinforcement of scheduling, aversive conditioning for oversleeping, group support, and graphing of sleep-wake time. The treatment of the irregular sleep-wake pattern requires a gradual reestablishment of a regular day-night cycle, the abolition of naps, the restriction of time in bed to the usual sleeping hours, and mild exercise during the day. If such a routine is carefully maintained, the sleep difficulties are usually resolved within a few weeks. Children who suffer from the delayed-sleep-onset syndrome should definitely not be allowed to sleep late in the morning, as this prevents an adjustment of synchronization with the environment. Initially such children should be allowed to have late bedtimes to train them to go to bed without a struggle. The times of morning awakenings should then be gradually but consistently advanced. Once the child becomes spontaneously sleepy in the evenings, the bedtimes are also advanced.

Another treatment technique, chronotherapy,[15] has been described in adult patients but could reasonably be tried in adolescents and perhaps younger children. The treatment attempts to entrain circadian rhythms to a twenty-four-hour day by delaying sleep/dark and wake/light times by three hours each day, until the desired clock hours of sleep and wakefulness are reached. Once bedtime reaches socially acceptable hours, patients must adhere rigidly to this schedule. In these patients, consistent wake-up times seem inadequate to reset bedtime, in contrast to those who habitually go to bed late and arise early during work days but sleep late on weekends. Ferber[18] has presented data using similar techniques to bring young children's sleep into phase with their adult caretakers' schedule. However, the general utility and limitations of these new techniques remain to be explored with children and adolescents.

Disorders Associated with Sleep, Sleep Stages, or Partial Arousals

The parasomnias include a few relevant to children and adolescents. Treatment for enuresis, sleep terrors, nocturnal head banging, sleepwalking, and bruxism will be reviewed here.

ENURESIS

Comprehensive management of enuresis includes parental counseling and perhaps individual psycho-

therapy to minimize anxiety, guilt, and poor self-esteem. The specific therapeutic interventions for the symptom can be divided into behavioral treatment, enuresis alarms, and drug treatment.

Behavioral treatment of enuresis. In a recent update of treatment of enuresis, Schmitt[52] reviewed in detail motivational counseling, bladder exercises, enuresis alarms, and medications as treatment for enuresis. Motivational counseling is based on the assumption that the key to overcoming enuresis lies in having the child actively take responsibility for the symptom. Schmitt provides detailed procedural notes in his review. In general, the approach aims at reassuring child and parents, reducing secondary friction in the family, and focusing on positive reinforcement for dry nights. Compared to other treatments, motivational counseling produced an 80 percent decrease in wet nights in 70 percent of ninety patients, and this approach was superior to urethral dilation, imipramine, or a bell-and-pad enuresis alarm.[34] Schmitt[52] also provides procedural details for bladder stretching. This technique involves urine-holding exercises with gradually increasing fluid intake. Stream interruption is also recommended as a way of increasing the child's ability to withstand bladder spasms. Schmitt cites a study that reported a 35 percent cure rate over six months. Both motivational counseling and bladder-exercise approaches involve commitment and active involvement of child and parents. Although the reported research findings are promising, the existing single studies do not allow an assessment of the generalizability and utility of these approaches. Furthermore, a recent study comparing three methods of teaching parents "dry bed training" found no difference between any of the three trained groups and a wait-list control.[32]

Enuresis alarms. More recently developed enuresis alarms are smaller, simpler, cheaper, and generally more reliable than the original "bell-and-pad" models. Although Schmitt[52] reports cure rates of 67 to 72 percent for these new models, even the most recent studies have used older models. Although criteria for success vary (two to six weeks dry), these studies report impressive success rates (73–84 percent). Speed of training varies with the criterion employed. Using a criterion of two weeks dry, Griffiths, Meldrum, and McWilliam[22] reported a range of two to twenty weeks of training (median four weeks). Success or failure is not related to either initial bladder capacity or change in capacity during treatment. Long-term follow-up has revealed relapse rates of 27 to 42 percent. Relapse usually occurs in the first twelve months and has been associated with an increased number of alarm signals[16] during training. Relapses are usually retreated successfully. Neither age nor sex affects treatment outcome, but a number of other factors are important.

Unsatisfactory housing and family difficulties markedly reduce the rate of initial success. Where parents and teachers give the child high ratings on emotional and behavioral disturbance, this is predictive of relapse and lack of long-term success.[4,16] Where similar scores are given on family difficulties, the same outcome is likely.

Thus recent research indicates that for most children (70–90 percent), enuresis alarm training has a high rate of success over short training periods and that the majority of these children (60–70 percent) will remain dry. The precise mechanism underlying the success remains unclear. While initial explanations were based on Pavlovian principles, the conditioned reflex mechanisms that are responsible are as yet unknown. It is known that enuretic children have small bladders, but current evidence indicates that bladder capacity does not change with successful treatment. Finally, a study with normal volunteer adults reported that sleep with the bell-and-pad device resulted in reductions of the number of shifts between sleep stages, time spent in wakefulness, the amount of movement, and the time spent in stage 1 sleep.[60] These effects have not been replicated in children, but such changes could be responsible for reducing the number of enuretic episodes.

Drug Treatment of Enuresis. There are over forty double-blind studies confirming the efficacy of tricyclic antidepressants in treating enuresis. Studies of other classes of drugs have generally shown no effects or were equivocal.[6] Of the tricyclics available, imipramine has been by far the most extensively studied and is currently the drug of choice. The usual dose of imipramine is 50 mg or 75 mg at bedtime. The effect of the drug is generally immediate, and initial success rates have been around 50 percent, with long-term cure rates approximately half this amount. Probably because of the single low dose, at bedtime, adverse effects are few; the most frequent is dry mouth. While there is some evidence for an association between plasma levels of imipramine and desipramine hydrochloride and response early in treatment, a high plasma level is not sufficient for efficacy; furthermore, tolerance has been shown to develop to the antienuretic effect of these tricyclics.[41] New-generation antidepressants may also be useful in treating enuresis. Simeon, Maguire, and Lawrence[57] reported on maprotiline. Its efficacy was similar to that of imipramine and adverse effects were infrequent and mild.

Imipramine increases functional bladder capacity, but the mechanism underlying this effect is unknown.[61] Proposals that it is due to the drug's peripheral anticholinergic effects[6] appear to be refuted by the failure of propantheline bromide[66] and methscopalamine[41] to improve enuresis. The efficacy of imipramine

and desipramine is unlikely to be due to their adrenergic action; indoramin (an alpha-adrenergic blocker) produced no improvement[53] and neither amphetamine[33] nor methylphenidate[9] has proven effective in enuresis. Based on an analysis of imipramine-induced changes in enuretic frequency and sleep stages, Kales and associates[31] hypothesized that imipramine results in a decrease in bladder excitability and/or an increase in bladder capacity, thus reducing enuretic events occurring early in the night. Later in the night, sleep is lighter, and the child may be more aware of stimuli from a full bladder. However, Mikkelsen and coworkers[35] reported that in their sample of forty boys, enuretic episodes were normally distributed throughout the night.

A number of studies[5,63] have demonstrated the efficacy of desamino-D-arginine vasopressin (DDAVP) in treating enuresis; the results were attributed to the drug's antidiuretic properties. In a more recent double-blind placebo controlled study, Aladjem and colleagues[1] reported that 10 mg DDAVP resulted in greater reductions in bed-wetting than those achieved with imipramine[41]; no side effects were observed. There appeared to be a better response in older children. However, once the DDAVP was discontinued, most children relapsed.

Summary. A controlled study comparing the effectiveness of an enuresis alarm with imipramine showed that the alarm therapy was significantly more effective.[65] These results should be interpreted with caution since the conditioning approach depends on the motivation, persistence, and consistency of both parents and child. The childhood conduct disorders and the high rate of family disturbances make the effective use of behavioral techniques in a psychiatric population more difficult than it might be in a general pediatric population. However, with careful training and appropriate support, behavioral approaches work. The current data on efficacy and maintenance of effect certainly make them the treatment of choice.

A final issue concerns the possibility that tricyclic antidepressants may cause changes of emotional or behavioral problems associated with enuresis. While most studies (see, for example, Rapoport et al.[41] and Wagner et al.[65]) reported no evidence of behavioral change, Werry and associates[68] reported that in the enuretic children treated with imipramine, there was a reduction in conduct problems and increased cooperativeness and happiness. In addition, in an open study of a new-generation antidepressant, maprotiline, a good level of efficacy with respect to bed-wetting as well as reductions in behavior problems and other sleep problems were reported.[57] Thus it appears that treatment of enuresis with antidepressants may also result in improvement of other psychiatric symptoms.

OTHER PARASOMNIAS

Other parasomnias such as sleepwalking, night terrors, nocturnal head banging, and bruxism occur much less frequently than enuresis and have not been the subject of controlled study. The available information relating to treatment is summarized in the following sections.

Sleepwalking (Somnambulism). Sleepwalking is usually outgrown in adolescence. Its onset in adolescence or persistence into adulthood reflects significant underlying psychopathology.[29] While some authors do not recommend the use of drugs in children with somnambulism, diazepam,[42] flurazepam,[44] imipramine, stimulants, and anticonvulsants have all been reported to be effective.[38] Others have reported successful treatment of a single case with behavior therapy[43] and with hypnosis.[12] Some cases may not respond to any known therapy.

Night Terrors (Pavor Nocturnus). Like sleepwalking, night terrors appear to have a genetic component and usually appear in childhood. These episodes are very disturbing for parents. Parents should be reassured that the episodes are usually "outgrown." The child should not be awakened from a sleep terror, and precautions must be taken to protect the child from harm during an attack. Medication is seldom required with these children, but in crises, or on special occasions, diazepam[21] can be used to suppress attacks. Imipramine has been used successfully in the treatment of night terrors in both children[39] and adults,[3] and flurazepam has also been reported as effective.[44]

Nocturnal Head Banging (Jactatio Capitis Nocturna). Head banging and body rocking usually occur in young children who suffer from mental retardation, pervasive developmental disorders, lack of environmental stimulation, or deafness, but may also be seen in normal children prior to the age of six years. Management of head banging and body rocking should aim at increasing contact between child and parent, sensory stimulation, and purposeful motor activity. With the young child, they become a management problem when they disturb the sleep of the other family members. Parents of normal children should be reassured that this behavior is usually not indicative of psychological disturbance and usually disappears with development. Behavioral methods also can be used to reduce the head banging. Medication should be used only for older children and for severe cases. Both diazepam and imipramine are reported to reduce head banging and rocking although this relief may be temporary.[19]

Bruxism. Sleep-related bruxism is of unknown etiology and occurs primarily in sleep stages 1 and 2. It has been suggested[20] that there may be no treatment for nocturnal bruxism, while diurnal bruxism may be related to stress and may respond to biofeedback therapy. A recent open trial of flurazepam[44] produced improvement in nine of fifteen children with sleep-related bruxism. If there is concern regarding damage to the teeth, the child should be referred to a dentist who may recommend use of a tooth guard at night.

Sleep Problems Associated with Child Psychiatric Disorders

Sleep disturbances are associated with a variety of child psychiatric disorders, including attention deficit disorders with hyperactivity, conduct disorders, depression, anxiety, and psychosis. A high proportion of child psychiatric referrals are reported to manifest sleep problems.[55,56] In such cases, the appropriate therapeutic strategy is first to treat the primary disorder. It is assumed that clinical improvement will be accompanied by a decrease in sleep problems. However, this is not always true; many sleep disturbances persist and require symptomatic therapy independent of the primary disorder.

Data from three single-blind studies show improvement of sleep problems incidental to pharmacotherapy for other disorders. In an open trial of bupropion in seventeen boys with attention deficit disorder with hyperactivity (ADDH) and/or conduct disorder (CD), there was significant clinical improvement, with reductions in reported sleep-onset insomnia, poor or restless sleep, and nightmares.[59] Similarly, in a single-blind trial of a tetracyclic antidepressant (maprotiline) in fifteen enuretic children with ADDH and CD, improvements were reported in a variety of other sleep problems: early-morning awakening, sleep-onset insomnia, poor or restless sleep, night awakening, nightmares, and bruxism.[57]

In a trial of alprazolam in twelve children with overanxious disorder, significant improvement in anxiety was paralleled by reduction in poor or restless sleep and sleep-onset insomnia.[58] These improvements of sleep problems were rapid and suggest a direct rather than an indirect effect of the medication on sleep behavior. However, unequivocal demonstration of the positive effects of these drugs on general sleep disturbances requires further study.

Conclusion

Recent research has established that children and adolescents suffer from a number of chronic and clinically significant sleep disorders that are more frequent in child psychiatry patients. Such disorders can interfere with the child's social, emotional, and cognitive development and, therefore, require a careful diagnostic evaluation and appropriate therapy. The successful management of any primary disorder is essential. Most sleep disturbances can be treated on an outpatient basis by environmental manipulation, behavior therapy, and/or pharmacotherapy. For more difficult cases, referral to a sleep disorders center may be necessary. The interaction between sleep and waking behavior is complex. Further research is needed with child populations to clarify the underlying mechanisms of sleep and sleep disorders and to determine and promote optimal sleep in individual children.

REFERENCES

1. ALADJEM, M., et al. "Desmopressin in Nocturnal Enuresis," *Archives of Diseases in Childhood,* 57 (1982):137–140.

2. ANDERS, T. F., CARSKADON, M. A., and DEMENT, W. "Sleep and Sleepiness in Children and Adolescents," *Pediatric Clinics of North America,* 27 (1980):29–43.

3. BEITMAN, B., and CARLIN, A. "Night Terrors Treated with Imipramine," *American Journal of Psychiatry,* 136 (1979):1087–1088.

4. BERG, I., FORSYTHE, I., and McGUIRE, R. "Response of Bedwetting to the Enuresis Alarm: Influence of Psychiatric Disturbance and Maximum Functional Bladder Capacity," *Archives of Diseases in Childhood,* 57 (1982):394–396.

5. BIRKASOVA, M., et al. "Desmopressin in the Management of Nocturnal Enuresis in Children: A Double-blind Study," *Pediatrics,* 62 (1978):970–974.

6. BLACKWELL, B., and CURRAH, J. "The Psychopharmacology of Nocturnal Enuresis," in I. Kolvin, R. C. MacKeith, and S. R. Meadow, eds., *Bladder Control and Enuresis.* London: Wm. Heinemann Medical Books, 1973, pp. 231–257.

7. BONNET, W. H., WEBB, W. B., and BARNARD, G. "Effect of Flurazepam, Pentobarbital and Caffeine on Arousal Threshold," *Sleep,* 1 (1979):271–279.

8. BOOTZIN, R. R., and NICASSIO, P. H. "Behavioral Treatments for Insomnia," in M. Hersen, R. M. Eisler, and P. Miller, eds., *Progress in Behavior Modification,* vol. 6. New York: Academic Press, 1978, pp. 1–45.

9. BREGER, E. "Hydroxyzine Hydrochloride and Methylphenidate Hydrochloride in the Management of Enuresis," *Journal of Pediatrics,* 61 (1962):443–447.

10. BUSBY, K., and PIVIK, R. T. "Failure of High Intensity Auditory Stimuli to Affect Behavioral Arousal in Children During the First Sleep Cycle," *Pediatric Research,* 17 (1983):802–805.

11. CAMPBELL, R. K. "The Treatment of Narcolepsy and Cataplexy," *Drug Intelligence & Clinical Pharmacy,* 15 (1981):257–262.

12. CLEMENT, P. W. "Elimination of Sleepwalking in a Seven-year-old Boy," *Journal of Consulting and Clinical Psychology,* 34 (1970):22–26.

13. COLE, J. O., HASKELL, D. S., and ORZACK, M. H. "Problems with the Benzodiazepines: An Assessment of the Available Evidence," *McLean Hospital Journal,* 6 (1981):46–74.

14. CONSENSUS DEVELOPMENT CONFERENCE SUMMARY, Vol. 4. Bethesda, Md.: U. S. Department of Health & Human Services, Public Health Service, 1983.

15. CZEISLER, C., et al. "Chronotherapy: Resetting the Circadian Clocks of Patients with Delayed Sleep Phase Insomnia," *Sleep,* 4 (1981):1–21.

16. DISCHE, S., et al. "Childhood Nocturnal Enuresis: Factors Associated with Outcome of Treatment with an Enuresis Alarm," *Developmental Medicine and Child Neurology,* 25 (1983):67–80.

17. DIXON, K., MONROE, L., and JAKIM, S. "Insomniac Children," *Sleep,* 4 (1981):313–318.

18. FERBER, R. "Sleeplessness in Infants and Toddlers," Paper presented at the annual meeting of the American Academy of Child Psychiatry, San Francisco, Calif., 1983.

19. FREIDIN, M. R., JANKOWSKI, J. J., and SINGER, W. D. "Nocturnal Head Banging as a Sleep Disorder: A Case Report," *American Journal of Psychiatry,* 136 (1979):1469–1470.

20. GLAROS, A. G. "Incidence of Diurnal and Nocturnal Bruxism," *Journal of Prosthetic Dentistry,* 45 (1981):545–549.

21. GLICK, B. S., SCHULMAN, D., and TURECKI, S. "Diazepam (Valium) Treatment in Childhood Sleep Disorders," *Diseases of the Nervous System,* 32 (1971):565–566.

22. GRIFFITHS, P., MELDRUM, C., and McWILLIAM, R. "Dry-bed Training in the Treatment of Nocturnal Enuresis in Childhood: A Research Report," *Journal of Child Psychology and Psychiatry,* 23 (1982):485–495.

23. GUILLEMINAULT, C., KOROBKIN, R., and WINKLE, R. "A Review of 50 Children with Obstructive Sleep Apnea Syndrome," *Lung,* 159 (1981):275–287.

24. HARRIS, J. C., and DeANGELIS-HARRIS, C. "Sleep and Its Disturbances in Children," in A. J. Moss, ed., *Pediatrics Update: Reviews for Physicians.* New York: Elsevier North Holland, 1981, pp. 13–23.

25. HAURI, P. "Treating Psychophysiologic Insomnia with Biofeedback," *Archives of General Psychiatry,* 38 (1981):752–758.

26. HAURI, P., and OLMSTEAD, E. "Childhood-onset Insomnia," *Sleep,* 3 (1980):59–65.

27. JOHNSON, L. C., and CHERNIK, D. A. "Sedative-hypnotics and Human Performance," *Psychopharmacology,* 76 (1982):101–113.

28. JONES, D.P.H., and VERDUYN, C. M. "Behavioural Management of Sleep Problems," *Archives of Disease in Childhood,* 58 (1983):442–444.

29. KALES, J. D., SOLDATOS, C. R., and KALES, A. "Childhood Sleep Disorders," *Current Pediatric Therapy,* 9 (1980):28–30.

30. KALES, A., et al. "Effectiveness of Hypnotic Drugs with Prolonged Use: Flurazepam and Pentobarbital," *Clinical Pharmacology and Therapeutics,* 18 (1975):356–363.

31. KALES, A., et al. "Effects of Imipramine on Enuretic Frequency and Sleep Stages," *Pediatrics,* 60 (1977):431–436.

32. KEATING, J. C., et al. "Dry Bed Training Without a Urine Alarm: Lack of Effect of Setting and Therapist Contact with Child," *Journal of Behavior Therapy and Experimental Psychiatry,* 14 (1983):109–115.

33. McCONAGHY, W. "A Controlled Trial of Imipramine, Amphetamine, Pad and Bell Conditioning, and Random

Awakening in the Treatment of Nocturnal Enuresis," *Medical Journal of Australia,* 2 (1969):237–239.

34. MARSHALL, S., MARSHALL, H. H., and LYON, R. P. "Enuresis: An Analysis of Various Therapeutic Approaches," *Pediatrics,* 52 (1973):813–817.

35. MIKKELSEN, I. J., et al. "Childhood Enuresis, Sleep Patterns and Psychopathology," *Archives of General Psychiatry,* 37 (1980):1139–1144.

36. OREM, J. "Control of the Upper Airways During Sleep and the Hypersomnia–Sleep Apnea Syndrome," in J. Orem and C. Barnes, eds., *Physiology in Sleep.* New York: Academic Press, 1981, pp. 273–313.

37. OUNSTED, M. K., and HENDRICK, A. M. "The First-born Child: Patterns of Development," *Developmental Medicine and Child Neurology,* 19 (1977):446–453.

38. PEDLEY, T. A., and GUILLEMINAULT, C. "Episodic Nocturnal Wanderings Responsive to Anticonvulsant Drug Therapy," *Annals of Neurology,* 2 (1977):30–35.

39. PESIKOFF, R. B., and DAVIS, P. C. "Treatment of Pavor Nocturnus and Somnambulism in Children," *American Journal of Psychiatry,* 128 (1971):778–781.

40. PRICE, V., et al. "Prevalence and Correlates of Poor Sleep Among Adolescents," *American Journal of Diseases of Children,* 132 (1978):583–586.

41. RAPOPORT, J. L., et al. "Childhood Enuresis II," *Archives of General Psychiatry,* 37 (1980):1146–1152.

42. REID, W. H., and GUTNIK, B. D. "Case Report: Treatment of Intractable Sleepwalking," *Psychiatric Journal of the University of Ottawa,* 5 (1980):86–88.

43. REID, W. H., AHMED, I., and LEVIE, C. A. "Treatment of Sleepwalking: A Controlled Study," *American Journal of Psychotherapy,* 35 (1981):27–37.

44. REIMAO, R., and LEFEVRE, A. "Evaluations of Flurazepam and Placebo on Sleep Disorders in Childhood," *Arquivas de Neuro-Psiquiatria,* 40 (1982):1–13.

45. RICHMAN, N. "A Community Survey of Characteristics of One- to Two-year-olds with Sleep Disruptions," *Journal of the American Academy of Child Psychiatry,* 20 (1981):281–291.

46. ———. "Annotations. Sleep Problems in Young Children," *Archives of Disease in Childhood,* 56 (1981):491–493.

47. ROSENFELD, A., et al. "Sleeping Patterns in Upper-Middle-class Families When the Child Awakens Ill or Frightened," *Archives of General Psychiatry,* 39 (1982):943–947.

48. ROTH, T., KRAMER, M., and LUTZ, T. "The Effects of Hypnotics on Sleep, Performance, and Subjective State," *Drugs Under Experimental and Clinical Research,* 1 (1977):279–286.

49. RUSSO, R., GURARAJ, V., and ALLEN, J. "The Effectiveness of Diphenhydramine HCl in Pediatric Sleep Disorders," *Journal of Clinical Pharmacology,* 16 (1976):284–288.

50. SCHMIDT, H. S., CLARK, R. W., and HYMAN, P. R. "Protriptyline: An Effective Agent in the Treatment of the Narcolepsy–Cataplexy Syndrome and Hypersomnia," *American Journal of Psychiatry,* 134 (1977):183–185.

51. SCHMIDT, H. S., WILLIAMS, M. B., and CLARK, R. W. "Treatment of Hypersomnia with Pemoline," in M. H. Chase, D. F. Kripke, and P. L. Walter, eds., *Sleep Research,* vol. 9. Los Angeles: Brain Information Service/Brain Research Institute, 1980, p. 221.

52. SCHMITT, B. D. "Nocturnal Enuresis: An Update on Treatment," *Pediatric Clinics of North America,* 29 (1982):21–37.

53. SHAFFER, D., HEDGE, B., and STEPHENSON, J. "Trial of an Alpha-adrenolytic Drug (Indoramin) for Nocturnal Enuresis," *Developmental Medicine and Child Neurology,* 20 (1978):183–188.

54. SIMEON, J. "Maprotiline Effects in Children with Enuresis and Behavioral Disorders," Paper presented at the American College of Neuropsychopharmacology, San Diego, December 15–18, 1981.

55. ———. "Sleep Studies in Children with Psychiatric Disorders," in L. Greenhill and B. Shopsin, eds., *The Psychobiology of Childhood: A Profile of Current Issues.* New York: Spectrum Publications, 1984, pp. 85–114.

56. SIMEON, J. G., FERGUSON, H. B., and VARGO, B. "Sleep Problems in Child Psychiatry," Paper presented at the annual meeting of the American Academy of Child Psychiatry, San Francisco, Calif., 1983.

57. SIMEON, J., MAGUIRE, J., and LAWRENCE, S. "Maprotiline Effects in Children with Enuresis and Behavioral Disorders," *Progress in Neuropsychopharmacology,* 5 (1981): 495–498.

58. SIMEON, J. G., et al. "Alprazolam Effects in Overanxious Children," Paper presented at the 14th International College of Neuropsychopharmacology Congress, Florence, Italy, July 1984.

59. SIMEON, J. G., et al. "Bupropion Effects in Children with Attention Deficit and Conduct Disorders," Paper presented at the 14th International College of Neuropsychopharmacology Congress, Florence, Italy, July 1984.

60. SIRELING, L. I., and CRISP, A. H. "Sleep and the Enuresis Alarm Device," *Journal of the Royal Society of Medicine,* 76 (1983):131–133.

61. STEPHENSON, J. D. "Physiological and Pharmacological Basis for the Chemotherapy of Enuresis," *Psychological Medicine,* 9 (1979):249–263.

62. SULLIVAN, C. E. "Breathing in Sleep," in J. Orem and C. D. Barnes, eds., *Physiology in Sleep.* New York: Academic Press, 1981, pp. 214–272.

63. TUREMO, T. "DDAVP in Childhood Nocturnal Enuresis," *Acta Paediatrica Scandinavica,* 67 (1978):753–755.

64. TURNER, R. M., and ASCHER, L. M. "A Within-subject Analysis of Stimulus Control Therapy with Severe Sleep-onset Insomnia," *Behavioral Research and Therapy,* 17 (1979):107–112.

65. WAGNER, W., et al. "A Controlled Comparison of Two Treatments for Nocturnal Enuresis," *Journal of Pediatrics,* 101 (1982):302–307.

66. WALLACE, I. R., and FORSYTH, W. I. "The Treatment of Enuresis. A Controlled Clinical Trial of Propantheline, Propantheline and Phenoburbitone and a Placebo," *British Journal of Clinical Practice,* 23 (1969):207–210.

67. WERRY, J., and CARLIELLE, J. "Common Sleep Problems in Children Under Five." Unpublished report, 1983. Available: Prof. J. S. Werry, Dept. of Psychiatry and Behavioral Science, School of Medicine, University of Auckland, Private Bag, Auckland, New Zealand.

68. WERRY, J., et al. "Imipramine in Enuresis: Psychological and Physiological Effects," *Journal of Child Psychology,* 16 (1975):289–300.

69. WITTIG, R., et al. "Narcolepsy in a 7-year-old Child," *Journal of Pediatrics,* 102 (1984):725–727.

70. YOUNGER, J. B. "The Management of Night Waking in Older Infants," *Pediatric Nursing,* 8 (1982):155–158.

54 / Advances in the Treatment of Disorders of Elimination

Jules R. Bemporad and Edward Hallowell

In her comprehensive chapter on encopresis, which appeared in volume 2 of this *Handbook,* Susan Fisher[13] wisely concludes by stating that "the wide range of therapeutic techniques reflects the different origins and meanings of the encopretic symptom, as well as the training and predilections of the . . . therapists (p. 567). The recent clinical literature on the treatment of encopresis exemplifies this diversity. Papers have been published proposing medical, behavioral, and psychotherapeutic approaches. While appearing contradictory at first, the differences among the several approaches reinforce the conclusion that encopresis is more a symptom than a disease entity and that it may occur in diverse personality types and situational contexts. Pediatricians are usually consulted for the milder forms of the condition, especially for younger children, while child psychiatrists tend to be sought out for treatment of the more entrenched symptoms in older children. It is therefore not surprising that the pediatric literature often recommends uncomplicated medical treatment and describes excellent results, while the psychiatric literature favors intensive family or individual therapy and admits to limited success. Between these two extremes are articles describing treatment with variants of behavior therapy, with mixed prognosis.

Differential Diagnosis of Encopresis

A major consideration in the assessment and treatment of functional fecal soiling is that this symptom may occur in a variety of children and situations, each requiring a specific therapeutic intervention.[8] Fecal incontinence may be seen in retarded or autistic children as part of an overall delay in development. Half of the encopretic children described in Shirley's pioneer study,[23] published in 1938, scored in the retarded range on intelligence tests. Usually the soiling for such children is not motivated by misapplied interpersonal manipulations or intrapsychic motives, and they appear to respond well to behavior modification, as reported by Doleys and Arnold.[12]

Some children with attention deficit disorder, with their hyperactivity and impulsiveness, may soil when deeply absorbed in interesting activities or when highly excited. These episodes of soiling are sporadic, without any meaningful pattern. In addition, the parents of these children do not seem obsessed by the soiling, nor do they consider it a hostile act against them. This form of the symptom usually resolves with supportive instructional therapy, parent counseling, and medication for the primary disorder.

Organically intact and psychologically normal children may occasionally soil involuntarily during instances of extreme stress. During the bombardment of London during World War II, Freud and Burlingham,[15] for example, described a high rate of soiling and wetting in children who were separated from their parents. Usually in such children the soiling will stop autonomously when the provoking stress is removed.

Other children will fail to achieve bowel or bladder continence due simply to a lack of training and a familial tolerance of soiling and wetting. Anthony[2] and Bellman[3] have described these children, and both authors stress that simple retraining, support, and reinforcement are sufficient treatment.

Finally, in a small number of children, fecal incontinence may be part of a more entrenched psychological battle between the child and the parents. Bemporad and associates[4,5] designated this form of soiling as chronic neurotic encopresis by virtue of the persistence of the soiling, the child's use of soiling as an age-inappropriate means of expressing feelings, and the occurrence of soiling in an ongoing struggle between family members. This form of encopresis proved much more resistant to treatment, necessitating family as well as individual therapy. Whereas other forms of soiling are usually given up by the child approaching puberty, this type of encopresis may persist into adolescence.[24] Among the children studied were those who had soiled persistently, usually in the presence of their parents, and defied all familial pressures and punishments as a consequence of soiling. They were found to have certain characteristics in common: a history of neurological delay making toilet training difficult; early or harsh bowel training; a family constellation consisting of a psychologically absent father and an erratic, unempathic mother who responded markedly to the child's soiling while ignoring other more appropriate attempts at communication; and the eventual formation of certain personality traits including withholding, passivity, and dependency.

In these cases, the soiling represents one manifestation of a long power struggle between a nonempathic mother and an angry child. The incontinence could be understood as the child's inappropriate way of punishing yet binding the mother in a hostile dependent relationship. Other symptoms were also exhibited by these children, some of which were related to their encopresis. The children would hide their soiled underwear, steal their siblings' underwear, or deposit feces in inappropriate places. In psychiatric evaluation, they would deny or minimize their soiling problem or claim no responsibility for it. Many of these behaviors could be understood in the framework of a sullen rebellion against parental intrusion into toilet habits, continuous threats of punishment, and lack of response to other attempts to communicate.

It is useful to differentiate between retentive and nonretentive encopresis. The retentive type is characterized by withholding of stools, which may lead to colonic enlargement, painful defecation, and abdominal cramps. In time, fecal material may leak around the fecal mass, resulting in chronic staining of underwear. Fleisher[14] found that this form of encopresis may begin with the parents' overzealous usage of laxatives, suppositories, or enemas when the infant appears to strain in order to pass bowel movements. Repeated regularly, this intervention is accompanied by excessive focusing of parental concern on the child's eliminatory functions and results in robbing the infant of learning to control his or her own bowels. Fleisher found that the child responds to the urge to defecate by tightening his or her muscles, leading to retention, which in turn leads to large, hardened stools which are painful to expel.

The clinical picture that emerges is one of large fecal masses that are withheld for days, followed by a painful expulsion, again followed by retention. As stated, there may be chronic leakage around the fecal mass, giving a picture of both soiling and withholding. Eventually these children develop many of the symptoms of the nonretentive encopretics if treatment does not intervene. Such children experience their bowel as "out of their control" and adopt a nonchalant attitude or frank denial of their problem. They may deposit their voluminous stools in inappropriate places, hide soiled underwear, avoid the toilet, and lie about bowel movements. The chronic leakage and its attendant odors may result in social teasing and ostracism as well as constant battles with the parents. Call[7] reported three such children; all were found to have serious difficulties in family relationships that appeared to maintain the symptoms.

While it appears that the retentive and nonretentive types are two separate initial forms of encopresis, if the bowel dysfunction is used in the service of parent-child disagreements, they evolve into almost identical syndromes in later childhood. Levine and Bakow[19] found that children with both forms of encopresis responded equally to treatment; it appeared that severity and not the type of encopresis was the more reliable prognostic indicator. Differentiation of these two clinical types may be important in treating milder cases, particularly in younger children. Nevertheless, the general goal of allowing children to develop age-appropriate control over their own bodily functions, free from the intrusion of others, remains the same.

This variety in the forms of soiling seen by clinicians may partially explain the disparity in treatment recommendations that continue to be espoused by different authors in the current literature. For convenience, this review of recent contributions on clinical management is organized into those that stress medical treatment, behavior modification, psychotherapeutic intervention, or a multimodal plan. As might be expected in a syndrome that so clearly involves both psychological and physical factors, most regimens of treatment are integrative, involving medical, behavioral, and psychodynamic measures.

Counseling-Medical-Behavioral Therapeutic Approaches

All authors agree on the importance of an initial medical evaluation to consider strictly organic etiologies such as Hirshsprung's disease, anal or rectal stenosis, disease of intestinal smooth muscle, or endocrine or pharmacological causes.

Beyond that point, the diversity among the modes of recommended approach begins. Reports of purely behavioral or purely psychodynamic approaches are now rare. More representative is the type of approach recommended by Levine and Bakow.[19] After an initial medical evaluation, there is a meeting with parents and child that fosters open discussion of the symptom in an attempt to remove blame and accusation. Levine and Bakow[19] stress the importance of "demystifying" the symptom, of explaining to the child that many other children have encountered the same problem and of depicting with pictures, in simple language, the rudiments of gastrointestinal anatomy and physiology. The therapist explains to the child that the treatment will be like an athlete's building up muscle, in this case gastrointestinal muscle. Concepts of autonomy, independence, effectiveness, control, and growing up are implied in the session with the child.

The initial meeting thus sets an affirmative tone of action and hope, rather than guilt and recrimination. Levine and Bakow then invoke the medical modality of an initial bowel catharsis, which is followed by daily doses of mineral oil or other laxatives. In addition, a behavioral regimen is set up: twice-daily timed, ten-minute periods on the potty with a reward like stars for successful completion. The potty or toilet is itself built to the child's needs by adding a stool or platform if the child's feet do not reach the floor. In the hubbub that usually surrounds the encopretic syndrome, practical details, such as the fact that it is difficult to have a bowel movement with one's feet off the floor, tend to be overlooked.

Using the regimen of initial counseling followed by behavioral and pharmacological therapy, Levine and Bakow found that 78 percent of 107 children studied showed marked improvement or complete remission. A follow-up study showed that symptom substitution did not ensue.[20]

Other authors from the pediatric and psychiatric literature recommend a similar approach with equally good results. Hein and Beerends[18] agree on the importance of the initial counseling session to correct the often bizarre misconceptions the child and parents may have about the symptom and to allow ventilation of the very strong emotions that inevitably surround the problem. The authors proceed to recommend a program of behavioral management similar to Levine and Bakow's, differing in details but agreeing on the optimistic, nonpunitive spirit of the program. Fleisher's approach[14] is similar as well, again noting the importance of taking emotional factors into account from the outset in order to bridge, as he puts it, the "empathy gap" that has so often arisen between parents and child because of the symptom.

Other authors recommend more complicated behavior regimens. In the three cases he reported, Butler[6] used overcorrection. That regimen includes "positive practice" wherein, if children soil, they must demonstrate appropriate potty behavior ten times immediately afterward, as if to "practice" what they have yet to learn. Wright's regimen,[25] which uses punishments as well as rewards, aims to place responsibility on the children in an effort to encourage them to take control. The use of enemas as a negative reinforcer is an element of his regimen with which most authors would disagree.

Recognizing the diversity of presentations within this syndrome, other authors stress the importance of a flexible, multimodal approach responsive to the needs of the individual case. Halpern,[17] in reviewing the literature, found physiological, interpersonal, intrapsychic, and behavioral conceptualizations as well as combinations thereof. From his review, as well as from his own series of ten patients with ten controls, he concluded that the eclectic approach worked best, starting with a trial of a quick-acting suppository plus support and education before considering more intensive physiological or psychological interventions. In many cases he found that quick symptom improvement changed the emotional climate so that permanent change ensued.

Cushmore[10] reported a modification of a strictly behavioral approach in which the mother plays the role of therapist. Standard techniques of operant conditioning are used. Of course, such an approach must be used judiciously so as not to exacerbate an already conflicted relationship with the mother.

Fritz and Armbrust[16] enlarged on the theme of family intervention in their extensive review. They stress the importance of reducing pressure on the child by immediate support for the entire family. They note that while the pediatric literature tends to stress somatic intervention and the psychiatric literature emphasizes dynamic intervention, approaches that synthesize the two work best. As other authors report, sometimes the initial supportive intervention changes the family atmosphere sufficiently so that more intensive measures are not needed.

A combination of behavioral and family therapy techniques appears in the British literature. Davis, Mitchell, and Marks[11] recommended that the child be taken out of school for rapid "retraining" that takes an average of five days. The mother is the retrainer while the physician is consultant. It was found that this approach worked well with cooperative parents. Failures occurred when features of a multiproblem family led to noncompliance. In Wright and Walker's behavioral regimen,[26] implemented by the family with the pediatrician as supervisor, primary responsibility is given to the child, while the parents adhere to a system of reward and punishments agreed on with the child in advance. Again, success for this kind of program depends on the ability of the parents to cooperate.

Reports of purely pharmacological treatments beyond laxatives are rare once it has been determined that the etiology is not organic. The pharmacological contribution to the treatment of encopresis centers mainly, as previously stated, on the use of mineral oil. Beyond this widely accepted mainstay, there is one report that imiprimine hydrochloride is useful in the primary treatment of the syndrome.[9] Controlled studies of this effect are as yet unpublished. Tricyclics have also been used to treat depression secondary to the encopresis. Musicco[21] reports the use of uridine-5-triphosphate to increase the contraction tone and activity of the smooth musculature of the lower bowel in a case where dynamic causes were present in combination with the organic factor of hypotonia of smooth musculature.

Other pharmacological approaches center on the adjunctive role laxatives play in the initial phases of therapy.

More Intensive Multimodal Therapeutic Approaches

All the programs of therapy mentioned so far report good results, typically 80 percent remission or marked improvement. But what of the resistant 20 percent? Levine and Bakow[19] noted that in their sample, the group that did not do well tended to share certain characteristics. A high percentage were learning disabled or hyperactive. In addition, they were described as "fearless," "moody," and "disobedient." In the more refractory cases other authors have noted the presence of severe family turmoil or neurological impairment in the child, or both. The pattern noted by Bemporad and associates[4] in chronic neurotic encopresis is frequently mentioned in connection with cases that require intensive treatment; it includes an erratic mother and an absent or passive father. Earlier, Anthony[2] called attention to disturbances in the "potting couple" of mother and child. In short, there appears to be if not a separate syndrome, a group of children in whom the encopretic symptom is most severe and who appear to require more intensive treatment than the outpatient paradigm offered by Levine and others. In these cases, a truly multimodal approach is essential, with particular attention to disturbances within the family system, even to the point of removing the child from the home for brief inpatient treatment.

Ringdahl[22] reports on such in-hospital treatment for thirteen children, all of whom had failed in outpatient therapy. A multimodal, intensive in-hospital approach was used including behavioral measures, milieu treatment, group therapy, family intervention, occupational therapy, and medication as well as individual work with the child. The mean length of stay was twenty-six days. Twelve of thirteen children achieved remission; the only failure was associated with an inability to engage the family in treatment.

Amsterdam[1] used a similar approach on an outpatient basis with five children who had failed to improve with less intensive therapy. Her strategy stresses family dynamics and aims particularly to effect change within the mother-child dyad. Behavioral methods, such as rewards, are used, but, unlike the simpler regimens, the methods are interpreted in an effort to enhance the child's sense of autonomy. The youngster is encouraged to negotiate and bargain in order to gain a sense of control. Boundaries between mother and child are set and the child is not subjected to punishments. Enemas in particular are avoided.

The approach is multisymptomatic in that the family issues are regarded as much of a symptom as the soiling. Particular emphasis is placed on the power struggle between mother and child. As boundaries are established, the child gains autonomy and the family system improves.

Summary

In summary, encopresis is best conceptualized as a symptom rather than a disease entity. Fecal soiling may occur for diverse reasons requiring diverse treatments. Most of the current literature recognizes the complexity of events that result in fecal incontinence and stresses a multimodal treatment approach. While most children appear to resolve their symptom by rather straightforward behavioral modification or direct counseling, about 20 percent of children require more intensive individual and family therapy.

REFERENCES

1. AMSTERDAM, B. "Chronic Encopresis: A System Based Psychodynamic Approach," *Child Psychiatry and Human Development,* 9 (1979):137–144.

2. ANTHONY, E. J. "An Experimental Approach to the Psychopathology of Childhood: Encopresis," *British Journal of Medical Psychology,* 30 (1957):146–175.

3. BELLMAN, M. "Studies on Encopresis," *Acta Paediatrica Scandinavica,* 170 (1966):1–151.

4. BEMPORAD, J. R., et al. "Characteristics of Encopretic Patients and Their Families," *Journal of the American Academy of Child Psychiatry,* 10 (1971):272–292.

5. BEMPORAD, J. R., et al. "Chronic Neurotic Encopresis

as a Paradigm of a Multi-Factorial Psychiatric Disorder," *Journal of Nervous and Mental Disease,* 166 (1978):472–479.

6. BUTLER, J. F. "Treatment of Encopresis by Overcorrection," *Psychological Reports,* 40 (1977):639–646.

7. CALL, J. D. "Psychogenic Megacolon in Three Preschool Boys," *American Journal of Orthopsychiatry,* 33 (1963):923–928.

8. CHESS, S., and HASSIBI, M. *Principles and Practice of Child Psychiatry.* New York: Plenum Press, 1978.

9. CONNELL, H. M. "The Practical Management of Encopresis," *Australian Journal of Pediatrics,* 8 (1972):273–278.

10. CUSHMORE, G. A. "The Reduction of Soiling Behavior in an 11 Year Old Boy with the Parent as Therapist," *New Zealand Medical Journal,* 84 (1976):238–239.

11. DAVIS, H., MITCHELL, W. S., and MARKS, F. "A Behavioral Programme for the Modification of Encopresis," *Child: Care, Health and Development,* 1 (1976):273–282.

12. DOLEYS, D. M., and ARNOLD, S. Treatment of Childhood Encopresis," *Mental Retardation,* 13 (1975):14–16.

13. FISHER, S. M. "Encopresis," In J. D. Noshpitz, ed., *Basic Handbook of Child Psychiatry,* vol. 2. New York: Basic Books, 1979, pp. 556–568.

14. FLEISHER, D. R. "Diagnosis and Treatment of Disorders of Defecation in Children," *Pediatric Annals* (November 1976):71–101.

15. FREUD, A., and BURLINGHAM, D. T. *War and Children.* New York: Medical War Books, 1943.

16. FRITZ, G. V., and ARMBRUST, J. Enuresis and Encopresis," *Psychiatric Clinics of North America,* 5 (1982):283–296.

17. HALPERN, W. I. "The Treatment of Encopretic Children," *Journal of the American Academy of Child Psychiatry,* 2 (1977):478–479.

18. HEIN, H. A., and BEERENDS, J. J. "Who Should Accept Primary Responsibility for the Encopretic Child?" *Clinical Pediatrics,* 10 (1978):67–70.

19. LEVINE, M. D., and BAKOW, H. "Children with Encopresis: A Study of Treatment Outcome," *Pediatrics,* 58 (1976):845–852.

20. LEVINE, M. D., MAZONSON, P., and BAKOW, H. "Behavioral Symptom Substitution in Children Cured of Encopresis," *American Journal of Diseases of Children,* 134 (1980):663–667.

21. MUSICCO, N. "Encopresis: A Good Result in a Boy with UTP (uridine-5-triphosphate)," *American Journal of Proctology,* 28 (1977):43–46.

22. RINGDAHL, I. C. "Hospital Treatment of the Encopretic Child," *Psychosomatics,* 21 (1980):65–71.

23. SHIRLEY, H. F. "Encopresis in Children," *Journal of Pediatrics,* 12 (1930):367.

24. SHOLEVAR, G. P. "Persistent Encopresis in Preadolescence," in G. P. Sholevar, R. M. Benson, and B. J. Blinder, eds., *Emotional Disorders in Children and Adolescents.* New York: SP Medical and Scientific Books, 1980, pp. 187–191.

25. WRIGHT, L. "Handling the Encopretic Child," *Professional Psychology,* 4 (1973):137–144.

26. WRIGHT, L., and WALKER, C. E. "Treatment of the Child with Psychogenic Encopresis," *Clinical Pediatrics,* 16 (1977):1042–1045.

55 / Attention Deficit Disorder: Clinical Evaluation and Treatment

Robert D. Hunt, Richard W. Brunstetter, and Larry B. Silver

Introduction

Perhaps the most common of all the clinical problems confronting the child psychiatrist is the group of dysfunctions subsumed under the diagnostic categories of attention deficit disorder with hyperactivity (ADDH), learning disability (LD), and conduct disorder. Although careful analysis of clinical populations does not demonstrate that these conditions occur in the aggregate often enough to warrant their designation as a specific syndrome—for example, "minimal brain dysfunction"—certainly in individual clinical instances they do occur together and their coexistence has great significance for the child's course and outcome.

LDs and conduct disorder are discussed elsewhere in this volume. Chapter 37 is concerned with diagnostic issues and etiology in regard to attention deficit disorder (ADD). This chapter addresses itself to evaluation and treatment.

Clinical Evaluation

Since ADDH is a multifaceted disorder, the diagnostic process requires evaluation of children and their environment from many perspectives. The physician must obtain information from the parents and teachers as well as the child. Collaboration with other physicians, educators, and psychologists is usually essential to effective diagnosis and treatment.[64]

FAMILY HISTORY

A family history of LD, childhood hyperactivity of the parent, or persisting symptoms of residual ADD may be obtained. These residual difficulties are characterized by persisting impulsivity; stimulus seeking and risk taking; impatience; irritability; explosiveness; disorderliness; inability to plan, follow, or execute plans; impaired interpersonal relationships; and diminished job performance. ADDH appears to be associated with a family history of alcohol and substance abuse.

NATAL AND PERINATAL HISTORY

Maternal consumption of excessive alcohol should be noted along with the use of other medications during pregnancy. Complications of pregnancy associated with bleeding, fetal anoxia or distress, or premature delivery should be documented.

LIFE EVENTS IN CHILDREN WITH ADDH

A childhood history of illness associated with high fever, encephalitis or meningitis, or seizure disorder should be noted. Lead consumption through eating of old paint still occurs in some cities. A history of psychological trauma with severe emotional neglect or abuse may be obtained from a parent, relative, school, or a child protection agency.

BEHAVIOR RATING SCALES

Systematic quantification of children's symptoms requires use of standardized behavioral rating scales. The most well standardized general behavioral rating assessment in child psychiatry is the Child Behavior Checklist (CBC) developed by Achenbach.[1] This scale has been standardized for children of both sexes from six to fourteen years of age; subscale norms exist for factors of internalizing (schizoid, depressed, uncommunicative, obsessive-compulsive, systematic complaints and externalizing, social withdrawal, hyperactive aggression, and delinquent behavior). A percentile rank for social adjustment reflects participation in school and extracurricular activities. Achenbach[3] has recently developed and standardized a similar behavior checklist to be completed by teachers. These questionnaires are particularly useful in the identification of associated disturbances in mood, anxiety, conduct, or neurotic symptoms of childhood

and provide an index of social and intellectual competence.

Behavior ratings of hyperactive and conduct disorder are best obtained using the behavior ratings scales developed by Keith Conners. The forty-eight-item Parents' Questionnaire has five behavior clusters or factors: conduct problems, learning problems, psychosomatic problems, impulsivity-hyperactivy, and anxiety. The Teachers' Questionnaire has twenty-eight items with three factors: conduct problems, hyperactivity, and inattention-passivity.[47,67] Behavioral factors on teachers' ratings of the Conners' scale were recently determined on a large normative population.[104] A Hyperactivity Index has been developed by Barkley,[9] for use with both parent and teacher Conners' questionnaires. Although many of the specific diagnostic items on DSM-III are not listed on the Conners' scales, their ratings correlate highly with DSM-III diagnosis ($r = 0.95$).[47]

These behavior ratings scales are extremely useful for both diagnostic assessment and the monitoring and coordinating of response to medication and other interventions. A comparison of the results of both scales and ratings from parents and teachers may identify setting-specific symptoms that indicate selective areas of conflict or difficulty. Pervasive pan-setting ADDH may be most biologically loaded and require the most aggressive treatment.

Prior to beginning medication Conners' scales should be obtained at least twice from both parent and teacher in order to provide more time to identify a stable baseline that reflects the child's behavior over a minimum of a two-week period. For teacher ratings, it is useful to know the size of the class, time of day (morning or afternoon), subject matter and difficulty, and whether or not this is a regular or special educational environment. For children in middle school, ratings from more than one teacher are often necessary to reflect differences in class time, size, and academic content.

A well-standardized and computerized form for obtaining a developmental history from parents is the Children's Personal Data Inventory (CPDI) developed by Shaywitz.[95] This scale encompasses demographic information, genetic background, pre- and perinatal events, developmental and social history, educational experiences, recent life stresses, and current areas of difficulty.

PSYCHIATRIC INTERVIEW

When evaluated in a psychiatrist's office, children with ADD frequently appear restless, fidgety, and squirmy. They may have difficulty staying seated. They frequently scan the office and are easily distracted and intrigued by what they see. They often seem oblivious to their difficulties and are inclined to report that things are going well at home and at school. Their speech may be somewhat rapid and crisp, but reflects no intrinsic difficulty with appropriate word usage or syntax. Their behavior and speech may indicate preoccupation with aggressive themes and a tendency to blame others. They frequently offer only a shallow, reflexive response to questions with little reflectivity and insight. Some children with ADDH convey feelings of inadequacy, low self-esteem, and regret concerning their difficulties in self-control and mastery. Others externalize and project their problems. While these personality characteristics are greatly affected by the family, the children's impulsivity becomes a significant force in shaping their character and emotional development.

Several standard psychiatric interviews' have recently been developed for children that provide an excellent method of confirming the diagnosis and screening for other psychiatric problems. Most of these interviews have separate schedules for parents and children. Since children often underestimate their degree of conduct and behavioral disturbance, both versions should be administered. These interviews are generally "scorable" for DSM-III diagnoses. The Schedule for Affective Disorders and Schizophrenia for School-Age Children (K-SADS)[84] requires somewhat more clinical judgment. The Diagnostic Interview for Children and Adolescents (DICA)[91] is more literally worded and can be used by less experienced clinicians; it consists of structured interviews that systematically survey parents and children for symptoms within the child.[111] The Diagnostic Interview Schedule for Children (DISC)[30] is being increasingly well standardized.

PHYSICAL AND NEUROLOGICAL EXAMINATION

A general physical examination is indicated in every child with ADDH. Measures of overall maturation, height and weight, and physical appearance are important. Visual and auditory acuity should be clinically assessed and followed up by laboratory measures if dubious. *Minor physical anomalies* occur at increased incidence in ADDH and may include abnormal size and symmetry of head; wiry, "electric" hair; and wide-set eyes (hyperteleorism) with increased epicanthal folds. Examination of the mouth may demonstrate malalignment of the teeth, a high arched or steepled palate. The hands may have have a short fifth finger; feet may exhibit irregular spacing of toes and webbing in the interdigital space.[4,107]

The neurological examination will assess gross and fine motor functioning and neuromaturational devel-

opment. An increase in overall activity level that occurs across all settings (in free play, interview, and classroom) should be noted. Gross motor skills are assessed by comparing a child's competence to those of age-matched controls in ability to stand on one foot, hop, skip, and stop and pivot. The ability to throw and catch a ball should be tested. Gait assessment should include tandem (heel-toe) gait and walking forward and backward on heels and toes. The quality of movement is assessed by noting flopping, uninhibited, poorly integrated motion. Disinhibition and overflow in latency-aged children is usually a sign of delayed maturation. A physical and neurological examination for soft signs (PANESS) appears to be a reliable indicator of neurological function and correlates well with behavioral and cognitive measures.[59]

Fine motor skills may be assessed through rapid finger tap and sequential apposition of fingers and thumb in which the rate and smoothness of performance are observed and overflow from right to left is monitored. Performance of a standard handwriting and drawing (Draw-A-Person, Bender Gestalt) sample provides another index of fine motor control and carefulness of work. Within a neuromaturational test battery a task such as peg-hole placement can be timed and compared to age-matched norms.[40]

LABORATORY ASSESSMENT

Blood should be drawn for a complete blood count to test for anemia, thyroid indices, liver function tests (if medication is prescribed), ceruloplasmin, and serum lead. Twenty-four-hour urinary catecholamine and copper measures may be useful.

Electroencephalograms with photic stimulation may be useful in children with ADDH. Petit mal, partial facial seizures, and temporal or frontal lobe excitability may underlie symptoms of ADDH in some children.

Assessment of Learning Difficulties

Clinicians can make an approximate assessment of cognitive competence and presence of learning difficulties through administration of screening tests. Visual-motor tasks might include the Draw-A-Person Test,[105] Kinetic Family Drawing,[56] the Bender Gestalt.[75] Simple age-standardized tasks are available for sampling vocabulary, spelling, reading ability, and comprehension. Problem-solving ability can be estimated. Tasks and questions such as those developed by Piaget may provide an index of reasoning and logic.

The assessment of a learning disability requires indices of overall intelligence (e.g., the revised Wechsler Intelligence Scale for Children[107] or Stanford-Binet[103]), actual academic achievement (e.g., the Wide-Range Achievement Test,[70] Woodcock-Johnson Psycho-Educational Battery,[56] or Peabody Individual Achievement Test),[33] social competence (e.g., the Vineland Social Maturity Scales),[32] and specific areas of learning. Perceptual and motor skills can be quantified in addition to clinical assessment through the use of tests such as the Porteus Maze,[80] Bender Gestalt Test,[12] or the Beery Test of Visual Motor Integration (VMI).[10]

Tests such as the Illinois Test of Psycholinguistic Ability (ITPA) or the McCarthy Scales of Children's Abilities[78] aid the school psychologist in assessing the mechanism of a learning disorder. The Detroit Tests of Learning Aptitude[53] measures nineteen different areas of learning aptitude and covers a broad range of abilities, providing both specific subtest scores and an index of general mental age. The Boehm Test of Basic Concepts[13] provides percentile scores of a child's development of verbal concepts. The limitations of psychological tests in differential diagnosis have been discussed by Gittelman.[42]

All these standardized tests have been used to define overall cognitive and social competence. Other measures have been developed that sample specific steps in information processing. These tests measure reaction time, selective attention, vigilance, acquisition learning, and short- and long-term memory, and address strategies of perception, encoding, and information retrieval.[64,69]

Treatment of ADDH

EDUCATION

For those ADDH children with learning disabilities, *special education* is frequently the primary treatment, and should begin early. Many ADDH children benefit from being in quieter, smaller classrooms with fewer distractions. Children should not repeat a grade unnecessarily or be promoted for purely social reasons. Instead, children should receive tutoring and/or periods in special education programs. The major tools of special education consist of repeated presentation of material after one-on-one teaching with few distractions and frequent reinforcement. Multisensory (visual, auditory, kinesthetic) presentation of material intensifies the learning process. Early remediation may allow children to move back into the mainstream of education. Ignoring a problem in school, under the label of mainstreaming, may assure eventual failure. Specific programs for enhancing motoric skills may be helpful.

PSYCHOTHERAPY

Individual Psychotherapy. Psychotherapy may change children's self-concept from that of inadequate underachievers who have compensated for deficits with clowning or misbehavior to one of more competent and more consistent individuals. For ADDH children psychotherapy has both educational and and interpretive components. Children can usually understand that they have a disorder that increases their distractibility and impulsivity. They must recognize these symptoms, develop internal controls, and anticipate situations that will be stressful. Parents and children can often learn to selectively use the medication to assist them in managing circumstances that create excessive arousal or demand increased control.

Psychotherapy can address specific issues within the intrapsychic life of children with ADDH. Themes of self-esteem, self-control, and other neurotic symptoms of childhood may require psychotherapy. These children often experience low self-esteem due to impaired academic and social performance. Some children blame themselves for their difficulties and have internalized a sense of being defective or "bad." The therapist can assist children in understanding that their tendency to be impulsive and restless is not their "fault." However, children can exert some measure of conscious, learned control over these impulses. The therapist must walk a fine line between freeing such children from internalized blame and assisting the children to maximize their self-control.[39,40]

Children may be envious and feel destructive anger toward others, including the therapist, who are more easily able to act appropriately and effectively. Often acting-out behavior becomes an internalized, ego-syntonic release of anxiety for ADDH children. Their predilection toward action may thwart the development of their own potential for reflection. As the therapist encourages the children to contain their behavior and reflect upon themselves, depression, which had previously been defended against through bravado and stimulus-seeking behavior, may surface. ADDH children may easily perceive the suggestions of teachers or the rules of home as excessively critical, controlling, and rejecting. A strong therapeutic alliance may be needed to enable children to perceive the suggestions of teachers or the rules of home (such as a behavioral-shaping program) as useful, rather than threatening, to their own interests. This intervention can assist the children to counter their own tendency for oppositional behavior. Psychotherapy and special education

ers to methylphenidate suggested a preference for that medication,[48] whereas Gittelman-Klein[43] reported nearly similar efficacy of imipramine and methylphenidate. Quinn and associates[88] treated seventy-six hyperactive children with 80 mg per day of either medication for ten weeks and noted preferential cognitive response to methylphenidate. Werry, Aman, and Diamond[113] treated thirty ADDH children in a crossover design with methylphenidate (0–4 mg/d) and imipramine (1–2 mg/kg/d) for four weeks at each dose. Both medications produced clinical improvement and facilitated performance on the Continuous Performance Task and the Porteus Maze. Huessy[60] has reported a rapid response to imipramine with minimal side effects in ADDH.

Clonidine. Recent studies of the noradrenergic agonist clonidine, in children with ADDH suggested its therapeutic usefulness may parallel results in subjects with Tourette's disorder. In a twelve-week, double-blind, placebo-crossover study, Hunt, Minderaa, and Cohen[67] found that clonidine has possible therapeutic utility in ADDH when compared to placebo. Parents' ratings on the Conners' scale showed that eight of the ten children clearly benefitted from clonidine. The mean behavior ratings for the group improved significantly by the end of active clonidine treatment ($p = 0.002$). Teachers' ratings also showed significant improvement on the hyperactivity index and on the total rating ($p = 0.01$). Children were not sedated or psychomotorically retarded; the initial sleepiness diminished after two weeks of treatment. While clonidine may be a useful alternative therapeutic agent for some children with ADDH, its relative effectiveness compared to methylphenidate on behavioral and cognitive measures requires further study.

Other medications that have been tried in ADDH include levodopa, lithium, carbama zepine, amitriptyline, thioridazine, haloperidol, chlorpromazine, and monoamine oxidase inhibitors. There is a need to further differentiate both the behavioral and cognitive effects of these medications to clarify their specific role and indications.

Diet. Diets restrictive of food additives, coloring, and sugar have been popular since Feingold's work[36] suggested that many ADDH children had a nonimmunological supersensitivity to these substances. Although parental testimony has frequently supported its claim of clinical benefit from avoidance diets, controlled studies have not supported their effectiveness. The National Institutes of Health consensus[83] found these diets to be safe but not usually helpful. These diets require considerable organization on the part of the family and self-control and cooperation of the part of the child. In total, controlled studies of dietary interventions suggest minimal sustained therapeutic utility.

Whether the offending dietary ingredient is sugar or a food dye or additive has [been] debated, as well as whether these ADDH [represent] a specific allergic or toxic response.[37,41]

Conners and associates[29] found small d[ifferences in] parents and teachers ratings in a few subje[cts involv]ing a challenge versus a control diet. Will[iams and] coworkers[116] found no effect of color-containi[ng food] in contrast to considerable benefit from medi[cation]. Administration of artificial coloring and flavori[ng to] twenty-two children selected for parents' report o[f re]sponse to the Feingold diet showed only two wh[ose] parental ratings demonstrated behavioral worsening.[109] However, following large doses of added food coloring versus placebo, diminished attention span and increased errors in learning were evident on the paired associate learning task.[101] Harley, Matthews, and Lichman[54] found that parents and teachers could not distinguish periods of additive-free versus routine diet in behavioral ratings of children who had been reported to be diet-sensitive. Similarly, control and additive-free diets had no measurable effect on retarded individuals observed in a residential setting.[55] When administered to normal, nonhyperactive children, the Feingold diet diminished fidgetiness, distractibility, and noise making in a small subset of the children, but adequate dietary controls were lacking.[58]

Although hypoglycemia has been postulated to cause symptoms of ADDH, subjective symptoms of light-headedness, diaphoresis, shakiness, and weakness did not correlate with the absolute level or rate of fall of blood sugar level in 192 adults receiving a five-hour glucose tolerence test.[72] Therapies based on optometric training, vestibular stimulation, and patterning or "neurological retraining" have no objectively demonstrated efficacy.[46]

Summary

Attention deficit disorder with hyperactivity is a serious disorder of childhood. Its impact on adjustment is profound and often persists into adulthood. ADDH and its frequently associated conditions, learning disability and conduct disorder, often resist efforts at amelioration and continue for many years to underlie increased vulnerability to a variety of adult dysfunctions, including substance abuse and occupational and marital instability. These conditions merit the most serious kind of consideration from the clinician. They challenge child psychiatrists to exercise to the fullest all their professional skills, including diagnosis and assess-

---

in a small classroom with few distractions may help improve ADDH children's academic skills, modulate their impulses, and sustain more consistent and intimate interpersonal relationships.

Family Psychotherapy. The family may need psychotherapy or counseling to help determine their behavioral expectations for their child. Parents need to rapidly, appropriately, and consistently provide consequences to their ADDH child's behavior and to avoid scapegoating, inappropriate punishment, or indulgence of their impulsive child. They often need assistance in managing their guilt and embarrassment at having a difficult child. It is easy for parents to become outraged at the child's "irresponsibility," "forgetfulness," "indifference," and imperviousness to parental authority and sanctions. Parents complain of feeling helpless, misunderstood, and isolated. They easily become furious and blame each other for being "too strict" or "too permissive." Such experiences exaggerate preexisting parental conflicts or intensify parents' intolerance of personality characteristics that they also see within themselves. Both processes may require therapeutic intervention.

BEHAVIOR MODIFICATION

Techniques of behavior modification or shaping have been developed for use at home and in the classroom. The underlying principles emphasize establishing clearly defined, limited goals reflecting specific behaviors to praise, punish, or ignore. Parent, teachers, and therapists must identify rewards that will motivate a specific child and develop a schedule of reinforcement to sustain performance on selected tasks. Behaviors to be encouraged should be specifically defined in positive terms. Baseline charting of the frequency and the severity of these behaviors should be performed prior to intervention. Behavior-shaping techniques are often very useful in children with ADDH if applied consistently. Difficulty of generalization from one setting to another and in sustaining the progress after the reinforcements are discontinued may limit their effectiveness.[81]

COGNITIVE TRAINING

A related psychotherapeutic method relies predominantly on teaching *self-monitoring and self-control* and altering internal self-messages. This treatment is an outgrowth of techniques of cognitive therapy. The essential intervention consists of teaching children to identify disruptive behaviors such as fidgetiness, talking out of turn, getting out of seat, using defiant or provocative speech, or teasing—behaviors to which these children are often oblivious, though they are ob-

vious to outside observers. Children are encouraged to label these actions, identify their antecedents, and tell themselves to inhibit them before they are acted out. Children who are learning not to talk in class until called on may be taught to notice when they feels like talking without raising their hand, and then to tell themselves, "I have to wait until I'm called on" or "Don't talk till teacher gives the okay." Children may also learn to substitute less disruptive behaviors: "I want to tap my pencil, but I'll write notes instead."[17]

MEDICATION

Effects of Stimulant Medications. Stimulants such as methylphenidate, amphetamine, and magnesium pemoline are useful in reducing the motor hyperactivity that frequently accompanies ADD; they narrow the spectrum of attention and reduce impulsivity, thus diminishing distractibility in class and improving persistence in vigilance and memory or associated learning tasks. Stimulants frequently improve behavior and ease social interaction at home and school. Many ADD children will experience an increased sense of control and mastery on medication. Diagnosis of underlying psychosis, multiple tics, and major side effects to stimulants in the past are contraindications to stimulant medication.[77]

Behavioral Monitoring. Prior to the initiation of medication, parents and teachers should be asked to complete a behavior rating scale, such as the Conners' Teachers' twenty-eight-item scale; such scales are useful in monitoring the effects of medication. These should be repeated on a weekly basis during initial treatment and monthly thereafter. Teachers should note class size, subject, and time of day. A systematic parent diary may add to the clinical assessment.

Dosage. Initial choice of medication is frequently methylphenidate at doses of approximately 0.1 to 0.2 mg per kg given before school. Medication dosage can gradually be increased toward a maximum of about 0.5 to 0.75 mg per kg, which may be given in divided doses, about 8:00 A.M. and noon. Eating meals before medication does not impair absorption of the medication. Weekly monitoring and rating of behavior by teacher and parents will assist in determining the optimal dose.

It is not yet certain whether the dosage required to produce optimal improvement in attention may be less than that needed to achieve maximal behavioral control. In a child with primarily attentional learning difficulties, a low dose (10–20 mg daily) may yield the best cognitive improvement, although some restlessness may remain.

Children can often learn to participate in the regulation of their medication by anticipating the demands of the next four hours and altering the dosage appropriately. While medication may be needed to sustain attention and quietness in a classroom, it may not be needed during free play or recreational activities. Medication is usually needed less consistently during the summer, allowing partial medication holidays. Except in severe cases, summer holidays are advisable and allow reassessment for continued treatment. Many ADD children can begin the academic year with a trial off medication or be tapered after initial adjustment to a new classroom. The empirical trial provides assessment of continued need for stimulants. In some ADD children, medication can be withdrawn before puberty; others require continued treatment into adolescence.

RESPONSE TO STIMULANTS

Considerable research suggests that medication alone does not improve academic grades or classroom learning. Stimulants do not always improve the scholastic performance of children with learning disabilities. Even in children with ADDH, behavioral and educational improvements do not always cooccur. While stimulants reduce motor behavior and improve reaction time, sustained vigilance, and recall of simple stimuli, they do not necessarily enhance the other processes of learning: identification of relevant concepts, reorganization, and encoding for appropriate conceptual retrieval. Short-term improvement does not always enhance long-term outcome. Improvement in cognitive laboratory measures does not always correlate with improved classroom learning. In one study following twelve weeks of flexible dose treatment with methylphenidate or thioridazine, few correlations were noted between classroom progress in academic areas and changes on behavioral or achievement ratings. Improvement in psychological test scores did not appear to correlate with each other, and improvement across behavioral ratings and psychological testing were generally unrelated.[43]

Stimulant medications have social effects: They decrease number of negative behaviors of the child, reduce the frequency of teachers' reprimands, and improve handwriting.[114] Charles and Schain,[21] in a four-year follow-up, reported that stimulants administered to ADDH children resulted in lessening of hyperactivity, but academic underachievement remained a greater problem than behavioral and social difficulties. The duration of treatment did not correlate with clinical improvement. Methylphenidate treatment improves both ADD children's behavior in class and the quality of their interaction with their teacher, and reduces their level of intensity and control.[115]

MULTIMODAL TREATMENT

The effectiveness of multimodal treatment was evident in the three-year prospective study by Satterfield, Cantwell, and Satterfield.[93] They utilized a combination of clinically optimal dose of methylphenidate with special education, tutoring, and family or individual psychotherapy as indicated. In an initial cohort of about one hundred carefully diagnosed ADDH children who were treated and monitored, this multimodal treatment produced both behavioral and academic improvement in those children who continued in treatment.

Several studies demonstrate an additive effect of combined interventions: medication, special education, and psychotherapy. Coupled with psychotherapy and special education, stimulants may improve academic adjustment and performance.[93] However, unless accompanied by appropriate psychotherapy, family counseling, or focused educational intervention, medications alone usually do not lead to improved academic learning, higher grades, or increase in achievement scores.[43,87] In kindergarten-age hyperactive children there was no difference between behavior modification and methylphenidate treatment.[26] Methylphenidate was more effective than behavioral self-control for children with ADDH.[7] Studies of the effectiveness of combined medication and behavioral modification suggest an additive effect of both interventions. Medication often has the most powerful short-term effect, but when used alone it does not enhance long-term development.[43]

While stimulants are usually beneficial for children with the combined behavioral and cognitive difficulties of ADDH, they are not useful in children with pure LDS uncomplicated by hyperactivity.[42] However, methylphenidate facilitated the performance of both hyperactive and nonhyperactive children on a visual search task with a short-term memory component, even at a high dose (1.25 mg/kg/d).[34]

SIDE EFFECTS OF STIMULANTS

Stimulant medications have multiple side effects and some specific contraindications. Transient side effects include anorexia, insomnia, stomachaches, afternoon withdrawal, and explosiveness.[19] Long-term side effects of stimulants may include growth suppression,[49,79] although this may be transient and depend on the dose and duration of medication. While stimulants have been reported to induce tics,[45,77] untreated ADDH children appear to be at increased endogenous risk for tics.[31] Hallucinosis and possible psychosis may follow stimulant treatment in vulnerable children.[119] Compliance with methylphenidate treatment is frequently low.[38,73,98] Weekend and summer drug holi-

may diminish concern about possible growth suppression. On stimulant medication, children may become more "rigid," irritable, and tense. In children with atypical development, childhood psychosis, and multiple tic syndrome, stimulants may lead to dramatic exacerbation of symptomatology. Since these children initially often have attentional problems and hyperactivity, physicians may mistakenly increase the medication rather than recognizing that the symptomatic exacerbation is a medication side effect.

PHARMACOKINETICS OF STIMULANTS

Approximately 200,000 to 400,000 children in the United States receive stimulant medication for attentional and behavioral control. Blood-level determination may have therapeutic utility in identifying children who absorb methylphenidate poorly or excrete it rapidly and thereby fail to achieve adequate levels.

Shaywitz and associates[96] reported that following a single oral dose of methylphenidate, the peak level was reached at 2.5 hours ($\pm$ 20 minutes). The peak blood levels achieved demonstrated a nearly threefold range across individuals receiving similar methylphenidate doses, but were highly replicable within individuals. The excretion half-life ($t^{1/2}$) of methylphenidate was 2.5 $\pm$ .5 hours. These results are compatible with other pharmacological studies of methylphenidate.[52,62,76] Eating prior to taking methylphenidate does not affect absorption.[20]

Substantial blood levels of methylphenidate persist for up to eight hours, although the clinical effect diminishes. This lack of a simple correlation between blood level and clinical effect probably reflects methylphenidate's release of stored catecholamines.

The two-hour blood levels of methylphenidate during chronic treatment were comparable to the levels obtained following an acute single dose of the drug. When the blood levels of these therapeutically treated children were compared to their behavioral improvement (Conners's Abbreviated Parent Teacher Behavior Rating Scale), those whose behavior ratings most improved during treatment had significantly higher two-hour methylphenidate blood levels. A minimum level of 7 ng per ml may be needed for behavioral response; however, some forms of learning may be impaired at higher doses in some children.[99,*] A linear dose-response relationship was found with performance on a cognitive task by Winsberg and associates.[118]

A similar pharmacokinetic profile was noted in studies of d-amphetamine.[23,35] Following a single dose of about 0.5 mg per kg, peak d-amphetamine concentra-

*J. Swanson, personal communication, 1985.

tions occurred after four hours. The elimina[tion half-]life ($t^{1/2}$) was about 6.8 $\pm$ 0.5 hours. Beha[vioral im]provement, rated on the Conners' abbreviate[d rating] scale, was significant from one to four hours [after med]ication. Retest of six children with [a single] d-amphetamine dose showed no significan[t change] in absorption or elimination one week late[r.]

Thus blood levels may provide informa[tion about] some children who are poor responders and [there is] variability in absorption, binding, or excr[etion.] hour blood levels may be clinically useful [in children] who do not respond, who have excessive si[de effects,] who suddenly require a major change in [dosage.]

OTHER TREATMENTS ATTEMPTED F[OR ADD]

Imipramine. Imipramine has been adm[inistered to] children for "hyperactivity," enuresis, sc[hool phobia,] depression, and petit mal seizures. In the [group of] children who have symptoms of ADDH, [it has usu-]ally been found to be more effective than [placebo but] somewhat less effective than methylpheni[date. Its clini-]cal utility may be time-limited and may d[ecline after] eight to twelve weeks. Imipramine has b[een found to] enhance performance on cognitive tests [such as the] Continuous Performance Test (CPT) by [shortening re-]sponse latency and diminishing errors. It[s effect on per-]formance on other measures of visu[al attention] (Matching Familiar Figures Test), sho[rt-term mem-]ory, and perceptual-motor tasks.

The major side effects of imipramine a[re seda-]tion, constipation, anorexia, and increa[sed] blood pressure. At high doses, elec[trocardiogram] (EKG) changes occur consisting of inc[reased PR in-]terval; imipramine toxicity may be assoc[iated with pro-]longed QRS interval, arrhythmias, and [reduced car-]diac contractility. EKG monitoring sh[ould be done] on a regular basis during imipramine t[reatment.]

In 1975, Quinn and Rapoport[87] re[ported imipra-]mine useful in treatment of children wi[th attentional/]behavioral problems. Huessy and Wrigh[t reported 80] percent improvement rate in a group [of hyperactive] children treated with an average dose o[f imipramine.] berg and associates[117] compared impr[amine with dex-]troamphetamine in a group of hyperkin[etic/impulsive] children and noted a preferential respo[nse to dexam-]pramine (69 vs. 44 percent for meth[ylphenidate). A] comparison of methylphenidate, d-am[phetamine, and] imipramine in children with "minima[l brain dysfunc-]tion" suggested that some children re[spond prefer-]entially to each treatment.[50] Imipra[mine was found] better than placebo in nineteen chil[dren for symp-]toms of hyperactivity, defiance, impa[tience, aggression,] and inattentiveness.[106] The response [rate for hy-]peractive children who were previous[ly...]

in a small classroom with few distractions may help improve ADDH children's academic skills, modulate their impulses, and sustain more consistent and intimate interpersonal relationships.

Family Psychotherapy. The family may need psychotherapy or counseling to help determine their behavioral expectations for their child. Parents need to rapidly, appropriately, and consistently provide consequences to their ADDH child's behavior and to avoid scapegoating, inappropriate punishment, or indulgence of their impulsive child. They often need assistance in managing their guilt and embarrassment at having a difficult child. It is easy for parents to become outraged at the child's "irresponsibility," "forgetfulness," "indifference," and imperviousness to parental authority and sanctions. Parents complain of feeling helpless, misunderstood, and isolated. They easily become furious and blame each other for being "too strict" or "too permissive." Such experiences exaggerate preexisting parental conflicts or intensify parents' intolerance of personality characteristics that they also see within themselves. Both processes may require therapeutic intervention.

BEHAVIOR MODIFICATION

Techniques of behavior modification or shaping have been developed for use at home and in the classroom. The underlying principles emphasize establishing clearly defined, limited goals reflecting specific behaviors to praise, punish, or ignore. Parent, teachers, and therapists must identify rewards that will motivate a specific child and develop a schedule of reinforcement to sustain performance on selected tasks. Behaviors to be encouraged should be specifically defined in positive terms. Baseline charting of the frequency and the severity of these behaviors should be performed prior to intervention. Behavior-shaping techniques are often very useful in children with ADDH if applied consistently. Difficulty of generalization from one setting to another and in sustaining the progress after the reinforcements are discontinued may limit their effectiveness.[81]

COGNITIVE TRAINING

A related psychotherapeutic method relies predominantly on teaching *self-monitoring and self-control* and altering internal self-messages. This treatment is an outgrowth of techniques of cognitive therapy. The essential intervention consists of teaching children to identify disruptive behaviors such as fidgetiness, talking out of turn, getting out of seat, using defiant or provocative speech, or teasing—behaviors to which these children are often oblivious, though they are ob-

vious to outside observers. Children are encouraged to label these actions, identify their antecedents, and tell themselves to inhibit them before they are acted out. Children who are learning not to talk in class until called on may be taught to notice when they feels like talking without raising their hand, and then to tell themselves, "I have to wait until I'm called on" or "Don't talk till teacher gives the okay." Children may also learn to substitute less disruptive behaviors: "I want to tap my pencil, but I'll write notes instead."[17]

MEDICATION

Effects of Stimulant Medications. Stimulants such as methylphenidate, amphetamine, and magnesium pemoline are useful in reducing the motor hyperactivity that frequently accompanies ADD; they narrow the spectrum of attention and reduce impulsivity, thus diminishing distractibility in class and improving persistence in vigilance and memory or associated learning tasks. Stimulants frequently improve behavior and ease social interaction at home and school. Many ADD children will experience an increased sense of control and mastery on medication. Diagnosis of underlying psychosis, multiple tics, and major side effects to stimulants in the past are contraindications to stimulant medication.[77]

Behavioral Monitoring. Prior to the initiation of medication, parents and teachers should be asked to complete a behavior rating scale, such as the Conners' Teachers' twenty-eight-item scale; such scales are useful in monitoring the effects of medication. These should be repeated on a weekly basis during initial treatment and monthly thereafter. Teachers should note class size, subject, and time of day. A systematic parent diary may add to the clinical assessment.

Dosage. Initial choice of medication is frequently methylphenidate at doses of approximately 0.1 to 0.2 mg per kg given before school. Medication dosage can gradually be increased toward a maximum of about 0.5 to 0.75 mg per kg, which may be given in divided doses, about 8:00 A.M. and noon. Eating meals before medication does not impair absorption of the medication. Weekly monitoring and rating of behavior by teacher and parents will assist in determining the optimal dose.

It is not yet certain whether the dosage required to produce optimal improvement in attention may be less than that needed to achieve maximal behavioral control. In a child with primarily attentional learning difficulties, a low dose (10–20 mg daily) may yield the best cognitive improvement, although some restlessness may remain.

Children can often learn to participate in the regulation of their medication by anticipating the demands of the next four hours and altering the dosage appropriately. While medication may be needed to sustain attention and quietness in a classroom, it may not be needed during free play or recreational activities. Medication is usually needed less consistently during the summer, allowing partial medication holidays. Except in severe cases, summer holidays are advisable and allow reassessment for continued treatment. Many ADD children can begin the academic year with a trial off medication or be tapered after initial adjustment to a new classroom. The empirical trial provides assessment of continued need for stimulants. In some ADD children, medication can be withdrawn before puberty; others require continued treatment into adolescence.

RESPONSE TO STIMULANTS

Considerable research suggests that medication alone does not improve academic grades or classroom learning. Stimulants do not always improve the scholastic performance of children with learning disabilities. Even in children with ADDH, behavioral and educational improvements do not always cooccur. While stimulants reduce motor behavior and improve reaction time, sustained vigilance, and recall of simple stimuli, they do not necessarily enhance the other processes of learning: identification of relevant concepts, reorganization, and encoding for appropriate conceptual retrieval. Short-term improvement does not always enhance long-term outcome. Improvement in cognitive laboratory measures does not always correlate with improved classroom learning. In one study following twelve weeks of flexible dose treatment with methylphenidate or thioridazine, few correlations were noted between classroom progress in academic areas and changes on behavioral or achievement ratings. Improvement in psychological test scores did not appear to correlate with each other, and improvement across behavioral ratings and psychological testing were generally unrelated.[43]

Stimulant medications have social effects: They decrease number of negative behaviors of the child, reduce the frequency of teachers' reprimands, and improve handwriting.[114] Charles and Schain,[21] in a four-year follow-up, reported that stimulants administered to ADDH children resulted in lessening of hyperactivity, but academic underachievement remained a greater problem than behavioral and social difficulties. The duration of treatment did not correlate with clinical improvement. Methylphenidate treatment improves both ADD children's behavior in class and the quality of their interaction with their teacher, and reduces their level of intensity and control.[115]

MULTIMODAL TREATMENT

The effectiveness of multimodal treatment was evident in the three-year prospective study by Satterfield, Cantwell, and Satterfield.[93] They utilized a combination of clinically optimal dose of methylphenidate with special education, tutoring, and family or individual psychotherapy as indicated. In an initial cohort of about one hundred carefully diagnosed ADDH children who were treated and monitored, this multimodal treatment produced both behavioral and academic improvement in those children who continued in treatment.

Several studies demonstrate an additive effect of combined interventions: medication, special education, and psychotherapy. Coupled with psychotherapy and special education, stimulants may improve academic adjustment and performance.[93] However, unless accompanied by appropriate psychotherapy, family counseling, or focused educational intervention, medications alone usually do not lead to improved academic learning, higher grades, or increase in achievement scores.[43,87] In kindergarten-age hyperactive children there was no difference between behavior modification and methylphenidate treatment.[26] Methylphenidate was more effective than behavioral self-control for children with ADDH.[7] Studies of the effectiveness of combined medication and behavioral modification suggest an additive effect of both interventions. Medication often has the most powerful short-term effect, but when used alone it does not enhance long-term development.[43]

While stimulants are usually beneficial for children with the combined behavioral and cognitive difficulties of ADDH, they are not useful in children with pure LDS uncomplicated by hyperactivity.[42] However, methylphenidate facilitated the performance of both hyperactive and nonhyperactive children on a visual search task with a short-term memory component, even at a high dose (1.25 mg/kg/d).[34]

SIDE EFFECTS OF STIMULANTS

Stimulant medications have multiple side effects and some specific contraindications. Transient side effects include anorexia, insomnia, stomachaches, afternoon withdrawal, and explosiveness.[19] Long-term side effects of stimulants may include growth suppression,[49,79] although this may be transient and depend on the dose and duration of medication. While stimulants have been reported to induce tics,[45,77] untreated ADDH children appear to be at increased endogenous risk for tics.[31] Hallucinosis and possible psychosis may follow stimulant treatment in vulnerable children.[119] Compliance with methylphenidate treatment is frequently low.[38,73,98] Weekend and summer drug holidays may diminish concern about possible growth suppression. On stimulant medication, children may become more "rigid," irritable, and tense. In children with atypical development, childhood psychosis, and multiple tic syndrome, stimulants may lead to dramatic exacerbation of symptomatology. Since these children initially often have attentional problems and hyperactivity, physicians may mistakenly increase the medication rather than recognizing that the symptomatic exacerbation is a medication side effect.

PHARMACOKINETICS OF STIMULANTS

Approximately 200,000 to 400,000 children in the United States receive stimulant medication for attentional and behavioral control. Blood-level determination may have therapeutic utility in identifying children who absorb methylphenidate poorly or excrete it rapidly and thereby fail to achieve adequate levels.

Shaywitz and associates[96] reported that following a single oral dose of methylphenidate, the peak level was reached at 2.5 hours ($\pm$ 20 minutes). The peak blood levels achieved demonstrated a nearly threefold range across individuals receiving similar methylphenidate doses, but were highly replicable within individuals. The excretion half-life ($t^{1/2}$) of methylphenidate was $2.5 \pm .5$ hours. These results are compatible with other pharmacological studies of methylphenidate.[52,62,76] Eating prior to taking methylphenidate does not affect absorption.[20]

Substantial blood levels of methylphenidate persist for up to eight hours, although the clinical effect diminishes. This lack of a simple correlation between blood level and clinical effect probably reflects methylphenidate's release of stored catecholamines.

The two-hour blood levels of methylphenidate during chronic treatment were comparable to the levels obtained following an acute single dose of the drug. When the blood levels of these therapeutically treated children were compared to their behavioral improvement (Conners's Abbreviated Parent Teacher Behavior Rating Scale), those whose behavior ratings most improved during treatment had significantly higher two-hour methylphenidate blood levels. A minimum level of 7 ng per ml may be needed for behavioral response; however, some forms of learning may be impaired at higher doses in some children.[99,*] A linear dose-response relationship was found with performance on a cognitive task by Winsberg and associates.[118]

A similar pharmacokinetic profile was noted in studies of d-amphetamine.[23,35] Following a single dose of about 0.5 mg per kg, peak d-amphetamine concentra-

*J. Swanson, personal communication, 1985.

tions occurred after four hours. The elimination half-life ($t^{1/2}$) was about 6.8 ± 0.5 hours. Behavioral improvement, rated on the Conners' abbreviated ten-item scale, was significant from one to four hours after medication. Retest of six children with the same d-amphetamine dose showed no significant difference in absorption or elimination one week later.[14]

Thus blood levels may provide information about some children who are poor responders and may reflect variability in absorption, binding, or excretion. Two-hour blood levels may be clinically useful in children who do not respond, who have excessive side effects, or who suddenly require a major change in dose.

OTHER TREATMENTS ATTEMPTED FOR ADDH

Imipramine. Imipramine has been administered to children for "hyperactivity," enuresis, school phobia, depression, and petit mal seizures. In the treatment of children who have symptoms of ADDH, it has generally been found to be more effective than placebo but somewhat less effective than methylphenidate. Its clinical utility may be time-limited and may diminish after eight to twelve weeks. Imipramine has been found to enhance performance on cognitive tests including the Continuous Performance Test (CPT) by increasing response latency and diminishing errors. It improves performance on other measures of visual searching (Matching Familiar Figures Test), short-term memory, and perceptual-motor tasks.

The major side effects of imipramine consist of sedation, constipation, anorexia, and increased pulse and blood pressure. At high doses, electrocardiogram (EKG) changes occur consisting of increased P-R interval; imipramine toxicity may be associated with prolonged QRS interval, arrhythmias, and decreased cardiac contractility. EKG monitoring should continue on a regular basis during imipramine treatment.

In 1975, Quinn and Rapoport[87] reported imipramine useful in treatment of children with learning and behavioral problems. Huessy and Wright[61] found a 67 percent improvement rate in a group of hyperactive children treated with an average dose of 50 mg. Winsberg and associates[117] compared imipramine and dextroamphetamine in a group of hyperkinetic, aggressive children and noted a preferential response rate to imipramine (69 vs. 44 percent for methylphenidate). A comparison of methylphenidate, d-amphetamine, and imipramine in children with "minimal brain dysfunction" suggested that some children responded preferentially to each treatment.[50] Imipramine was found better than placebo in nineteen children with symptoms of hyperactivity, defiance, impaired sociability, and inattentiveness.[106] The response of fifty-eight hyperactive children who were previously good responders to methylphenidate suggested a preference for that medication,[48] whereas Gittelman-Klein[43] reported nearly similar efficacy of imipramine and methylphenidate. Quinn and associates[88] treated seventy-six hyperactive children with 80 mg per day of either medication for ten weeks and noted preferential cognitive response to methylphenidate. Werry, Aman, and Diamond[113] treated thirty ADDH children in a crossover design with methylphenidate (0–4 mg/d) and imipramine (1–2 mg/kg/d) for four weeks at each dose. Both medications produced clinical improvement and facilitated performance on the Continuous Performance Task and the Porteus Maze. Huessy[60] has reported a rapid response to imipramine with minimal side effects in ADDH.

Clonidine. Recent studies of the noradrenergic agonist clonidine, in children with ADDH suggested its therapeutic usefulness may parallel results in subjects with Tourette's disorder. In a twelve-week, double-blind, placebo-crossover study, Hunt, Minderaa, and Cohen[67] found that clonidine has possible therapeutic utility in ADDH when compared to placebo. Parents' ratings on the Conners' scale showed that eight of the ten children clearly benefitted from clonidine. The mean behavior ratings for the group improved significantly by the end of active clonidine treatment ($p = 0.002$). Teachers' ratings also showed significant improvement on the hyperactivity index and on the total rating ($p = 0.01$). Children were not sedated or psychomotorically retarded; the initial sleepiness diminished after two weeks of treatment. While clonidine may be a useful alternative therapeutic agent for some children with ADDH, its relative effectiveness compared to methylphenidate on behavioral and cognitive measures requires further study.

Other medications that have been tried in ADDH include levodopa, lithium, carbama zepine, amitriptyline, thioridazine, haloperidol, chlorpromazine, and monoamine oxidase inhibitors. There is a need to further differentiate both the behavioral and cognitive effects of these medications to clarify their specific role and indications.

Diet. Diets restrictive of food additives, coloring, and sugar have been popular since Feingold's work[36] suggested that many ADDH children had a nonimmunological supersensitivity to these substances. Although parental testimony has frequently supported this claim of clinical benefit from avoidance diets, controlled studies have not supported their effectiveness. The National Institutes of Health consensus[83] found the diets to be safe but not usually helpful. These diets require considerable organization on the part of the family and self-control and cooperation of the part of the child. In total, controlled studies of dietary interventions suggest minimal sustained therapeutic utility.

Whether the offending dietary ingredient is a form of sugar or a food dye or additive has been widely debated, as well as whether these ADDH children have a specific allergic or toxic response.[37,41,86,112]

Conners and associates[29] found small differences in parents and teachers ratings in a few subjects following a challenge versus a control diet. Williams and coworkers[116] found no effect of color-containing diets in contrast to considerable benefit from medication. Administration of artificial coloring and flavoring to twenty-two children selected for parents' report of response to the Feingold diet showed only two whose parental ratings demonstrated behavioral worsening.[109] However, following large doses of added food coloring versus placebo, diminished attention span and increased errors in learning were evident on the paired associate learning task.[101] Harley, Matthews, and Lichman[54] found that parents and teachers could not distinguish periods of additive-free versus routine diet in behavioral ratings of children who had been reported to be diet-sensitive. Similarly, control and additive-free diets had no measurable effect on retarded individuals observed in a residential setting.[55] When administered to normal, nonhyperactive children, the Feingold diet diminished fidgetiness, distractibility, and noise making in a small subset of the children, but adequate dietary controls were lacking.[58]

Although hypoglycemia has been postulated to cause symptoms of ADDH, subjective symptoms of light-headedness, diaphoresis, shakiness, and weakness did not correlate with the absolute level or rate of fall of blood sugar level in 192 adults receiving a five-hour glucose tolerance test.[72] Therapies based on optometric training, vestibular stimulation, and patterning or "neurological retraining" have no objectively demonstrated efficacy.[46]

Summary

Attention deficit disorder with hyperactivity is a serious disorder of childhood. Its impact on adjustment is profound and often persists into adulthood. ADDH and its frequently associated conditions, learning disability and conduct disorder, often resist efforts at amelioration and continue for many years to underlie increased vulnerability to a variety of adult dysfunctions, including substance abuse and occupational and marital instability. These conditions merit the most serious kind of consideration from the clinician. They challenge child psychiatrists to exercise to the fullest all their professional skills, including diagnosis and assessment, case management and consultation, psycho-pharmacology, and individual and family intervention. Particularly important is the need to monitor progress over an extended period of time. While improvement may occur with psychotropic medication, the patient may remain vulnerable to successive developmental stresses and require continued treatment for these and for specific subsequent difficulties.

ACKNOWLEDGMENTS

Dr. Hunt's research is supported by a grant from the MacArthur Foundation and the Mental Health Clinical Research Center. The authors gratefully acknowledge the assistance of Cathy Radmer, Research Assistant, with editing and preparation of this manuscript.

REFERENCES

1. ACHENBACH, T. M. "The Child Behavior Profile: I. Boys Aged 6–11," *Journal of Consulting and Clinical Psychology,* 46 (1978):478–488.
2. ———. *Research in Developmental Psychology.* New York: Free Press, 1978.
3. ———. "The Child Behavior Profile: An Empirically Based System for Assessing Children's Behavioral Problems and Competencies," *International Journal of Mental Health,* 7 (1979):24–42.
4. ADAMS, R. M., KOESIS, J. J., and ESTES, R. E. "Soft Neurological Signs in Learning Disabled Children and Controls," *Journal of Diseases of Childhood,* 12 (1974):614–618.
5. AMERICAN PSYCHOLOGICAL ASSOCIATION. *Standards for Educational and Psychological Tests,* 3rd ed. Washington, D.C.: American Psychological Association, 1974.
6. ANASTASI, A. *Psychological Testing,* 4th ed. New York: Macmillan, 1976.
7. ANDERSON, E. E., CLEMENT, P. W., and OETTINGER, L., Jr. "Methylphenidate Compared with Behavioral Self-control in Attention Deficit Disorder: Preliminary Report," *Journal of Developments in Biological Psychiatry,* (1981):137–141.
8. AULT, R., CRAWFORD, D., and JEFFREY, W. "Visual Scanning Strategies of Reflective, Impulsive, Fast-accurate, and Slow-inaccurate Children on the Matching Familiar Figures Test," *Child Development,* 43 (1972):1412.
9. BARKLEY, R. A. *Hyperactive Children: A Handbook for Diagnosis and Treatment.* New York: Guilford Press, 1981.
10. BEERY, K. E., and BUKTENICA, N. *Developmental Test of Visual-Motor Integration.* Chicago: Follett, 1967.
11. BENDER, L. *A Visual Gestalt Test and Its Clinical Use.* New York: American Orthopsychiatric Association Research Monograph, no. 3., 1938.
12. ———. *Psychopathology of Children with Organic Brain Damage.* Springfield, Ill: Charles C Thomas, 1956
13. BOEHM, A. E. *Boehm Test of Basic Concepts Manual.* New York: Psychological Corporation, 1971.
14. BROWN, G. L., et al. *Clinical Pharmacology of d-amphetamine in Hyperactive Children.* New York: Spectrum Publications, 1979.
15. BUROS, O. K., ed. *The Seventh Mental Measurements Yearbook.* Highland Park, N.J.: Gryphon Press, 1972.
16. BUSH, W. J., and WAUGH, K. W. *Diagnosing Learning Abilities.* Columbus, Oh.: Merrill, 1976.
17. CAMERON, M. I., and ROBINSON, V. M. "Effects of Cognitive Training on Academic and On-task Behavior of Hyperactive Children," *Journal of Abnormal Child Psychology,* 8 (1980):405–419.
18. CAMPBELL, S. B., DOUGLAS, V. I., and MORGENST-ERN, G. "Cognitive Styles in Hyperactive Children and the Effect of Methylphenidate," *Journal of Child Psychology and Psychiatry,* 12 (1971):55–57.
19. CANTWELL, D. P. *The Hyperactive Child: Diagnosis, Management, and Current Research.* New York: Spectrum Publications, 1975.
20. CHAN, A. U., et al. "Methylphenidate Hydrochloride Given with or Before Breakfast: II. Effects on Plasma Concentration of Methylphenidate and Ritalinic Acid," *Pediatrics,* 72 (1983):56–59.
21. CHARLES, L., and SCHAIN, R. "A four-Year Follow-up Study of the Effects of Methylphenidate on the Behavior and Academic Achievement of Hyperactive Children," *Journal of Abnormal Child Psychology,* 9 (1981):495–505.
22. CHARLES, L., SCHAIN, R., and ZELNICKER, T. "Optimal Dosages of Methylphenidate for Improving the Learning and Behavior of Hyperactive Children," *Journal of Developments in Biological Psychiatry,* 2 (1981):78–81.
23. CHENG, L. T., et al. "Amphetamine: New Radio-immunoassay," *FEBS Letters,* 36 (1973):339–342.
24. COHEN, D. J., and DOUGLAS, V. I. "The Effect of Methylphenidate on Attentive Behavior and Autonomic Activity in Hyperactive Children," *Psychopharmacologia,* 22 (1971):282–294.
25. ———. "Characteristics of the Orienting Response in Hyperactive and Normal Children," *Psychophysiology,* 9 (1972):238–245.
26. COHEN, N. J., et al. "Evaluation of the Relative Effectiveness of Methylphenidate and Cognitive Behavior Modification in the Treatment of Kindergarten-aged Hyperactive Children," *Journal of Abnormal Child Psychology,* 9 (1981):43–54.
27. CONNERS, C. K. "A Teacher Rating Scale for Use in Drug Studies with Children," *American Journal of Psychiatry,* 126 (1969):152–156.
28. ———. *Food Additives and Hyperactive Children.* New York: Plenum Press, 1980.
29. CONNERS, C. K., et al. "Food Additives and Hyperkinesis: A Controlled Double-blind Experiment," *Pediatrics,* 58 (1976):154–166.
30. COSTELLO, A. J., et al. "Report of the NIMH Diagnostic Interview Schedule for Children (DISC)," 1984 (manuscript).
31. DENCKLA, M. B., et al. "Motor Proficiency in Dyslexic Children With and Without Attention Disorders," *Archives of Neurology,* 42 (1985):228–231.
32. DOLL, E. "Measurement of Social Competence," in *Manual for the Vinland Social Maturity Scale.* Princeton, N.J.: Educational Testing Service, 1953.

33. DUNN, L. M., and MARKWARDT, F. C. *Peabody Individual Achievement Test.* Circle Pines, Minn.: American Guidance Service, 1970.

34. DYKMAN, R. A., ACKERMAN, P. T., and MCCRAY, D. S. "Effects of Methylphenidate on Selective and Sustained Attention in Hyperactive, Reading-disabled and Presumably Attention-disordered boys," *Journal of Nervous and Mental Disease,* 168 (1980):745–752.

35. EBERT, M. H., VAN KAMMEN, D. P., and MURPHY, D. L. "Plasma Levels of Amphetamine and Behavioral Response," in L. A. Gottschalk and S. Merlis, eds., *Pharmacokinetics of Psychoactive Drugs: Blood Levels and Clinical Response.* New York: Spectrum Publications, 1976, pp. 157–169.

36. FEINGOLD, B. *Why Your Child Is Hyperactive.* New York: Random House, 1975.

37. FERGUSON, H. B., RAPOPORT, J. L., and WEINGARTNER, H. "Food Dyes and Impairment of Performance in Hyperactive Children (Letter)," *Science,* 211 (1981):410–411.

38. FIRESTONE, P. "Factors Associated with Children's Adherence to Stimulant Medication," *American Journal of Orthopsychiatry,* 52 (1982):47–57.

39. FREEMAN, D. F., and CORNWALL, T. P. "Hyperactivity and Neurosis," *American Journal of Orthopsychiatry,* 50 (1980):704–711.

40. GARDNER, R. A. "The Objective Diagnosis of Minimal Brain Dysfunction," Summit, N.J.: Creative Therapeutics, 1979.

41. GARFINKEL, B. D., WEBSTER, C. D., and SLOMAN, L. "Responses to Methylphenidate and Varied Doses of Caffeine in Children with Attention Deficit Disorder," *Canadian Journal of Psychiatry,* 26 (1981):395–401.

42. GITTELMAN, R. "The Role of Psychological Tests for Differential Diagnosis in Child Psychiatry," *Journal of Child Psychiatry,* 19 (1980):413–438.

43. GITTELMAN-KLEIN, R., and KLEIN, D. F. "Methylphenidate Effects in Learning Disabilities: Psychometric Changes," *Archives of General Psychiatry,* 33 (1976):655–664.

44. GLASSER, A. J., and ZIMMERMAN, I. L. *Clinical Interpretation of the Wechsler Intelligence Scale for Children.* New York: Grune & Stratton, 1967.

45. GOLDEN, G. S. "Gilles de la Tourette's Syndrome Following Methylphenidate Administration," *Developmental Medicine and Child Neurology,* 16 (1974):76–78.

46. ———. "Neurobiological Correlates of Learning Disabilities," *Annals of Neurology,* 12 (1982):409–418.

47. GOYETTE, C. H., CONNERS, C. K., and ULRICH, R. F. "Normative Data on Revised Conners Parents and Teacher Rating Scales," *Journal of Abnormal Child Psychology,* 6 (1978):221–236.

48. GREENBERG, L. M., et al. "Clinical Effects of Imipramine and Methylphenidate in Hyperactive Children," in C. K. Conners, ed., *Clinical Effects of Stimulants in Children.* The Hague: Excerpta Medica, 1974, p. 144.

49. GREENHILL, L. L., et al. "Growth Disturbances in Hyperkinetic Children (Letter)," *Pediatrics,* 66 (1980): 152–154.

50. GROSS, M. D. "Imipramine in the Treatment of Minimal Brain Dysfunction in Children," *Psychosomatics,* 14 (1973):283.

51. GUALTIERI, C. T. "Imipramine and Children: A Review and Some Speculations About the Mechanism of Drug Action," *Diseases of the Nervous System,* 38 (1977): 368–375.

52. GUALTIERI, C. T., et al. "Clinical Studies of Methylphenidate Serum Levels in Children and Adults," *Journal of the American Academy of Child Psychiatry,* 21 (1982):19–26.

53. HAMMOND D. *Detroit Tests of Learning Aptitude.* Austin, Tx.: Pro-Ed Press, 1985.

54. HARLEY, J. P., MATTHEWS, C. G., and EICHMAN, P. L. "Synthetic Food Colors and Hyperactivity in Children: A Double-blind Challenge Experiment," *Pediatrics,* 61 (1978): 975–983.

55. HARNER, I. C., and FOILES, R. A. "Effects of Feingold's K-P Diet on a Residential Mentally Handicapped Population," *Journal of the American Dietetic Association,* 6 (1980): 55–58.

56. HARRIS, D. *Children's Drawing as Measures of Intellectual Maturity.* New York: Harcourt Brace Jovanovich, 1963.

57. HESSLER, G. L. "Use and Interpretation of the Woodcock-Johnson Psycho-Educational Battery," in F. Nudren, ed., *Teaching Resources.* New York: New York Times Press, 1977, pp. 1–384.

58. HOLBORO, P. L. "Ascorbic Acid, Dietary Restrictions, and Upper Respiratory Infection" (letter), *Pediatrics,* 65 (1981):1191–1192.

59. HOLDEN, E. W., TARNOWSKI, K. J., and PRINZ, R. J. "Reliability of Neurological Soft Signs in Children: Reevaluation of the PANESS," *Journal of Abnormal Child Psychology,* 10 (1982):163–172.

60. HUESSY, H. R. "Imipramine for Attention Deficit Disorder," *American Journal of Psychiatry,* 140 (1983):272.

61. HUESSY, H. R., and WRIGHT, A. "The Use of Imipramine in Children's Behavior Disorders," *Acta Paedopsychiatrica,* 37 (1970):194.

62. HUNGUND, B. L., et al. "Pharmacokinetics of Methylphenidate in Hyperkinetic Children," *British Journal of Clinical Pharmacology,* 8 (1979):571–576.

63. HUNT, R. D. "Attention Deficit Disorder: Diagnosis, Assessment and Treatment," in E. Kestenbaum and D. Williams, eds., *Clinical Assessment of Children and Adolescents—A Biopsychosocial Approach.* New York: New York University Press, forthcoming.

64. HUNT, R. D., and COHEN, D. J. "Recognizing Psychiatric Problems in Early and Middle Childhood," in H. Leigh, ed., *Psychiatric Problems in Primary Practice.* Menlo Park, Calif.: Addison-Wesley, 1983, pp. 399–467.

65. HUNT, R. D., ANDERSON, G. A., and COHEN, D. J. "Noradrenergic Mechanisms in Attention Deficit Disorder and Hyperactivity," in L. Bloomingdale, ed., *Attention Deficit Disorder and Hyperactivity,* vol. 3. New York: Spectrum Publications, forthcoming.

66. HUNT, R. D., MINDERAA, R. B., and COHEN, D. J. "Clonidine Benefits Children with Attention Deficit Disorder and Hyperactivity: Report of a Double-blind Placebo-crossover Therapeutic Trial," *Journal of the American Academy of Child Psychiatry,* 24 (1985): 617–629.

67. HUNT, R. D., MINDERAA, R. B., and COHEN, D. J. "Clonidine's Effect in Children with Attention Deficit Disorder: Report of a Double-Blind Placebo-Crossover Trial and Summary of Clinical Experience," *Psychopharmacology Bulletin,* in press.

68. HUNT, R. D., et al. "Possible Change in Noradrenergic Receptor Sensitivity Following Methylphenidate Treatment: Growth Hormone and MHPG Response to Clonidine Challenge in Children with Attention Deficit Disorder and Hyperactivity," *Life Sciences,* 35 (1984):885–897.

69. HUNT, R. D., et al. "Strategies for the Study of Neurochemical Aspects of Cognitive Dysfunction: Their Application in Attention Deficit Disorder," in submission.

70. JASTAK, J. F., and JASTAK, S. R. *The Wide Range Achievement Test* (manual). Wilmington, Del.: Guidance Associates, 1965

71. JOHNSTON, M. V., and SINGER, H. S. "Brain Neuro-

transmitters and Neuromodulators in Pediatrics," *Pediatrics,* 70 (1982):576–569.

72. KAUFMAN, A. S., and HOLLENBECK, G. P. "Factor Analysis of the Standardized Edition of the McCarthy Scales," *Journal of Clinical Psychology,* 29 (1973):358–362.

73. KAUFFMAN, R. E., et al. "Medication Compliance in Hyperactive Children," *Pediatric Pharmacology,* 1 (1981):- 2317.

74. KIRK, S. A., and KIRK, W. D. *Psycholinguistic Learning Disabilities: Diagnosis and Limitations.* Urbana, Ill.: University of Illinois Press, 1971.

75. KOPPITZ, E. *Human Figures Drawing Test.* New York: Grune & Stratton, 1968.

76. KUPIETZ, S. S., WINSBERG, B. G., and SVERD, J. "Learning Ability and Methylphenidate (Ritalin) Plasma Concentration in Hyperkinetic Children. A Preliminary Investigation," *Journal of the American Academy of Child Psychiatry,* 21 (1982):27–30.

77. LOWE, T. L., et al. "Stimulant Medications Precipitate Tourette's Syndrome," *Journal of the American Medical Association,* 247 (1982):1729–1731.

78. MCCARTHY, D. *McCarthy Scales of Children's Abilities.* New York: Psychological Corporation, 1972.

79. MILLICHAP, J. G. "Growth of Hyperactive Children Treated with Methylphenidate," *Journal of Learning Disorders,* 11 (1978):567–570.

80. MINN, L. "Perceptual Training: Misdirections and Redirections," *American Journal of Orthopsychiatry,* 40, (1970):30–38.

81. MURRAY, M. E. "Behavioral Management of the Hyperactive Child," *Journal of Developments in Biological Psychiatry,* 1 (1980):108–111.

82. NAGEL-HEIMKE, M., et al. "The Influence of Methylphenidate on the Sympathoadrenal Reactivity in Children Diagnosed as Hyperactive," *Klinik Paediatrica,* 196 (1984):- 78–82.

83. "National Institutes of Health Consensus Development Conference Statement: Defined Diets and Childhood Hyperactivity," *American Journal of Clinical Nutrition,* 37 (1983):- 161–165.

84. ORVASCHEL, H. "Psychiatric Interviews Suitable for Use Research with Children and Adolescents," in J. Rapoport, C. K. Conners, and N. Reatig, eds., *Psychopharmacology Bulletin,* 21 (1985):737–747.

85. ORVASCHEL, H., et al. "Retrospective Assessment of Child Psychopathology with the Kiddie-SADS-E," *Journal of the American Academy of Child Psychiatry,* 21 (1982):392– 397.

86. O'SHEA, J. A., and PORTER, S. F. "Double-blind Study of Children with Hyperkinetic Syndrome Treated with Multiallergen Extract Sublingually," *Journal of Learning Disabilities,* 14 (1981):189–191.

87. QUINN, P. O., and RAPOPORT, J. L. "One-year Follow-up of Hyperactive Boys Treated with Imipramine and Methylphenidate," *American Journal of Psychiatry,* 132 (1975):- 241–245.

88. QUINN, P. O., et al. "Imipramine and Methylphenidate Treatments in Hyperactive Boys: A Double-blind Comparison," *Archives of General Psychiatry,* 30 (1974):789–793.

89. RABIN, A. J. "Diagnostic Use of Intelligence Tests," in B. B. Wolman, ed., *Handbook of Clinical Psychology.* New York: McGraw-Hill, 1965.

90. RAPOPORT, J. L., et al. "Dextroamphetamine: Its Cognitive and Behavioral Effects in Normal and Hyperactive Boys and Normal Men," *Archives of General Psychiatry,* 37 (1980):933–943.

91. REICH, W., et al. "Development of a Structured Psychi-

atric Interview for Children: Agreement on Diagnosis Comparing Child and Parent Interviews," *Journal of Abnormal Child Psychology,* 10 (1982):325–336.

92. ROACH, E. F., and KEPHART, N. C. *The Purdue Perceptual Motor Learning Task.* Columbus, Oh.: Merrill, 1966.

93. SATTERFIELD, J. H., CANTWELL, D. P., and SATTERFIELD, B. T. "Multimodality Treatment: A One-year Follow-up of 84 Hyperactive Boys," *Archives of General Psychiatry,* 36 (1979):965–974.

94. SATTERFIELD, J. H., SCHELL, A. M., and BARB, S. D. "Potential Risk of Prolonged Administration of Stimulant Medication for Hyperactive Children," *Journal of Developments—Biological Psychiatry,* 1 (1980):102–107.

95. SHAYWITZ, S. E. "The Yale Neuropsycho-educational Scales," *Schizophrenia Bulletin,* 8 (1982):360–424.

96. SHAYWITZ, S. E., et al. "Psychopharmacology of Attention Deficit Disorder: Pharmacokinetic, Neuroendocrine, and Behavioral Measures Following Acute and Chronic Treatment with Methylphenidate," *Pediatrics,* 69 (1982):- 688–694.

97. SHEN, Y. C., and WANG, Y. F. "Urinary 3-methoxy-4-hydroxyphenylglycolsulfate Excretion in 73 Schoolchildren with Minimal Brain Dysfunction Syndrome," *Biological Psychiatry,* 19 (1984):861–870.

98. SLEATOR, E. K., ULLMAN, R. K., and VON NEUMANN, A. "How Do Hyperactive Children Feel About Taking Stimulants and Will They Tell the Doctor?" *Clinical Pediatrics,* 21 (1982):474–479.

99. SPRAGUE, R. L., and SLEATOR, E. K. "Methylphenidate in Hyperactive Children: Differences in Dose Effects on Learning and Social Behavior," *Science,* 198 (1977):1274– 1276.

100. STERNBERG, L., EPSTEIN, M. H., and ADAMS, D. "Performance Characteristics of Retarded and Normal Students on Pattern Recognition Tasks," *Contemporary Educational Psychology,* 2 (1977):209–218.

101. SWANSON, J., and KINSBOURNE, M. "Stimulant-related State-dependent Learning in Hyperactive Children," *Science,* 192 (1976):1254–1256.

102. SYKES, D. H., DOUGLAS, V. I., and MORGENSTERN, G. "The Effect of Methylphenidate (Ritalin) on Sustained Attention in Hyperactive Children," *Psychopharmacologia,* 25 (1972):262–274.

103. TERMAN, L. A., and MERRILL, M. *Stanford-Binet Intelligence Scale. 1972 Norms.* Boston: Houghton Mifflin, 1973.

104. TRITES, R. L., BLOUIN, A. G., and LAPRADE, K. "Factor Analysis of the Conners Teacher Rating Scale Based on a Large Normative Sample," *Journal of Consulting and Clinical Psychology,* 50 (1982):615–623.

105. URBAN, W. *Draw A Person,* Los Angeles: Western Psychological Services, 1963.

106. WAIZER, J., et al. "Outpatient Treatment of Hyperactive School Children with Imipramine," *American Journal of Psychiatry,* 131 (1974):587.

107. WALDROP, M., and HALVERSON, C. F. "Minor Physical Anomalies and Hyperactive Behavior in Young Children," in J. Hellmuth, ed., *Exceptional Infant,* vol. 11: *Studies of Abnormalities.* New York: Brunner/Mazel, 1971, pp. 343– 389.

108. WECHSLER, D. *Manual for the Wechsler Intelligence Scale for Children—Revised.* New York: Psychological Corporation, 1974.

109. WEISS, B. "Food Additives and Environmental Chemicals as Sources of Childhood Behavior Disorders," *Journal of the American Academy of Child Psychiatry,* 21 (1982):144–152.

110. WEISS, G. "Controversial Issues of the Pharmacotherapy of the Hyperactive Child," *Canadian Journal of Psychiatry,* 26 (1981):385–392.

111. WELNER, Z., et al. "Parent-Child Agreement, Reliability, and Validity Studies of the Diagnostic Interview for Children and Adolescents (DICA)," 1985 (manuscript).

112. WENDER, P. H. "New Evidence on Food Additives and Hyperkinesis: A Critical Analysis," *American Journal of Diseases of Children,* 134 (1980):1122–1125.

113. WERRY, J. S., AMAN, M. G., and DIAMOND, E. "Imipramine and Methylphenidate in Hyperactive Children," *Journal of Child Psychology and Psychiatry,* 21 (1980):27–35.

114. WHALEN, C. K., HENKER, B., and DOTEMOTO, S. "Teacher Response to the Methylphenidate (Ritalin) Versus Placebo Status of Hyperactive Boys in the Classroom," *Child Development,* 52 (1981):1005–1014.

115. WHALEN, C. K., HENKER, B., and FINCK, D., "Medication Effects in the Classroom: Three Naturalistic Indicators," *Journal of Abnormal Child Psychology,* 9 (1981):419–433.

116. WILLIAMS, J. I., et al. "Relative Effects of Drugs and Diet on Hyperactive Behaviors: An Experimental Study," *Pediatrics,* 61 (1978):811–817.

117. WINSBERG, B. G., et al. "Effects of Imipramine and Dextroamphetamine on Behavior of Neuropsychiatrically Impaired Children," *American Journal of Psychiatry,* 128 (1972):1425.

118. WINSBERG, B. G., et al. "Methylphenidate Oral Dose Plasma Concentrations and Behavioral Response in Children," *Psychopharmacology,* 76 (1982):329–332.

119. YOUNG, J. G. "Methylphenidate-induced Hallucinosis: Case Histories and Possible Mechanisms of Action," *Developmental and Behavioral Pediatrics,* 2 (1981):35–37.

120. ZAHN, T. P., RAPOPORT, J. L., and THOMPSON, C. L. "Autonomic and Behavioral Effects of Dextroamphetamine and Placebo in Normal and Hyperactive Prepubertal Boys," *Journal of Abnormal Child Psychology,* 8 (1980):145–60.

121. ZAHN, T. P., et al. "Minimal Brain Dysfunction, Stimulant Drugs, and Autonomic Nervous System Activity," *Archives of General Psychiatry,* 32 (1975):381–387.

56 / Learning Disabilities: Current Therapeutic Methods

Larry B. Silver and Richard W. Brunstetter

Introduction

This chapter reviews recent advances since the publication of the initial four volumes of the *Basic Handbook of Child Psychiatry.*[34,35] A basic definition and description of learning disability can be found in the Introduction section of chapter 38 in this volume.

Clinical interventions with children and adolescents who have LDs must be based on an assessment of the total person in his or her total environment. This concept is important for two reasons: (1) LDs are not just school disabilities; they can interfere with all aspects of psychosocial development, with peer interactions, and with family and out-of-school activities; and (2) there are related clinical disorders that are commonly present with such children and adolescents; if present, each must be diagnosed and treated.*

The Clinical Picture

As noted, the areas of specific LD are discussed in chapter 38 of this volume. Twenty-five to 40 percent of LD children will also be hyperactive and/or distract-

*The views expressed in this chapter are those of the authors and may not reflect those of the National Institute of Mental Health.

ible (DSM-III, Attention Deficit Disorder). Many will develop secondary emotional, social, and family problems.[36]

HYPERACTIVITY

It is presumed that the increased motor activity these children so commonly display is related to some form of central nervous system (CNS) dysfunction. It should be differentiated from anxiety-based increased motor activity. With the child who expresses his or her anxiety at least in part by an increase in motor activity, the behavior usually relates to a specific life-space experience. The history will convey that the hyperactivity began during the first grade, or that it happens only in school but not at home. With physiologically based hyperactivity, there is usually a pervasive history of such activity since birth. In some cases, a parent might even report that prior to birth the child kicked more than usual *in utero.* And ever since birth he or she squirmed in mother's arms, rolled in the crib, ran before walking, and has been in almost constant motion. The hyperactivity does not relate to any specific event; it is not limited to school hours; it occurs all the time and anyplace. There may be instances where this distinction between anxiety and neurophysiologically based increased motor behavior is difficult to delineate. Both may be present. Or the history and observations do not clarify the problems. An empirical trial on stimulant medication may be useful.

DISTRACTIBILITY

Some children with LDs have difficulty filtering out less relevant sensory inputs; thus most or all stimuli reach the cortex and compete for full attention. For some children, the distractibility is greater in dealing with visual inputs; for others, auditory inputs; and for some, both. As with hyperactivity, it is presumed that this distractibility is due to some form of CNS dysfunction.

Children with this disability might try to attend to a task and work, but each passing visual and/or auditory stimulus continues to capture their attention. With each such distraction, there is the need to reattend; thus the children display a *short attention span.*

The distractibility caused by external stimuli appears to be clinically different from a type of internal distractibility. Children with this problem have difficulty inhibiting their thoughts, a condition sometimes referred to as cognitive disinhibition. They are distracted because the internal thoughts are competing for their attention. It is helpful to differentiate the two clinical problems; as will be discussed later, distractibility in response to external stimuli often improves with the use of psychostimulants whereas disinhibition may or may not.

SOCIAL, EMOTIONAL, AND FAMILY PROBLEMS

Many children and adolescents with specific LDs become frustrated; they experience repeated failures and have difficulty coping with a number of situations. As a result, there is a high incidence of associated social and emotional problems.[36] Not infrequently, the youngsters' behavior may lead to stress within the family.[33] More than that, too often the LDs are not recognized or treated, and the children continue to experience repeated frustrations and failures. Ultimately the children or adolescents may be referred for evaluation, but this is often delayed until conspicuous emotional problems have developed. Occasionally a clinician will overlook the importance of previously unrecognized LDs and regard such persons as having primary emotional difficulties. To do so, however, is to miss a significant etiological factor, and the outcome will be an inadequate treatment plan. It is of critical importance to differentiate between children or adolescents whose emotional problems are a *consequence* of the academic difficulties.

These children have difficulty with all stages of psychosocial development.[11,32] The LDs, hyperactivity, and or distractibility may interfere with mastery of many different developmental tasks.[37] The children's

difficulties, in turn, weigh heavily on the parents, who may become frustrated, helpless, and dysfunctional.[11,28,37]

The multiple types of social, emotional, and family difficulties are reported and discussed in chapter 20 in volume 2 of this *Handbook.*[34]

LDs can interfere with normal psychosocial development. Infancy may be very difficult. Babies with motor delay or difficulties may be floppy, poorly coordinated, and have difficulty with sucking and eating. It is not yet known what impact perceptual disabilities may have during the early months of life. It is possible that an infant's auditory or visual perceptual problems interfere with the earliest interactions with the environment and with significant parenting objects.

If the young child's interactions with the outside world are unsuccessful, the child might have difficulty mastering separation. Peer interactions may be poor. Activities may be unmastered. A parent may sense this difficulty and protect the child, thus delaying the separation process; the result may be a child who prefers to stay at home. The struggle to master separation may show up as negativism, power struggles, and the need to be in control.

The older child might have problems with individuation. He or she may have difficulty mastering group interactions or sports; this might lead to a poor self-image and, possibly, to feelings of disappointing a parent. Identifying with the parent of the same sex may be hard to do.

During adolescence the fact that an LD is a total life disability takes on even greater meaning. It affects every kind of personal involvement and interaction. Even when the problems had been recognized and treated during childhood, as adolescents the youngsters must now handle new challenges. Those whose problems had gone unrecognized until adolescence have a double problem—they must deal with the consequences of their existing disabilities while trying to compensate for the academic and emotional price they have already paid.

The adolescent with LDs has special problems. Early adolescence is characterized by a strong need *not* to be different. As a child, a person may have cooperated peacefully with a special education routine; as an adolescent, however, he or she may suddenly refuse to continue in special programs and insist on being in regular classes. Medication may be refused.

Moving from a dependent to an independent relationship may be difficult both within the family and with peers and other adults. An adolescent who is insecure, who has a poor self-image, and does not do well with his or her peers may not be able to move away comfortably from the family. Instead, some adolescents may embrace their dependency. They turn away from outside companions, retreat into the home, and put on an appearance of being contented, even preferring to be alone or to watch television. Others find these excessive dependency feelings upsetting and fight them internally or by lashing out at others. Negativism, power struggles with adults, and unacceptable clothing, hairstyles, and choice of friends may be ways of expressing fear of and discomfort with dependence. If adolescents have experienced failures at school, with friends or within the family, then at best it will be difficult for them to finalize their own identity in positive terms.

In addition to limitations with specific developmental tasks, LD adolescents may find it difficult to take part in sports, dancing, and most of the other activities in which their peers are involved. Often they lack social skills. Making small talk, maintaining eye contact, listening to others, waiting for someone to finish talking before they speak—all of these abilities are critical to social acceptance and the adolescent may not have mastered one or many of them. LD youths may misunderstand what is said, make inappropriate remarks, or forget what a conversation is about. They may be bossy, aggressive, and belligerent, or so quiet and passive that they fade away in any group.

None of these patterns is likely to lead to easy peer acceptance, and instead of steering in the right direction, some adolescents withdraw into the house, becoming absorbed with television, listening to the stereo, or reading. Others will be so desperate for social acceptance that they may act inappropriately and get into trouble: Girls may become sexually active in an effort to get attention and "love"; boys may try acting "tough," hanging out on the fringes of a gang or getting involved in petty crime.

Clinical Interventions

The following types of clinical interventions will be discussed: (1) school-based programs, (2) family counseling and other interventions, (3) individual psychotherapeutic and behavioral interventions, (4) psychopharmacological therapies, and (5) current controversial therapies.

SCHOOL-BASED PROGRAMS

The child psychiatrist or other mental health professional may refer a child or adolescent to the school's special education program, may be a consultant for that program, or may be asked by the parents to assist in the evaluation. It is important to clarify all clinical problems and, when possible, to determine whether the emotional or family difficulties are a cause or a consequence of the academic problems. It is essential that this clinician advocate for the appropriate special educational evaluation, diagnosis, and treatment.

If the school concurs with the diagnosis, the child or adolescent will be classified as learning disabled (under P.L. 94-142, Education for All Handicapped Children Act).

Three kinds of programs are generally available in schools, be they public or private special educational settings. Which one is selected will depend on the degree of the child's disability, the level of his or her current academic performance, and the availability of programs.

The best program is the one that is judged to offer what the child needs academically and behaviorally in the *least restrictive environment* possible. This judgment has to be made for each child individually. The least restrictive environment is not necessarily the program closest to a regular program. For some children and adolescents, the least restrictive environment that will do the job might be the most restrictive environment available. For example, a child with multiple LDs who is several years behind in basic skills might feel most relaxed and safe in a small, self-contained, special education classroom. The freedom and rough-and-tumble of a regular classroom might so overwhelm the child that his or her involvement would be completely inhibited.

The core of special educational therapy is the corrective or remedial interventions provided by a professional qualified in special education. Remedial speech and language therapists plus physical and/or occupational therapists also may be part of the treatment team. For younger children, the focus will be on remedial approaches designed to minimize or overcome the specific LDs. At the same time grade-expected skills will be taught through the use of the individual's learning strengths. By early adolescence, additional strategies for learning are added to the treatment approaches.

The least disruptive level of placement is in a regular classroom program with a daily thirty to sixty minutes of supplemental special educational help. For a program like this to work, the special educators must communicate actively with the classroom teachers. If such communication breaks down, the classroom teacher will not understand the disabilities and may continue to expect too much of the child or to penalize him or her because of learning problems.

A program designed to function at the second level of intensity is often called mainstreaming. Children or adolescents are assigned to a special education class for part of each day. With this as home base, they are then "mainstreamed" into regular classroom programs for as much of the day as they can handle. At first, this might be just gym class, music, or art. Later, it might include English, science, or math. As with the supplemental help model, it is critical that the resource room special educator communicate with regular classroom teachers.

If a more intensive, third-level program is needed, the child might be assigned full time to a self-contained classroom. Such a program is designed and staffed exclusively for LD children or adolescents. These special classes usually have no more than eight to twelve students and are taught by a certified special education teacher assisted by an aide.

FAMILY COUNSELING AND OTHER INTERVENTIONS

With the family, the first task is to educate them as fully as possible as to their son or daughter's LDs and to explain how these might affect all aspects of school, family, and peer interactions.[33] If the family is too dysfunctional for this approach, it might have to be delayed until family treatment or behavioral therapy has stabilized the situation.

The educational process should be done by the primary clinician. Parents need to understand their child's strengths as well as the nature of the disabilities. They must know how to build on these strengths rather than to magnify the weaknesses. Such knowledge helps them plan home activities, chores, outside activities, sports, and camping ventures in a way that is most likely to be successful and to lead to positive psychological and social growth. Of equal importance, such knowledge and strategies help parents feel less helpless and more in control.

One approach is that of preventive family counseling.[37] The full evaluation should be reviewed in detail with the parents. They need to know their child's intellectual potential, level of academic performance, and why he or she is underachieving. Any existing emotional, social, or family problems must be clarified. A treatment plan should be presented, specifying what the parents must do. Next, the full evaluation should be shared with the child. He or she must understand the nature of the academic difficulties. Youngsters may be confused by their failures and might fear that they are bad or dumb or retarded. They must also understand the treatment plan.

Parents have a critical role to play in helping their child or adolescent.[37] The specific LDs will be apparent at home. Parents need to tell their child that they understand. They should reassure their daughter or son that they are glad that she or he is getting help. They should ask for their child's own views on how the adults can help best. With knowledge, parents can both avoid problems and assist their child. For example, in talking to a child with an auditory figure-ground problem—that is, one who has difficulty selecting what sounds to focus on—they may need to establish eye contact before speaking. They will have to go into the room where the child is and call out his or her name, speaking to the child only after he or she has looked up. If the child has difficulty with sequencing—that is, getting the steps of a task in the right order—they might need to help their child get started. They do not do the job for the child, but help him or her get organized. If they want the table set, for instance, they might offer a concrete model by doing one sample setting (plate here, fork, knife, and spoon there, glass here). If the child has trouble dressing in the morning because it is difficult to remember the sequence, a parent can set the clothes out on the bed in their proper order. If the child has fine motor problems and difficulty with buttons or shoe laces, slip-over tops or loafers might be tried. Such behaviors communicate acceptance and encourage independent growth.

Parents might make a list of the areas in which their child is strong and weak. Next to each strength, they can write out all of the things he or she is capable of doing. Next to the weaknesses, write out all of the things that they notice with which the disability interferes. Then, by thinking creatively, they can build on the child's strengths while helping to compensate for the weaknesses. For example, what household chores can the child do? If gross motor problems result in frequent accidents when the child takes out the trash, can some other task be assigned? The special educator might help by offering suggestions. The goal is to find the right chores rather than to excuse the child from family participation.

The same technique can be applied outside the home in sports, at clubs, and in other activities. Each sport requires different strengths. If the child has sequencing, fine motor, and visual motor disabilities, games with elaborate rules, or those that require eye-hand coordination skills, like baseball and basketball, may be difficult. The child's poor performance will also add to the social and peer problems. But let us say that he or she has good gross motor strengths. Swimming, diving, soccer, horseback riding, skiing, bowling, or certain field and track events, all of which rely on gross motor abilities and require minimal eye-hand coordination, may be successes. The same ten-year-old who stopped playing baseball because he could not catch, throw, or hit well, and who did no better at basketball might do very well in soccer or become an excellent swimmer. Let the child find success and peer acceptance with these sports.

Some children find all sports difficult. But it might be possible to improve some of the required skills through practice. Perhaps the children his or her own age will not take the time or have the patience to help, but a parent or an older brother or sister can go into the yard (or anyplace else where other children will not see) and practice catching, throwing, or hitting.

Because of their difficulty following directions or because they simply play so badly, some children never learn the basic rules of a game. Once again, someone in the family may need to sit down and teach the child how to play baseball or hopscotch from the ground up, going back over the rules repeatedly until the child catches on.

This approach can be used with the child's outside activities as well. Whether it be cub scouts, a local youth center, or any other activity, the goal for parents is to build on strengths rather than to magnify weaknesses. By working with the coordinator or leader of these activities, tasks can be selected that maximize success and avoid failure.

If properly informed, the club, group, or activity leaders can be helpful in facilitating peer interactions. Such people should understand that this child does not always hear every instruction given; they must be cued in advance to check with the child and to repeat things if necessary. This child may appear quiet or indifferent because language does not come easily. The leaders need to know that the child is not retarded, bad, or lazy; the disability is simply invisible. The same advice holds for Sunday school and religious education programs. The staff must know a good deal about the child so that they can design appropriate classroom and activity programs.

Choosing a camp, whether day or sleep-away, requires the same attention. Parents may consider a camp designed for children with special needs, or they might turn to a carefully selected regular camp. They need to think about whether this child would be better in a large or small camp. What strengths and abilities does the child have, and how do they match with the offerings of a particular camp? Some camps focus on drama or arts and crafts. Are these activities that will build on strengths or will they set the child up for failure? Some camps are sports-oriented and competitive and woe to the child who drops a ball and causes his or her cabin to lose a game. But other camps focus on noncompetitive activities or on gross motor sports. A clumsy, nonathletic son or daughter might do very well at a camp where the emphasis is on horseback riding or on waterfront activities. Swimming, rowing, and sailing all are gross motor activities. Communicating with parents is important while at camp. If reading or writing skills are limited, then one might turn to the use of a tape recorder and the child and family can mail each other tapes.

Before selecting a camp, parents need to talk with the director at length. Is that person flexible? Can he

or she describe programs that might work for their particular child? Nor should the parents hesitate to educate the counselors. They are usually young people who appreciate the information, and the child will benefit from the understanding of such important figures.

These examples are meant to illustrate a style of thinking and problem solving that can be helpful to families. The primary clinician must be sure that the parents know both their child's areas of strength and of learning disability. Once they are informed, these caring adults can then use appropriate strategies to build on the strengths in order to maximize psychosocial growth and peer successes.

INDIVIDUAL PSYCHOTHERAPEUTIC AND BEHAVIORAL INTERVENTIONS

Types of Intervention. If the clinician believes that the emotional problems are secondary to frustrations and failures caused by the LDs, the initial phase of treatment should focus on the cause; that is, on establishing the necessary educational programs and clarifying the nature of the problem with both the individual and family. If the secondary psychological problems have become so established that they now have a life of their own, they must be given separate attention.

When intrapsychic difficulties exist, psychodynamically oriented psychotherapy may be necessary. If the patterns of learned and/or reinforced behaviors are dysfunctional or if performance anxiety is high, a behavioral management plan or behavioral therapy approach may be needed. For youngsters whose interpersonal skills are poor, group therapy or a social learning skills group might be useful. And when there is family dysfunction, family therapy may be indicated. More often than not, a multimodel approach is used. Whichever interventions are needed, the primary clinician must be the one to coordinate the efforts with the school and to provide initial preventive family counseling.

If the child or adolescent's emotional problems are in part a reflection of the LDs, psychotherapy alone may not succeed. One or two hours a week of therapy can not undo twenty or more hours a week of school experiences that reinforce the poor self-image or that beget anxiety or depression. In all such instances, the educational needs must be addressed. Even if psychotherapy is needed, it might be better to delay its initiation until all negotiations with the school are complete. To start therapy before this might give the school personnel grounds for saying that the academic problems are emotionally based and thus not the school's responsibility.

When any therapy is initiated, be it individual, behavioral, group, or family, the clinician must understand the nature of the LDs and how they might interfere with the therapeutic process. This concern is especially cogent if the disabilities are in the auditory and language areas and the therapeutic interaction consists primarily of listening and talking. Sequencing or memory disorders, on the other hand, might decrease the individual's ability to understand the concepts involved in a behavioral management approach. If distractibility is also present, it will make for further problems in attending.

Where the child appears to misunderstand the clinician's comments or questions or has difficulty with word finding or organizing thoughts, the clinician should explain that these are understandable disabilities. Clinicians can enable a therapeutic alliance to get underway by asking how they can help the child and by modifying the style of interaction. Clinicians might need to talk more slowly, to make comments that are shorter or more simple, or to use paper and pencil to write out or illustrate for the patient the ideas or concepts that are being developed. Such additional efforts might help the patient organize and/or integrate the treatment process.

The use of play as a vehicle for therapy might pose problems to these children. Reading cards or instructions, following sequences, doing motor tasks (e. g., building with blocks)—any or all of these might be difficult.

There are times when the therapist doing dynamic therapy concludes that the child is blocking or resisting, or when the behavioral therapist decides that the child is not responding to a particular reinforcement system. Before such a conclusion is reached, however, the possible interference of the LDs must be considered. Often the special educator can define the LDs and can suggest alternative models for interacting or for accomplishing specific tasks.

PHARMACOTHERAPY

If the child with a learning disability is also hyperactive or distractible, stimulant medication may well be of help.[34] Such medication will usually make the child more available for attending and learning and may improve some forms of fine motor difficulties; however, it does not treat the underlying LDs.[4] Educational therapy is still essential.

Piracetam has been suggested as having a specific ability to improve cognitive and memory functioning.[29,38,40,41] As of this writing, the data remain unclear.

CURRENT CONTROVERSIAL THERAPIES

Most of the controversial therapies are discussed in chapter 20 of volume 2 and chapters 24 and 37 in volume 3 of this *Handbook*.[34,35] Only updates or newer concepts will be reviewed at this time.

Ophthalmology versus Optometry. The differences in view between these two disciplines are not new but have escalated. The clinician and families may be confused by optometrists' and ophthalmologists' different methods of treating LDs. Ophthalmologists believe that when a child or adolescent with LDs is referred to them they should check for problems with vision— nearsightedness, farsightedness, astigmatism—for eye-muscle imbalance, and for any ocular disease. If they find any of these problems, they prescribe treatment. If they do not find any of these problems, they believe that the child should be referred to a special educator or some other appropriate specialist for treatment of his or her LDs.

Optometrists look for the same problems that ophthalmologists do. But, after they have ruled out problems or treated the problems they found, many optometrists believe they can also treat the LDs. Most optometrists evaluate the child's visual abilities and then prescribe glasses or the use of visual training or eye-muscle training techniques, if they believe these are indicated. Another group of these specialists use a developmental vision approach, and see a broader role for the optometrist in learning problems.[17,25] They feel that learning in general, and reading in particular, requires high levels of visual perception. They point out that visual perception processes are also related to the child's sensorimotor coordination. They employ a wide variety of educational and sensorimotor-perceptual training techniques in an attempt to correct children's visual perceptual and educational problems. It is this subgroup of optometrists who have been active with children with LDs.

The American Academy of Pediatrics, the American Academy of Ophthalmology and Otolaryngology, and the American Academy of Ophthalmology issued a joint statement that criticizes this approach.[1] This joint communiqué emphasizes the need for a multidisciplinary approach to LDs. No single professional can evaluate and treat the whole child. The statement further cautions that there are no peripheral eye defects that can produce dyslexia and associated LDs.

Despite the absence of supporting data, visual training programs continue to be widely used. Optometrists believe that visual deficits cause reading disabilities. Metzger and Serner[24] recently reviewed the ophthalmologic, optometric, and psychological literature on this theory and concluded that, "there is no evidence that reading disabilities result from problems in the visual system." They also reviewed the literature on the efficacy of visual training and found that the reported studies were without proper research design or controls.

Vestibular Dysfunction Therapy. Recently, Levinson published two books on the causative role of the vestibular and vestibular-cerebellar systems with dyslexia.[19,21] He proposes the treatment of dyslexia with anti-motion sickness medication.

The role of the vestibular system in the higher cortical functions required for academic performance is not yet known. Some of the symptoms generally associated with learning disabilities (for example, faulty eye-movements, poor postural coordination, poor balance, and poor spatial orientation) could be indicative of vestibular disorder. Such symptoms are, however, only indirect evidence for vestibular dysfunction. The most prominent objective sign of vestibular involvement is nystagmus. Levinson uses "blurring speed" (the speed at which words passing across the visual field can no longer be recognized) as evidence for abnormal vestibular function. This test involves passing stimuli across the subject's visual field at varying speeds; thus, it constitutes visual stimulation, not vestibular.

A recent study by Polatajko[27] investigated the relationship between children's vestibular function and academic learning using well defined criteria for learning disabilities and exact measurements of vestibular activity. No significant differences either in the intensity of vestibular responsivity or in the incidence of vestibular dysfunction were found between the normal and learning disabled children. There was no evidence that children having low, average, or high vestibular responsivity differ significantly on measures of academic performance. Nor was there any significant correlation between measures of vestibular function and measures of academic performance. No evidence at this time supports either the vestibular theories or the proposed treatment approaches.

Megavitamins. The use of massive doses of vitamins to treat emotional and thinking disorders began with the treatment of schizophrenia. Hoffer, Osmond, and Smythies[15] suggested that schizophrenia was caused by an improper breakdown of certain chemicals normally found in the brain. Then Hoffer and Osmond[14] proposed that administration of large quantities of certain B vitamins could stop this faulty breakdown. To date, no documented biochemical studies on schizophrenic patients have confirmed this theory. A five-year study carried out by the Board of Directors of the Canadian Mental Health Association strongly suggested that this treatment had no therapeutic effect.[4] After reviewing the history and literature relating to this subject, the members of an American Psychiatric Association task force produced a report in which they concluded that there is no valid basis for the use of megavitamins in the treatment of mental disorders.[3]

Dr. Allan Cott wrote the first paper suggesting megavitamin treatment for children with LDs.[8] His assertion was that megavitamins can help these children; this, however, has not been confirmed by other researchers. Despite these negative results, the approach remains popular.

Trace Elements Certain trace elements, including copper, zinc, manganese, magnesium, and chromium, along with more common elements such as calcium, potassium, sodium, and iron, are necessary nutrients— that is, their presence is essential for maintenance of normal physiological function. Deficiencies in specific trace elements have been proposed as a cause of LDs.[3] In many parts of the United States, children are treated with trace-element replacement therapy. To date, no research has shown that such treatment can correct learning disabilities.

Refined Sugars. Clinical observations and parent reports suggest that refined sugars promote adverse behavioral reactions in children. Hyperactive behavior is most commonly reported.[29] Conners and Blouin[6] studied the relationship of sugar intake to either conduct disorders, learning disorders, or attention deficit disorder in children. Behavioral and classroom measures were made after intake of sucrose, fructose, and placebo. The results did not distinguish the normal effects of increased calorie intake versus sugar effects. They could not conclude that deviant behavior was increased by sugar. Another study, by Rapoport,[30] reached the same conclusions. There was no significant effect of sugar on any of the behavioral measures either when the individual sugars were compared with placebo or when both sugars were combined.

Hypoglycemia. Cott[8] proposed that learning disabilities could be due to hypoglycemia. The treatment proposed is to place the child or adolescent on a hypoglycemia diet. Clinical studies on learning disabled students using a formal glucose tolerance test are not conclusive.[30] If hypoglycemia is suspected, a full evaluation including the glucose tolerance test should be done.

Food Additives and Preservatives. In 1975 Feingold proposed that synthetic flavors and colors in the diet were related to hyperactivity in children.[9] He reported that the elimination of all foods containing artificial colors and flavors as well as salicylates and certain other additives stopped the hyperactivity.

Following the introduction of this clinical concept, two different types of clinical study were done by research teams: dietary crossover and specific challenge. These studies were reviewed by the American Council on Science and Health.

In the dietary crossover studies, hyperactive children were randomly assigned either to the elimination diet or to a control diet and then crossed over to the other treatment. Conners, et al.[7] and Conners[5] noted ambiguous findings. Improvement in behavior was noted in a few children but only by the teachers when the control diet was given before the elimination diet; the findings were not noted when the order was reversed. Harley et al. [13] noted the same order-related results.

The diet crossover studies showed that a different research approach was needed. In the specific challenge studies, the strategy was changed from testing the general efficacy of the overall elimination diet to considering the specific involvement of the artificial colors or flavors with the hyperkinetic syndrome. In this design, the children are maintained on Feingold's elimination diet throughout the study. Periodically, the child is given (challenged with) foods that contain the suspected offending chemical (e.g., artificial food colors). Measures are taken to note if the hyperkinetic state was precipitated or aggravated by this challenge. This design was used by Williams et al., [39] Goyette et al., [12] Harley et al., [13] Levey et al., [22] and others.

In 1982 the National Institutes of Health held a Consensus Development Conference on "Defined Diets and Childhood Hyperactivity." [26] This conference was sponsored by the National Institute of Child Health and Human Development. The panel of experts concluded that "these studies did indicate a limited positive association between the 'defined diets' (i.e., Feingold diet) and a decrease in hyperactivity." The panel noted that there was insufficient evidence available to permit identification beforehand of this small group of individuals who may respond or to determine under what circumstances they may derive benefits. The panel believed that the defined diets should not be universally used in the treatment of childhood hyperactivity at this time.

Two later literature reviews also concluded that the Feingold diet is not effective in treating hyperactivity in most children. Although a small number of patients (one to two percent) appear to respond positively to the diet for reasons that are not yet clear, there is no way for the physician to identify in advance which patients might be part of this small percentage.

Conclusion

The clinical picture of a child or adolescent with learning disabilities is most apparent in the academic setting. He or she has difficulty with one or more required learning skills and has fallen behind in many subject areas. Educational and psychological testing will identify the presence and types of the specific LDs.

It is important that the clinician understand that these LDs can interfere with or be reflected in all aspects of family and peer interactions. Preventive family counseling is needed.

When evaluating the associated emotional, social, and family problems, it is critical to determine whether these problems are *causing* the academic difficulties or are their *consequences*. Each conclusion leads to a different treatment approach. If treatment is indicated, the clinician must be aware that the LDs can also interfere with the therapeutic process. Adaptations in technique may therefore be needed.

REFERENCES

1. AMERICAN ACADEMY OF PEDIATRICS, Joint Organizational Statement. "The Eye and Learning Disabilities," *Pediatrics,* 49 (1972):454–455.

2. AMERICAN COUNCIL ON SCIENCE AND HEALTH, *Diet and Hyperactivity: Is There a Relationship?* prepared by M. J. Sheridan for the American Council on Science and Health, New York, 1979.

3. AMERICAN PSYCHIATRIC ASSOCIATION, Task Force on Vitamin Therapy in Psychiatry. *Megavitamin and Orthomolecular Therapy in Psychiatry.* Washington, D.C.: American Psychiatric Association, 1973.

4. CANADIAN MENTAL HEALTH ASSOCIATION, Board of Directors. Quoted in Ban, T. A., "The Niacin Controversy: The Possibility of Negative Effects," *Psychiatric Opinion,* 10 (1973):19–24.

5. CONNERS, C. K. *Food Additives and Hyperactive Children.* New York: Plenum Press, 1980, pp. 28–40.

6. CONNERS, C. K., and BLOUIN, A. G., "Nutritional Effects on Behavior of Children," *Journal of Psychiatric Research,* 17 (1982/83):193–199.

7. CONNERS, C. K., et al. "Food Additives and Hyperkine-

sis: A Controlled Double-Blind Experiment," *Pediatrics,* 58 (1976):154–166.

8. COTT, A. "Orthomolecular Approach to the Treatment of Learning Disabilities," *Schizophrenia,* 3 (1971):95–107.

9. FEINGOLD, B. F. *Why Your Child is Hyperactive.* New York: Random House, 1975.

10. GADOW, K. D. "Pharmacotherapy for Learning Disabilities," *Learning Disabilities,* 2 (1983):127–140.

11. GARDNER, R. A. "The Guilt Reaction of Parents of Children with Severe Physical Disease," *American Journal of Psychiatry,* 126 (1969):636–644.

12. GOYETTE, C. H.; CONNERS, C. K.; PETTI, T. A.; and CURTIS, L. E. "Effects of Artificial Colors on Hyperkinetic Children: A Double-blind Challenge Study," *Psychopharmacology Bulletin,* 14 (1978):39–40.

13. HARLEY, J. P., et al. "Hyperkinesis and Food Additives: Testing the Feingold Hypothesis," *Pediatrics,* 61 (1978):818–828.

14. HOFFER, A., and OSMOND, H. *The Chemical Basis of Clinical Psychiatry.* Springfield, Ill.: Charles C Thomas, 1960.

15. HOFFER, A., OSMOND, H., and SMYTHIES, J. "Schizophrenia: A New Approach: I. Results of a Year's Research," *Journal of Mental Science,* 100 (1954):29–54.

16. KAVALE, K. A., and FORNESS, S. R. "Hyperactivity and Diet Treatment: A Meta-analysis of the Feingold Hypothesis," *Journal of Learning Disabilities,* 16 (1983):324–330.

17. KEOGH, B. B. "Optometric Vision Training Programs for Children with Learning Disabilities: Review of Issues and Research," *Journal of Learning Disabilities,* 7 (1974):219–231.

18. LEVINE, M. D. "Reading Disability: Do the Eyes Have It?" *Pediatrics,* 73 (1984):869–870.

19. LEVINSON, H. N. *A Solution to the Riddle Dyslexia.* New York: Springer-Verlag, 1980.

20. LEVINSON, H. N. *A Solution to the Riddle Dyslexia.* New York: Springer-Verlag, 1981.

21. LEVINSON, H. N. *Smart But Feeling Dumb.* New York: Warner Books, 1984.

22. LEVY, F.; DUMBRELL, S.; HOBBES, G. "Hyperkinesis and Diet: A double-blind Crossover Trial with Tartrazine Challenge," *Medical Journal of Australia,* 1 (1978):61–64.

23. MATTLES, J. A. "The Feingold Diet: A Current Reappraisial," *Journal of Learning Disabilities,* 16:(1983)324–323.

24. METZGER, R. L., and WERNER, D. D. "Use of Visual Training for Reading disabilities: A Review," *Pediatrics,* 7 (1984):824–829.

25. MILKIE, G. M., and MILLER, S. C. "Visual Training/Vision Therapy: An Optometric Approach to the Treatment of Vision Problems Interfering with Learning," in G. Leisman, ed., *Basic Visual Processes and Learning Disabilities.* Springfield, Ill.: Charles C Thomas, 1976.

26. National Institutes of Health. *Defined Diets and Childhood Hyperactivity.* National Institutes of Health Consensus Development Conference Summary. Vol. 4, No. 3, 1982.

27. POLATAJKO, H. J. "A Critical Look at Vestibular Dysfunction in Learning-Disabled Children," *Developmental Medicine and Child Neurology,* 27 (1985):283–292.

28. POZNANSKI, E. "Psychiatric Difficulties in Siblings of Handicapped Children," *Clinical Pediatrics,* 8 (1969):232–234.

29. PRINZ, R. J.; ROBERTS W. A.; and HARTMAN, E. "Dietary Correlates of Hyperactive Behavior in Children," *Journal of Consulting and Clinical Psychology,* 48 (1980):760–769.

30. RAPOPORT, J. "Effects of Dietary Substances in Children," *Journal of Psychiatric Research,* 17 (1982/83):187–191.

31. RUDEL, R. G., and HELFGOTT, E. "Effect of Piracetam on Verbal Memory of Dyslexic Boys," *Journal of the American Academy of Child Psychiatry,* in press.

32. SILVER, L. B. "Emotional and Social Problems of Children with Developmental Disabilities," in R. E. Weber, ed., *Handbook on Learning Disabilities.* Englewood Cliffs, N.J.: Prentice-Hall, 1974, pp. 97–120.

33. ———. "Acceptable and Controversial Approaches to Treating the Child with Learning Disabilities," *Pediatrics,* 55 (1975):406–415.

34. ———. "Minimal Brain Dysfunction," in J. D. Noshpitz, ed., *Basic Handbook of Child Psychiatry,* vol 2. New York: Basic Books, 1979, pp. 416–439.

35. ———. "Therapeutic Interventions with Children Who Have Perceptual and Other Learning Problems," in J. D. Noshpitz, ed., *Basic Handbook of Child Psychiatry,* vol. 3, ed. S. I. Harrison. New York: Basic Books, 1979, pp. 605–614.

36. ———. "The Relationship Between Learning Disabilities, Hyperactivity, Distractibility, and Behavioral Problems: A Clinical Analysis," *Journal of the American Academy of Child Psychiatry,* 20 (1981):385–397.

37. ———. *The Misunderstood Child. A Guide for Parents of Learning Disabled Children.* New York: McGraw-Hill, 1984.

38. SIMEON, J.; WATERS, B.; and RESNICK, M. "Effects of Piracetum in Children with Learning Disorders," *Psychopharmacology Bulletin,* 16 (1980):65–66.

39. WILLIAMS, J. I., et al, "Relative Effects of Drugs and Diet on Hyperactive Behaviors: An Experimental Study," *Pediatrics,* 61 (1978):811–817.

40. WILSHER, E. R., and MILEWSKI, J. "Effects of Piracetam on Dyslexics' Verbal Conceptualizing Ability," *Psychopharmacology Bulletin,* 19 (1983):3–4.

41. WILSHER, C. R., ATKINS, G., and MANFIELD, P. "Piracetam as an Aid to Learning in Dyslexia. Preliminary Report," *Psychopharmacologia,* 65 (1979):107–109.

57 / Treatment of Psychotic Children

Marian K. DeMyer

Accounts of treatment of psychoses of childhood in the last decade have focused largely on the autistic child; treatment of schizophrenia in childhood has been discussed much less often. Thus far nearly all research in treatment has been carried out with preadolescent autistic patients; currently, however, there are signs of increasing interest in adolescent patients.[44]

Pretreatment Evaluation

If diagnosticians are to understand individual children and their parents and to prescribe a sensible treatment program, a comprehensive evaluation must be carried out. The clinical features of pervasive developmental disorder (PDD) or schizophrenia in childhood should be observed during several visits over a period of several weeks. The child with PDD is afflicted with a brain syndrome of variable and often unknown etiology (see chapter 39). Because any one of a number of biochemical or anatomical disorders may be present, the same work-up must be performed as with any other child suspected of developmental brain disorder. Schizophrenia in childhood, while less well researched for concomitant neurobiological factors, merits the same diagnostic approach. Table 57–1 lists the procedures that should be performed in every case and those elective procedures that should be done depending on specific findings from the routine evaluation. Such a thorough evaluation also assures the parents that their child has been studied properly and sets the stage for their cooperation in following treatment recommendations.

The goal of developmental testing is to provide a profile of scores as well as an overall IQ or developmental quotient, which is one of the best predictors of outcome.[19] Most autistic children can do only simple tasks and therefore require items designed for infants or children far below their chronological age; for example, the Wechsler Intelligence Scale for Children designed for six- to fifteen-year-old subjects is often too difficult in whole or in part for an autistic child in that age range. Autistic children frequently have splinter abilities (most often in fitting and assembly tasks such as block design), and verbal autistic children may have relatively good digit span scores. Nearly all do poorly on language comprehension and on items requiring creative speech. It is important that the IQ measure be based on a battery of scores and not on one type of performance, as either an over- or underestimate of IQ can result. The intellectual performances of schizophrenic children should also be carefully evaluated, because they likewise often have cognitive disabilities involving abstract thinking.[9]

A careful and detailed history of the child's behavior in the home, of parents' attempts to deal with the problems, and of intrafamily relationships will aid diagnosticians in assessing relative strengths and weaknesses and guide them in presenting findings and treatment recommendations in the most effective way. Diagnosticians must always remember that being the parent of a psychotic child is inherently an anxiety-producing situation. Assessing the mental health of the parents should be an ongoing process, and clinicians should proceed carefully before designating the mother (who may be quite anxious) as mentally ill or characterizing the marriage as conflict ridden.

TABLE 57–1

Diagnostic Procedures for Initial Evaluation

Minimal Acceptable Work-Up

Description of child's behavior in the home and
    parents' methods of handling
Family and marital relationships
Medical history of parents, child, pregnancy, delivery
Family pedigree
Complete physical and neurological examination
Electroencephalogram (EEG)
Computed brain tomography (CT scan)
Urinary screen for inborn errors of metabolism
Developmental testing (IQ, developmental level,
    mental age)
Screen for toxoplasmosis, other, rubella, cytomegalic
    inclusion disease, herpes simplex (TORCH screen)

Elective Procedures in Selected Cases

Lysosomal enzyme battery
Electroretinogram (ERG)
Brain-stem auditory evoked response (BAER)
Visual evoked response (VER)
Somatosensory evoked response (SSER)
Cerebrospinal fluid examination
Skin biopsy with electron microscopy for
    degenerative disease
Chromosome analysis
Nuclear magnetic resonance brain imaging (MRI)

Presenting Diagnostic Findings to Parents

The clinician's repeated observations over several visits will confirm the presence of psychosis and help determine whether there is a diagnosable neurological condition. Often the degree of cognitive deficit may take several months or a year to specify. The parents should be made aware of the extent and severity of the disorder and given the diagnostic term that best fits their child. This encounter with the name of the illness can come as a severe stress to them. Parents describe their reaction as shocklike; it can interfere with their ability to "hear what the doctor says."[16] Such a reaction frequently necessitates follow-up visits. In cases of PDD particularly, the parents should be told that some event has impaired the development of the brain of their child and that they are not responsible for the behavioral symptoms. If the evaluation has uncovered a putative cause, this can be pointed out to the parents, although in many cases of PDD, as well as most other developmental brain disorders, no putative cause is apparent. The cognitive deficits need to be discussed in a tentative fashion particularly if the child is under six years of age because in this age range accelerated cognitive development may occur. Many parents are extremely resistant to accepting the fact that their autistic child is mentally retarded, especially if the child has a splinter skill. These discussions should begin at the diagnostic summation interview but will need to continue in the school setting as it is there that the degree of cognitive difficulty will become increasingly apparent.

The attitude of the physician who has major responsibility for diagnosis can make an enormous difference to parents in lifting depression and guilt and helping them accept treatment recommendations. Above all the physician should be warm, kind, supportive, and helpful, neither minimizing the seriousness of the problem nor denying the possibility of amelioration of symptoms. The parents may not remember all that was said by the physician but they will forever remember the physician's attitude. [17]

IMPORTANCE OF INVOLVING PARENTS EARLY

Because autism affects infants and is a chronic, lifelong condition in most cases, the parents must be considered at every step of treatment. The goal of most parents and of society is to keep the autistic child in the home as long as possible. To attain this goal it is important that therapists at once encourage the parents to become partners in treatment (albeit in a special way) and also see to it that parents have a realistic appreciation of the basic biological intelligence of their child and of the resources available in the community. In order to avoid the burnout syndrome, parents also need considerable psychological and practical support from professional and educational resources and regular periods of respite from the stress of caring for an autistic child. [17]

From the outset all professionals who diagnose and treat autistic children must educate, support, and take the side of both the parents and all their children, for autism forces a family to adopt a life-style that is generally far different from what family members would otherwise choose. The natural proclivities of the parents and the myths frequently published in newspapers and aired on television make parents hope that there is some quick and easy treatment that will be the key to unlock the silence and the social wall behind which their child has supposedly "retreated." When that quick cure is not forthcoming, as it generally is not, parents feel frustrated and increasingly burdened. They react as do many people under stress, by becoming angry, anxious, critical, depressed, unsure if they have chosen the right doctor, the right school, the right

program for their child. In short, the parents become "difficult"; at this point parents and professionals can become adversaries if professionals are unaware of parental expectations.

Beginning with the first evaluation, the parents must enter an educational process that will instruct them about autism in general and about their child in particular. In turn, the parents can also educate the clinicians who evaluate and treat their child about idiosyncracies and difficulties the child presents in the home. Clinicians must educate the parents about cognitive disabilities, any medical conditions the child might have, more effective child-care techniques, and appropriate treatments and educational strategies.

Treatment Recommendations

What kinds of treatment should the up-to-date clinician prescribe for the psychotic child? All treatment advice should be individualized because different autistic children need different strategies. [34]

If the evaluation reveals neurological pathology that is not static or if the child has seizures, a neurologist should follow the child as well as a child psychiatrist. In the decades from the 1940s through most of the 1960s, both autism and child schizophrenia were largely thought to be environmentally determined, and separation of the parent and child was often recommended as the way to give the best chance for improvement. Thus inpatient care for the child and separate psychotherapy for the parents, especially the mother, were recommended. [16] Currently the pendulum has swung the other way, and too often inpatient care is difficult to find even for highly aggressive or self-destructive psychotic children. [17] Young children are seldom treated in an inpatient setting, but special programs can be found in many public and some private schools. While psychotherapy can be tried for some higher-functioning young children, for the most part the treatment of this age group is educational. Later in life when autistic individuals are more motivated and capable of verbalizing their problems, individual psychotherapy may be the treatment of choice. For some individuals group therapy may help. The child with schizophrenia may be helped by sensitively applied psychotherapy but, like the autistic child, also generally needs a special education program.

The welfare of the school-age child and the quality of family life in large measure hinge on the adequacy of the school program and whether the parents perceive the program to be a good one. [17] Most psychotic children learn best in a structured situation and a school that provides a five-day-a-week program. Many children also need a summer program to maintain gains made during the regular term. Teachers must understand the various levels of abilities (or "scatter") that exist in many psychotic children so that appropriate material—neither too hard nor too easy—can be presented to the child. These levels should be determined at the beginning of each school year and serve as a measuring guide for progress in learning. Wing and Wing[50] stressed that the school environment should be highly structured, should not be permissive, and that emphasis should be placed on effective training. In such an atmosphere a satisfactory relationship will develop between teacher and child. Because parents put great store in the school program, they are observant and quick to perceive any practice they feel is not in the best interest of their child. Teachers should be aware of this attitude and work with the parents to develop a tandem effort and to avoid adversary relationships.

OPERANT CONDITIONING OR BEHAVIOR MODIFICATION

The symptoms of autism affect nearly every aspect of development, and thus, to be successful, therapeutic procedures must affect many aspects of behavior—for example, interpersonal relationships, language, cognition, emotions, self-help skills, eating, toileting, and sleeping. In the last decade many advances have been made, but medical science still has much to learn before child psychoses can be treated successfully. If the underlying brain dysfunction can be prevented, such will probably be the treatment of choice ultimately. To date, perhaps the most significant developments have occurred in the continued growth of behavioral/education programs. Since the first report by Ferster and DeMyer in 1961,[23] over three hundred papers have appeared on the subject; a generous share of them deal with efforts to develop verbal skills in autistic children through the use of operant conditioning procedures.[18]

TREATMENT FOR SPEECH DEFICIENCIES

The magnitude of the speech problem is illustrated by the statistic that about 50 percent of autistic children never learn to speak and many of those who achieve any speech may be limited to uttering a few communicative words or phrases or noncommunicative echolalia. Howlin[32] reviewed the history of operant language training beginning in the early 1960s. Early treatment focused largely on teaching vocalization and words; current practice is to teach more complex forms and transformational rules. Although simi-

lar training procedures have been used across studies, the results of many studies have differed and the majority of successful reports have been accounts of single cases. Howlin reviewed seventy studies involving over two hundred children with sufficient information to evaluate their language level at onset of therapy and found that initial language level was the best predictor of outcome. Mute children had the worst prognosis, and only 17 percent developed phrase speech. In contrast, almost half of the children who used single words and over 80 percent of echolalic children developed phrase speech.

Even the projects that have been very systematic[36,37] and have achieved increased speech for many children have rarely been able to help the child produce spontaneous and rule-governed speech.[13,43] Frequently autistic children fail to generalize speech from the teaching situation to other settings or fail to maintain what they have learned after hundreds of training hours.

One of the most widely used methods to enhance the autistic child's communication has been sign language. As Bonvillian, Nelson, and Rhyne[5] pointed out, sign training and behavior modification programs are not mutually exclusive, and many teachers of sign employ operant methods. Two common sign methods are the American Sign Language system, in which signs are put in English word order, and Signing Exact English, which puts English syntax into a signing mode.[28]

In reviewing twenty studies on teaching signing to autistic patients, Bonvillian, Nelson, and Rhyne[5] found that most investigators emphasized simultaneous communication modes—that is, they taught speech and sign together. Most autistic children can acquire at least a few signs and 20 percent learn to produce combinations of signs. While generalization of signing is reported in some cases, this achievement is often failed and special efforts must be made to facilitate its generalization and maintenance.[10,28] It is interesting to note that children who learned to sign were often those who had learned to point in their natural environment. Even when given simultaneous sign and auditory training, mute children generally did not learn phrase speech; those who started the program with echolalia were helped more. Barrera and Sulzer-Azaroff[2] demonstrated with three high-functioning, echolalic girls that simultaneous training was more efficacious than verbal training alone.

Multisensory training in communication can involve the clinician using intrusive play, imitating the teacher's movements, and pairing objects in the child's natural environment with signs and words.[4,48] Beisler and Tsai[3] reported on a practical program to increase communication skills using intensive modeling by the teacher of the child's activities and verbalizations and employing a reinforcement system that fulfilled the "intent of the child's communication." Within six weeks the children were able to demonstrate significant increases in several aspects of verbal skills. Expressive language was not among these gains although the mean length of utterances was longer and "post-treatment comments of parents were favorable." Other favorable results were the self-reinforcing nature of the modeling activities, increase in the children taking turns and reduction of inattention, self-stimulation, and tantrum behaviors.

Pronouns give special trouble to autistic children because of the complex rules that underlie their acquisition. Fay[22] has advised that autistic children should be encouraged to use proper names as long as necessary. When training in use of pronouns is introduced, emphasis should be put on comprehension of you/me and you/I. Pointing, gesturing, and touching can be used to teach the referents of pronouns. A third person present in the training session also helps. After first- and second-person pronouns are learned, third-person and plural forms can be introduced. These latter forms are extremely difficult for most autistic children to learn.

Other novel methods have been used to teach speech. A mother[30] taught communicative speech to her musical, echolalic autistic child by singing communicatively to him. Eventually the mother changed from singing her utterances to speech delivered "with very exaggerated pitch and cadence" and then later to normally delivered speech. This child learned to communicate with speech at home and school although he "still runs around the house on his toes, flapping his hands and repeating the same sentence over and over, but when we tell him to stop he argues with us about it" (p. 456). The mother cautions that the technique is not to be considered "a panacea or a cure" but it is something to consider for other musical, echolalic children.

How much can parents be expected to participate in actual operant condition therapy? Many parents can participate for a short while if they have close guidance, but left to themselves they frequently do not persist.[29,31,41] However, some parents show great aptitude and motivation. It should be remembered that introducing special procedures on the homefront poses many problems for the family; thus for most families therapy will need to be conducted by professionals and reinforced in the home.[45]

Smith and associates[46] discussed the point that children may perceive operant conditioning methods of teaching speech as stressful and they thus may be unmotivated. They hypothesized that autistic subjects may suffer from "input overload" because they may not be able to "mask out ambient environmental sounds." To reduce stress the children may block all auditory stimuli. This situation would be expected to prevent autistic children from using their own vocalizations as feedback—to engage in "self-talk." To test this idea, the investigators used earphones with a built-in FM receiver and a microphone (the "Phonic Ear") suspended near children's mouth. The device allowed the children to listen to their own voice while blocking out environmental sounds and vice versa. Both children tested by Smith and coworkers increased their utterances while using the Phonic Ear.

However, in a delayed auditory feedback study,[40] five high-functioning autistic adolescents showed no differences from normal controls under stressful, disruptive auditory conditions except for providing themselves with about eight decibels higher self-speech feedback. The autistic youngsters "did not tune out the external auditory input" (p. 186). The authors say that language therapists have found they provide a louder voice in their language training for many autistic individuals even though hearing tests were in the normal range.

These two studies with divergent findings illustrate the need for studying larger samples of autistic patients over a wider age and ability range and to integrate procedures if we are to learn more about their puzzling auditory reactions. There are reports that about 50 percent of young autistic children appear clinically to be hypersensitive to certain sounds.[16] Such findings raise important questions, such as whether this phenomenon exists mainly in early childhood or in lower-functioning autistics.

How valid is the criticism that behavior modification methods to teach verbal skills are perceived as stressful by autistic subjects? Operant conditioning or behavior modification therapy are terms that refer to a technique of reinforcing (rewarding) certain acts to make it more likely that the acts will occur again. To a large extent every teacher and every therapist uses such methods, whether or not they understand behavior modification principles.

Consider this illustrative vignette. If we want to eliminate some unpleasant behavior such as screaming, for example, we could proceed with the operant training in the classroom, the language therapist's office, or in the backyard of the children's home. If children scream to be swung, they should be swung only when not screaming. If we wish to teach children to raise their hand as a signal they would like to swing, then we will raise their hand for them (when not screaming) and then immediately reinforce (swing) them. Eventually the children will be reinforced (swung) only when they voluntarily raise their hand. If this method is applied consistently, wonder of all wonders, children who previously have used screaming to express most of their needs are able to sign a message in a calm way. There generally is a period of stress (extra tantrums) when no reinforcement is provided at points along the way but smiles of pleasure and calmness nearly always accompany the mastery of tasks. Churchill[12] reported that successful completion of tasks was accompanied by signs of pleasure and diminution of "crazy" behavior in autistic children.

If, however, the operant trainer picks tasks that are impossible for the children to perform and delivers aversive stimuli (punishment) when they are not accomplished, then certainly the children would be unduly stressed. The power and beauty of operant conditioning is that it requires the teacher-therapist to devise specific goals that are possible for that particular child to perform. The rule in operant training is to require children to perform a behavior that is only slightly better or one step nearer to the goal behavior than their current behavior. For example, the therapists seeking to train children to name objects might first reinforce mute autistic children if they say "uh" as a label for "ball," whereas in an echolalic child the therapist might reinforce only the single word "ball" in order to eliminate extraneous echolalia.

Every child is different and every autistic child has certain blocks in learning language. Some cannot even learn to label objects while others may finally learn complex speech. The success of speech therapy depends to a large extent on how complete the damage is to the central nervous system centers subserving speech. (Consult *The Language of Autistic Children* by Churchill[13] for the various modal and crossmodal deficiencies that underlie the speech deficiencies of autistic children.) In those children who do have the capacity for developing speech, part of the success of that development depends on the capacity of the central nervous system to elaborate anatomically as occurs with advancing age and part would depend on the skill of the therapist. It is my impression that nature deserves most of the credit for children who progress to creative communicative speech. However, the search for more efficient types of speech training should be pursued.

OTHER SYMPTOMS

Most efforts to decrease emotional distance and to increase positive social behaviors have come from studies carried out by adult therapists and their systematic use of reinforcement contingencies. However, Strain, Kerr, and Ragland[47] trained an "age-peer" (another child) to approach autistic children in a prescribed and sustained fashion. All autistic children so approached demonstrated increased social responsivity, which unfortunately was neither maintained nor generalized when the age-peer ceased the social approaches.

Although eye and face gaze behaviors are frequently thought to be reduced in autistic children, some research supports the idea that their eye gaze is qualitatively different rather than less in amount.[14] It is not necessary to develop face gaze before shaping other behaviors. Nevertheless, many investigators have developed methods for teaching eye contact before teaching other activities. First any spontaneous eye contacts by the child are reinforced, then verbalizations such as "Look at me" are introduced. Ultimately eye or face gaze can be chained to other behaviors.[13]

Mutual play with objects has been shown by Tiegerman and Primavera[48] to increase interaction between adults and autistic children. As Clark and Rutter[15] pointed out, when autistic children are left to do just what they please, they are most likely to engage in stereotypies, but when social demands are made, they are likely to respond socially. In general, when a certain performance is demanded, if that performance is possible—that is, within the child's mental age level—the child is more likely to perform and also to interact with the adult requesting the performance.

Another characteristic of autism, the tendency toward self-stimulation, seems to interfere with the acquisition of learning. Chock and Glahn[11] found this interference to be more of a problem in mute than in echolalic children. Physical punishment has been used to decrease such behaviors but these investigators have used effectively the word "No" and other prompts as less restrictive procedures.

The most difficult cases of self-stimulation to control are those in which the patients inflict severe self-injury, an activity that demoralizes families and interferes significantly with treatment procedures. Durand[21] found that a combination of haloperidol and mild punishment had more satisfactory results than either procedure applied singly in the case of a severely self-injurious retarded seventeen-year-old male.

Operant conditioning procedures also can be used effectively to toilet train autistic youngsters when they are ready neurologically for such control (see Foxx and Azrin[25] for details of training methods), to improve attending to various activities in home and schoolroom, and to improve eating behavior. Unfortunately, it is often of no benefit in cases of severe sleep disturbances, which can also be resistive to most medication.

The cognitive deficits of autistic children have been shown to be severe or profound in 40 percent of cases and moderate or mild in 35 percent. On perceptual-motor subtests, about 25 percent probably test in the normal or near-normal IQ range. It has always been the hope that increases in communication skills and social relationships would increase cognitive skills beyond what could be expected with the passage of time. DeMyer and associates[19] found that treatment (primarily of behavior modification type) seemed to be of some differential benefit to those with IQs over 60 at the beginning of therapy but not for those with IQs under 40. Unfortunately, in most cases even those children whose social skills improve remain mentally retarded. IQs measured in the pre-school years are predictive of outcome. The under-40 IQ children seldom make accelerated progress in mental age. Those children who do make such accelerated cognitive progress come from the over-60 IQ group, but not all in this higher-functioning group have a good prognosis for normal or near-normal cognitive function. About 1 to 2 percent of children diagnosed as autistic by an experienced clinician will function as normal adults. About 5 to 15 percent will be borderline normal and another 16 to 25 percent have a fair outcome. Unfortunately, over 50 percent have a poor outcome. [16]

ADOLESCENCE

With the advent of sexual maturity and growth in size to nearly adult levels, new treatment problems may arise. Compulsive, open masturbation, a not infrequent problem, can often be managed by teaching individuals to masturbate in their room. Increased aggression or even continuance of prior levels of aggression in adolescents of nearly adult size may make institutionalization mandatory. Frequently parents lose hope as they see a lack of progress sufficient enough for their psychotic child to support independent or even semiindependent living, and they seek an institutional placement. There is some evidence that, given enough supportive services, parents can maintain adolescents fairly comfortably in the home. However, as age and illness take their toll on the parents, invariably the moderate- to low-functioning psychotic person grown to adulthood must be cared for in some kind of institution.

In the last decade particularly, an important support service for parents of autistic children has been the National Association for Autistic Citizens (NAAC, 1234 Massachusetts Avenue, N.W., Suite 1017, Washington, D.C. 20005). The organization has been effective through local meetings and because of its influence in passage of legislation to provide special education facilities for autistic individuals. Parents generally find much help from hearing how practical child-care methods can alleviate symptoms in the child and stress in the family. They find that such practical advice comes from other parents and professionals who have a great deal of experience in dealing with the day-to-day behavior of psychotic children.

PHARMACOTHERAPY

Over the years since neuroleptic agents were introduced in the 1950s for the treatment of psychotic conditions, these agents have been tried repeatedly with psychotic children. Indeed, increasingly well controlled medication trials have interested many investigators. The number of these studies reached a peak between 1970 and 1974, when about thirty accounts appeared in the literature. In contrast, about half that number appeared from 1975 through 1979 and less than a handful from 1980 through the first half of 1984. This dramatic decline is probably due to several factors: (1) while there is evidence that some medications help some psychotic children, most often the improvement is modest and the medications frequently lose their efficacy after variable periods; (2) antipsychotic medications reduce the severity of delusions and hallucinations in childhood schizophrenia but are generally not of great value for cognitive and interpersonal symptoms; (3) side effects can be troublesome and potentially serious; and (4) medication studies are difficult to do properly and take much funding, which has diminished considerably in the last decade.

Several recent reviews* have discussed the problems of psychopharmacological research with psychotic children and described the relative efficacy of the various agents. These reviews can be consulted for original citations of early studies. Chlorpromazine hydrochloride, studied rather extensively for autistic populations in the 1950s and 1960s, was found to be oversedating but of some benefit for children who were hyperactive and anxious. During the 1970s and continuing into the 1980s, haloperidol was the subject of numerous trials. It has been compared to thioridazine hydrochloride, chlorpromazine, fluphenazine hydrochloride, operant conditioning, and placebo. In general, haloperidol was found to be better than placebo in reducing stereotypies, agitation, and social withdrawal; it was about equal in effectiveness to the other nonsedating neuroleptics but quicker in onset of action. Stimulants such as amphetamines were generally not helpful and seemed to cause an increase of disorganization in some children. The use of operant conditioning was better than haloperidol in eliciting imitative speech, but the introduction of haloperidol to the treatment regimen facilitated an increase of imitative speech. There was some evidence that 1 to 2 mg haloperidol per day was the optimal dose for most children. However, in clinical practice the dosage must be adjusted to the response of the individual child.

In comparison to trifluperidol (a close analogue of haloperidol) and chlorpromazine, thiothixine was demonstrated in one study to be as effective but possessing fewer side effects, while in another study side effects were similar for all three medications. Fish, Shapiro, and Campbell[24] gave evidence that severity of symptoms can influence the effectiveness of trifluoperazine hydrochloride. Children with greater language impairment showed greatest improvement over controls while taking the medication. In contrast, the more mildly impaired children did better without medication and with a structured nursery school program.

*See references 6, 7, 18, 33, and 38.

Other agents may have some limited uses. Imipramine hydrochloride was not found generally useful but may be of some benefit in retarded, mute, anergic, and borderline psychotic children, and lithium carbonate may help children who are aggressive and explosive. Molindone hydrochloride has been reported to lessen withdrawal and increase responsivity.

While nonsedating antipsychotic drugs may facilitate reduction of certain symptoms, they are not curative. Moreover, the side effects can be considerable. Among significant side effects are weight gain, ocular changes, tardive dyskinesia, and impaired learning, although Campbell and associates[8] have reported that haloperidol may facilitate learning. After withdrawal of neuroleptic medication, about 42 percent of those treated will develop temporary involuntary movements of their extremities, which in many cases are unlike the adult pattern of affecting predominantly the face and upper trunk. The sedative tranquilizers may produce seizures especially in children with a history of seizures or with focal neurological disorders. Thioridizine may be less likely than other medications to cause such extrapyramidal movements or seizures. Extrapyramidal symptoms generally rapidly abate when diphenhydramine hydrochloride (Benadryl) is administered. Werry[49] advises child psychiatrists to exploit the potential role of psychotropic drugs in the study of biological factors in child psychopathology.

No discussion of drug treatment would be complete without some mention of megavitamin therapy. Results of studies have been contradictory although some recent evidence supports vitamin B_6 (pyridoxine) combined with magnesium as having mild therapeutic effects in about 34 percent of autistic children.[35] However, Sankar[42] found no vitamin deficiencies in a group of 125 children admitted to an inpatient unit, which suggests that whatever therapeutic value pyridoxine and magnesium might possess may be due to other than nutritional properties. It is well to remember that in high doses (200 mg/kg/day in animals) pyridoxine is neurotoxic; indeed, in humans as little as 500 mg per day total dose over a period of months can be toxic.

The latest medication on the horizon for PDDs is fenfluramine hydrochloride. Ritvo's group[26] hypothesized that this substituted phenylethylamine reduces brain serotonin levels as it does blood levels. (See chapter 39 for a discussion of elevated blood levels of serotonin in autistic and mentally retarded patients). Controlled trials are now underway in several centers. Hopefully, fenfluramine will live up to its early promise of reducing agitation, screaming, stereotypies, and facilitate better use of the autistic child's cognitive abilities without introducing disabling side effects. Fenfluramine is not currently approved for children, and it should not be prescribed until its efficacy and toxicity are better elucidated in these multicenter studies.

In summary, pharmacotherapy for psychotic children at this point is largely a trial-and-error process. The nonsedating tranquilizers such as haloperidol and thiothixine are generally believed to relieve symptoms such as agitation, stereotypies, and hyperactivity better than sedating tranquilizers and stimulants.[1] However, as many a clinician can attest, stimulants such as methylphenidate may bring considerable help to individual cases and should be tried when antipsychotic medication fails. In most cases, psychoactive medication should be prescribed when environmental manipulation does not reduce symptoms and should be used in a pediatric population for the shortest feasible time because of its potential for adversely affecting the developing child. Neuroleptics can be expected to reduce or eliminate delusions and hallucinations for schizophrenia in childhood for variable periods.

Although most of the treatment literature of child psychosis is focused first on behavioral methods for autistic children and second on medication, we must not forget that many practitioners use methods reflecting a psychodynamic and psychoanalytic framework. However, little in the recent literature describes these types of treatment advances. Goldfarb[27] exemplifies one of the very few recent contributors telling how forty schizophrenic children changed for the better over three years of residence in a psychoanalytically oriented treatment and education program. Noteworthy was his finding that these children, despite their improvement, remained "quite aberrant by ordinary clinical criteria" and that they did not improve on five rating items that reflected neurobiological dysfunction. It is hoped that in the next decade psychotherapists and biological and operant therapists will pool their efforts to enhance and deepen our understanding of the basic deficits of psychotic children and thus allow us to upgrade the therapeutic efficacy of treatment programs.

REFERENCES

1. AMAN, M. G. "Stimulant Drug Effects in Developmental Disorders and Hyperactivity—Toward a Resolution of Disparate Findings," *Journal of Autism and Developmental Disorders*, 12 (1982):385–398.

2. BARRERA, R. D., and SULZER-AZAROFF, B. "An Alternating Treatment Comparison of Oral and Total Communication Training Programs with Echolalic Autistic Children," *Journal of Applied Behavior Analysis*, 16 (1983):379–394.

3. BEISLER, J. M., and TSAI, L. Y. "A Pragmatic Approach to Increased Expressive Language Skills in Young Autistic Children," *Journal of Autism and Developmental Disorders,* 13 (1983):287–303.

4. BENAROYA, S., et al. "Sign Language and Multisensory Input Training of Children with Communication and Related Developmental Disorders: Phase II," *Journal of Autism and Developmental Disorders,* 9 (1979):219–220.

5. BONVILLIAN, J. D., NELSON, K. E., and RHYNE, J. M. "Sign Language and Autism," *Journal of Autism and Developmental Disorders,* 11 (1981):125–137.

6. CAMPBELL, M., COHEN, I. L., and ANDERSON, L. T. "Pharmacotherapy for Autistic Children: A Summary of Research," *Canadian Journal of Psychiatry,* 26 (1981):265–273.

7. CAMPBELL, M., COHEN, I. L., and SMALL, A. M. "Drugs in Aggressive Behavior," *Journal of the American Academy of Child Psychiatry,* 21 (1982):107–117.

8. CAMPBELL, M., et al. "The Effects of Haloperidol on Learning and Behavior in Autistic Children," *Journal of Autism and Developmental Disorders,* 12 (1982):167–175.

9. CAPLAN, J., and WALKER, H. A. "Transformational Deficits in Cognition of Schizophrenic Children," *Journal of Autism and Developmental Disorders,* 9 (1979):161–177.

10. CARR, E. G., and KOLOGINSKY, E. "Acquisition of Sign Language by Autistic Children. II: Spontaneity and Generalization Effects," *Journal of Applied Behavior Analysis,* 16 (1983):297–314.

11. CHOCK, P. N., and GLAHN, T. J. "Learning and Self-Stimulation in Mute and Echolalic Autistic Children," *Journal of Autism and Developmental Disorders,* 13 (1983):365–381.

12. CHURCHILL, D. W. "Effects of Success and Failure in Psychotic Children," *Archives of General Psychiatry,* 25 (1971):208–214.

13. ———. *The Language of Autistic Children.* New York: John Wiley & Sons, 1978.

14. CHURCHILL, D. W., and BRYSON, C. Q. "Looking and Approach Behavior of Psychotic and Normal Children as a Function of Adult Attention or Preoccupation," *Comprehensive Psychiatry,* 13 (1972):171–177.

15. CLARK, P., and RUTTER, M. "Autistic Children's Responses to Structure and to Interpersonal Demands," *Journal of Autism and Developmental Disorders,* 11 (1981):201–217.

16. DEMYER, M. K. *Parents and Children in Autism.* Washington, D.C.: Victor H. Winston & Sons, 1979.

17. DEMYER, M. K., and GOLDBERG, P. "Family Needs of the Autistic Adolescent," in E. Schopler and G. B. Mesibov, eds., *Autism in Adolescents and Adults.* New York: Plenum Press, 1983, pp. 225–250.

18. DEMYER, M. K., HINGTGEN, J. N., and JACKSON, R. K. "Infantile Autism: A Decade of Research," *Schizophrenia Bulletin,* 7 (1981):338–451.

19. DEMYER, M. K., et al. "The Measured Intelligence of Autistic Children," *Journal of Autism and Childhood Schizophrenia,* 4 (1974):42–60.

20. DEMYER, W., and DEMYER, M. K. "Infantile Autism," *Neurologic Clinics,* 2 (1984):139–152.

21. DURAND, V. M. "A Behavioral/Pharmacological Intervention for the Treatment of Severe Self-Injurious Behavior," *Journal of Autism and Developmental Disorders,* 12 (1982):243.

22. FAY, W. H. "Personal Pronouns and the Autistic Child," *Journal of Autism and Developmental Disorders,* 9 (1979):247–259.

23. FERSTER, C. B., and DEMYER, M. K. "The Development of Performances in Autistic Children in an Automatically Controlled Environment," *Journal of Chronic Disease,* 13 (1961):312–345.

24. FISH, B., SHAPIRO, J., and CAMPBELL, M. "Long-term Prognosis and the Response of Schizophrenic Children to Drug Therapy: A Controlled Study of Trifluoperazine," *American Journal of Psychiatry,* 123 (1966):32–39.

25. FOXX, R. M., and AZRIN, N. H. *Toilet Training the Retarded: A Rapid Program for Day and Nighttime Independent Toileting.* Champaign, Ill.: Research Press Company, 1973.

26. GELLER, E., et al. "Preliminary Observations on the Effect of Fenfluramine on Blood Serotonin and Symptoms in Three Autistic Boys," *New England Journal of Medicine,* 307 (1982):165–169.

27. GOLDFARB, W. *Growth and Change of Schizophrenic Children: A Longitudinal Study.* Washington, D.C.: Victor H. Winston & Sons, 1974.

28. GUSTASON, G., PFETZING, D., and ZAWOKLOW, E. *Signing Exact English.* Rossmoor, Calif.: Modern Signs Press, 1972.

29. HARRIS, S. L., WOLCHIK, S. A., and WEITZ, S. "The Acquisition of Language Skills by Autistic Children: Can Parents Do the Job?" *Journal of Autism and Developmental Disorders,* 11 (1981):373–384.

30. HILL, L. F. "A Mother's Report of Effective Language Training," *Journal of Autism and Developmental Disorders,* 11 (1981):455–456.

31. HOLMES, N., et al. "Parents as Co-Therapists: Their Perceptions of a Home-Based Behavioral Treatment for Autistic Children," *Journal of Autism and Developmental Disorders,* 12 (1982):331.

32. HOWLIN, P. A. "The Effectiveness of Operant Language Training with Autistic Children," *Journal of Autism and Developmental Disorders,* 11 (1981):89–105.

33. ITIL, J., and SOLDATOS, C. "Epileptogenic Side Effects of Psychotropic Drugs," *Journal of the American Medical Association,* 244 (1980):1460–1463.

34. JANICK, M. P., LUBIN, R. A., and FRIEDMAN, E. "Variations in Characteristics and Service Needs of Persons with Autism," *Journal of Autism and Developmental Disorders,* 13 (1983):73–85.

35. LELORD, G., et al. "Effects of Pyridoxine and Magnesium on Autistic Symptoms—Initial Observations," *Journal of Autism and Developmental Disorders,* 11 (1981):219–230.

36. LOVAAS, O. I. *The Autistic Child: Language Development Through Behavior Modification.* New York: John Wiley & Sons, 1977.

37. LOVAAS, O. I., et al. "Some Generalizations and Follow-up Measures on Autistic Children in Behavior Therapy," *Journal of Applied Behavior Analysis,* 6 (1973):131–165.

38. MIKKELSEN, E. J. "Efficacy of Neuroleptic Medication in Pervasive Developmental Disorders of Childhood," *Schizophrenia Bulletin,* 8 (1982):320–332.

39. MIRENDA, P. L., DONNELLAN, A. M., and YODER, D. E. "Gaze Behavior: A New Look at an Old Problem," *Journal of Autism and Developmental Disorders,* 13 (1983):397–409.

40. NOBER, E. H., and SIMMONS, J. Q. "Comparison of Auditory Stimulus Processing in Normal and Autistic Adolescents," *Journal of Autism and Developmental Disorders,* 11 (1981):175–189.

41. RUNCO, M. A. and SCHREIBMAN, L. "Parental Judgments of Behavior Therapy Efficacy with Autistic Children: A Social Validation," *Journal of Autism and Developmental Disorders,* 13 (1983):237–248.

42. SANKAR, D. V. S. "Plasma Levels of Folates, Ribofla-

vin, Vitamin B₆, and Ascorbate in Severely Disturbed Children," *Journal of Autism and Developmental Disorders,* 9 (1979):73–82.

43. SCHAEFFER, B., et al. "Spontaneous Verbal Language for Autistic Children Through Signed Speech," *Sign Language Studies,* 17 (1977):287–328.

44. SCHOPLER, E., and MESIBOV, G. B. *Autism in Adolescents and Adults.* New York: Plenum Press, 1983.

45. SCHOPLER, E., MESIBOV, G., and BAKER, A. "Evaluation of Treatment for Autistic Children and Their Parents," *Journal of the American Academy of Child Psychiatry,* 21 (1982):262–267.

46. SMITH, D. E. P., et al. "The Effects of Improved Auditory Feedback on the Verbalization of an Autistic Child," *Journal of Autism and Developmental Disorders,* 11 (1981):-449–454.

47. STRAIN, P. S., KERR, M. M., and RAGLAND, E. U. "Effects of Peer-Mediated Social Initiations and Prompting/Reinforcement Procedures on the Social Behavior of Autistic Children," *Journal of Autism and Developmental Disorders,* 9 (1979):41–54.

48. TIEGERMAN, E., and PRIMAVERA, L. "Object Manipulation: An Interactional Strategy with Autistic Children," *Journal of Autism and Developmental Disorders,* 11 (1981):-427–438.

49. WERRY, J. S. "An Overview of Pediatric Psychopharmacology," *Journal of the American Academy of Child Psychiatry,* 21 (1982):3–9.

50. WING, J. K., and WING, L. A. "A Clinical Interpretation of Remedial Teaching," in J. K. Wing, ed., *Early Childhood Autism: Clinical, Educational and Social Aspects.* London: Pergamon Press, 1966, pp. 185–203.

58 / The Treatment of Eating Disorders

L. K. George Hsu

While the two eating disorders, anorexia nervosa and bulimia nervosa, share many common clinical features, the treatment needs of the patients are largely different. For the sake of clarity, the management of each will be addressed separately.

The Treatment of Anorexia Nervosa

The list of therapies that have been advocated for anorexia nervosa is lengthy,[28] but, as Bruch[9] pointed out more than ten years ago, these accounts of treatment efforts often reflect the exasperated frustration of being trapped in a battle of wills. Worse, the goals of the several therapies often are not clearly formulated, and short-lived gains are sometimes mistaken for lasting improvement. Thus, for instance, a suicide following weight gain in the hospital can hardly be regarded as indicating success in treatment.[3] Objective data are lacking to establish the long-term efficacy of any of the treatments[40,62]; so glaring a gap in our knowledge cannot be made up by bold assertions unsupported by critical and carefully conducted treatment research.[39,47] At present, the etiology of anorexia nervosa remains largely unknown (see chapter 40), and no single treatment method ensures long-term cure. As a result, treatment approaches are necessarily prag-

matic[62] and should be designed to address the major areas of dysfunction in this disorder.[36] Moreover, the treatment needs of individual patients may differ, and the needs of any given patient may change over the course of what is usually a long illness. Flexibility and sensitivity on the part of the physician are therefore essential, and treatment goals should always be clearly defined. Physicians who are confronted with an unwilling patient in danger of starving herself * to death are thus called upon to make a series of clinical decisions:

1. How can the patient and the family be engaged in treatment?
2. What investigations should be performed?
3. What are the major treatment goals?
4. Where should the patient be treated?
5. How can weight gain and the development of normal eating attitudes and behavior be induced?
6. How can relapse be prevented?

In the following section, the voluminous literature on the treatment of anorexia nervosa is reviewed according to this scheme.

ENGAGING THE PATIENT

The patient's denial of illness and her unwillingness to cooperate with treatment have been recognized since

---

*Females outnumber males by a 10 to 1 ratio for the eating disorders. Hence, the feminine pronoun is used throughout this chapter.

Gull[34] first described the condition in 1874. Engaging the patient as a collaborator is one of the most difficult of the many treatment tasks, and recently several authors have specifically addressed this issue.[12,28,36] The treatment alliance is probably best established by openly acknowledging the significance and meaning of the youngster's striving for thinness and control. At the same time the clinician addresses the negative and possibly dangerous effects of what the patient is doing —specifically, the depression, malnutrition and starvation, fatigue, insomnia, restlessness, social withdrawal, and constant preoccupation with food and exercising. The benefits of treatment should also be emphasized with the reassurance that treatment is not aimed at destroying the patient's specialness or control. An explanation of the effects of starvation and of the course and outcome of the illness may serve to dispel many misunderstandings. Several authors recommend a joint meeting with the patient and the family to discuss the illness and the specific recommendations for treatment.[12,16,28] Sometimes the cooperation of the family is a major determinant of whether the patient does or does not receive treatment. Garfinkel and Garner[28] also recommend books for the patient and the family to read.

Unfortunately, very little data exist as to what percentage of patients refuse treatment and what their outcome is. In Crisp's series, 30 percent of patients whose outcomes appeared to be poor nonetheless declined his offer of treatment.[42]

PHYSICAL AND PSYCHOLOGICAL EVALUATION

A full psychiatric evaluation to establish the presence of the characteristic "weight phobia," "fear of fatness," or "pursuit of thinness" is essential as atypical cases do not demonstrate this cardinal feature.[15,28,63] The psychiatric examination should determine also the presence or absence of other psychiatric symptoms, such as depression or obsessive-compulsive features. A careful history of family psychiatric illness is necessary also for treatment formulation.

Extensive endocrine and metabolic disturbances are seen in anorexia nervosa (see chapter 40), and careful evaluation may be necessary to rule out a primary organic syndrome. This is particularly important if the characteristic weight phobia is absent at the time of examination. An occasional (usually a chronic) patient may deny the weight phobia until she has actually gained weight. In all these cases, a careful physical evaluation is necessary. In addition to the physical and neurological examination, Casper[12] recommends a full range of investigations, including blood hematology and chemistry, urine analysis, plasma cortisol, liver and renal function tests, thyroid status; electrocardio-

gram (EKG) and electroencephalogram (EEG); skull and chest x-ray; and most of the pituitary hormone levels. In practice, the extent of the investigations will probably be determined by the actual indications based on the findings of the detailed physical and neurological examinations; at a minimum it should consist of the following: hematology including sedimentation rate (which is low in anorexia nervosa and may be helpful in distinguishing this condition from other causes of cachexia),[35] liver function tests, Tine test, and EKG and EEG. Consultation with an internist is advisable if abnormalities are found in the course of these investigations.

MAJOR TREATMENT GOALS

Practically all recent writers agree that the treatment goals should consist of both weight restoration and psychological improvement of major areas of personality dysfunction.* Since the work of Keys and his associates,[27,44] the psychological effects of starvation have been clearly established. During World War II, thirty-six male conscientious objectors between twenty and thirty-three years of age volunteered to participate in an experiment at the University of Minnesota to study the physiological and psychological effects of starvation. Prior to the experiment none of these subjects had any history of overtly abnormal eating attitudes or behavior, and all were of normal weight. They were placed on semistarvation diets for six months, which resulted in an average loss of 24 percent of original body weight. As time went on, many "anorectic" features appeared, such as intense preoccupation with food, "food fads," mixing unusual food combinations, "dawdling" over meals, hoarding food, cutting food into small pieces, compulsive gum-chewing, and increases in both smoking and consumption of coffee and tea. In four subjects bulimia occurred and was followed by remorse. A few of the men started stealing, and some reported vivid food-related dreams. Depression, poor concentration, narrowing of interests, social withdrawal, and irritability appeared in many of the subjects. Compared with their prestarvation baseline scores on the Minnesota Multiphasic Personality Inventory, the subjects showed elevation of the depression, hypochondriasis, and hysteria scales. It is thus suggested that many of the features of anorexia nervosa are a direct result of starvation, and the Minnesota study highlights the importance of nutritional rehabilitation in the treatment of this condition. That such anorexia nervosa symptoms improve with nutritional rehabilitation has been repeatedly demonstrated.[28,49,56]

*See references 9, 12, 16, 28, 36, and 62.

Practically all recent writers agree also that it is essential to treat the major areas of dysfunction such as the pursuit of slimness, the lack of a sense of competence, the misguided striving for individuality, and related family issues.[9,12,16,28] These writers agree also that both individual and family therapy should be instituted as part of the treatment.

The needs of chronic patients who have had many hospitalizations are complex, and the treatment goals more difficult to formulate. Injudicious or coercive treatment may precipitate depression and suicide.[16] For such patients, the greatest care and clinical acumen are needed in the formulation of treatment goals.

THE TREATMENT SETTING

Weight restoration and improvement in nutritional status are achieved most efficiently and rapidly within a structured inpatient treatment setting.[36] There appears to be general agreement among clinicians that inpatient treatment is necessary when weight loss is severe or when other physical or psychological complications are present.* However, there is less agreement as to whether an outpatient or inpatient treatment setting is the most effective in the long run or as to what the criteria should be for discharge to outpatient care, once the patient has been hospitalized. While there is relatively little dispute regarding the short-term benefits of inpatient treatment, the long-term gains are still in question.[42,49] There are, however, no studies that compare the relative effectiveness of inpatient versus outpatient treatment and what population of outpatients eventually requires inpatient treatment.[36] For practical reasons, most clinicians agree that inpatient care is necessary if the patient weighs less than 70 percent of her average weight.[12,28,50] In describing the way they work, however, Reinhart, Keima, and Succop[57] stated that "hospitalization is used only for brief separation of the child who is not eating from an anxious and frightened environment" (p. 117). Their claims of good results in almost all of their patients with an outpatient approach are notoriously difficult to evaluate.[62] At the minimum, inpatient treatment for an emaciated patient may be life-saving,[9,28] the amelioration of starvation symptoms with nutritional rehabilitation may make meaningful psychotherapy possible,[12,28,36] major complications may be treated, and the weight gain and improved eating behavior may encourage the establishment of a treatment alliance with the patient and the family.[47] Crisp[16] has long advocated that restoration to the patient's average weight for height at the onset of illness will allow the patient and the family to reex-

perience the existential issues that precipitated the psychobiological regression; such a restoration should therefore be a major goal of inpatient treatment. Others have aimed at restoration to an age-appropriate weight,[12,36] a low-average weight,[28] or gaining 50 percent of the weight needed to achieve an age-appropriate weight.[13] In the absence of controlled trials, the relative merits of each treatment approach cannot be evaluated. Outpatient therapy may be appropriate for those who are cooperative and whose illness is less severe (i.e., of shorter duration and without bulimia and vomiting)[36] and for patients who are reluctant to enter the hospital.[61]

WEIGHT RESTORATION

As Garfinkel and Garner[28] have pointed out, a variety of treatment methods are currently being recommended for weight restoration. Minor variation aside, they fall into five main categories, and are often used in various combinations: (1) nursing care and high-calorie diet with total or modified bed rest, (2) behavior modification, (3) coercive methods such as tube feeding and parenteral hyperalimentation, (4) psychotherapy, and (5) pharmacotherapy.

Within the hospital setting, a patient will usually eat the prescribed amount of food and gain weight provided the following conditions are fulfilled:

1. Weight restoration must occur in conjuction with other treatments, such as individual and family therapy,[12,16,28,50] so that the patient does not feel that eating and weight gain are the only goals of treatment.

2. The patient must trust the treatment team and believe that she will not be allowed to become overweight.[16,28,62]

3. The patient's fear of loss of control must be contained. This may be accomplished by having the patient eat frequent, smaller, balanced meals (around 400 to 500 calories per meal four to six times per day), so as to produce a gradual but steady weight gain (on average 0.2 kg per day).[16,28]

4. A member of the nursing staff must be present during mealtimes to encourage the patient to eat and to discuss the fears and anxiety over eating and weight gain.[16,28,62]

5. Gradual weight gain, rather than the amount of food eaten, must be regularly monitored (the patient should be weighed at regular intervals, the frequency varying from once a day to once a week, depending on the preference of the treatment team) and made known to the patient (information feedback), and some form of negative and positive reinforcement must exist, such as the use of a graduated level of activity and bed rest, whether or not these reinforcements are formally conceptualized as behavior modification techniques.[28,36] In this way the patient may learn that she can control not only her behavior but also the consequences of her behavior.

6. If they are suspected, the patient's self-defeating behav-

---

*See references 9, 12, 13, 16, 28, 50, and 61.

iors such as surreptitious vomiting or purging, must be confronted and ultimately controlled. [16,28,60]

7. The dysfunctional conflict between the patient and the family around eating and food must not be reenacted in the hospital with the treatment team. [36] If reenactment is allowed (such as in a therapeutic lunch session with the family), [47] its special purpose should be clearly defined and the fact that the treatment team itself does not reenact such dysfunctional conflict patterns with the patient should be reinforced. [16]

Using these principles, clinicians treating large numbers of anorectic patients have reported encouraging results for the vast majority of patients. [16,28,62] Two conclusions can be drawn from these results. First, in the vast majority of cases, a carefully planned, structured inpatient treatment program implemented by a competent treatment team is effective in bringing about weight restoration, and, second, pharmacotherapy and formal behavior therapy, coercive treatments, and overrestrictive measures such as locked rooms and depriving patients of bathing are usually unnecessary. Such measures should be used only in extremely refractory cases or where definite clinical indications are present, such as the symptoms of a major depression.

In this connection, it should be pointed out also that the rate of weight increase and the amount of food eaten or the number of mouthfuls of food eaten are not among the primary goals of treatment. Rapid weight gain in particular may induce a fear of loss of control in the patient and precipitate a depression. Increasing the amount or the number of mouthfuls of food eaten is hardly conducive to the development of normal eating habits and may inadvertently encourage the patient to overeat.

The development of more normal eating habits is encouraged by having the patient eat regular balanced meals. [12,28] Many clinicians give increasing responsibility to the patient as she improves, including allowing her to choose her own food, to eat in the hospital cafeteria rather than on the unit, and to eat outside of the hospital. There is no general agreement about when during the course of inpatient treatment this increase in autonomy and responsibility should take place. Thus, for instance, Collins, Hodas, and Liebman [13] discharged their patients after they had gained 50 percent of what was needed to achieve target weight, while Crisp [16] discontinued bed rest and increased the range of patients' activity very gradually, only *after* they had achieved their target weight. While no data exist to suggest the superiority of either practice over the other, both Morgan and Russell [49] and Hsu, Crisp, and Harding [42] found improved eating habits to correlate with normal weight maintenance.

The use of liquid food supplements during the early stages of refeeding has been advocated by several authors. [12,36,62] This may well be necessary for a small number of patients who are extremely fearful of certain foods and who are thus unable to tolerate a balanced meal consisting of solid food. However, it is probably more conducive to the development of normal eating habits if balanced regular meals are introduced as early as possible in the course of treatment. [28] The help of a dietitian in the actual planning of the meals is advisable.

Weight fluctuation usually is an early sign of vomiting or laxative abuse. Vomiting may be treated by closely monitoring the intake and output, by requiring the patient to be at bed rest after each meal, and by not allowing access to the bathroom for a suitable period of time (usually one hour) after each meal. [28,36,60] Laxative abuse may be treated similarly, with diarrhea being an additional warning sign. If constipation persists despite improved eating behavior, it should be treated with stool softeners and not by laxatives. [36]

PSYCHOTHERAPY

With the possible exception of Russell, [62] who advocated only nursing support, practically all researchers emphasize the importance of psychotherapy in the treatment of anorexia nervosa. Bruch, [7,9,11] Palazzoli, [51] Crisp, [16] Garner and Bemis, [30] and Halmi [36] have all found the traditional psychoanalytic approach rather ineffective. Bruch has written extensively on the theory and practice of psychotherapy in anorexia nervosa, [7,9,10,11] and her style of therapy arises directly out of her conceptualization of the illness. She found the traditional interpretive psychoanalytic approach had the effect of reinforcing the patient's pervasive feeling that someone else "knew what she herself did not know or feel." Emphasis was therefore placed on fact-finding and paying careful attention to and evoking awareness of the patient's own feelings, sensations, and ideas. Treatment is initiated by giving the patient a dynamic explanation of the meaning of the illness and explaining that the preoccupation with eating and weight is a cover-up for underlying problems and severe self-doubts. The patient is then invited to express her feelings and wants, and her right, even duty, to do so is spelled out. Such issues as the need to behave, to do what is expected, and to be perfect; the self-doubt and self-belittling; and the sense that her worth depends on other's approval and hence the basic mistrust despite the need to please are all addressed and then systematically worked through, with the ultimate goal being personality reorganization. Bruch emphasized also family therapy, not only to support and alleviate the family's anxiety so that treatment is not prematurely terminated but also to reevaluate family interactions and experiences. However, Bruch stated repeatedly that family therapy alone is unlikely to be sufficient. Crisp [16] shared this view and suggested that psychotherapy be directed as well at the anorectic patient's psychobiological regression, which serves to protect both the patient and the family from adolescent turmoil. However, Crisp has not described his psychotherapeutic techniques in detail.

Garner and Bemis [30] and Garfinkel and Garner [28] have described a cognitive-behavioral approach to the treatment of anorexia nervosa. Their careful and unassuming description of the treatment deserves special attention. In essence, their technique involves teaching the patients to examine the validity of their beliefs on a moment-to-moment basis. Beliefs such as selective abstraction, overgeneralization, magnification, dichotomous thinking, personalization, and superstitious thinking are examined first by helping the patient to define and operationalize them. Then they are challenged by the use of a variety of techniques, such as decentering, the "what-if" technique, and evaluation and modification of automatic thoughts and underlying assumptions. These authors identified a number of similarities between their own approach and Hilde Bruch's treatment methods. [30] Such similarities are interesting since each model is derived from different theoretical orientations regarding the nature of the illness and its etiology.

Minuchin and his coworkers approached the condition from a systems perspective (see chapter 40) and employ structural family therapy as their primary treatment design. In essence, the structural approach aims at changing the dysfunctional family structure that governs the transactions of the family members. [46,47] In anorexia nervosa, this structure includes enmeshment, rigidity, overprotectiveness, and failure of conflict resolution. The therapist is active and often directive and uses a variety of techniques such as joining, reducing resistance, relabeling, and enactment to change the structure, initially through unbalancing and dissolving the homeostatic dysfunctional pattern and later through reorganizing the family structure around more open and healthy communication. Throughout treatment, the therapist focuses on the interactional process as well as the content of communication, and in practice, many strategic and behavioral techniques are employed as well. Palazzoli [51,52] also conceptualized anorexia nervosa as a "systemic" illness, and prescribed strategic and at times paradoxical interventions for the family. These interventions are calculated to change the family epistemology without resorting to explanations, criticisms, or any other verbal interventions. Such strategies are therefore not formulated primarily for the purpose of promoting insight, awareness, emotional release, or personal growth, but instead are plans of action designed to replace old dysfunctional interaction patterns. Very little has been written about the use of other family therapy techniques such as psychoanalytic or behavioral approaches in the treatment of anorexia nervosa.

BEHAVIOR THERAPY

In 1972 Stunkard [66] described behavior modification as a new therapy for the eating disorders, and during the 1970s many articles appeared on the use of behavior therapy for the treatment of anorexia nervosa. [28] Operant strategies have proven effective in the short term, and weight gain is usually impressive.* Elkin and associates [23] found that information feedback, reinforcement, and meal size all produced weight gain and increased caloric consumption. Even physicians who do not conceptualize treatment in terms of behavior modification, such as Crisp [15] and Russell, [63] have used feedback in the form of weight charts, and this has become a central part of behavior therapy programs. [28] A variety of positive reinforcements may be employed, such as increased physical activity, visiting privileges, and social activities; each, or all of these, can be made contingent upon weight gain. With some of the more severely ill and resistant patients, negative reinforcements such as bed rest, isolation in bedroom, and tube or intravenous feeding may be resorted to. An individualized approach is clearly necessary as patients differ in their preferences; hence a detailed individual behavioral analysis is essential before the treatment program is implemented. The reinforcement for weight gain is usually given on a daily basis, and its timing is also important. One-half to one-quarter of a pound (0.1 to 0.2 kg) each day is a reasonable and safe amount of weight gain to expect. While increased meal size may be effective in inducing weight gain and caloric intake, it may also inadvertently heighten the patient's anxiety about loss of control and may indeed encourage overeating. Similarly, reinforcing caloric intake and the number of bites of food taken during each meal is unlikely to encourage normal eating behavior and should therefore be abandoned. Attempts at desensitization of the anxiety related to eating have not been particularly effective.

Most clinicians now include some form of behavior modification with the medical management of anorexia nervosa patients. [12,13,28,36] It is important to heed the advice of Garfinkel and Garner, [28] who caution that behavioral techniques should not be applied mechanically without regard to individual differences between patients or without careful consideration of possible unintended negative effects.

PHARMACOTHERAPY

Medication has been used in anorexia nervosa chiefly to induce weight gain and to treat the associated

*See references 1, 2, 3, 5, 22, 29, 38, and 53.

depression. As already mentioned, with a combination of good nursing care, behavioral management, and psychotherapy, the in-hospital weight gain is usually satisfactory. At the end of three months of inpatient treatment in a double-blind trial against placebo,[37] some evidence accumulated to suggest that both cyproheptadine hydrochloride and amitriptyline hydrochloride produced significant effects on both weight gain and depressed mood as measured by the Hamilton Rating Scale. In another double-blind trial, lithium carbonate was found to induce a more rapid weight gain than placebo.[33] In any case, the clinical relevance of rapid weight gain per se is uncertain, as it may have the effect of heightening the patient's fear. The long-term benefits of these medications are unknown. Chlorpromazine hydrochloride was first recommended in the late 1950s by Sargant and his associates, and in all probability it is still one of the most widely used medications.[21] Through its sedative effects it seems to reduce anxiety and resistance to eating and to promote bed rest.[19] It may also have a direct effect on weight gain.[58] Chlorpromazine, however, has significant side effects, including the occurrence of hypotension, hypothermia, and grand mal seizures. No controlled trial of the effectiveness of chlorpromazine exists, and the early studies used it in conjunction with bed rest and nursing care[20] or bed rest and psychotherapy.[14] In Dally and Sargant's series[19,20] it had no apparent long-term benefit; more recently Dally[17] has used it in only 50 percent of his patients.

Earlier, efforts had been made to use insulin based on the mistaken notion that anorectic patients have a true loss of appetite; such methods are now generally abandoned.[18] Minor tranquilizers also have been used and may reduce the anxiety related to eating and weight gain, but these agents are potentially addictive and their long-term effects uncertain.[28]

Antidepressants have been recommended on the grounds that depression is prominent in anorexia nervosa and that the condition may actually be a variant of major depression (see chapter 40). With the exception of the double-blind trial by Halmi, Eckert, and Falk,[37] most studies involve only a small number of patients and are uncontrolled. The efficacy of antidepressants in anorexia nervosa must therefore be regarded as preliminary, and they should be used clinically only when depression is clearly present.

In summary, the effectiveness of medication for this illness appears to be marginal in the short term and unknown in the long term. When the use of medication is being considered, the physician should formulate treatment goals clearly and consider whether the possible benefits (which are often short term and can usually be achieved without medication) will outweigh the side effects.

OTHER FORMS OF TREATMENT

Since many anorectic patients are still in their school years, the fact that hospitalization may take several months mandates the presence of psychoeducational support within the hospital. A special education teacher who works in close liaison with the school is probably the most effective means toward this end. The patient's perfectionistic, overachieving attitude should be dealt with in psychotherapy, although some limits may have to be set on how much time may be spent in doing schoolwork.[12,28] Vocational guidance may be necessary for the older teenager who is unsure about career choices. Expressive arts therapy, using drama, music, or painting, may be helpful where the patient has difficulty verbalizing feelings. Since many patients with this condition are socially inept and unassertive, social skills training may be useful either individually or in a group context. Pillay and Crisp[54] did not find social skills training beneficial, but their failure may have had more to do with the content and methods of their particular programs. Group therapy may sometimes exacerbate the intense competitiveness between anorectic patients and should be led by a skillful therapist.[28] All of these adjunctive treatments are best implemented as part of a structured treatment program for anorexia nervosa.

OUTPATIENT TREATMENT AND THE
PREVENTION OF RELAPSE

Relapse is common in anorexia nervosa, and about one-third to one-half of the patients will relapse within a year of discharge from the hospital.[40] Prevention of relapse is therefore one of the most difficult treatment tasks. Unfortunately, virtually no research has been conducted in this area, and the physician can be guided only by clinical judgement.

Following discharge, most clinicians recommend continuing long-term outpatient care. It has been found that in those patients who do recover, the course of the illness usually lasts about four years,[16] and continuing support is therefore necessary. The individual psychotherapeutic approaches described earlier form the mainstay of outpatient treatment. Body weight should be monitored regularly, and weight loss serving as a cover-up for underlying emotional issues should be confronted rather than avoided. Group therapy for support and assertiveness training for other forms of social skills training may all be helpful, but data in this area are lacking.[28]

Family therapy may continue also. Many self-help organizations have been formed, and membership in such groups may offer support and encouragement for the patient to continue with treatment. If a severe relapse occurs, further hospitalization may be necessary.[61]

Patients who are less severely ill may be treated as outpatients. These patients have been found to have a better outcome.[42]

The Treatment of Bulimia Nervosa

Clinicians treating a bulimic patient are to a large extent confronted with the same set of questions encountered in the treatment of anorexia nervosa. However, relatively little has been written about the treatment of bulimia nervosa. Here too the initial step consists of seeking to engage the patient as a collaborator, and a similar approach may be adopted that expresses both an understanding of the patient's need to gorge and remain slim and an awareness of the price paid through depression, shame, guilt, and physical ill-health. Treatment options may then be outlined.

The treatment goals in bulimia usually are as follows: (1) the elimination of the binge-vomit behavior, (2) the establishment of normal eating habits, and (3) the development of strategies and skills to cope with the kinds of life situations that had previously precipitated the binge-vomit episodes.

Patients will usually bargain for weight reduction, but it would appear that control of the bulimia and concurrent weight loss are difficult, if not impossible, to achieve.[45,65] For most of these patients Russell[63] recommends inpatient treatment in order to break the vicious cycle of bingeing and vomiting. There is no evidence, however, that this approach produces a long-term cure, and Russell himself has expressed some pessimism regarding the treatment outcome. Several researchers have conducted their treatment programs in an outpatient setting, and their preliminary results are encouraging.* Inpatient treatment is therefore usually held in reserve for patients who are suicidal, who feel that they have completely lost control over their eating and vomiting, whose metabolic disturbances require immediate inpatient treatment, or whose diagnosis is sufficiently unclear so as to require inpatient evaluation. It is not known how many bulimic patients drop out of treatment. Two surveys[26,43] found that only about one-third of the women studied had sought counseling or medical advice, and it is unclear how many completed treatment.

Two promising treatment approaches for bulimia have recently emerged: cognitive behavior therapy and the use of antidepressants. These approaches are par-

*See references 4, 24, 45, 55, 65, 69, and 71.

ticularly interesting in that they are derived from different conceptualizations of the disorder and are directed at different target areas.

COGNITIVE BEHAVIOR THERAPY

Several studies involving more than a few patients have found cognitive behavior therapy to be effective in the treatment of bulimia. The approach may be applied individually[24,25] or in a group.[4,45,65] Minor differences aside, these studies used a number of similar techniques to help the patient to gain control over and to be responsible for her eating behavior:

1. A treatment contract was developed, including an agreement to maintain current weight.
2. Dietary advice on eating balanced meals was provided.
3. Body weight was measured at each session.
4. A dietary journal was used to record intake daily and to note down feelings and thoughts in temporal sequence to the details of food consumed.
5. Strategies were developed to help patients avoid binge eating.
6. Alternative strategies were developed to help patients cope with those life situations that precipitate a binge.

Treatment results in these studies are encouraging; over 80 percent of patients responded to time-limited outpatient treatment with a significant decrease in the number of binge-eating episodes. Furthermore, improvement was largely maintained at short-term follow-up. All of these approaches are directed primarily at control of the bulimia. In a single case study, Rosen and Leitenberg[59] used response prevention (i.e., preventing vomiting after binge eating) and successfully treated a woman with bulimia. It would appear that preventing the bulimia and encouraging normal eating habits are probably more conducive to the development of a healthy pattern of eating.

PHARMACOTHERAPY

Early uncontrolled trials found phenytoin to be effective in treating bulimia.[31,32] In a double-blind, cross-over study, Wermuth and associates[70] found this agent to be significantly more effective than placebo; on the other hand, it produced moderate to marked improvement in only eight of nineteen patients (42 percent). Again, using a double-blind controlled six-week trial, Pope and colleagues[55] found imipramine hydrochloride to be vastly superior to placebo. Eight of nine patients on imipramine showed marked or moderate improvement, while only one of ten patients on placebo manifested a moderate degree of improvement. A significant reduction in depression, measured by the Hamilton Rating Scale, also occurred in the imipramine group. At one to eight months follow-up, eighteen of twenty patients who completed a trial of imipramine and/or another antidepressant showed moderate to marked improvement. In an open trial, Walsh and coworkers[69] found monoamine oxidase inhibitors to be effective in six bulimic patients. The improvement was accompanied by a reduction in Eating Attitudes Test score and a minimal body-weight change. It is unclear, however, whether these two studies also used dietary advice and other forms of self-monitoring of eating behavior. Brotman, Herzog, and Woods[6] carried out a retrospective study and found the response to antidepressants to be less encouraging; in particular, only about half of the patients responded, and 40 percent of those who did respond were found to have relapsed subsequently at follow-up. However, blood levels were not obtained and it is not known if the patients were receiving adequate doses of antidepressants. In their prospective observations, Brotman, Herzog, and Woods[6] found antidepressants to be effective but not strikingly so, although in their series blood levels of the antidepressants were not monitored. In an eight-week double-blind trial, Sabine and colleagues[64] failed to demonstrate any benefit of mianserin hydrochloride over placebo; however, the dropout rate was high in both groups, and it was unclear whether therapeutic drug levels were achieved in those receiving mianserin. In an open, uncontrolled trial, this author[41] used lithium carbonate to treat fourteen bulimic patients; twelve patients responded with a marked to moderate reduction in binge-eating episodes. Improvement was largely maintained at six- to sixteen-month follow-up. Behavior therapy and some form of self-monitoring were employed with more than half of the patients in this study. Despite the relatively small number of patients involved and the various methodological problems, all the findings just cited suggest strongly that antidepressants may be effective in the treatment of bulimia. Although their mode of action remains unknown, it seems that they do decrease the dysphoria that is usually an identified antecedent to binging.

In summary, it would appear that most normal-weight bulimic patients may be treated successfully as outpatients. While both cognitive behavior therapy and the use of antidepressants appear to be effective, the relative effectiveness of the two approaches are unknown. It would seem that even in those patients who are treated with antidepressants, some form of behavioral self-monitoring is probably still necessary.

Outcome of the Eating Disorders

Several review articles have recently appeared on the outcome of anorexia nervosa.[28,40,68] In terms of body weight, the long-term outcome is generally encouraging, with about 75 percent of patients achieving a normal weight; in terms of social and sexual adjustment, however, the outcome is less favorable. About 5 percent of patients die from the illness.

Regarding bulimia nervosa, long-term outcome studies are lacking. Over the short term (i.e., one to three years after treatment), the results appear to be encouraging in that most patients who improve with treatment are able to maintain their improvement. In both disorders, formal evaluation of treatment effectiveness is still lacking and is urgently needed.

REFERENCES

1. AGRAS, S. and WERNE, J. "Behavior Modification in Anorexia Nervosa," in J. P. Brady and H. K. H. Brodie, eds., *Controversy in Psychiatry*. Philadelphia: W. B. Saunders, 1978, pp. 655–675.

2. BHANJI, S., and THOMSON, J. "Operant Conditioning in the Treatment of Anorexia Nervosa," *British Journal of Psychiatry,* 124 (1976):166–172.

3. BLINDER, B. J., FREEMAN, D. M. A., and STUNKARD, A. J. "Behavior Therapy of Anorexia Nervosa: Effectiveness of Activity as a Reinforcer of Weight Gain," *American Journal of Psychiatry,* 126 (1970):1093–1098.

4. BOSKIND-LODAHL, M., and WHITE, W. C. "The Definition and Treatment of Bulimarexia in College Women—A Pilot Study," *Journal of the American College Health Association,* 27 (1978):84–97.

5. BRADY, J. P., and REIGER, W. "Behavior Treatment of Anorexia Nervosa," in T. Thompson and W. S. Dockens III, eds., *Proceedings of the International Symposium in Behavior Modification.* New York: Appleton-Century-Crofts, 1972.

6. BROTMAN, A. W., HERZOG, D. B., and WOODS, S. W. "Antidepressant Treatment of Bulimia," *Journal of Clinical Psychiatry,* 45 (1984):7–9.

7. BRUCH, H. "Perceptual and Conceptual Disturbances in Anorexia Nervosa," *Psychosomatic Medicine,* 24 (1962):187–194.

8. ———. "Psychotherapy in Primary Anorexia Nervosa," *Journal of Nervous and Mental Disease,* 150 (1970):51–67.

9. ———. *Eating Disorders.* New York: Basic Books, 1973.

10. ———. "Psychological Antecedents of Anorexia Nervosa," in R. A. Vigersky, ed., *Anorexia Nervosa.* New York: Raven Press, 1977, pp. 1–10.

11. ———. "Anorexia Nervosa: Therapy and Theory," *American Journal of Psychiatry,* 139 (1982):1531–1538.

12. CASPER, R. C. "Treatment Principles in Anorexia Nervosa," *Adolescent Psychiatry,* 10 (1982):431–454.

13. COLLINS, M., HODAS, G. R., and LIEBMAN, R. "Interdisciplinary Model for the Inpatient Treatment of Adolescents with Anorexia Nervosa," *Journal of Adolescent Health Care,* 4 (1983):3–8.

14. CRISP, A. H. "A Treatment Regime for Anorexia Nervosa," *British Journal of Psychiatry,* 112 (1965):505–512.

15. ———. "Diagnosis and Outcome of Anorexia Nervosa," *Proceedings of the Royal Society of Medicine,* 70 (1977):464–470.

16 CRISP, A. H., et al. "Clinical Features of Anorexia Nervosa," *Journal of Psychosomatic Research,* 24 (1980):197–191.

17. DALLY, P. "Anorexia Nervosa: Do We Need a Scapegoat?" *Proceedings of the Royal Society of Medicine,* 70 (1977):7–11.

18. DALLY, P., and GOMEZ, J. *Anorexia Nervosa.* London: Heineman, 1980.

19. DALLY, P. J., and SARGANT, W. "A New Treatment of Anorexia Nervosa," *British Medical Journal,* 1 (1960):1770–1774.

20. ———. "Treatment and Outcome of Anorexia Nervosa," *British Medical Journal,* 2 (1966):793–795.

21. DALLY, P. J., OPPENHEIM, G. B., and SARGANT, W. "Anorexia Nervosa," *British Medical Journal,* 2 (1958):633.

22. ECKERT, E. D., et al. "Behavior Therapy in Anorexia Nervosa," *British Journal of Psychiatry,* 134 (1979):55–59.

23. ELKIN, M., et al. "Modification of Caloric Intake in Anorexia Nervosa," *Psychological Reports,* 32 (1973):75–78.

24. FAIRBURN, C. G. "A Cognitive Behavioral Approach to the Management of Bulimia," *Psychological Medicine,* 11 (1981):707–711.

25. ———. "Binge Eating and Its Management," *British Journal of Psychiatry,* 141 (1982):631–633.

26. FAIRBURN, C. G., and COOPER, P. J. "Self-induced Vomiting and Bulimia Nervosa: An Undetected Problem," *British Medical Journal,* 1 (1982):1153–1155.

27. FRANKLIN, J. C., et al. "Observations on Human Behavior in Experimental Semi-starvation and Rehabilitation," *Journal of Clinical Psychology,* 4 (1948):28–45.

28. GARFINKEL, P. E., and GARNER, D. M. *Anorexia Nervosa: A Multidimensional Perspective.* New York: Brunner/Mazel, 1982.

29. GARFINKEL, P. E., MOLDOFSKY, H., and GARNER, D. M. "The Outcome of Anorexia Nervosa: Significance of Clinical Features, Body Image and Behavior Modification," in R. A. Vigersky, ed., *Anorexia Nervosa.* New York: Raven Press, 1977, pp. 315–329.

30. GARNER, D. M., and BEMIS, K. "A Cognitive Behavioral Approach to Anorexia Nervosa," *Cognitive Therapy and Research,* 6 (1982):1–27.

31. GREEN, R. S., and RAU, J. H. "Treatment of Compulsive Eating Disturbances with Anticonvulsant Medication," *American Journal of Psychiatry,* 131 (1974):428–432.

32. ———. "The Use of Diphenylhydantoin in Compulsive Eating Disorders: Further Studies," in R. A. Vigersky, ed., *Anorexia Nervosa,* New York: Raven Press, 1977, pp. 377–382.

33. GROSS, H. A., et al. "A Double-blind Controlled Trial of Lithium Carbonate in Primary Anorexia Nervosa," *Journal of Clinical Psychopharmacology,* 1 (1981):376–381.

34. GULL, W. "Anorexia Nervosa (Apepsia Hysterica, Anorexia Hysterica)," *Transactions of Clinical Endocrinological Metabolism,* 49 (1874):805–809.

35. HALMI, K. A. "Anorexia Nervosa: Recent Investigations," *Annual Review of Medicine,* 29 (1978):137–148.

36. ———. "Treatment of Anorexia Nervosa," *Journal of Adolescent Health Care,* 4 (1983):47–50.

37. HALMI, K. A., ECKERT, E., and FALK, J. R. "Cyproheptadine for Anorexia Nervosa," *Lancet,* 1 (1982):1357–1358.

38. HALMI, K. A., POWERS, P., and CUNNINGHAM, S. "Treatment of Anorexia Nervosa with Behavior Modification," *Archives of General Psychiatry,* 32 (1975):93–96.

39. HOGAN, C. C. "Psychodynamics," in C. P. Wilson, ed., *Fear of Being Fat.* New York: Jason Aronson, 1983, pp. 115–128.

40. HSU, L. K. G. "Outcome of Anorexia Nervosa—A Review of the Literature (1954–1978)," *Archives of General Psychiatry,* 37 (1980):1041–1046.

41. ———. "Treatment of Bulimia with Lithium," *American Journal of Psychiatry,* 141 (1984):1260–1262.

42. HSU, L. K. G., CRISP, A. H. and HARDING, B. "Outcome of Anorexia Nervosa," *Lancet,* 1 (1979):61–65.

43. JOHNSON, C. L., et al. "Bulimia: A Survey of 509 Cases of Self-reported Bulimia" in P. L. Darby, et al., eds., *Anorexia Nervosa: Recent Developments in Research.* New York: Alan R. Liss, 1982, pp. 159–172.

44. KEYS, A., et al. *The Biology of Human Starvation, vols. 1 and 2.* Minneapolis: University of Minnesota Press, 1950.

45. LACEY, J. H. "Bulimia Nervosa, Binge Eating, and Psychogenic Vomiting: A Controlled Treatment Study and Long-term Outcome," *British Medical Journal,* 1 (1983):1609–1613.

46. MINUCHIN, S. *Families and Family Therapy.* Cambridge, Mass.: Harvard University Press, 1974.

47. MINUCHIN, S., BAKER, L., and ROSMAN, B. L. *Psychosomatic Families: Anorexia Nervosa in Context.* Cambridge, Mass.: Harvard University Press, 1978.

48. MINUCHIN, S., et al. "A Conceptual Model of Psychosomatic Illness in Children," *Archives of General Psychiatry,* 32 (1975):1031–1038.

49. MORGAN, H. G., and RUSSEL, G. F. M. "Value of Family Background and Clinical Features as Predictors of Long-term Outcome in Anorexia Nervosa," *Psychological Medicine,* 5 (1975):355–371.

50. MORGAN, H. G., PURGOLD, J., and WOLBOURNE, J. "Management and Outcome in Anorexia Nervosa: A Standardized Prognosis Study," *British Journal of Psychiatry,* 143 (1983):282–287.

51. PALAZZOLI, M. S. *Self-Starvation.* New York: Jason Aronson, 1974.

52. PALAZZOLI, M. S., et al. "Family Rituals: A Powerful Tool in Family Therapy," *Family Process,* 16 (1977):445–453.

53. PERTSCHUK, M. J. "Behavior Therapy: Extended Follow-up," in R. A. Vigersky, ed., *Anorexia Nervosa.* New York: Raven Press, 1977, pp. 305–313.

54. PILLAY, M., and CRISP, A. H. "The Impact of Social Skills Training for Anorexia Nervosa," *British Journal of Psychiatry,* 139 (1981):533–539.

55. POPE, H. G., et al. "Bulimia Treated with Imipramine: A Placebo-controlled, Double-blind Study," *American Journal of Psychiatry,* 140 (1983):554–558.

56. QUAERITUR. "Treatment of Anorexia Nervosa (Letter)," *Lancet,* 1 (1971):908.

57. REINHART, J. B., KEIMA, M. D., and SUCCOP, R. A. "Anorexia Nervosa in Children: Outpatient Management," *Journal of the American Academy of Psychiatry,* 11 (1972):114–132.

58. ROBINSON, R. G., McHUGH, P. R., and FOLSTEIN, M.

F. "Measurement of Appetite Disturbances in Psychiatric Disorders," *Journal of Psychiatric Research,* 12 (1975):59–68.

59. ROSEN, J. C., and LEITENBURG, H. "Bulimia Nervosa: Treatment with Exposure and Response Prevention," *Behavior Therapy,* 13 (1982):117–124.

60. RUSSELL, G. F. M. "Anorexia Nervosa—Its Identity as an Illness and Its Treatment," in J. H. Price, ed., *Modern Trends in Psychological Medicine,* vol. 2. London: Butterworths, 1970, pp. 131–164.

61. ———. "General Management of Anorexia Nervosa and Difficulties in Assessing the Efficacy of Treatment," in R. A. Vigersky, ed., *Anorexia Nervosa.* New York: Raven Press, 1977, pp. 277–289.

62. ———. "The Present Status of Anorexia Nervosa," *Psychological Medicine,* 7 (1977):353–367.

63. ———. "Bulimia Nervosa: An Ominous Variant of Anorexia Nervosa," *Psychological Medicine,* 9 (1979):429–448.

64. SABINE, E. J., et al. "Bulimia Nervosa: A Placebo-controlled Double-blind Therapeutic Trial of Mianserin," *British Journal of Clinical Pharmacology,* 5 (Supplement) (1983):195–202.

65. STEVENS, E. V., and SALISBURG, J. D. "Group Therapy for Bulimic Adults," *American Journal of Orthopsychiatry,* 54 (1984):156–161.

66. STUNKARD, A. "New Therapies for the Eating Disorders," *Archives of General Psychiatry,* 26 (1972):391–398.

67. STURZENBERGER, S., et al. "Anorexia Nervosa—An Affective Disorder?" *Archives of General Psychiatry,* 34 (1977):1087–1093.

68. SWIFT, W. J. "The Long-term Outcome of Early Onset Anorexia Nervosa," *Journal of the American Academy of Child Psychiatry,* 21 (1982):38–46.

69. WALSH, B. T., et al. "Treatment of Bulimia with Monoamine Oxidase Inhibitors," *American Journal of Psychiatry,* 139 (1982):1629–1630.

70. WERMUTH, B. M., et al. "Phenytoin Treatment of the Binge-eating Syndrome," *American Journal of Psychiatry,* 134 (1977):1249–1253.

71. WHITE, W. C., and BOSKIND-WHITE, M. "An Experimental-behavioral Approach to the Treatment of Bulimarexia," *Psychotherapy: Theory, Research and Practice,* 18 (1981):501–507.

59 / Treatment of Adolescent Substance Abuse

John E. Meeks

Introduction

Psychiatrists have had great difficulty in dealing effectively with substance abuse. In 1937 Knight[4] said of alcoholism, "among psychiatrists themselves, however, there has been no unanimity of opinion as to either etiology or treatment" (p. 538). Almost fifty years later the same statement could be made in regard to drug dependency in general.

A wide range of treatment methods have been utilized. Medications have been given, ranging from LSD and antidepressants to disulfiram (Antabuse). Psychotherapy in many forms, including psychoanalysis, has been utilized to a somewhat more limited extent due to the difficulty of gaining the drug-dependent patient's cooperation. However, psychiatrists who have worked in institutional settings—hospitals, drug treatment centers, and other residential placements—have garnered considerable experience with the management of these patients.

Paralleling and, in some locations, replacing psychiatric care for these patients is treatment extended by self-help groups such as Alcoholics Anonymous (AA),

Narcotics Anonymous (NA), and Straight, Incorporated. From a statistical point of view, these treatment groups probably care for the vast majority of people with substance abuse problems. Unfortunately, the programs in these highly effective organizations tend to emphasize acts of faith derived from prior successful intervention with the substance-abusing adolescent or adult. Although this gives the program the power of intense conviction, it also tends to produce a degree of inflexibility. In addition, the programs are not designed for drug-dependent individuals who have serious psychiatric problems or, indeed, even for some substance-abusing adolescents who are not psychiatrically disturbed. This represents a more serious drawback in programs for adolescents than in those designed for adult abusers. Many adult programs are characterized by self-referral at the outset and subsequent easy exodus. These qualities protect them from much potential mismatching of adult patient and program. Teenagers, on the other hand, are often required to remain in the assigned program whether or not it is a good match for their needs.

The treatment approach presented in this chapter will propose and expand on a program combining elements of traditional psychiatric treatment with techniques derived from the recovery principles of AA and its associated groups.

Clinical Evaluation

Drug-abusing adolescents are a heterogeneous lot. With each patient there are a number of issues that must be addressed by the evaluating psychiatrist. The first concerns the role of chemical agents in producing the presenting clinical picture. The basic question is whether or not the adolescent has arrived at a point where drugs have become the primary source of pleasure, the sole basis for maintenance of self-esteem, and the chief motivation for activity. In short, the evaluation seeks to determine whether drugs have become more important than people in the adolescent's life.

It is important to underline that gaining a clear and accurate picture of an adolescent's drug use is quite difficult. First of all, for internal psychological reasons that will be discussed more fully later, adolescents tend to deny and minimize the extent of drug use. In addition, in an effort to escape treatment at the earliest possible moment, they may lie about the seriousness of their drug involvement. Finally, youngsters deeply involved in drugs have become so accustomed to deceit that, when faced with an adult asking questions regarding drug habits, lying is almost habitual. For these reasons at various points in the course of the patients' treatment it is usually necessary to obtain several drug histories. As a rule, as youngsters progress and become more hopeful of the possibility of sustaining a drug-free life, these accounts become more accurate.

The drug history should contain a good deal of data. For example, at what age did the youngster begin to use drugs? This is important information since those who begin drug use at a very early age are more likely to be psychiatrically impaired than those who begin in midadolescence. The age may be obtained with more reliability by inquiring "How young were you?" in lieu of asking "How old were you?" In addition, the regular and substantial use of drugs causes a disruption of the learning process and socialization patterning, which further disturbs the developmental process. Youngsters who begin drug use in their elementary school years are usually quite disturbed, and the drug use deepens and widens their disability.

What kind of drugs have the youngsters used and at what times in their lives? The choice of specific drug seems to be less important than had been initially assumed. Some youngsters do have clear drug preferences, which may suggest important areas of conflict or personality deficiency. For example, those with a strong preference for amphetamines or other stimulants may be more depressed and ambitious than their peers who prefer marijuana. However, the vast majority of adolescents who are heavily involved in drugs tend to use alcohol and marijuana. In part, this is because of the ready availability of these two substances, and in part it is due to their general acceptability within the culture.

In addition to describing the choice of specific agents, it is useful to observe the longitudinal pattern of unfolding drug involvement. Some youngsters show a clear progression with movement toward more drugs and heavier use, while others maintain a more steady pattern. Rapid progression in drug ingestion is a cautionary sign that suggests a more malignant course. The specific drug history will also influence the expected process of detoxification, potential side effects, and, to some extent, the likelihood of relapse. For example, marijuana is retained within the body for several weeks because of its affinity to body fat. In order to experience a truly drug-free state, a patient would have to be abstinent for a month. However, for the same reason, withdrawal symptoms are subtle and very gradual in onset.

In general, withdrawal effects are the mirror image of drug effect. That is, withdrawal from stimulants tend to produce states of drowsiness, apathy, fatigue, and depression, while withdrawal from depressant drugs such as barbiturates, alcohol, and benzodiazepines tends to cause restlessness, insomnia, nightmares, irritability, and even seizures. In adolescents these effects are often masked by behavior, as are other kinds of adolescent distress. The youngster in detoxification is reluctant to ascribe discomfort to drug withdrawal since that would suggest to everyone that he or she was, in fact, addicted. Major physical withdrawal complications such as seizures or delerium tremens are reported rarely in adolescents.

In the case of phencyclidine (PCP) and the hallucinogenics, the management problems relate not to withdrawal but to extended states of intoxication, which may last days to weeks with behavioral features that resemble psychosis. The management of states of intoxication and withdrawal symptoms in adolescents is supportive. Vitamins, especially vitamin C, and careful nutrition support the rapid return to normal functioning that characterizes adolescents once abstinence is achieved. Small doses of benzodiazepines rapidly tapered over seventy-two hours, may be needed occasionally for extreme restlessness or agitation in youngsters withdrawing from heavy doses of central nervous system–depressant drugs.

From a long-range treatment perspective, there do not appear to be important dynamic differences between youngsters who use particular agents. Switching from one agent to another is common. Sometimes the change is prompted by a desire to try something new, the urgings of a friend, or simple availability. The basic focus seems to be on the state of intoxication rather than fine distinctions between drug effects.

In addition to a careful assessment of drug use, all youngsters deserve a thorough psychiatric evaluation. This should include a detailed developmental and family history, a careful mental status, psychological testing, and, in particular, an in-depth evaluation of their patterns of peer relationship. For some adolescents, the detailed assessment of friendship patterns is particularly informative both in helping to understand the genesis of the severe drug use and, to some extent, in planning their treatment and predicting the prognosis. A rather high percentage of substance-abusing adolescents are shy, isolated individuals who, prior to their discovery of chemical assistance, were unable to feel comfortable in groups. With the drugs, they have found a way not only to calm their social anxiety but to have access to an endless source of conversation and a sense of commonality with their drug-using friends. All this permits them, often for the first time in their lives, to achieve a sense of belonging. Associated with this peer group membership is a strongly welcomed sense of independence from their parents. As a consequence of their previous overattachment to their parents, they often exaggerate their emancipation and present themselves as extremely maverick and unconventional (as they cling desperately to their new "friends"). As Wikler[9] and others have pointed out, the addict is addicted not only to the chemical agent but to a life-style that includes a particular array of social settings along with the drug-using friends. To state it another way, the disturbance is far more pervasive than merely the fact that the adolescents take drugs. What it comes down to is that they frequently view themselves as being part of "the drug scene," and this becomes an important portion of their identity.

For many of these youngsters psychological testing may be necessary to determine the presence and degree of any subtle brain damage produced by the drug use as well as to dismiss or confirm the existence of learning disabilities and other cognitive defects that often predate substance abuse. Often enough these cognitive defects have gone unrecognized and untreated, resulting in repeated failures with predictable damage to self-esteem. Many youngsters who are heavy users of drugs have themselves recognized defects in their recent memory, ability to concentrate, and other higher mental functions. As a result they have deep fears that they have injured their brains. Here too, as in other psychiatric syndromes, psychological testing may also be valuable in helping to sort out basic psychopathological dynamics and areas of strength that could be built on in psychotherapy.

As is true for any adolescent patient, family and developmental history are crucial. In most instances, the adolescent who has turned heavily to drug use has experienced important developmental vulnerabilities that have increased the attractiveness of this practice. Eventually these problems will need to be addressed, even though this may have to be delayed until the acute drug problem is remedied. The sequence of treatment here is important. Adolescents may view excessive attention to the underlying psychological etiology at the time of intensive treatment for the drug problem itself merely as further permission and justification for continuing the self-destructive drug use.

The family history is important because of the frequency with which extensive patterns of depression and chemical abuse are encountered in immediate and distant family members. A history of chemical dependency in the parent or other family members, and the adolescent's exposure to that behavior, should be carefully documented. It is important also to evaluate the extent to which the parents have been drawn into typical patterns of "enabling" the adolescent's continued drug use. In many cases, there exist family attitudes and reactions toward the substance-abusing adolescent that permit or even encourage continued drug use.[8]

The Question of Abstinence

When it comes to the treatment of youngsters who use drugs excessively, there are two schools of thought. One perspective recommends treating the drugs as one symptom of a general psychiatric problem, pointing out the negative impact of the chemical agents on the adolescent's life and on the therapy process but maintaining a primary focus on more basic psychological issues including the patient's feelings, relationship to the therapist, and general adaptation. The theoretical position is that as the supportive therapy relationship begins to meet some of the patient's emotional needs and the interpretive work relieves some of his or her conflicts, the drugs will be easier to forgo.

The second line of thought states that drug abusers are incapable of forming a genuine therapeutic relationship. Hence when most of the patient's emotional investment is directed toward obtaining and continuing to use the chemical substance, abstinence is necessary for treatment to proceed constructively. Therapists committed to this viewpoint suggest that with the first type of psychotherapist, much of the motivation for continuing in therapy is that patients learn many good reasons why they have a right to continue using drugs.

The difficulty in resolving this issue is probably related to the fact that there is a wide range of individuals with substance abuse problems. Indeed, it would be unusual these days to encounter a seriously disturbed adolescent who is not also involved in self-medication with a variety of psychoactive street drugs. For many of these teenagers, this is only a stop-gap measure, and, when effective psychotherapy is offered, they are quite prepared to turn away from the drugs and to a person. The confusing aspect is that this group of patients includes a number of adolescents who at least for a period of time use drugs very heavily and who talk as though they are deeply invested in the drug culture.

On the other hand, it is true also that many of the adolescents who are deeply dependent on drugs to maintain their functioning cannot relate to a therapist. These drug-dependent youngsters secretly view everyone who opposes their drug use as an enemy, including their therapist and their parents. Such adolescents are probably treatable only within an abstinent framework where some of their underlying depression, yearnings for human contact, and defective self-regard can be expressed openly and therapeutically encountered.

Although it may not be possible always to separate these two groups of patients without a trial of treatment, a careful diagnostic study as described previously can offer many clues. The profile of an adolescent who might respond to traditional psychotherapy without an insistance on early abstinence would include the following factors:

1. Late beginning of drug use—preferably not before middle adolescence.
2. History of maintaining relationships and continued contact with at least some "straight" friends.
3. Clear presence of a continuing interest in conventional ambitions even if these have been somewhat disrupted by drug use.
4. Continuation of basic positive relationships with parents.
5. Ambivalence about drug use and some recognition of its destructive impact on his or her life.
6. Motivation for therapy and evidence of positive attachment to the therapist.

Obviously, the obverse of these findings would present adolescents who had started drugs early, seemed totally committed to a deviant life-style, rejected "materialistic" goals, were vague or nihilistic about their future, were alienated from their family, and showed little positive interest in psychotherapy. These adolescents would probably require specialized inpatient drug treatment or an outpatient program that had the capacity to monitor and enforce abstinence.

Outpatient Therapy of Adolescent Substance Abuse

The outpatient psychotherapy of drug-using adolescents poses many problems. The degree of supervision, structure, and limit setting that are often necessary for successful treatment may be difficult to provide in outpatient settings. However, as described previously, a number of adolescents who use drugs are still candidates for traditional psychotherapy and should be approached in that way. It is important, however, to maintain a high index of suspicion, particularly if the patient's performance seems unusually erratic and there are many inexplicable mood changes and regressions in the therapeutic effort. Careful attention to the possibility that these alterations are the result of a return to heavy drug use must be kept in the forefront of therapeutic consideration. Obviously, if this drug use is occurring without open discussion in the therapy session then the treatment approach is severely compromised.

However, a certain number of seriously involved drug-abusing adolescents can be treated in an outpatient setting if the treatment plan is designed for their specific needs. The treatment should include their participation in group work with other youngsters with similar problems, attention to defective socializing skills, monitoring of abstinence through drug urine checks, close contact with the parents, and drug counseling and education presented by individuals properly trained in those skills.

For adolescents with serious chemical dependency, group work is of special importance. As mentioned earlier, many of them have poor peer relations, and what little they do have tends to center around obtaining and using drugs as the primary interactional mode. Hence an extremely important part of a well-designed treatment plan for these adolescents is support, reinforcement, and social stimulation of a group oriented toward abstinence and emotional growth. As a rule, some educational groups and recreational activities are useful. These patients have limited positive skills in the use of leisure time and yet desperately need social contacts. For this reason, provision of adequate opportunities for interaction is also necessary. This means that if they are to have any hope of offsetting the temptations of substance abuse and the seductions to reentry into the drug-oriented peer group, the youngsters will need to be involved in a treatment activity of some kind for three or four days of the week.

Group work of this kind often is greatly strengthened by the use of trained drug counselors, particularly those who are recovered from a drug problem of their own. Recovered counselors provide an understanding and sensitivity to the drug-abusing adolescent that is difficult for the nonaddicted professional to gain. This sensitivity, by the way, includes a healthy skepticism and alertness to the possibility that the adolescent is leaning again toward drug use. In the author's experience the recovered drug counselor has a generous dose of what Levine[5] used to call benevolent skepticism. There are also obvious potential dangers to the use of such staff. Drug abuse is a chronic illness, and the recovering addict functioning as a counselor may relapse. Most programs require an extended period of successful drug-free life as a qualification for employment.

The random use of drug urine screens not only provides information that can be utilized in case youngsters have succumbed to drug use but also, perhaps of greater importance, provides structure, a clear statement of the desire for abstinence, and a face-saving excuse for adolescents who really wish to remain abstinent anyway. These youngsters can tell their drug-using friends, "I'd be glad to smoke with you but those clowns at my program will be checking my urine."

In addition to the formal group therapy and drug counseling just described, it is usually wise to arrange for drug-using adolescents to become involved in NA and/or AA and to encourage this as strongly as possible. Finding the proper group, one that is running reasonably smoothly and yet contains a population with which the specific adolescents will feel at home, requires some research. It is another area where the recovered drug counselors can be extremely helpful.

Even for severe drug abusers, individual psychotherapy is an important element in the treatment.[10] Most of these youngsters, even when they become free of drug use, continue to have serious individual and family problems. As they gain control over their compulsive drug use, their interest and ability in addressing these problems increase. In addition, there is an appropriate depression and grieving that results from giving up the "pseudosolution" of drug use. Though it has been viciously destructive to their lives, in many cases adolescents still view the drug as a lost "friend" and support. As time passes, the psychotherapy of these patients becomes more and more traditional except for one important factor. The therapist must recognize that substance abuse is a chronic illness and that faced with new or unusual stresses, even including developmental advances, there is a significant risk that even well-treated youngsters may once again relapse into chemical use. This should not be viewed as a failure of treatment. The therapist needs to be very clear on this

point, since often the family and the adolescents will need strong support to view the occurrence as a temporary setback rather than as proof that patients had made no genuine gains.

Family therapy is a crucial part of outpatient treatment.[8] Therapists who work with chemically dependent people have noted a particular pattern of family involvement in the substance abuse as such. While usually condemning the drug use, the family behaves in ways that permit or even encourage the patient to continue using drugs. Firm limits are not set. Subtle messages of pessimism and acceptance of the addictive state are given verbally and nonverbally to the patient. This complex of behaviors is known as enabling. Its importance is shown not only with substance-abusing adolescents but in studies of wider populations of adolescents.[6] Since youngsters are living at home in outpatient therapy, a close working alliance with the parents in support of youngsters treatment is particularly important.

Education and orientation are an important first step in engaging these families as allies in the treatment effort. Many drug treatment programs offer extended "marathon" training and treatment groups to families soon after an adolescent's admission. Parents also benefit from reading factual and understandable books about the problem and its treatment. One that has gained wide acceptance is *Getting Tough on Gateway Drugs: A Guide for the Family* by DuPont.[3]

Multiple family groups consisting of the parents and the children of two or three families are an effective treatment modality for this group of patients. The mutual support, confrontation around enabling behavior, and sense of shared accomplishment are effective antidotes to the tendency toward nihilism, cynicism, rejection, and regression that are ever present dangers in these cases. Some families also benefit by joining Al-Anon, Tough Love, or other community parent peer groups that provide support and information to the parents.

Inpatient Treatment of Adolescent Substance Abuse

Many adolescents who seriously abuse substances will require a period of inpatient treatment. In outpatient programs, patients can be asked to abstain and can be monitored for compliance. However, many seriously drug involved youngsters would not even pretend that they intended to abstain even though objective judgment would suggest that they are destroying their lives through massive drug use. However, in spite of their conscious rejection of treatment, these adolescents often utilize an inpatient experience in an extremely constructive fashion. It is as though they had no hope that any positive life experience outside of the drug culture was conceivable. However, if they are forced to have a positive experience without drugs, they can then recognize the many negative elements that they had been denying and utilize treatment constructively.

There are two kinds of inpatient drug treatment programs. One is the hospital program, which tends to be relatively brief, highly intense, and oriented primarily toward detoxifying the patient, breaking through massive resistance, and introducing family and patient to the possibility of effective treatment. This type of program usually requires two to three months of inpatient care followed by referral either to a structured outpatient program or to one of the longer term residential programs to be described.

The other is the long-term residential drug center. These centers tend to be modeled along the lines of the therapeutic community concept in drug treatment. They aim toward a total reorientation of the client's life based on a residential stay of one to several years. In contrast to the hospital programs, which are heavily staffed with professionals, in these programs the residents take important treatment responsibility for one another and provide most of the direct care.

In the hospital programs, family treatment is crucial. Ultimately, the family will either be charged with the direct care of the adolescent if he or she is referred to outpatient therapy or it will need to throw its strong support behind the residential treatment program (often in the face of the adolescent's strong resistance) if that is the course of action recommended following the hospitalization. Many hospital programs have found that families are best involved with an initial intense educational and therapeutic exposure lasting two to four days, as was mentioned earlier. This total immersion in a "marathon" has the effect of quickly bonding the families. It brings them to recognize the similarity of their problems, provides extensive factual information about drug use, and introduces them to the concept of enabling within a supportive framework. Following this extensive introduction, families are often more cooperative, have a better understanding of treatment issues and goals, and in general feel less guilty and more prepared to provide help and assistance to drug-involved adolescents. Following the marathon, the strategy invoked may be either single-family or multigroup-family treatment, depending on the availability of personnel and their skills and training.

Adolescents in inpatient treatment require even more thorough evaluation than that described earlier. Since they do represent the more severe end of the drug-using spectrum, many of these youngsters may experience severe reactions to drug withdrawal. Compared to adult addicts, in the past there was a tendency to perceive withdrawal for adolescent drug abusers as a relatively symptom-free experience. However, growing evidence suggests that adolescents simply deal with the pangs of withdrawal through atypical behavior patterns. This is similar to the alloplastic expression of symptoms adolescents display in regard to other psychic pain. During withdrawal adolescents may become massively depressed or irritable and angry, may complain only of multiple psychosomatic disabilities, or may become extremely paranoid and suspicious. Invariably, however, they fail to relate any of these feelings to the absence of drug intake. Although we still have a great deal to learn about the meaning of these various manifestations of withdrawal in adolescents, the therapist should be aware of them and alert to the possibility that some early untoward responses to hospitalization may in fact be disguised symptoms of drug withdrawal.

Effective inpatient treatment programs provide a variety of services to adolescent drug users, including active and ongoing drug education groups. These education groups are designed to cover in a predetermined number of sessions (sixty in most facilities) important information about drug use, including its pharmacology, possible side effects, effect on human relationships and on learning behavior, and any other information that adolescents need to know about drugs and their impact on people. The tone of these sessions is matter of fact and nonjudgmental, and no effort is made to introduce scare tactics or horror stories of negative outcome of drug use. In fact, as the program continues, one can rely on the adolescents themselves to provide numerous cautionary tales. It is important also to keep this program interesting by having guest speakers, employing films and videotapes, and providing opportunities for discussion. Since adolescents may enter and exit the program at any point, depending on their admission date, the presentations must be so designed that each session is self-contained. In other words, the adolescents come and go as they need the services of the hospital, but the sequence repeats itself regularly every sixty days.

Most effective programs are organized in the form of a therapeutic community supported by confrontational groups of some kind. The goal is to provide constructive and usable feedback to teenagers regarding the impact of their attitudes and behavior on those around them. These portions of the program are important also in teaching adolescents how to be self-assertive and confrontative with others without becoming violent or abusive in the process.

Many programs find that a number of drug-abusing adolescents desperately need social skills training. Accordingly, the settings often provide groups designed to help youngsters identify and express feelings, begin to trust others, acquire simple living skills, learn the usages of basic courtesy, get some sense of expected behavior in dating situations, and have some chance for assertiveness training. [1,2,7] These assist adolescents in becoming more effective at having needs met by people rather than by depending on chemicals.

Finally, traditional psychotherapy, both individual and group, is an important element of the treatment process. However, it is essential that psychotherapy be focused in support of the overall effort to help adolescents gain control of their dangerous substance abuse. For this reason it is important that psychotherapy be directed by mental health professionals who truly understand the nature of addiction, including the fact that even if it was initially an effort at self-medication, at some point it becomes the primary illness.

Summary Comments

The treatment of adolescents who are seriously involved with chemical abuse is a relatively recent undertaking. It is an area where two ideologies—the views of the Alcoholics Anonymous and other recovery groups and those of traditional psychiatry—have clashed to some extent. But it has become increasingly clear that adolescent victims of drug dependency need the expertise that has been acquired from both of these sources. This is crucial because in many cases, adolescents who severely abuse substances behave like addicts and require specific treatment for their substance abuse. At the same time, few of such adolescents appear even remotely normal when drugs are removed from their lives. This is partly a result of the preexisting emotional problems that made them more vulnerable to substance abuse and partly a consequence of the impact of drug use on psychological development during the teenage years.

REFERENCES

1. BRADY, J. P. "Social Skills Training for Psychiatric Patients, I: Concepts, Methods and Clinical Results," *American Journal of Psychiatry,* 141 (1984):333.

2. ———. "Social Skills Training for Psychiatric Patients, II: Clinical Outcome Studies," *American Journal of Psychiatry,* 141 (1984):491.

3. DuPont, R. L., JR. *Getting Tough on Gateway Drugs: A Guide for the Family.* Washington, D.C.: American Psychiatric Press, 1984.

4. KNIGHT, R. P. "The Psychodynamics of Chronic Alcoholism," *Journal of Nervous and Mental Disease,* 86 (1937):538.

5. LEVINE, M. "Principles of Psychiatric Treatment," in F. Alexander and H. Ross, eds., *The Impact of Freudian Psychiatry.* Chicago: University of Chicago Press, 1952.

6. McDERMOTT, D. "The Relationship of Parental Drug Use and Parents' Attitudes Toward Drug Use to Adolescent Drug Use," *Adolescence,* 19 (1984):89.

7. STRAVYNSKI, A., MARKS, I., and YULE, W. "Social Skills Problems in Neurotic Outpatients," *Archives of General Psychiatry,* 39 (1982):1378.

8. WEGSCHEIDER, S. *Another Chance.* Palo Alto, Calif.: Science and Behavior Books, 1981.

9. WIKLER, A. "Conditioning Factors in Opiate Addiction and Relapse," in H. Schaffer and M. E. Burdass, eds., *Classic Contributions in the Addictions.* New York: Brunner/Mazel, 1981, pp. 339–351.

10. ZINBERG, N. E. "Addiction and Ego Function," *Psychoanalytic Study of the Child,* 30 (1975):567.

60 / Alternative Mental Health Services for Youth

Milton F. Shore

Introduction

The late 1960s and early 1970s was a time of turbulence and upheaval in the United States. Part of the temper of the times was the almost religious fervor of an ideology that challenged established social structures and institutions. This ideology arose in response to what was perceived as massive dehumanization; the new outlook was characterized by attitudes that were antiwar, antiauthority, antibureaucracy, antigovernment, and antiprofessional. The ideological push was particularly visible among many young people who felt that society was not being responsive to their needs and concerns. In particular, many of the young felt even more threatened and became increasingly alienated from various social settings and, especially, from established helping services. A great many retreated into drugs, alcohol, and indiscriminate sexual behavior. Some ran away from home; they ended up hungry and penniless, and driven to engage in antisocial behavior in order to survive. Others developed a counterculture and established alternative social arrangements such as cults and communes.

It was out of this matrix of social turmoil that alternative mental health services for youth arose. Although opposition to tradition had become a rallying cry, there were serious and important questions being raised about the delivery of mental health services. These were especially cogent in respect to certain unserved and underserved populations, particularly in the highly industrialized nations. Indeed, some of the issues raised by the new movement had already been addressed by a few traditional organizations. These agencies were identified with the public health philosophy of the community mental health movement; they, too, spoke for placing helping services in storefronts, encouraged outreach programs, and developed new emergency mental health units.

Alternative mental health services for youth began in the late 1950s when some mental health professionals became interested in children from middle-class families who had run away from home, only to become involved in drugs, illicit sexual behavior, and delinquency. It was not until 1967, however, that the first center for runaways was set up in the Haight-Ashbury Region in San Francisco.

There was an explosive growth of drug problems among the young; this created a demand that services be developed to stem the tide of personal breakdown and social disorganization. The result was the sudden proliferation of alternative services of different types and highly varying quality—telephone hot lines, free clinics, street clinics, rap groups, drop-in centers, crisis centers, walk-in clinics, information centers, runaway houses, shelters, specialized crisis foster homes—that sprang up all over the country and that tended to be located in storefronts, churches, abandoned buildings, old schools, donated houses, and even mobile vans.

The services offered in these settings ranged widely —counseling; cognitive therapy; housing; referral; advice; supportive therapy; advocacy; outreach; concrete legal, medical, educational, and employment help; recreation; psychodrama; social work assistance; and even yoga and bodybuilding. (It is of considerable interest that long-term individual psychotherapy, which has been associated with more traditional approaches, was rarely offered in these settings.)

Characteristics of Alternative Services

Although the types, functions, and settings for alternative services varied widely (both in the United States and in Europe), all were characterized by four main features: accessibility, flexibility, comprehensiveness, and advocacy.

ACCESSIBILITY

In order to reach a group that was or that felt underserved and that was suspicious of those services that were available, accessibility had to be increased.

Thus a major theme of the alternative mental health services was to make the help they offered easily accessible. Traditionally, mental health services tended to be located in formal institutional settings such as hospitals and/or schools; in contrast to this, alternative services were usually established in the local community within walking distance of their clientele, or where public transportation was easily available. The setting itself was informal, and usually equipped with used furniture (often donated by interested community residents). Staff members were young and casually dressed; this was part of a deliberate attempt to reduce the status barriers that they believed existed in the usual doctor-patient relationship. The involved professionals were critical of the lack of mental health services at other than daytime hours; the alternative services were accordingly open twenty-four hours a day, seven days a week; if the center itself was not open at certain times telephone hotlines were available. To encourage their use, the services were tendered free of charge; insurance forms or other third-party reimbursements were eliminated. The availability of care was fostered as well by the fact that there were no scheduled appointments; the client was offered the opportunity to walk in any time of the day or night. Moreover, there were no restrictions by diagnostic group—anybody who sought help was seen. Thus many adolescents on drugs, suicidal individuals, draft evaders, gays, psychotic youth, unwed pregnant teenagers, and others in trouble with the law or with any degree of emotional upset felt free to contact these services. Contacts were fostered as well by eliminating any formal records and by maintaining strict confidentiality even to the point of permitting total anonymity. Thus youngsters below legal age had access to help without obtaining parental permission.

FLEXIBILITY

Alternative mental health services prided themselves on being extremely flexible. The lack of time restrictions (a person could walk in and be seen or talked to anywhere from a few minutes to many hours) made it possible to resolve many difficult situations on the spot. There were no intake procedures and no concern about diagnosis; the focus was on immediate problem solving. Those who could not come in to the "clinic" were seen in other settings—on street corners or at home. Schedules were adjusted to meet immediate needs, and emphasis was placed on moving from one service element to another as needs arose.

COMPREHENSIVENESS

Alternative mental health services were comprehensive along two dimensions: They used a variety of mental health approaches—individual psychotherapy, group therapy, family therapy, Gestalt therapy, and even transcendental meditation; in addition, they offered a comprehensive range of resources—medical (internists and gynecologists), educational (tutors), legal (lawyers), employment (vocational counselors), recreational (group workers), social services (social workers), and/or counseling (mental health workers). These were often located within the same physical setting, and the basic philosophy was a multidimensional, multidisciplinary, holistic approach. The several services and approaches were mixed and matched in various combinations in order to meet the immediate needs at a given point in time.

ADVOCACY

In the course of the last two decades, a major new element introduced into the mental health delivery system has been mental health advocacy. The advocacy role of alternative mental health services took many forms: Those providing these services regarded the interpretation of problems of youth to parents and the society and, more specifically and concretely, to other more formal and traditional youth-serving agencies as one of their major responsibilities. Based on their belief of a right to service, alternative services undertook vigorous case advocacy, actively seeking services for those adolescents who came to them. For example, after referrals had been made by a worker, there would often be a follow-up to check that the person had, indeed, followed through. (In one European country adolescents were sent to various agencies anonymously in order to check on whether an agency was carrying out its stated mission. Agencies were then rated as to their responsiveness to young people's problems.) When services were not available, the alternative program would press for and even act to facilitate their establishment. Alternative services also encouraged their clients to engage in political action. Thus they constantly fostered consumer input and activity. A

major focus was the empowerment of those who were outside the mainstream and in need of help. Teenagers were encouraged to establish self-help groups and to participate in building resources that could help others. Many of the ideas generated by the alternative service movement have now become a large, and active, part of the consumer movement in mental health—for example, the skyrocketing rise in the number and size of self-help and mutual help groups.

Legitimization of Alternative Services

Alternative mental health services for youth began as a reaction to established traditional approaches; during the 1970s, however, they gained legitimacy in a number of ways.

Because of the high visibility of drug abuse among runaways, local, state, and federal governments began to fund alternative youth services in great part through drug abuse agencies. However, a major step in the national acceptance of alternative services occurred in 1974 with the passage of the Runaway Act (now called the Runaway and Homeless Youth Act) as part of the Juvenile Justice and Delinquency Act of that year. The act is administered through what is now the Department of Health and Human Services (formerly the Department of Health, Education, and Welfare). It has funded a number of runaway centers across the country. Currently, many alternative services have in fact accepted public funds, but there has been concern expressed by some that they might lose their autonomy. Moreover, they feared that any association with government might prevent many disturbed youth from seeking help. Nevertheless, with survival at stake and private funds inadequate to run the programs (even with the very large number of volunteers available), it was necessary for many of these services to accept government funding. At the same time, public funding agencies changed their requirements. They sought ways to make the money more available to those groups that had shown themselves capable of reaching the many young people who were not being served by other agencies in the community.

In 1975 the American Psychiatric Association Joint Information Service did a national survey of alternative services; this involved studying fourteen selected programs in depth.[4] They concluded that the services were, on the whole, of high quality and that they were staffed by extremely dedicated individuals who understood how mental health services might be provided to many adolescents who were extremely difficult to help.

The survey teams noted that the staff did not reject mental health professionals if these professionals expressed an interest and desire to help the programs undertake new directions. Indeed, there was a great wish for training on the part of these committed staff members, with many programs developing carefully thought out steps, selection procedures, and innovative staff strategies for dealing with suicides, drug addiction, abortion, family violence, homosexuality, and other behaviors.

In 1973 the World Health Organization Regional Office for Europe undertook a study of alternative youth services [6] that formed the basis for two European conferences. [7,8] The situation was not altogether comparable because, unlike the United States, Eastern and Western European countries had highly developed national health and welfare services. Instead of regarding these services out of the mainstream, the European countries considered them to be a natural development of ways of reaching youth who were responding to the extreme stress of a rapidly paced, impersonal, industrial society. The government agencies, therefore, referred to these arrangements as "youth advisory services" and encouraged and funded them nationally, frequently through the ministries of recreation, education, and/or social welfare rather than through the governmental health ministry. Because of this encouragement by the larger society, many of these programs were afforded an opportunity to develop along unusually innovative lines. [5]

Adding to the legitimacy of alternative mental health services for youth was the interest of many young mental health professionals who identified with their ideology and offered their time and their expertise, often gratis, to these programs. Many of these highly trained younger people served as important links between the more traditional academic settings in which they had been prepared and the new, sometimes daring, direction of the alternative setting.

The importance and value of alternative services was also recognized in 1978 when the President's Commission on Mental Health set up a special study of this area. The report [1] covers the breadth and scope of alternative services, summarizing the statistics available at that time. Recommendations were made for expanding the scope, number, and breadth of alternative services and for strengthening their financial base.

Effectiveness of Alternative Service

How effective have alternative services been? Unfortunately, there is a paucity of hard data regarding the effectiveness of most of our mental health programs. Since they are more diverse, more informal, and more wide-ranging, the evaluation of alternative services is even more difficult. Nonetheless, evidence suggests that alternative services were able to reach many youths who felt alienated and who would not have made use of any of the existing mental health services. Studies of those who called in to hotlines, for example, suggested that the issues for which the adolescents sought help ranged from such minor difficulties as loneliness and boy-girl relationships, to the most severe problems involving pyschosis, drug overdose, and violence. Most of those using alternative services had multiple problems. A study of information given by hotlines found that these communications were of high quality, pertinent, and of great value. [2] Indeed, the quality of care at these alternative services has been high enough to qualify many of them as settings for the placement of trainees from well-known academic programs in the core mental health disciplines.

Contribution of Alternative Services

A number of the alternative youth programs established in the 1960s and 1970s no longer exist. Some have been absorbed by or become part of more established agencies; others have disappeared for other reasons. A number of alternative mental health services are still in operation, although over the decade even these have changed their focus or their *modus operandi*. In any case, alternative mental health services for youth have made a significant contribution to the field of mental health. Their language has now become part of the terminology of mental health service delivery—hotlines, crisis centers, rapping, and so forth. Traditional services have accepted the challenge of flexibility and comprehensiveness and developed programs for youth, especially for the so-called unreachable, underserved groups. These include outreach, educational and vocational services, shelters, and others. The influence on other developmental levels has been great for we now have shelters for battered women, hotlines for the aged, and rape crisis centers.

Another contribution has been a new direction for mental health. There has been a notable expansion of the boundaries of interaction between the mental health field and the educational, legal, medical, and social service systems. Major efforts are being made to coordinate and integrate different service elements, often under the auspices and lead of mental health. New holistic and ecological models have arisen and are being put into practice.

A third contribution has been the expansion of the range of mental health services from preventive and health-promoting activities through therapeutic and rehabilitative care. Networks of service have been fostered. Self-help groups have emerged and become an important part of the mental health service network. Peer counseling and nonprofessional helping services have expanded into schools and agencies. Students in mental health training now have more experience in working with others and are more aware of the challenges of working with difficult groups. There is a greater focus on consumer orientation, and major efforts are being made to adapt and change services in order to meet consumer needs in a better way.

The alternative mental health services movement has also confronted mental health professionals with the need to rethink a number of issues. These include the role of the professional, of the community, and of the consumer in the mental health service delivery system. For example, recent research has shown that even disturbed young people, given the opportunity to assist and help others, can show major personal growth and development.[3] (This is particularly likely to work if they are carefully supervised and appropriately reimbursed.) This "helper principle," particularly in adolescence, seems to be an important new direction for the young.

Above all, alternative mental health services for youth have served to reinforce the need for mental health workers to think about more general issues of social policy and service delivery. Mental health professionals are recognizing more and more the role that social policy plays in molding the nature of mental health practice. Fee for service, third-party payments, the profit motive, the legal status of adolescents, all are factors that play a major role in determining whether, and how, health and mental health services become available to the young, and what these services must be. We need to study various social policy issues in order to identify and to change those forces that serve to limit and constrain our efforts to help these distressed and disturbed young persons and their families.

REFERENCES

1. "Alternative Services—A Special Study," in *The President's Commission on Mental Health,* vol. 2. Washington, D.C.: U.S. Government Printing Office, 1978, pp. 376–410.

2. BLEACH, G., and CLAIBORN, W. L. "Initial Evaluation of Hotline Telephone Crisis Centers," *Community Mental Health Journal,* 10 (1974):387–394.

3. GARTNER, A., KOHLER, M. and RIESSMAN, F. *Children Teach Children.* New York: Harper & Row, 1971.

4. GLASSCOTE, R. M., et al. *The Alternate Services: Their Role in Mental Health.* Washington, D.C.: Joint Information Services, 1975.

5. SHORE, M. F. "Innovative Mental Health Programs for Youth in Six European Countries," *Journal of Clinical Child Psychology,* 4 (Spring) (1975):7–9.

6. WORLD HEALTH ORGANIZATION, Regional Office for Europe. *Patterns of Youth Advisory Services.* Copenhagen: World Health Organization, 1977 (Document ICP/MNH 016 III).

7. ———. *Youth Advisory Services.* Copenhagen: World Health Organization, 1976 (Document ICP/MNH 016 III (1)).

8. ———. *Objectives of Youth Advisory Services.* Copenhagen: World Health Organization, 1978 (Document ICP/MNH 035 III).

SECTION VI

Prevention

Irving N. Berlin / Editor

Introduction

Irving N. Berlin

In Volume IV of the *Basic Handbook of Child Psychiatry,* we described definite areas of primary and secondary prevention with infants, young mothers, and specific age groups in our population. The role of crisis intervention as a preventive effort was presented.

In this volume, the section on prevention deals with the increased knowledge base arising from epidemiological studies. This allows us to examine data that can be utilized to understand mental health problems in various populations. The collaborative neurological study, the Isle of Wight study, the twenty-five-year Children of Kaui epidemiological research project, and other such undertakings all point to a methodology for examining specific developmental, neurological, or psychiatric phenomena in a population over time. Among other issues, Richard W. Brunstetter emphasizes that these studies may assist in determining possible specific preventive interventions which could lead us to greater effectiveness in averting disability in certain populations.

The research in early infant intervention programs with a "high-risk" population is described by Stanley Greenspan and Karl R. White. I describe the implications of working with the parents of children and adolescents with chronic disease in order to reduce invalidism, to enhance their functioning, and to achieve more normal development.

Shirley B. Lansky and Nancy U. Cairns describe therapeutic efforts that are necessary in work with children and adolescents who are recovering from cancer

or are in a state of extended remission. Dealing with the fear of recurrence and helping families to live more normally in the face of uncertainty over long periods of time are mental health problems that have important implications for the prevention of both disequilibrium in the families and developmental disorders for the child and adolescent patients.

Dorothy Otnow Lewis reviews the recent biological and neurophysiological variables that may influence delinquent behaviors. Along with this, the simultaneous review of data about psychosocial developmental issues which affect violent behavior in adolescence is of great interest to us. These findings are especially notable in light of the new understanding of developmental disturbances and treatment methods for addressing the problems of borderline and narcissistic personalities (based on self psychology as defined by Kohut, Kernberg, Masterson, and others).

Notman and associates review the current programs that seek to enhance the health and capacity for nurturance of pregnant teenagers. I present some pilot efforts to prevent some of the depression, alcoholism, inhalant abuse, and suicide that are prevalent among adolescents in some American Indian communities.

Taken together, this update on prevention illustrates the directions of new research and the possible effectiveness of interventive measures that may significantly avert difficulties for the child and adolescent populations.

61 / Epidemiology and Child Psychiatry

Richard W. Brunstetter

Epidemiology is the study of the rates of occurrence of disorders within populations or subpopulations whose common features may be of causal significance. It is a science basic to public health and prevention. Until recently it has been more widely applied within the realm of general medicine than it has in psychiatry. The past decade, however, has witnessed the advent of DSM-III and the development of standardized instruments and computerized approaches to data analysis. As a result, many of the methodological problems that impeded progress in the past have begun to be solved. To date, there have been fewer studies carried out in child psychiatry than in general psychiatry but even here the work of such individuals as Lee Robins[15] and Michael Rutter[22] and the landmark investigations on the Isle of Wight[22] and Kauai[29] have begun to demonstrate the impact that the powerful tools available to epidemiology can have on the field.

Basic Concepts

Before proceeding further, a definition of certain key terms may be helpful.

- *Incidence* is the number of new cases occurring in a population in a given period of time, usually a year.
- *Prevalence,* on the other hand, is the total number of cases—new and continuing—in existence at a given point or over a given period of time.
- *Risk factors,* derived from the study of variations in rates of incidence and prevalence in subgroups, are defined here as the characteristics associated with an increased likelihood that a particular disorder will occur.

Epidemiological studies make frequent use of screening instruments to ascertain the possible presence of a disorder prior to more detailed study.

- *Sensitivity* refers to how well the instrument avoids failing to identify cases (false negatives).
- Specificity, on the other hand, is the capacity to avoid the mistaken identification of a case that more detailed study reveals not to be a true example of the condition (false positives).

In order to gather information about the occurrence of disorders, a variety of questionnaires and other non-clinical survey devices are widely used in epidemiology. With all such instruments the issue of validity is of critical importance.

- *Validity,* or the degree to which judgments drawn from data arrived at through the use of the instrument correspond to the real situation, is an issue of critical importance with all such instruments.
- *Face validity* refers to the seeming inherent plausibility of a finding.
- *Construct validity* is the consistent relationship of the instrument to the theoretical structure from which it is derived.
- *Consensual validity,* however, rests on the agreement of acknowledged experts that a thing is so.
- *Predictive validity* confirms a finding by means of correlation with some other set of parameters, such as treatment outcome or genetic loading.

Development of Psychiatric Epidemiology and Current Status

The President's Commission on Mental Health[14] of 1978 gave considerable impetus to the development of epidemiological research in psychiatry. The need for a much more comprehensive and detailed picture of the nature and extent of the problem of mental disorders in the country was so evident that the recommendation for a much-expanded program in this area was readily accepted. Furthermore, developments in diagnosis and in survey methodology had been accumulating at an increasingly rapid pace throughout the previous decade and the field was ready for advancement. Weissman and Klerman[28] summarized the current state of psychiatric epidemiology in 1978. They traced the history of the field from its early beginnings and described how investigators sought to enumerate cases both as they occurred in clinical settings and from case records. The fallacies in this approach soon became evident, however, and efforts were then initiated to move away from studies of treated prevalence toward surveys of the population at large. In this way all of those cases that were untreated or that received help through other care systems could be included.

Among the important investigations of this post–World War II era the best known are probably the Stirling County study[9] and the Midtown Manhattan study.[26] These investigations were very carefully carried out and paid rigorous attention to issues of sampling and to the construction of standardized instruments. In general, however, they focused on psychosocial variables and used either DSM-I diagnoses or derived from a unitary concept of mental impairment that avoided the idea of discrete medical disorders. Furthermore, the sample sizes, although impressive for the time, were not large enough to allow for generalization; more than that, they were somewhat misleading in that only noninstitutionalized persons were interviewed. Although the findings varied widely and clearly needed verification, nevertheless the studies raised profound questions because for the first time they afforded some insight into the state of affairs outside of the clinical setting. In midtown Manhattan, where 1,860 door-to-door interviews were completed, an astonishing 81 percent of the population from twenty to fifty-nine years of age had symptoms that were mildly to severely incapacitating; 23.4 percent were substantially impaired.

The next generation of epidemiological studies had to wait for a major shift in psychiatric conceptualization and the development of instruments that grew out of that shift. For the first time the large-scale determination of diagnoses in a population was possible without the necessity of relying on clinicians. The psychodynamic constructs that dominated post–World War II psychiatric thinking had deemphasized specific diagnoses of discrete disorders in favor of a continuum of stress and impairment; the target manifestations were those that were shaped largely by psychosocial factors. But in the 1960s and early 1970s, investigatory work from a variety of different sources began to challenge the assumption of a universal psychodynamic etiology. In particular, genetic studies of schizophrenia and bipolar disorder and psychopharmacological advances made it clear that different disorders responded to different treatments and had different outcomes. The contributions of the group from Washington University in St. Louis that resulted in the 1972 formulation by Feighner and Associates[4] of the Research Diagnostic Criteria grew out of this earlier work, as did the monumental contributions of Robert Spitzer and his associates in the development of DSM-III. For the first time a classificatory system based on operationalized definitions of discrete disorders was available. No longer did the entities under consideration merge imperceptibly into one another as varying expressions of one underlying psychopathological process. Rather, the several conditions were separate illnesses defined by careful clinical description, genetic studies, a characteristic course, and their differential response to treatment. In this form, they lent themselves much more readily to epidemiological investigation.

What was lacking still, however, was a standardized technique for applying these formulations. This eventually took the form of a structured interview that could be used to make diagnoses in large-scale community surveys without having to depend on the judgment of clinicians. The lack of such an instrument had impeded the progress of the field for generations. However, in the upsurge of activity following the work of the President's Commission on Mental health, the National Institute of Mental Health (NIMH) undertook to sponsor the development of just such an instrument. Building on previous efforts, such as the Schizophrenia and Affective Disorder Scale (SADS-L), and drawing heavily on the contributions of a growing number of individuals, in the late 1970s NIMH did develop, standardize, and field-test an instrument known as the Diagnostic Interview Schedule (DIS)[18] which could be administered door to door by lay interviewers and which yielded DSM-III diagnoses.

Building on all of these developments, the latest advance in psychiatric epidemiology has been the conceptualization of the Epidemiology Catchment Area (ECA) program. Since 1978 NIMH has funded a large-scale collaborative epidemiological study using the DIS. This effort aims at determining for the first time the incidence and prevalence of DSM-III disorders in community and institutional population across the country. Five sites are involved: Johns Hopkins in Baltimore, Washington University in St. Louis, Yale University, Duke University, and the University of California at Los Angeles. All told, when the project is completed, nearly twenty thousand respondents will have been interviewed and then reinterviewed a year later.

Based on the results of the first wave of interviews from three of the sites, preliminary findings of the ECA project have recently appeared.[10,19,25] The results are impressive. Nearly one in four respondents report the occurrence of a diagnosable mental disorder at some time during their life. Most such disorders do not receive professional treatment. In contrast to previous reports, the findings suggest that disorders are not more common in men than in women. Instead there is a differential distribution. Depression and phobias are more common in women, whereas alcoholism and antisocial problems rank first among men. The prevalence of schizophrenia is about 1 percent and of affective disorders about 8 percent. Phobia and obsessive-compulsive disorder are much more common than had been previously thought.

Epidemiological Investigations in Child Psychiatry

The 1980s represent a critical period in the development of child psychiatry. The field has come a long way from the beginnings of the discipline in the community-based guidance clinics of the 1920s and 1930s. Five decades of growth and change have brought the academic component of the profession to a new level. Today child psychiatry is firmly established within schools of medicine as a part of departments of psychiatry. The next step is to meet the challenge of developing the kind of broad-based research endeavor that is appropriate to the academic realm.

Accordingly, the last ten years have seen a major shift in the direction of child psychiatric research activity, particularly within academic settings. It has been a difficult shift to make, for the profession is firmly rooted in its clinical traditions. But it is an important one if the promise of the insights and understanding that have been gained over the years is to be translated into a solid knowledge base. Epidemiology has much to offer to child psychiatry at this point in its development. The questions with which epidemiology concerns itself and the methods it employs are closely related to clinical psychiatry. But the systematization of observation and the attention to scientific design bring orderliness and a new kind of power to the pursuit of an understanding of the causes of disorders. The epidemiological approach fits well with the clinically based academic child psychiatry program, and the rigor of its thought enhances teaching and enriches practice. Over the past ten years several schools—perhaps most notably Columbia under David Shaffer,[23] St. Louis with Felton Earls[2,3] and Pittsburgh with Anthony Costello—have made this transition successfully and with real benefit to their programs.

One of the most powerful inducements to pursue child psychiatric work has always been the sense that the origins of disorder were to be found in childhood and that etiological investigation could be conducted more readily through study of the early years of life. The combination of epidemiology and child psychiatry fosters that search for cause by focusing on rates of disorder in high-risk groups. A particularly powerful method available to child psychiatry has been the combination of epidemiological and longitudinal approaches that Rutter[21] has emphasized. The span of a longitudinal study of childhood disorders is inherently shorter and more manageable than is the duration of investigations of adult disorders, which must pursue the question of outcome over decades. Three landmark investigations, the Collaborative Perinatal Study,[12] the

Isle of Wight study,[22] and the Kauai study,[29] illustrate the effectiveness of this method. Each has contributed significantly to our knowledge of the causes of disorders in childhood and the kinds of preventive interventions that might be helpful.

THE COLLABORATIVE PERINATAL STUDY

In the 1950s the newly established National Institute of Neurological and Communicative Disorders and Stroke (NINCDS) undertook a major prospective study, the Collaborative Perinatal Study. It was designed to test the hypothesis that abnormalities and complications of pregnancy, delivery, and the neonatal period were causative factors in many neurological disorders, mental retardation, and some milder states of dysfunction. Beginning in 1957, study teams were established at fourteen leading centers around the country. Over the next decade data were gathered on over 55,000 pregnancies and on the neurological and psychological fate of the children born. In addition to prenatal studies of the mother, information was collected at the time of birth, at four and eight months, one year, and three years, and finally at seven years of age. The result was an unprecedented data base drawn from a national sample that, for the first time, was large enough to answer questions about both relatively uncommon conditions as well as those that occur frequently. The data base exists on computer tapes at the NINCDS and is used regularly by researchers to investigate a whole series of questions about what Pasamanick and associates[13] referred to as the "continuum of reproductive casualty."

Nichols and Chen's[12] use of the Collaborative Perinatal Study data to study predictors of minimal brain dysfunction illustrates the methodology and the kinds of answers that can be obtained in this way. They studied the 38,624 children who were available for psychological examination at age seven. Excluding children whose examinations were not complete as well as those with IQs less than 80 and limiting the sample to the white/black ethnic groups and those who were enrolled in the first and second grades reduced the sample size to 28,889 children. Computer runs were performed on seven behavioral items (hyperactivity, short attention span, impulsivity, emotional liability, etc.), six cognitive and perceptual-motor variables (such as the Bender-Gestalt score, Draw-A-Person, Illinois Test of Psycholinguistic Abilities, low verbal IQ, etc.), three academic measures drawn from the Wide Range Achievement Test and ten neurological signs and symptoms (poor coordination, impaired position sense, abnormal gait, etc). Pearson product-moment correlation matrices were calculated for all twenty-six variables and for age-sex groups as well as for each individual center. Factor analysis of the matrices showed four emerging factors: hyperkinetic-impulsive behavior, learning difficulties, neurological soft signs, and social immaturity.

The combination of symptoms said to constitute the syndrome of minimal brain dysfunction (MBD) did not associate well enough to support the concept of a syndrome. Children were said to have "symptoms" in regard to a particular factor if they exceeded a predetermined cutoff score—specifically, the extreme 8 percent of the total group was defined as having the symptom and the extreme 3 percent were said to have it to a severe degree. In this way three symptom groups were defined among the total cohort of 29,889 children: the HI's (hyperactive-impulsive–5.85 percent, 2,337 children), the LD's (learning difficulties—6.54 percent, 2,499 children) and the NS's (neurological "soft signs"—6.15 percent, 2,331 children). Only fifty-four children were found to have symptoms in all three areas. The investigation itself consisted of calculating correlation coefficients for each of the MBD symptoms and for 331 antecedent variables selected from among the more than 5,000 measures contained in the overall data base on the basis of anticipated significance. The 331 antecedent variables included 56 demographic and maternal history items (socioeconomic index, father's education, mother's education, marital status, etc.), 62 pregnancy and delivery variables (low hemoglobin, jaundice, vomiting, highest fetal heart rate, type of delivery, etc.), 82 neonatal and infancy measurements (head circumference, one-minute Apgar test, five-minute Apgar, major and minor malformations), 31 preschool factors (language reception, language expression, Porteus maze, etc.), and 100 medical history and concomitant condition variables (refractive error, asthma, hernia, heart infection, undescended testicle, etc.). The results of this analysis yielded 366 significant associations between 188 antecedent variables and the MBD symptoms.

Although space does not permit a detailed presentation of these findings, they may be summarized as follows: Learning difficulties were related to low socioeconomic status and tended to run in families with patterns suggestive of environmental effect. Generally speaking, the forerunner characteristics of hyperactive—impulsive behavior were not evident in early life but were identifiable by the preschool period. Genetic, demographic, pregnancy, and infant development factors were positively associated. Like the HI group, the neurological "soft sign" children were more readily detectable in the preschool period than earlier on. Overall many of the 366 significant associations found—for example, frequent changes of residence, family configuration, maternal smoking, and specific physical abnormalities—offer promising leads for future investigations and for preventive interventions.

THE ISLE OF WIGHT STUDIES

A group of English investigators has made a unique contribution to the development of epidemiological approaches to child psychiatry. Among them, the leading figure is Michael Rutter of the Maudsley Hospital in London. In the early 1960s, Rutter and his staff undertook a comprehensive survey of the handicapped child population on the Isle of Wight, an island community of 100,000 located about four miles off the southern coast of England.[22] The purpose of the study was to define the need for services for physically and psychiatrically handicapped children in the community. This is a common use of epidemiological data. However, at the time it was—and still continues to be—one of the very few attempts to define the nature and extent of psychopathology in an entire population. The information gained from the study has been used over and over again to address a whole series of questions about the causes of mental disorder.

Children who were nine, ten, or eleven years of age were chosen as the target population for study. In June 1964 there were 3,519 such youngsters on the island. A two-stage design was employed. Children with suspected handicaps in the medical, social, intellectual, educational, neurological, or psychiatric spheres were identified by a screening procedure. Then, through a much more detailed examination, a professional determined the actual presence or absence of the handicap. In addition, control groups were selected at random and studied intensively in a manner comparable to the group of children with positive findings.

Only the ten- and eleven-year-olds were screened for psychiatric disorder. Of the 2,199 children available for study, 285 showed positive findings; on clinical examination along with parent and teacher interviews, 118, or 5.4 percent, were in fact found to have a disorder. Since the screening procedure had been shown to miss about a fifth of the cases actually present in a population, the prevalence of psychiatric disorder in this population was thus in the neighborhood of 6.8 percent. The most common problems were neurotic and antisocial disorders. There were thirty-four boys and nine girls with antisocial disorders; an additional twenty-two boys and five girls showed mixed antisocial and neurotic pictures. There were twenty-six girls and seventeen boys in the purely neurotic group. The breakdown of neurotic disorders showed thirty cases of anxiety with general fearfulness and worrying and, in a third of the cases, specific fears or phobias. There were seven children with obsessional symptoms, three with tics, three with depression, and only two who were considered to be hyperkinetic. As might be expected in such a small population, only two cases of psychosis were discovered.

In order to evaluate the persistence of symptom states, the Isle of Wight children were restudied four years later.[20] Overall, the contributions of this investigation are several. Methodologically, it pioneered the development of the two-stage technique (i.e., mass screening followed by detailed clinical study of positives) and its application to an entire community. Regarding content, for the first time it gave us a picture of the distribution of disorders in a nonclinical population. It is of interest that only 10 percent of the psychiatrically disturbed children were receiving treatment. This finding alone makes evident the importance of carrying out population-wide determinations of incidence and prevalence. Previous studies that had relied on distributions in clinic populations would offer only distorted pictures of the population at large since they would be dealing with only a small fraction of the cases.

THE KAUAI LONGITUDINAL STUDY

The Kauai Longitudinal Study[29] is a twenty-year investigation of the developmental course of a cohort of 660 children of multiethnic backgrounds born in 1955 on an outer island of the Hawaiian archipelago. It is similar in design to the anterospective Collaborative Perinatal Study but with a more frankly behavioral focus. Assessment began early in pregnancy and included measures of perinatal stress followed by a series of subsequent evaluations of physical, intellectual, and social development at two, ten, and eighteen years of age. A particularly valuable feature was the appraisal of the quality of the family environment. Within this isolated and relatively circumscribed community, the attrition rate was remarkably low: 88 percent of the original cohort participated in the eighteen-year follow-up. Because of the nature of the study, data analysis was able to address both forward- and backward-looking questions. Among those questions considered were: What was the ultimate significance of risk factors present early in life? and What factors could be seen in retrospect to have played a role in the lives of children whose outcome at age ten or eighteen was pathological? Each question of this kind is critical both to epidemiology and to child psychiatry, and the strength of the Kauai study is the fascinating responses it provides to such inquiries.

The effect of perinatal stress and family environment were evaluated prospectively. Based on a pediatric scoring of approximately sixty potential complications, infants were assigned a stress rating from 0 to 3, with 2 and 3 representing "moderate" and "severe" degrees of stress respectively. Ten percent of the children were considered to be moderately stressed, three percent severely stressed. When the effect of stress on adjustment at age two, ten, and eighteen was evaluated, it was clear that the passage of time tended to soften the impact. The effect was less pronounced at ten than it had been at two, although beyond that point it tended to persist. Four out of five children with severe perinatal stress showed significant learning behavior or physical problems at age eighteen. The incidence of mental problems in this group was five times what it was in the control group. However, the effect of stress was modified by environment.

At birth, pediatricians were asked to identify children whom they felt were suffering from chronic conditions likely to lead to MBD. Judgments were made of family stability based on interviews early in life; these were subsequently correlated with significant differences in outcome for this MBD group. Where family stability was judged to be lacking, a total of eighteen percent by age ten were judged to have long-term mental health problems. When the family life was stable, however, pathology was present in only 2 to 3 percent, a proportion that did not differ from that of the control group. This finding of an interactive effect between biological and environmental stressors is one of the most significant contributions of the Kauai study.

At age ten, three groups of children with pathological outcomes were identified. The groups were children with learning disabilities (22), children in need of long-term mental health services (25), and children in need of short-term mental health services (60). The antecedents of these conditions were then studied. The learning-disabilities group were not drawn from among those considered to have suffered severe perinatal stress, but they did show a higher proportion of moderate complications, low birth weight, and congenital stigmata. Problems were evident early in life. At one and again at two, they were noted to be fretful and not affectionate, and their mothers were judged to be erratic and worrisome to a greater degree than was true in the control group. Finally, a very significant finding had to do with the relative intractability of this condition. Between the ages of ten to eighteen, four out of five of the learning-disabilities children continued to have difficulties, with a tendency to develop secondary symptoms in the areas of acting-out behavior and sexual misconduct. The 4 percent of the children who at age ten were considered to be in need of long-term mental health care were principally those with acting-out disorders; at birth nearly half of them had been thought to have potential "MBD." Moderate to severe perinatal stress and low birth weight were common historical antecedents, and temperamental problems tended to be evident at ages one and two. These disorders, too, were likely to persist; indeed, between age ten and eighteen, only one out of three showed improvement. In contrast, the larger group (10 percent) of those thought to be in need of short-term mental health care had a much more benign origin and course. They did not differ from the control group in the incidence of perinatal stress. Moreover, their principal symptoms were related to anxiety and insecurity, and correlated with temporary reductions in emotional support (which were present in three out of four cases). In spite of the fact that treatment was relatively uncommon in this group, between ages ten and eighteen improvement was evident in 60 percent of the cases.

In summary, the Kauai study demonstrates the importance particularly of the interaction between perinatal stress and family instability. More than that, it speaks for the persistence of learning difficulties and acting-out behaviors over time from their earliest manifestations in temperamental problems to antisocial symptoms in late adolescence. In contrast, there is a milder group of emotional disturbances that is less rooted in biology and more likely to improve over time. Social class and "non-rewarding patterns of child-caretaker interaction" are strong predictors of serious difficulties at age eighteen.

Future Directions

The epidemiology of childhood psychiatric disorders is now in a position somewhat similar to where the studies of adult disorders stood prior to the inception of the ECA investigations. The acquisition of specific information about the incidence and prevalence of disorders in the general population and the collection of accurate data regarding risk factors are vital next steps in constructing a science of child psychiatry. The methodological developments necessary to taking those steps are already underway. Over the past three years, staff of NIMH working in association with expert consultants in the field of child mental health have developed a survey instrument known as the Diagnostic Interview Scale—Children (DIS-C). It is based on Barbara Herjanic's Diagnostic Interview for Children and Adolescents (DICA) instrument from St. Louis but is considerably modified; again, however, it is designed for administration in the field by lay interviewers and will yield DSM-III diagnoses. Currently it is being tested in Pittsburgh on known clinical populations by Anthony Costello. An improved version should be ready soon, and it will then be available for use in the ECA program. In the realm of childhood disorders, the questions of incidence and prevalance are more difficult than they are with adult disorders because childhood conditions are less clearly defined and more confounded by Axis II developmental issues. Nevertheless, even though the first data in these areas will necessarily undergo many modifications, they represent important advances and begin a process that is long overdue.

The ultimate goal of any epidemiological endeavor is prevention. Just as Snow's assigning responsibility to the Broad Street pump was instrumental in the control of cholera epidemics in nineteenth-century London, so is there the hope that by identifying important risk factors in childhood psychiatric disorders, interventions that will significantly reduce their incidence may begin. Preventive approaches seem the only possible answer to such disorders, for, once they have fully developed, the ability of the United States—or any nation—to provide effective treatment is far below what is needed. As a first step in the planning of preventive strategies, the studies of Langner, Gersten, and Eisenberg[8] in New York City illustrate a sophisticated statistical approach to the delineation of risk factors. Over a ten-year period the staff of the Family Research Project surveyed two samples of children—one a representative Manhattan sample of 1,034 children, the other a racially balanced group of 1,000 members of Aid to Needy children households. Mothers were also interviewed in depth. Data were collected on 654 behavioral items; eventually, by dint of selection and by collapsing, eighteen dimensions of child behavior were factored out. They included: conflict with parents, dependence, fighting, regressive anxiety, mentation problems, competition, delinquency, self-destructive tendencies, undemandingness, conflict with siblings, isolation, repetitive motor behavior, noncompulsiveness, sex curiosity, training difficulties, weak group membership, delusions-hallucinations, and late development. These dimensions were then converted into profiles and the incidence of the profile types was determined within the populations. The distribution was as follows: 16 percent were considered sociable; 12 percent, competitive-independent; 34 percent, dependent; 16 percent, moderate backward isolate; 12 percent, aggressive; 4 percent, severe backward isolate; 1 percent, organic; and 2 percent, other. These profiles were tested for reliability and validity in a number of ways, and then the examination of independent variables or predictors was begun.

From parent interviews, factor analysis was used to create eight dimensional groupings of parental characteristics and marital state as well as an additional five groupings of child-rearing behavior. Another forty-five demographic variables were added to these for consideration, and correlations were established between these independent variables and the behavioral dimensions just described. These were ascertained at the time of the initial survey and also when it was repeated five years later. Thus it was possible to determine both the current state of affairs and the forecasting power of the predictor. Interestingly, "Parents Punitive" was by far the most powerful long-term predictor of undesirable outcome, particularly in regard to aggression and antisocial behavior. This suggests that if any serious effort is to be made to prevent the occurrence of conduct disorders and delinquency, we will need to intervene programmatically into this dimension of child rearing. In contrast, at the time of the initial survey "Mother Excitable-Rejecting" was strongly associated with undesirable outcomes but its predictive power at resurvey declined to only a tenth of what it had been previously. "Parental Coldness" showed a similar temporal pattern. "Race, Ethnic Background, and Social Class" were strongly associated with the occurrence of psychopathology.

The implications of such studies both for future etiological research and for the planning of preventive interventions are obvious. Less obvious perhaps is the beneficial effect that investigations of this type must have on the whole profession of child psychiatry. Work with patients cannot be rigidly determined by the kind of broadly defined information that epidemiology yields, but it certainly should be informed by it at every turn. Furthermore, within the community planning process, the credibility of the profession and, ultimately, its effectiveness will be progressively increased as its secure knowledge base is strengthened by studies such as the ones cited here.

REFERENCES

1. BOYD, J. H., and WEISSMAN, M. "Epidemiology of Affective Disorders: A Reexamination and Future Directions," *Archives of General Psychiatry*, 38 (1981):1039–1046.
2. EARLS, F. "Epidemiology and Child Psychiatry: Historical and Conceptual Development," *Comprehensive Psychiatry*, 20 (1979):256–269.
3. ———. "Epidemiologic Methods for Research in Child Psychiatry," in F. Earls, ed., *Studies of Children*, Monographs in Psychosocial Epidemiology #1. New York: Neale Watson Academic Publications, 1980, pp. 1–33.
4. FEIGNER, J. P., et al. "Diagnostic Criteria for Use in Psychiatric Research," *Archives of General Psychiatry*, 26 (1972):57–63.
5. GOULD, M. S., WUNSCH-HITZIG, R., and DOHREN-WEND, B. "Estimating the Prevalence of Childhood Psychopathology," *Journal of the American Academy of Child Psychiatry*, 20(1981):462–476.
6. HIRSCHFELD, R. and CROSS, C. K. "Epidemiology of Affective Disorders: Psychosocial Risk Factors," *Archives of General Psychiatry*, 39 (1982):35–46.
7. KELLAM, S. G., et al. "Why Teen-agers Come for Treatment," *Journal of the American Academy of Child Psychiatry*, 20 (1981):477–495.
8. LANGNER, T. S., GERSTEN, J. C., and EISENBERG, J. G. "The Epidemiology of Mental Disorder in Children: Implications for Community Psychiatry," in G. Serban and B. Astrachan, eds., *New Trends of Psychiatry in the Community*. Ballinger, 1977, pp. 69–109.
9. LEIGHTON, D. C. et al. "Psychiatric Findings of the Stirling County Study," *American Journal of Psychiatry*, 119 (1963):1021–1026.
10. MYERS, J. K., et al. "Six-month Prevalence of Psychiatric Disorders in Three Communities," *Archives of General Psychiatry*, 41 (1984):959–967.
11. NEEDLEMAN, H. L. and BELLINGER, D. D. "The Epidemiology of Low Level Lead Exposure in Childhood," *Journal of the American Academy of Child Psychiatry*, 20 (1981): 496–512.
12. NICHOLS, P. L. and CHEN, T. C. *Minimal Brain Dysfunction: A Prospective Study.* Hillsdale, N.J.: Lawrence Erlbaum Associates, 1981.
13. PASAMANICK, B., et al. "A Survey of Mental Disease in an Urban Population," *American Journal of Public Health*, 47 (1956):923–929.
14. Report of the President's Commission on Mental Health, vol. 1. Washington, D.C.: U.S. Government Printing Office, 1978.
15. ROBINS, L. N. *Deviant Children Grown Up*. Baltimore, Md.: Wilkins & Wilkins, 1966.
16. ———. "Psychiatric Epidemiology," *Archives of General Psychiatry*, 35 (1978):697–701.
17. ———. "Epidemiological Approaches to Natural History Research: Antisocial Disorders in Children," *Journal of the American Academy of Child Psychiatry*, 20 (1981):556–580.
18. ROBINS, L. N., et al. "National Institute of Mental Health Diagnostic Interview Schedule: Its History, Characteristics, and Validity," *Archives of General Psychiatry*, 38 (1981):381–389.
19. ROBINS, L. N., et al. "Lifetime Prevalence of Specific Disorders in Three Sites," *Archives of General Psychiatry*, 41 (1984):949–958.
20. RUTTEV, M. *Changing Youth in a Changing Society.* Cambridge, Mass.: Harvard University Press, 1980.
21. ———. "Epidemiological/Longitudinal Strategies and Causal Research in Child Psychiatry," *Journal of the American Academy of Child Psychiatry*, 20 (1981):513–544.
22. RUTTER, M., TIZARD, J., and KINGSLEY, W. eds. "Psychological and Medical Study of Childhood Development" in *Education, Health and Behaviour*. New York: John Wiley & Sons, 1970.
23. SHAFFER, D. "Epidemiology and Child Psychiatry: Introduction," *Journal of the American Academy of Child Psychiatry*, 20 (1981):439–461.
24. SHAFFER, D., and FISHER, P. "The Epidemiology of Suicide in Children and Young Adolescents," *Journal of the American Academy of Child Psychiatry*, 20 (1981):545–565.

25. SHAPIRO, S., et al. "Utilization of Health and Mental Health Services," *Archives of General Psychiatry,* 41 (1984): 971–989.

26. SROLE, L., et al. *Mental Health in the Metropolis: The Midtown Manhattan Study,* vol. 1. New York: McGraw-Hill, 1962.

27. STEIN, Z., and SUSSER, M. "Methods in Epidemi-

ology," *Journal of the American Academy of Child Psychiatry,* 20 (1981):444–461.

28. WEISMAN, M. M. and KLERMAN, G. K. "Epidemiology of Mental Disorders: Emerging Trends in the United States," *Archives of General Psychiatry,* 35 (1978):705–712.

29. WERNER, E. E. and SMITH, R. S. *Kauai's Children Come of Age.* Honolulu: University Press of Hawaii, 1977.

62 / An Overview of the Effectiveness of Preventive Early Intervention Programs

Karl R. White and Stanley I. Greenspan

Introduction

Preventive interventions for infants and young children involve an enormous range of activities. Parents are taught to "stimulate" their infants through various activities that involve the senses and the motor systems. Infants are brought into a day-care center where curricula are implemented that focus on the infant's emerging cognitive skills. Parents are counseled regarding their own feelings and the emotional needs of their babies. Visiting nurses help parents with a range of challenges, from planning appropriate nutrition to supporting a new baby's cognitive and motor skills. Preschool programs for two- to four-year-olds often involve cognitive and social games and, on occasion, various degrees of guidance and family counseling. More recently, comprehensive "clinical" approaches have tried to include the ingredients of many of these approaches but with a simultaneous focus on the child and the family in the context of the child's physical, cognitive, and emotional development, and the child's and family's individual differences.

Preventive interventions are also being used increasingly with children at risk of or with established handicaps. Here, too, a wide variety of programs are included under the rubric of "early intervention." Such programs include: vestibular stimulation for cerebral-palsied children, language therapy for hearing-impaired children, auditory and kinesthetic stimulation for low-birth-weight infants, teaching self-help skills to mentally retarded children, and diet therapy for "hyperactive children." Intensity of such programs ranges from a few seconds of vestibular stimulation

once a day to forty hours per week of intensive educational programming beginning at birth. Objectives range from prevention, to complete resolution, to slowing the rate of deterioration, to helping families to cope.

Such a broad range of programs, each with different goals and strategies, did not emerge accidentally. The diversity of programs evolved purposefully from the experience, clinical intuition, and perceptions of thousands of professionals in psychology, medicine, education, social work, and nutrition who have been concentrating on the needs and deficiencies of infants, young children, and their families. Concerned parents responded eagerly to the first demonstration programs. Building on the efforts of Head Start and similar "Great Society" programs of the 1960s, and motivated by the hope that later problems could be reduced or prevented with early attention, legislators, parents, and professionals have cooperated in the expansion of all types of preventive intervention programs.

Because of problems in defining exactly what preventive intervention is and is not, exact estimates of the number of children participating in preventive intervention programs are difficult. It is safe to say, however, that while many who require preventive services are not served, millions of children are cared for each year. For example, thirty-one states now mandate services for preschool disabled children, and similar legislation is pending in several more. Head Start serves more than 400,000 children each year. The U.S. Department of Education's Handicapped Children's Early Education Program has funded more than three hundred demonstration projects in the last fifteen years; twenty-two of these have been approved for national dissemination, resulting in more than two thousand replications in other sites.

As the needs of infants, young children, and their families have become better understood and programs have proliferated, there has been increasing concern about the match between the program and the child's needs and the efficacy of existing approaches. Legislators and funding agencies are becoming increasingly cost conscious. Although hundreds of research studies have been conducted, much confusion remains.

Given the challenges these programs are facing, the basic question is whether or not the types of preventive interventions currently being offered are likely to be successful. To answer this question, one must also ask what types of programs are most effective with what types of children. For example, is a program that focuses only on teaching cognitive skills likely to succeed when there are multiple problems in the family, including severe social and emotional difficulties? Similarly, is a program that can offer only outreach once every two weeks likely to be helpful for a family that is in constant crisis? Is it efficacious to work with a baby's emotional functioning and to disregard motor or cognitive lags? How long must a program last or how early must it start to produce clinically important results? And what evaluation measures are most likely to document progress in relevant areas of human functioning? In light of mounting evidence that many "high-risk" families are in fact multirisk ones, these issues are extremely important. [28,29,31]

The answers to such questions are frequently neither straightforward nor definitive. Zigler [72,73] has highlighted their importance and complexity and suggested strategies for beginning to resolve them. As new research and conceptual frameworks become available, techniques tend to swing back and forth on a pendulum activated by popularity, prejudice, and prevailing practice. If the field is to move forward, it is critically important that such questions be further addressed. This chapter summarizes and discusses the results of the most comprehensive review of preventive intervention conducted to date.

The Efficacy of Preventive Early Intervention Programs: An Integrative Review

The more one understands about the heterogeneous nature of children served and the variety of programs, the clearer it becomes that it is overly simplistic, inap-

propriate, and probably misleading to answer questions about the efficacy of preventive intervention with a simple yes or no. Furthermore, as one reviews the literature, it becomes clear that the types of programs that would probably be most successful (e.g., comprehensive approaches to infants and families) have been researched very infrequently.

As shown later, a critical issue in interpreting previous research is the degree to which program goals and activities match the population's needs. It may, for example, turn out that many poorly supported conclusions are true but that the research designs to date have been inappropriate for the questions asked. For example, one cannot reasonably test the effectiveness of a cognitive program on families who need much more. This review will show that the seeming limitations of interventions may often be a product of inappropriate research designs and that new research is needed to answer many important questions.

PREVIOUS REVIEWS OF PREVENTIVE INTERVENTION RESEARCH

Dozens of researchers have completed reviews of preventive intervention efficacy research. In an analysis of sixty-four previous reviews, Bush and White [12] found that most reviewers (87 percent) concluded that preventive intervention was effective. Previous reviewers who have studied the variables associated with the most effective interventions have frequently reached the following conclusions:

1. Interventions that involve parents are most effective.*
2. The earlier the age at which intervention begins, the greater the benefits.†
3. Intensity/duration of the intervention is positively correlated with benefits.‡
4. More highly trained intervenors are more effective than intervenors with less training.§

Reviewers agreed less about whether preventive intervention resulted in long-term benefits—only twenty-three of the sixty-four reviews addressed this issue, and only five of the twenty-three reviewers concluded that there was convincing evidence for long-term impact.

Unfortunately, all of the reviews analyzed by Bush and White failed to consider large numbers of preventive intervention efficacy studies, and most suffered from serious methodological problems. For example, even though literally hundreds of early intervention studies have been conducted, the median number of efficacy studies cited in the sixty-four reviews was only 16.5, and the largest number of efficacy studies cited by

*See references 5, 10, 11, 18, 19, 27, 34, 39, 49, 53, and 63.
†See references 10, 13, 32, 47, 48, 62, and 63.
‡See references 5, 10, 27, 55, 62, and 65.
§See references 10, 32, 41, 47, and 49.

any one review was 60. Only two reviewers explained the criteria and/or procedures used for locating/including research studies. Less than 10 percent systematically analyzed how subject or study characteristics covaried with outcomes, and less than 15 percent systematically considered the methodological quality in conjunction with outcomes for the studies they cited.

A particularly comprehensive review of preventive intervention efficacy research is currently in progress at the Early Intervention Research Institute at Utah State University. [15,70] White & Casto, 1985. Initial results from this analysis provide important information that extends and clarifies previously available information. The following sections provide a brief description of the procedures used in that integrative review and summarize those findings that are most relevant to this chapter. (A more extensive discussion of the procedures and results of this integrative review is contained in Casto, White, and Taylor. [15])

PROCEDURES

Based on a search of relevant computerized data bases (e.g., *Educational Resources Information Center, Psychological Abstracts, Dissertation Abstracts, Smithsonian Science Information Exchange*), citations in previous reviews, references of articles already obtained, and letters to prominent preventive intervention researchers, over 1,500 articles related to intervention efficacy were identified. Most were program descriptions, philosophical articles, or position papers, but approximately 425 were research reports describing the results of over 200 efficacy studies. When multiple articles were available about the same study, information from all of the articles was considered in the analysis of that particular study.

To make sense of this voluminous body of literature, meta-analysis techniques described by Glass[21,22] were used. Briefly described, meta-analysis requires the collection of a representative or comprehensive sample of research in a particular area; quantitative coding of study and subject characteristics and study outcomes for each study; and the use of descriptive and correlational statistical procedures to examine study outcomes and how those outcomes covary with subject and study characteristics. Studies were included in the analysis if effects were reported for an educational, preventive, or therapeutic intervention with at-risk, handicapped, or disadvantaged children beginning before sixty-six months of age, and some type of research design was used that allowed estimates of program impact to be made (i.e., true-experimental, quasi-experimental, or pretest/posttest designs). Case studies, anecdotal reports, and interventions limited solely to surgical or dietary procedures were excluded. Thus

far data from 162 studies described in 316 research articles have been analyzed.

Based largely on what previous reviewers considered to be the most important concomitant variables of early intervention efficacy,[12] ninety-seven variables in the following five categories of subject and study characteristics were coded for each study included in the analysis.

1. The type of subjects included in the research (e.g., type and severity of handicap).
2. The type of intervention used (e.g., home-based vs. center-based).
3. The type and quality of research design employed (e.g., whether data collectors were blind).
4. The type of outcome measured and the procedures used (how long after the intervention was completed was the test administered).
5. The conclusions of the study (e.g., the magnitude of the effect size).

The magnitude of each intervention's effect was estimated using a standardized mean difference effect size (ES), defined as $(X_E - X_C) \div SD_C$.[23] This "effect size" measure is essentially a *z* score and has been widely advocated in recent years to describe the impact of educational programs.[16,21,36,66] In cases where pretest/posttest designs were used without a control group, pretest scores were used as the best estimate of how a control group of subjects would have performed had they not received the treatment.

Occasionally the articles reported insufficient information to code an item. For example, it was possible to code "type of design used" for every study, but "educational level of mother" was reported or could be estimated for only 29 percent of the ES's. It is also important to note that one study could yield multiple ES's. For example, four ES's would be coded for a study that compared an experimental group to a control group on language and motor functioning immediately after completion of the intervention program and again one year later. Standardized mean differences between experimental and control groups would be computed for (1) language measured immediately, (2) motor measured immediately, (3) language measured one year later, and (4) motor measured one year later. For any given study, only one ES was computed for each twelve-month period and for each outcome domain.

RESULTS AND DISCUSSION
Characteristics of the Data Set. Analyses of the 162 preventive intervention efficacy studies resulted in 1,665 ES's. Of these, 899 were from studies that compared some type of intervention program to a no-treatment group (hereafter referred to as intervention vs.

control studies). Only 143 of these intervention versus control ES's came from studies done with handicapped children (mostly mentally retarded or developmentally delayed). There were also 766 ES's from studies that compared one type of intervention with another type of intervention (hereafter referred to as intervention A vs. B studies). Such a study might have compared children in a center-based program in which parents were not involved to children in the same center-based program whose parents were involved.

The consideration of results from both intervention versus control and intervention A versus B studies provided information used to "cross-validate" findings. For example, one can examine whether parental involvement leads to more effective programs by comparing the average ES of all intervention versus control studies that used parents extensively to those that did not use parents. Another way is to examine intervention A versus B studies that did a direct comparison of using parents extensively versus not using parents at all within the same study. If the results of both comparisons are consistent, the evidence is stronger.

The effect sizes included thus far in the analysis came from studies conducted from 1937 to 1984—71 percent since 1970. Studies were reported mostly in educational and psychological journals (49 percent of the ES's), but with substantial numbers from medical journals, books, documents in the Educational Resources Information Center, government reports, and dissertations. Not surprisingly, the most frequently measured outcome (41 percent of all ES's and 68 percent of all studies) was some measure of IQ. Language, academic functioning, and motor skills accounted for most other outcomes. Only 31 percent of the studies measured any type of social/emotional outcome, and only 5 percent of all ES's were measures of the impact of intervention on someone other than the target child (e.g., parents, siblings).

In examining the results of the meta-analysis, it is important to remember the predominance of IQ measures in previous preventive intervention efficacy research. Although IQ is an important and legitimate variable to consider,[71] many other important variables, such as family functioning, mental health, social competence, and daily living skills, have been measured very infrequently. Thus previous research is heavily weighted by measures of IQ, and it is often difficult to draw conclusions about the impact of preventive intervention on many other important outcomes.

Overall Results. One way of answering the question "Is preventive intervention effective?" is to examine the average ES from all intervention versus control studies. As shown in figure 62–1, the distribution of such ES's reveals that the average impact of early inter-

vention is almost half of a standard deviation. The distribution of ES's is slightly skewed, having a mean of 0.44, a median of 0.38, and a standard deviation of 0.68. For most educational and psychological outcomes, an effect size of 0.38 represents an important and clinically significant effect.[66] An effect size of this magnitude is equivalent to a gain of 6.5 points on the Stanford Binet IQ, twelve months' worth of reading gain at the third grade, or an increase from the thirty-fifth percentile to the fiftieth percentile of children that age on a measure of self-concept.

However, these results are based on a very heterogeneous group of studies. It includes studies with medically at-risk, disadvantaged, and handicapped children; and interventions ranging from vestibular stimulation with cerebral-palsied children, to rocking premature infants on waterbeds; to language therapy with hearing-impaired children; to comprehensive educational, therapeutic, and psychological interventions with at-risk children and families. Intensities range from a few seconds of vestibular stimulation several times a day over a period of three weeks, to forty-plus hours a week of intervention with parents and children from birth to five years of age. To understand the impact of preventive intervention, it is necessary to examine various subgroups of the data and to investigate how the apparent impact of early intervention for any subgroup may be influenced by other subject and study characteristics (e.g., do children who start intervention programs earlier make larger gains than children who start later?) Such analyses are also important to determine the credibility of results (e.g., if ES's from poor-quality studies were ten times as large as those from high-quality ones, and most of the ES's were from poor studies, one would justifiably be less trusting of an overall average).

Data for handicapped and disadvantaged children are reported separately in table 62–1, revealing an ES slightly higher for handicapped than for disadvantaged children. When analyses for these two groups are limited to good-quality studies, the average ES remains essentially the same for disadvantaged subjects and is somewhat reduced for handicapped subjects. Notice that there are only twenty-three ES's from good-quality studies done with handicapped children.

Table 62–2 shows the results when data are analyzed to determine whether there are enduring effects for disadvantaged and handicapped populations. Unfortunately, there are not enough data to draw conclusions about handicapped populations—no data collected later than twenty-four months after the intervention ended, no data from good-quality studies collected later than twelve months after the intervention ended, and only three ES's from good studies where the data were collected at any time other than immediately after

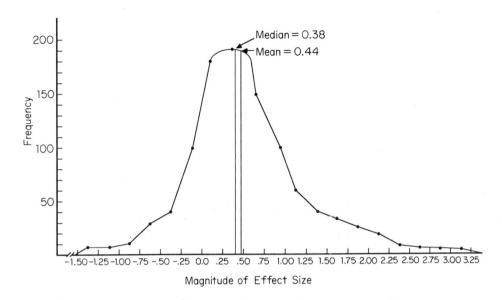

FIGURE 62–1

Frequency Distribution of Effect Sizes from Intervention Versus Control Studies

the intervention ended. Thus the question of whether early intervention for handicapped children results in long-term benefits is essentially unanswered and unaddressed.

For disadvantaged children, far more data are available. However, it is important to remember that most of these data are based on measures of IQ and academic achievement. As shown in table 62–2, the more time that has elapsed since the completion of the intervention program, the less benefit is observed. The average for 415 ES's measured immediately after the conclusion of the intervention was 0.63. There is an immediate drop of approximately one-third of a standard deviation for outcomes measured one month after intervention. The average for 135 ES's measured more than thirty-six months after the intervention was completed is essentially zero.

When data are limited to only high-quality studies with disadvantaged children, the same trend is observed, but a small residual effect remains (note: Some caution is necessary because these data are based on far fewer effect sizes). The immediate benefit is about one-half a standard deviation, and the average of fifty-four ES's measured up to thirty-six months (i.e., combining all of the ES's taken between one and thirty-six months after the intervention was completed) is 0.27. Benefits measured after thirty-six months averaged 0.10 for twenty-five ES's. Although there is a clear decline, a small residual effect remains when only good-quality studies are considered.

One study stands out in stark contrast to the trend reported in table 62–2 for effects to "wash out" substantially over time. The nineteen-year follow-up of the Perry Preschool Project children shows that in respect

TABLE 62–1

Average Effect Size for Intervention Versus Control Preventive Intervention Efficacy Studies for Subgroups of Data

	Handicapped			Disadvantaged		
	$\overline{ES}$	$S_{\overline{es}}$	N_{es}	$\overline{ES}$	$S_{\overline{es}}$	N_{es}
All studies	0.56	0.06	143	0.42	0.02	751
Only good quality studies	0.39	0.13	23	0.41	0.03	188
Only good quality studies with immediate posttest	0.43	0.15	20	0.51	0.04	121

$\overline{ES}$ = mean effect size.
$S_{\overline{es}}$ = standard error of the mean for $\overline{ES}$.
N_{es} = number of ES's on which a calculation is based.

TABLE 62–2

Average Effect Sizes for Various Times at which Outcome Data were Collected for Handicapped and Disadvantaged Children

Time of measurement in months since completion of intervention	All studies				Good-quality studies		All studies				Good-quality studies	
	$\overline{ES}$	$S_{\overline{es}}$	N_{es}	$(N_{studies})$	$\overline{ES}$	N_{es}	$\overline{ES}$	$S_{\overline{es}}$	N_{es}	$(N_{studies})$	$\overline{ES}$	N_{es}
0 months (immediate)	0.56	0.06	122	(45)	0.43	20	0.63	0.03	415	(69)	0.51	121
1–12 months	0.25	0.34	6	(5)	0.13	3	0.33	0.05	93	(20)	0.19	16
12–24 months	0.52	0.34	2	(2)	–	–	0.29	0.04	75	(23)	0.33	23
24–36 months	0.94	0.39	4	(2)	–	–	0.27	0.06	28	(7)	0.27	15
36–60 months	–	–	–	–	–	–	0.02	0.07	52	(8)	−0.01	13
60+ months	–	–	–	–	–	–	−0.05	0.05	83	(6)	0.22	12

$\overline{ES}$ = mean effect size.
$S_{\overline{es}}$ = standard error of the mean for $\overline{ES}$.
N_{es} = number of ES's on which a calculation is based.
$(N studies)$ = number of studies on which a calculation is based.

to high-school graduation rates, employment, criminal records, and placement of children in special education programs, there are substantial differences that favor experimental group children over randomly assigned control group children.[6] (See references 67 and 68 for earlier follow-up reports of this data set.)

The interpretation of these trends is not self-evident. First, the best studies show some long-term impact, although this effect is fairly small, except for the Perry Preschool Project, which shows strong differences. Second, the apparent "washout" in many studies may be a function of inadequate research designs, or the fact that IQ or academic achievement may be a poor long-term outcome variable in comparison to broader social, emotional, and functional cognitive adaptation (as

measured in the Perry Preschool Study). Third, it may be that programs that do not work with family coping capacities are unlikely to have substantial long-term benefits. Alternatively, it may be that without family-oriented services to maintain cognitive gains, programs must continue in order to combat the environmental challenges faced by many families. To use a medical analogy, antibiotics must be continued as long as exposure to the bacteria is present.

CONCOMITANTS OF EFFECTIVE INTERVENTION

As noted earlier, Bush and White[12] identified four conclusions that had been drawn frequently in previous reviews of the preventive intervention efficacy liter-

TABLE 62–3

Average Effect Sizes for Different Levels of Parent Participation in the Intervention

Parent Participation	All studies				Good studies		Adjusted for differences on age at start, quality of outcome measure, and time of measurement	
	$\overline{ES}$	$S_{\overline{es}}$	N_{es}	$(N_{studies})$	$\overline{ES}$	(N_{es})	All studies $\overline{ES}$	Good studies $\overline{ES}$
Minor or not at all	0.42	0.03	558	(56)	0.40	(130)	0.47	0.39
Major or only	0.41	0.04	176	(20)	0.42	(54)	0.39	0.43

$\overline{ES}$ = mean effect size.
$S_{\overline{es}}$ = standard error of the mean for ES.
N_{es} = number of ES's on which a calculation is based.
$(N_{studies})$ = number of studies on which a calculation is based.

ature: Better intervention programs involve parents, use highly trained primary intervenors, and begin earlier; in addition, the more intense the intervention, the more a child gains. Data from the meta-analysis are useful in determining whether these frequently advocated positions can be empirically supported by currently available research. (Note: Because of space limitations, only a brief summary can be reported here. A more complete description is contained in Casto, White, and Taylor[15].) The analyses reported are limited largely to preventive intervention studies with disadvantaged and at-risk children, since so few data addressing the four issues are available from good-quality studies with handicapped children.

For people concerned about the efficacy of early intervention with handicapped children, data from studies with disadvantaged and at-risk children are relevant for two reasons. First, for many years reviewers and advocates have relied heavily on efficacy studies from the disadvantaged and at-risk literature to draw conclusions about the efficacy of early intervention for the handicapped.* Therefore, before deciding whether generalization to handicapped populations is warranted, it is important to understand what can be confidently concluded from the disadvantaged/at-risk literature. Second, there is evidence that if intervention is not available, many at-risk preschool children will eventually be classified as handicapped.[26,38,58] Even though the disadvantaged literature is relevant to questions about early intervention with handicapped children, direct generalizations are often inappropriate.

Before examining each area, it should be highlighted that these important questions are often difficult to answer definitively. A number of factors combine to cause this. To begin with, there are a variety of measurement problems that make it difficult to measure the effects of intervention. Furthermore, more often than not the fact that some questions remain unresolved may be due to research design and measurement limitations rather than to deficiencies in the programs per se. What will be evident is the need for new research designed to answer the critical questions of what types of programs work best for what types of problems.

Involvement of Parents in Intervention Programs.

One of the most frequent conclusions in the preventive intervention efficacy literature is that programs that involve parents are more effective than programs that do not.† Although intuitively logical, there is little empirical support for this position from current studies. As shown in table 62–3, there is almost no difference in outcomes for intervention versus control studies that used parents extensively (ES = 0.41 based on

176 ES's) and those that used parents very little or not at all (ES = 0.42 based on 586 ES's). When ES's were limited to only high-quality studies, the results were very similar (0.42 vs. 0.40). These initial analyses suggest that parental involvement may not be the "key to effective intervention" that many have claimed. However, these apparent relationships may be an artifact of the age at which intervention begins or of some other associated variable.

To investigate whether such confounding might be a problem, ES's for each category of parental involvement were statistically adjusted for any differences in age at which the intervention began, quality of the dependent variable, and time at which the dependent variable was measured (e.g., immediately after intervention vs. thirty-six months after intervention). Regression equations (identical to those used to compute adjusted means in analysis of covariance) were used to estimate what the average ES for substantial parental involvement versus little or no parental involvement would have been if the values for each ES on age at start, quality of dependent variable, and time of data collection had been the same for every effect size. As seen in the last two columns of table 62–3, only very minor adjustments resulted from such analyses for the average ES of all studies or good studies.

Other data from the meta-analysis were used to examine further questions about the effect of parental

TABLE 62–4

Average Effect Sizes for Within-Study Comparisons of Different Levels of Parental Involvement

Degree of Parental Involvement[a] (More versus less)	$\overline{ES}$	$S_{\overline{es}}$	N_{es}
All comparisons			
Parent vs. no parent			
or			
More vs. less	0.08	0.05	134
Gordon study only			
More involvement			
vs.			
Less involvement	0.18	0.06	70
All comparisons except Gordon study			
Parent vs. no parent			
or			
More vs. less	−0.06	0.09	64

[a]ES's from nine studies.

$\overline{ES}$ = mean effect size.
$S_{\overline{es}}$ = standard error of the mean for ES.
N_{es} = number of ES's on which a calculation is based.

*See references 2, 9, 47, 48, and 63.
†See references 11, 17, 24, 35, and 69.

TABLE 62–5

Average Effect Sizes for Different Levels of Training for the Primary Intervenor

Training of Primary Intervenor	All studies				Good studies		Adjusted for differences on age at start, quality of outcome measure, and time of measurement	
	$\overline{ES}$	$S_{\overline{es}}$	N_{es}	$(N_{studies})$	$\overline{ES}$	(N_{es})	All studies $\overline{ES}$	Good studies $\overline{ES}$
Certified	0.47	0.03	386	(41)	0.41	(123)	0.43	0.43
Not certified	0.23	0.04	266	(30)	0.40	(63)	0.26	0.38

$\overline{ES}$ = mean effect size.
$S_{\overline{es}}$ = standard error of the mean for ES.
N_{es} = number of ES's on which a calculation is based.
$(N_{studies})$ = number of studies on which a calculation is based.

TABLE 62–6

Average Effect Sizes for Different Ages at which Intervention was Begun

Age at Start	All studies				Good studies		Adjusted for differences on age at start, quality of outcome measure, and time of measurement	
	$\overline{ES}$	$S_{\overline{es}}$	N_{es}	$(N_{studies})$	$\overline{ES}$	(N_{es})	All studies $\overline{ES}$	Good studies $\overline{ES}$
0–6 months	0.43	0.04	135	(12)	0.47	(62)	0.42	0.47
6–18 months	0.42	0.07	71	(14)	0.55	(22)	0.37	0.55
18–36 months	0.69	0.07	93	(14)	0.35	(7)	0.67	0.35
36–48 months	0.38	0.05	171	(20)	0.37	(70)	0.39	0.36
48–66 months	0.33	0.04	264	(22)	0.26	(25)	0.42	0.26

$\overline{ES}$ = mean effect size.
$S_{\overline{es}}$ = standard error of the mean for ES.
N_{es} = number of ES's on which a calculation is based.
$(N_{studies})$ = number of studies on which a calculation is based.

involvement. Studies in which both the parent and the child received treatment had slightly smaller effect sizes than studies in which only the child received treatment (0.36 vs. 0.47). Interventions delivered in the home or in home/center models had slightly smaller effects than those delivered solely in the center (0.36 vs. 0.46). These findings were maintained when the analyses were limited to high-quality studies or when adjustments were made for possible confounds.

Additional information about the effect of parental involvement was obtained by examining the results of nine studies that had made direct comparisons between different levels of parental involvement.* As summa-

rized in table 62–4, in these studies the experimental groups that utilized parents were only slightly more effective than those that did not (ES = 0.08). However, only one of the nine studies showed a moderately large effect.[25] The other eight studies actually showed a slight advantage for programs that did not use parents. Taken together, these data suggest that programs for disadvantaged and at-risk children that involve parents extensively can be effective, but there is no clear empirical support that they are more effective than programs that do not involve parents. Does this mean that preventive intervention programs should not involve parents? Not necessarily!

Before using these preliminary data to draw conclusions about whether parents should be involved in

*See references 1, 7, 25, 42, 46, 50, 52, 54, and 55.

TABLE 62–7

Average Effect Sizes for Within-Study Comparisons of Age at Which Intervention Begins[a]

	ES	$S_{\overline{es}}$	N_{es}
Effect sizes from unconfounded studies	−.04	.08	17
Effect sizes confounded with other variables (e.g., intensity, setting)	.16	.06	101

[a]Data based on 8 studies. Comparisons of earlier versus later.

$\overline{ES}$ = mean effect size.
$S_{\overline{es}}$ = standard error of the mean for ES.
N_{es} = number of ES's on which a calculation is based.

early intervention programs, it is important to note the limitations of the available data. First, most of the arguments in support of involving parents in early intervention programs have come from studies done with disadvantaged and at-risk children.[11,25,57] Such children often come from large families with a high incidence of single parents and poverty and low levels of parent education—all of which may hinder effective parent participation. In addition, the programs generally did not have the resources for or the aims of a "comprehensive approach" involving the extensive outreach and crisis intervention.[28,30] In other words, most of these studies focused solely on achieving cognitive enrichment as opposed to attaining more comprehensive goals, including improvement in the family's psychosocial functioning. Thus it may be that effective tests of parent involvement have not been done. Second, many of the outcomes included in this meta-analysis (over 40 percent) are from measures of IQ. It may well be that the involvement of parents leads to gains in other areas that have not been investigated. Finally, very few of the ES's (less than 2 percent) came from studies in which the investigators verified that parents were actually involved to the degree intended, or described quantitatively in what way parents were involved. Thus it may be that many investigators were examining "intended" rather than "actual" parent involvement.

Training of the Primary Intervenor. As shown in table 62–5, initial analyses showed a substantial advantage for programs that utilized certified intervenors versus those that used uncertified intervenors. However, when analyses were limited to studies of good methodological quality, these differences largely disappeared. There were also no differences between types of intervenors when the data for good studies were adjusted for differences in age at start, quality of dependent variable, and time of measurement.

Only three studies[3,42,61] made direct comparison between the utilization of certified versus noncertified intervenors. The fourteen ES's from these three studies yielded an average advantage of 0.16 favoring certified intervenors. Thus there is some evidence to suggest a small advantage for certified intervenors, but, given the currently available research, these differences are neither substantial nor compelling. Furthermore, what constituted a trained person is not clear. For example, very few of the intervenors were trained to deal with family coping challenges. Type of training may be even more important than the presence of training.

Age at Which Intervention Begins. As shown in table 62–6, a number of studies compared experimental to control group children beginning at different ages. In all these instances the average ES's are very similar. When analyses are limited to only good-quality studies and adjustments are made for time at which the outcome was measured and quality of dependent variable, there does appear to be a slight advantage (about one-fifth of a standard deviation) for those programs that begin earlier.

As shown in table 62–7, the seventeen ES's from five studies that made direct comparisons of starting children at two different ages with all other variables held constant* show 0.04 of a standard deviation advantage for those children who begin later. Studies that have examined the effect of age at start but have been substantially confounded with other variables, such as duration or setting,[4,25,59,64] show an average ES of 0.16 favoring children who began earlier.

Taken together, the available data suggest a very slight advantage for starting intervention programs for children earlier. However, available evidence is contradictory, and the five studies that have made the most direct comparisons did not find an advantage for beginning intervention programs earlier. Unfortunately, none of these were good-quality studies.

Intensity/duration of Intervention. Available data provide some, but not compelling, evidence that programs of longer duration or greater intensity are more effective. (See, e.g., Brittain[10]; Ramey and Bryant[55]; Ramey, Bryant, and Suarez[56]; and Swan[65].) It is important to note that although intensity and duration are related, a program in which a child's home is visited once each month for thirty minutes for five years has the same duration but very different intensity from a program in which the child is receiving six to eight hours of daily therapeutic programming for a period of five years. Because of inadequate reporting of available research, it was often impossible to adequately distinguish intensity from duration.

As shown in table 62–8, the average ES for disadvan-

*See references 8, 14, 25, 39, and 51.

TABLE 62–8

Average Effect Sizes for Interventions Different Duration

Duration of Intervention in Weeks	All studies				Good studies		Adjusted for differences on age at start, quality of outcome measure, and time of measurement	
	$\overline{\text{ES}}$	$S_{\overline{\text{es}}}$	N_{es}	(N_{studies})	$\overline{\text{ES}}$	(N_{es})	All studies $\overline{\text{ES}}$	Good studies $\overline{\text{ES}}$
0–24 weeks	0.66	0.56	71	(21)	0.49	(17)	0.57	0.40
25–52 weeks	0.40	0.72	378	(49)	0.42	(80)	0.48	0.46
53–104 weeks	0.36	0.55	168	(25)	0.45	(52)	0.36	0.49
105+ weeks	0.40	0.53	94	(10)	0.32	(36)	0.40	0.35

$\overline{\text{ES}}$ = mean effect size.
$S_{\overline{\text{es}}}$ = standard error of the mean for ES.
N_{es} = number of ES's on which a calculation is based.
(N_{studies}) = number of studies on which a calculation is based.

taged children in programs of short duration is about the same as that in programs of longer duration. Similar results are obtained when comparing different levels of intensity.[70]

Several studies have made direct comparisons between programs of varying duration and intensity. These comparisons were of two types: first, those studies that compared two different durations with all other major variables either balanced or held constant[33,45]; and second, those studies in which different levels of duration/intensity were confounded with other important variables—for example, a two-year program that was home-based compared to a one-year program that was center-based.* As shown in table 62–9, the results of both types of comparisons indicate an advantage for programs of longer duration/intensity. Again, however, data are rather limited. Only two studies have been identified in which there were no major confounding variables, and neither of those was a good-quality study.

Conclusions

Based on the analysis of 162 preventive intervention efficacy studies, there is compelling evidence that such interventions for disadvantaged, at-risk, and handicapped children across a range of outcome variables and for many different types of children and intervention programs have an immediate, positive effect of almost one-half of a standard deviation. When the analyses are limited to only high-quality

*See references 20, 25, 37, 44, 52, and 59.

studies, these estimates of program impact are reduced only slightly. Effects of that size are enough to move a child from the thirty-fifth to the fiftieth percentile of his or her age group on whatever measure is being considered. Furthermore, this estimate of program impact may well be low since most investigators have focused primarily on outcomes of cognitive functioning and have largely ignored outcomes such as social competence, family functioning, and adaptability, which are more closely linked with the goals of most intervention programs.

The evidence for long-term impact is less compelling. Only a few studies have examined effects more than three years after intervention is completed. For this group, with one dramatic exception, the effects of early intervention are substantially reduced. The ex-

TABLE 62–9

Average Effect Sizes for Within-Study Comparisons of Differences in Duration/Intensity

	$\overline{\text{ES}}$	$S_{\overline{\text{es}}}$	N_{es}
Effect sizes from unconfounded studies[a]	0.66	0.12	27
Effect sizes from studies confounded with other variables (e.g., setting, age at start)[b]	0.27	0.05	141

[a]Date based on two studies.
[b]Data based on eight studies.

$\overline{\text{ES}}$ = mean effect size.
$S_{\overline{\text{es}}}$ = standard error of the mean for ES.
N_{es} = number of ES's on which a calculation is based.

ception, the Perry Preschool Project, is one of the best designed of all available studies; major differences were found on variables such as employment, high-school graduation, teenage pregnancy, and need for special education services. These results may be indicative of what can be expected of all preschool intervention programs for disadvantaged children when such a broad array of important societal outcomes are measured; whether or not this is so will have to await further research and replication. Based on this exemplary study, for the time being we can cautiously conclude that preventive intervention with disadvantaged children does seem to result in important long-term effects. At the same time we must remember that several other programs (albeit not as methodologically strong) have failed to find such compelling long-term differences.

For handicapped children, the long-term effects of intervention are less clear since the issue remains largely uninvestigated. There are inherent differences between handicapped and disadvantaged children; hence it would be extremely risky to generalize findings for disadvantaged children to programs for the handicapped.

With respect to the concomitants of effective intervention, the analyses of previous research also contained some surprises. Contrary to what has long been assumed, there is no compelling empirical evidence, from available limited studies, that either intervention programs which start earlier or programs which involve parents are more effective. Most disturbing is the fact that even though these issues are hotly debated, few data exist with which these questions can even be addressed. Those data that do exist are so laden with methodological problems that conclusions concerning the relation of these variables to intervention effectiveness must be temporary and speculative. The best we can recommend at this point is to proceed on the basis of intuition and clinical experience while at the same time renewing our efforts to investigate such variables empirically.

Data regarding the effect of intensity/duration of the intervention and degree of training of the primary intervenor are also sparse. What few data are available suggest very tentatively that more highly trained intervenors and more intensive interventions of longer duration are slightly more effective. However, the data are somewhat inconsistent, very few direct comparisons exist, and methodological problems abound. Even more disturbing is the fact that so few "comprehensive" programs that simultaneously address physical, cognitive, emotional, and family functioning have even been attempted. This gap in our research must be addressed. In the meantime, case studies and clinical wisdom should be used to guide program design and implementation.

The most urgent need is for research that can inform practitioners and policy makers about the most effective form of preventive intervention. Past research has focused to an inordinate extent on justifying the existence of preventive intervention programs; relatively little effort has been devoted to investigating the efficacy of alternative forms of intervention objectively (e.g., in what way should parents be involved, or are there situations where it is appropriate not to involve them too intensively? How early should different types of intervention begin?). The question of whether any type of preventive intervention should be given is primarily one of values; at this time such issues can be informed by but will not be resolved by data. On the other hand, questions about what type of intervention is most effective are eminently addressable by methods of scientific inquiry and should be pursued vigorously. As a European researcher once noted to one of our colleagues, Milton Shore:

You Americans have a funny way of looking at evaluation. First, you confuse research and politics. There are some things that are not research questions; that is, issues such as should there be equity in health care? These are basic questions of social philosophy that the country must answer. Research can determine if this equity is taking place. But one does not research whether or not people should have a place to live or food to eat. In addition, in the United States you evaluate programs to decide whether or not to withdraw financial support. This differs from the attitude in much of Europe, where the basic thrust of a program is assumed to be correct and the evaluation is used to improve it, or to determine why it did not accomplish what it set out to do. (P. 401)[60]

REFERENCES

1. ABBOTT, J., and SABATINO, D. "Teacher-Mom Intervention with Academic High-Risk Preschool Children," *Exceptional Children,* 41 (1975):267–269.

2. ALLEN, K. E. "Early Intervention for Young Severely and Profoundly Handicapped Children: The Preschool Imperative," *AAESPH Review,* 3 (1978):30–41.

3. BARBARACK, C. R., and HORTON, D. M. *Educational Intervention in the Home and Paraprofessional Career Devel-*

opment: A Second Generation Mother Study with an Emphasis on Cost and Benefits Final Report. Demonstration and Research Center for Early Education, George Peabody College for Teachers, Nashville, Tenn. (ERIC Document Reproduction Service No. ED 052 814), 1970.

4. BELLER, E. K. "The Evaluation of Effects of Early Educational Intervention on Intellectual and Social Development on Lower Class Disadvantaged Children," in E. Grotberg, ed., Critical Issues in Research Related to Disadvantaged Children, Proceedings of six Head Start seminars, Princeton, N.J., 1969.

5. ————. "Early Intervention Programs," in J. Osofsky, ed., Handbook of Infant Development. New York: John Wiley & Sons, 1979, pp. 2–38.

6. BERRUETO-CLEMENT, J. R., et al. Changed Lives: The Effects of the Perry Preschool Program as Youths Through Age 19. Monograph 8. Ypsilanti, Mich.: High/Scope Press, 1984.

7. BIDDER, R. T., BRYANT, G., and GRAY, O. P. "Benefits of Downs Syndrome Children Through Training Their Mothers," Archives of Disease in Childhood, 50 (1975):383–386.

8. BRAUN, S. J., and CALDWELL, B. M. "Emotional Adjustment of Children in Day Care Who Enrolled Prior to or After the Age of Three," Early Child Development and Care, 2 (1973):13–21.

9. BRICKER, W., and BRICKER, D. "The Infant, Toddler and Preschool Research and Intervention Project," in T. Tjossem, ed., Intervention Strategies for High-Risk Infants and Young Children. Baltimore, Md.: University Park Press, 1976, pp. 545–572.

10. BRITTAIN, C. V. "Some Early Findings of Research on Preschool Programs for Culturally Deprived Children," Children, 13 (1966):130–134.

11. BRONFENBRENNER, U. A Report on Longitudinal Evaluations of Preschool Programs, vol. 2, Is Early Intervention Effective?" Washington, D.C.: Office of Child Development (ERIC Document Reproduction Service No. ED 093 501), 1974.

12. BUSH, D. W., and WHITE, K. R. "The Efficacy of Early Intervention: What Can Be Learned from Previous Reviews of the Literature?" Paper presented at the annual meeting of the Rocky Mountain Psychological Association, Snowbird, Utah, 1983.

13. CALDWELL, B. M. "The Rationale for Early Intervention," Exceptional Children, 36 (1970):717–726.

14. CALDWELL, B. M., and SMITH, L. E. "Day Care for the Very Young: Primary Opportunity for Primary Intervention," American Journal of Public Health, 60 (1970):690–697.

15. CASTO, G., WHITE, K., and TAYLOR, C. Final Report 1982–1983 Work Scope. Logan, Utah: Early Intervention Research Institute, Utah State University, 1983.

16. COHEN, J. Statistical Power Analysis for the Behavioral Sciences. New York: Academic Press, 1977.

17. COMPTROLLER GENERAL. Early Childhood and Family Development Programs Improve the Quality of Life for Low Income Families, Report to the Congress (#HRD-79-40). Washington, D.C.: U.S. General Accounting Office, 1979.

18. DENHOFF, E. "Current Status of Infant Stimulation or Enrichment Programs for Children with Developmental Disabilities," Pediatrics, 67 (1981):32.

19. DUDZINSKI, D., and PETERS, D. L. "Home-based Programs: A Growing Alternative," Child Care Quarterly, 6 (1977):61–71.

20. DUSEWICZ, R. A., and O'CONNELL, M. A. "The Pennsylvania Research in Infant Development and Educational Project: A Five-Year Perspective," Paper presented at the annual meeting of the American Educational Research Association, Washington, D.C., 1975.

21. GLASS, G. V. "Primary, Secondary, and Meta-analysis of Research," Educational Researcher, 5 (1976):3–8.

22. ————. "Integrating Findings: The Meta-analysis of Research," Review of Research in Education, 5 (1978):351–379.

23. GLASS, G. V., McGAW, B., and SMITH, M. L. Meta-analysis in Social Research. Beverly Hills, Calif.: Sage, 1981.

24. GOODSON, B. D., and HESS, R. D. Parents as Teachers of Young Children: An Evaluative Review of Some Contemporary Concepts and Programs. Stanford, Calif.: Stanford University, Department of Psychology (ERIC Document Reproduction Service No. ED 136 967), 1975.

25. GORDON, I. J. "Stimulation Via Parent Education," Children, 16 (1969):57–58.

26. GOTTLIEB, M. "Exceptional Children Intervention Programs: From Conception to Cradle," Allied Health and Behavioral Sciences. 1 (1978):31–46.

27. GRAY, S. W. "Selected Longitudinal Studies of Compensatory Education: A Look From the Inside," Paper presented at the annual meeting of the American Psychological Association, Washington, D.C. (ERIC Document Reproductive Service No. ED 033-762), 1969.

28. GREENSPAN, S. I. "Psychopathology and Adaptation in Infancy and Early Childhood: Principles of Clinical Diagnosis and Preventive Intervention," Clinical Infant Reports, 1 (1981).

29. ————. "Infant Developmental Morbidity and Multiple Risk Factor Families: Clinical Impressions and an Approach to Services, Public Health Reports, 97 (1982):16–23.

30. GREENSPAN, S. I., and WIEDER, S. "Dimensions and Levels of the Therapeutic Process," Psychotherapy, 21 (1984):5.

31. GREENSPAN, S. I., et al., eds. Clinical Infant Reports, No. 3, Infants in Multi-risk Families: Case Studies of Preventive Intervention. New York: International Universities Press, 1985.

32. GUSKIN, S. L., and SPICKER, H. H. "Educational Research in Mental Retardation," in N. R. Ellis, ed., International Review of Research in Mental Retardation, vol. 3. New York: Academic Press, 1968, pp. 217–278.

33. HEBER, R., et al. Rehabilitation of Families at Risk for Mental Retardation. Madison: University of Wisconsin, 1972.

34. HEINZ, R. S. Practical Methods of Parent Involvement, Paper presented at the annual meeting of the National Association for the Education of Young Children, Atlanta (ERIC Document Reproduction Service No. ED 188 776), 1979.

35. HEWETT, K. D. Partners with Parents: The Home Start Experience With Preschoolers and Their Families. Washington, D.C.: U. S. Department of Health, Education, and Welfare, (DHEW Publications No. DHEW OHDS 78-31106), 1977.

36. HORST, D. P., TALLMADGE, G. K., and WOOD, C. T. A Practical Guide to Measuring Project Impact On Student Achievement. No. 1, Stock No. 017-080-01460-2, Washington, D.C.: U.S. Government Printing Office, 1975.

37. HOWARD, J. L., and PLANT, W. T. "Psychometric Evaluation of an Operant Head Start Program," Journal of Genetic Psychology, 111 (1967):281–288.

38. HUNT, J. M. "Implications of Plasticity and Hierarchial Achievements for the Assessment of Development and Risk of Mental Retardation," in D. Sawin, et al., eds., Exceptional Infant, vol. 4, PsychoSocial Risks in Infant-Environment Transactions. New York: Brunner/Mazel, 1980, pp. 7–54.

39. JASON, L. "Early Secondary Prevention with Disadvantaged Preschool Children," American Journal of Community Psychology, 3 (1975):33–46.

40. ———. "A Behavioral Approach in Enhancing Disadvantaged Children's Academic Abilities," *American Journal of Community Psychology,* 5 (1977):413–421.

41. JOHNSON, N. M., and CHAMBERLIN, H. R. "Early Intervention: The State of the Art," in American Association of University Affiliated Programs for Persons with Developmental Disabilities, *Developmental Handicaps: Prevention and Treatment.* Washington, D.C.: AAUAP, 1983.

42. KARNES, M. B. "Evaluation and Implications of Research with Young Handicapped Low-Income Children," in J. C. Stanley, ed., *Compensatory Education for Children Ages Two to Eight: Recent Studies of Educational Intervention.* Baltimore, Md.: Johns Hopkins University Press, 1973, pp. 109–143.

43. KARNES, M. B., TESKA, J. A., and HODGINS, A. S. "The Effects of Four Programs of Classroom Intervention on the Intellectual and Language Development of Four-Year-Old Disadvantaged Children," *American Journal of Orthopsychiatry,* 40 (1970):58–76.

44. KARNES, M. B., et al. "Educational Intervention at Home by Mothers of Disadvantaged Infants," *Child Development,* 41 (1970):925–935.

45. LEVENSTEIN, P. "Cognitive Growth in Preschoolers Through Verbal Interaction with Mothers," *American Journal of Orthopsychiatry,* 40 (1970):426–432.

46. MCCARTHY, J. L. G. "Changing Parent Attitudes and Improving Language and Intellectual Abilities of Culturally Disadvantaged Four-Year-Old Children Through Parent Involvement" (Ph.D. diss. Indiana University, Bloomington, 1968).

47. MCDANIELS, G. "Successful Programs for Young Handicapped Children," *Educational Horizons,* 56 (1977):27–31.

48. MCNULTY, B. A., SMITH, D. B., and SOPER, E. W. *Effectiveness of Early Special Education For Handicapped Children.* (Report commissioned by the Colorado General Assembly.) Denver: Colorado Department of Education, 1983.

49. MILLER, J. O. *Review of Selected Intervention Research With Young Children.* Urbana, Ill.: ERIC Clearinghouse on Early Childhood Education (ERIC Document Reproduction Service No. ED 027 091), 1968.

50. MILLER, L. B., and DYER, J. L. "Four Preschool Programs: Their Dimensions and Effects," *Monographs of the Society for Research in Child Development,* 40 (1975).

51. MORRIS, A. G., and GLICK, J. A. *A Description and Evaluation of an Educational Intervention Program in a Pediatric Clinic,* Washington, D.C.: Department of Health, Education, and Welfare (ERIC Document Reproduction Service No. ED 160 190), 1977.

52. NEDLER, S., and SEBRA, P. "Intervention Strategies for Spanish-Speaking Preschool Children," *Child Development,* 42 (1971):259–267.

53. PARKER, M., and MITCHELL, D. *Parents as Teachers of Their Handicapped Children: A Review,* Occasional Paper No. 1, Project PATH, Waikato University, Hamilton, New Zealand. (ERIC Document Reproduction Service No. ED 201-125). 1980.

54. RADIN, N. "Three Degrees of Parent Involvement in a Preschool Program: Impact on Mothers and Children," Paper presented at the annual meeting of the Midwestern Psychological Association, Detroit, Michigan (ERIC Document Reproduction Service No. ED 052 831), 1971.

55. RAMEY, C. T., and BRYANT, D. M. *Enhancing the Development of Socially Disadvantaged Children with Programs of Varying Intensities.* Chapel Hill, N.C.: Frank Porter Graham Child Development Center, University of North Carolina at Chapel Hill, 1983.

56. RAMEY, C. T., BRYANT, D., and SUAREZ, T. "Preschool Compensatory Education and the Modifiability of Intelligence: A Critical Review," in D. Detterman, ed., *Current Topics in Human Intelligence.* Forthcoming.

57. RESCORLA, L. A., PROVENCE, S., and NAYLOR, A. "The Yale Child Welfare Research Program: Description and Results," in E. Zigler and E. Gordon, eds., *Day Care: Scientific and Social Policy Issues.* Boston: Auburn House, 1982, pp. 183–199.

58. SCOTT, K., and MASI, W. "The Outcome from and the Utility of Registers of Risk," in T. Field, et al., eds., *Infants Born At Risk.* Jamaica, N.Y.: Spectrum Publications, 1979, pp. 485–496.

59. SCOTT, R. "Research and Early Childhood: The Home Start Project," *Child Welfare,* 53 (1974):112–119.

60. SHORE, M. F. "Marking Time in the Land of Plenty: Reflections on Mental Health in the United States," *American Journal of Orthopsychiatry,* 51 (1981):391–402.

61. SHORTINGHUIS, N. E., and FROHMAN, A. "A Comparison of Paraprofessional and Professional Success of Preschool Children," *Journal of Learning Disabilities,* 7 (1974): 62–65.

62. SPICKER, H. H. "Intellectual Development Through Early Childhood Education," *Exceptional Children,* 37 (1971):629–640.

63. STONE, N. W. "A Plea for Early Intervention," *Mental Retardation,* 13 (1975):16–18.

64. STRICKLAND, S. P. "Can Slum Children Learn?" *American Education,* 7 (1971):3–7.

65. SWAN, W. W. "Efficacy Studies in Early Childhood Special Education: An Overview," *Journal of the Division of Early Childhood,* 4 (1981):1–4.

66. TALLMADGE, G. K. *Ideabook: The Joint Dissemination Review Panel.* Washington, D.C.: U.S. Office of Education, 1977.

67. WEBER, C. U., FOSTER, P. W., and WEIKART, D. P. *An Economic Analysis of the Ypsilanti Perry Preschool Project.* Monograph 5. Ypsilanti, Mich.: High/Scope Press, 1978.

68. WEIKART, D. P., BOND, J. T., and MCNEIR, J. T. *The Ypsilanti Perry Preschool Project: Preschool Years and Longitudinal Results.* Monograph 3. Ypsilanti, Mich.: High/Scope Press, 1978.

69. WEIKART, D. P., et al. *The Ypsilanti Preschool Curriculum Demonstration Project.* Monograph 4. Ypsilanti, Mich.: High/Scope Press, 1978.

70. WHITE, K. R., and CASTO, G. "An Integrative Review of Early Intervention Efficacy Studies with At-Risk Children: Implications for the Handicapped," *Analysis and Intervention in Developmental Disabilities,* 5 (1985):7–31.

71. ZIGLER, E., and BALLA, D. "Selecting Outcome Variables in Evaluations of Early Childhood Special Education Programs," *Topics in Early Childhood Special Education,* (1982):11–22.

72. ZIGLER, E., and BERMAN, W. "Discerning the Future of Early Childhood Intervention," *American Psychologist,* 38 (1983):894–906.

73. ZIGLER, E., and TRICKETT, P. K. "IQ, Social Competence, and Evaluation of Early Childhood Intervention Programs," *American Psychologist,* 33 (1978):789–798.

63 / Conducting Research with Preventive Intervention Programs

Stanley I. Greenspan and Karl R. White

One of the clearest findings from the analysis of previous investigations into the efficacy of preventive interventions is the need for more extensive and higher-quality research. Many previous reviewers have also lamented the ubiquity of methological flaws in preventive intervention research[2,3,19] and offered caveats or skepticism about whatever conclusions were drawn. Fortunately (for the future), many of the most serious problems with previous studies and evaluation efforts can be resolved. In the following sections we outline suggestions for improving the quality and credibility of preventive intervention research in two main areas: selecting outcome measures and assessing the impact of intervention and design and analyses of intervention research. Obviously the two areas are somewhat interactive.

Selecting Outcome Measures and Assessing the Impact of Intervention

In recent years there has been a growing awareness that efforts to evaluate the efficacy of preventive intervention programs have been too narrowly focused.[18,19,22] Forty-one percent of all outcomes included in the integrative review described in chapter 62 were confined to measures of IQ and more than 75 percent to measures of the child's cognitive, language, or motor functioning. Clearly, past efforts have been too narrow. However, assessing the impact of preventive intervention has suffered from several other problems as well. In the next sections we outline our recommendations to substantially improve the quality of such assessments.

SYMMETRY BETWEEN GOALS AND OUTCOMES

The specific nature of the interventive program being evaluated should in large part dictate the outcome measures that are selected. Because resources for evaluation are always limited, investigators should make sure that the outcomes assessed are clearly indicated by the goals, activities, and underlying theory of the program or have been identified as important by other investigators.

For example, some interventions have focused primarily on enhancing social and emotional functioning but have limited their assessment to measures of IQ. Because there is a substantial interrelationship between the multiple lines of development, differences in IQ may have been found, but they would likely be much smaller than would have been the case if the measures assessed had been directly related to the intervention.

In other cases investigators may serendipitously discover differences that are not expected on certain variables. Suppose an investigator finds dramatically lowered divorce rates among families who have participated in an intervention program versus rates among nonparticipants. Even if the program did not include activities that one would expect to impact on divorce rates, other investigators with similar problems would be well advised to determine if similar reductions in divorce rates were occurring in their programs. Many of the most important scientific findings have been accidental, but only by replication can it be determined whether such findings are valid or merely artifacts.

In selecting outcome measures then, two sources of information should guide researchers: (1) what would be predicted by the goals, activities, and underlying theory of the program and (2) in what areas have other investigators with similar types of interventions found important differences. Using a particular type of outcome because of its popularity, availability, or psychometric properties without primary reference to the criteria just mentioned is likely to be disappointing.

USING MULTIPLE SOURCES OF DATA

In evaluating the effectiveness of preventive intervention, researchers must account for the fact that human development is comprised of multiple interwoven lines. Consequently, evaluations of preventive interventions must examine a number of dimensions. This is not to suggest that every intervention program must measure an extraordinarily large number of variables. It may appropriately be argued that interventions should be evaluated as part of a larger, more general hypothesis wherein the intervention is thought to enhance a particular aspect of functioning that should be measured in great detail. For example, a program that attempts to enhance an infant's motor abilities should presumably focus on very subtle features of fine and gross motor coordination. Yet to the degree that motor functioning is part of the infant's overall capacities and intricately related to cognitive, emotional-social, and family functioning, these other parameters cannot be ignored—although it would be inappropriate to measure them in the same degree of detail as that directed toward motor functioning.

If investigators concentrate only on areas of functioning central to their hypothesis about the intervention, salient dimensions of a child's functioning will be ignored. Critical mistakes may then be made about the clinical value of the intervention. For example, a program that enhances cognitive skills but disturbs the formation of human relationships might be deemed ineffective because the hazards outweigh the benefits. Yet if the impact of the program on the formation of human relationships were not studied, such a finding might be missed.

Consider the following hypothetical example about a program that isolates infants from their family in order to promote motor and cognitive development. The youngsters initially achieve some benefit from the extra practicing of sensory, cognitive, and motor skills. However, within each family an original sense of disorganization, helplessness, and apathy continues, and even worsens, because of the additional stress related to their being isolated from the infant. In time the family's ability to support what is happening in the intervention program may become even less than what it was before the program began. These negative emotional, social, and family factors may eventually erode a youngster's gains. While this scenario is hypothetical, it is not totally unreasonable to assume that families feel strongly about their members. Even seemingly "uncaring" families, in fact, do care, but in ways that may be different from those of other families.

The importance of measuring outcomes in a variety of salient areas is also demonstrated by a medical example. It is inconceivable to study the impact of a drug that allegedly improves kidney functioning without looking at its effect on the number of red and white blood cells, pulmonary functioning, and other relevant bodily systems. A "review of systems" is routine.

Similarly, our evaluation strategies for preventive intervention should include a review of systems.

Evaluations must be based on a theoretical understanding of the salient functions that characterize the infants, young children, and families who are the objects of study. These functions include the general physical, sensory, motor, cognitive, social-emotional, family-caregiver, and the broader social and cultural context. At times interventions in only one area will lead to growth in other areas. On the other hand, interventions that attend to one area may lead to regressions or deficits in other areas.

The narrowness of assessments in previous preventive intervention research is emphasized by the data from the integrative review reported earlier. In tables 63–1 and 63–2 we can observe the number and percentage of effect sizes in relation to the type of measures used, the duration of the intervention, and interval elapsing between the time of intervention and the time when outcome was assessed. It might have been thought that studies of shorter duration would focus more on cognitive variables and those of longer duration on psychosocial and familial variables and also that longer-term follow-ups would focus more on measures of family functioning, school progress, or social/emotional functioning. As can be seen in the tables, however, this is not the case. The studies focus predominantly on limited-outcome measures (primarily IQ, language, and academics) regardless of the duration of the intervention or the time of follow-up.

SENSITIVITY OF OUTCOME MEASURES

Another and more subtle problem of preventive intervention research relates to the sensitivity of the outcome instruments. In a few specific areas, a great deal is known about the relationship between early and later development, and differentiated instruments have been designed for different ages. For example, the growth of intelligence can be measured with a variety of reasonably differentiated instruments. Even here, however, instrumental versus functional intelligence is rarely dealt with.

In areas such as human feelings, relationships, and the organization and representation of the self, there is an even more pronounced lack of available landmarks, normative data, and differentiated reliable instruments. Therefore, any statement about functioning must always be modest and certainly take on no "life of its own" independent of the sensitivity of the measure. For example, in comparison to overall adaptive skills, it is debatable whether a modest gain of IQ points is functionally important in the life of an individual child. Unfortunately, because of the "precision" with which our instruments can measure a theoretical construct such as IQ, many people assume that any difference which can be reliably measured must be important. We would do well to rely more heavily on

TABLE 63-1

Number and Percentage of Effect Sizes Categorized by "Type of Measure" and "Duration of Intervention"[a]

Duration of Intervention in weeks	Type of Measure									
	IQ	Motor	Language	Social/ Emotional	ITPA[b]	Academic	Attitude	Parent- Skill	Health	School Progress
1–24	106/ 6.5%	42/ 2.6%	36/ 2.2%	44/ 2.7%	7/ 0.4%	3/ 0.2%	5/ 0.3%	9/ 0.6%	8/ 0.5%	2/ 0.1%	290/ 17.9%
24–52	281/ 17.3%	43/ 2.6%	118/ 7.3%	37/ 2.3%	44/ 2.7%	122/ 7.5%	10/ 0.6%	7/ 0.4%	6/ 0.4%	5/ 0.3%	720/ 44.3%
52–104	175/ 10.8%	28/ 1.7%	28/ 1.7%	27/ 1.7%	29/ 1.8%	71/ 4.4%	0/ 0.0%	6/ 0.4%	1/ 0.1%	10/ 0.6%	379/ 23.3%
104+	92/ 5.7%	10/ 0.6%	41/ 2.5%	19/ 1.2%	3/ 0.2%	35/ 2.2%	2/ 0.1%	4/ 0.2%	6/ 0.4%	19/ 1.2%	235/ 14.5%
Total	654/ 40.3%	123/ 7.6%	223/ 13.7%	127/ 7.8%	83/ 5.1%	231/ 14.2%	17/ 1.0%	26/ 1.6%	21/ 1.3%	36/ 2.2%	1624/ 100.0%

[a] N = 624.
[b] Illinois Test of Psycholinguistic Abilities.

TABLE 63-2

Number and Percentage of Effect Sizes Categorized by "Type of Measure" and "Time of Measure"[a]

Months After Intervention Completed, Outcome Was Measured	Type of Measure										
	IQ	Motor	Language	Social/emotional	ITPA[b]	Academic	Attitude	Parent-skill	Health	School Progress	
Immediate	339/ 21.1 %	103/ 6.4 %	159/ 9.9 %	90/ 5.6 %	70/ 4.4 %	46/ 2.9 %	12/ 0.7 %	23/ 1.4 %	19/ 1.2 %	10/ 0.6 %	929/ 58.0 %
1–12	101/ 6.3 %	16/ 1.0 %	18/ 1.1 %	14/ 0.9 %	9/ 0.6 %	31/ 1.9 %	5/ 0.3 %	2/ 0.1 %	1/ 0.1 %	4/ 0.2 %	201/ 12.5 %
12–24	77/ 4.8 %	0/ 0.0 %	17/ 1.1 %	2/ 0.1 %	2/ 0.1 %	40/ 2.5 %	0/ 0.0 %	1/ 0.1 %	1/ 0.1 %	4/ 0.2 %	144/ 9.0 %
24–36	42/ 2.6 %	1/ 0.1 %	9/ 0.6 %	0/ 0.0 %	0/ 0.0 %	33/ 2.1 %	0/ 0.0 %	0/ 0.0 %	0/ 0.0 %	2/ 0.1 %	87/ 5.4 %
36–60	42/ 2.6 %	0/ 0.0 %	9/ 0.6 %	4/ 0.2 %	2/ 0.1 %	31/ 1.9 %	0/ 0.0 %	0/ 0.0 %	0/ 0.0 %	8/ 0.5 %	97/ 6.1 %
60+	44/ 2.7 %	0/ 0.0 %	10/ 0.6 %	14/ 0.9 %	0/ 0.0 %	50/ 3.1 %	0/ 0.0 %	0/ 0.0 %	0/ 0.0 %	6/ 0.4 %	145/ 9.0 %
Total	645/ 40.2 %	120/ 7.5 %	222/ 13.8 %	124/ 7.7 %	83/ 5.2 %	231/ 14.4 %	17/ 1.1 %	26/ 1.6 %	21/ 1.3 %	34/ 2.1 %	1603/ 100.0 %

[a] N = 603.
[b] Illinois Test of Psycholinguistic Abilities.

clinical wisdom and experience in making such judgments.

FOLLOW-UP

Previous research has paid too little attention to collecting longitudinal data. In many studies either the efficacy of the intervention or the relationship between early constitutional differences and later development are assessed after a relatively short time; this overlooks the time it takes for personality to differentiate. Individual differences in cognition or affect may in some instances remain obscure until early latency and the emergence of the capacity for more complex cognitive and affective skills. Subtle constitutional differences or the consequences of interventions in the first year of life may not be apparent until sometime later.

Compounding these problems is another concern—these instruments that attempt to assess cognitive or emotional functioning have been shown to be valid and reliable in discriminating among groups, yet somehow they become the main measures for individually oriented longitudinal research. It is evident that the use of such cross-sectional instruments may have limited validity when employed for evaluating individuals over time. Using the same test over an extended period of time may also cause a confounding of the results due to an interaction between specific historical events and each test session (e.g., what may have happened to the infant just prior to the test session). Even repeating the measures and using "the best performance" for a given test will not overcome these contextual contaminants.

Interestingly, clinicians rarely consider one source of data as sufficient. In clinical assessment, multiple techniques are used together with a detailed history of development along multiple lines and in the context of familial and social cultural factors, plus any other relevant and available data. Yet many longitudinal outcome studies, relying on a limited number of cross-sectional instruments that are valid only for large groups, draw conclusions about individuals. Judgments of developmental progress need to be based on multiple sources of data related to a conceptual understanding of the multiple lines and tasks of developmental phases.

Still another problem is the tendency "to go where the light is"—to measure what is known rather than develop conceptually consistent categories of functioning on a developmental continuum. A clear longitudinal concept of a personality function, its variables at different ages, and assessments of these variables over time is needed. Frequently, assessments cross from one area of development to another because of the availability of given assessment instruments suited to certain times in life. For example, although the relationship

between early motor maturity and IQ may not be clear, it is not unusual to measure an infant's motor maturity at six months and his or her IQ at five or six years, abilities that are both easily measured at the respective ages. Because of the cross-over effect there may be a relationship, but it could be a spurious one. Assessments must be made longitudinally along conceptually consistent categories.

AREAS OF FUNCTIONING TO BE ASSESSED

The ideal assessment protocol would define a limited number of key outcome criteria and specify reliable and valid instruments in each important area. The variables (e.g., mother-infant interaction) assessed to plan interventions would differ from variables employed to assess outcome, avoiding the possibility of "teaching the test." A minimum number of "domains" should always be considered for both clinical planning and outcome assessment. Specific instruments selected will depend on the age, subject's level of functioning, and goals of the program.

The descriptions for each of the following areas illustrate some of the dimensions of development that should be studied but do not include all possible variables. In areas where there are no existing standardized instruments, new clinical rating scales and instruments will need to be developed. It is important to be conceptually consistent in the variables studied over time rather than merely using the same test. The latter procedure often provides a confusing picture of development because "tests" often measure different variables (discontinuous from earlier measurements) at different times in an individual's development.

Prenatal and Perinatal Variables. Although the extent of their impact is unknown, prenatal and perinatal variables all have some effect on the infant's constitutional status and developmental tendencies. The prenatal variables include familial genetic patterns; mother's status during pregnancy (her nutrition, physical health, and illness); personality functioning, mental health, and degree of stress; characteristics of familial and social support systems available; characteristics of the pregnancy and the delivery process (e.g., complications, the length of various stages); and the infant's status after birth (along a number of dimensions). Perinatal variables include maternal perceptions of the infant and reports of the emerging daily routine, and direct observations of the infant and of the maternal-infant interaction.

Parent, Family, and Environmental Variables. This category includes evaluations of parents, other family members, and individuals who relate closely to the family along a number of dimensions. These assessments include each member's personality organization and developmental needs, his or her child-rearing capacities, and the family's interaction patterns. Evaluations of the support system (e.g., extended family, friends, and community agencies) used by or available to the family and of the total home environment (both animate and inanimate components) are also important.

Caregiver-Child Relationship. Evaluations in this area focus on the interaction between the infant and his or her important nurturing figure(s). Included are the quality of mutual rhythms, feedback, and capacity for joint pleasure, as well as the flexibility of the nurturing couple in tolerating tension and being able to return to a state of intimacy. Later in development the infant's capacities to experience differentiation, form complex emotional and behavioral patterns, and construct representations are important.

Infant Variables—Physical, Neurological, and Physiological. In this category the variables include the infant's genetic background and status immediately after birth, including physical integrity (size, weight, general health), neurological integrity, physiological tendencies, rhythmic patterns, and levels of alertness and activity. Special attention should be paid to the infant's physical integrity and how this could foster or hinder his or her capacities to experience internal and external stimulation, regulate internal and external experience to reach a state of homeostasis, begin to develop human relationships, interact in cause-and-effect reciprocal patterns, form complex behavioral and emotional patterns, and construct representations to guide behavior and feelings.

Infant Developmental Variables—Sensory, Language, Motor, and Cognitive. The variables in this category include the development, differentiation, and integration of the infant's motor and sensory systems. Also included is the relationship of the infant's sensorimotor development to his or her cognitive development.

Infant Variables—Formation of Object and Human Relationships. These variables define the interrelationships and capacities for relationships among the infant, his or her parents, and other family members. These early relationships facilitate in the infant a capacity for a range of emotions (dependency to assertiveness) in the context of a sequence of organizational stages. These stages are characterized by emerging capacities, which range from purposeful interactions of complex, organized social and emotional patterns, to constructing representations, and to differentiating internal representations along self versus nonself, time, and space dimensions.[7,8]

The variables that focus on the mother and other caregivers involve their capacity to reach out and foster attachment; provide physical comfort and care; perceive basic states of pleasure and discomfort in the infant; respond with balanced empathy (i.e., without either overidentification or isolation of feeling); perceive and respond flexibly and differentially to the infant's cues; foster organized complex interactions; and support representational elaboration and differentiation.

Design and Analysis of Intervention Research

The best way to design an intervention research study depends in large measure on the question being asked. In some cases program managers are interested only in whether clients are satisfied with the services they are receiving. In other cases it is important to know whether children and families in a particular program are any different from what they would have been had they been in some alternative program or in no program at all. The suggestions summarized in the following sections apply to the latter category, or what we will refer to as comparative research.

USE OF RANDOMIZED DESIGNS

It is often argued that random assignment to groups in early intervention efficacy research is difficult if not unethical or impossible.[2,3,19] Although admittedly it is difficult, it is not impossible to assign children randomly to treatment/no treatment or to alternate treatment conditions. This is evidenced by the fact that in the meta-analysis described in chapter 62, more than 50 percent of the effect sizes for disadvantaged children and 20 percent of the effect sizes for handicapped children came from randomized designs (see, e.g., Gordon,[5] Gray and Klaus,[6] Ramey and Haskins,[17] and Williams and Scarr[21]). In fact, random assignment to groups is especially feasible and advantageous in those cases where the number of families in need of services far exceeds the capacity of the agency to provide them (an almost ubiquitous occurrence, if one is to believe funding requests to state and federal agencies), or in those cases where alternative treatment programs are being considered (e.g., half day versus full day).

IMPARTIAL DATA COLLECTION

Another relatively simple procedure that would substantially improve quality and credibility of research would be to use data collectors who are uninformed and unaware of the purpose of the experiment and/or the group membership of subjects. Only 21 percent of the effect sizes included in the meta-analysis came from studies in which the data collector was definitely "blind." Unfortunately, many people tend to see what they expect to see. The educational and medical literature is rife with examples of weak or ineffective treatments advocated by well-intentioned people who believed that their treatment was making a difference when in fact it was not. The use of "blind" data collectors eliminates this threat to result credibility.

EVALUATION OF THE INTERVENTION PROCESS

Virtually all of the existing preventive intervention efficacy research has failed to determine the extent to which the intended treatment was actually implemented and how it was experienced. For example, in programs that intend to utilize parents as intervenors in their child's program, is there any evidence that parents actually do become involved to the degree intended by the program designer? At what degree of intimacy do parents or children relate to the intervention? How intensely do they carry out the intervention? Unless such information is obtained, there is a real danger that comparisons are being made between programs that were intended to be different but that were not. The failure to verify that intended treatments were actually implemented may be responsible in part for the failure of previous research to detect differences between alternative intervention programs (e.g., programs that involved parents versus those that did not).

Another reason for evaluating the intervention process is to determine what specific part of the program is facilitating or hindering progress. A process evaluation would lead us to ask, more generally, what the relationships are among aspects of the intervention approach, its context, the disorder, and the outcomes. When looking at the intervention approach, we must separate its technical components from the components of the process. The clinician may be using the appropriate "technique," but the clinical process that is expected may or may not necessarily follow. "Process," therefore, refers to operative experiences that occur in the intervention. It does not refer to client characteristics, therapist characteristics, or technical factors alone, but rather to the "experiences" generated by these and other factors. In most therapies, such experiences may be usefully conceptualized as a series of sequential process steps.[9,10] These process steps, which can be rated reliably,[10] are outlined in table 63–3.

Components of the Intervention Process

ASSESSING PROGRAM COMPREHENSIVENESS

As pointed out in chapter 62, comprehensive programs have been implemented so infrequently that research comparing them with other programs is nonexistent. However, there are strong theoretical reasons and much clinical experience to suggest that such programs have the best chance for success, particularly in families we will refer to as multirisk—where both child and parent(s) are suffering from or at risk for physical, emotional, and/or cognitive impairment. In order to properly evaluate a program, one must consider how closely it approximates a comprehensive model and meets the hypothesized needs of the population it serves. The following model may prove useful in this endeavor.

A comprehensive intervention approach would involve a regular pattern of services including: (1) organizing existing service systems (e.g., food, housing, and medical care) on behalf of the family's survival needs; (2) providing a constant emotional relationship with the family; and (3) most important, intervening at pivotal junctures when the infant's development may be in jeopardy, to provide highly technical patterns of care in order to deal with the infant's and family's individual vulnerabilities and strengths. As a part of this service pattern it is often useful to provide partial or full therapeutic day care for the child, innovative outreach to the family, and ongoing training and supervision to the program staff.

To be effective, such a comprehensive intervention must occur over a sufficiently long period as to allow the family's own strengths to take over and to sustain it. In other words, a crisis intervention approach for a few months is not sufficient. Instead, intervention activities must continue to be available to the families for several years or more. When the helping relationship is offered over a sufficient period of time, the frequently observed tendency of multiproblem families to deteriorate further upon the birth of each subsequent baby begins to be reversed.

A useful way of visualizing this model is to consider it from a developmental perspective. The tasks implicit within each stage of development (see Greenspan[7]) require that certain components of the service system must be available to assure appropriate support for the functions of that stage. One might visualize comprehensive preventive intervention as a pyramid (see figure 63–1). Specialized services, be they physical therapy, occupational therapy, psychological counseling, or parent-infant interactional guidance, will not be

TABLE 63–3

Dimensions of the Therapeutic Relationship

Steps in the Therapeutic Process		
Regularity and Stability	Attachment	Process
1. Willingness to meet with an interviewer or therapist to convey concrete concerns or hear about services.	1. Interest in having concrete needs met that can be provided by anyone (e.g., food, transportation, etc.).	1. Preliminary communication, including verbal support and information gathering.
2. Willingness to schedule meetings again.	2. Emotional interest in the person of the therapist (e.g., conveys pleasure or anger when they meet).	2. Ability to observe and report single behaviors or action patterns.
3. Meeting according to some predictable pattern.	3. Communicates purposefully in attempts to deal with problems.	3. Focuses on relationships involved in the behavior-action pattern.
4. Meeting regularly with occasional disruptions.	4. Tolerates discomfort or scary emotions.	4. Self-observing function in relationship to feelings.
5. Meeting regularly with no disruptions.	5. Feels "known" or accepted in positive and negative aspects.	5. Self-observing function in relationship to complex and interactive feeling states.
		6. Self-observing function for thematic and affective elaboration.
		7. Makes connections between the key relationships in life, including the therapeutic relationship.
		8. Identification of patterns in current, therapeutic, and historical relationships to work through problems and facilitate new growth.
		9. Consolidation of new patterns and levels of satisfaction and preparing to separate from the therapeutic relationship.
		10. Full consolidation of gains in the context of separating and experiencing a full sense of loss and mourning.

SOURCE: S. I. Greenspan and S. Wieder, "Dimensions and Levels of the Therapeutic Process," *Psychotherapy: Theory, Research, and Practice*, 21 (1984): 7.

successful unless they are based on a foundation that deals with concrete survival issues and the formation of a regular, stable working relationship.

In addition, however, the ingredients of the service pyramid must be sensitive to the changing developmental needs of infants and families. Greenspan[7] has conceptualized the developmental process as going from a period in which the infant achieves homeostasis to a period where he or she is capable of representation, differentiation, and consolidation. As shown in figure 63–2, within the pyramid there are different service patterns that are appropriate for each stage of development.

KEY ATTRIBUTES OF COMPREHENSIVE INTERVENTION PROGRAMS

Based on the rationale just outlined, there are ten key attributes that, to varying degrees, should be present in any comprehensive preventive intervention program. Depending on the population being served, any particular program might emphasize one specific aspect to a different degree. In addition, in any given program families will participate in some aspects more than others. Nonetheless, the following attributes are useful in conceptualizing how comprehensive preventive intervention programs should be designed.

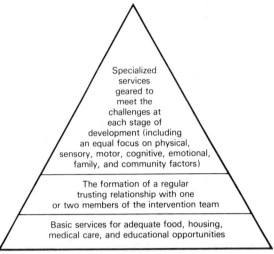

FIGURE 63–1

The Service Pyramid

1. Attention to multiple lines of development. Program activities must recognize and account for the fact that human development proceeds simultaneously in different areas (e.g., cognitive, emotional, motor). Services/ activities in each area must be individually tailored, integrated with work in other areas, and generally interdisciplinary.

2. Establishment of personal relationship. Consistent attention must be given to helping each family establish a personal, ongoing relationship with one or more program staff members. "Turnover" in the staff member responsible for each family must be minimized.

3. Attention to the child's development. Regular, specific activities must focus on the child's ongoing physical, cognitive, and emotional development. Often this will occur as a part of a "therapeutic day care" program or outreach programs.

4. Attention to parent's development. Intervention program staff must regularly assess and respond to needs, unique abilities, and/or difficulties or maladjustments on the part of parents.

5. Attention to parent/child interaction. In addition to focusing on the individual development of child and parents, the intervention must foster appropriate growth-promoting interaction between parents and child.

6. Ability to respond to "crisis" situations. The program must be capable of responding to unforeseen urgent needs, be they physical (e.g., loss of housing), emotional (e.g., threatened suicide), medical emergencies, or otherwise.

7. Assistance in accessing community resources. The intervention functions as a part of the broader community and must assist in providing the family with needed health, education, and social service resources.

8. Duration of program. Program staff must be prepared to continue intensive services for an extended period (often two or more years) until the family is able to be self-supporting and regenerative.

9. Outreach. Program staff must seek out those families who are most in need of program services since they will usually not seek out assistance.

10. Ongoing training and supervision of staff. Due to the interdisciplinary and emerging nature of preventive in-

tervention, it is essential that program staff continually seek to upgrade and refine their skills.

DETECTING OUTLIERS

Practitioners in early intervention programs frequently note that some children respond and others do not. One reason for identifying children who do not respond to intervention programs is that such children may mislead researchers about the efficacy of early intervention for other children. All too often we make the error of assuming that our therapeutic intent for a particular infant or family is in fact what they experience. For example, we plan a preventive intervention approach that will offer an enriched social, emotional, and cognitive experience to an infant of a depressed, low-income mother. We do so in the hope that these experiences will promote development and prevent later educational lags. We set up a clinical trial design, randomly assigning twenty children to the intervention group and twenty to a comparison group (where they receive routine community care). Three years later, when we do our evaluation, we find no differences between the groups and are amazed that the enormous energy that went into the intervention did not appear to pay off. If, however, we look, case by case, at each of the participants, we find that in the course of the intervention program, Mrs. Jones actually came in only one out of every four visits. When she did come for her visit she was suspicious of the intervention team, refused to practice any of the exercises they suggested, and built up more and more anger against "all of you who are accusing me of being a bad mother." She came in once every fourth time because she seemed to enjoy ventilating her annoyance at the team. Often, suspicious of the team's efforts, she did just the opposite of what had been suggested. Needless to say, the clinicians working with Mrs. Jones were quite discouraged and often felt "helpless in the face of such a resistant mother."

This scenario may seem quite extreme but experience suggests that such situations do occur. The real issue is that for some families, the experience of the program is quite different from its intent. To borrow another analogy from medicine, if we want to assess the effectiveness of a new drug for heart disease, we first must know whether patients in the experimental trial are taking the medicine regularly.

It is not enough simply to indicate that such situations may be occurring and to look only at the scores of those children who made the most progress. Such an approach would capitalize too much on chance variation. Rather, since it is a fact that some children respond better than others, those situations that may be contributing to this must be identified independent of the results of outcome measures and empirically tested over time.

		Representation, Differentiation, and Consolidation	
24–40 months	Services to permit, as appropriate more independent functioning and new relationships (e.g., nursery schools).	Facilitation of representational capacity and reality orientation.	Work on capacity to shift between fantasy and reality and integrate wide range of affective and thematic issues.
		Representational Capacity	
17–30 months	Services to permit direct psychotherapeutic work with toddler on as intensive basis as necessary.	Engagement of evolving representational (symbolic) capacities across a wide thematic and affective range.	Work on capacity to use and elaborate fantasy.
		Behavioral Organization, Initiative, and Internalization	
9–18 months	New services to permit direct exploratory work with the toddler now useful. Remedial educational approach should also be available.	Secure availability while admiring and supporting greater behavioral organization initiative and originality.	Further work on self-observing capacity permits integration of affective polarities around dependency and aggression and passivity and assertiveness.
		Somatopsychological Differentiation	
3–10 months	Services include educative and psychotherapeutic and, as necessary, auxiliary caretaker to facilitate reading of infant's communications.	Reading and responding contingently to range of affective and behavioral cues.	Includes work on capacity for self-observation to facilitate empathetic reading of the "other."
		Attachment	
2–8 months	Special services to support consistent affective caretaker-infant relationship.	Rich investment in human world wooed and is wooed.	Evolves an attachment that survives negative feelings.
		Homeostasis	
0–2 months	Health, mental health, social service, educational, legal.	Protection, care, engagement in world.	Has a pattern that is predictable, regular, comforting.
	INTERAGENCY COLLABORATION	BASIC REQUIREMENTS	THERAPEUTIC RELATIONSHIP

FIGURE 63–2

Schematic Illustration of Levels of Development and Corresponding Service System Requirements and Expected Shifts in the Therapeutic Relationship

Conclusions: Optimism or Pessimism?

Most of the existing reports of research on the efficacy of preventive interventions have not been comprehensive in either intervention intent or outcome measures. It is, therefore, difficult to draw conclusions about the long-term effectiveness of any given approach or about ingredients that would favor one type of intervention over another. For example, the "staying power" of the intervention cannot be readily assessed because the way in which an intervention manifests itself would be in the overall functioning of a child, not necessarily in the child's motor or intellectual functioning alone. Similarly, the effect of family involvement cannot be ascertained unless one knows more about the quantity and quality of the family involvement. Family approaches that go beyond engaging the family in the instructional curriculum and that also pay attention to the emotional aspects of the family have not been adequately studied.

After reviewing the state of the art, (see chapter 62 also), should we be optimistic or pessimistic; is the glass half empty or half filled? Even for programs that do not take a comprehensive view of the infant and family, there are a preponderance of positive effect sizes at program termination, as described in chapter 62. The fact that it cannot yet be demonstrated how long these effect sizes last beyond the end of the program, or that one type of program is better than another, should not suggest that the glass is half empty. It is our view that we should take a rather optimistic view toward the existing data for a number of reasons. The data are based on rather limited intervention and evaluation technology. Arguably, the limitations in intervention and evaluation technology may well bias results toward the unfavorable rather than toward the favorable. Therefore, any positive trend, particularly one as dramatic as the effect sizes reported in the last chapter, should lead researchers to be very optimistic indeed.

For example, any time we attempt to promote growth and development in an organism, we are involved with many factors. If we decide to pay attention only to one dimension of that organism while simultaneously ignoring all other relevant dimensions that obviously interact with the key dimension, we are leaving a great deal to chance. We know, for example, that the emotional milieu in which children live will greatly determine their interest in their world; this includes the degree to which they practice using motor skills, sensory apparatus, and their emerging intellect in order to meet challenges. Children who are apathetic and depressed because of extreme social and emotional deprivation will often lag behind as well in their sensorimotor and cognitive growth. In animal studies, severe emotional deprivation compromises the growth of the brain and the degree to which neuronal connections form. There is, therefore, little question that each of the relevant aspects of functioning—familial, emotional-social, cognitive, sensorimotor, and physical—are connected to one another.

A problem in one area invariably affects the other areas. Children with physical or learning deficits have a harder time emotionally and socially, just as children with severe emotional difficulties are often limited cognitively. For example, if it is difficult for a child to figure out sequences of sounds or visual stimuli, how much more challenging will it be for her to figure out complex emotional sequences and patterns? Therefore, programs that leave most of the variables up to chance and focus only on teaching the A-B-C's, so to speak, are essentially fighting an uphill battle. The fact that there is a generally positive showing raises enormous optimism. Programs that are truly comprehensive in nature and pay equal attention to emotional-social, cognitive, and family development may expect even greater gains.

Similarly, it could be assumed that because functioning is interrelated, it follows then that an intervention that focuses on one dimension of development at one time will necessarily express itself on that same dimension later on in life. Some studies suggest that the broader effects of an intervention on overall adaptation may be far more useful than isolated tests such as those of (IQ type) intelligence. For example, the results from the well-designed Perry Preschool Project indicate that even though IQ gains were negligible, more children stayed within the structure of the school system and society; there was less need for special education, less delinquency, and less teenage pregnancy, and there were fewer dropouts from school.[1] These findings of movement along interpersonal and family functioning lines are also supported by data from other clinically oriented programs that have broad psychosocial perspectives.* Thus it appears that for studying program effectiveness, broad measures of adaptation may be more useful than cross-sectional IQ tests. Clinical intuition suggests the same conclusion. It is, in fact, amazing that after intervention we do see gains on narrowly defined outcomes such as intelligence test scores alone.

It may therefore be argued that the limited technology used in the past has biased us in a negative direction. The fact that findings are positive at program termination should lead to enormous enthusiasm to conduct further research on the more challenging questions of what works best, for how long, and for what types of problems.

In future studies we would be well advised to employ a comprehensive methodology in our approaches to both intervention and evaluation. The fact that overall efficacy has now been well established at program termination allows us to turn to more difficult questions regarding what kinds of approaches work best with what kinds of children, with what kinds of difficulties, with what kinds of effects. And these effects must be looked at over a full range of functioning.

*See references 4, 7, 11, 12, 13, 14, 15, 16, and 20.

REFERENCES

1. BERRUETO-CLEMENT, J. R., et al. *Changed Lives: The Effects of the Perry Preschool Program on Youths Through Age 19.* Monograph 8. Ypsilanti, Mich.: High/Scope Press, 1984.

2. BRICKER, D., BAILEY, E., and BRUDER, M. B. "The Efficacy of Early Intervention and the Handicapped Infant: A Wise or Wasted Resource," *Advances in Developmental and Behavioral Pediatrics,* 5 (1984):373–423.

3. Dunst, C. J., and Rheingrover, R. M. "An Analysis of the Efficacy of Infant Intervention Program with Organically Handicapped Children," *Evaluation and Program Planning,* 4 (1981):287–323.

4. Fraiberg, S. H. *The Magic Years: Understanding and Handling the Problems of Early Childhood.* New York: Scribner's, 1965.

5. Gordon, I. J. "Stimulation via Parent Education," *Children,* 16 (1969):57–58.

6. Gray, S. W., and Klaus, R. A. "The Early Training Project: A Seventh-Year Report," *Child Development.* 41 (1970):909–924.

7. Greenspan, S. I. "Psychopathology and Adaption in Infancy and Early Childhood. Principles of Clinical Diagnosis and Preventive Intervention," *Clinical Infant Reports,* vol. 1. New York: International Universities Press, 1981.

8. ———. "The Development of Psychopathology; Perspectives from Clinical Work with Infants, Young Children and Their Families," in D. Finesilver, ed., *Toward a Comprehensive Model for Schizophrenic Disorders.* Hillsdale, N.J.: The Analytic Press, 1985, pp. 157–209.

9. Greenspan, S. I., and Sharfstein, S. S. "Efficacy of Psychotherapy: Asking the Right Questions," *Archives of General Psychiatry,* 38 (1981):1213–1219.

10. Greenspan, S. I., and Wieder, S. "Dimensions and Levels of the Therapeutic Process," *Psychotherapy,* 21 (1984):5.

11. Greenspan, S. I., et al., eds. *Clinical Infant Reports,* No. 3, "Infants in Multi-risk Families, Case Studies of Preventive Intervention." New York: International Universities Press, 1984.

12. Olds, D. "The Prenatal/Early Infancy Project: An Ecological Approach to Prevention of Developmental Disabilities," in J. Belsky, ed., *In the Beginning.* New York: Columbia University Press, 1982, pp. 270–285.

13. Olds, D., et al. "Improving Maternal Health Habits, Obstetrical Health, and Fetal Growth in High-Risk Populations: Results of a Field Experiment of Nurse Home-Visita-

tion," Rochester, N.Y.: University of Rochester, Department of Pediatrics, 1984 (manuscript).

14. Olds, D., et al. "The Prevention of Child Abuse and Neglect in a High-Risk Population: Results of a Field Experiment of Nurse Home-Visitation," Rochester, N.Y.: University of Rochester, Department of Pediatrics, 1984 (manuscript).

15. Provence, S., and Naylor, A. *Working with Disadvantaged Parents and Their Children: Scientific and Practice Issues.* New Haven: Yale University Press, 1983.

16. Provence, S., Naylor, A., and Patterson, *The Challenge of Daycare.* New Haven: Yale University Press, 1977.

17. Ramey, C. T., and Haskins, R. "The Causes and Treatment of School Failure: Insights from the Carolina Abecedarian Project," in M. Begab, ed., *Psychosocial Influences and Retarded Performance: Strategies for Improving Social Competence,* vol. 2. Baltimore: University Park Press, 1981, pp. 89–112.

18. Ramey, C. T., McPhee, D., and Yeates, K. O. "Preventing Developmental Retardation. A General Systems Model," in L. A. Bond and J. M. Jeffe, eds., *Facilitating Infant and Early Childhood Development.* London: University Press of New England, 1982, pp. 343–401.

19. Simeonsson, R. J., Cooper, D. H., and Scheiner, A. P. "A Review and Analysis of the Effectiveness of Early Intervention Programs," *Pediatrics,* 69 (1982):635.

20. Wieder, S., et al. "Identifying the Multi-Risk Family Prenatally: Antecedent Psychosocial Factors and Infants Developmental Trends," *Infant Mental Health Journal,* 4 (1984):165–201.

21. Williams, M. L., and Scarr, S. "Effects of Short-Term Intervention on Performance in Low-Birth-Weight, Disadvantaged Children," *Pediatrics,* 47 (1971):289–298.

22. Zigler, E., and Balla, D. "Selecting Outcome Variables in Evaluations of Early Childhood Special Education Programs," *Topics in Early Childhood Special Education,* 1 (1982):11–22.

---

64 / Working with Parents of Children with Chronic Disease

Irving N. Berlin

Introduction

Chronic diseases in children produce a state of major stress for both child and family. Asthma, diabetes, eating disorders, ulcerative colitis, rheumatoid arthritis, rheumatic heart disease, seizures, anorexia, blood and kidney disorders, and others affect many children and adolescents. In recent years some of the tumors, cancers, and blood dyscrasias like leukemia and renal disease, once rapid killers, have responded to new treatment. These diseases may be cured, or they may stay

in remission for long periods of time; in any case, their impact on patient and family may be similar to that of a chronic disease.[9,46]

The early onset of a persistent condition like asthma, diabetes, or seizures may be frightening to the child; to add to the hazards, the parents may find that their own anxiety about the disease makes it difficult for them to provide their child with the necessary comfort and reassurance.[2]

A very disconcerting aspect of many chronic diseases is that children may use their illness to avoid meeting normal expectations, such as doing chores at home or learning effectively in school. Parents who feel anxiety or guilt, or both, about their child's disease will find it difficult to be firm in their expectations that the child function to the maximum capacity which that particular condition permits. Some children and adolescents learn early that they can exacerbate their illness—in asthma, by overexercise with resultant wheezing or by initiating wheezing as a result of anxiety or anger; or in diabetic illness by either overeating or not eating enough. Thus they create a crisis that frightens the parents and increases their guilt, with subsequent parental inability to be firm in their expectations.[51,64,65]

Rarely are parents helped by their physicians to understand that a considerable burden of guilt feelings is normal for parents whose children suffer from chronic disease. The parents may experience an acute sense of disappointment if the disease interferes with the child's achieving what father and mother have set out as their educational, vocational, or professional hopes. So often, parents yearn to have the child either succeed where they had failed or continue in their footsteps. It is also predictable that, at times, the parents will feel that life would be easier if the child were dead or had never been born. To most parents, such feelings are intolerable and serve as a continuous spur to feelings of guilt.*

Parents' Concerns and Needs

Rothenberg[53] described a psychological syndrome that characterizes many children with chronic disease. He gave it an acronym, FAGS: fear, anxiety, guilt, and shame. I have found that the parents often suffer with a similar syndrome. In the child, the fear is related to the unknown aspects of the illness; will it be crippling, will it kill me, will I ever be normal or ever get well? The anxiety results from the continued worry about the effects of the illness on social relationships, school functions, and about the parents' real feelings toward the child. The guilt represents youngsters' feelings that what has brought the illness into being is some "badness" in them, be it oedipal feelings about either parent, occasional death wishes toward a parent, masturbation, normal anger, sibling jealousies and hatred, and so forth. The shameful feelings arise from not being normal and acceptable in the eyes of their peers, teachers, and friends. Will they be shunned?

The parents experience some variant of the same syndrome. Their fear represents the unknown effects of the illness on their child, the incapacity or crippling

*See references 3, 10, 19, 26, 30, and 36.

effects it may engender, and the possibility of death. The anxiety is related to the long-term effects on the child's functioning and future capacity for effective living, to the uncertainty of outcome in most chronic diseases, and to concerns about how they can help the child with the imposed burdens. The guilt, as mentioned previously, comes from the normal, occasional death wishes toward the child and an understandable desire to be rid of a chronic burden. The shame often stems from each parent's concern that it may be his or her own hereditary stock that is tainted and that, albeit unknowingly, he or she may nonetheless be responsible for the illness.[23,33,47]

The Physician's Potential Help to Parents

In the course of making the diagnosis of the illness, the physician has an unrivaled opportunity to deal with many of these issues during the initial visits. First, the physician needs to be aware that the diagnosis of a chronic illness creates enormous stress for the child/adolescent and parents. Indeed, initially they may be in a state of shock and unable to hear accurately the doctor's account of the nature of the illness, its causes, the prescribed treatment, or the limitations the illness may place on the child's normal functioning. Thus it is important that the doctor conduct several discussions with the patient and parents. There needs to be clarification of any hereditary factors. Any measures that can be taken to reduce the effect of the illness on the child's life must be clearly spelled out. Which medications will be employed, the reasons for their use, and their possible side effects need to be carefully explained. Usually literature is available for reading at home to help the parents and patient better understand the many aspects of the disease, its origin, course, medication, and any interferences it may offer with normal living.[18,50,64]

After several weeks, the physician needs to talk again with the patient and family both in order to answer any questions they may have and also to hear from them what they now understand about the disease from the previous discussions. Often parents and child will ask to have separate sessions with the physician so that private anxieties and doubts can be raised. It is, in general, important to the child that there be family discussions and that there be no secrets shared with the parents alone.[38,43,49]

Often, with adequate treatment, many illnesses will not seriously interfere with development. However, if the physician does not deal with the parents' feelings about the illness, their guilt, their desire to be rid of the problem, their questions concerning the cause of the illness, and so forth, the parents will end up infantilizing the patient. This is likely to occur despite the doctor's warnings and the prognosis that very little disturbance in development, learning, and peer interaction is likely to occur.

It is this issue—the ability of parents to be clear about their role in aiding the child or adolescent to avoid regression and to continue as normal a life as possible—that becomes critical to the patient's future functioning and development. [5,11,12]

Many children and adolescents exploit their illness to the detriment of their treatment and development. [16,20,62] The physician must always be aware of the tendency of the stressed child or adolescent to regress and the natural temptation to avoid difficult or demanding aspects of chores or schooling by using the illness as an excuse for not performing optimally and for failing to achieve as much as possible within the realistic constraints of the disease.

When such exploitation does occur, it usually indicates unresolved parent-child conflicts that the disease tends to aggravate, complicate, and prolong. It also reveals a problem in communication between parents and child. Parental encouragement of the child's or adolescent's questions and open discussion about fears and doubts are important to the patient's optimal functioning.*

Developmental Issues— Normal Developmental Crises

For the child with chronic disease, working through each developmental stage with its particular stresses and crises is an achievement. The child's successful working at and living through a developmental stage may depend on the degree to which each parent has experienced severe conflict and major problems at that stage. [21] Thus parents who have had severe difficulties during the stage of attachment and bonding are likely to be severely disturbed; such psychological burdens are prone to affect their management of their child and in that way to complicate further development. The temperamental match between child and parents may also be an important factor in how each participant deals with a chronic illness and how well the parents are able to understand their child's needs. [63] For a child who had already achieved only a marginal adjustment,

*See references 1, 4, 17, 26, 32, 34, 39, 41, 49, and 55.

the added stress of a chronic illness may well result in a psychotic picture or in some form of severe conduct disorder.

The separation-individuation process of the preschool child may be seriously interfered with by parents whose need for symbiotic attachment prevents separation and the necessary independent and exploratory play of the practicing phase. As a result, the establishment of object constancy (one of the end results of this stage of development) may be tenuous. Thus children who develop a chronic illness may be caught in a very tight symbiotic relationship that not only infantilizes them but provides a reason for preventing individuation and independence. This in turn permits the children to regress to an unhealthy dependence and to exploit their parents and the other people about them. In adolescence, especially, there may be failure to move toward any pattern of independent living and productivity. Thus children seem destined to repeat the developmental failures experienced by their parents. [2]

In the therapeutic situation, the ability of the child to work through developmental failures or arrests often depends on the parents being helped to work through similar problems from the same developmental stages, or at least to understand and to empathize with their child's problems so they can facilitate the youngster's efforts to change. [42]

The severely abused child provides a clear example of parental developmental problems being visited upon the child. Severe mistreatment engenders a serious impairment of the child's ability to trust, to separate and individuate, and to work through oedipal and adolescent developmental issues. The ensuing depression, anger, and acting out add to the youngster's inability to relate to caretakers with any trust or intimacy. In such a case, the initiation of a chronic illness may precipitate a psychotic depression, suicide attempts, or self-destructive, hostile behavior. Any of these will mitigate against the patient's cooperating with caretakers in a quest for effective control of the disease.

Adolescent issues in dealing with sexuality, independence, and intimacy need to be worked through with the help of the parents; lacking such help, the ensuing burdens may interfere with the adolescent's development. Envy of the adolescent, who is moving toward formal operational thinking and can conceptualize in ways the parent cannot, may inhibit the adolescent's learning. Parents who have long had grave problems with intimacy may resent their adolescent being helped in treatment to experience relationships and closeness they have never known. Thus therapy for the adolescent may be interfered with by the parents, unless they, too, have been brought into the process and are beginning to experience new feelings and to understand the need to facilitate their child's development. [37]

Development and Time of Onset as Factors in Control and Treatment of Chronic Disease

The impact of a chronic disease on children and their family will, to a large extent, be determined by the age and developmental state of the children. The younger the children, the greater the demand on the their capacity to cope and the more deforming the effect on subsequent development. Regression is a common response to a major stress, and in young children the regression may be very severe. The behavioral aspect may take the form of a loss of recently acquired developmental skills such as bowel and bladder control, speech, and beginning investigativeness; and the relationship dimension may take the form of withdrawal, isolation, increased dependence on the parent, and loss of capacity to socialize with other children. During the separation-individuation stage, increased symbiosis and regression from independent behavior may occur. [10]

Preschool children are especially vulnerable, and their obvious regression due to stress results in very protective and nurturant attitudes on the part of family members. Similarly, the young primary-school child is more likely to display overt reactions to stress, especially in the form of regression in self-care and in the capacity to learn. [57]

In the oedipal child, the onset of an illness may be perceived as punishment for the normal oedipal fantasies and wishes. The oedipal conflicts may therefore fail to be resolved and the long-range result may be strained relationships with one or both parents.

In the preadolescent and young adolescent periods, the regression may manifest itself as a loss of independent functions, a failure in one's striving for independence, and an inhibition in the enjoyment of such capacities as learning and exploring the world. [45] There may be a giving up of intimate friendships because of a fear of not being acceptable; this often results from the development of a distorted body image. A feeling of not being lovable, especially of not being desirable as a sexual partner, is also common. [58,61]

The family's behavior in response to their child's chronic illness may be determined by the child's vulnerability to stress. It may also be determined by the parents' need to protect the child or adolescent because of his or her immaturity or because of the special character of the adolescent problems that may have developed during the process of separation and becoming independent.*

*See references 5, 7, 14, 35, and 53.

Working with Parents in the Initial Stages of a Chronic Disease

It is evident from work with families whose young children develop chronic disease that the most effective preventive work can be done during the crisis period when the family is still under great stress due to the diagnosis of a chronic disease. In a university setting, efforts to involve the consultation-liaison child psychiatrist with the family at this early stage have proven very effective. It is important for the pediatrician to provide sanctioned intervention; this is best done in meetings with the family, the patient, and the psychiatrist. In my experience, this seems to smooth the transition from pediatrician to mental health professional in working through the crises provoked by the diagnosis of a chronic disease.

As consultant, the mental health professional needs to take an active role in explaining the kinds of feelings and anxieties that such a diagnosis may engender. It is relieving to the child and family to hear that their fears are understood and can be talked about. Sometimes the primary physician does not spell out clearly the seriousness of the illness or the major restrictions in activities necessary; these may then need to be clarified, leaving some room for hope and optimism. The frequent, regular appointments suggested by the mental health professional in the beginning make it evident that there are important matters to be discussed. [6]

Early in the disease, it is especially important that parents are helped to understand the implications of the condition in terms of disability, duration, possible interferences with normal developmental tasks, and so forth. When the child psychiatrist or other mental health professional can review—and sometimes interpret—the pediatrician's opinions and their implications for the child, then it becomes possible to elicit the parents' reactions and to discuss how they may foresee and deal with specific issues and problems. It is also possible to help the parents recognize their own needs to overprotect and infantilize the patient, as a means of reducing their guilt or making sure the child is well taken care of. In most chronic illnesses, it is important for the child to maintain usual patterns and current level of learning as much as possible.

Perhaps the most significant kind of primary prevention occurs when the parents are helped to work through their guilt and also helped to expect that the child will function at optimal capacity within the limitations imposed by the disease. These expectations need to be restated repeatedly to the parents, and then followed through with observations of the way in which the patient and family interact. When the child is not permitted to use the illness to avoid continued growth and development, then the psychologically healthy aspects of the child's and parents' personalities are marshaled in the service of mental and physical health. Thus maintaining the patient and family as fully functional as possible reduces exploitation, guilt, regression, and the psychological disorders that accompany conflictful behavior in child and parents. When they occur, such conflicts may interfere with a satisfactory adaptation in the present and optimal development in the future.[42]

The physician in private practice needs to become aware of his or her ability to perform this vital task of primary prevention. Where neither time nor ability to perform such a service permit the necessary involvement, then it becomes important to find a mental health professional, usually a psychiatric nurse or social worker hired by the physician, or to make an early referral to a collaborating mental health professional.

CASE VIGNETTE

Sandy was a five-and-one-half-year-old boy with chronic asthma. He had learned that an acute asthmatic attack evoked panic in his parents, and he began to use labored breathing as a means of getting his own way with them.[11,60] On enrollment in the first grade, his difficulty in breathing seemed to flare up when he was faced with a demand that he perform in reading. In fact, however, because of the advanced teaching and learning at home, he was well able to do this. He resisted the teacher's insistence that he read aloud in the group. With the parents' permission, the school nurse was called. She discussed Sandy's problem with his pediatrician and learned of his concern about the child's manipulation. This school nurse had previously worked in a child psychiatric setting and understood the parents' problems. She called the parents for a conference and discussed her concerns in terms of Sandy's already delayed development in sensorimotor activities and socialization, the possible future deleterious effects on his learning, and his current manipulation. The nurse then described what she believed the parents could do to help ensure the youngster's optimal function and development. They met weekly, four times, to discuss the parents' anxieties when their firmness at home began to produce wheezing. The pediatrician came to one of the meetings and prescribed a regimen for the parents when this occurred. In school, if wheezing began, Sandy was sent to the nurse, asked to lie down, and was given some aminophylline. Sometimes only the adrenaline mist was used.[20] Within a half hour, he was returned to the classroom and required to complete his reading task. Within a period of six weeks, the prompt response of parents, teacher, and nurse to breathing problems decreased their frequency markedly and increased Sandy's total, normal functioning in school and at home. The nurse's continued telephone contact with parents, her encouragement at moments of doubt, and her compliments at their ability to contain these breathing problems with less anxiety and more matter-of-fact handling were important factors in greatly reducing the manipulative behavior. There was marked improvement in Sandy's capacity to play games without labored breathing, in his learning in school, and in less disruptive behavior at home. The prospects for his further normal development were greatly improved.[18]

Problems Parents Experience

Not infrequently, parents will not agree with the physician's assessment that only a minimal degree of dysfunction or disability is present, nor do they share the opinion that the expectations made of the child should be quite normal. In those instances, some couples' therapy or counseling with a qualified child mental health professional is important.

A disagreement between parents usually reflects other areas of conflict. It often represents the abdication by one parent of a consistent parental role. As a rule, it is the father who withdraws and expects the mother, despite her anxiety, to be able to handle the situation.

I have found that short of long-term therapy, the most effective strategy is to depict for the parents the age-specific developmental tasks. It is then possible to delineate with each parent the role he or she could play in helping the child toward the most normal developmental adjustment that can be attained. It is of critical importance to help both parents recognize the value and excellence of the job they are already doing to promote their child's current adaptation and development. In each particular case of chronic disease, the mental health professional needs to obtain from the physician a picture of the existing degree of disability and an account of which activities can be safely encouraged. In the course of such brief treatment, clear action goals need to be outlined for each parent and to be reviewed on a weekly basis. In my experience home visits, usually at dinnertime, make it possible to see for oneself both the degree of the child's manipulative behavior and the interactions of parents, siblings, and patient. Repeated visits demonstrate how the various agreed-on tasks are being carried out. Where problem-solving efforts have been decided on in which each parent consents to carry out a task, such observations help clarify the obstacles to their realization. Over time, both parents learn to function in a more mutually supportive and effective way, with reduced manipulation by the child. In many instances the parents' new learning in the service of aiding more normal development is reflected in their increased capacity to talk together with reduced stress about many other family issues.[6]

CASE VIGNETTE

Annie, age eight, was a recently diagnosed juvenile diabetic.[22,66] An effort was made to treat the disease primarily by means of dietary management and to keep insulin treatment to a minimum; this was interfered with, however, by the father giving in to his daughter's requests for sweets. Despite several minor hyperglycemic crises, the father was convinced that if the mother were not so reluctant to give more insulin shots, his daughter could have her sweets.[56] When several conferences with the pediatrician and reiteration of the importance of dietary treatment did not alter the father's behavior, the family was referred to a child psychiatrist.[59] The child psychiatrist took several sessions to reeducate the parents and child about the course of the disease and the possible serious sequelae if the prescribed regimen were not followed. In couples' therapy, the father's reluctance to admit that his daughter had a chronic illness, his concern that it was his fault because there was diabetes in several immediate family members, and his anxiety about unresolved oedipal problems began to emerge.[29] There were oedipally tinged conflicts between the parents, which took form in the father's slavish compliance with every wish of their daughter; these were also clarified, as were the needs for parental collaboration on behalf of the daughter's continued normal development and the realization of her full intellectual potential. There were three months of weekly sessions; after parental collaboration had been effected, the last three sessions were held with the daughter present. The daughter's natural tendency to manipulate was discussed and the problems in the parents' working together were clarified. The impact of the parents' collaboration on the increased normality of their daughter's functioning proved the effectiveness of their mutual efforts.[25,27] In the three final family sessions, a clarification of the purpose of the parents' newly found, joint efforts in helping Annie occurred. The much more effective treatment of the diabetes was credited to the parents' unity and to Annie's responsiveness to their mutual support; this resulted in the parents and Annie feeling much closer to each other. The parents' increased collaboration on Annie's behalf also led to a more unified and effective handling of their rebellious, fourteen-year-old adolescent son.

Problems in Brief Interventions

The intervention process with parents is more important and, as a rule, easier to carry out in the case of the younger child who becomes ill with a chronic disease. By early and midadolescence, certain personality and developmental patterns will already have consolidated, and the young person will often require intensive psychotherapeutic help to continue both development and personality growth.

When the parents are seriously mentally ill or very disorganized and primitive in their pattern of living, effective cooperation in the treatment of their child's chronic disease becomes very difficult. In my experience, these families require concrete help such as frequent home visits by a visiting nurse or frequent phone calls to remind them of their resolve not to yield to the child's manipulative behavior. They also need a very goal-oriented approach that requires only small increments of behavioral change.[6]

CASE VIGNETTE

Debbie, a twelve-year-old anorexic, was referred for psychiatric evaluation prior to her discharge from the pediatric ward.[44] Her mother had several hospitalizations for schizophrenia; she was constantly on the ward and repeatedly interfered with the nurses' efforts with her daughter.[24,48] The family had recently moved from Appalachia and were on welfare. The father and the oldest son worked together to repair their rented, run-down house and to repair old cars when such work was available. Living arrangements in the home were chaotic; unless the mother was at home and in sufficiently integrated condition to supervise the family, no one cleaned house or helped with washing clothes, cleaning the yard, and so on.

In interviews Debbie and her parents were anxious about Debbie's entrance into high school and the reported sexual acting-out behavior of "many" students. The mother was apprehensive that despite her cadaverous appearance, Debbie would be molested. We worked with Debbie alone and in family therapy; we worked with the parents in couples' therapy as well as family therapy.[52] The problem of keeping appointments was overcome when the two cotherapists and a visiting nurse made an evening home visit after each missed appointment. After three such occasions, Debbie, the parents, and, later, the two brothers and a sister came on time for their various appointments.

The visiting nurse played a vital role in helping the family obtain needed services from welfare and health agencies. When we talked with the nurse about the need for the father and older brother, Dan, to find work, she went with Dan to vocational rehabilitation to assist in his enrollment in a welding and auto mechanics course. With much urging in treatment and with reminders by the visiting nurse who saw the family at least once a week at home, the father began to look for a job in earnest and finally found one as laborer in a construction project. At this point, the mother looked both more disoriented and fragile; at the same time, however, with Debbie's help, she gradually began to clean up the house, throw out broken furniture, and paint some of the rooms.[15,28,31]

In her own treatment, Debbie began to deal with her sexual fears as well as her fear of father's reprisals if she had a boyfriend. Ultimately she was able to raise these issues in family therapy.

When we invited ourselves to dinner with the family, its unappetizing quality resulted in no one eating very much. With the nurse's help, the mother took an afternoon nutrition class, and our second experience of dinner together was much improved and more enjoyable. When eating with the family, it was clear that no one was really concerned with Debbie's not eating or about her weight loss.

The parents were concerned that Debbie might find someone who would give her a good life, not only economically but also in terms of closeness, tenderness, and sexual enjoyment. There was a good deal of anxiety related to her loss to the family if this should happen. The parents had had their first child nine months after they were married. The mother would not talk about her feelings toward sexual relations except, as an aside, that it was for the man's pleasure.

While the treatment took three years and dealt with many issues individually for Debbie, the parents, and the family, improvement in the family's functioning with jobs, school, and home improvement began with open, direct, frequent interventions and support that enabled such changes to occur. After the first six months the mother did not have another psychotic episode and both parents worked toward allowing Debbie to develop as a more normal adolescent. After three years, Debbie, quite pretty and at normal weight, had a boyfriend, with no objections from her father. The father had become quite effective on the job and his skill as an electrician was being utilized. Dan was working as a mechanic on a used car lot, and the mother became proud of her home management and often brought samples of her cakes (she had learned cake decoration) to family meetings to show and "brag on" to the cotherapists. It is clear that aspects of the parents' developmental problems, the disorganized nature of the family, and the problems of living with mother's psychosis all needed to be handled along with Debbie's individual treatment. The practical issues of altering living patterns for parents and older brothers had required support and actual help in dealing with agencies in order to get family members moving. The constant reexamination of weekly accomplishments helped the family maintain their efforts. Each family member became pleased and proud of his accomplishments, but the first praise and encouragement came from the visiting nurse and the therapists. While the dynamics of symbiotic attachment between mother and daughter, problems in separation-individuation, and oedipal problems were all identified, they were dealt with only in the psychotherapy with Debbie. Our work and collaboration prevented continued family disorganization, stopped its dependence on society, prevented recurrent maternal psychosis, and interrupted Debbie's drift toward becoming a chronic anorexic.

Parental Empathy

Many parents who are disturbed by their child's chronic illness are not themselves psychologically minded. They may be too disturbed to be dealt with in brief family therapy, or their concrete level of thinking makes it difficult for them to understand necessary therapeutic concepts. Many disorganized families come from environments where they resort to often-stated, simplistic solutions to life problems on the one hand and massive denial on the other, which makes problem solving very difficult. It may be difficult to state the problem in terms that are comprehensible to the parents, but it is essential to strive to do so. In her paper on the use of parental empathy, Anna Ornstein points to a method that may be effective with many such parents. [6,42] The work with parents is focused on helping them feel sympathetic to the pain of the child, understand its origin, and become willing to act in such a way as to reduce the suffering.

Such is the case of Debbie and her very disorganized parents: One parent was seriously mentally ill; the other was very confused, simple-minded, and overwhelmed by the move from the Kentucky hills to a large, West Coast city.

Mother had loudly upbraided the nurses who tube-fed her very weak, anorexic daughter. Despite her schizophrenic decompensation, however, when she was required to recognize her daughter's anguish, she somehow was able to do so and became less demanding and vituperative toward the nurses.

With the emergence of the parents' fear that their daughter's return to school would result in a sexual assault, the girl's fears and reluctance to attend school were greatly magnified. The parents were asked to control their fears of the daughter's going off to school; they were assured that she was attending a good academic high school with the opportunity to learn and prepare for a desirable job or profession. With the help of role playing, the parents learned how to convey these ideas with some conviction. During home visits at dinnertime, it became clear that at best the food was poorly prepared and that no one cared about Debbie's starvation. One of our hypotheses was her anorexia stemmed from several sources. For one thing, there were sexual fears and anxieties that her father would kill any boyfriend of hers; for another, there was her hope that her very disturbed mother might become concerned about her starvation and feed her. When her mother paid her daughter little attention, it only reinforced Debbie's desire to punish herself. In addition to deserving her father's unexpressed anger at her for growing into womanhood, she was unworthy of her mother's love.

We were able to ask the mother to help us by experimenting with preparing better meals and, especially, by providing the specific foods that Debbie enjoyed. We asked her to let her daughter know in words that she was cooking for her. Gradually, the mother began to understand both Debbie's and her own need to be fed. Thus both mother and daughter began to work together to cook more appetizing meals.

Debbie was attracted to a boy in her class and, despite the fact that she was obviously fearful of her father's anger, she brought this up in family therapy. The father was asked to observe Debbie's anxious demeanor. We wondered if he were angry even at nice young men who liked Debbie, and whether this attitude was fair. The father recognized he could allay Debbie's fears and help her toward the normal, adolescent goals that we had discussed so many times. He grudgingly said if this were a nice boy he'd like to meet him and would then approve of their going out together.

Thus, at every step, we were able to help the parents become aware of their ability to understand their child's pain and to encourage them to try to alleviate it.

Special Problems of the Adolescent

Some of the most difficult problems occur in working with families whose adolescents have developed chronic disease—especially young adolescents just beginning to make friends and to find a compatible peer group. The chronic disease alters their self-image; they are certain that with their disease, no one could care about them. The turmoil of adolescence arises from a mix of hormonal and environmental changes; to this there are now added a variety of other stresses: alterations in cognitive capacities, the need to individuate and separate from parents, the development of the sense of a sexual self, and the need to develop a capacity for intimacy. Taken together, they all become urgent issues. In the face of all this, the stress brought on by a chronic disease may prove overwhelming. Thus there may be severe depression and suicidal feelings. Half-formed plans for further schooling, going to work, or possible marriage all need to be laid aside for a while.

Some adolescents will already have become expert at challenging adults and manipulating them to their ends. In the face of the illness, they may either abandon such efforts to obtain more parental support, or such behavior may become aggravated due to the anger directed at fate and the need to blame someone for the disease.

The necessity for individual help, counseling, or treatment for the adolescent has been noted.

In many situations, some alienation will have already occurred because of the adolescent's constant demands, frequent and unpredictable alterations in affect, and efforts to manipulate. When the illness then supervenes, parents who had hoped the adolescent would soon be independent may resent the increased dependency that is now thrust upon them. Indeed, in the face of the changed conditions, parents may have difficulty in clarifying their new role.

One of the foci of the work with parents of adolescents is the restatement and clarification of the developmental goals of adolescence, the review of how or in what ways the chronic disease may interfere or delay realization of these goals, and how, in each area of development, the parents can help toward goal attainment.

Summary and Discussion

The chronic illness of a child always affects the homeostasis within the family. The more developmental problems and failures, the greater the difficulties confronting the family.

One of the critical developmental issues centers around the child or adolescent's tendency to use the illness to manipulate and exploit the family and to avoid the pain of learning and growing in the context of the invalidism and incapacity. Thus very early discussions with the family (and sometimes family therapy or couples' therapy) that focus on and anticipate the manipulation may prevent its occurrence or may at least cut it short so that no pervasive patterns are developed.

The physician has an important role in preparing the patient and family to deal with the stress of a diagnosis of chronic disease. Because of the pressure of time or the failure to understand the human needs involved, this responsibility may not be discharged in an optimal fashion.

The role of mental health professionals then becomes critical. The work with parents to help their child to live as effectively as possible without becoming manipulative is a very important dimension of primary or secondary prevention.

Those parents whose own developmental problems make it difficult to deal with their child who is going through a similar developmental stage will ultimately require extra help to deal with some of their past difficulties, if they are to understand their child's problems and pain empathically.

Similarly, the parents' guilt about wanting to be rid of a burdensome child with chronic disease may well require clarification and understanding from a mental health professional. Only if it is possible to relieve the guilt will they be free to take seriously their obligation to help the child or adolescent to function more effectively and develop with less difficulty.

Where things go well, as the parents act to promote optimal growth, family strife is reduced and manipulation by the patient becomes unnecessary. The result of effective therapeutic work with the parents is the prevention of serious and prolonged regression, of the manipulation that can so readily interfere with the child's functioning and development, and, finally, of the serious family problems that all too often compound the effects of the chronic illness on both family and child.

REFERENCES

1. ANDERSON, B. J., and AUSLANDER, W. F. "Research on Diabetes Management and the Family: A Critique," *Diabetes Care*, 3 (1980):696–702.

2. ANTHONY, E. J. "A Working Model for Family Studies: A Developmental-Transactional Model," in E. J. ANTHONY and C. KOUPERNIK, eds., *The Child in His Family: The Im-pact of Disease and Death.* New York: John Wiley & Sons, 1973, pp. 3–20.

3. ANYAN, W. R., JR., and SCHOWALTER, J. E. "A Comprehensive Approach to Anorexia Nervosa," *Journal of the American Academy of Child Psychiatry,* 22 (1983):122–127.

4. BELMONTE, M. M., GUNN, T., and GONTHIER, M. "The

Problem of 'Cheating' in the Diabetic Child and Adolescent," *Diabetes Care,* 4 (1981):116–20.

5. BENEDEK, T. "Parenthood as a Developmental Phase: A Contribution to the Libido Therapy," *Journal of the American Psychoanalytic Association,* 7 (1959):389–417.

6. BERLIN, I. N. "A Developmental Approach to Work with Disorganized Families," *Journal of the American Academy of Child Psychiatry,* 18 (1979):354–365.

7. ——. "Opportunities in Adolescence to Rectify Adolescent Failures," in S. C. Feinstein et al., eds., *Adolescent Psychiatry.* Chicago: University of Chicago Press, 1980, pp. 231–243.

8. ——. "Family Treatment of Severe Adolescent Problems," in J. H. Masserman, ed., *Current Psychiatric Therapies.* New York: Grune & Stratton, 1981, pp. 61–69.

9. ——. "Family Treatment of Chronic Illness in a Child: Mutual Developmental Problems," in A. E. Christ and K. Flomenhaft, eds., *Psychosocial Family Interventions in Chronic Pediatric Illness.* New York: Plenum Press, 1982, pp. 13–28.

10. BERLIN, I. N., and BERLIN, R. "Parents on the Developmental Advocates of Children," in I. N. Berlin, ed., *Advocacy for Child Mental Health.* New York: Brunner/Mazel, 1975, pp. 37–45.

11. BHAT, B. R., et al. "Study of Social, Educational, Environmental and Cultural Aspects of Childhood Asthma in Clinic and Private Patients in the City of New York," *Annals of Allergy,* 41 (1978):89–92.

12. BINGER, C. M., et al. "Childhood Leukemia: Emotional Impact on Patient and Family," *New England Journal of Medicine,* 280 (1969):414–418.

13. BRUCH, H. "Anorexia Nervosa Therapy and Theory," *American Journal of Psychiatry,* 39 (1982): 1531–1538.

14. BRUMBERG, J. J., "Chlorotic Girls, 1870–1920: A Historical Perspective on Female Adolescence," *Child Development,* 53 (1982):1468–1477.

15. CAILLE, P., et al. "A Systems Theory Approach to a Case of Anorexia Nervosa," *Family Process,* 16 (1977):455–465.

16. CEASER, M. "The Role of Maternal Identification in Four Cases of Anorexia Nervosa," *Bulletin of the Menninger Clinic,* 41 (1977):475–486.

17. CONRAD, D. E. "A Starving Family," *Bulletin of the Menninger Clinic,* 41 (1977):487–495.

18. CREER, T. L., and BURNS, K. L. "Self-Management Training for Children with Chronic Asthma," *Psychotherapy and Psychosomatics,* 32 (1979):270–278.

19. DEBUSKEY, M., ed. *The Chronically Ill Child and His Family.* Springfield, Ill.: Charles C. Thomas, 1970.

20. DOLOVICH, J., and HARGREAVE, F. E. "Strategies in the Control of Asthma," *Medical Clinics of North America,* 65 (1981):1033–1043.

21. ERIKSON, E. H. "Eight Ages of Man," in *Childhood and Society.* New York: W. W. Norton, 1963, pp. 247–274.

22. GALATZER, A., et al. "Crisis Intervention Program in Newly Diagnosed Diabetic Children," *Diabetes Care,* 5 (1982):414–419.

23. GARDNER, R. "The Guilt Reaction of Parents of Children with Severe Physical Disease," *American Journal of Psychiatry,* 126 (1969):636–644.

24. GOLDSTEIN, M. J. "Family Factors Associated with Schizophrenia and Anorexia Nervosa," *Journal of Youth and Adolescence,* 10 (1981):385–405.

25. HAMBURG, B. A., and INOFF, G. E. "Relationships Between Behavioral Factors and Diabetic Control in Children and Adolescents: A Camp Study," *Psychosomatic Medicine,* 44 (1982):321–339.

26. HARPER, G. "Varieties of Parenting Failure in Anorexia Nervosa: Protection and Parentectomy, Revisited," *Journal of the American Academy of Child Psychiatry,* 22 (1983):134–139.

27. HAUSER, S. T., et al. "Ego Development and Self-Esteem in Diabetic Adolescents," *Diabetes Care,* 2 (1979): 465–471.

28. HEDBOM, J. E., HUBBARD, F. A., and ANDERSEN, A. E. "Anorexia Nervosa: A Multidisciplinary Treatment Program for Patient and Family," *Social Work in Health Care,* 7 (1981):67–86.

29. HINKLE, L. E., and WOLF, S. "A Study of Experimental Evidence Relating Life Stress to Diabetic Mellitus," *Journal of the Mount Sinai Hospital,* 1 (1952):337.

30. KAPLAN, D. M. "Early Interventions for Families with Chronically Ill Children," in A. E. Christ and K. Flomenhaft, eds., *Psychosocial Family Interventions in Chronic Pediatric Illness.* New York: Plenum Press, 1982, pp. 37–48.

31. LAGOS, J. M. "Family Therapy in the Treatment of Anorexia Nervosa: Theory and Technique," *International Journal of Psychiatry in Medicine,* 11 (1981):291–302.

32. LIEBMAN, R., SARGENT, J., and SILVER, M. "A Family Systems Orientation to the Treatment of Anorexia Nervosa," *Journal of the American Academy of Child Psychiatry,* 22 (1983):128–133.

33. LISS, J., and SHARMA, C. N. "Multi-Generational Dynamics in a Case of Ulcerative Colitis," *Psychiatric Quarterly,* 44 (1970):461–475.

34. LITT, I. F., and CUSKEY, W. R. "Compliance with Salicylate Therapy in Adolescents with Juvenile Rheumatoid Arthritis," *American Journal of Diseases of Children,* 135 (1981):434–436.

35. LITT, I. F., CUSKEY, S. R., and ROSENBERG, A. "Role of Self-Esteem and Autonomy in Determining Medication Compliance Among Adolescents with Juvenile Rheumatoid Arthritis," *American Academy of Pediatrics,* 69 (1982):15–17.

36. McCOLEUM, A. T. *The Chronically Ill Child.* New Haven: Yale University Press, 1982.

37. MATTSON, A., and AGLE, D. P. "Group Therapy with Parents of Hemopheliacs: Therapeutic Process and Observations of Parental Adaptations to Chronic Illness in Children," *Journal of the American Academy of Child Psychiatry,* 11 (1972):558–571.

38. MILLER, L. V., GOLDSTEIN, J., and NICOLAISEN, G. "Evaluation of Patient's Knowledge of Diabetes Self-Care," *Diabetes Care,* 1 (1978):275–180.

39. MINUCHIN, S. "The Use of an Ecological Framework in Treatment of a Child," in E. J. Anthony and C. Koupernic, eds., *The Child in His Family.* New York: Wiley Interscience, 1970, pp. 41–58.

40. MINUCHIN, S., et al. "A Conceptual Model of Psychosomatic Illness in Children," *Archives of General Psychiatry,* 32 (1975):1031–1038.

41. MORGAN, H. G., and RUSSELL, G.F.M. "Value of Family Background and Clinical Features as Predictors of Long-Term Outcome in Anorexia Nervosa: Four-Year Follow-up Study of 41 Patients," *Psychological Medicine,* 5 (1975):355–371.

42. ORNSTEIN, A. "Making Contact with the Inner World of the Child: Toward a Theory of Psychoanalytic Psychotherapy with Children," *Comprehensive Psychiatry,* 17 (1976): 3–36.

43. PAGE, P., et al. "Patient Recall of Self-Care Recommendations in Diabetes," *Diabetes Care,* 4 (1981):96–98.

44. PLANK, E. N. *Working with Children in Hospitals.* Chicago: Year Book Medical Publishers, 1971.

45. PLOWDEN REPORT, Central Advisory Council for Education (England). *Children and Their Primary Schools,* vol. 1. London: Her Majesty's Stationery Office, 1966.

46. POZNANSKI, E. O., et al. "Quality of Life for Long-Term Survivors of End-Stage Renal Disease," *Journal of the American Medical Association,* 239 (1978):2343–2347.

47. PRUGH, D. G., and JORDAN, K. "The Management of Ulcerative Colitis in Childhood," in J. G. Howell, ed., *Modern Perspectives in International Psychiatry.* Edinburgh: Oliver and Boyd, 1969, pp. 494–524.

48. RAMPLING, D. "Single Case Study, Abnormal Mothering in the Genesis of Anorexia Nervosa," *Journal of Nervous and Mental Disease,* 168 (1980):501–504.

49. REINHART, J. B. "Disorders of the Gastrointestinal Tract in Children: Consultation-Liaison Experience," *Psychiatric Clinics of North America,* 5 (1982):387–397.

50. RICHARDS, W., et al. "A Self-Help Program for Childhood Asthma in a Residential Treatment Center," *Clinical Pediatrics,* 20 (1981):453–457.

51. ROBERTS, M. C., and WURTELE, S. K. "Research Note: On the Noncompliant Research Subject in a Study of Medical Noncompliance," *Social Science and Medicine,* 14A (1980):171.

52. ROSE, J., and GARFINKEL, P. E. "A Parents' Group in the Management of Anorexia Nervosa," *Canadian Journal of Psychiatry,* 25 (1980):228–233.

53. ROTHENBERG, M. B. "The Effect of a Child's Chronic Illness on the Family," in A. E. Christ and K. Flomenhaft, eds., *Psychosocial Family Interventions in Chronic Pediatric Illness.* New York: Plenum Press, 1982, pp. 163–178.

54. SHAFI, M., SALGUERO, C., and FINCH, S. M. "Psychopathology and Treatment of Anorexia Nervosa in Latency-Age Siblings," Paper presented at the annual meeting of the American Academy of Child Psychiatry, New Orleans, 1972.

55. SIMONDS, J. F. "Emotions and Compliance in Diabetic Children," *Psychosomatics,* 20 (1979):544–551.

56. SIMONDS, J. F., et al. "The Relationship Between Psychological Factors and Blood Glucose Regulation in Insulin-Dependent Diabetic Adolescents," *Diabetes Care,* 4 (1981):610–615.

57. STEELE, B. F. "Parental Abuse of Infants and Small Children," in E. J. Anthony and T. Benedek, eds., *Parenthood: Its Psychology and Psychopathology.* Boston: Little, Brown, 1970, pp. 449–477.

58. STEIN, S. P., and CHARLES, E. "Emotional Factors in Juvenile Diabetes Mellitus: A Study of Early Life Experiences of Adolescent Diabetics," *American Journal of Psychiatry,* 128 (1971):56.

59. STERKY, G. "Family Background and State of Mental Health in a Group of Diabetic School Children," *Acta Paediatrica,* 52 (1963):377.

60. SUBLFIT, J. L, et al. "Noncompliance in Asthmatic Children: A Study of Theophylline Levels in a Pediatric Emergency Room Population," *Annals of Allergy,* 43 (1979):95–97.

61. SULLIVAN, B. J. "Self-Esteem and Depression in Adolescent Diabetic Girls," *Diabetes Care,* 1 (1978):18–22.

62. TARNOW, J. D., and TOMLINSON, N. "Juvenile Diabetes: Impact on the Child and Family," *Psychosomatics,* 19 (1978):487–491.

63. THOMAS, A., and CHESS, S. *Temperament and Development.* New York: Brunner/Mazel, 1977.

64. TETREAULT, A. I., "Evaluation of Developmental Health Counseling: Healthfulness of Self-Support Behavior," *Nursing Research,* 26 (1977):386–390.

65. TROUT, J. D. "Birth of a Sick or Handicapped Infant: Impact on the Family," *Child Welfare,* 52 (1983):337–348.

66. WINTER, R. J. "Special Problems of the Child with Diabetes," *Pediatrics,* 8 (1982):7–13.

65 / Childhood Cancer: Survival

Shirley B. Lansky and Nancy U. Cairns

Introduction

It is anticipated that in the next decade, one twenty-year-old out of every one thousand will be a survivor of childhood cancer.[17] This statistic represents truly astounding progress over the past quarter of a century in the treatment of this illness. Advances in surgery, radiotherapy, and chemotherapy have dramatically improved the prognosis for childhood cancer. Whereas twenty or thirty years ago such a child faced virtually certain death, many of those diagnosed now have an excellent chance of long-term, disease-free survival. The quality of survival has therefore become increasingly important, and the mental health community faces both the opportunity and obligation to address the needs of these children.

Long-term survival is not achieved without problems. Even under the best of circumstances, the patients and their families have gone through a severely traumatic period. Living under a lethal threat has altered life-style, relationships, and future plans, and has brought about some more subtle intrapsychic change as well. This chapter identifies the problems encountered by the child and family and offers suggestions for intervention/prevention strategies. It also suggests areas in which research is needed to answer questions as to long-term effects of both the disease and the treatment on the child's physical and emotional development.

574

Before discussing the long-term survivor, it is important to review the problems encountered by the child and family as they move through the course of the diagnosis and treatment. Adequate care during this period is the best foundation for the child and family's long-term adaptation.

Diagnosis and Referral to a Tertiary Care Center

Most children suspected of having cancer are now referred to a tertiary care center for diagnostic procedures and initiation of treatment. At this time, the child and family face the double burden of fear of the diagnosis and fear of a large medical center. There are many tasks for them during this initial period. They must absorb information about the illness and prognosis, learn about various tests and treatment procedures, and master the names and side effects of numerous chemotherapeutic agents. Most of the parents have had no previous experience with severe illness and complicated medical care. While learning about the disease and treatment ultimately gives them a sense of mastery, in the early stages the parents find that this education produces anxiety.

Meanwhile, at a time when making a positive diagnosis and the institution of therapy are of primary concern to the physician, the parents may have more immediate concerns, such as comforting the child and coping with this major disruption in their lives. Ultimately, the priorities of the child, the parents, and the physician must be brought into synchrony, an outcome that is not readily accomplished.

One example of the disparity between parents', child's, and physician's priorities is that the family will often protest the number of diagnostic procedures which the physician sees as necessary to establish an accurate diagnosis and institute appropriate treatment. Both the child and the parents are usually very frightened by the many procedures, particularly those that are invasive and cause pain. This is a period when a child psychiatrist can intervene effectively by serving as an interpreter between the oncologist and the family as well as by focusing on the family's anxiety.

When a surgical procedure is planned, detailed information about events leading up to and following the operation is very helpful to the child and parents. Children may have to face amputation or other procedures that result in disability or visible deformity; in such instances education about the procedure and its consequences should begin very early. Children are best able to handle this kind of trauma when they have several days to respond to the information, ask questions, and seek support from others in the family and from friends. Other amputees can assist immeasurably in the child's preparation for surgery and are usually more than willing to do so. It is important to provide opportunities for the child to discuss the changes that will result from surgery and to rehearse or role-play talking with friends and returning to school and community after surgery. In addition, the child psychiatrist assists in dispelling unrealistic fantasies (e.g., "the prosthesis will work as well as your own leg") and helping the child mourn the loss.

The problems most often encountered on inpatient oncology services relate to difficult and demanding patients and parents and their resistance to the treatments. One such problem is frequently encountered and, once established, is particularly difficult to change. It is called symbiotic regression.[10]

A symbiotic relationship between the sick child and a parent (usually the mother) leads them to isolate themselves in the child's hospital room. They resist contact with medical caregivers, other patients and families, and even with their own families. This maladaptive behavior progresses to a hostile-dependent relationship between the two, characterized by extremely regressive behavior on the part of the child and severe separation anxiety for both. Their pathological clinging interferes with the child's medical care because the pair resists any intrusion in their relationship, including that of physicians and nurses. As noted, once it develops, this pattern is difficult to reverse; thus early identification of warning signals and encouragement of separation are of paramount importance.

The Return Home

The return home can be a literal event or a figurative one. For some children, there is an actual period of hospitalization whereas others receive induction therapy as outpatients. In both situations, the end of induction therapy is a transition period for both patient and family. By this time the effect of the disease and treatment has caused a marked change in the patient's self-concept and in how others relate to him or her. Friends and relatives will have been informed about the disease, but their previous experiences with cancer, usually in adults, will color their interpretation of the limited information they receive.

On their arrival home, the family must establish a new routine that accommodates the care of the sick child into their everyday activities. Despite the staff's and parents' best efforts, children are often overindulged in the hospital, and they then have difficulty settling back into a normal routine in which they have assigned chores, fixed bedtimes, and the usual limits placed on their behavior. The parents' compassion for the child's suffering, fear of possible death, and guilt over the illness compound their difficulties in reestablishing a normal pattern of discipline. The same factors may produce altered sleep patterns and sleeping arrangements for the child. For example, in some families the child with cancer sleeps with the parents. Initially this practice begins because of the child's anxiety and the parents' fear for the child's safety at night. Once begun, the practice is difficult to interrupt and interferes with the child's growing need for independence and increasing autonomy.

Another task involves reintegration into the community.[9] Upon their return home the child and family may face social isolation. Friends and relatives may avoid the family because they do not understand the diagnosis and treatment or are overwhelmed by the emotional connotations of cancer. Among the lay public it is common to associate all cancer with pain, mutilation, and inevitable death. The emotional reaction of those who hold this view may interfere with their ability to talk to the patient and the family. Many believe that cancer is contagious and thus avoid exposure to anyone with the disease. If the child and family recognize these possible causes of isolation, they can help dispel the misconceptions. Families and children who take an assertive approach to educating others are usually successful in renewing their friendships and family ties.

The opposite side of the isolation problem is intrusive interference on the part of family and friends. Criticism and unwanted advice can be offered in a misguided attempt to help the family. Such advice often concerns issues the family has already identified and attempted to resolve—such as place and type of treatment, discipline, open discussions with the child, division of responsibilities, or school. When close relatives (such as grandparents) interfere, a conference with the doctors will usually assist the parents in affirming the decisions they have already made.

News coverage of cancer treatment is the impetus for much unsolicited advice. Newspapers, magazines, fund-raising events, and television talk shows disseminate information about cancer research ("breakthroughs") and unconventional treatments in such a dramatic way that it is difficult for the general public to evaluate the reports. The result is that relatives and friends may encourage the family to change the child's treatment by transferring to another, more prestigious cancer center or by seeking a "miracle cure." Those who suggest alternative treatment approaches to the family are well-meaning and often very persuasive. In refusing to subject their child to unproven methods, the family may experience guilt and anxiety about their decision and about their relationship with the persuader.

SCHOOL

The patient's most frequent encounter with the community occurs at school. School is a particularly important task for the child with cancer. Just as the success of psychosocial rehabilitation of the adult cancer patient is measured by return to employment, so can the child's rehabilitation be assessed by progress in school.

Children with cancer have a very high rate of absenteeism and outright school refusal. In a study of a large sample of such children, the rate of classical school phobia was 11 percent.[13] Even in those children who do not have a full-blown school phobia, there is a higher than expected rate of absenteeism.[12] The high rate of nonattendance is not directly related to serious medical problems, as absences occur even when the child is in remission and doing well. Besides absenteeism, other problems noted in the school records of these children are behavior problems and decline in grades.

The presence of this high rate of absenteeism and frequent school problems in this population is quite disturbing. It cannot be safely assumed that the newly diagnosed child with cancer will return smoothly to school and be able to maintain a prediagnosis level of attendance and achievement. Throughout the treatment period, the importance of school must be addressed and a program of surveillance and active intervention maintained.

Cost of Treatment

Because of its intensity and duration, the cost of treatment contributes significantly to the overall stress on the family. The cost of treatment can be divided into direct medical charges and nonmedical out-of-pocket expenses. The nonmedical costs have a greater immediate impact on the family's budget.[14] The expenditures are generally in six categories: extra food, transportation, family care, lodging, extra clothing, and miscellaneous items. In a survey of these out-of-pocket expenses, half the families reported that at least 26 percent of their weekly family budget went toward these items; an additional problem was the loss of parents' pay. Four factors influenced nonmedical expenses. For obvious reasons, hospitalization (as opposed to outpatient treatment or no contact) and distance from the treatment center were associated with higher expenses. As the child's ability to perform normal activities deteriorated, expenses increased. Costs also increased with family size; the more children in the family, the greater the expense of caring for them in the parents' absence. Single-parent families bore a particularly heavy burden, presumably because single mothers have to turn to paid helpers to care for siblings while the patient is being treated at the medical center. These out-of-pocket expenses are not covered by third-party carriers and are therefore not reimbursed. Most of them are not even deductible for income tax purposes.

Direct medical costs for cancer treatment are staggering. In 1976 approximately $15 billion per year were spent for cancer treatment in the United States. This sum represented one-sixth of the total cost of health care in this country.

In a group of fifteen children who died of cancer, based on an average duration of illness of thirty-two months, the mean treatment charges for the course of the illness were $33,000. The major source of payment of these bills was insurance. However, up to three years after the child's death, half the families still had longstanding medical debts to pay. In the past, it has been said that an illness should be considered catastrophic if it costs more than 15 percent of the yearly gross family income. Half of the affected families experienced costs related to their child's illness that amounted to at least one-third of their monthly income.[11] This total financial burden was made up of medical charges not covered by third-party carriers, nonmedical out-of-pocket costs, and loss of pay. Clearly no family can plan for this type of financial assault, and at best this economic impact must add significantly to the family's overall distress. Many will be faced with the possibility of bankruptcy when they are trying to ensure the best care available. Because of the depletion of resources over an extended period, even when the financial hardship is less extreme, it has long-lasting deleterious effects on all members of the family. Ultimately parents and siblings are deprived of basic necessities because such a large proportion of the family budget goes toward the care of the sick child. It is interesting to note that a similar study was done in a country that has a National Health Service. The conclusions were the same: The out-of-pocket costs of childhood cancer were devastating for the families.[2]

There are no simple solutions for the financial plight of these families. The best one can do is to forewarn them about the magnitude of the expenses they will encounter.

Completion of Therapy

When a child has cancer, the moment at which therapy is discontinued is another nodal point of stress. Initially the family looks forward to the completion of therapy as the end of all their difficulties. By the time they arrive at this point, however, they may be very anxious about taking the child off chemotherapy. Since the diagnosis was determined, the members of the medical team have been stressing the importance of medications in keeping the child in remission. The routine of taking pills or receiving intravenous medication has become important in maintaining the parents' and child's security and optimism. Consequently, there is an understandable fear that discontinuing therapy will bring about a relapse of the cancer. Thus it is imperative that the physician outline the reasons for discontinuing therapy, the probability of relapse with or without treatment, and the risks of continuing therapy any longer than necessary. For those parents who need more reassurance, a brief description can be provided of treatments that can be utilized if a relapse occurs.

Long-Term Survival

The issues facing long-term survivors and their families can be divided roughly into medical and psychosocial problems. However, as in any consideration of psyche and soma, the division is an arbitrary one with many obvious linkages between the two. For purposes of discussion, however, we will maintain the psyche/soma distinction while pointing out some of the important interrelationships between the two. The medical/physical problems to be considered include: the possibility of late recurrence of the initial disease, long-term sequelae of the disease and treatment, the possibility of developing a second malignancy, and concerns about fertility and progeny. The psychosocial issues include: fear of recurrent disease and/or late sequelae, coping with disability and "differentness," emancipation from the family despite the fact that dependency needs are intensified by the illness, achieving and maintaining academic and vocational success, and normal experiences with peers including heterosexual relationships culminating in intimacy and marriage.

MEDICAL LATE EFFECTS OF CANCER AND CANCER THERAPY

The late effects of cancer therapy are wide-ranging. There are obvious physical disabilities that result from the effects of surgery or drug toxicity on major organ systems. The other end of the spectrum includes those subtle neurologic deficits that result from prophylactic central nervous system (CNS) treatment. In the first category, a wide variety of physical sequelae have been reported. One major problem is vital organ failure.[1,4] Children are being seen who have developed cardiac abnormalities, liver failure, severe pulmonary dysfunction, and impairment of renal function. These effects may show up quite late; some cases have occurred as long as nine years following treatment. The combination of irradiation and certain of the anthracycline chemotherapeutic agents can cause a hepatopathy that may progress on to cirrhosis. The lungs are also susceptible to the effects of these agents causing pneumonopathies of varying degrees of severity.

Scoliosis and other skeletal abnormalities as well as growth and development alterations can originate from two sources: (1) when given for a long time, radiation and chemotherapeutic agents can affect bone growth directly[3]; and (2) irradiation of the pituitary and thyroid can lead to hypofunction with secondary curtailment of growth.

Another type of long-term impairment occurs in leukemia patients who receive prophylactic CNS therapy. Two abnormalities may appear in a significant percentage of such patients who have had CNS prophylaxis in the form of intrathecal (IT) chemotherapy and/or radiotherapy. The first consists of abnormalities found on computed tomography (CT) scans and, to a lesser extent, neurological examination. CT scan abnormalities include dilated ventricles, subarachnoid dilation, hypodense areas, and calcifications.[18] These findings usually occur in asymptomatic children. It is interesting that in research at the National Cancer Institute, these same abnormalities have been induced in primates with radiation alone.* Then there are a group of children who have the severe problem of leukoencephalopathies. Additionally, some investigators are reporting a high rate of seizures associated with methotrexate therapy.

The second type of abnormality in recipients of CNS prophylaxis shows up in the results of psychological testing.[15] Formerly, the intellectual capacities of these children were thought not to be affected. More recent longitudinal studies, however, have indicated that some patients experience impairments or deficits in intellectual and academic functioning. While subtle and difficult to pinpoint, after therapy is discontinued these changes nonetheless continue to affect the patient's performance over a period of years. For the most part, attempts at correlating CT scan findings with psychological test results or academic achieve-

ment have been unsuccessful. Studies have suggested that the highest incidence of cognitive deficit occurs in patients receiving cranial irradiation at an early age; however, the number of subjects is small. Thus, while we have many bits and pieces of information, this area remains highly problematic and there are many more questions than answers.

Finally, some oncologists who see large numbers of children who have had acute leukemia have suggested that they look different. They seem to be short and overweight and to have rather coarse facies. It is too early to know whether or not this set of observations will ultimately be described as a syndrome, but the issue is important.

Another late effect that is particularly frightening for this group of children is the possibility of a second malignancy. In former Hodgkin's disease patients, the incidence of second primary malignancies has been variously reported to range from as low as 3 percent to as high as 12 percent. A study reported by Li[16] in 1977 found that among 410 patients who had survived six to twenty-one years after a childhood cancer, there were fifteen second malignant neoplasms. Most of these neoplasms arose within sites of previous radiation therapy. The author concluded that over a twenty-year interval, there was a 12 percent cumulative probability of developing a new malignancy. Li's study dealt with long-term survivors of Wilm's tumor, neuroblastoma, soft tissue sarcoma, and lymphoma. Studies currently underway will provide further data concerning children who are now surviving other forms of cancer, such as brain tumors and Hodgkin's disease. While both radiotherapy and chemotherapy have been implicated in the development of second primary neoplasms, one cannot assume a simple cause-and-effect relationship between treatment and the eventual appearance of a second cancer. There is abundant evidence that underlying genetic predispositions also have a profound influence.

The issues of sexuality and fertility are areas in which medical and psychosocial concerns are particularly enmeshed. While decreased fertility has been reported in cancer survivors, there are also reports of normal rates of reproduction and normal progeny of former patients.

Some cancer treatments do indeed cause sterility, but many do not.[6] Nonetheless, the concern is universal. Many adolescents equate fertility with sexuality; they may interpret information about impairment of fertility as inability to perform sexually. This issue becomes further complicated because of the altered peer relationships that inevitably accompany the diagnosis of a chronic disease in adolescence.

Another question is whether there is any risk of malignancy among the offspring of cancer survivors. A recently completed collaborative study would indicate

*D. G. Poplack, personal communication, 1984.

that the rate is quite low. Among 2,328 parents who had had a malignancy, eight offspring were diagnosed with cancer. Thus cancer occurred at a rate of 0.3 percent in this group, as compared with a 0.2 percent rate in the control group. The incidence of birth defects in the infants was similar to that in the general population.

MEDICAL MANAGEMENT OF LONG-TERM SURVIVORS

In sum, there are potentially serious sequelae for which the patient is at risk over an extended period. This poses serious questions regarding how aggressive one should be in terms of periodic checkups and the optimal interval between visits. As caregivers deal with the life-and-death issues, the concerns about toxicity, as well as social and psychological crises among children during active treatment for cancer, it is sometimes difficult to give full attention to the problems of long-term survivors. In the face of the increasing numbers of survivors each year, a critical management issue has emerged: Who will provide ongoing care, and how detailed should each visit be? Busy pediatric oncologists now have to conduct two types of clinics. In the first, they are dealing with the acute-care patient's problems of therapy and immediate toxicity. In the second, they see long-term survivors. Often it is difficult for the oncologist to "shift gears" and come to grips with the unique problems posed by this group of adolescents and young adults.

Still another problem arises where adult survivors who were diagnosed at a very young age have little recall of the disease or treatment process. They may know that they are somehow special—perhaps stigmatized—because of this disease. Yet they do not often have enough information to seek adequate health maintenance care to deal with the risk of serious late effects. The family physician or internist from whom these patients seek medical care may also lack information about what types of toxicities to investigte.

PSYCHIATRIC/PSYCHOSOCIAL ISSUES IN LONG-TERM SURVIVAL

As the months pass and the child remains free of disease, the anxiety felt when therapy is completed tends slowly to dissipate. As concern about recurrent disease diminishes, other worries take its place. These include: fears about the long-term sequelae of the illness and treatment, about the chance of developing a second malignancy, and about possible effects on the patient's sexuality and progeny. At the same time, the problems that arose during diagnosis and treatment (e.g., difficulty with school attendance and achieve-ment, altered peer relationships, and hostile dependency between parent and child) do not always disappear simply because active anticancer treatment is no longer needed.

There have been some reports of a high incidence of psychiatric problems in survivors of childhood cancer.[5] Other authors, however, observed that former patients' vocational experiences and marital status are comparable to those of their agemates in the general population.[7] Overall, to date the data suggest that most children cured of their cancer move back into the mainstream of life. While this knowledge is certainly reassuring, it offers no grounds for complacency; one should also be aware that many youngsters may display residual deficits and require special services.

ACADEMIC AND VOCATIONAL CONCERNS

Following treatment for the acute leukemias and lymphomas, CNS toxicity may impair some children's ability to achieve academically. During the years they receive treatment, these children's needs for remedial and/or special education may or may not be addressed. An additional source of problems in school achievement affects virtually all cancer patients, even those receiving no CNS treatment. During each of their years of maintenance therapy, cancer patients average twenty or more days absent. Even in the absence of intellectual impairment, the cumulative effect of this high rate of absenteeism can seriously limit the child's educational attainments.

Difficulty in school may be followed by difficulty in acquiring vocational skills and getting jobs. Patients with physical disabilities may need vocational rehabilitation and retraining. It is by no means certain that former cancer patients obtain these services when they need them. It has been reported that the majority of adult cancer patients are unaware of their eligibility for vocational rehabilitation services; this lack of awareness is very likely shared by patients who were treated as children. The Candlelighters, a group of parents of children with cancer, has raised the general issue of cancer patients' employability and eligibility for the armed services. Other authors suggest that potential employers discriminate against cancer survivors because they fear absenteeism, high turnover, and excessive health care and insurance costs. These issues require extensive study as well as efforts to ensure that cancer survivors have adequate access to vocational rehabilitation resources.

PEER RELATIONSHIPS

For children from five to eighteen years old, paramount among their developmental tasks is the need to establish and maintain meaningful and satisfying relationships with peers. Peer relationships can be drastically interrupted by the demands of the disease and the treatment process. Some of these children are particularly vulnerable to this interruption in normal development, and they never seem quite to compensate for it. Such a disruption of peer relationships is most severe when it occurs in conjunction with overprotection by parents. When they reach late adolescence and early adulthood, such youngsters may experience prolonged dependency on their family of origin along with an exaggerated need for security. They often describe their mother as their "best friend." These survivors may live at home much longer than one expects, decide against college or vocational training, accept employment that does not challenge or satisfy them in order to have security, and generally avoid any risks. Obviously, their dependency must alter their opportunities and aspirations for the future.

Still another consequence is that this population may not progress to intimate heterosexual relationships. Childhood cancer patients experience concerns about their attractiveness and, ultimately, their acceptability as sexual partners. These issues arise naturally in response to the obvious physical changes such as hair loss, weight change, and abnormal growth and development that may accompany cancer and its treatment. Another relevant factor is the sense of physical weakness and vulnerability that life-threatening illness imposes. Additional concerns about infertility (which is often misconstrued as impotence or frigidity) increase the chances that the child will develop a very distorted self-image as a sexual object. These fears about their bodies further influence cancer survivors' interaction with others. Obvious disfigurement such as that resulting from amputation or easily visible scarring has been reported as being associated with decreased likelihood of marriage (and gainful employment) for this group.[8]

In coping with the disease and treatment, the child and the family experience emotional turmoil, financial hardship, and other difficulties. Considerable information is available about the impact of medical and nonmedical costs on the family budget. However, little is known about the long-term effects of this financial privation on the parents and siblings of the cancer survivor. Similarly, there is evidence that during the course of the cancer patient's treatment the parents experience heightened marital stress and the siblings endure anxiety and lack of emotional nurturance from their parents. There is a dearth of information, however, about the later adaptation of parents and siblings of cancer survivors in the years following active treatment.

Summary

In summary, surviving cancer is accompanied by medical, social and psychological concerns that may significantly affect the survivors' quality of life. Anxiety about recurrent disease or a second primary malignancy, residual physical, intellectual or emotional impairment, decreased fertility, fears for progeny, and a host of other difficulties may bring long-term survivors to the attention of psychiatrists and other physicians long after they have completed their antitumor therapy. There is inadequate information as to the kind and degree of both medical and psychological problems these survivors and their families can expect. As the number of long-term survivors continues to rise, so will both the need and the opportunity to assess the many associated unknowns.

REFERENCES

1. BIANCANIELLO, T., et al. "Doxorubicin Cardiotoxicity in Children," *Journal of Pediatrics,* 97 (1980):45–50.

2. BODKIN, C. M., PIGOTT, T. J., and MANN, J. R. "Financial Burden of Childhood Cancer," *British Medical Journal,* 284 (1982):1542–1549.

3. D'ANGIO, G. J. "The Child Cured of Cancer: A Problem for the Internist," *Seminars in Oncology,* 9 (1982):143–149.

4. ———. "Early and Delayed Complications of Therapy," *Cancer,* 51 (1983):2515–2518.

5. GOGAN, J. L., et al. "Pediatric Cancer Survival and Marriage," *American Journal of Orthopsychiatry,* 19 (1978):423–430.

6. GREENE, P. E., and FERGUSSON, J. H. "Nursing Care in Childhood Cancer," *American Journal of Nursing,* (March 1982):443–446.

7. HOLMES, H. A., and HOLMES, F. F. "After Ten Years What Are the Handicaps and Life Styles of Children Treated for Cancer," *Clinical Pediatrics,* 14 (1975):819–823.

8. KOOCHER, G. P., and O'MALLEY, J. E. *The Damocles Syndrome.* New York: McGraw-Hill, 1981.

9. LANSKY, S. B., and CAIRNS, N. U. "Affective, Social, and Cognitive Issues and Interventions," in T. Vietti, D. Ferbach, and W. Sutow, eds., *Clinical Pediatric Oncology.* St. Louis: C. V. Mosby, 1984, pp. 303–318.

10. Lansky, S. B., and Gendel, M. "Symbiotic Regressive Behavior Patterns in Childhood Malignancy," *Clinical Pediatrics,* 17 (1978):133–138.

11. Lansky, S. B., Black, J., and Cairns, N. U. "Childhood Cancer: Medical Costs," *Cancer,* 52 (1975):762–766.

12. Lansky, S. B., Zwartges, W., and Cairns, N. U. "School Attendance Among Children with Cancer," *Journal of Psychosocial Oncology,* 2 (1983):75–82.

13. Lansky, S. B., et al. "School Phobia in Children with Malignancies," *American Journal of Diseases of Children,* 129 (1975):42–48.

14. Lansky, S. B., et al. "Childhood Cancer: Nonmedical Costs of Illness," *Cancer,* 43 (1979):403–408.

15. Lansky, S. B., et al. "Central Nervous System Prophylaxis: Studies Showing Impairment in Verbal Skills and Academic Achievement," *American Journal of Pediatric Hematology/Oncology,* 6 (1984):183–190.

16. Li, F. P. "Follow-up of Survivors of Childhood Cancer," *Cancer,* 29 (1977):1776–1778.

17. Meadows, A. T., Krejmas, N. L., and Belasco, J. B. "The Medical Cost of Cancer: Sequelae in Survivors of Childhood Cancer," in J. Van Eys and M. Sullivan, eds., *Status of the Curability of Childhood Cancers.* New York: Raven Press, 1980, pp. 263–275.

18. Ochs, J. J., et al. "Computed Tomography Brain Scans in Children with Acute Lymphocytic Leukemia Receiving Methotrexate Alone as Central Nervous System Prophylaxis," *Cancer,* 45 (1980):2274–2278.

66 / New Perspectives on Juvenile Delinquency

Dorothy Otnow Lewis

Introduction

Delinquency is a legal term, not a psychiatric term. Over the years it has come to designate children whose behaviors have ranged from truancy to rape and murder. Although the term is commonly associated with the current DSM-III diagnosis of conduct disorder, research over the past decade suggests that many children labeled delinquent suffer from neuropsychiatric impairments such as attention deficit disorder (or its synonyms), psychosis, and seizure disorders.

Over the past ten years there have been two major trends in juvenile justice that have influenced the ways in which delinquency has been regarded. First, there has been a federally mandated movement to separate juvenile delinquents from adult offenders. Within the juvenile population there has been a parallel effort to separate status offenders from those whose offenses, if committed by adults, would be classified as felonies.

In response to rising crime rates in the 1960s and 1970s, many states have lowered the age at which a juvenile who commits a serious felony can be processed within the adult system. Procedures vary from state to state. For example, in some states like New York, juveniles as young as thirteen years of age who commit certain offenses are automatically under the jurisdiction of the adult courts unless waived down to the family court. In other states (e.g., Connecticut), such a young offender is initially screened by the juvenile justice system from which at the discretion of a judge he or she may be transferred to the adult criminal justice system. Whichever system is used, both reflect the current tendency to ignore the issue of stages of child development and to treat antisocial children, especially violent children, as adults.

This tendency to dispense with psychological considerations and treat children as adults for the purpose of law enforcement is in part a reflection of impatience and disappointment with sociological and psychoanalytic theories of delinquency so prevalent from the 1930s onward. Before considering recent developments in the understanding of juvenile delinquency, it is useful to summarize some of the older theories that were so influential in the middle of the twentieth century.

Both the psychoanalytic and sociological theories of delinquency stood in contrast to the earlier pessimistic theories of Cesare Lombroso. He believed that criminals represented a phenomenon of biological degeneration and that antisocial behaviors were transmitted genetically from generation to generation.[2] Psychoanalytic thought, on the other hand, emphasized the importance of interpersonal and intrapsychic experiences in the development of behavior disturbances. Aichorn[1] described the "defective superego" of delinquents resulting from pathological family interactions. One of the most popular psychoanalytic theories was that of "superego lacunae" proposed by Johnson and Szurek.[22] According to this view, delinquent children were considered to be acting out their parents' unconscious antisocial wishes. Thus they were not totally without conscience, but rather lacked guilt in certain circumscribed areas of behavior. Others called attention to "ego deficiencies" in delinquent children.[16] Unfortunately, overenthusiasm regarding the effectiveness of psychoanalytic understanding of deviant behavior led to extravagant claims for the efficacy of psychiatric treatment.[61] It was asserted that child guidance clinics, with their psychodynamic orientation and focus on familial problems, would diminish if not eradicate delinquency.[17] There has been a recent interest in what have been termed borderline states and delinquency[47]; however, lack of agreement regarding the definition of "borderline" in children and adolescents and an absence of controlled research makes the work in this area hard to evaluate.

While psychiatry was thus devoting attention to the individual child, sociology focused on social factors associated with deviance. Influential sociologists hypothesized that antisocial behavior resulted primarily from the frustrations of socioeconomically deprived individuals who lacked legitimate access to the material goods and social status of the more affluent members of society.[41] Others asserted that antisocial behavior often reflected an adherence to different social norms from the majority of society.[63] Thus within a delinquent subculture antisocial behavior was considered the norm and adherence permissible. Still others claimed that delinquency was more a reflection of who got caught than of who committed delinquent acts.[6]

The most influential tradition that affects the way in which many clinicians view delinquency today has been the typological. In the 1940s Hewitt and Jenkins[20] tried to document the existence of three types of delinquents, socialized, unsocialized, and overinhibited. Initially these groupings were based on clinical judgment and on Jenkins's perception of the association of particular traits within certain types of delinquents. The way Jenkins explored the nature of delinquency ultimately influenced the current DSM-III classification of conduct disorders. The traits upon which he based his categorizations were in part descriptions of manifest behaviors (e.g., aggressive stealing, running away, using obscenities) and in part judgments of affective states (e.g., emotional immaturity, overdependence, revengefulness). In general, he minimized the importance of neuropsychiatric traits or factors that would have required specialized clinical expertise to identify (e.g., illogical thought processes, impaired short-term memory, paranoid ideation, learning disabilities). More recently, Quay reinvestigated the question of typologies of delinquency.[54,55] Using more sophisticated statistical analyses than had Jenkins, he nonetheless arrived at similar categories. A study of the factors coded by Quay and his colleagues

reveals, however, that he used the same kinds of data as had Jenkins and also ignored the same kinds of neuropsychiatric and psychoeducational information. Thus it is not surprising that the results of these two investigators corresponded so well.

In keeping with the typological tradition, Offer and his colleagues[48] recently studied a sample of fifty-five delinquents "who were in need of hospitalization and who were not retarded, brain damaged, psychotic, or epileptic" (p. 18). These delinquents received extensive physical, neurological, and psychological evaluations and were interviewed and observed at length. Their parents and their therapists also completed a variety of questionnaires. These procedures generated literally hundreds of pieces of data on each subject. When these data were analyzed statistically, four types of delinquents were identified: (1) the impulsive, (2) the narcissistic, (3) the depressed borderline, and (4) the empty borderline. Impulsive delinquents were characterized by more violent and nonviolent antisocial behavior than other delinquents, were considered quite disturbed by the therapist, were called socially insensitive by teachers, and were deemed "unlikable" by most staff. Narcissistic delinquents were characterized as seeing themselves as well adjusted. Others, however, saw them as "resistant, cunning, manipulative, and superficial" (p. 51), perjorative terms similar to some of those used previously by Jenkins. Empty-borderline delinquents were "passive, emotionally depleted" and "not well liked" (p. 52). Their delinquency was interpreted as an effort to avoid psychotic disintegration. Finally, depressed-borderline delinquents were discussed as more motivated at school than other delinquents, more able to engage therapeutically, and more capable of internalizing parental value systems and of experiencing guilt. Delinquency in this group was thought to function "as a relief" to neurotic conflicts. Clearly these delinquents were better liked.

Thus the Offer typologies, by eliminating brain-injured, retarded, epileptic, and psychotic signs and symptoms from paramount consideration, bear a strong resemblance to the earlier typologies of Jenkins and Quay. These kinds of typologies have influenced the DSM-III category of conduct disorder with its socialized, undersocialized, and aggressive, nonaggressive subtypes.

Epidemiology of Juvenile Delinquency

During the 1960s all forms of violent crime by youth increased disproportionately to the growth of the youth population. By the 1970s, however, the per-capita rates of rape and murder by juveniles had stabilized. Nevertheless, in 1981 almost 40 percent of arrests for property crimes and almost 20 percent of arrests for violent crimes were of youngsters under eighteen years of age.[13] Males under age eighteen years committed over eight times as many violent crimes and approximately four times as many nonviolent crimes as females. These data are especially disturbing for urban dwellers, where the rate of violent crime is almost ten times that of rural areas and five times that of suburban areas.

In one of the most important epidemiological studies of delinquency of this century, Wolfgang[74] found that 35 percent of the boys in a Philadelphia birth cohort were arrested at least once before age eighteen. Of this delinquent group, however, only 18 percent (or 6 percent of the initial sample) went on to become chronic offenders. It was this subgroup, however, that was responsible for more than half of the reported delinquencies in the area. These recidivist youngsters tended to come from socioeconomically deprived minority backgrounds, were below-average achievers at school, and began their delinquencies early in childhood. According to this study the best predictor of ongoing delinquency was the number of previous arrests. On the basis of these findings, Wolfgang recommended that minority delinquents from socioeconomically deprived backgrounds with more than three offenses receive special attention because it was they who were at greatest risk for ongoing delinquency.

Wolfgang's study used hospital, police, and school records. As such, it was not clinical and shed no light on possible underlying psychopathology. Robins's thirty-year follow-up study of antisocial youngsters seen in a child guidance clinic documented the close association between severe psychopathology and early antisocial behavior.[56] Ostensibly a report of adult sociopathy in formerly antisocial children, Robins's study actually documents the pervasiveness of a variety of nonantisocial symptoms in her adult subjects. "It is interesting that highly antisocial children not appearing in Juvenile Court had a significantly high rate of adult psychosis, a total of 28% vs. 8% of children appearing in court" (p. 210). In fact, of all children referred to the clinic for antisocial behaviors, only 28 percent were later diagnosed sociopathic and "this sociopathic group averaged almost 8 nonsociopathic symptoms each" (p. 119). Similarly, subjects later diagnosed as schizophrenic had a median number of six antisocial symptoms in childhood compared with nine antisocial symptoms for those later called sociopathic. Thus a study that purported to document adult sociopathy in antisocial children actually shed light on the severe nonsociopathic, psychotic, and organic symptomatology in antisocial youngsters.

Areas of Current Research

BIOCHEMICAL APPROACHES

With the advent of the antipsychotic and antidepressant medications in the mid-1950s came a new interest in the biochemical underpinnings of human behavior. Special interest has focused on the neurotransmitters, particularly dopamine (DA), norepinephrine (NE), and serotonin (5HT). Some of the most interesting biochemical studies related to human antisocial behavior have been performed on animals depleted of specific neurotransmittor substances. For example, there is evidence that DA-depleted rats have somewhat less social and physical interaction with each other than do nontreated control rats.[5] The relationship of aggressive behavior to NE metabolism is another area of active investigation.[5]

One of the most interesting areas of biochemical investigation related to human behavior is the study of the correlation of aggressive animal behavior with neurochemical changes in the brain induced by social deprivation. Several investigators have documented an increase in aggressive activity in animals such as dogs and rats that are raised in social isolation.[39,44,59] According to Sahakian, Robbins, and Iversen,[23] "Children reared in social impoverishment—any situation where the child is without a good caretaker, for example an inferior institution, a broken home with no loving caretaker, or an abusive home situation—show a behavioral syndrome similar to that seen in socially deprived experimental animals" (p. 175). According to these researchers, rats reared in social isolation show bouts of hyperactivity and an inability to follow through on directed responses. Others have reported an increase in aggression in socially isolated animals.[70,72] Several studies of biochemical correlates of social deprivation have reported an association between increased aggression and decreased turnover rate of brain 5HT.[14,70] Others have found a lower concentration of 5HT in the brains of genetically hyperaggressive rats compared with strains of more docile rats.

These studies, which correlate social with biochemical factors in animal experiments, are especially intriguing; they bear a potential relevance to some of the environmental factors we already recognize to be associated with human aggressive antisocial behaviors. If experimental factors can lead to biochemical and behavioral changes in animals, then we may suspect a similar relationship among life experience, biochemical phenomena, and behavioral consequences in humans. Thus factors such as social deprivation or parental abuse, which have hitherto been regarded as exerting exclusively psychodynamic influences, may also have physiological effects on the development of aggressive behavior.

PHYSIOLOGICAL PERSPECTIVES

Simultaneous with an interest in biochemical phenomena and behavioral deviance, there has been a rebirth of interest in physiological factors and delinquency. Mednick,[21,38] Hare,[19] and others have hypothesized that antisocial youngsters behave as they do at least in part because of an inherent autonomic hyporeactivity. According to this theory, children with normal autonomic responses can be trained to inhibit their antisocial impulses more easily than hyporesponsive children. Normal children recover quickly from fear; receive a quick, large positive reinforcement when they inhibit their aggressive impulses; and thereby learn easily to control these impulses. Mednick[38] has hypothesized that antisocial children are born with an autonomic nervous system that recovers slowly and therefore they receive a slow, small reinforcement for the inhibition of antisocial or aggressive acts. Such children are slow to learn to inhibit aggressive behaviors. According to Mednick, this theory is supported by a number of studies indicating especially that sociopathic individuals have a slower electrodermal recovery than do nonpsychopathic individuals.[64] Mednick has gone on to cite studies of biological offspring of criminal fathers, indicating that they have a slower electrodermal recovery than do the offspring of noncriminal fathers.

These findings are both intriguing and puzzling. In fact, a wide variety of neurological and psychiatric disorders characterizes delinquent children. This in turn raises a critical question: Why would youngsters with so many different kinds of vulnerabilities resemble each other in respect to autonomic responsiveness?

Other physiological studies have focused on possible hormonal factors and delinquency. Longitudinal studies of girls with adrenogenital syndrome who have been treated with cortisone replacement suggest that such girls are more energetic and physically active than a comparison sample of normal untreated girls.[12] There is also evidence that boys treated with cortisone for adrenogenital syndrome are more physically active and athletic than are normal males.[12]

Other studies have focused on the relationship of testosterone levels and aggressive behavior in males. In one of the first systematic studies of male aggression and testosterone, Persky, Smith, and Basu[53] reported a positive correlation between self-assessed aggression and plasma levels of testosterone. Others have failed to replicate these findings.[11,24,42] Mattsson[37] performed one of the few hormonal studies using juvenile delinquent subjects; he found that incarcerated recidivist males had slightly higher testosterone levels than did normal male adolescents. The finding of some correlation between testosterone levels and violence has led to trials of testosterone-suppressing agents in the treatment of sex offenders and other violent male offenders.[7,43]

GENETIC PERSPECTIVES

Along with the studies of physiological concomitants of aggression, there has been renewed interest in the study of possible genetic factors associated with antisocial behavior. Hutchings and Mednick[21] reported that the adopted-away offspring of criminal fathers were more likely to become antisocial than were the adopted-away children of noncriminal fathers. The children at greatest risk for antisocial behavior were those with criminal biological fathers and criminal adoptive fathers, a finding that suggests an interplay between genetic and environmental factors.

Relying as they do on registered parental criminality, such studies must be interpreted with caution. They do not take into consideration the likelihood that parental criminality as reflected in police records may simply be the most obvious sign of other types of neuropsychiatric disorders that in certain circumstances are manifested by antisocial behaviors (e.g., schizophreniform disorders, depression, attention deficit disorder, psychomotor epilepsy, learning disabilities). Hence when considering genetic factors, it makes more clinical sense to conceptualize an inherent vulnerability to a variety of disorders of adaptation, any one of which, under certain circumstances, may express itself in antisocial acts.

MEDICAL HISTORIES AND NEUROLOGICAL DISORDERS

There has been considerable disagreement in the past regarding the medical status of delinquent youngsters. Glueck and Glueck[15] and others[62] asserted that medical problems were irrelevant factors. More recent epidemiological evidence suggests that delinquents have especially adverse medical histories. In a study of hospital records of delinquents and nondelinquents, delinquents made greater numbers of hospital visits than nondelinquents, used all services more frequently, and suffered more accidents, injuries, and illnesses.[25] Subsequent studies comparing incarcerated delinquents with less aggressive nonincarcerated delinquents revealed that the incarcerated youngsters suffered significantly more head and face injuries, were significantly more likely to have had perinatal difficulties, and were somewhat more likely to have been recognized by a hospital as having been physically abused.[27] A recent study compared black and white delinquents and nondelinquents.[28] The findings revealed that white delinquents had significantly more adverse medical histories than did white nondelinquents. The medical histories of black delinquents, however, were only slightly more adverse than were those of their black nondelinquent counterparts.

The relationship of adverse medical factors and delinquency is complex. Clearly most individuals with perinatal problems, head injury, or signs of neurological impairment are not delinquent, much less violent. The nature of the parenting visited on delinquent youngsters accounts in great measure for the adversity of their medical histories. Nevertheless, recent studies of violent juveniles suggest that they suffer from a multiplicity of neurological impairments which seem to contribute to their impulsivity, their difficulties concentrating and completing schoolwork, and their inability to make appropriate judgments under stress. A recent clinical study of incarcerated juveniles found that the more violent youngsters were significantly more likely to demonstrate both major and minor signs of neurological impairment than their less violent counterparts.[32]

Within the spectrum of neurological vulnerabilities, hyperkinesis or its synonyms (e.g., attention deficit disorder) is one of the most common neurobehavioral phenomena reported to exist in the delinquent population. Whether it is a sequela of perinatal trauma, is secondary to head injury, or, as some have suggested, is inherited, it clearly impedes school functioning, peer relationships, and overall social adjustment.

One of the less well recognized neurological disorders found more often in the delinquent than in the nondelinquent population is psychomotor epilepsy. Although its relevance to directed violence remains an area of heated debate, there is some evidence that psychomotor seizures are more prevalent in samples of violent delinquents than in their less violent counterparts.[35] In a recent study,[35] only five of eighteen youngsters with psychomotor seizures committed violent acts during these seizures; all five had also committed other violent acts when they were not experiencing seizures. These findings suggest that psychomotor epilepsy is probably but one kind of central nervous system (CNS) dysfunction that, like other forms of CNS abnormalities, in certain contexts makes a youngster more vulnerable to committing impulsive acts.

PSYCHIATRIC AND PSYCHOEDUCATIONAL CHARACTERISTICS OF SERIOUSLY DELINQUENT YOUTH

As they approach adulthood, the great majority of children who come in conflict with the law seem to grow out of these maladaptive behaviors.[57,74] Indeed, in many respects those who commit only one or two delinquent acts are similar to children who are never designated delinquent.[57] This finding probably explains why much of the delinquency literature that focuses on large numbers of nonviolent delinquents ignores issues of severe psychopathology other than characterologic disorders.

More recent evidence suggests that seriously delinquent recidivist youth are in fact more psychiatrically impaired than are their less antisocial peers. In a recent study, Ouston[51] found that 45 percent of boys with three or more convictions had been recognized as deviant by the age of ten as compared with 23 percent of delinquents who had only two offenses and with 22 percent of nondelinquents.

A clinical study of the psychiatric status of incarcerated delinquents revealed that the more violent youngsters were significantly more likely to suffer from psychotic symptoms, particularly paranoid ideation, and that these symptoms often contributed to their propensity to lash out at others.[32] Much of the literature on adult offenders reports that female criminals are more psychiatrically disturbed than males. However, a clinical study comparing incarcerated male and female delinquents found that the two groups were remarkably similar; both demonstrated a wide variety of signs and symptoms of psychotic and organic dysfunction.[31] Given this finding, it seems likely that the very same kinds of deviant behaviors that in females are recognized as evidence of severe psychopathology are considered in males to be simply antisocial.

There is ample evidence that delinquents as a group score lower on tests of intelligence than do nondelinquents.[51] These findings may reflect test bias, cultural deprivation, the consequences of CNS injury, innate intellectual limitations, or combinations thereof. It is likely that intelligence also plays a role in determining which delinquent youngsters will be caught. Clearly, however, intelligence alone does not account for most antisocial behavior. Most intellectually limited, even retarded, children are not antisocial. It would seem that low intelligence in certain cases is but one of the many biopsychosocial vulnerabilities of some delinquent children.

One of the most frequently replicated findings in the literature is that of severe learning disabilities.[66,69,71] This degree of learning difficulties is, by definition, greater than what would be expected in terms of IQ. There is evidence that the more violent the youngster, the greater the learning disorder tends to be.[32] Such severe learning disorders cannot be explained simply in terms of inadequate educational opportunities. Because of ongoing frustration in the classroom, often the learning-disabled youngster drops out of school. The theory that learning disorders in delinquent youngsters are a reflection of their conscious or unconscious resentment of the educational system is no longer considered an adequate explanation for the high prevalence of these kinds of problems in the delinquent population. We do know that repeated failure and frustration are associated with dropping out of school early. Thus by the age of thirteen or fourteen years learning-impaired youngsters may no longer have the kind of organization in their life that the school, even the most inadequate of schools, provides for other youngsters through their sixteenth year. At the same time such adolescents are too young and untrained to acquire the kind of steady employment that might take the place of hours missed from school. Rarely do such multiply handicapped youngsters come from a sufficiently competent family to help them organize their activities in the absence of the structure of the schoolroom. Left to their own devices, they are particularly susceptible to the influences of a nonsupportive social environment.

PARENTS OF DELINQUENTS

For many years investigators have recognized that delinquency in children is related to severe intrafamilial disturbance. Glueck and Glueck[15] spoke of under-the-roof chaos. They described the parents of delinquents as being unable to provide the kind of discipline or affection necessary for their children to adapt appropriately to society's demands. Broken homes, originally thought to be etiologically important, are in and of themselves no longer thought to be especially criminogenic. Rather the family discord that so often precedes family dissolution is now thought to be an important factor contributing to children's maladaptive behaviors.[58]

Explanations of the causal relationship between parental characteristics and children's delinquency are often vague and general. Recently Patterson[52] has described parents of delinquents as lacking "house rules" or predictable family routines, as failing to monitor their children's behaviors, and as inconsistent in their responses to either good or bad behavior. He described them as lacking the ability to deal effectively with crises and to resolve interpersonal conflicts effectively.

Studies in Great Britain and in the United States suggest that boys are more vulnerable than girls to the stresses of parental discord and more likely to develop antisocial behaviors.[57] Moreover, boys growing up in households with antisocial brothers are at a greater risk for becoming delinquent than are girls.[49]

An increasing body of knowledge suggests that the reason why many of the parents of delinquents are unable to provide structure, discipline, and, perhaps most important, consistent affection is that many of

them are severely psychiatrically impaired.* There is evidence that the children of schizophrenic parents are at greater risk of delinquency than are the children of demographically similar, nonpsychotic parents. This is true particularly for minority families. Family studies of hyperkinetic children[9] suggest that familial as well as environmental factors are associated with children's antisocial behaviors. Mendelson[40] and his associates found that extremely antisocial children often had fathers who, in their own childhoods, had had learning disorders as well as behavior problems.

Finally, both parental sociopathy and alcoholism have been reported to be associated with delinquency in children.[56] In light of the aforementioned evidence of other kinds of parental disorders, however, it is likely that many of the parents of delinquent children suffer from a variety of conditions ranging from CNS dysfunction to psychoses. These illnesses are often overlooked either because the research methodology rarely includes the necessary sophisticated neuropsychiatric assessment of parents or because the more obvious addictive or antisocial characteristics of such parents obfuscate the existence of underlying psychopathology.

CHILD ABUSE AND HOUSEHOLD VIOLENCE

In spite of the commonly held notion that violence begets violence, only in the recent past has the close association between family violence and juvenile delinquency received the close attention it deserves.

According to the 1982 report of the National Center on Child Abuse and Neglect, approximately 0.34 percent of children suffer demonstrable physical harm at the hands of parents or other caretakers.[46] On the other hand, studies from all over the United States report an extraordinarily high prevalence of childhood physical abuse among the delinquent populations.† For example, of one hundred juvenile offenders in Philadelphia, 82 percent reported abuse or neglect and 43 percent recalled having been knocked unconscious by a parent.[67] Others have studied subsequent rates of delinquency in children known to have been abused.[8,65] Alfaro[3,4] found that approximately 10 percent of abused or neglected children from a county in New York were subsequently adjudicated as delinquent or ungovernable.

Violent forms of delinquency are especially likely to be associated with a history of having been abused and having witnessed violence. A study of ninety-seven incarcerated males revealed that 75 percent of the more violent boys had been severely abused compared with 33 percent of the less violent boys.[32] The medical his-

*See references 26, 29, 30, 50, and 73.
†See references 3, 4, 23, 45, and 68.

tories of violent delinquents reflected in hospital records indicate that the more serious their delinquency, the more likely that abuse will have been noted in their hospital chart.[27] Moreover, when hospital records were compared with other sources of data regarding abuse, it became clear that abuse was underreported in medical charts.[34] Similarly, delinquents' accounts of adverse medical events have been compared with several other information sources, such as social histories, probation records, hospital charts, and parent interviews. It turns out that delinquents often minimize adverse medical events, including injury at the hands of parents.

Clearly, brain dysfunction alone does not create violence in most instances. Since so many severely abused delinquents do have evidence of brain dysfunction, it is hard to know whether, in the absence of CNS impairment, physical abuse in and of itself can evoke violent antisocial behaviors.

There are several ways in which the effects of battering can be understood. First, physical abuse as well as neglect will often lead to CNS damage. This damage, in turn, can make children less able to control their impulses, focus their attention, relate sensitively to others, and adapt appropriately. Second, by virtue of modeling, identification, or simple imitation, children learn to behave in aggressive ways. Finally, it would seem that the rage engendered in a child by severe abuse gives rise to a chronically angry individual whose fury is frequently displaced onto others in the environment such as animals, younger children, and peers as well as authority figures.

One of the reasons that there are so many theories about the origins of delinquency is because no single factor is sufficient to account for the complex of behaviors called delinquency. Certain constellations of biopsychosical factors are extremely characteristic of delinquents, especially of violent recidivists. Not only are many delinquent youngsters multiply handicapped by virtue of CNS dysfunction, episodic psychosis, perceptual motor impairment, and learning disabilities, but they also have been the victims of extreme abuse and they have witnessed violence toward others. It would seem that when children with such vulnerabilities are also exposed to extreme violence as victim or observer, the consequence is often the creation of an aggressive delinquent child.

RACE

In both the United States[74] and Great Britain[57] there have been studies that indicate a higher prevalence of delinquency in the black population than in the white. Many reasons have been put forth to explain these data, with explanations ranging from socio-

cultural values of minorities to discrimination by police regarding who gets arrested. There is considerable evidence to support the idea that commitment of a child to reformatory or jail often reflects racial bias. One study compared all adolescents from a small Connecticut city who in a given year were sent either to corrections or to a psychiatric hospital. The two groups turned out to be quite similar symptomatically and behaviorally.[33] Of note, the hospitalized adolescents as a group were as aggressive as the incarcerated group. When all the clinical and demographic variables were tabulated, the most important factor distinguishing the two groups was race. White violent psychiatrically disturbed adolescents tended to be hospitalized; black violent psychiatrically impaired adolescents were sent to correctional school.

DIAGNOSIS

At one time or another the great majority of seriously delinquent children receive the diagnosis conduct disorder. This diagnostic label is often affixed to a behaviorally disturbed child regardless of underlying neuropsychiatric status. In the case of delinquents, their conduct is often so disruptive and unpleasant that it obfuscates underlying psychiatric signs and symptoms.

A recent study[36] comparing psychiatrically hospitalized children who had ever been diagnosed as conduct disordered with patients never so diagnosed revealed numerous similarities and few differences. For example, these groups were equally likely to suffer from psychotic symptoms and organic symptoms. In this study the major factor distinguishing children diagnosed as conduct disordered from those never so diagnosed was violence. Regardless of their other symptomatology, children who acted aggressively tended to be called conduct disordered. Indeed, approximately half of the children diagnosed as conduct disordered had at other times been diagnosed psychotic.

TREATMENT ISSUES

To date no treatment programs for delinquents are universally considered effective.[18] Some programs have used behavioral models; others have focused on group therapy; still others have attempted to coordinate multiple community services for the care of the delinquent and the family. Almost all programs have had a modicum of success. None have provided outstanding results.

One of the main reasons why no single treatment modality has proved especially beneficial is that delinquency is not a single disorder. It should be recognized rather as a final common pathway, an outcome of the interplay of a wide variety of intrinsic vulnerabilities and past and current experiences. In order for treatment to be of benefit to seriously delinquent children, each of their vulnerabilities must be identified with as much specificity as possible and addressed as such. This principle applies whether dealing with learning disorders, psychosis, or intrafamily distress secondary to a severely disturbed parent.

Finally, although seriously delinquent youngsters demonstrate a wide variety of neuropsychiatric and psychoeducational deficits, they are rarely flamboyantly impaired. Their pathology is situated on the border of numerous conditions (e.g., attention deficit disorder, psychosis, epilepsy, retardation). Most of these conditions, moderate or mild, are nevertheless chronic. Hence the success of even the finest interventions may be undone if children are suddenly extruded from a program with little follow-up from those who had cared for them.

Basic to treatment is the recognition that seriously delinquent children have many different needs. Accordingly an attempt at intervention must be multifaceted and as various as the problems. Finally, in many cases, treatment must be sustained over a period of several years if youngsters are ever to function in a socially adaptive fashion.

REFERENCES

1. AICHORN, A. *Wayward Youth.* New York: Viking Press, 1935.

2. ALEXANDER, F., and SELESNICK, S. T. *The History of Psychiatry.* New York: Harper & Row, 1966.

3. ALFARO, J. D. *Report on the Relationship Between Child Abuse and Neglect and Later Socially Deviant Behavior.* Albany, N.Y.: New York State Assembly, 1978.

4. ———. "Report on the Relationship Between Child Abuse and Neglect and Later Socially Deviant Behavior," in R. J. Hummer and Y. E. Walker, eds., *Exploring the Relationship Between Child Abuse and Delinquency.* Montclair, N.J.: Allanheld, Osman and Co., 1981.

5. ALPERT, J. E., et al. "Disorder of Attention, Activity, and Aggression," in D. O. Lewis, ed., *Vulnerabilities to Delinquency.* New York: Spectrum Publications, 1981, pp. 109–172.

6. BECKER, H. S. *Outsiders: Studies in the Sociology of Deviance.* New York: Free Press, 1963.

7. BLUMER, D., and MIGEON, C. "Hormone and Hormonal Agents in the Treatment of Aggression," *Journal of Nervous and Mental Disease,* 160 (1975):127–137.

8. BOLTON, F. G., REICH, J. W., and GUTIERRES, S. E. "Delinquency Pattern in Maltreated Children and Siblings," *Victimology,* 2 (1977):349–357.

9. CANTWELL, D. P. "Hyperactivity and Antisocial Behavior," *Journal of the American Academy of Child Psychiatry,* 17 (1978):252–262.

10. COHEN, A. K. *Delinquent Boys: The Culture of the Gang.* New York: Free Press, 1955.

11. DOERING, C. H., et al. "A Cycle of Plasma Testosterone in the Human Male," *Journal of Clinical Endocrinology and Metabolism,* 40 (1975):492–500.

12. EHRHARDT, A. A. "Prenatal Hormonal Exposure and Psychosexual Differentiation," in E. J. Sachar, ed., *Psychoendocrinology.* New York: Grune & Stratton, 1975, pp. 67–82.

13. *FBI Uniform Crime Reports.* Washington, D.C.: U.S. Government Printing Office, 1981.

14. GERATTINI, S., GIACOLONE, E., and VALZELLI, L. "Biochemical Changes During Isolation-induced Aggressiveness in Mice," in S. Garattini and E. Sigg, eds., *Aggressive Behavior.* New York: John Wiley & Sons, 1969.

15. GLUECK, S., and GLUECK, E. *Unraveling Juvenile Delinquency.* Cambridge, Mass.: Harvard University Press, 1950.

16. GROSSBARD, H. "Ego Deficiency in Delinquents," *Social Casework,* 43 (1962):171–178.

17. HAKEEM, M. "A Critique of the Psychiatric Approach," in J. S. Roueck, ed., *Juvenile Delinquency.* New York: Philosophical Library, 1958.

18. HAMPARIAN, D. H. "Control and Treatment of Juveniles Committing Violent Offenses," in L. Roth, ed., *Clinical Treatment and Management of the Violent Person.* DHHS Publication No. (ADM) 85–1425, 1985, pp. 164–187.

19. HARE, R. D. *Psychopathy: Theory and Research.* New York: John Wiley & Sons, 1970.

20. HEWITT, L., and JENKINS, R. L. *Fundamental Patterns of Maladjustment: The Dynamics of Their Origin.* Springfield, Ill.: State of Illinois, 1946.

21. HUTCHINGS, B., and MEDNICK, S. A. "Registered Criminality in the Adoptive and Biological Parents of Registered Male Criminal Adoptees," in S. A. Mednick, et al., eds., *Genetics, Environment and Psychopathology.* Amsterdam: North Holland/Elsevier, 1974.

22. JOHNSON, A. M., and SZUREK, S. A. "The Genesis of Antisocial Acting Out in Children and Adults," *Psychoanalytic Quarterly,* 21 (1952):323.

23. KRATCOSKI, P. C. "Child Abuse and Violence Against the Family," *Child Welfare,* 61 (1982):435–444.

24. KREUZ, L. E., and ROSE, R. M. "Assessment of Aggressive Behavior and Plasma Testosterone in a Young Criminal Population," *Psychosomatic Medicine,* 34 (1972):321–332.

25. LEWIS, D. O., FELDMAN, M., and BARRENGOS, A. "Race, Health, and Delinquency. *Journal of the American Academy of Child Psychiatry,* 24 (1985):161–167.

26. LEWIS, D. O., and SHANOK, S. S. "Medical Histories of Delinquent and Nondelinquent Children: An Epidemiological Study," *American Journal of Psychiatry,* 134 (1977): 1020–1025.

27. ———. "Delinquency and the Schizophrenic Spectrum of Disorders," *Journal of the American Academy of Child Psychiatry,* 17 (1978):263–276.

28. ———. "Perinatal Difficulties, Head and Face Trauma and Child Abuse in the Medical Histories of Seriously Delinquent Children," *American Journal of Psychiatry,* 136 (1979):419–423.

29. LEWIS, D. O. SHANOK, S. S., and BALLA, D. A. "Toward Understanding the Fathers of Delinquents: Psychodynamic, Medical and Genetic Perspectives," in E. Rexford, ed.,

A Developmental Approach to Problems of Acting Out. New York: International Universities Press, 1978, pp. 137–152.

30. ———. "Parents of Delinquents," in D. O. Lewis, ed., *Vulnerabilities to Delinquency.* New York: Spectrum Publications, 1981, pp. 265–295.

31. LEWIS, D. O., SHANOK, S. S., and PINCUS, J. H. "A Comparison of the Neuropsychiatric Status of Female and Male Incarcerated Delinquents: Some Evidence of Sex and Race Bias," *Journal of the American Academy of Child Psychiatry,* 21 (1982):190–196.

32. LEWIS, D. O., et al. "Violent Juvenile Delinquents: Psychiatric, Neurological, Psychological and Abuse Factors," *Journal of the American Academy of Child Psychiatry,* 18 (1979):307–319.

33. LEWIS, D. O., et al. "Race Bias in the Diagnosis and Disposition of Violent Adolecents," *American Journal of Psychiatry,* 137 (1980):1211–1216.

34. LEWIS, D. O., et al. "The Medical Assessment of Seriously Delinquent Boys: A Comparison of Pediatric, Psychiatric, Neurological, and Hospital Record Data," *Journal of Adolescent Health Care,* 3 (1982):160–164.

35. LEWIS, D. O., et al. "Psychomotor Epilepsy and Violence in an Incarcerated Adolescent Population," *American Journal of Psychiatry,* 139 (1982):882–887.

36. LEWIS, D. O., et al. "Conduct Disorder and Its Synonyms: Diagnoses of Dubious Validity and Usefulness," *American Journal of Psychiatry,* 141 (1984):514–519.

37. MATTSSON, A., et al. "Plasma Testosterone, Aggressive Behavior, and Personality Dimensions in Young Male Delinquents," *Journal of the American Academy of Child Psychiatry,* 19 (1980):476–491.

38. MEDNICK, S. D., and CHRISTIANSEN, K. O. *Biosocial Bases of Criminal Behavior.* New York: Gardner Press, 1977.

39. MELZAK, R. "Early Experience: A Neurophysiological Approach to Heredity and Environment Interactions," in G. Newton and S. Levine, eds., *Early Experience and Behavior.* Springfield, Ill.: Charles C Thomas, 1968.

40. MENDELSON, N., JOHNSON, N., and STEWART, M. A. "Hyperactive Children as Teenagers: A Follow-up Study," *Journal of Nervous and Mental Disease,* 153 (1971):273–279.

41. MERTON, R. K. *Social Theory and Social Structure.* New York: Free Press, 1957.

42. MEYER-BAHLBERG, H.F.L., et al. "Aggressiveness and Testosterone Measures in Man," *Psychosomatic Medicine,* 36 (1974):269–274.

43. MONEY, J., et al. "Combined Antiandrogenic and Counseling Programs for Treatment of 46 XY and 47 XYY Sex Offenders," in E. J. Sachar, ed., *Hormones, Behavior, and Psychopathology.* New York: Raven Press, 1976, pp. 105–120.

44. MORGAN, M. "Effects of Post-weaning Environment on Learning in the Rat," *Animal Behavior,* 21 (1973):429.

45. MOUZAKITAS, C. M. "An Inquiry into the Problem of Child Abuse and Juvenile Delinquency," in R. J. Hunner and Y. E. Walker, eds., *Exploring the Relationship Between Child Abuse and Delinquency.* Montclair, N.J.: Allanheld, Osman & Co., 1981.

46. National Center on Child Abuse and Neglect. *Executive Summary: National Study of the Incidence and Severity of Child Abuse and Neglect* (DHHS Publication No. OHDS 81-30329). Washington, D.C.: U.S. Government Printing Office, 1982.

47. NIELSON, G. *Borderline and Acting-Out Adolescents: A Developmental Approach.* New York: Human Sciences Press, 1983.

48. OFFER, D., MAROHN, R. C., OSTROV, E. *The Psycho-* *logical World of the Juvenile Offender.* New York: Basic Books, 1979.

49. OFFORD, D. R. "Family Backgrounds of Male and Female Delinquents," In J. E. Gunn and D. P. Farrington, eds., *Abnormal Offenders: Delinquency and the Criminal Justice System.* Chichester, U.K.: Wiley, 1982, pp. 129–151.

50. OFFORD, D. R., ALLEN, N., and ABRAMS, N. "Parental Psychiatric Illness and Broken Homes and Delinquency," *Journal of the American Academy of Child Psychiatry,* 17 (1978):224–238.

51. OUSTON, J. "Delinquency, Family Background and Educational Attainment," *British Journal of Criminology,* in press.

52. PATTERSON, G. R. *Coercive Family Processes.* Eugene, Ore.: Castalia Publishing Co., 1982.

53. PERSKY, H., SMITH, K. P., and BASU, G. K. "Relation of Psychologic Measures of Aggression and Hostility to Testosterone Production in Man," *Psychosomatic Medicine,* 33 (1971):265–277.

54. QUAY, H. C. "Dimensions of Personality in Delinquent Boys as Inferred from Factor Analysis of Case History Data," *Child Development,* 35 (1964):479–484.

55. ———. "Classification in the Treatment of Delinquency and Antisocial Behavior, in N. Hobbs, ed., *Issues on the Classification of Children,* vol. 1. San Francisco: Jossey-Bass, 1975, pp. 377–392.

56. ROBINS, L. *Deviant Children Grown Up.* Baltimore: Williams & Wilkins, 1966.

57. RUTTER, M., and GILLER, H. *Juvenile Delinquency: Trends and Perspectives.* New York: Guilford Press, 1984.

58. RUTTER, M., and MADGE, N. *Cycles of Disadvantage.* London: Heinemann, 1976.

59. SAHAKIAN, B. J. "The Neurochemical Basis of Hyperactivity and Aggression Induced by Social Deprivation," in D. O. Lewis, ed., *Vulnerabilities to Delinquency.* New York: Spectrum Publications, 1981, pp. 173–186.

60. SAHAKIAN, B. J., ROBBINS, T., and IVERSEN, S. "The Effects of Isolation Rearing on Exploration in the Rat," *Animal Learning and Behavior,* 5 (1977):193.

61. SCHMIDEBERG, M. "The Psychoanalysis of Delinquents," *American Journal of Orthopsychiatry,* 23 (1972): 13–21.

62. SCOTT, P. D. "Medical Aspects of Delinquency," in T. Silverstone and B. A. Barraclough, eds., *Contemporary Psychiatry: Selected Reviews from the British Journal of Hospital Medicine.* Kent, U.K.: Headley Brothers Ltd., 1975, pp. 287–295.

63. SHAW, R. C., and McKAY, H. D. *Juvenile Delinquency and Urban Areas.* Chicago: University of Chicago Press, 1942.

64. SIDDLE, D.A.T., et al. "Skin Conductance Recovery in Antisocial Adolescents," in K. O. Christiansen and S. A. Mednick, eds., *Biosocial Bases of Criminal Behavior.* New York: Gardner Press, 1977.

65. SILVER, L. B., DUBLIN, C. C., and LOURIE, R. S. "Does Violence Breed Violence? Contributions from a Study of the Child Abuse Syndrome," *American Journal of Psychiatry,* 126 (1969):404–407.

66. SLAVIN, S. H. "Information Processing Deficits in Delinquents," in L. J. Hippchen, ed., *Ecology—Biochemical Approaches to the Treatment of Delinquents and Criminals.* New York: Van Nostrand Reinhold, 1977, pp. 75–102.

67. STEELE, B. F. "Violence Within the Family," in R. E. Helfer, and C. H. Kempe, eds., *Child Abuse and Neglect: The Family and the Community.* Cambridge, Mass.: Ballinger, 1976.

68. STEELE, B. F., and POLLOCK, C. B. "A Psychiatric Study of Parents Who Abuse Infants and Small Children," in R. E. Helfer and C. H. Kempe, eds., *The Battered Child,* 2nd ed. Chicago: University of Chicago Press, 1974.

69. TARNAPOL, L. "Delinquency and Minimal Brain Dysfunction," *Journal of Learning Disabilities,* 3 (1970):200–207.

70. VALZELLI, L. "5-Hydroxytryptamine in Aggressiveness," in E. Costa, G. Gessa, and M. Sandler, eds., *Advances in Biochemical Psychopharmacology.* New York: Raven Press, 1974.

71. VIRKUNNEN, N., and NUUTILA, A. "Specific Reading Retardation, Hyperactive Child Syndrome, and Juvenile Delinquency," *Acta Psychiatrica Scandinavica,* 54 (1976):25–28.

72. WELCH, A., and WELCH, B. "Isolation, Reactivity and Aggression: Evidence for an Involvement of Brain Catecholamines and Serotonin," in B. Eleftheriou and J. Scott, eds., *The Physiology of Aggression and Defeat.* New York: Plenum Press, 1971.

73. WEST, D. J., and FARRINGTON, D. P. *Who Becomes Delinquent?* London: Heinemann, 1973.

74. WOLFGANG, M. E., FIGLIO, R. M., and CELLIN, T. *Delinquency in a Birth Cohort.* Chicago: University of Chicago Press, 1972.

67 / Preventive Programs with Pregnant Teenagers and Young Mothers

Malkah T. Notman, Carol C. Nadelson, Maria Sauzier, and Margaret P. Gean

Introduction

In 1976 the United States had the fourth highest adolescent pregnancy rate of all the industrialized nations in the world.[32] According to figures from the mid to late 1970s, a higher proportion of adolescents in the United States became mothers each year than in any developed country except for Czechoslovakia, East Germany, Yugoslavia, Romania, Hungary, and Bulgaria.[32] It is estimated that half the population of fifteen- to nineteen-year-olds and a fifth of the thirteen- and fourteen-year-olds are sexually active. Of the 10 million adolescent females ages fifteen to nineteen in the United States, over 1 million become pregnant each year[22]; of these, 22 percent end in out-of-wedlock births, 10 percent are legitimized by marriage, 13 percent end in miscarriage, and 38 percent end in abortion.[22] Between 1975 and 1978, 60 percent of births to white teenagers and 90 percent of births to black teenagers were conceived out of wedlock. These figures represent a 250 percent and a 50 percent increase in the past twenty-five years, respectively.

According to a 1981 report from the Guttmacher Institute,[32] although an increasing proportion of adolescents are sexually active, the percentage of these using effective means of contraception has not risen as rapidly. Thus more teens are at risk for becoming pregnant than in the past, and 80 percent of premarital pregnancies among teens are unintended. Even though teenagers represent about one-fifth of those sexually active women who are capable of becoming pregnant, they account for almost half of the out-of-wedlock births and one-third of the abortions. According to Kirby, Alter, and Scales,[43] despite the availability of comprehensive sex education programs in schools, fewer than 10 percent of today's youth receive such programs. It is interesting to note that 80 percent of Americans favor sex education and that this is recognized as a primary preventive step. However, while knowledge of sexuality does make a difference, it is not the only variable in preventing teenage pregnancy.[55] Demographic and family characteristics, social and peer pressure, available options to repeating a cycle of early pregnancy, and incomplete education are all important. These are discussed later.

Of those teenagers who become pregnant and continue to term without marrying, many now keep their babies. In the past, families rather than social institutions had provided care for these children. This pattern, however, has been changing, and, as more women enter the workforce and grandmothers and other family members are less available, it will continue to change.

Earlier literature inevitably linked adolescent pregnancy with psychopathology. In girls it was discussed as a form of delinquency and was compared to boys stealing cars; it was described as "acting out," a manifestation of intrapsychic disturbance. More recently, cultural and social variables, as well as differences in emotional and personality constellations, have been taken into account before concluding that psychopathology is a causal factor.[54]

In describing a group of disturbed teenage mothers, Fraiberg[27] pointed to the relationship of this group to "the larger population of teenage mothers in which we can find a fair amount of adequate or excellent mothering" (p. 9). She stated further, "the adolescent and mothering conflicts which we encountered are not typical but are exaggerated and heightened conflicts in which universal problems of adolescent maturation become distorted by disorder in the adolescent personality and the inability of the primary family of the girl to provide the vital pathway to resolution of conflict"[27] (p. 9).

Psychodynamic and Developmental Issues

In order to understand some of the psychodynamic issues that are involved in the motivation for pregnancy, developmental determinants must be considered. The adolescent girl is caught up in the process of changing ties to her parents and turning to peers and other adults for support as she moves toward the assumption of an adult identity and adult roles. For some, the process of distancing themselves from their parents may be marked by rebellion and challenge.

The changes of menarche are both welcomed and regarded with apprehension. The integration of a concept of femininity is a complex process and, especially for those with earlier conflict around feminine identity, adolescent pubertal changes can have a particularly strong impact. Peers are extremely important in this process and peer pressures are influential. Despite her own ambivalence, a girl may become involved sexually because her self-esteem depends in part on peer approval. If her group pressures her to have sexual experiences, she may succumb despite her own contrary convictions and desires. When asked about the circumstances of her pregnancy, one fourteen-year-old said that she had been the only girl on the block who didn't have a baby. When she was teased about this by her friends, she said yes to the next boy who pressured her for sex. For their part, boys are sometimes pressured to prove that they are "masculine" and, in addition, have their own needs to consolidate a masculine identity.

Some teenagers turn to heterosexuality as a means of distancing themselves from the regressive pull toward dependency on and attachments to their parents that they perceive as unacceptable. For many, it is not the actual pregnancy they seek; this is a by-product of the adolescent denial, poor planning, lack of future orientation or realistic sense of the implications or consequences of sexuality. Likewise, the closeness of a sexual relationship and/or a baby may be seen as providing love and a less lonely life. One fifteen-year-old said, "I wanted something of my own." The baby may not be perceived as a separate person but as an integral and lifelong companion. Schaffer and Pine[63] point to the function of a pregnancy as expressing a longing to be cared for, both as mother and baby. For a teenager, pregnancy may also be motivated by the need to replace a loss, cope with an uncertain identity, hold onto a love object, or regain closeness with the mother. Identification with the mother can also be an important motivation for pregnancy. In contrast to this, Deutsch[20] has noted what she defined as a flight from incestuous fantasies by means of intimacy with the man encountered. The acting-out of unconscious oedipal fantasies, a wish for revenge, and defective ego function have also been mentioned in the literature.[19,20,63]

Blos and others[9,10,54,63] have stressed the importance of attachment of the girl to the preoedipal mother-child relationship and the strength of this pull. Whether seeking some reestablishment of this contact through a pregnancy is to be considered "infantile" or "regressive" or whether it should be regarded as part of the uneven process of growth and development (without the pejorative implications of a term such as regressive) is a subject for further discussion.

Family and Social Issues

Family studies provide another perspective. These suggest that the covert messages expressed by a family may be very important determinants of teenage pregnancy. The teenager may consciously or unconsciously carry out the family wish and provide a baby, especially as a replacement for a lost sibling or for the mother's loss of reproductive capacity, or in some other way to express a family dynamic.[57]

Once pregnancy occurs, the relationship with the family, especially with the mother, also appears to influence the subsequent course of action—for example, whether or not an abortion is obtained. This relationship is an important variable, as are social class and economic situation. One study[39] that compared teenagers who chose abortion with those who chose to carry the baby to term found that those who chose abortion reported greater conflict with their mothers. This suggests that they may also have experienced greater autonomy, as reflected by their greater freedom to act.

Other aspects of family and societal dynamics are stressed by Kennel and Klaus,[41] among others. They indicate that in some subcultures an adolescent may be fully integrated into the role of a sexually functioning woman and a pregnancy may be consistent with perceived expectations. The importance of maternal support systems, and the devaluing of fathers and men, is emphasized by Sauzier[62] in her study of a Boston high school and its pregnant adolescent population.

Recently attention has focused on those families who incorporate an adolescent mother and child into the household. Smith[64] developed a typology of these families suggesting that they may structure themselves in several different ways: They may share roles, they may block the assumption of the maternal role by the biological mother, or they may bind the adolescent to the multiple tasks and obligations associated with being a mother, thus supporting the relinquishing of adolescent developmental tasks and restricting the young mother's social, educational, and economic options. When the maternal role is blocked for the teenage mother, it may occur, in part, as a result of her abdication of the role or because another family member has taken it on. This interferes with the young mother's development of her competence as a mother.

In any case, adolescent development is complicated by the addition of a child. Fraiberg's study[27] of a group of disturbed adolescents, each of whom became pregnant when attachment and detachment from the primary family figures had produced considerable conflict, suggested that these unresolved conflicts became the focus of new conflicts that embraced the child. She reported disorders of attachment in the babies. They represented a symbol of hope and self-renewal for the mother and they seemed to help solve past interpersonal problems. However, these babies were often poorly developed and neglected. Many of the typical conflicts of adolescents with their own mothers had become intensified and magnified for each of the girls before they became pregnant.

When considering teenage pregnancy, we have gradually come to understand the complexity of etiology and outcome. To understand it, we must deal with its multidetermined character, attend to the heterogeneity of our culture, and consider the diversity of motivations of individuals and their families. At the same time, even though pregnant teenagers are more likely to be without support and adequate resources, we must recognize that negative consequences are not inevitable.

The Use of Contraception

Many teenagers have to cope with the unavailability of contraception, their own ambivalence or lack of knowledge about contraception, or an environment in which

pregnancy may even be supported as a means of demonstrating adulthood or the attainment of some measure of independence; there are also family, peer, and social pressures.

Studies have documented that most adolescents do not use contraceptives, especially with their first sexual intercourse.[57] The reasons for contraceptive nonuse are complex. Discomfort and conflict regarding sexuality as well as concerns about disturbing a relationship make it difficult to plan contraception. Contraceptive availability is another factor. Obtaining contraceptives may necessitate informing parents or other authorities, or negotiating a medical care system that may be hostile or inaccessible to the teenager. While much has been said about the importance of contraceptive education, there does not seem to be a consistent correlation between a girl's prior exposure to sex education courses and her sexual knowledge, nor between contraceptive information and knowledge and contraceptive use.[56,57,63] Further, stopping contraceptive use is frequent and peer pressure, social demands, and fear of damage because of real or fantasied side effects from pills or intrauterine devices are often important factors. Guilt about sexual activity, fear of discovery of contraceptive use, impulsivity, and characteristics of adolescence such as inability to plan for the future and denial are prominent determinants. Conscious and unconscious wishes for pregnancy must also be considered; one form of denial, the feeling that "it can't happen to me," also contains an ambivalent wish to become pregnant and thus demonstrate "femininity."

Cobliner[17] points to the cognitive state of adolescent development in the midteens and to the effects of the teenager's cognitive capacity on contraception and planning. He describes figurative family characteristics of adolescence that narrow the subject's reality appraisal by an attention to the immediate effects of action to the exclusion of their foreseeable long-range effects. Cvetkovitch and Grote[19] also implicate the more "primitive" cognitive development of adolescents in the nonuse of contraception. These factors can be offset by support of long-range thinking and planning that may not be present in the teenager's family setting.

Why Prevention?

Any discussion of preventive programs requires clarification of several questions. First, it is important to define what is to be prevented, and why: teenage sexuality, teenage pregnancy, repeat teenage pregnancy, and/or the consequences of teenage pregnancy? Each question involves value judgments and reflects current theories as well as social, economic, and political trends.

The negative consequences of teenage parenthood also need definition. The traditional concern centered on the medical dangers for mother and child[34]; more recent literature focuses on the psychological, educational, vocational, and economic consequences.[29,32] Societal issues, such as the impact of demographic trends and the cost of social support programs, are also of concern.[51] Currently the focus is on the long-term consequences of teenage pregnancy, particularly regarding the potential for child abuse, the development of children with lower IQ scores, and the transmission of a cycle of poverty.[11] This has replaced the older debate about the extent of psychopathology inherent in teenage pregnancy.

Addressing these issues before attempting to provide services is essential. It is important not to impose on the teenager the expectations and patterns of those providing services. In a society or subculture with accepting or neutral attitudes toward illegitimacy, for example, the teenage parent can rely on an active familial support system; this might not be available to one whose out-of-wedlock pregnancy leads to extrusion and isolation from the family. This availability of a supportive network affects not only the teenager but her child as well. In any discussion of the prevention or reduction of negative consequences of teenage pregnancy, it therefore becomes particularly important to clarify value judgments.

Prevention of Medical Consequences

Among the many concerns about adolescent pregnancy, a particularly important issue has been the increased incidence of complications of pregnancy. Age alone does not constitute a risk factor. Those obstetric complications such as toxemia, anemia, prolonged labor, fetal and perinatal morbidity and mortality, low birth weight for gestational age, and prematurity, which used to be attributed to age, are now linked to the absence of prenatal care and to poor nutrition. These, in turn, are related both to socioeconomic status and illegitimacy rather than to age.[16,31,59]

Studies that correct for prenatal care and race show that adolescent patients ages fifteen and older fare medically as well as, or better than, older primaparas.[46,50] Those under age fifteen do show a slight increase in medical complications, but it is not clear whether this is due to biological or social factors.[71] Prevention of the medical complications associated

with teenage pregnancy is possible and has been achieved by programs with strong community or outreach components.[4]

Social and Economic Consequences of Pregnancy for Teenagers

Waters[69] spoke of a "syndrome of failure" in the course of which poor adolescents deprive themselves of their chances to escape poverty. The essential features of this cycle are the recurrent inability of the adolescent to carry out the tasks inherent in her developmental phase, and includes failure to remain in school, to establish a vocation and become self-supporting, and to limit family size. Ultimately, these young women are unable to remain in stable marriages and rear children who reach their own full potential.

FAILURE TO FULFILL THE FUNCTIONS OF ADOLESCENCE

As described, the developmental issues of adolescence are numerous and complex. Whether or not one adheres to the theory of adolescent crisis,[5,28] adolescence is a time of rapid but uneven psychologic growth toward goals partly defined by social norms, including separation and individuation, education, economic autonomy, productivity, and intimacy. Teenage pregnancy and parenting radically alter the sequence expected by our culture. Parenthood is seen as an independent variable by these teenagers, one that does not necessarily interfere with schooling or imply marriage.[30] For them, identity formation and an adult role may be acquired through parenthood, especially motherhood.[2,61]

FAILURE TO REMAIN IN SCHOOL

There is a strong correlation between the educational level attained by the mother and the age at which she first gives birth to a child.[53] This correlation is stronger for white than for black teenagers. Quite aside from any question of pregnancy, achievement levels, goals, and interests are important predictors of those who will make it through school. In general, pregnancy rates are higher among the more marginal students; abortion rates are higher among those teenagers who excel in school.[13,39]

In addition, leaving school increases the adolescent's social and emotional isolation. For teenagers who experience high levels of guilt or shame about their pregnancy, dropping out may be a confirmation of their worthlessness. It is only since 1971 that pregnant teenagers have been legally allowed to remain in school.[26]

FAILURE TO ACHIEVE VOCATIONAL GOALS AND BE SELF-SUPPORTING

Studies correlating welfare dependency with other variables describe many of the factors found in teenage parenthood: early first birth, low level of education, large family size, and high divorce rate.[13,51] There is a lifelong correlation between income and the adolescent's age at the birth of her first child.[67]

Most teenagers come from homes where parents hope and expect their children will do better than they; this wish for upward mobility is transmitted to the child. During adolescence, however, this often leads to unrealistic fantasies, common to all adolescents. Within this developmental ambience, those who do become parents tend to minimize the obstacles that pregnancy and parenthood will present in reaching goals.

Marriage for teenagers is a special issue. Teenage marriage has a poor outlook as the majority of these end in divorce, except in those subcultures where it is accepted and expected. Those teenage mothers who do get married have a poorer educational and vocational prognosis. They have more children, they bear them earlier, and they often lose the support of their family of origin.[29,52]

FAILURE TO LIMIT FAMILY SIZE

Early first birth is followed by continued increased fertility, even if one corrects for race and religion.[13,68] Subsequent children of adolescent parents fare much worse in all areas. More medical problems and increased mortality due to lack of prenatal care have been documented.[38] Emotional problems and child abuse are also more frequent, presumably because an already stressed system becomes overloaded.[42] The psychological health of teenagers who become pregnant more than once has been studied in several surveys, with no consistent results. Some authors do find psychopathology in that particular subgroup; others do not and see attempts to prevent repeated pregnancies as an imposition of middle-class values on teenagers from different backgrounds (e.g., rural Appalachians in Kentucky).[2,6]

Those services that stop with the birth of the infant have no effect on the rates of either school dropout or repeat pregnancies.[14] It is therefore crucial to follow the adolescent for a few years after the birth of her first child, providing support, advocacy in the school system, birth control options, nutritional counseling, and child development education.

The Consequences for the Children of Adolescents

The lack of prenatal care, so frequent in adolescent pregnancy, is correlated with potential problems for the baby, including low birth weight and prematurity. These have been linked by some studies to a number of negative long-term outcomes—for example, lower IQ rates—particularly for male children.[4,33] The most important corrective factors are the availability of another adult caretaker (e.g. grandmother or spouse), and lack of economic stress.[4,30,40] Inner-city black teenagers usually have had strong extended family ties and have made use of this network for baby care.[26] The majority of "other" adults are maternal grandmothers, but paternal relatives as well as the fathers may take on a sizable portion of the burden of child care. Populations that view teenage pregnancy as an aberration tend to exclude the teenager and her child from the family system or press her to marry, thus increasing the likelihood of the negative effects of teenage parenthood. Without intervention there is a considerable risk that the new infants will, in time, also become teenage parents. The maternal and paternal grandmothers of teenage parents were often teenage mothers themselves.

Many of the negative consequences affect the later years of the mother, the father, the firstborn and subsequent children. These long-term effects may become apparent only many years after the teenagers have graduated from programs that were geared to their needs during the pregnancy. Early preventive intervention is thus of primary importance.[23]

Implications for Intervention Programs

Without intervention the negative consequences of teenage pregnancy and parenthood can be overwhelming and have the potential of entrapping parents and offspring in a continuing cycle of poverty.[69] Prenatal care tends to start late[46] because many teenagers and even their families manage to deny the pregnancy during the first few months. Many factors aid such denial: irregular menstrual periods, a body still in the process of changing, and an absent or weak self-concept as an adult woman capable of reproduction. Nutritional habits among teenagers are generally poor and do not necessarily change even after counseling. Experimentation with or addiction to alcohol, cigarettes, and other drugs is common. These are physiological dangers related to developmental issues and are not related to physical maturity.

These problems are in turn strongly influenced by the socioeconomic status of the pregnant teenager. Disadvantaged people use preventive health care less frequently and have more nutritional deficits than more affluent subgroups of the population.[46,59] Because the majority of teenagers who become parents are disadvantaged, efforts to improve pregnancy outcome need to be available locally. These should include screening and outreach components, offer multiple services, and be staffed by professionals who can work with the sociocultural norms of their client population. The following program is an example of those offered to pregnant and parenting teenagers in a Boston public high school,[62] and illustrates how a small core staff (one nurse and one child psychiatrist, both full-time) can provide multiple services to a large population by acting as advocates who coordinate the services available in other systems.

The program's philosophy defines pregnant and parenting teenagers as presenting with a broad spectrum of psychological, social, and medical needs. Some require only support and advocacy, others need psychiatric treatment. All need an advocate-counselor who acts as a model and provides nurturance and gratification of basic needs and fosters knowledge and ego development.

Teenagers in this urban integrated school with an enrollment of eight hundred students are referred to the program by teachers, peers, or themselves. They are first seen, in the school, by a nurse who has special training in mother-infant development and intervention. Permission from parents or guardians is sought but is not a prerequisite to involvement. A psychiatric evaluation is performed by the child psychiatrist, who offers treatment to those who require it. Infants and children up to the age of three are screened by the child psychiatrist with Bayley examinations,[7] in the school as well as in their home. These assessments are used not only for screening purposes but also as tools offering guidelines in child development.

Intervention consists of advocacy, counseling, and Bayley examinations in the infant's home. The nurse becomes the teenager's advocate and helps her negotiate dealing with the school (e.g., leave of absence, home tutoring, transferral to special school, etc.) and with the medical system (e.g., prenatal visits, postnatal care, birth control, pediatric appointments, etc.). If necessary, arrangements with the state welfare system are provided (e.g., obtaining public assistance, housing, or a day-care slot before returning to school) and with the legal system (e.g., in Massachusetts only a judge can

allow a teenager to decide about obtaining an abortion without the consent of her parents). In addition, the nurse offers counseling and education in a variety of areas such as nutrition, medical care, child development, home safety, and so forth. These topics are covered in weekly group sessions led by the nurse and the psychiatrist, in the school. Supportive counseling is offered in individual meetings, in the school or at home, as well as in less traditional settings such as on the way to a hospital appointment or while waiting for the judge. All teenagers are seen in the hospital after labor and delivery.

The teenager's family is involved in a variety of ways during home visits. All available family members, including fathers, assist at Bayley examinations, which provide the focus for child development education. Teenagers with hostile families or families resistant to intervention can bring their infants to the school and receive counseling there.

Teenage fathers are seen in group sessions in the school, discussing psychological as well as practical issues (e.g., assisting at birth, contraception, marriage, vocational training, legal and financial responsibilities, etc.). Couples' meetings are arranged when indicated.

The teenagers and their children are followed by this program until the child reaches the age of three. The goals are to help the parents gain a high-school diploma and prepare for gainful employment. This requires help with the caretaking of the child and the prevention of further pregnancies until these goals have been achieved.

Pregnant teenagers require a multitude of services: pregnancy tests, counseling around decisions to be made after a positive test, availability of abortion and adoption centers, and nutritional advice. Prenatal medical and psychological care must also be readily available. Group therapy with peers in similar life stages can be a most effective supportive and educational tool. The group leader should be capable of teaching, empathizing, and setting limits; in effect, providing the teenager with the role model of a good parent. In addition, pregnant teenagers need educational counseling. They are often marginal students who are not invested in pursuing a high-school diploma,[13,39] which they may regard as having little value.[2] For inner-city teenagers, graduating from high school does in fact have a major effect on their lifelong earning capacity. Encouraging this achievement requires contact with the school system, advocacy for the teenager, discussions with the teenager's family and determining family members' views, hopes, and fears, in addition to evaluating and counseling the teenagers themselves. In some areas, placement in an alternative school geared to the needs of pregnant teenagers may be indicated. Depending on how an illegitimate pregnancy is viewed in their milieu, some teenagers are proud to continue attending their usual high school, while others prefer to be less visible to avoid the shame of public knowledge. Without intervention, these teenagers might spend a few months away from home, living, for example, with a relative in another city, isolated from peers and missing school.[26]

Parenting teenagers have additional needs. They, too, require educational and vocational counseling to enhance motivation and follow-through, as well as health care for mother and child, birth control counseling, child development education, and nutritional information. The teenager's cultural and familial norms must also be attended to. When another adult caretaker is involved, the mother's chances of continuing her education and finding employment are greater, and the long-term outcome for the child is better.[4,30] These family ties should therefore be fostered and acknowledged as important. Giving a teenager instructions about a particular feeding pattern, for example, will be effective only if the other caretaker agrees to follow the same pattern. The teenager cannot be relied on to transmit instructions that would require changing familial habits. Balancing caretaking and control issues between two caretakers may be quite difficult and may require family meetings. Home visits should be an integral part of all programs for parenting teenagers; such programs give valuable insight about boundaries, both psychological and physical, and about the family hierarchy. They also provide information about practical matters such as eating and sleeping habits. Parenting teenagers also need an advocate to help negotiate all the systems they may encounter (school, vocational training, employment, day care, medical care for herself and her child, etc.). They may also require financial support from state or federal agencies, or help with legal issues.

In addition to the teenager's extended family, which may be involved in the child's care, the father of the child also requires services. He may be the biological or the social father of the child, and his involvement may be financial, affective, or practical. In subgroups where teenage pregnancy is viewed as acceptable, the mother and father will often have had a stable relationship before the pregnancy. Some fathers are very supportive, to the point of assisting at the birth. Others are troubled by the financial responsibility and the fear that this will interfere with their fulfilling their own adolescent needs. Most are proud of being a father, and many would like that status legitimized by marriage. They, too, have medical and psychological needs, require birth control information, and sometimes need to participate in couple counseling. Group meetings can be very helpful too but should be oriented to concrete issues and practical help of a vocational or educational nature, as often male teenagers do not find it easy to sit and talk for extended periods of time.

All these services should be available for the first three to four years of the baby's life. The most stressful period seen is often around the age of two and one-half to three years, when the toddler attempts to negotiate separation-individuation issues that have not been adequately mastered by his or her mother. This stresses not only the teenager but also the extended family that is helping with the care of the child. It is at this time that the teenager may need to renegotiate her relationship with her own mother, and she may find herself more isolated than when her child was an infant. If she is living alone, isolated and with no medical or emotional care, this may lead to another pregnancy. Continued access to an intervention program is crucial throughout these difficult years.[14,15]

Intervention Programs

The distinction between prevention and intervention is not a rigorous one. Intervention programs prevent some of the problems of teenage pregnancy. Though this review of intervention programs focuses on those designed specifically for teenagers, it should be noted that many other services are available for high-risk parents independent of age. These programs are often the most suitable as well as the only programs available in some areas. As with teenage-focused programs, these cover a range from early intervention for the children's cognitive problems that are secondary to environmental understimulation or congenital medical problems, to comprehensive full day-care services that also have parent groups and parent participation in the child care. The use of visiting nurses, homemakers, parent aides, and therapeutic psychiatric intervention offers opportunities for growth and support during early parenting years. Continuation of services over a several-year period is essential for maintaining the gains. At age three, many children can begin preschool programs to ensure ongoing healthy development.

Specialized services for pregnant teenagers and teenage parents have gradually been evolving over the last twenty years. By the mid-1970s, there were approximately 1,200 such programs in the United States.[37] Most current programs offer either a particular type of support such as educational or medical services and child development information, or they are matched to specific phases of teenage pregnancy and provide prenatal care with a high emphasis on medical care, nutrition, and continuing education or else postnatal care. The emphasis is generally on family planning, child development, and continued growth of the teenage parent.

The teenage father has recently received increased attention. Rivara[60] notes that less than half of the programs he surveyed provided services for fathers, and those programs that did reached only about 20 percent of these fathers. The literature on fathers is frequently directed toward assessing the importance of the father's relationship with the teenage mother, the impact of this relationship on parenting, and the limited techniques to effectively engage these young men.

Very little information is available about special groups who become pregnant or who are at risk for pregnancy. Hein, Coupey, and Cohen[35] review a small number of teenagers with limited cognitive capacities and emphasize that typical adolescent developmental tasks must be addressed in dealing with these young people with an appreciation for the adolescent's intellectual skills. A program that addresses the special needs of youngsters in a developing country is described by McNeal and associates[47] from work with adolescent mothers in Jamaica. Other specialized programs are reflected in the work of Field and coworkers,[25] who studied the impact of intervention on lower socioeconomic black mothers who had preterm infants. Better outcomes were reported when interventions were used.

SEX EDUCATION IN SCHOOLS

One of the major problems of teenage pregnancy is its impact on formal education and subsequent earning power. Dunn[21] delineates the rationale for sex education in schools and emphasizes the priority given to reducing teenage pregnancy. Within school systems there are many approaches to providing sex education. Orr[58] states that 36 percent of public high schools in the United States offer formal sex education courses, as do 38 percent of Catholic high schools and 24 percent of other nonpublic schools. She gives details about the content of courses and indicates that about 42 percent of the school programs require some parental involvement. Thus as many as three-quarters of high-school students are reported to receive some form of sex education; the programs are, however, highly variable. Maslach and Kerr[48] emphasize the need to have related topics included in courses, such as the physical as well as emotional aspects of intercourse, and information for teenagers' parents regarding their children's sexuality. A study by Jay and colleagues[36] compares the effects of peer counselors versus nurse counselors on compliance of teenagers in the use of oral contraceptives. Their fourth-month follow-up indicated there was greater compliance by the teenagers who had peer counselors, and they suggest this as an additional technique.

Block and Block[8] compare two programs aiming to prevent teenage pregnancy, one high-school and one junior-high-school program. An outreach method was used. The students were found to be better informed after exposure to the curriculum. Mecklenberg and Thompson,[49] of the Adolescent Family Life Program, note that demonstration projects are needed to help develop an array of strategies for the varying needs of different adolescents.

PRENATAL PROGRAMS

Taylor and associates[66] addressed the question of whether hospital-based prenatal care resulted in a different pregnancy outcome than school-based prenatal care. They found that the care provided by the school resulted in earlier and more frequent prenatal visits. However, on follow-up, they found that those who were given specialized adolescent prenatal care in the hospital reported outcome success that was similar to that achieved in the school-based program. Another comparison between specialized teenage prenatal services and regular obstetric clinics was carried out by Felice and coworkers.[24] Their study used birth weight of infants as an outcome measure. They found that pregnancies followed in the specialized teenage obstetrical unit reported low birth weight in only 9 percent of the infants followed, as compared to 20.9 percent low-birth-weight infants among those followed in the regular obstetrical clinic. A study by Aries and Klerman[1] compared comprehensive adolescent pregnancy programs with regular health care at a hospital. They found that, except for postdelivery educational status, the two groups had similar medical and social outcomes. In further pursuing their findings, however, they noted that the two programs served very different clients. The authors emphasized the need for a "good fit" to accommodate the requirements of different teenagers, suggesting the desirability of multiple models for delivery of services. Copeland[18] focused on what teenagers felt should be included in prenatal classes and found that their highest priority was information about labor and delivery.

A less frequently addressed issue is the decision on the part of some teenagers to give their children up for adoption. Klerman[44] reviews this subject from the public health perspective, including the recommendations from the Office for Adolescent Pregnancy Programs that support adoption as an alternative for adolescent parents. She notes the limited data available for the birth parents regarding the process of deciding on and implementing adoption. Outcomes for children adopted in infancy seem more positive than for those who stay with teenage parents. Leynes[45] discusses factors that influence the way adolescent pregnant teenagers plan for their babies, including consideration of adoption. She found that those adolescent mothers who released their children for adoption were psychologically healthier than those who did not. The adolescent's age and socioeconomic status, the influence exerted by parents and male partners, as well as an evaluation by a psychiatrist and level of function as measured on the DSM-III, Axis V, were used to define psychological health. The mothers who released their infants for adoption did undergo some psychological upheaval after deciding on adoption. The mothers who kept their babies, however, were noted to have more need for support services.

A number of programs focus on enhancing the adolescent's development after her child's birth. The Cincinnati Maternal and Infant Care Project reports that teenage mothers are able to use postnatal classes both to realize their own educational and employment goals and to limit the size of their family. Weekly postnatal classes were economically feasible to assist this high-risk population of mothers.[3] A follow-up telephone study after three years reported that high and low class attenders, in spite of their similar aspirations, showed striking differences in outcome. Those who attended more frequently were more able to complete school and prevent unwanted pregnancy.

A study by Cappleman and colleagues[12] on the effects of a home-based intervention program for infants of adolescent mothers found that only 11 percent of the children remained at risk biomedically and environmentally after this method of intervention, while 50 percent of the children in a control group remained at risk. Sung and Rothrock[65] discuss some of the issues involved in setting up separate schools for pregnant teenagers as a way to focus on their specialized needs. The program described by these authors encouraged completion of high school, entry into employment, and avoidance of repeated pregnancies.

An initial report of a comprehensive teenage pregnancy program by Salguero and associates[61] describes a population of at-risk, inner-city adolescent mothers. The investigators looked at three risk groups and found that 27.5 percent were at high risk and 24.5 percent at moderate risk for failure to thrive, child abuse, and neglect. Therapeutic interventions were offered, and the importance of comprehensive programs attending to the range of needs of adolescent parents was emphasized.

In summary, there are several consistent themes in the programs described. The most striking one is the finding that if specialized services are provided that take into account the developmental needs of adolescents, many, if not all, of the risk factors associated with teenage pregnancy can be eliminated. Many studies compare traditional prenatal and postnatal care with specialized programs and find that routine care is not adequate to prevent problems associated with high risk.

Another notable finding is the need for variety in the types of programs offered. No one program meets the needs of all pregnant and parenting teenagers. Additionally, it is important for programs to provide comprehensive services including medical care, developmental information, educational assistance, and parenting skills. It is also critical to have programs that do not stop too early in delivery of services, but follow mother and child for the first three years of the child's development. Since the vast majority of teenage pregnancies occur in lower socioeconomic groups, awareness of the need for specialized services to provide less risky outcomes for these parents and their children seems to be warranted. If this is not addressed because of societal or national priorities, the problem will continue to compound and laboriously achieved gains can be lost.

Conclusion

Adolescent pregnancy is a complex phenomenon with determinants at many levels. Although in many subcultural groups it can be considered nonpathological, there are profound consequences for development in terms of education of the mother and welfare of the child. Many of the negative consequences can be prevented if the priorities of society allow for sufficient supportive resources.

REFERENCES

1. ARIES, N., and KLERMAN, L. "Evaluating Service Delivery Models for Pregnant Adolescents," *Women & Health,* 6 (1981):91–107.

2. AUG, R., and BRIGHT, T. "A Study of Wed and Unwed Motherhood in Adolescents and Young Adults," *Journal of the American Academy of Child Psychiatry,* 9 (1970):577–594.

3. BADGER, E., and BURNS, D. "Impact of a Parent Education Program on the Personal Development of Teenage Mothers," *Journal of Pediatric Psychology,* 5 (1980):415–422.

4. BALDWIN, W., and CAIN, V. "The Children of Teenage Parents," *Family Planning Perspectives,* 12 (1980):34–43.

5. BARGLOW, P., and SCHAEFER, M. "The Fate of the Feminine Self in Normative Adolescent Regression, in M. Sugar, ed., *Female Adolescent Development.* New York: Brunner/Mazel, 1979.

6. BARGLOW, P., et al. "Some Psychiatric Aspects of Illegitimate Pregnancy in Early Adolescence," *American Journal of Orthopsychiatry,* 38 (1968):672–687.

7. BAYLEY, N. *Bayley Scales of Infant Development.* New York: Psychological Corp., 1969.

8. BLOCK, R., and BLOCK, A. "Outreach Education: A Possible Preventer of Teenage Pregnancy," *Adolescence,* 15 (1980):657–660.

9. BLOCK, R., SALTZMAN, S., and BLOCK, S. "Teenage Pregnancy. A Review," *Advances in Pediatrics,* 28 (1981): 75–98.

10. BLOS, P. *On Adolescence.* New York: Macmillan, 1962.

11. BLUM, R., and GOLDHAGEN, J. "Teenage Pregnancy in Perspective," *Clinical Pediatrics,* 20 (1981):335–340.

12. CAPPLEMAN, M., et al. "Effectiveness of a Home-based Early Intervention Program with Infants of Adolescent Mothers," *Child Psychiatry and Human Development,* 13 (1982):56–65.

13. CARD, J., and WISE, L. "Teenage Mothers and Teenage Fathers: The Impact of Early Childbearing on the Parents' Personal and Professional Lives," *Family Planning Perspectives,* 10 (1978):199–205.

14. CARTOOF, V. "Postpartum Services for Adolescent Mothers," *Child Welfare,* 57 (1978):660–666.

15. ———. "Postpartum Services for Adolescent Mothers: Part 2," *Child Welfare,* 58 (1979):673–680.

16. CLARK, A. "Adolescent Obstetrics: Obstetric and Sociologic Implications," *Clinical Obstetrics and Gynecology,* 14 (1971):1026–1036.

17. COBLINER, W. "Prevention of Adolescent Pregnancy: A Developmental Perspective," *Birth Defects,* 17 (1981):35–47.

18. COPELAND, D. "Unwed Adolescent Primigravidas Identify Subject Matter for Prenatal Classes," *Journal of Gynecological Nursing,* (July–August 1979):248–253.

19. CVETKOVITCH, G., and GROTE, B. "On the Psychology of Adolescents' Use of Contraception," *Journal of Sex Research,* 11 (1975):256–270.

20. DEUTSCH, H. *The Psychology of Women,* vol. 2. New York: Grune & Stratton, 1945.

21. DUNN, P. "Reduction of Teenage Pregnancy as a Rationale for Sex Education: A Position Paper," *Journal of School Health,* (1982):611–613.

22. EDITORS. "Pregnancy Seen in Teens Least Able for Motherhood," *Psych. News.* 15,20, Aug. 20, 1982.

23. ELSTER, A., et al. "Parental Behavior of Adolescent Mothers," *Pediatrics,* 71 (1983):494–503.

24. FELICE, M., et al. "The Young Pregnant Teenager," *Journal of Adolescent Health Care,* 1 (1981):193–197.

25. FIELD, T., et al. "Teenage, Lower-class, Black Mothers and Their Preterm Infants: An Intervention and Developmental Follow-up," *Child Development,* 51 (1980):426–436.

26. FISHER, S., and SCHARF, K. "Teenage Pregnancy: An Anthropological, Sociological and Psychological Overview," in S. Feinstein, ed., *Adolescent Psychiatry,* vol. 8. Chicago: University of Chicago Press, 1980, pp. 393–403.

27. FRAIBERG, S. "The Adolescent Mother and Her Infant," *Adolescent Psychiatry,* 10 (1982):7–23.

28. FREUD, A. "Adolescence," *Psychoanalytic Study of the Child,* 13 (1952):255–278.

29. FURSTENBERG, F. *Unplanned Parenthood: The Social Consequences of Teenage Childbearing.* New York: Free Press, 1976.

30. FURSTENBERG, F., and CRAWFORD, A. "Family Support: Helping Teenage Mothers to Cope," *Family Planning Perspectives,* 10 (1977):322–333.

31. GRANT, J. and HEALD, F. "Complications of Adolescent Pregnancy: Survey of the Literature on Fetal Outcome in Adolescence," *Clinical Pediatrics,* 11 (1972):567–570.

32. GUTTMACHER INSTITUTE. *Teenage Pregnancy: The Problem that Hasn't Gone Away.* New York: Alan Guttmacher Institute, 1981.

33. HARDY, J., et al. "Long-range Outcome of Adolescent Pregnancy," *Clinical Obstetrics and Gynecology,* 21 (1978):1215–1232.

34. HASSAN, II., and FALLS, F. "The Young Primipara: A Clinical Study," *American Journal of Obstetrics and Gynecology,* 88 (1964):256–262.

35. HEIN, K., COUPEY, S., and COHEN, M. "Special Considerations in Pregnancy Prevention for the Mentally Subnormal Adolescent Female," *Journal of Adolescent Health Care,* 1 (1980):46–49.

36. JAY, S., et al. "Effect of Peer Counselors on Adolescent Compliance in Use of Oral Contraceptives," *Pediatrics,* 73 (1984):126–131.

37. JEKEL, J. "Evaluation of Programs for Adolescents," *Birth Defects* (orig. article series), 17 (1981):139–153.

38. JEKEL, J., et al. "A Comparison of the Health of Index and Subsequent Babies Born to School-age Mothers," *American Journal of Public Health,* 65 (1975):370–374.

39. KANE, F., et al. "Motivational Factors in Abortion Patients," *American Journal of Psychiatry,* 130 (1973):290–293.

40. KELLAN, S., ENSMINGER, M., and TURNER, R. "Family Structure and the Mental Health of Children," *Archives of General Psychiatry,* 34 (1977):1012–1022.

41. KENNELL, J., and KLAUS, M. "Mother-infant Interaction: Implications for Adolescent Mothering," *Birth Defects,* 17 (1981):123–129.

42. KINARD, E., and KLERMAN, L. "Teenage Parenting and Child Abuse: Are They Related?" *American Journal of Orthopsychiatry,* 50 (1980):481–488.

43. KIRBY, D., ALTER, J., and SCALES, P. *An Analysis of U.S. Sex Education Programs and Evaluation Methods.* Bethesda, Md.: MATHTECH, 1979.

44. KLERMAN, L. "Adoption: A Public Health Perspective," *American Journal of Public Health,* 73 (1983):1158–1160.

45. LEYNES, C. "Keep or Adopt: A Study of Factors Influencing Pregnant Adolescents' Plans for Their Babies," *Child Psychiatry and Human Development,* 11 (1980):105–112.

46. McANARNEY, E., et al. "Obstetric Neonatal and Psychosocial Outcome of Pregnant Adolescents," *Pediatrics,* 61 (1978):199–207.

47. McNEIL, P., et al. "The Women's Center in Jamaica: An Innovative Project for Adolescent Mothers," *Studies in Family Planning,* 14 (1983):143–149.

48. MASLACH, G., and KERR, G. "Tailoring Sex Education Programs to Adolescents: A Strategy for the Primary Prevention of Unwanted Adolescent Pregnancies," *Adolescence,* 18 (1983):449–456.

49. MECKLENBURG, M., and THOMPSON P: "The Adolescent Family Life Program as a Preventive Measure," *Public Health Reports,* 98 (1983):21–29.

50. MEDNICK, B., BAKER R., and SUTTON-SMITH, B. "Teenage Pregnancy and Perinatal Mortality," *Journal of Youth Adolescence,* 8 (1979):343–357.

51. MOORE, K. "Teenage Childbirth and Welfare Dependency," *Family Planning Perspectives,* 10 (1978):233–235.

52. ———. "Teenage Motherhood: Its Social and Economic Costs," *Children Today,* 8 (1979):12–16.

53. MOORE, K., and WAITE, L. "Early Childbearing and Educational Attainment," *Family Planning Perspectives,* 9 (1977):220–225.

54. NADELSON, C. "The Pregnant Teenager: Problems of Choice in a Developmental Framework," *Psychiatric Opinion,* 12 (1975):6–12.

55. NADELSON, C., and NOTMAN, M. "Sexual Knowledge and Attitudes of Adolescents: Relationship to Contraceptive use, *Obstetrics and Gynecology,* 55 (1980):340–345.

56. ———. "Behavioral-psychological Aspects of Pregnancy," in Z. DeFries, ed., *Sexual Behavior in College Students.* Westport, Conn.: Greenwood, forthcoming.

57. NOTMAN, M. "Teenage Pregnancy: The Nonuse of Contraception," *Psychiatric Opinion,* 12 (1975):23–27.

58. ORR, M. "Sex Education and Contraceptive Education in U.S. Public High Schools," *Family Planning Perspectives,* 14 (1982):304–313.

59. OSOFSKY, H., et al. "Nutritional Status of Low Income Pregnant Teenagers," *Journal of Reproductive Medicine,* 6 (1977):29–33.

60. RIVARA, F. "Teenage Pregnancy: The Forgotten Father," *Journal of Developmental and Behavioral Pediatrics,* 2 (1981):142–145.

61. SALGUERO, C., et al. "Studies of Infants at Risk and Their Adolescent Mothers," in S. Feinstein, ed., *Adolescent Psychiatry,* vol. 8. Chicago: University of Chicago Press, 1980, pp. 404–421.

62. SAUZIER, M., "Importance of Maternal Support Systems," Grand Rounds presentation, Tufts-New England Medical Center Hospital, 10 February 1983.

63. SCHAFFER, C., and PINE, F. "Pregnancy, Abortion and the Developmental Tasks of Adolescence," *Journal of Child Psychiatry,* 14 (1975):511–536.

64. SMITH, L. "A Conceptual Model of Families Incorporating an Adolescent Mother and Child into the Household, *Advances in Nursing Science,* (October 1983):45–60.

65. SUNG, K., and ROTHROCK, D. "An Alternate School for Pregnant Teenagers and Teenage Mothers," *Child Welfare,* 59 (1980):427–436.

66. TAYLOR, B., et al. School-based Prenatal Services: Can Similar Outcomes Be Attained in a Non-school Setting?" *Journal of School Health,* 53 (1983):480–486.

67. TRUSSEL, T. "Economic Consequences of Teenage Childbearing," *Family Planning Perspectives,* 8 (1976):184–195.

68. TRUSSEL, T., and MENKEN, J. "Early Childbearing and Subsequent Fertility," *Family Planning Perspectives,* 10 (1978):209–218.

69. WATERS, J. "Pregnancy in Young Adolescents: A Syndrome of Failure," *Southern Medical Journal,* 62 (1969): 655–658.

70. ZUCKERMAN, B., et al. "Neonatal Outcome: Is Adolescent Pregnancy a Risk Factor?" *Pediatrics,* 71 (1983):489–493.

---

68 / Prevention of Psychiatric Disorder in American Indian Children and Adolescents

Irving N. Berlin

Introduction

For many years the traditional Indian cultural heritage and Anglo influences and pressures have been locked in chronic conflict. The ensuing tensions seriously affect the mental health of American Indian children and adolescents.* There have been longstanding efforts on the part of the U.S. Government to contain Indians on reservations as one means of forcing acculturation by eliminating their usual means of economic survival and forcing them to remain in one place and farm, for example, rather than hunt. These efforts lead to enforced education of Indian children and the forced assumption of another life-style. Cumulatively, these have proven destructive to many tribes. The outcome has been disruption of the traditional religious influences on daily living, fragmentation of the old methods of economic survival, dispersal of the extended family structure, and devaluation of the general philosophy of living. In many tribes the destruction of the extended family in particular has interfered with the transmission of Indian heritage and tradition from elders to young family members.* Models of effective living and coping by elders and adults are often missing, and traditional puberty rites and other ceremonies may be lost. The disruption of traditional religious and philosophical influences on daily living has a considerable impact on the child and adolescent; it leaves these young people at a loss for their place and role in the

*See references 1, 4, 8, 30, and 37.

*See references 38, 39, 61, 65, 83, 94, and 95.

life and tradition of the tribe.[83,106,107] For most tribes the concomitant loss of economic vitality means that many adolescents and young adults must leave the reservation to find work.

The confluence of many of these factors appears to contribute significantly to the enormous increase in alcoholism among adults and adolescents along with parallel increases in child abuse, neglect, adult depression, and failures in the nurturance of the infant and small child. In many tribes the traditional distribution of roles was for the elders to use their wisdom in child rearing, while the young adults provided for the tribes' economic needs. Thus because traditional roles have been upset, many aspects of infant, child, and adolescent development appear to have been disrupted. A coincident increase has occurred in adolescent suicides and suicide attempts, alcohol and substance abuse, violent deaths by auto accidents, and homicides. Recent studies also indicate a major increase in childhood depression, poor academic performance, and very early solvent sniffing with consequent serious brain damage in many young persons.*

It is very important to note that not all Native American people have responded to these stresses in the same way. Members of some tribes exhibit few manifestations of severe family problems and have few adolescents with major psychosocial problems and little child abuse. It is obviously desirable to investigate what differences exist. One of the important variables seems to be the degree to which tribal members adhere to their traditions and provide a means for communicating their heritage and ensuring participation by young people in religious activities.†

Concerns with Maldevelopment

Two meetings were convened recently on the problems of childhood and adolescence among American Indians, cosponsored by the American Academy of Child Psychiatry and various American Indian mental health professional organizations and the Council of American Indian Tribal Judges. These assemblies have provided an opportunity for tribal leaders to express concern about the increasing problems of adolescents and among families. The tribal courts were especially troubled by the marked increase in child abuse. Two subsequent meetings on the American Indian child sponsored by Save the Children Foundation also focused on the great increase in family problems and aspects of adolescent disturbances.[2,76,131]

*See references 81, 88, 90, 91, 118, 120, 129, 133, and 155.
†See references 6, 12, 52, 63, 95, 100, and 143.

Normal Development

Within the various Indian tribes, the normal developmental tasks of children and adolescents appear to be similar, yet the means for carrying them out may be different. The primary tasks are related to preserving the continuity and traditions of the tribe. The child-rearing tasks are variously shared by the elders, young adults, and older children of an extended family or clan. The several developmental duties are parceled out in a variety of ways, and the appropriate models of adult functioning are provided, especially through the religious rites of the clan. Where there is an extended family, modeling of the expected next steps in development may be carried out by older children. In his description of several Indian tribes, Erikson recounts how autonomy and independence are fostered. It is clear from many descriptions as well as from my observations in various American Indian and Native Alaskan communities that infants are cherished and handled with tenderness. Members of the extended families provide a good deal of visual and other sensorimotor stimulation. There is a security that comes from opportunities for attachment and from the fostering of separation/individuation; this is usually built into the traditional child-rearing practices. In some instances, extended families are able to make up for some young parents' depression and alcoholism. The degree to which the extended family can be effective depends on how well the tribes' and families' human and economic resources permit both responsible and responsive parenting.[47,49,50]

In some tribes, there are enough adolescents who become involved in religious rites and ceremonies to provide an environment of clear expectations for the younger children. In these same tribes, religious leaders and native healers are potent forces in daily life and are available to troubled individuals and families.[72,101,141]

Prevalent Interferences with Normal Development

A number of researchers and behavioral scientists have described the problems in child-rearing resulting from the alcoholism that is so pervasive among young and middle-aged Indian mothers.[63] Some authors have also described the depression noted in single young mothers where there is serious disruption of the extended family and no one to help them with caring for the young child.

Interferences with attachment and bonding in infants have been noted where the parents, especially single young mothers, are depressed and alcoholic. The infants' constant irritability, crying, and problems in sleeping attest to the difficulties brought on by failure of the nurturing person to provide predictable and persistent satisfaction of the infants' needs.

In the preschool child, the working through of the separation and individuation process may be seriously interfered with because of the parents' depressed and alcoholic state. This in turn affects the development of curiosity and competence in sensorimotor spheres, bowel training, speech, locomotion, eye-hand coordination, and of object constancy. It is during this period that most child abuse occurs, with resulting major developmental delays and arrests.[56,77,121]

The school-age child who has not suffered previous serious developmental problems requires attention and recognition of his or her efforts to be successful as a student from parents or other important adults. The Plowden Report[128] makes this issue clear. Thus alcoholic parents and the lack of extended family to replace the parents' encouragement of learning may devalue the importance of education of the child.[115]

In some tribes, there is evidence that children do well in the first three grades and begin to do poorly thereafter. This reversal may be the result of several factors. Learning in the first three grades is not very competitive; it becomes competitive as math, English skills, history, and so forth begin to require more effort. At this point Indian noncompetitive traditions, especially the belief that it is bad to stand out, are in conflict with the teacher's demands for excellence. Children raised to speak their native language now face demands for a more extensive use and understanding of English. This also serves as an increasing handicap. Where subject matter is taught in both the native language and English, there seem to be fewer difficulties. However, the content of the curriculum is usually not very relevant to Indian children and their families. The subject matter is not very interesting to children whose lifestyle does not stress formal education; ultimately this acts to increase their learning difficulties.*

Major Problems in Adolescent Development

Adolescent development seems especially stressful for American Indian children. The traditional tasks of adolescents—to learn to become adults who are useful to their tribes and who thus provide a continuity of

tradition—may seem irrelevant where one's heritage is not valued or emphasized in the family. The fact that employment is not available on or near the reservation adds to adolescents' hopeless feeling about establishing themselves as adults. The usual developmental work of separation from the family, individuation, learning about sexuality, and experiencing intimacy in one's peer group are difficult to accomplish when there are few adult models who have successfully mastered these tasks. The widespread depression among these young people is symptomatic of their hopeless and helpless feelings. Thus drugs, inhalants, and alcohol are resorted to in order to escape the sense of a hopeless future. Suicide attempts are becoming more frequent and the suicide death rate is growing among American Indian adolescents, as is violent death by auto accidents and homicide.*

Suicide as a Major Adolescent Problem of American Indians

The data on Indian suicide indicate that about 60 percent of those who commit suicide have lost a parent figure in their first two years of life. Seventy percent have had a parent who was recently arrested for alcoholism and related minor crimes. Sixty-five percent of those who commit suicide had themselves been arrested in the year before, suggesting feelings of anger and a need to act out. On some reservations 50 percent of adolescent suicides have occurred in jail. The youngsters were apprehended for a minor offense; in the face of the accompanying feelings of losing face and being a disgrace in the eyes of family and tribal elders, they hanged themselves in their cells. Over 50 percent of the suicides were precipitated by the recent loss of a family member known to be supportive to the adolescent.

While females do not engage in suicidal behavior as frequently as do males, the number of suicide attempts among young women has increased tenfold in a decade. Investigators believe this is related to the young women's sense of aloneness. The girls feel helpless as they face the problems of growing up and becoming an adult with marriage and family as ultimate goals. Most suicide attempts occur after these young women are discarded by a boyfriend for someone else. About 70 percent of the males who commit suicide and 50 percent of the females who attempt suicide have been abused and neglected as young children; they grow up with a distrust of adults, an inability to turn to others for help, and a poor self-image.†

In boarding schools, female adolescents who do well

---

*See references 27, 31, 66, 68, 96, 97, 98, 103, 109, and 127.

†See references 13, 19, 26, 42, 55, 149, and 150.

†See references 37, 45, 53, 93, 101, 111, 112, 116, 124, 125, and 136.

academically and stand out in social life as, for example, cheerleaders and school officers have been maligned and maltreated by their agemates for discarding their tradition of not standing out and acting better than others. Paradoxically, this has led to some mass suicide attempts. However, albeit dramatic, these are isolated events. Other mass suicides appear to be the result of contagion among peers who drink and use drugs together. The suicide of one young male heightens the awareness of others in the group that their lives lack purpose or a future.[21,22]

The majority of these adolescents have parents who are alcoholic and who provide no support or evidence that adulthood has much purpose.*

Adoption as an Identity Crisis

The Indian adoption rate is three times that of the Anglo population. Usually it is the Indian children who are adopted by Anglo families, with resulting separation from family and culture. When these Indian children reach eighteen and leave their adoptive families, they find that they are neither Indian, with a family and tribe to which to return, nor Anglo, with some better opportunities for jobs. The suicide rate among these adolescents is twice that of the tribes with the highest adolescent suicide rate.†

The Role of Boarding Schools in Creating Psychiatric Problems

Boarding schools, which were initially set up by the Bureau of Indian Affairs (BIA) with the clear purpose of acculturating Indian children, must be taken into account as an important contributor to the foregoing problems. Although most Indian children now go to school on or near their reservations, the current young and middle-aged adults, for the most part, attended boarding schools; several Indian researchers have called these boarding-school attendees the "missing generations." Their acculturation was never truly accomplished, yet they were sufficiently divorced from their own traditions to prevent their learning and integrating their values and heritage or passing these on to their children. Recently some tribes have attempted to break this circle of devaluation of heritage and tradition. However, on my recent visits to some boarding schools that still exist, I have been struck by their alarming similarity to those attended by the "missing generations."

The boarding-school experiment has gone wrong for a number of reasons, and will continue to do so unless basic changes are made.

The children are isolated for many years, not only from their families but often from anyone who speaks their language. They are placed in a setting in which their need to affirm the values of their culture is ignored. Since a good number of the children come from already disorganized tribes, in many cases the effect of this approach is devastating to normal development. As children or adolescents, they are unable to identify with a family or adults whose traditions serve as guidelines for their behavior or future living in the community.

This unpromising atmosphere is further complicated by poor teaching by ill-prepared teachers who are often overwhelmed by student-teacher ratios of forty or fifty to one. The curricula offered are usually primitive and boring and constructed with little or no awareness of needs and opportunities at various stages of development. The adolescents acquire neither the tools of the Anglo culture nor the traditions of their own culture.

The less than optimal environment of the boarding schools worsens when tribes realize that they can rid themselves of troublesome acting-out and antisocial adolescents by sending them away to school. Administrators and teachers begin to regard their students as difficult children, rejected even by their own tribes, and it becomes common for dormitories to be run by small circles of antisocial-hostile older students. Administrators tolerate this as a means of providing discipline. Over the years the basic function of the boarding school has shifted subtly in the minds of students and teachers, from a place of education to a holding, way station until graduation. Instead of counseling from teachers and mental health professionals, troubled students can get alcohol and drugs from dormitory student leaders.

It seems unlikely that the basic failures of the boarding schools can be remedied. The Kennedy study in 1969 recommended closing all boarding schools, and the data base of this study was confirmed by a Bureau of Indian Affairs' study in 1975.[4,85]

When I discussed my observations of boarding schools with various tribal leaders, they were surprised to learn how bad the schools are. Most had themselves experienced boarding-school education and felt that the food, clothing, shelter, and opportunity to learn stood in marked contrast to the poverty and lack of schooling at home. Of course, they were describing a period when the child-adolescent population was relatively small, as were the boarding schools themselves. In 1960 there were 552,800 American Indians and Na-

*See references 5, 22, 73, 102, 140, and 151.
†See references 18, 24, 51, 58, 59, 62, 69, 74, 114, 138, and 142.

tive Alaskans; in 1970, 827,108; in 1980, 1,801,217. The current birth rate of 30.2 per 1,000 population among American Indians is twice the 15.9 per 1,000 population rate of all other races in the United States. The infant mortality rate in 1956 was 62.7 per 1,000 live births as compared to 14.6 per 1,000 live births in 1980—a decrease of 77 percent in infant mortality.*

In 1940 there were fifty-five BIA boarding schools. Few were located on a reservation. There are now thirty-two BIA boarding schools, most on or near reservations.

Prevention of Developmental Disorders

PRIMARY PREVENTION

As many tribal leaders and judges see it, the tribes' most critical task is to find ways to help adolescents with their hopelessness and depression and, especially, to help disturbed female adolescents with the tasks of child rearing.

In a few tribes, a major effort is currently underway to help adolescents with alcoholic parents find new adult models in their communities. Attempts are also being made to find employment opportunities on or near reservations so that these young people can feel more effective as individuals and more nurturant as parents.

One of the most effective pilot projects involved the identification of female adolescents who were getting into trouble in school or into difficulties with the law or dropping out of school. These teenagers were then assigned to volunteer tribal elders who served as their sponsors and to whom the courts gave responsibility for their management. The elder's task was to be available to the adolescent as a listener and advocate, to convey to her the tribes' concern, and to impart ways in which knowledge of their mutual heritage and traditions could help the youngster become important to the continuity of the tribe.[21,43]

Using a similar model, Shore and coworkers succeeded in greatly reducing adolescent suicide in a Northwest tribe. Whenever an adolescent was jailed for a minor offense, an elder, often a healer, came to the jail on the reservation or in town and remained in the jail cell with the adolescent until he was released. The elder conveyed the group's need of that young person as a member of his family, clan, and tribe and remained

involved with him as a listener, facilitator, and conveyer of tribal traditions.[43]

Similar efforts were made to tie female adolescents who made suicide attempts, usually from broken or nonfunctional families, to respected adult or elder females. These mature women maintained a concern with the youngsters' education, their problems in dating boys or, if pregnant, their nutrition and subsequent child-rearing methods. Within the several tribes where these pilot efforts were undertaken, they seem to have been effective in reducing child abuse and neglect.

In several tribes efforts were made to provide work through light industry and training in the group's health, welfare, and other social organizations. These adolescents were clearly involved in the tribes' religious activities, and there was little alcoholism and destructive behavior. These adolescents appeared to become nurturant parents and mutually supportive and caring partners.*

The adolescent mother is a special concern of tribal leaders and educators. Young unwed mothers are noted to be at high risk for neglecting or abusing their infants and young children. Several important pilot projects have demonstrated how effective early intervention can be.

In one project special opportunities were offered to a group of vulnerable female adolescents.[21,82] These young women came from broken homes or alcoholic families, they appeared depressed, they were poor learners, and they were beginning to get into trouble with alcohol or substance abuse. The adolescents were paid to work in a nearby day-care center and required to participate in a child development seminar in order to get their school credits. They quickly identified with the most needy and disturbed young children. In their seminars, they inquired about the causes of the disturbances. Thus as they learned to care for and nurture these young children, they also learned about the developmental processes and the kinds of parent-child relationships (either hostile, overactive behavior, or withdrawal and depression) that resulted in behavioral disturbances. The disturbed behavior and difficulties in relating to adults or peers of these abused children particularly troubled the young women. A number of them went on to take college courses in early childhood education in order to prepare for preschool teaching; others became interested in helping parents and turned to social work education and training.

On these same reservations, pregnant adolescents were given similar opportunities to do paid work in infant and child care and to attend child development seminars. Both groups of young women spent a good deal of time recounting their own childhood experi-

---

*These figures are based on Indian Health Service, Office of Program Statistics, and U.S. Bureau of Census, 1984.

*J. D. Kinzie, personal communication, 1975.

ences and sharing their observations on what made for good and poor marriages. The pregnant adolescents were able to place their babies in the infant nurseries and day-care centers; in this way they could continue to work, care for their babies, and finish their education. The rate of child abuse and neglect among this female adolescent population was very low.

It was astounding to the high-school teachers and child-care professionals that some male adolescents volunteered for both the work and the seminars. These young men were especially helpful with the very withdrawn or overly aggressive little boys. It became clear that very little had been done to involve the boyfriends and infants' fathers in child care. When an opportunity was made available, some fathers became very much involved.

The early findings in these pilot efforts were very encouraging.*

Several infant stimulation programs were developed for the mothers of newborns. The mothers were encouraged to learn how to care for and stimulate their infants. One of the attractions of these programs was the opportunity afforded to these young women to care for several babies and to recognize the infants' differences in temperament and style of learning and interaction. As a consequence of these experiences, new mothers were able to view their own infants more objectively and learned to tune into their babies and to comfort and care for them with minimum loss of patience or temper. Older mothers with a new baby often yielded to the public health nurses' urging to participate in the infant stimulation programs because of the opportunities for socialization and sharing of experiences with other mothers. Mothers often socialized outside the program and formed baby-sitting cooperatives to provide each member with free time. In one tribe where there were several infant stimulation programs, mothers came from great distances in transportation provided by public health nurses. In observing the young women and their babies in these settings, it was evident that they were very nurturant and cheerful, and obviously enjoyed the program. One of the programs run by a tribal elementary school also provided stimulation programs for infants who were handicapped, retarded, blind, deaf, cerebral palsied, and so forth. They were integrated with the normal infants. These mothers enjoyed the social aspects greatly as they were helped to stimulate and help their babies cope with the effects of the developmental deficits. Grandmothers were invited to participate in this program, especially with the handicapped infants. A nurse reported with pleasure that one of these older women had boasted to the other grandmothers that she was learning to become a healer

of handicapped babies. In another program on the same reservation, the female healers were invited to participate and to teach some of their healing methods to the mothers. Several healers became important leaders in this undertaking and were eager learners of stimulation methods. They then taught these to new mothers who could not attend the programs because of great distance and large families. Thus they extended the benefits of the program at the same time they enhanced their own reputations.*

The Educational Process as Secondary Prevention

THE PRESCHOOL

In a number of Indian and Native Alaskan communities, one role of Head Start programs has been to provide an opportunity to identify preschool children with a variety of developmental problems. These difficulties usually resulted from problems in early nurturance and centered primarily in the areas of trust and socialization. The concentrated attention from teachers and tribal aides in these programs seemed to alter these young children's withdrawn, mistrusting attitudes and to bring about increased socialization with evident pleasure in play. Elders provided similar models for nurturing young children as described in other programs.

It is evident that good preschools can provide both the diagnostic opportunities to identify disturbed children early and some of the remediation necessary for at least those children who are not severely disturbed.

The traveling teams of the Indian Children's Program of the Indian Health Service in the Southwest regularly consult with Head Start and other preschools. The teams seek to help diagnose severe disturbance and arrange some treatment for the child as well as offering assistance to the parents.

It is clear that as the extended family becomes progressively more fragmented, preschools present important socializing opportunities for all young children as well as sites for exploration and the satisfaction of curiosity.

One of the critical needs of the infant stimulation programs and preschools is a trained corps of native child-care diagnosticians and specialists in early intervention. One junior college on a reservation is beginning such a training program, but because of limited federal support, the scarcity of programs in

*See references 39, 40, 79, 82, 113, 132, and 137.

*See references 9, 21, 28, 29, 89, 92, 99, and 117.

which to work has not made it an attractive training opportunity. Resources for the treatment of the more severely disturbed preschoolers are scarce, and there are very few trained child mental health specialists among the American Indian and Alaskan Native populations.*

The Role of Schools in Secondary Prevention

In contrast to the boarding schools described previously, one of the boarding schools I visited did provide the kind of education that tended to prevent mental illness and to promote mental health in its students. In each dormitory there were three to four counselors for thirty to forty children. There were a number of counselors from each tribe represented in the student body. Each child or adolescent was evaluated by a team consisting of psychologist, pediatrician, and educational specialist in order to determine the child's assets and needs in health, academics, and psychosocial areas. Teachers and dormitory counselors were alert to signs of depression as well as interferences with living and learning in the school. Regular group discussions were held in each class led by a teacher-counselor team in order to discuss problems in the school that impaired learning. Most counselors and teachers were young Indian adults concerned with preserving native traditions and heritage. One of the most interesting classes in each grade was concerned with descriptions of the differences and similarities among the traditions of the various tribes. The myths and tales recounted to the children by the tribal elders were of special interest both to the young children and to the high-school seniors who were examining the traditional symbolic meaning of these stories. There was a high level of interest in Indian culture. Various healers who used religious ceremonies for their work came from the various tribes to talk with the children and adolescents as did some of the religious leaders.[23,57]

The ever-present problem of Indian children and youth not "standing out" or being competitive was dealt with by the young adults in terms of working out individualized learning goals. They also stressed how important it was for young Indians to be competent and well educated in order to carry out the many important tribal tasks.

The curriculum was designed to use practical approaches to learning math, English, and history. There were two American history textbooks in use; one was

*See references 21, 86, 87, 99, and 119.

a standard text and one was written by Indian scholars. World history was taught as a way of learning and understanding the various forces important in bringing about critical events.

The Use of Problem-solving Learning to Enhance Mental Health

Problem solving is a crucial issue in learning. Little research has focused on the question of how to teach problem solving; Native Americans could be leaders in this area.

In the few cases where problem solving is encouraged through project learning, it often meets resistance from various political forces in a tribe. Yet becoming a problem-solving person is vital to mental health and essential for the prevention of a state of hopelessness and helplessness so characteristic of depression and other mental illness.[25,32,48,146]

Educators and investigators concerned with cognitive development consider most aspects of education as an opportunity to learn how to think in problem-solving terms. This means being able to define a problem, gather data about it, and evaluate the findings or data in terms of solutions that may emerge with regard to that problem.[32] Pilot projects demonstrate that it is important to involve children early. The use of collaborative projects such as documenting who the leading Indian chiefs were in the 1800s and discovering their important statements can be started as early as the third grade.[146] There is increasing data that, in Piagetian terms, environmental experience (i.e., how and what learning has been encouraged at home and in school) will determine when, during the concrete operational stage, the concept of conservation will emerge. For some children the concept of conservation is present by age eight to twelve, for some not until age fifteen or sixteen.[126,127] One of the major concerns of developmentalists is that many adolescents never move from the concrete operational level to the stage of formal operational thinking with the associated capacity to understand abstract concepts, such as those in science. Again, achievement of these developmental stages appears vulnerable to environmental and educational limitations. There is current interest in the possibility that learning to think in problem-solving terms and achieving the ability to deal with abstract ideas seem to enhance the kinds of choices one makes in work, family relationships, and civic responsibilities.

All this, in turn, seems related to feelings of adequacy and competence.[20,135]

Tertiary Prevention

Early and effective treatment of psychiatric disorders in children and adolescents is rarely possible. Mental health and social service agencies are small and seldom staffed with enough competent professionals or paraprofessionals, especially those trained to work with children, adolescents, and families. Many native paraprofessionals can do an excellent job when well trained, but they become ineffective when overwhelmed by a huge caseload.[10,11,15,54]

The available data about the use of mental health and health outpatient services and the rare inpatient facilities indicate a much higher utilization rate by American Indians than by comparable non-Indian populations. Many health supportive activities that have been effective in reducing neonatal morbidity and many diseases may have been important influences in acquainting Indians with medical personnel; medical facilities are viewed as helpful.

In most tribes, it is the medicine men who are the important healers. For some years there has been an effort to help these medicine men learn to understand and use psychiatric thinking about serious mental illness and modern treatment methods. It was hoped that such efforts would enlist an important influence in the management of mental illness. Referrals from medicine men are also more meaningful to Indian patients and to some extent reduce their suspicions of the Anglo mental health professionals. Such referrals also indicate that the medicine at the mental health clinic is potent. This kind of collaboration between medicine men and women on the one hand and mental health professionals and paraprofessionals on the other has been very important in a number of communities.[3,14,71,72]

The Indian community represents a multiplicity of cultures, each with different values, its own systems of healing, and its own cultural definitions of illness, especially mental illness.[134] One of the major issues in mental health treatment is the application of knowledge gained from an Anglo culture to so varied an array of societies.

An understanding of the traditions and values of each tribe makes it easier to begin a psychotherapeutic process. Given such an understanding, it becomes possible to use traditional values to reinforce both the therapeutic process and the therapeutic relationship. Where a good collaboration with the medicine men and women exists, consultation may be especially important for adolescents who question their traditions or are disturbed by a lack of traditional guidelines for living; they become aware of the respect for the medicine man and the collaboration that can occur on the adolescents' behalf.

On most reservations there are very few mental health professionals or paraprofessionals trained to work with children and adolescents. This creates serious problems. For example, for most mental health workers without special training it is very difficult to deal with an adolescent whose family, teachers, or peers express concern about suicidal intent.[44,110,139,145]

To date, tertiary prevention has not been very effective on American Indian reservations because the existing services are usually minuscule compared to the need. In some tribes there is also a reluctance to utilize existing alcohol treatment or mental health facilities because such use exposes the problems within the family or clan to others in the tribe. It is, therefore, not encouraged by responsible elders.

The Use of Mental Health Consultation in Various Indian Communities

Mental health consultation to a variety of Indian community agencies has been effective. It has been especially helpful with schools, courts, and welfare departments. The consultation process often permits broad education of agency staff as well as problem solving with the individual staff member about students, clients, probationers, or parents. The case consultation method frequently enhances the workers' capacity to deal with troubled children, youth, and parents. By working with the administration of an agency, policy changes can be brought about that encourage agency workers to be more involved with mental health problems. Such consultation may have widespread effects. In many American Indian communities, mental health consultation has been a major factor contributing to an increase in the number of agency workers who are then able to carry out mental health activities in their normal work setting.

Whenever possible, the effort is to influence agency and, sometimes, tribal policy in the direction of enacting or approving programs to enhance the mental health of children, adolescents, and families. Such consultation efforts by the Indian Children's Program of the Indian Health Service in Albuquerque has permitted a small professional staff to work effectively in a large region with many tribes and pueblos. [16,17,64,78]

Summary and Conclusions

At all levels, prevention needs to be designed to deal with the effect of dislocation, impotence, and dependence of many of the American Indian tribes and Native Alaskan communities and tribes. The descriptions of primary and secondary prevention of psychiatric disorder in Indian children and adolescents in many ways offer an account of intervention strategies that strive to accomplish this. The interference with traditional ways of living has resulted in disorganization and fragmentation of the extended family and clan and has obstructed communication of tribal heritage and traditions to younger generations. Many of the pilot projects cited are in themselves important in enhancing self-regard and the capacity to parent. However, unless these programs occur with tribal sanction, involve Indian personnel as project workers, and seek to enhance the teaching and continuity of tradition, they tend to be short-lived.

A major educational effort is required to focus tribal attention on the many ubiquitous mental health problems that cry out for intervention. Among these are the prevalent and severe alcoholism in adults; the violence, suicide, depression, and substance abuse in children and adolescents; the failure in attachment and bonding in infants and children; and child neglect and abuse. Tribes and communities need also to be educated about the number of pilot programs that have been effective in dealing with these critical problems.

It is important that there be a meaningful change in the way teaching and learning occur in schools and in the community, as well as in boarding schools. The basic thrust must be toward a new emphasis on problem-solving learning in school. The most effective curriculum has been one that is problem oriented, stresses traditional values and history, and uses native languages in teaching and learning.

There is a clear opportunity to do research on the epidemological factors that increase the prevalence of psychiatric disorder in some tribes and keeps it at a low rate in other tribes. There is also need for a major investment in prevention of disorders as well as an increase in treatment personnel and facilities.

Recently the Indian Health Services have made a commitment to increase prevention efforts. Currently their efforts are focused on some of the early developmental problems. An increased use of mental health consultation would enhance the treatment and prevention capabilities of a number of tribes that are beginning to initiate more traditional ways of living. The return to more traditional ways of relating to the extended family and clan, which are so important to the tribal heritage, and increased concern with traditional religion are not easily conceptualized or made operational. Some of the more disorganized tribes may not be able to move in this direction. It is also clear that a number of tribes are making a serious effort to return to more traditional ways.

An increase in employment for adolescents and adults in order to enhance mental health and a sense of self-worth is a major goal of intervention. That goal is now being implemented with some effectiveness by several tribes individually and by consortia of tribes. The examples provided by these tribes may encourage other tribes to attempt to increase employment.

The serious concern of many tribes about vulnerable adolescent females who become pregnant has been effectively addressed by means of some of the pilot projects discussed briefly in this chapter.

Out of the turmoil and problems described in many American Indian and Alaska Native tribes and communities, there is emerging a variety of important primary and secondary prevention efforts. In time, these will become models for other Indian and Alaska Native communities who have yet to come to grips with the serious problems on their reservations.

These examples, as well as the enhancement of mental health treatment services and mental health consultation, may act as a continuing means of education and stimulus to all Indian people troubled by mental health problems.

REFERENCES

1. ABLON, J., METCALF, A., and MILLER, D. "An Overview of Mental Health Problems of Indian Children," Report to the Joint Commission of the Mental Health of Children, Washington, D.C., 1967.
2. AMERICAN ACADEMY OF CHILD PSYCHIATRY. Group leader's workshop notes, "Strengthening the American Indian and Alaska Native Family," Washington, D.C.: American Academy of Child Psychiatry, 1979.
3. ATTNEAVE, C. "Medicine Men and Psychiatrists in the Indian Health Service," *Psychiatric Annals,* 4 (1974):49–55.

4. ———. "The American Indian Child," in J. D. Noshpitz, ed., *Basic Handbook of Child Psychiatry,* vol. 1. New York: Basic Books, 1979, pp. 239–248.

5. BEBBINGTON, P. E. "The Epidemiology of Depressive Disorder," *Culture, Medicine and Psychiatry,* 2 (1978):297–341.

6. BEISER, M. "Etiology of Mental Disorders: Socio-cultural Aspects," in B. Wolman, ed., *Manual of Child Psychopathology.* New York: McGraw-Hill, 1972, pp. 150–188.

7. ———. "A Hazard to Mental Health: Indian Boarding Schools" (editorial), *American Journal of Psychiatry,* 131 (1974):305–306.

8. ———. "Mental Health of American Indian and Alaska Native Children: Some Epidemiological Perspectives," *White Cloud Journal,* 2 (1981):37–47.

9. ———. "Evaluating Primary Prevention Programs: Models and Measures," in S. M. Manson, ed., *New Directions in Prevention Among American Indian and Alaska Native Communities.* Portland, Ore.: Oregon Health Sciences University, 1982, pp. 301–321.

10. BEISER, M., and ATTNEAVE, C. L. "Mental Health Services for American Indians: Neither Feast nor Famine," *White Cloud Journal,* 1 (1978):3–10.

11. ———. "Mental Disorders Among Native American Children: Rates and Risk Periods for Entering Treatment," *American Journal of Psychiatry,* 139 (1982):193–198.

12. BEISER, M., and McSHANE, D. "Epidemiology of Mental Disorder in American Indian Children," NIMH Grant Number 1 RO1 MH36678-01, Washington, D.C.: National Institute of Mental Health. 1981.

13. BENJAMIN, E. F. "An Investigation of the Self Concept of Alaskan Eskimo Adolescents in Four Different Secondary School Environments" (Ph.D. diss., Oregon University), 1973. (*Dissertation Abstracts International,* 34 [1973]:2377).

14. BERGMAN, R. L. "A School for Medicine Men," *American Journal of Psychiatry,* 130 (1973):663–666.

15. ———. "Paraprofessionals in Indian Mental Health Programs," *Psychiatric Annals,* 4 (1974):76–84.

16. BERLIN, I. N. "Consultation and Special Education," in I. Philips, ed., *Prevention and Treatment of Mental Retardation.* New York: Basic Books, 1966, pp. 279–293.

17. ———. "Mental Health Consultation to Child-Serving Agencies as Therapeutic Intervention," in J. D. Noshpitz, ed., *Basic Handbook of Child Psychiatry,* vol. 3. New York: Basic Books, 1979, pp. 353–364.

18. ———. "Anglo Adoption of Native-Americans: Repercussions in Adolescence," *Journal of the American Academy of Child Psychiatry,* 17 (1978):387–388.

19. ———. "Opportunities in Adolescence to Rectify Development Failures," in S. C. Feinstein, et al., eds., *Adolescent Psychiatry,* vol. 8. Chicago: University of Chicago Press, 1980, pp. 231–243.

20. ———. *Problem Solving and Creativity: A Family School Collaboration.* Albuquerque, N.M.: University of New Mexico Press, 1981.

21. ———. "Prevention of Emotional Problems Among Native-American Children: Overview of Developmental Issues," *Journal of Preventive Psychiatry,* 1 (1982):319–330.

22. ———. "Suicide Among American Indian Adolescents," in N. Gale, ed., *Linkages.* Washington, D.C.: National American Indian Court Judges Association, 1984, pp. 1–8.

23. BERLIN, R., and BERLIN, I. N. "Parent's Advocate Role in Education as Primary Prevention," in I. N. Berlin, ed., *Advocacy for Child Mental Health.* New York: Brunner/Mazel, 1975, pp. 145–157.

24. BLANCHARD, E. "The Question of Best Interest," in *The Destruction of American Indian Families.* New York: Association of American Indian Affairs, 1977, pp. 31–43.

25. BLOCK, J. *Mastery Learning: Theory and Practice.* New York: Holt Rinehart & Winston, 1971.

26. BLOS, P. "Second Individuation Process of Adolescence," *Psychoanalytic Study of the Child,* 22 (1967):162–186.

27. BRYDE, J. F. *The Indian Student: A Study of Scholastic Failure and Personality Conflict.* Vermillion, S. D.: University of South Dakota Press, 1970.

28. CALDWELL, B. M. "What Does Research Tell Us About Day Care?" *Children Today,* 1 (1972):1–4.

29. CALDWELL, B. M., and RICHMOND, J. B. "The Children's Center in Syracuse, N.Y.," in L. L. Dittman, ed., *Early Child Care: The New Perspective.* New York: Atherton Press, 1968, pp. 162–178.

30. CLEVENGER, J. "Native Americans," in A. Gaw, ed., *Cross-Cultural Psychiatry.* Littleton, Mass.: John Wright, 1982, pp. 149–158.

31. CLIFTON, R. A. "Self-concept and Attitudes: A Comparison of Canadian Indian and Non-Indian Students," *Canadian Review of Sociology and Anthropology,* 12 (1975):577–584.

32. COCHE, E., and DOUGLAS, A. "Therapeutic Effects of Problem Solving Training and Play Reading Groups," *Journals of Clinical Psychology,* 33 (1977):820–827.

33. COCKERHAM, W. C. "Drinking Attitudes and Practices among Wind River Reservation Indian Youth," *Quarterly Journal of Studies on Alcohol,* 36 (1975):321–326.

34. ———. "Patterns of Alcohol and Multiple Drug Use among Rural White and American Indian Adolescents," *International Journal of the Addictions,* 12 (1977):271–285.

35. CONRAD, R. D., and KAHN, M. "An Epidemiological Study of Suicide among the Papago Indians," *American Journal of Psychiatry,* 131 (1974):69–72.

36. DELK, J. L., et al. "Drop-outs from an American Indian Reservation School: A Possible Prevention Program," *Journal of Community Psychology,* 2 (1974):15–17.

37. DENNIS, W. *The Hopi Child.* New York: John Wiley & Sons, 1965.

38. DEVEREUX, G. *Mohave Ethno-Psychiatry.* Washington, D.C.: Smithsonian Institution Press, 1961.

39. DINGES, N. "Preventive Intervention: Isolated Navajo Families," Final report to the Juvenile Problems Division. Washington, D.C.: National Institute of Mental Health, 1976.

40. ———. "Mental Health Promotion with Navajo Families," in S. M. Manson, ed., *New Directions in Prevention among American Indian and Alaska Native Communities.* Portland, Ore.: Oregon Health Sciences University, 1982, pp. 119–143.

41. DINGES, N. G., and HOLLENBECK, A. R. "The Effect of Instructional Set on the Self-Esteem of Navajo Children," *Journal of Social Psychology,* 104 (1978):9–13.

42. DINGES, N. G., TRIMBLE, J. E., and HOLLENBECK, A. R. "American Indian Adolescent Socialization: A Review of the Literature," *Journal of Adolescence,* 2 (1979):259–296.

43. DINGES, N., YAZZIE, M., and TOLLEFSON, G. "Developmental Intervention for Navajo Family Mental Health," *Journal of Personnel and Guidance Psychology: Special Issue,* 52 (1974):390–395.

44. DINGES, N. G., et al. "The Social Ecology of Counseling and Psychotherapy with American Indians and Alaskan Natives," in A. Marsella and P. Pedersen, eds., *Cross-Cultural Counseling and Psychotherapy: Foundations, Evaluations, Cultural Considerations.* New York: Pergamon Press, 1981, pp. 50–71.

45. DIZMANG, L. J., et al. "Adolescent Suicide at an Indian

Reservation," *American Journal of Orthopsychiatry,* 44 (1974):43–49.

46. DLUGOKINSKI, E., and KRAMER, L. "A System of Neglect: Indian Boarding Schools," *American Journal of Psychiatry,* 131 (1974):670–673.

47. DREYER, P. H. "The Meaning and Validity of the 'Phenomenal Self' for American Indian Students," *National Study of American Indian Education Research Reports,* 1 (1970):1–27.

48. ELKIND, D. "Recent Research in Cognitive Development in Adolescence," in S. E. Drogastin and C. H. Elder, eds., *Adolescence in the Life Cycle.* New York: Halstead, 1975, pp. 49–62.

49. ERIKSON, E. H. "Observations on Sioux Education," *Journal of Psychology,* 7 (1939):101–156.

50. ———. *Childhood and Society,* 2nd ed. New York: W. W. Norton, 1963.

51. FISCHLER, R. "Protecting American Indian Children," *Social Work,* 25 (1980):341–349.

52. FOULKS, E. F., and KATZ, S. "The Mental Health of Alaskan Natives," *Acta Psychiatrica Scandinavica,* 49 (1973):91–96.

53. FREDERICK, C. "Suicide, Homicide, and Alcoholism among American Indians," DHEW Pub. No. ADM 76-42. Washington, D.C.: U.S. Government Printing Office, 1975.

54. FRITZ, W., and D'ARCY, C. "Comparisons: Indian and Non-Indian Use of Psychiatric Services," *Canadian Journal of Psychiatry,* 27 (1982):194–203.

55. FUCHS, E., and HAVINGHURST, R. J. "The Self Esteem of American Indian Youth: The Personal Social Adjustment of American Indian Youth," National Study of American Indian Series, Final Report. Chicago: University of Chicago, 1970.

56. GELLES, R. J. "Violence Toward Children in the United States," *American Journal of Orthopsychiatry,* 48 (1978):580–592.

57. GOLDSTEIN, G. S. "The Model Dormitory," *Psychiatric Annals,* 4 (1974):85–92.

58. GOLDSTEIN, J., FREUD, A., and SOLNIT, A. *Beyond the Best Interests of the Child.* New York: Free Press, 1973.

59. ———. *Before the Best Interests of the Child.* New York: Free Press, 1979.

60. GOLDSTEIN, G. S., et al. "Drug Use among Native American Young Adults," *International Journal of the Addictions,* 4 (1979):855–860.

61. "A Good Day to Live for One Million Indians," *Report of Special Populations Subpanel on Mental Health of American Indians and Alaska Natives.* Washington, D.C.: U.S. Dept. of Health, Education and Welfare, Public Health Service, Indian Health Service, 1978, pp. 1–69.

62. GOODLUCK, C. T., and ECKSTEIN, F. "American Indian Adoption Program: An Ethnic Approach to Child Welfare," *White Cloud Journal,* 1 (1978):4–7.

63. GREEN, B. E., SACK, W. H., and PAMBRUN, A. "A Review of Child Psychiatric Epidemiology with Special Reference to American Indian and Alaska Native Children," *White Cloud Journal,* 2 (1981):23–36.

64. GREENE, B. E. "Child Psychiatric Consultation to an Indian Tribal Court," in S. M. Manson, ed., *New Directions in Prevention among American Indian and Alaska Native Communities.* Portland, Ore.: Oregon Health Sciences University, 1982, pp. 253–263.

65. HALLOWELL, A. I. "Ojibway Personality and Acculturation," in P. Bohanon and F. Plog, eds., *Beyond the Frontier.* New York: National History Press, 1967, pp. 227–237.

66. HAMMERSCHLAG, C., ALDERFER, C. P., and BERG, D.

"Indian Education: A Human Systems Analysis," *American Journal of Psychiatry,* 130 (1973):1098–1102.

67. HARVEY, E. B., GAZAY, L., and SAMUELS, B. "Utilization of a Psychiatric-Social Work Team in an Alaskan Native Secondary Boarding School," *Journal of Child Psychiatry,* 15 (1976):558–574.

68. HOLLISTER, W. G. "Concept of Stress in Education: A Challenge to Curriculum Development," in E. M. Bower and W. G. Hollister, eds., *Behavioral Science Frontiers in Education.* New York: John Wiley & Sons, 1967, pp. 128–142.

69. ISHISAKA, H. "American Indians in Foster Care: Cultural Factors and Separation," *Child Welfare,* 57 (1978):-299–308.

70. JENSEN, G. F., STAUSS, H. H., and HARRIS, V. W. "Crime, Delinquency, and the American Indian," *Human Organization,* 36 (1977):252–257.

71. JILEK, W. "From Crazy Witchdoctor to Auxiliary Psychotherapist: The Changing Image of the Medicine Man," *Psychiatrica Clinica,* 4 (1971):200–220.

72. ———. *Indian Healing.* Blaine, Wash.: Hancock House Publishers, 1982.

73. JOHNSON, D. L., and JOHNSON, C. A. "Totally Discouraged: A Depressive Syndrome of the Dakota Sioux," *Transcultural Psychiatric Research,* 1 (1965):141–143.

74. JONES, D. M. "Child Welfare Problems in an Alaskan Native Village," *Social Service Review,* 43 (1969):297–309.

75. KAUFMAN, A. "Gasoline Sniffing among Children in a Pueblo Indian Village," *Pediatrics,* 51 (1973):1060–1064.

76. KELSO, D. R., and ATTNEAVE, C. L. *Bibliography of North American Indian Mental Health.* Westport, Conn.: Greenwood Press, 1981.

77. KEMPE, C. H., and SILVER, H. D. "The Problem of Parental Criminal Neglect and Severe Physical Abuse of Children," *American Journal of Diseases of Children,* 98 (1959):-528.

78. KINZIE, J. D., SHORE, J. H., and PATTISON, E. M. "Anatomy of Psychiatric Consultation to Rural Indians," *Community of Mental Health Journal,* 8 (1972):196–207.

79. KLEINFELD, J. "Getting It Together at Adolescence: Case Studies of Positive Socializing Environments for Eskimo Youth," in S. M. Manson, ed., *New Directions in Prevention among American Indian and Alaska Native Communities.* Portland, Ore.: Oregon Health Sciences University, 1982, pp. 341–364.

80. KLEINFELD, J., and BLOOM, J. "Boarding Schools: Effects on the Mental Health of Eskimo Adolescents," *American Journal of Psychiatry,* 134 (1977):411–417.

81. KLEINFELD, J. S., and BUFFLER, P. A. "Sociocultural Stress and the American Native in Alaska: An Analysis of Changing Patterns of Psychiatric Illness and Alcohol Abuse among Alaska Natives," *Culture, Medicine and Psychiatry,* 3 (1979):111–151.

82. KOHLER, M. "The Rights of Children: An Unexplored Constituency," *Social Policy,* 1 (1971):36–43.

83. KRAUSE, R. F., and BUFFLER, P. A. "Socioculture Stress and the American Native in Alaska: An Analysis of Changing Patterns of Psychiatric Illness and Alcohol Abuse among Alaska Natives," *Culture, Medicine and Psychiatry,* 3 (1979):111–151.

84. KRUSH, T. P., and BJORK, J. "Mental Health Factors in an Indian Boarding School," *Mental Hygiene,* 49 (1965): 94–103.

85. KRUSH, T. P., BJORK, J., and SINDELL, P. "Some Thoughts on the Formulation of Personality Disorder: Study of an Indian Boarding School Population," *Hearings Before the Special Subcommittee on Indian Education,* Ninetieth

Congress, vol. 5. Washington, D.C.: U.S. Government Printing Office, 1969, pp. 2218–2241.

86. LEFLEY, H. P. "Effects of an Indian Culture Program and Familial Correlates of Self Concept among Miccosukee and Seminole Children" (Ph.D. diss., University of Miami, 1973), (*Dissertation Abstracts International,* 34 [1973]:414–415.

87. ———. "Effects of a Cultural Heritage Program on the Self-Concept of Miccosukee Indian Children," *Journal of Educational Research,* 67 (1974):462–466.

88. ———. "Acculturation, Child-Rearing, and Self-Esteem in Two North American Indian Tribes," *Ethos,* 4 (1976):385–401.

89. ———. "Self-Perception and Primary Prevention for American Indians," in S. M. Manson, ed., *New Directions in Prevention among American Indian and Alaska Native Communities.* Portland, Ore.: Oregon Health Science University, 1982, pp. 65–90.

90. LEIGHTON, A. "Cosmos and the Gallup City Dump," in B. H. Kaplan, ed., *Psychiatric Disorder and the Urban Environment.* New York: Behavioral Publications, 1971, pp. 293–321.

91. LEIGHTON, D., and KLUCKHOHN, C. *Children of the People.* Cambridge, Mass.: Harvard University Press, 1948.

92. LEON, R. L. "Some Implications for a Preventive Program for American Indians," *American Journal of Psychiatry,* 125 (1968):128–132.

93. LEVY, J. E. "Navajo Suicide," *Human Organization,* 24 (1965):308–318.

94. LEVY, J. E., and KUNITZ, S. J. "Indian Reservations, Anomie, and Social Pathologies," *Southwestern Journal of Anthropology,* 27 (1971):97–128.

95. LEVY, J. E., et al. "Hopi Deviance in Historical and Epidemiological Perspective," Unpublished manuscript, 1982.

96. McDERMOTT, J. F. "Social Class and Mental Illness in Children: The Diagnosis of Organicity and Mental Retardation," *Journal of American Child Psychiatry,* 6 (1967):309–320.

97. McSHANE, D. "A Review of Scores of American Indian Children on the Wechsler Intelligence Scale," *White Cloud Journal,* 1 (1980):3–10.

98. ———. "Otitis Media and American Indians: Prevalence, Etiology, Psychoeducational Consequences, Prevention and Intervention," in S. M. Manson, ed., *New Directions in Prevention among American Indian and Alaska Native Communities.* Portland, Ore.: Oregon Health Sciences University, 1982, pp. 265–294.

99. MANSON, S. M., ed. *New Directions in Prevention among American Indian and Alaska Native Communities,* Portland, Ore.: Oregon Health Sciences University, 1982.

100. MANSON, S. M., and SHORE, J. H. "Psychiatric Epidemiological Research among American Indians and Alaska Natives: Some Methodological Issues," *White Cloud Journal,* 2 (1981):48–56.

101. MANSON, S. M., SHORE, J. H., and BLOOM, J. D. "The Depressive Experience in American Indian Communities: A Challenge for Psychiatric Theory and Diagnosis," in B. Good and A. Kleinman, eds., *Culture and Depression: Toward an Anthropology of Affects and Affective Disorder.* Berkeley: University of California Press, 1985, pp. 331–368.

102. MARSELLA, A., KINZIE, J. D., and GORDON, P. "Ethnic Variations in the Expression of Depression," *Journal of Cross-Cultural Psychology,* 4 (1973):435–458.

103. MARTIG, R., and DeBLASSIE, R. "Self Concept Comparisons of Anglo and Indian Children," *Journal of American Indian Education,* 12 (1973):9–16.

104. MAY, P. A. "Arrests, Alcohol and Alcohol Legalization among an American Indian Tribe," *Plains Anthropologist,* 20 (1975)129–134.

105. ———. "Contemporary Crime and the American Indian: A Survey and Analysis of the Literature," *Plains Anthropologist,* 27 (1982):225–238.

106. MEDICINE, B. "The Changing Dakota Family and the Stresses Therein," *Pine Ridge Research Bulletin* (Indian Health Service), 3 (1969):18–31.

107. ———. "Native American Resistance to Integration: Contemporary Confrontations and Religious Revitalization," *Plains Anthropologist,* 26 (1981):277–286.

108. MESTETH, L. "Gas and Glue Sniffing among the School Age Population," *Pine Ridge Research Bulletin* (Indian Health Service), 4 (1968):36–40.

109. MICKELSON, N. L., and GALLOWAY, C. G. "Verbal Concepts of Indian and Non-Indian School Beginners," *Journal of Educational Psychology,* 67 (1973):55–56.

110. MILLER, D. "Treatment of the Seriously Disturbed Adolescent," in S. C. Feinstein, et al., eds., *Adolescent Psychiatry,* vol. 8. Chicago: University of Chicago Press, 1980, pp. 469–481.

111. MILLER, M. "Suicides on a Southwestern American Indian Reservation," *White Cloud Journal,* 1 (1979):14–18.

112. MILLER, S., and SCHOENFIELD, L. S. "Suicide Attempt Patterns among the Navajo Indians," *International Journal of Social Psychiatry,* 17 (1971):189–193.

113. MILLER, W. T. "A Special Problem in Primary Prevention: The Family that Cares About Their Children but Is Not Able to Rear Them," *Journal of Clinical Child Psychology,* 10 (1981):38–41.

114. MINDELL, C., and GURWITT, A. "The Placement of American Indian Children: The Need for Change," in S. Unger, ed., *The Destruction of the American Indian Family.* New York: Association on American Indian Affairs, 1977, pp. 61–66.

115. MINDELL, C., and MAYNARD, E. "Ambivalence Towards Education among Indian High School Students," *Pine Ridge Research Bulletin* (Indian Health Service), 1 (1967):26–31.

116. MINDELL, C., and STUART, P. "Suicide and Self-Destructive Behavior in the Oglala Sioux: Some Clinical Aspects and Community Approaches," *Pine Ridge Research Bulletin* (Indian Health Service), 1 (1968):14–23.

117. MOHATT, G., and BLUE, A. W. "Primary Prevention as It Relates to Traditionality and Empirical Measures of Social Deviance," in S. M. Manson, ed., *New Directions in Prevention among American Indian and Alaska Native Communities.* Portland, Ore.: Oregon Health Sciences University, 1982, pp. 91–118.

118. ———. "Relationships Between an Empirical Measure of Traditionality and Social Deviance," in S. M. Manson, ed., *New Directions in Prevention among American Indian and Alaska Native Communities.* Portland, Ore.: Oregon Health Sciences University, 1982, pp. 91–115.

119. NELSON, L. G., et al. "Screening for Emotionally Disturbed Students in an Indian Boarding School: Experience with the Cornell Medical Index Health Questionnaire," *American Journal of Psychiatry,* 120 (1964):1155–1159.

120. NURGE, E. *The Modern Sioux: Social Systems and Reservation Culture.* Lincoln, Neb.: University of Nebraska Press, 1970.

121. OAKLAND, L., and KANE, R. L. "The Working Mother and Child Neglect on the Navajo Reservation," *Pediatrics,* 51 (1973):5.

122. OETTING, E. R., and GOLDSTEIN, G. S. "Drug Use

among American Indian Adolescents," Final Report, National Institute of Drug Abuse, Rockville, Maryland, 1975.

123. ———. "Drug Abuse among Indian Adolescents," Report to the National Institute of Drug Abuse, Grant no. 2 R01 DA0154. Fort Collins, Colo.: Colorado State University, 1978.

124. OGDEN, M., SPECTOR, M. I., and HILL, C. A. "Suicides and Homicides among Indians," *Public Health Reports,* 35 (1970):75–80.

125. PETERS, R. "Suicide in American Indian and Alaska Native Tradition," *White Cloud Journal,* 2 (1981):9–20.

126. PHILIPS, S. "Participant Structures and Communicative Competence: Warm Springs Children in Community and Classroom," in C. Cazden, V. John, and D. Hymes, eds., *Functions of Language in the Classroom.* New York: Columbia University Press, 1972, pp. 370–394.

127. PIAGET, J., and INHELDER, B. *The Psychology of the Child.* New York: Basic Books, 1969.

128. PLOWDEN REPORT. Central Advisory Council for Education (England). *Children and Their Primary Schools,* vol. 1. London: Her Majesty's Stationery Office, 1966.

129. RED HORSE, J. "Family Structure and Value Orientation in American Indians," *Social Casework,* 61 (1980):462–467.

130. ———. "American Indian Community Mental Health: A Primary Prevention Strategy," in S. M. Manson, ed., *New Directions in Prevention among American Indian and Alaska Native Communities.* Portland, Ore.: Oregon Health Sciences University, 1982, pp. 217–232.

131. REPORT OF THE THIRD NATIONAL INDIAN CHILD CONFERENCE. "The Indian Family—Foundations for the Future." Albuquerque, N.M.: Dept. of Health and Human Services, Indian Health Service, Office of Mental Health Programs, 1981.

132. ROBBINS, M. "Project Nak-nu-we-sha: A Preventive Intervention in Child Abuse and Neglect among a Pacific Northwest Indian Community," in S. M. Manson, ed., *New Directions in Prevention among American Indians and Alaska Native Communities.* Portland, Ore.: Oregon Health Sciences University, 1982, pp. 233–248.

133. ROSENTHAL, B. G. "Development of Self Identification in Relation to Attitudes Toward the Self in Chippewa Indians," *Genetic Psychology Monographs,* 90 (1974):43–143.

134. SANUA, V. "Familial and Sociocultural Antecedents of Psychopathology," in H. Triandis and J. Draguns, eds., *Handbook of Cross-Cultural Psychology: Psychopathology,* vol. 6. Boston: Allyn & Bacon, 1980, pp. 175–236.

135. SARANSON, I. G., and GANZER, V. J. *Modeling: An Approach to the Rehabilitation of Juvenile Offenders.* Washington, D.C.: U.S. Dept. of Health, Education and Welfare, Social Rehabilitation Service, 1971.

136. SHORE, J. H. "American Indian Suicide: Fact and Fantasy," *Psychiatry,* 38 (1975):86–91.

137. ———. "Preventive Mental Health Programs for American Indian Youth—Success and Failure," in D. V. Siva Sankar, ed., *Mental Health in Children.* New York: PJD Publications, 1975, pp. 61–71.

138. ———. "The Destruction of Indian Families—Beyond the Best Interests of Indian Children," *White Cloud Journal,* 1 (1978):13–16.

139. SHORE, J. H., and KEEPERS, G. "Examples of Evaluation Research in Delivering Preventive Mental Health Services to Indian Youth," in S. Manson, ed., *New Directions in Prevention among American Indian and Alaska Native Communities.* Portland, Ore.: Oregon Health Sciences University, 1982, pp. 325–337.

140. SHORE, J. H., and MANSON, S. M. "Cross-Cultural Studies of Depression among American Indians and Alaska Natives," *White Cloud Journal,* 2 (1981):5–12.

141. ———. "Overview: American Indian Psychiatric and Social Problems," *Transcultural Psychiatric Research Review,* 20 (1983):159–180.

142. SHORE, J. H., and NICHOLLS, W. M. "Indian Children and Tribal Group Homes: New Interpretation of the Whipper Man," *American Journal of Psychiatry,* 132 (1975):454–456.

143. SHORE, J. H., et al. "Psychiatric Epidemiology of an Indian Village," *Psychiatry,* 36 (1973):70–81.

144. SHORE, J. H., et al. "A Suicide Prevention Center on an Indian Reservation," *American Journal of Psychiatry,* 128 (1972):76–81.

145. SHORE, J. H., et al. "Towards an Understanding of American Indian Concepts of Mental Health: Some Reflections and Directions," in A. Marsella and P. Pederson, eds., *Intercultural Applications of Counseling and Therapies.* Beverly Hills, Calif.: Sage Publications, forthcoming.

146. SURE, M., SPIVAK, G., and JAEGER, M. "Problem Solving Thinking and Adjustment among Disadvantaged Preschool Children," *Child Development,* 4 (1971):1791–1803.

147. STRATTON, R., ZEINER, A., and PAREDES, A. "Tribal Affiliations and Prevalance of Alcohol Problems," *Journal of Studies on Alcohol,* 39 (1978):1166–1177.

148. SWANSON, D. W., BRATUDE, A. P., and BROWN, E. M. "Alcoholism in a Population of Indian Children," *Diseases of the Nervous System,* 32 (1971):834–842.

149. TEFFT, S. K. "Anomie, Values and Culture Change among Teen-Age Indians: An Exploration," *Sociology of Education,* 40 (1967):145–157.

150. TOEWS, J. "Adolescent Development Issues in Marital Therapy," in S. C. Feinstein, et al., eds., *Adolescent Psychiatry,* vol. 8. Chicago: University of Chicago Press, 1980, pp. 244–252.

151. TOWNSLEY, H. C., and GOLDSTEIN, G. S. "One View of the Etiology of Depression in the American Indian," *Public Health Report,* 92 (1977):458–461.

152. TRIMBLE, J. E. "Value Differentials and Their Importance in Counseling American Indians," in P. Pedersen, et al., eds., *Counseling Across Cultures,* 2nd ed. Honolulu: University Press of Hawaii, 1981, pp. 203–226.

153. ———. "American Indian Mental Health and the Role of Training for Prevention," in S. M. Manson, ed., *New Directions in Prevention among American Indian and Alaska Native Communities.* Portland, Ore.: Oregon Health Sciences University, 1982, pp. 147–171.

154. TRIMBLE, J. E., and MEDICINE, B. "Development of Theoretical Models and Levels of Interpretation in Mental Health," in J. Westermeyer, ed., *Anthropology and Mental Health.* The Hague: Mouton, 1976, pp. 161–200.

155. UNGER, S. *The Destruction of American Indian Families.* New York: Association of American Indian Affairs, 1977.

156. WESTERMEYER, J., WALKER, D., and BENTON, E. "A Review of Some Methods for Investigating Substance Abuse Epidemiology among American Indians and Alaska Natives," *White Cloud Journal,* 2 (1981):13–21.

SECTION VII

Impact of Current Events

Lawrence A. Stone / Editor

Introduction

Lawrence A. Stone

The mission of this section of Volume V is to remind child mental health practioners that contemporary issues profoundly affect current and future generations of children; it is, therefore, necessary for child psychiatry to study, investigate, and comprehend these issues. The topics in this section were chosen because they represent an array of contemporary issues that are playing significant roles in life today. These examples do not create an exhaustive roster, but they add to the subjects presented in Volume IV, and soon even more will need to be added.

Today's world is one of rapid change in all areas. Not only the number but the rapidity of the changes affects the nature of both our lives and our environment. The proliferation of information and misinformation is enormous and in itself creates new problems of information overload. The basic social perceptions of the nature of life are likewise changing. The search for new definitions and dimensions of life are being pursued in radically new arenas—for example, genetic engineering, *in vitro* fertilization, and embryo transplants; has involved significant departures from previous standards—for example, legal definitions of life, death, and parenting; and has produced knowledge and questions about life on earth and in outer space not even dreamed of a few years ago. *Time* magazine's naming a computer as "Man of the Year" for 1982 seems to say something about current confusions and perceptions about the nature of "modern man." Child psychiatry must raise wide-ranging queries into the affect on the child's perceptions of the computer as an early object choice and an identification model.

There has been widespread parental emotional abandonment of children and societal destruction of childhood. As adults become increasingly enmeshed in the megatrends of their own world, the microneeds of the child and adolescent remain increasingly unserved. Likewise, when societal preoccupations become so entwined in "life is a war" or "life is a game," the result is a demanding defensiveness or a devouring narcissistic entitlement. In these states of mind, adults create pressures that obliterate the natural processes of childhood growth and development, either by forcing a premature maturation and thus producing a pseudoadult or by modeling primary process behavior and thus creating an infantile adult.

Many of the areas covered by the Current Events chapters have also been included in other sections. There are, however, so many more current events that no single volume could begin to cover all of their significance to the mental health of children, adolescents, and their families. Let us consider as examples some recent events and wonder about their meanings and their place in our spectrum of current events that affect the lives of children and the world in which they live.

An ordinary thirteen-year old girl, Samantha Smith, hitherto unknown outside her circle of family and friends, entranced the world with a letter that brought her an international visit with heads of state and that miraculously established her as a symbol of hope for universal peace. Shortly thereafter she died in a plane crash, a tragedy that startled the world, seized its attention, and produced an international affective response from young and old, individuals and governments. In quite a different saga of children in the contemporary world, a two-year-old child, taught and coached by her father, was apprehended by police for stealing a sizable amount of money from a public place.

Numerous statistical trends, representing aspects of life today need to be made known and efforts made to comprehend their meanings. There are significant increases in youth violence, suicide, substance abuse, homosexual exposure, and pregnancy, along with child abuse, including multiple forms of sexual abuse, and incest. There are more chronically mentally disabled young people trying unsuccessfully to make it in the world, and even more of them are having children. Family structures are being changed by adult life-style choices, or by death, trauma, divorce, and work, as well as by increasing numbers of child runaways, kidnappings, or child snatching.

The diversity of new life circumstances created by changes in customs and technologies is great. Another example illustrating a multiplicity of factors of contemporary living is the "marriage" of two lesbians, who first announced their love for each other on television. Thereafter, artificial insemination, using the sperm of one woman's brother, was carried out on the other, who gave birth to a daughter. The couple then separated and went through a legal battle to establish an out-of-court settlement of visitation rights.

Influences from the mass media are visible in the

increasing number of episodes involving children; Rambo Kids and young Ninja Warriors, Joy Ride Gangs, and Dragon Masters are acting out popularized roles involving violence, sexual assault, property destruction, and suicide. The National Coalition on Television Violence has been formed, following in the footsteps of a similiar organization dealing with movie violence and sexuality. In parallel with these efforts, the Parents Music Resource Center was established. It points out that the average teenager listens to rock music four to six hours daily and that rock music often has a dangerous negative theme, with lyrics advocating aggressive and hostile rebellion, abuse of drugs and alcohol, irresponsible sexuality, sexual perversions, violence, and suicide. Not only does this music have direct effects on young people, but many relatively uninvolved children are being pressured to choose sides for or against rock music as if they were experts on its effects.

Trends toward the "legalization of society" are taking form as the number of litigious issues grows. These in turn have produced forensic psychiatry as a new subspeciality, and the role of witness has become a growing part of the psychiatrist's professional work. Overall, commercialization has brought enormous concerns to all medical practitioners. These concerns manifest themselves in renewed interest in private practice rather than in academics or research and in a burgeoning of new information about marketing strategies and consumer issues. The proliferation of corporate medicine and for-profit hospital chains adds new complexities to the practice of modern medicine.

Thus, in reviewing current events, these and many other aspects of contemporary life challenge child psychiatry to investigate, to comprehend, and to strive to develop new methods for helping children progress in the direction of healthy growth and development within the Real world in which they live. The Current Events material in Volumes IV and V seeks to chronicle many of the phenomena that child psychiatry must address in its research and investigations and include in its overall body of knowledge to teach. It is imperative, however, that this body of knowledge be added to systematically and refined steadily. While this information must be used now, there must also be an appreciation of the scientific principles under which all medical knowledge must function. The accumulation of information, the formation of theories, the development of techniques of therapy, and the validation processes will take time. Solid scientific data will lag because of the rapidity of change and the magnitude of variables. Because of this, child psychiatry must thoughtfully incorporate information pertaining to current events into training programs, provide knowledgeable supervision, and develop consultants with specialized expertise in order to produce practitioners with the maximum available experience and skill to function effectively when encountering problems related to these areas, and to enhance their overall care of children, adolescents, and families.

69 / Children, Adolescents, and the Threat of Nuclear War

Frederick J. Stoddard and John E. Mack

Introduction

Our world has sprouted a weird conception of security and a warped sense of morality—weapons are sheltered like treasures, while children are exposed to incineration.

—Bertrand Russell

For many adults and children the continuous imminent threat of nuclear annihilation has been at the periphery of awareness. In recent years, however, there is increasing evidence that the nuclear threat is consciously on the minds of a large number of children and adolescents, that it is troubling to them. Young people are growing up in a situation in which they perceive that their lives and worlds may come to an end at any moment. Questions have been raised about the impact of this awareness on their psychological and moral development. President Reagan in 1982 expressed concern about "the effects the nuclear fear is having on our people," and he described upsetting letters "often full of terror" he was receiving from schoolchildren telling of their fear of a nuclear holocaust. [33] Social psychologist M. Brewster Smith noted how little research had been done on this subject, considering the "human centrality and scientific interest of the issue." [38] The subject of nuclear war has not before been included in any textbook of child psychiatry or psychology, due perhaps to the stressful and politically sensitive nature of the topic.[2]

Those who seek to understand the psychological impact of the nuclear threat on children and adolescents have the special difficulty of trying to bridge the gap between a phenomenon in the outside world and the inner life of young people. How many of the attitudes and feelings expressed by the young reflect the messages they are getting from their parents and other members of our culture? For example, we know that children and adolescents tend naturally to displace and project their internal conflicts onto external events. How do we identify this phenomenon when it happens? At the same time, as child psychiatrists, how do we distinguish fears that are realistic and appropriate in relation to an external threat from those anxieties that are the result of emotional conflict or other private distortions? It is evident that children are aware of large-scale irrationality or "psychopathology" emanating from society itself at a national or international level. But what is the impact of this perception on their emotional lives? Although we cannot answer these questions fully, we do begin to address each of them at different points in this chapter.

The subject of the impact of the nuclear threat on children and adolescents has begun to be studied from several perspectives. These include: (1) the experiences of young people who have endured actual atomic war, even though this would not be comparable to thermonuclear war with present arsenals; (2) semistructured or unstructured interviews and group discussions about nuclear war with children and adolescents; and (3) questionnaire studies of children and adolescents. All of this work has implications for child psychiatry, for new directions for child psychiatric research, and for possible public policy initiatives.

The possible psychological effects of actual nuclear war on children have received little attention despite some psychiatric literature on war and children and the known emotional devastation to children and families following the destruction of Hiroshima and Nagasaki by atomic bombs. Recent government documents project the physical and psychological trauma from thermonuclear war to be far more severe than what occurred in 1945. Although most child psychiatrists have little experience with the emotional effects of war or disasters on children, they have all taken part in consultation-liaison work on pediatric units. In wartime situations, the psychiatric care of children as well as other types of medical care is generally inadequate. It would be literally impossible were thermonuclear war actually to occur. Prevention is our only effective intervention, and it is important for child psychiatrists to contribute to this effort.

The larger question of the effect of the threat of nuclear war on children's and adolescent's thinking and psychological development is beginning to be studied.[14,15] To date, four types of investigation have been carried out: interviews with children and families, an interview study with adolescents, detailed questionnaires given to particular communities, and surveys given to a broad sample of young people. In addition, there are media accounts, films, and anecdotes reported by teachers and others. The public anxiety that surrounded the showing in 1983 of the television film *The Day After,* which graphically presented some effects of nuclear war, made clear how limited is our knowledge of the actual state of children's awareness of the nuclear threat and the impact of that awareness on their emotional lives.

Psychological Effects of Nuclear War on Children and Adolescents

This discussion of the psychological effects of nuclear war on children and adolescents is presented at a time when the prevailing scientific judgment is that following nuclear war, life might be extinguished due to freezing temperatures (the so-called nuclear winter), caused by dust and ash obscuring the sun.[13,44] If, however, life were temporarily sustained or a "limited" war should occur, some of the effects of devastating physical and emotional trauma to be described would probably take place. Psychiatric[41,42] and medical-surgical[1,11] care of even one or two children with acute burns or other severe trauma is so trying on the medical personnel, and so specialized and expensive, that most children who survived would receive little or no care. In addition, due to their relatively larger exposed body surface areas compared to that of adults, children would be more vulnerable to severe injury and high mortality.

The recollections that follow were written six years later by a girl who was in the sixth grade at the time of the Hiroshima bombing.[31] Her words illustrate more graphically than any statistics the psychological trauma she remembered:

Old Mrs. T., one of our neighbors, had come over to borrow our stone mortar. My mother was talking to her on the veranda, holding the top of the mortar. I was in the living room, leaning against a post and folding things out of paper for my three-year-old brother. I had roasted some beans for my brother that morning, and he was eating them one by one, out of a dish. He saw our neighbor sitting on the veranda, and went over to her, holding the dish out and saying, "Have some beans."

The bomb was dropped at that very moment. The paper sliding doors began to burn. I automatically thought, "Water!" and ran to the kitchen. That instant I was knocked down by the ceiling boards, plaster, pictures and things that came falling down. By the time I could get up, the fire had already been put out by the blast following the flash.

There were a few moments of ominous silence.

"Megumi-chan! Megumi-chan!" I came to my senses at the sound of my mother's voice and rushed into the air-raid shelter in the back garden. My mother, brother, and old Mrs. T., and the old lady from next door, and her daughter-in-law were there.

My mother put her arms around me and cried. I saw that my mother, brother, and old Mrs. T. had all been burned so badly on the right side of their bodies that the burns were blistered and raw looking. I was shocked and ran back into the house to get some medicine. This was the first time I saw how badly the house had been damaged.

Once we calmed down a little, we started worrying about the people in our family who had gone out to work. Yukiyo [one of my older sisters] had been injured, or not allowed to leave, or . . . worse . . . Fate chose the last. The life of a 19-year-old sister and that of the Credit Association Building ended together.

My father got home about ten that evening. I was so happy that I hugged him tight and cried. It was all I could do to say, "Father, Yukiyo hasn't . . ." He must have known already. There were tears running down his cheeks.

The morning of the seventh came . . . and I went out with my father to look for Yukiyo.

We thought that Yukiyo might have returned to the main office. We walked in, but I immediately staggered back, covering my eyes. Was this the meaning of "hell on earth"? There were burned bodies, eyes lifeless, all over the floor and on the counters. My father walked among them shouting, "Yukiyo, where are you? Is Yukiyo Sera here?" But we could not find her.

From Yokogawa we went on to the Tokaichi area. There were many bodies on the ground that had been burned black. There were the bodies of a soldier and his horse, and of a mother and her baby. But we didn't find any sign of Yukiyo.

We learned that the juice of cucumbers was good for burns, but at the time cucumbers were very difficult to get. The local doctors, whose homes and clinics had been destroyed, set up an emergency treatment center at the Ohshiba Primary School. But, of course, none of them knew the best way to treat the bomb sickness, when its true nature was unknown.

Whenever he heard an airplane, my three-year-old brother would run out into the street, his arms and legs all in bandages and shout, "Bring back my sister! Bring back my sister!"

October came and it was cooler in the mornings and evenings, but my brother got worse. He could not get out of bed after the tenth. We went to the country to look for more nutritious food for him, but all we could find were a few eggs. My little brother, who had cursed the airplanes that had taken the life of his loving sister, and who had feared even to look at the sky, died in my mother's arms on October 22, without having known even a single pleasant moment and without a chance to be treated by a doctor. The neighbors cremated him on the river bed. It was done simply and plainly. Just a little bit of white smoke rose up . . ." (pp. 255–260)*

Megumi Sera's story describes the death, shock, burns, radiation sickness, grief, and unavailability of resources following a nuclear explosion more poignantly than seems possible in other ways. Similar unforgettable images are expressed in stories and pictures

*Reprinted from "Children Who Survive Nuclear War, A View from the Burn Unit" in *Children of Hiroshima*, Ed. A. Osada, (Cambridge Ma.: Oelgeschlager, Gunn, and Hain Publishers, Inc. 1982), 255–260.

by many other children who survived.[22] There is no reason to think that many children would survive very long after a thermonuclear war, but there might be periods of minutes to weeks during which many children would experience ghastly physical and psychological suffering.

In both Hiroshima and Nagasaki children were relatively spared because of rapid massive evacuations. Even though most were evacuated, among all children enrolled in primary schools in Nagasaki the *acute mortality rate* was about 7.6 percent (1,653 children). Many died of severe burns and radiation sickness, while others survived and were known as A-bomb Orphans. Psychiatric care for the dying and injured was unavailable, but volunteers provided important support. It is noteworthy that children also offered critically important help to the adults as well as the reverse.[10] One can imagine the degree of societal collapse affecting everyone. One report described it well: ". . . communities disintegrated. The social services collapsed. Many people went mad or committed suicide. . . . Fear of malformed offspring often prevents marriages, and unusual susceptibility to disease and fatigue often threatens employment. . . ."[10]

A publication[30] from the U.S. Congress described the extent of possible thermal radiation and fires from a one-megaton bomb and from a 25-megaton bomb (1 megaton = 1 million tons of TNT). The Hiroshima bomb was only about 13,000 tons, with effects that were relatively trivial compared to those which would follow a nuclear war today. The United States and Soviet Union together have over 50,000 nuclear weapons, many of which are seventy or more times as destructive as those used on Japan. What sort of care would be necessary for the millions of children who might be injured, in shock, or orphaned in the event of nuclear war? Acute treatment would be needed to care for massive burns, dehydration, infection, grief reactions, depressions, delirium, brain damage, and severe posttraumatic disorders.[26,27,43] Such care would be impossible even in a minimally devastating situation; the medical personnel as well as children and other adults would be suffering equally. Yet this situation may occur unless steps are taken by government leaders of the nuclear powers to prevent it from happening.

The Psychological Effects of the Nuclear Threat on Children and Adolescents

Although the nuclear age began in 1945 with the New Mexico explosion followed by primitive atomic bombs over Hiroshima and Nagasaki, there is no evidence of research on the psychological effects of the nuclear threat on children until the time of the Berlin blockade and Cuban missile crises of 1961 and 1962. In addition, except for reports of the aftereffects of the atomic bombings on children in Japan, until the 1960s there were no case reports suggesting that children were aware of the threat.

EXPERIENCES AND COMMUNICATIONS OF YOUNG AND PREADOLESCENT CHILDREN

Up to 1984 few children have presented to child psychiatrists complaining of "nuclear fears." As a result, clinical case material from young children has rarely been obtained. Clinicians do not ordinarily inquire into their patients' feelings about the threat of nuclear war.[45] Revealing and powerful though it is, the material that follows is based mainly on reports obtained from children or parents outside of clinical settings. In addition, many of the reports are from children or parents who have shown a particular awareness of the nuclear threat and are able to share their thoughts and feelings about it. This information must, therefore, be regarded as suggestive, although it is consistent with what has been discovered in questionnaire studies.

In an effort to identify awareness of the nuclear threat among preschool children, an educator explored this subject with four groups of nursery-school and day-care children. Teacher and parent questionnaires were administered. Among the ninety-two children, eleven showed in their drawings or verbal statements that they were aware of and frightened by the nuclear threat.[16] Parents have also provided us with anecdotes illustrating their children's awareness of the threat of nuclear war. A five-year-old in Holland asked, "Daddy, when the bomb comes, will the rabbit die too?" A six-year-old boy said that whenever a plane flies over, he thinks it is the end of the world. A seven-year-old said, "I heard the world is going to end. I saw a film about it." A ten-year-old asked his father what it was like to be forty-two. His father said he would have to wait. The boy said he did not expect to live that long so he wanted to know now.

The following are more detailed examples:

A six-year-old asked his mother to make cookies for a Saturday several days off because he was going to have some friends over. He had overheard his father talking on the telephone about the possibility of ships armed with cruise missiles coming to Boston Harbor. His father was trying to prevent this from happening. Ordinarily he shielded his little boy from his activities related to the prevention of nuclear war. It turned out that the child wanted to have his friends over in order to prepare a letter to their congressman, Tip O'Neill, to keep "the death ships" out of Boston. The father was surprised that the boy had absorbed so much of what was going on.

A colleague, the father of a six-year-old boy, reported the following discussion with his son:

BOY: "I'm scared about a nuclear war—we talked about it with Billy's Dad. He said that there might be a space war. . . . I'm scared about a nuclear war on earth . . . and I don't want to talk about it any more. I feel like it might happen at any minute."
FATHER: "Where have you learned about this—anywhere besides Bill's Dad—like TV?"
BOY: "Yeah, cartoons and stuff tell all about it, but I don't want to talk about it any more."
FATHER: "I know you don't want to talk with me about it any more, but I do want you to know that I and other parents and grownups are working to stop any war from happening. Also, our talking about it could help to make it feel less scary."
BOY: "Talking about it isn't helping now."
FATHER: "Talking seems to have helped some kids with scared feelings—but this isn't helping you."
BOY: "Nope" (firmly).
FATHER: "Are you feeling anything can help you feel less scared?"
BOY: (Looking over a bridge over a large river, quietly answers) 'You'd have to jump off a bridge."
FATHER: "You mean the thing is just scary and there's no way not be be scared unless you're dead?"
BOY: "Yeah. And I don't want to talk about talking about it any more."
FATHER: "Okay, but if you do ever want to, you can."
BOY: "Okay."

Several aspects of this interchange are salient: (1) the child's accurate understanding of the nuclear threat; (2) his intense fear of it, which he felt could only be decreased by "jumping off a bridge"; (3) his hostility, influenced both by his feeling unprotected as well as his anger toward his father, which may be influenced by other developmentally related conflicts.

In the fall of 1983, a discussion occurred among a therapy group of hospitalized boys two days before the film *The Day After* was to be shown. Each boy had been severely burned a year or more before and was recovering from reconstructive surgical procedures. These boys were aroused by an advertisement for the movie showing a rocket with a bomb in it taking off. They were overwhelmed with fear, which appeared related only partially to their own burn experiences. The overwhelming nature of the film presentation of nuclear war—incomprehensible to children of that age and, perhaps, to some degree at any age—forced them to withdraw, distort, or use a grandiose flight of fantasy to cope with the threat as portrayed on the film.

Jody, an eleven-year-old girl, was brought to one of us (J.M.) for child psychiatric consultation. Jody's parents requested the consultation because she had asked if she would have time to commit suicide in the interval between learning that nuclear bombs were on the way and their actual detonation.

Jody's fears were greater at night. "Sometimes it just seems like everything is dark and dismal and I am sure the Russians are going to launch a bomb," she told her therapist. "All kids are scared to death that they won't live to be thirty," she said, "but most would rather watch *The Dukes of Hazzard* and other programs which would take their minds off such troubling matters." She explained to her therapist that she is a person who likes to know about the world. She said, "I like knowing what is going on. I like reading the news and finding out what is happening. I don't like being told that 'Oh, it's all okay,' and all of that, because sometimes it's not. When you know things, when I am thinking reasonably, I am less scared." She said that the reason that most of the kids were not as upset as she was had to do with the fact that "it is not happening right now," that "if it is not happening right now, then they don't understand." For herself, she likes to be "in charge of the situation—to have control."

Jody was clear about the distinction between reasonable fears, such as fear of nuclear war, and unreasonable ones, such as fear of skeletons, monsters in the cellar, and images in ghost stories and other products of her imagination that follow, for example, seeing scary television programs. After several sessions, Jody seemed not to be so troubled by the nuclear problem. Her parents had always felt the emphasis should be on ordinary troubles in the family. Therapy was discontinued after a few meetings.

A year and a half later the therapist spoke with Jody's mother in order to learn of Jody's progress. Her mother said she did not talk about nuclear war fears, but she was buried instead in violent videos. The mother called the therapist back a few days later. She told him that after his follow-up call Jody revealed that she had a nightmare about nuclear war and could not sleep. She asked her mother whether Canada would be destroyed by a nuclear war. "Probably," her mother replied. "What about South America or Australia?" Jody asked. "Probably not," her mother said. Jody asked if they could move to Australia. Her mother said, "Oh, Jody, I am not going to let anything happen to you." Jody said, "You can't stop it from happening." Then she revealed that she was having many frightening dreams and thinking about dying in a nuclear war much of the time. However, she felt "There is nothing you or anybody can do about it, so why talk about it?"

Jody's case illustrates the isolation many older children feel from their parents in relation to this issue, their ability to distinguish imaginary or neurotic distortions from fears related to real danger, and the resentment they feel when parents, out of their need to quiet their children's apprehensions, offer transparently false reassurances.

A children's group to discuss nuclear issues was organized in 1980, and fourteen children ages eight to thirteen met weekly for six months.[12] Girls tended to be critical of all weaponry while the boys enjoyed war play but sharply distinguished that from the buildup of nuclear weapons, of which they were highly critical. On reading and speaking with knowledgeable officials, they felt angry, lied to by adults, and so deeply distressed that they sought to write a book for children.

They wished their poems and essays to speak for themselves rather than have them interpreted by adults.*

From stories, artwork, and direct reports, we know that images of nuclear destruction have intruded into the consciousness of children in ways we do not understand and did not expect. An elementary school teacher in New Hampshire showed an eleven-year-old boy's story to one of us (J.M.) in which almost everyone but the storyteller was killed in a nuclear war. The class and writing assignment had had nothing to do with war or nuclear war. In the story, just before death reached him, the boy was miraculously saved by a great powerful Lord of the Cosmos. The passages that followed took place forty thousand years later. Filled with cosmic images of birth, death, and rebirth, the story evolved into an apocalyptic moral drama between monumental forces of good and evil. Myth piled upon epic myth, reflecting this child's effort to find some frame in which to contain the overwhelming fact of imminent nuclear planetary death that is part of the reality with which he and every other child must grow up. A systematic study of children's poetry, diaries, compositions, drawings, and other imaginative creations would be an informative way to discover how the nuclear threat is experienced on an everyday basis by children in the United States and other countries.

The reports, cases, and writings available to date suggest a developmental progression in cognitive awareness of the nuclear threat. While even a few preschool children may speak of nuclear war, their awareness seems only partial, and it may be that parental reassurance can protect very young children from their fears. However, when a better grasp of cause and effect, a sharpened sense of reality versus fantasy, and awareness of parental vulnerability occur—probably as early as five or six for some children—they may feel overwhelmed by their experience of the threat of nuclear war. Children from six to twelve may be less capable of denying or sublimating the knowledge of this threat or of developing effective ways of coping emotionally with what they sense, or know. Some children may develop a profound feeling of despair about the present as well as the future. Many express the fear that they will survive and be left alone without their parents. Children's despair may contribute to inhibiting curiosity about the world and interfere as well with the establishment of trust or confidence in parents and other adults. On the other hand, supportive parents may be able to help their children develop creative ways of expressing their feelings of despair, helplessness, and anger. For many children, the nuclear threat has contributed to nightmares and, in more vulnerable chil-

*Regrettably, space considerations preclude the inclusion of these poems and essays.

dren, even to depressive and suicidal thoughts, feelings, and actions.

How may the fear of nuclear annihilation relate to more familiar fantasies of annihilation known to emerge in a child's psychological development? These include fantasies of abandonment or violence by mother, father, or sibling that would be annihilating; fears of death from illness or accident; or terrifying fantasies aroused by other separations or losses in relation to some other treasured object, person, or environment. Growing awareness of the nuclear threat may intensify age-related conflicts and stresses and interface with ego and moral development. Although fear of nuclear annihilation may be experienced in some ways as similar to other fears, awareness of the terrible differences seems to become distinct as children grow more conscious of the real possibility of extinction of their own and everyone else's future world.

FAMILY ISSUES

In most instances parents and other adults do not engage in discussions with children about nuclear war. The gulf that Jody described between herself and her parents ("There is nothing . . . anybody can do about it, so why talk about it?") is also implicit in other reports. This avoidance has also characterized the child psychiatry and family therapy professions. The family therapy literature contained nothing on this subject until two short papers by Robert Simon and Steven Zeitlin appeared in the family therapy journal *Networker* in 1984. Simon writes that "nuclear fears" have become a "kind of family secret."[37,47] During the weeks after the showing of the television film *The Day After,* a study in the town of Ridgewood, New Jersey, found that 43 percent of the parents said that they never discussed nuclear issues in the family with their children, and 41 percent stated that they discussed such issues only occasionally.[23]

Zeitlin has documented that parents often do not want to face the issue themselves or hear their children's reproaches on the subject of the nuclear threat.[47] Children protect their parents from the *parents'* vulnerability. According to Zeitlin, they feel they have to show their parents that they can handle the issue themselves so as not to disturb their parents by discussing it.

STUDIES OF ADOLESCENTS

Interview Study.　Only one formal interview project has been reported.[19] Thirty-one high-school students from the Boston area were interviewed regarding the impact on their lives of the threat of nuclear annihilation along with their perceptions of the surrounding

political context. The issues that were discussed included: the extent of awareness of the nuclear threat; perceptions of personal and national security; assignment of responsibility and blame; views on the U.S.-Soviet relationship and leadership; and visions of the future. Widespread fear, sadness, helplessness, cynicism, and anger were present among the seventeen girls and fourteen boys ages fourteen to nineteen. Each teenager thought that nuclear war would come in his or her lifetime. Some seemed to live on two levels, planning as if there were a future while believing nuclear annihilation to be inevitable. Civil defense was dismissed by all as useless, while none believed a nuclear war could remain limited. Both superpowers were held responsible for the arms race, which was seen as dangerously out of control with a momentum of its own. Some regarded technology as having wrested control from man. Many expressed the desire for more knowledge, especially about the Soviet Union. In offering solutions to the impasse, these students emphasized better communication between the leaders of the superpowers and expressed the desire for a greater chance to participate in the decision-making process. They also viewed this as a way of overcoming their sense of terror and helplessness.

Questionnaire Studies.　Several questionnaire studies will be described. We believe it is of central importance that these studies consistently find *many* children and adolescents growing up in fear of nuclear annihilation. There are limitations to the data about what children and adolescents think and feel about the threat of nuclear war. The samples are not always representative, and some investigations may at times reflect a researcher bias. Questionnaire studies on an emotionally laden topic such as this suffer from the fact that some of the complex thoughts and feelings which they elicit cannot be categorized. Some teenagers, for example, seem *not* to be involved by the nuclear threat. Does this mean that they are truly not involved, or are they in fact defending themselves emotionally? Some children's concerns seem to be below the surface. For example, after one eleven-year-old boy was interviewed by a teacher about the nuclear issue, he said that until that time he had not known "how much it was on my mind." In responding to a question as to whether the nuclear threat had affected his plans for the future, a ninth grader wrote "No, No, No" in letters over an inch high. How are we to categorize such a response —as a yes or a no? Another limitation in the research is that there have been no studies devoted just to pre-teenage children.

One study of a broad sample of adolescents addresses their concerns about nuclear war, among other things, and does not have a researcher bias. The only survey of its kind, it was conducted by Jerald G. Bachman and his colleagues at the Institute for Social Research of the University of Michigan.[3] From 1975 to 1982 they administered questionnaires to over 119,000 seniors from 130 public and private schools across the country; a sample of over 20,000 of the youths were asked about their concerns about nuclear war. To the multiple choice question: "of all the problems facing the nation today, how often do you worry about the chance of nuclear war," Bachman found a fourfold increase from 1975 to 1982 in the number of those who worry "often." During this period Bachman and his coworkers also found a 61 percent increase among those who agreed or mostly agreed with the statement "nuclear or biological annihilation will probably be the fate of all mankind within my lifetime." Psychiatrist Daniel Offer has been using self-administered questionnaires since 1962 to assess teenagers' views of themselves and their worlds. He found that the samples of young people in the early 1960s expressed more hope and greater belief in the future than did those questioned from 1979 to 1981.[29] This may or may not be related to the nuclear issue; Offer did not ask specifically about it. Summarizing the available data in December 1982; survey specialist Daniel Yankelovich reported a mood of despair and gloom in Western Europe and the United States.[46] He related this mood to "a sense of the future as being very threatening, as perhaps there not being a future, a future of grimness, of shortages, of greater difficulty, a closing of horizons."

The first ground-breaking explorations were carried out near the time of the Berlin and Cuban missile crises and offer data for historical comparison. Between 1962 and 1963, Sibylle Escalona examined 311 children ranging from ten to seventeen years old, from widely different socioeconomic groups. She found that 70 percent mentioned the issue of war and peace and, of the 70 percent, 35 percent considered a destructive war very possible, or certain. She observed that "the profound uncertainty about whether or not mankind has a foreseeable future exerts a corrosive and malignant influence upon important developmental processes in normal and well-functioning children." More recently she concluded, "growing up in the full knowledge of the fact that there may be no future, and that the adult world seems unable to combat the threat, can render the next generation less well capable of averting actual catastrophe than it would be if the same threat existed in a different social climate."[15] Milton Schwebel sent questionnaires to three thousand high-school juniors and seniors from various socioeconomic backgrounds. The results showed they knew and cared about the threat of nuclear war and were concerned about the widespread death and destruction that would occur. This knowledge provoked two opposing atti-

tudes: One group confronted their fear and were forced to live with its "erosive effects," while the other defended themselves against it by suppressing, avoiding, and denying.[35]

In 1982 the American Psychiatric Association (APA) published a report that included a study on the impact of nuclear developments on children and adolescents.[4,32] In 1978, 1979, and 1980, 1,151 questionnaires were administered to children from the fifth through the twelfth grades in the Boston, Los Angeles, and Baltimore areas. Approximately 40 percent of the total group reported they were aware of nuclear developments before they were twelve. Although the majority of the overall group thought that civil defense would not work, a considerable percentage considered it essential. Approximately 50 percent of the 1979 sample of 389 students reported that nuclear advances had affected their thoughts about marriage and their plans for the future. Among the more detailed responses of teenagers from the Boston area were vivid expressions of terror and powerlessness, grim images of nuclear destruction, doubt about whether they will ever have a chance to grow up, an accompanying attitude of "live for now," and anger toward the adult generation.

In the past few years additional questionnaire studies have been undertaken with groups of adolescents in the Greensboro-Guilford County area in North Carolina[48,49]; Newton, Massachusetts[24]; Akron, Ohio[20]; Lansing, Michigan[34]; Salt Lake City, Utah[6]; Toronto, Ontario; and other cities and communities. The results of these studies create a picture of increasing worry about the future, a sense of powerlessness, and, on the part of a significant percentage of the young people questioned, a feeling that nuclear war is inevitable in their lifetimes. The Greensboro-Guilford County study also demonstrated that adolescents questioned had a striking lack of basic information about nuclear weapons–related matters.

Much misinformation was related about what the world would be after a nuclear attack; at the same time, the great majority expressed the wish for more information.

Psychologist Ronald M. Doctor and his coworkers administered a questionnaire developed with pediatrician John Goldenring to 913 high-school juniors and seniors in the Los Angeles, San Fernando Valley, and San Jose areas.[18] In general, when questions are asked about the nuclear issue, the examiner's agenda may be disclosed, which would introduce a methodological bias into the study. In order to overcome this problem, these researchers embedded the nuclear war question in twenty items. When the results were tabulated, 58.2 percent of the sample were worried or very worried about nuclear war. Specifically, this concern ranked fourth, behind a parent dying, getting bad grades, and being a victim of a violent crime. When asked their "greatest worry," the students ranked nuclear war second behind their parents dying.

Developmental Considerations. As Escalona had done before, Beardslee and Mack raised questions about the impact of the nuclear threat on personality and moral[4,5] development. The formation of stable ideals or values depends on a sense of human continuity and confidence in the future, and the investigators were concerned especially about the effect of such a frightening presence on aspects of personality formation. They asked what happens to the formation of such ideals when the adult generation toward whom young people turn as models, and to whom their futures are entrusted, cannot protect them and may even be seen as jeopardizing the future.

At each stage of development the child mitigates disappointments by looking ahead and building a vision of the future in which he or she may possess what cannot now be had or in which it is possible to become what he or she is incapable of being now. A healthy ego ideal builds out of possible goals or standards that are both realizable and worth struggling to achieve. But the building of such values, or of an ego ideal, depends on a present life which is perceived as stable and enduring and a future upon which the adolescent can, at least to some degree, rely.

But what happens to the ego ideal if society and its leaders are perceived cynically and the future itself is uncertain. Furthermore, how does it affect the ego ideal when the reason for that uncertainty is readily perceived to be the folly or "stupidity" of the adults around the adolescent who, because of perceived incompetence, greed, aggressiveness, lust for power, ineffectualness, can leave their children no future other than a planet contaminated by radiation and on the verge of incineration through the holocaust of nuclear war? In such a world, planning seems pointless, and ordinary values and ideals appear naive. In such a context, impulsivity, a value system of "get it now," the hyperstimulation of drugs and the proliferation of apocalyptic cults that try to revive the idea of an after life while extinguishing individuality or discriminating perception seem to be natural developments.[4]

At a lecture in 1984 Milton Schwebel described effects on development that he saw occurring as a result of the nuclear threat[36]:

(1) It complicates the child's coping with the discovery of death. Children generally learn in stages about the deaths of living things, including their parents and themselves, and are told that these will be far-off events. But when it is feared that total death may come at any moment, this changes the meaning of death and the way the child learns to handle the notion of death itself.[25]

(2) Children develop inappropriate defenses to deal with the fear of nuclear death. The subject is taboo and they see adults being passive and doing nothing about it. Older children and adolescents may use denial, fatalism, illusions of power, and immediate forms of gratification (premature use of alcohol, drugs, sex, and possibly suicide). Furthermore, they see that adults are not dealing effectively with the threat and they are thus denied the usual strengthening impact of constructive

identifications. (3) In adolescence, the threat interferes with the establishment of identity. Identity depends on the continuity of the sense of self. What happens to this sense when the future is seen as uncertain or ephemeral? (4) The threat of annihilation interrupts the development of human relationships. It tells us that life is brief and long-term relationships may therefore seem foolish, especially as annihilation of human life will occur by human intention. If the world and life itself can be thrown away, then how can relationships be seen as valuable or worth preserving over the long term? (5) A threat to the future of such magnitude can induce a sense of powerlessness that may in turn interfere with ego mastery. If no one can affect this central threat, then how powerful can anyone feel oneself to be in the real world?

QUESTIONS OF SOCIAL CONTEXT AND CLASS DIFFERENCE

As Robert Coles has pointed out, when trying to assess the meaning of the nuclear threat for a particular child or adolescent, it is important to know as much as possible about the social and family background of the young person and the relationship of this issue to other emotionally important areas. Coles believes that the nuclear threat is a worry of educated middle- and upper-class youth but is much less important than economic concerns, jobs, and food to youth from blue-collar families.[9] Preliminary work has been done by Coles himself, who has talked with young people in various regions of the country, and by psychologist Scott Haas, who has compared the attitudes of high-school students in western Connecticut, Massachusetts, and Manchester, New Hampshire, toward the nuclear threat. Their work suggests that there may be socioeconomic or class differences in the relative importance and meaning of the nuclear issue for different groups of adolescents.[21] In questionnaires and discussions with working-class high-school students in the industrial city of Manchester, Haas has found that they ranked the nuclear issue behind jobs and the economy. However, in relation to the nuclear issue, Haas's subjects expressed a deep sense of powerlessness and hopelessness. They gave a picture of a world out of their control, in a constant state of war, dominated by technology and manipulated by large corporations and organizations that are indifferent to their wishes yet upon whom they must depend for their livelihoods.

The experience of one educaator, who was invited to teach a short course about nuclear issues in a Boston largely black, inner-city high school, suggests that the bravado and seeming indifference of working-class teenagers toward the nuclear issue may be quite superficial.[39] After a minimum of classroom discussion and an opportunity to see a film of Soviet children talking about *their* fears of nuclear war, the students in the class began to discuss quite openly their anxieties about nuclear annihilation. The stereotyped anti-Soviet cliches that had characterized their initial discussions were replaced by an acknowledgment of fearfulness and a desire to know more about the nuclear reality and to find common ground with Soviet adolescents.

STUDIES FROM OTHER COUNTRIES

Surveys done in countries other than the United States confirm the findings of investigations performed here, but with certain differences. Data are available from the Soviet Union and Finland. Surveys are also now being done in Holland, Australia, Great Britain, and other countries.

During the summer of 1983 Chivian, Waletzky, and Mack surveyed 293 children ages nine to seventeen[7,8] at a Soviet pioneer camp in the Caucasus on the Black Sea. About 60 percent were girls. The children were asked to rank their degree of worry about a list of concerns from "not at all worried" to "very worried." Almost all of the Soviet children were "very worried" about nuclear war. The following tables compare the Soviet sample (mean age 12.7 years) with an age matched subsample of American children (mean age 13.2 years). The investigators used the same instrument used by Goldenring and Doctor to ask several additional questions:

These data on a small Soviet sample suggest that, like American children, many Soviet children are worried about nuclear war, pessimistic (or realistic) about whether survival would be possible, and optimistic—more than the U.S. sample—that such a war could be prevented. The optimism may be due to the fact that Soviet children receive information in a more controlled fashion and participate actively in peace efforts.

In 1982 a much larger study[40] was carried out in Finland. By means of a postal survey, 6,851 twelve to eighteen-year-olds were sampled nationwide in a completely random fashion. In each of the age groups, the fear of war exceeded all other fears. In the twelve-year-old group, 79 percent mentioned war as their greatest fear. Thirty-seven percent of girls and 15 percent of boys responded that they had experienced strong anxiety about war during the preceding month. The threat of war also emerged in nightmares: 13 percent of girls and 6 percent of boys had had such nightmares during the preceding month. Thirty-six percent of the youth were optimistic that they could do something to prevent war. Children in the youngest age group expressed more fears about war than did the older adolescents, and girls expressed greater anxiety about war than did boys. The data suggest that the threat of war forms an important part of Finnish children's social and psychological experience.

Do you think a nuclear war between the U.S. and U.S.S.R. will happen during your lifetime?

	Soviet	American
Yes	11.8%	38.4%
No	54.5%	16.9%
Uncertain	33.7%	44.8%

If there were a nuclear war, do you think that you and your family would survive?

	Soviet	American
Yes	2.9%	16.4%
No	80.7%	41.3%
Uncertain	16.4%	40.8%

If there were a nuclear war, do you think that the U.S. and the U.S.S.R. would survive it?

	Soviet	American[a]
Yes	6.1%	21.9%
No	78.9%	37.8%
Uncertain	15.0%	39.8%

Do you think nuclear war between the U.S. and U.S.S.R. can be prevented?

	Soviet	American[a]
Yes	93.3%	65.2%
No	2.9%	14.5%
Uncertain	3.9%	19.9%

[a]American children were asked only about the survival of the United States.
NOTE: Reprinted from Chivian, E., and Goodman, A. "What Soviet Children are Saying About Nuclear War," in International Physicians for the Prevention of Nuclear War *Report*, 2 (1):10–12, 1984.

SUMMARY OF RESEARCH ON EFFECTS OF THE NUCLEAR THREAT

1. Many children in different parts of the United States, the Soviet Union, Finland, and other countries are concerned about the threat of nuclear war and experience troubling fears, sadness, powerlessness, and anger.
2. The meaning of this concern varies according to the developmental level and socioeconomic situation of the young person.
3. In the period from 1975 to 1983, as the nuclear arms competition has appeared to become increasingly out of control, worry about the nuclear threat has increased among adolescents in the United States.
4. An important aspect of children's worry and sense of helplessness is the perception that nuclear weapons decision making has slipped out of human control and has been taken over by the momentum of technological developments.
5. Children and adolescents seem less well defended psychologically than adults and more vulnerable to the implications of what nuclear weapons can do and what nuclear war would mean for them, their families, and the world.
6. There are great variations in the amount and quality of information that children and adolescents receive. The chief sources of information for young people in the

United States appear to be television and the reports of their peers.

7. Many children feel they have no one with whom they can discuss the nuclear problem. Children in the Soviet Union and Finland seem to feel more protected, perhaps because of the possibility of shared activity and their leaders' visible public profession of efforts to prevent nuclear war and promote peace.

8. Many children and adolescents express uncertainty about whether there will be a future. This sense of futurelessness has raised questions about the possible corrosive effects of the nuclear threat on personality and moral development, but there is no systematic data on this subject.

Issues for Child Psychiatry

It is important for the profession of child psychiatry to come to terms with the reality of the nuclear threat and its impact on ourselves, our families, and our patients and their families. The problem is powerful but so intangible that we have great difficulty coping with it. We know we are unable to protect our children, and at the same time we sense the deep impact that the nuclear threat may be having on the emotional lives of many young people. Upon facing the threat we risk becoming demoralized, isolated, and "burned out" by the immensity of the issue. For emotional, professional, and political reasons, we shy away from the subject and immerse ourselves in our profession's struggle to prove itself scientifically. By discussing the nuclear issue among ourselves and at professional meetings, we may begin to see its importance. Once we have faced this issue as child psychiatrists we may better understand our patients' concerns and provide counsel and support to their parents, teachers, and others.

The information presented here suggests that awareness of the nuclear threat as an issue in child psychiatric work may provide understanding of an important source of fear, anxiety, depression, and pessimism among some child patients and their families. In addition, within the general hospital it would be useful for child psychiatrists to recognize that traumatized, grieving, homeless, burned, and dying children provide an example, a glimpse on a small scale, of the human suffering that countless children would experience should nuclear war occur. Such information should be shared within and outside the medical profession. Schools in the United States—a far too small percentage—offer courses in which information on nuclear war is presented.

The desire or need for psychiatric consultation may arise in various settings—among teachers, for example,

and in parent groups in schools; again, it may appear within the context of other group structures such as academic courses, discussions in group therapy, or distress experienced within student activist groups. An indication that the nuclear threat may be affecting the thinking of a teenager can be quite subtle, taking the form, for example, of moody withdrawal or compulsive preoccupation with violent video games or rock tapes that contain apocalyptic images. Where such suggestive data are noted, further questioning of the child is very appropriate. Other examples, suggestive of anxiety related to the nuclear threat, may include direct requests for information or expressions of interest, fear, or despair after exposure to lectures, news programs, films such as those in the series *Star Wars, The Day After,* or *Testament.* Nightmares with nuclear and other world annihilation images, and self-destructive ideas or actions connected with the sense of futurelessness, also require further investigation. In most instances "treatment" begins with providing children and adolescents an opportunity to observe or meet with adults behaving responsibly in relation to the nuclear problem, as Escalona suggested two decades ago.

In those rare instances when fears or worries about the nuclear threat are communicated in clinical practice, the concerns need to be assessed in relation to other developmental issues, such as the sense of helplessness and despair that occurs for a variety of reasons in adolescence. At the same time the child psychiatrist needs to be open to the possibility that, in the case of the older child or adolescent, the despair or moral confusion is genuinely related to the failure to feel protected in anticipating a future clouded by the nuclear predicament. In addition to providing an opportunity to talk about the nuclear issue with responsible and concerned adults, the facilitation of group discussions with peers or the encouragement of older children and adolescents to take part actively in projects to prevent nuclear war may often be constructive interventions.

When child psychiatrists are involved in forming public policy, they must address several implications of the nuclear issue. In other sections of this book dealing with the federal government's activities and policies pertaining to child mental health, no mention is made of this subject. Despite constantly expanding funding for weapons development, no federal funds have been allocated to examine the implications of the nuclear threat for the emotional lives of children and adolescents. Educational programs in high schools and junior high schools are needed to provide accurate information about a number of areas. These include: nuclear science and technology; the historical, political, and cultural realities of the arms race; and objective studies of the history and psychology of "enemies." Opportunities should be provided in homes, schools, and communities that would permit children and adolescents to talk about their questions and worries about nuclear war with responsible adults. In this way the youngsters can participate appropriately in the national dialogue regarding nuclear weapons. There is an urgent need to broaden the conceptions and discussions of national security to include a consideration of health issues. In the case of children and adolescents exposed to the threat of nuclear weapons, this involves both their physical and psychological health and well-being.

REFERENCES

1. ABRAMS, H. L., and VON KAENEL, W. E. "Medical Problems of Survivors of Nuclear War: Infection and the Spread of Communicable Disease," *New England Journal of Medicine,* 305 (1981): 1226–1232.

2. ADELSON, J. Prepared statement for Hearing before the Select Committee on Children, Youth, and Families. U.S. House of Representatives, 87th Congress, 20 September, 1983, "Children's Fears of War." Washington, D.C.: U.S. Government Printing Office, 1983, pp. 108–109.

3. BACHMAN J. G. "American High School Seniors View the Military: 1976–1982," *Armed Forces and Society,* 10 (1983): 86–104.

4. BEARDSLEE, W. R., and MACK, J. E. "The Impact on Children and Adolescents of Nuclear Weapons," in *Psychosocial Aspects of Nuclear Developments.* Task Force Report #20, Washington, D.C.: American Psychiatric Association, Spring 1982.

5. ———. "Adolescents and the Threat of Nuclear War: The Evolution of a Perspective," *Yale Journal of Biology and Medicine,* 56 (1983): 79–91.

6. BORGENICHT, L. "Threat in the Nuclear Age: Children's Responses to the Nuclear Arms Debate" (abstract:). Hearing Before the Select Committee on Children, Youth, and Families, U.S. House of Representatives, 87th Congress, 20 September 1983, "Children's Fears of War." Washington, D.C.: U.S. Government Printing Office, 1983, pp. 123–134.

7. CHIVIAN, E., and GOODMAN, J. "What Soviet Children Are Saying About Nuclear War," *International Physicians for the Prevention of Nuclear War Report,* 2 (1984): 10–12.

8. CHIVIAN, E., et al. "Soviet Children and the Threat of Nuclear War, A Preliminary Study," *American Journal of Orthopsychiatry,* 55 (1985): 484–502.

9. COLES, R. "Children and the Nuclear Bomb," in *The Moral Life of Children.* Boston: Atlantic Monthly Press, 1986, pp. 243–280.

10. Committee for the Compilation of Materials on Damage Caused by the Atomic Bomb on Hiroshima and Nagasaki. *Hiroshima and Nagasaki: The Physical, Medical and Social Effects of the Atomic Bombings.* New York: Basic Books, 1981.

11. CONSTABLE, J. "Surgical Problems Among Survivors," *Bulletin of the Atomic Scientists,* (1981): 222–225.

12. DOLMETSCH, P., HAMBURG, P., AND THE CHILDREN'S GROUP ON NUCLEAR ISSUES. Untitled manuscript.

13. EHRLICH, P. R., et al. "Long-term Biological Consequences of Nuclear War," *Science,* 222 (1983): 1293–1300.

14. ESCALONA, S. "Children and the Threat of Nuclear War," in M. Schwebel, ed., *Behavioral Science and Human Survival.* Palo Alto, Calif.: Science and Behavioral Books, 1965, pp. 201–209.

15. ———. "Growing Up with the Threat of Nuclear War: Some Indirect Effects on Personality Development," *American Journal of Orthopsychiatry,* 52 (1982): 608–618.

16. FRIEDMAN, G. "Preschoolers' Awareness of Nuclear Threat," *Newsletter of the California Association on the Education of Young Children,* 12 (1984): 4–5.

17. GOLDBERG, S. et al. "The Effect of the Nuclear Threat on Children: A Pilot Study," Paper presented at Research Symposium on the Impact of the Threat of Nuclear War on Children and Adolescents, 4th Congress of International Physicians for the Prevention of Nuclear War, Helsinki, Finland, June 4–8, 1984.

18. GOLDENRING, J. and DOCTOR, R. "Research Symposium: The Impact of the Threat of Nuclear War on Children and Adolescents," Paper presented at the 4th International Congress of the International Physicians for the Prevention of Nuclear War, Helskinki, Finland, June 4–8, 1984.

19. GOODMAN, L. A., et al. "Threat of Nuclear War and the Nuclear Arms Race: Adolescent Experience and Perceptions," *Political Psychology,* 4 (1983): 501–530.

20. HANNA, S. D. "The Psychosocial Impact of the Nuclear Threat on Children," manuscript, 1982.

21. HAAS, S. D. "Class and Nuclear War" and "Working Class Kids' View of War and Peace," manuscripts, 1984.

22. JAPAN BROADCASTING CORPORATION. *Unforgettable Fire: Pictures Drawn by Atomic Bomb Survivors.* New York: Pantheon, 1977.

23. JOHNSON, N. *Arms Control and the Nuclear War: A Sense of Attitudes in an American Town.* Washington, D.C.: Center for Public Policy Research, 1984.

24. KLAVENS, J. Questionnaire on the impact of nuclear advances, 1982.

25. KOOCHER, J. "Children's Concept of Death," in R. Bibace and M. Walsh, eds., *New Directions for Child Development: Children's Conceptions of Health, Illness and Bodily Functions, No. 14.* San Francisco, Jossey-Bass, 1981.

26. LIFTON, R. J. *Death in Life: Survivors of Hiroshima.* New York: Vintage, 1967.

27. LINDEMANN, E. "Symptomatology and Management of Acute Grief," *American Journal of Psychiatry,* 101 (1944): 141–148.

28. LOWN, B. "Physicians and Nuclear War," *Journal of the American Medical Association,* 246 (1981): 2332–2333.

29. OFFER, D. "Adolescent Self-Image: Empirical Studies and Theoretical Implications," Paper presented at The Cambridge Hospital Symposium on Self-Esteem: Development and Sustenance, Boston, 10 December 1982.

30. OFFICE OF TECHNOLOGY ASSESSMENT, U. S. Congress. *The Effects of Nuclear War.* Washington, D.C.: U.S. Government Printing Office, 1979.

31. OSADA, A., ed. *Children of Hiroshima.* Cambridge, Mass.: Oelgeschlager, Gunn, & Hain, 1982.

32. *Psychosocial Aspects of Nuclear Developments.* Task Force Report #20. Washington, D.C.: American Psychiatric Association, 1982.

33. REAGAN, R. Address to the Nation on Nuclear Strat-

egy Toward the Soviet Union, *New York Times,* 23 November, 1982.

34. SANDLER, R. "The Impact of the Threat of Nuclear War on Adolescents in a United States Mid-Western Urban School," Paper presented at Research Symposium on the Impact of the Threat of Nuclear War on Children and Adolescents, 4th Congress of International Physicians for the Prevention of Nuclear War, Helsinki, Finland, June 4–8, 1984.

35. SCHWEBEL, M. "Nuclear Cold War: Student Opinion and Professional Responsibility," in M. Schwebel, ed., *Behavioral Science and Human Survival.* Palo Alto, Calif.: Science and Behavioral Books, 1965, pp. 210–223.

36. SCHWEBEL, M. "Children's Reactions to the Nuclear Threat: Trends and Implications," paper presented at Symposium of the New York University School of Social Work on the Impact of the Nuclear Threat on the Mental Health of Children and Parents, 13 April 1984.

37. SIMON, R. "The Nuclear Family," *Networker,* March–April (1984): 22 ff.

38. SMITH M. B. "The Threat of Nuclear War: Psychological Impact," Paper presented to the Physicians for Social Responsibility Symposium, Eugene, Oregon, 9 October 1982.

39. SNOW, C. "Nuclear Nightmares in Inner City Schools," *World Paper,* July (1984): 15.

40. SOLANTAUS, T., RIMPELA, M., and TAIPALE, V. "The Threat of War in the Minds of the 12–18 Year Olds in Finland" *Lancet,* (1984): 784.

41. STODDARD, F. J. "Body Image Development in the Burned Child," *Journal of the American Academy of Child Psychiatry,* 21 (1982): 502–507.

42. ———. "Coping with Pain: A Developmental Approach to Treatment of the Burned Child," *American Journal of Psychiatry,* 139 (1982): 736–740.

43. TERR, L. C. "Chowchilla Revisited: The Effects of Psychic Trauma Four Years After a School Bus Kidnapping," *American Journal of Psychiatry,* 140 (1983): 1542–1550.

44. TURCO, R. P., et al. "Nuclear Winter: Global Consequences of Multiple Nuclear Explosions," *Science,* 222 (1983): 1283–1292.

45. WILKESON, A. "Nuclear Numbing and the Practice of Psychiatry," Paper presented at the annual meeting of the American Psychiatric Association, Los Angeles, May 6–11, 1984.

46. YANKELOVICH, D. "Changing Social Values," Paper presented at the Research Workshop in Preventive Aspects of Suicide and Affective Disorders Among Adolescents and Young Adults, Harvard Medical School and Harvard School of Public Health, Boston, 3 December 1982.

47. ZEITLIN, S. "Nuclear Secrets: What Do We Tell Mom and Dad?" *Networker,* March–April (1984): 30 ff.

48. ZWEIGENHAFT, R. L. "The Psychological Effects of Living in a Nuclear Age," Report of the War Planning Evaluation Committee of the Greensboro-Guilford (North Carolina) County Emergency Management Agency, 1983.

49. ———. "Providing Information and Shaping Attitudes About Nuclear Dangers: Implications for Public Education" *Political Psychology,* (1985): 461–480.

70 / **Video Games and Computer-Assisted Instruction**

Richard A. Gardner

Introduction

As far as children's lives are concerned, probably the most frequent contacts with the computer involve the video game and the video arcade. These have become, without doubt, the most popular forms of indoor entertainment currently engaged in by children and adolescents. Computer games have become favorite Christmas presents. More serious use of home personal computers by children has also become a national pastime. A parental threat to deprive the child of the opportunity to play with or use the computer or to visit a video arcade can be a very potent disciplinary measure. So rapid has been the growth of computer availability and so widespread its infiltration into children's lives that the editors of this volume saw fit to include a chapter about its effects on children. Here I will describe the two forms of computer utilization to which children are most frequently exposed, namely the video arcade and computer-assisted instruction (CAI). Throughout I will refer to studies that have been conducted to assess the effects and value of this novel influence on the lives of children. It is important for the reader to appreciate that our experience with these instruments is just beginning and the conclusions of many of these studies are highly biased. It is only with long-term, follow-up studies that we will really know how useful and/or how detrimental these instruments are.

Video Games and Video Arcades

The video game and video arcade have become as much a part of childhood as Little League, television viewing, scouting, and birthday parties. Kegan[13] states, "*Time* magazine reported that the amount of money spent on video games in 1982 was twice the amount spent in all of the casinos in Nevada, twice the gross receipts of the American movie industry, and three times the combined television revenues of professional baseball, basketball, and football." According to Smith,[28] the pinball machine has been replaced by the computerized game. We see a host of other machines: submarine fights, cruising astroids, invaders from outer space, and cowboy gunfights. Guns are somewhat in disrepute, however, but the same hostile outlets are probably provided by other items on the games: rockets, beam projectors, destruction of aliens, knocking down walls, and so forth.

Video games have become standard Christmas presents, and video arcades are to be seen everywhere. And this popularity is not restricted to the United States. All over the western world the same phenomenon is evident. The video game can be seen as a marriage between television and the computer. And, like many marriages, it represents the union of the best and the worst.

THE PSYCHOLOGICAL EFFECTS OF VIDEO GAMES AND VIDEO ARCADES ON CHILDREN

Because video games have been with us such a short time, extensive studies have not yet been reported regarding the long-term psychological effects of their utilization. However, some studies have been completed and some conclusions formulated. At this point, the results seem mixed. In time we will be in a better position to assess the effects of these ingenious devices on our children.

Whether the games are to be regarded as an asset or a liability, the data suggest that children involved with video games generally spend less time watching television. In the study by Greenfield[11] most of the children claimed that video games displaced the time they spent watching television. She points out that one of the significant differences between video games and television is that video games are interactive; the player has some control over the game. The degree of control is even greater with the laser disc, which provides the child with the opportunity to interact and manipulate animated cartoons. With this device, the child can actually control the outcome of the story, a far cry from a television where the viewer must passively accept whatever happens. This, Greenfield believes, is an element in the attraction of these games. Nearly all the children she studied claimed that they preferred video games over television, and their interactive quality was a common reason given. Greenfield also points out that video games are not an expensive form of entertainment for the child who gains significant skill. Although the child may spend $15 to $20 acquiring proficiency,

after that he or she may play as long as an hour or two for only a quarter.

Most will agree that video games keep children off the streets and probably keep some of them out of trouble. Obviously, children cannot simultaneously play video games and engage in antisocial activities or general troublemaking behavior. By the same token, such involvement could also preclude desirable behavior, and, in fact, many parents fear that the lure of video games is so great that their children will become truant from school. Brooks[2] found no evidence that this was the case. Some parents fear that the video arcade setting will increase the chances that their children will become involved in drug and alcohol abuse. Again, Brooks found no evidence for this. In fact, most of the children he studied claimed that video games diminished their desire for the use of alcohol or drugs because such substances compromised their efficiency when playing the games. However, addiction to the games per se is merely another kind of addiction, and that is a factor which must be seriously considered. Some children do become addicted to these games, and this cannot but interfere with their educational activities. Even if video games and arcades are not associated with a higher truancy rate, they cut into time spent at homework, sports, and other activities that require more originality and creativity.

The violent themes so ubiquitous in video games have been the object of criticism by those who believe that such emphasis contributes to antisocial behavior. There is no question that violent themes do pervade video games. Spaceships are destroyed by the thousands, cities are blown up, and people are killed. However, the player's main concern is a high score, most children pay practically no attention to the destructive factor that pervades the games. Cacha[4] believes that the violence portrayed in many video games is antithetical to the values and the educational models of our society. She thereby concludes that they contribute to violence. I find this a dubious assertion. As mentioned, children who are absorbed in video games cannot at the same time be committing antisocial acts. As I have described elsewhere,[10] I believe violent types of antisocial behavior are generated primarily by faulty upbringing in disturbed homes, not by visualizing hostile games on a TV screen. By extension, the same thinking applies to playing these games.

It remains to be determined whether video games increase isolation or provide a greater degree of interpersonal involvement. Undoubtedly there are tens of thousands of young people who are sequestered in their homes playing and devising video games. However, many of these children communicate with one another, both directly by means of a modem (an instrument that connects the computer to a telephone) and indirectly through a national computer network to which they may purchase access. In the video arcades, as well, there is often a fair degree of socialization. Many of the games involve cooperation among members of teams or at least require that one play against another partner (also an interpersonal event). In the same arcades, however, there are children who are essentially "alone in a crowd"—they have little or no social involvement with the dozens of peers who surround them. Smith[28] emphasized this point, noting that some of these children are so absorbed that they are not likely to talk very much with one another.

Mitchell[18] followed twenty families over a two-month period after they had purchased an Atari video game in the Christmas season of 1981. Interestingly, although these games are often played alone, in the families studied, as the games became a focus of family attention, they increased family interaction. Some of these families had previously watched television to a significant degree, but mostly in a passive and silent manner.

Studies have also been carried out on the effects of these games on children's self-esteem. Mitchell[18] claims that one of the attractions of the Atari game was that it allowed children to excel over their parents. Kegan[13] emphasizes the ego-enhancing feeling that comes to youngsters when they pass from the phase in which the game appears overwhelming to the phase in which there is a sense of control and efficiency. Children who may not have acquired any particular skill in school work, sports, music, or other areas in which members of their peer group may gain competence can in this realm, and with relatively little effort, equal the proficiency of their peers. With the video game everybody starts at the same level, and the degree of practice necessary to achieve proficiency is generally far less than that necessary for other more demanding endeavors. Donchin[7] emphasizes that video games enable novices to become experts in a relatively short period of time, and this is one of their significant attractions. Smith,[28] however, points out that there is also an ego-debasing factor in video games. Ultimately, he states, the child loses: "No matter how far along the player can go, the toy's program can take it further, better, and faster." He admits, however, that this does not seem to discourage the players, so one can only wonder about how ego-debasing the experience really is.

Not surprisingly, those who sell video games claim that they have an intrinsic educational value, that they improve both logical thinking and eye-hand coordination. Greenfield[11] also emphasizes that many of the games involve the development of various cognitive skills. What may initially appear to be random targets are generally appreciated to have certain patterns. Furthermore, skill in such games also involves parallel

mental processing in that the child must learn to consider a number of variables simultaneously. This is different from reading where one acquires information seriatim. For example, in the game Tranquility Base the child tries to land a spaceship on a rough terrain. There are six basic variables involved in making a successful landing: altitude, gravity, thrust, direction, amount of fuel, and terrain. To land a spaceship safely, the child must simultaneously integrate all these variables. The game teaches this complex cognitive task.

Smith[28] is less enthusiastic. He claims that although video games may teach children a little more eye-hand coordination, they do not teach much else. Moreover, they restrict imagination. The child does not have the faintest idea how the game works; in fact, most of the games have a warning on the back that they should not be opened. While children play computer baseball, computer football, and computer soccer, they are not playing the real game, and thus they are losing out on learning how to play these games in reality.

Video games have also been said to have therapeutic benefits. Slaby[27] describes the value of the games as part of the treatment of chronically ill mental patients. Part of their therapeutic effect is the pleasure they provide for these patients. They also make for a certain degree of interpersonal stimulation in a very regulated way. The individual can play the game alone or in close association with others, as he or she prefers. Such an activity can also improve attention, which is commonly impaired in psychotic patients. In an organization set up for the rehabilitation of ex-offenders and delinquents, Stone[29] found the games useful in reducing recidivism. She also found the computers to be useful as a step toward the education of many of these people, most of whom were not functioning beyond the second-grade level. Lynch[16] has found video games helpful in the rehabilitation of brain-injured patients. These devices help improve attention span and require scanning of a visual display with quick reaction to changes. This is the kind of experience many brain-injured patients need.

Computer-Assisted Instruction: The Computer in the Classroom

The computer is causing another revolution in the field of education. Early programs in the schools relied on large mainframe computers that were connected to school-based terminals by long-distance telephone. The new microprocessor-based equipment is self-sufficient and provides a school with much more autonomy with regard to programs utilized. Unless otherwise mentioned, I will be discussing the use of these small microprocessor units in the schoolroom. As is true of many innovations, computers have enjoyed an onrush of enthusiasm, overoptimistic anticipations regarding their value, the resistance and even the fear with which all new approaches are met, the backlash resulting from the inevitable disillusionment, and a variety of other reactions that shift the pendulum back and forth regarding their acceptance and use. These vicissitudes notwithstanding, most educators agree that we have reached the point of no return, that computers are finding their place, and that they are very much here to stay.

THE CAPACITY OF THE COMPUTER TO ENHANCE EDUCATIONAL MOTIVATION

The computer's capacity to enhance the child's motivation to learn is well known and is one of the strongest arguments given for its utilization in the classroom. There are a number of ways this happens.

Fun. The game approach to learning is likely to be successful in that it involves the element of fun. Accordingly, computer-assisted instruction (CAI) may represent a significant breakthrough in the educational process. It is not that teachers were not previously aware of this factor; it is only that we now have an instrument that is predictably able to provide more fun more consistently than previous methods. In addition, no human being can keep up a level of fun as persistently and as predictably as a computer. Even the most dedicated teachers are at times in a bad mood, and at that point, their educational value can be compromised. The computer is always in the mood to offer its educational program. In addition, the computer's ability to combine graphics, color, music, and voice in an optimum fashion can also enhance the child's enjoyment of the lesson.

Challenge. Malone[17] points out that the properly programmed computer can sensitively monitor the response of each child and create an individualized hierarchy of challenges that a teacher is not likely to offer. The computer can keep the challenge at just the proper level to increase the likelihood of ongoing interest. Motivation is reduced when challenge becomes either too great or too little. The concept of challenge includes not only a goal, but uncertainty about its outcome. If the child knows the outcome in advance with certainty, or if the goal is too easy, the challenge is reduced. Self-esteem is closely tied up with success in meeting a challenge. Perkins[20] points out that each level of challenge can be carefully delineated and mastered. This produces immediate success, which in turn enhances self-esteem and motivation.

Fantasy. Computer programs can introduce a fantasy element, especially when the educational instrument takes on a gamelike quality. To do this, animals, figurines, and a wide variety of appealing creatures are used. Fantasy is enriching, it is pleasurable, and it thereby increases motivation. The program can enhance curiosity by including variety and surprise. Of course, teachers can do this as well, but computers have prodigious memories and may thus have a greater storehouse and repertoire of such surprises available in their programs.

Esteem Enhancement. The educational computer alerts the child to the error at the very moment it is being made. This reduces the likelihood of frustration and increases the probability of feelings of success. Related to self-esteem is the element of control that the computer provides. CAI is a much more active process than learning from a textbook or even from a teacher. There is a give-and-take that absorbs the child; this sense of control enhances self-esteem. Malone[17] points out that with the computer, the players can control the fantasy, the level of difficulty, the choice of topic, and even the outcome or the alternatives. One cannot do this with a book. The student's decisions are an important determinant of what comes thereafter. Furthermore, the computer's "voice" is intended to be benevolent and accepting. It is never harsh or critical, it never gets irritable, and it never ever yells at the child. Thus the child is protected from the ego-debasing results of these common teacher reactions. In fact, it is reasonable to say that no teacher can ever be as patient as a computer. The instrument never gets tired and will tolerate the same mistakes endlessly, offering its corrections with the same good humor and the same precision. Such saintlike patience is never seen in a human being.

Interaction. Related to control is interaction. There is an active involvement between the child and the computer, almost to the point of a human involvement. This give-and-take enhances motivation. Some programs actually "speak" to the child. The requirements for frequent responses and choices shift each player from a passive role to one of active participation; this serves to enhance attention, concentration, and interaction. With some devices keyboards are not used; instead the whole unit is held by the child, which further enhances involvement and interaction.

USES OF THE COMPUTER IN THE EDUCATIONAL PROCESS

Computers are much more expensive than books. In order to justify their cost, their proponents must demonstrate compellingly that computers can do things that books and teachers cannot do or, at least, are unable to do as well. This is a crucial question, and it is often asked by the more conservative educators who take issue with those who have embraced the use of computers in education in what they consider to be an exaggerated and overenthusiastic way.

Individualized Instruction. The computer can provide a degree of individualized instruction that far surpasses the kind of teaching that any single teacher can offer. It can truly be adapted to each student's individual interests and level. By instruction through complex, multilevel branching programs, a student is given access to information both horizontally and vertically. The program can go into any direction at any place and to whatever depth the student wants to take it. Even within a particular area, the computer can provide different types of learning experiences. For example, it can emphasize graphics, or the written word, or even auditory learning. It is capable of providing the same information in different formats: didactic, allegorical, logical sequencing of yes/no answers, and so on. The organization of the material allows the child to move ahead at his or her own pace in a way that is not possible when a teacher teaches a classroom of children. Even when the class is divided into subgroups working at different levels, there are individual variations within each group that cannot be handled by a teacher.

The computer can also be used to save the student the time it would take to read material that he or she might already know. If, when reading a book, one wishes to skip over material one suspects one already knows, there is still a scanning process necessary and, inadvertently, one may skip information that one does not know. Computer program questions can take this into account. For example, a question can be asked and the student responds. The computer will indicate whether or not the answer is correct and, if it is, will then ask whether or not the student wishes a further explanation. If the student says yes, then more material is provided. If the student says no, then he or she can go on to the next question. If, however, the answer is wrong, the student might be given a second guess. And if the answer is wrong once again, the assumption is made that the student will want to know both the source of the error and how to correct it. Accordingly, the explanation is automatically provided. This arrangement offers the student the opportunity to learn about the *nature* of his or her errors. In order to do the same thing, a book would have to describe each of the possible errors; much space would be taken up. The computer can bring to the screen the information relevant to just that error the particular student has made.

Immediate Positive Feedback. When a student takes a written examination, there is usually a time lag between when the test is returned to the teacher and when the student learns which questions were answered incorrectly. With the computer, there is immediate recognition of whether one is right or wrong, and the positive and negative feedback are thus given immediately. The response is provided exactly when there is the greatest curiosity about whether one's answer was correct. As a result, there is a greater likelihood that the student will learn.

The Word Processor. The word processor may prove to be one of the most widespread and useful ways in which computers are used in the educational process. It is basically a typewriter with a screen on which the typewritten letters are immediately displayed. Attached is a printer that enables the student to print what has been typed. One of its greatest advantages over traditional typewriters is the ease with which corrections are made. Errors can be deleted immediately without laborious erasing. Words and paragraphs can be shifted into new places at the touch of a few keys. It makes writing a game. Many children who viewed writing compositions as a tedious bore may now vie with one another for the utilization of the word processor.

Asbell[1] points out that since the 1930s, over six hundred studies have demonstrated that children learn better with typewriters. The typewriter enables them to avoid the labor of pencil-and-paper writing. She believes that the failure of educational systems to utilize typewriters has been unfortunate. In order to avoid the extra expenditure of purchasing typewriters, generations of children have been deprived of a powerful tool for easy writing. The struggle to write with pencil and paper at an age when this may be difficult has soured millions of children on writing and compromised their education. The computer not only makes writing even easier and more pleasurable than the typewriter, but adds other benefits the typewriter lacks. It offers the visual screen, visual and auditory positive feedback, graphics, easy opportunity for correction of errors, and greater speed.

Asbell also describes the pioneering work of Dr. John Henry Martin, a former school superintendent in Mount Vernon, New York, who has introduced a method of teaching reading he calls "Writing to Read." Rather than following the traditional method in which children learn to read first and then write, he reverses the sequence and teaches children first how to write the phonemes with which they are already familiar on the basis of their knowledge of verbal language. Once the children have mastered ten of the forty-two phonemes in the English language, they are encouraged to write their own words. Both visually and auditorily the computer teaches the child to tap the letter or letters that corresponds to each of the phonemes in a word. Children are happy to convert their thoughts into written words, and, with the help of the computer, they get the immediate feedback of seeing what they have written on the screen. Without the restriction of having to compare their spelling with a standard, they are much more likely to enjoy the thrill of quick transition of their verbal language into written form. Afterward, they usually learn quickly the necessary revisions to correct their spelling. There is every indication that this method will enhance early reading and provide children with the many psychological benefits to be derived from such early opportunity to learn about the world.

Drill and Practice. One of the simplest and most common uses of the computer is for drill and practice. It can be used alone for this purpose or as a supplement to other forms of instructional material such as a workbook. Budoff and Hutten[3] claim that computers are more efficient than workbooks for this purpose. Computers provide immediate feedback and can free the teacher for other forms of instruction. The associated programs generally employ a highly rigid format. Searles[25] claims that because computers increase students' efficiency and learning speed at the drill-and-practice level, they have more time to spend on higher intellectual levels of study, including analysis, synthesis, and judgment.

Tutorial Teaching. In tutorial teaching the student moves from one step to the next by answering questions. These may be branched to remedial or review sections as well as to more advanced levels, depending on the student's performance throughout the tutorial. Tutorial instruction is less formal and rigid than drill and practice.

Problem Solving. Problem-solving programs were developed to help children become problem developers and problem solvers. They teach children conceptualizations and abstractions as well as higher levels of sophisticated cognitive thinking. Problem-solving programs have been utilized with medical students to teach diagnosis. A student gives the computer the patient's presenting symptoms and then an interchange takes place between the student and the computer, the final goal of which is to provide the student with a diagnosis. On the basis of the presenting symptoms, the computer can select the most likely diseases that the patient might have. It then might ask for the results of certain laboratory tests, and, when these are provided, the diagnosis can be further defined. As the years go by the data bank for such diagnoses is rapidly expanding, making the information more accurate. Such computer learning is not only useful in medical education but for practicing physicians as well.

Simulations. Simulation provides the student with the opportunity to learn a complex task in a dynamic fashion. For example, pilots can be taught to fly air-

planes from simulated cockpits. The computer introduces many if not all of the variables that would be encountered in an actual flight situation. However, the techniques and skills developed with the simulated computer cockpit offer a much safer way to learn, especially for the beginner. Just as simulated cockpits help pilots learn how to fly, simulated road conditions can help students learn how to drive. Businesses use simulated business problems that require consideration of multiple, dynamic factors that may affect price, demand, sales, and so on. The simulated computer experience much more closely approximates what one experiences in real life than does any textbook description. Recently the National Board of Medical Examiners announced that beginning in 1987, certain sections of their medical licensing examinations will be conducted with computers. Their Computer-Based Teaching (CBX) program will utilize simulated "patients" with whom the testee will interact for the purposes of diagnosis and treatment. The testee must initiate all diagnostic and therapeutic choices and then must manage the consequences of these choices.

Computerized Data Banks. Computer-based resource units have also proved useful in the educational process. They circumvent the laborious task of searching in libraries through books and other documents. The student can have direct access to a wealth of data and need not go through the hunting process. Unfortunately, my own personal experience with such data banks has been that the individuals who are programming the material are often naive about the subject matter. Accordingly, their categorizations are often inaccurate and include irrelevant material. More than that, I am sure that significant material is lost as well because it was not filed under the proper category. However, another factor that contributes to such errors is that, in certain cases, the computers may not be sophisticated enough to make the proper selections or to differentiate between terms. Probably the most commonly utilized data bank in medicine is Medline. Attorneys are finding Lexis Nexis to be extremely valuable in researching the legal literature. Data banks on drug side effects as well as computerized information on antidotes to poisons are increasingly useful to physicians. There are data banks for prescriptions as well, and these lead readily to identifying drug abusers who manage to obtain prescriptions from a number of physicians simultaneously.

Programming. It is important for the reader to appreciate that none of the aforementioned uses of the computer require any knowledge of computer languages or programming on the part of the user. Programming is generally done by others, and even knowledge of computer language is becoming progressively less necessary for its utilization. The term computer language generally refers to the intermediary language between the language employed by the user and the basic electronic language of the computer. This machine language is usually referred to as bits (contraction of "binary digit"—the smallest unit of information in a computer: zero or one, on or off) and bytes (8 bits, enough to store any conventional character, e.g., numbers and letters). BASIC, FORTRAN, and PASCAL are three commonly utilized computer languages. The intermediary languages increase the efficiency of communication between the user and the basic electronic systems that do the computer's work. Studying computer languages and programming is certainly worthwhile, but only a small fraction of those who use computers are knowledgeable in these areas. However, learning how to program expands one's capacity to utilize the computer. Furthermore, programming can be a useful intellectual exercise, one that has educational value in its own right, especially with regard to learning logical reasoning. Seidman[26] confirmed this in a study in which he demonstrated that learning the LOGO language (a language commonly used for educational computers) enhanced children's reasoning capacity.

THE DRAWBACKS OF COMPUTER-ASSISTED INSTRUCTION

As is true for all innovations, only time and experience will provide us with accurate information regarding both the advantages and disadvantages of CAI. At the present time an obvious drawback is the expense of the equipment. Accordingly, it is still available only to a small percentage of the school population. However, there is good reason to believe that within a few years prices of both equipment and software will come down to a level where most students in the United States should have access to this equipment. Another problem at this time is the expense of creating programs for subjects like English and social studies as well as designing full courses, especially at the higher grade levels. The expense of formulating such programs is so great that there are very few programs available in these categories. Accordingly, most of the programs that have been created for CAI are for drilling purposes at the lower grade levels. Hence even though the price of the equipment will be less, the software problem is not going to be resolved quickly. Perhaps more efficient programming techniques might provide the answer.

The computer does not involve the human element in education. An important factor in the educational process is the child's identification with and emulation of a teacher. One of the reasons why children learn is that they want to gain the approval and respect of an admired mentor. They want to join in the fun of learning in order to gain the gratifications that the teacher is offering. Although to some extent this may be possible with a computer, it is obviously limited to a significant degree. Furthermore, teachers who are more committed and involved generally do not rely upon the computer as much as those who are less gifted. In fact, the less committed teacher may resort to computer utilization as a way of avoiding his or her teaching responsibilities, and indeed, this is one of the computer's grave dangers. It is reasonable to say that no matter how advanced computers may become, no matter how efficient, they are still machines and will never substitute completely for teachers in the educational process. Even the use of video discs, wherein teachers are portrayed on a screen, does not substitute for a real interacting human being.

For the most part, CAI is an asocial educational experience. There are few group activities involved in its utilization; cooperation and the development of interpersonal relationships do not occur to a significant extent. Computers probably contribute to children becoming undersocialized. One does not learn from others with the computer; one learns from a machine. In some families all family members spend a significant amount of time *separately* at their respective computers. Although they are all brought together by this common interest, they are all isolated from one another as well. The computer is therefore a mixed blessing. Because the obsession with computers is so widespread at this point, this phenomenon is also ubiquitous.

One often-quoted advantage of CAI is that the machine has "infinite patience and tolerance." Although this may be a virtue for the child who is normal or above average in intelligence, such tolerance for error may not be to the advantage of the slow learner, the minimally brain damaged child, or the retarded child. One could argue that such a child might be more motivated by some impatience and some intolerance from time to time, that complete patience and acceptance of error may not motivate that child to learn. No one would claim that impatience to the point of producing fear is desirable, but perhaps a slight degree of impatience could serve as a motivating factor. The machine will tolerate high error rates, and the poor student does not get the feeling that there are negative consequences to being continuously wrong. However, there may be some consequences in that the teacher can be apprised of the student's poor performance. A related phenomenon is the dependency element. Just as calculators circumvent the child's need to learn how to calculate, a computer can circumvent the necessity of the child's learning how to perform a variety of other functions. Programs that scan the material for incorrect spelling may reduce the child's motivation to learn how to spell correctly. This is a definite compromise in the educational process.

Perkins[20] raises the question as to whether the rewards provided by CAI might contaminate the educational process in that the child will learn for the sake of the rewards rather than for the intrinsic joy of learning. This, of course, is the same danger we have with grades in the traditional educational programs. I do not believe that this will prove to be a significant drawback. Many of the programs do not provide any rewards at the higher levels, and even those provided at the lower levels are, I believe, small compared to the fun and challenge elements.

Perkins also raises the question as to whether material learned on a computer can easily be transferred into real-world situations. He suspects that there might be some contextual welding in which the skill becomes "welded" to accidental features of the learning context. This "extra baggage" might impede transfer of learning from experience with the computer to encounter with the real world and might even contaminate it. Again, whether this phenomenon will prove to be a contaminant remains to be seen.

Another drawback to CAI is that it does not examine exactly *how* the student came upon a correct answer. It can only assess whether the answer is right or wrong, true or false. It does not allow for "wrong" answers that might in themselves be creative. Here it is likely that the computer will never supplant the human being.

Computer-Assisted Instruction for the Disabled

Considering the promise that CAI has shown for the education of normal children, it is not surprising that its application in the education of disabled children has also been explored. The results are promising, and we have good reason to believe that this methodology will become an intrinsic part of the education of such children. However, only with time and experience will we know exactly how important a part CAI will play in the education of these children.

LEARNING-DISABLED CHILDREN

Even the most hyperactive children and those with severe attentional deficits generally have no problem concentrating for long periods on their favorite television programs. The television screen appears to be a powerful motivator of attention, and this principle should prove useful in helping learning-disabled (LD) children attend to academic material. CAI appears to be well fitted to this task.

Especially because of their anticipation of failure, LD children often have severe motivational problems. It is reasonable to hope that the special attractions of the computer might offset this motivation-reducing element. In addition, CAI enhances the efficiency of learning, and this factor might also improve LD children's motivation. Torgeson and Young[30] found CAI to enhance children's attention as well as improve their motivation to drill and practice. Lynch[16] also found computers useful in the education of brain-injured adult patients, especially those with language disabilities.

Lally[15] used a talking computer to teach mildly retarded children how to read. The computer displayed a word and simultaneously "spoke" it verbally. It also gave the children positive reinforcement ("that's right") every time they were able to respond correctly to the computer's requests. A group who learned to speak a selected set of words with the aid of a speaking computer did significantly better than a group who learned without it.

Budoff and Hutten[3] point out that when CAI is used for LD children, teachers must be trained to provide specially tailored programs for each child. General programs for such children have not yet been developed to a significant degree. The differences between LD children are greater than the differences among normal children. CAI learning can also decrease the reliance on tutors who are frequently used to supplement the education of LD children. Cartwright, Cartwright, and Robine[5] found that teachers being trained to provide special education for LD students learned more quickly and more efficiently with CAI learning than did a control group utilizing traditional tutorial methods.

CEREBRAL-PALSIED AND OTHER PHYSICALLY HANDICAPPED CHILDREN

Foulds[9] described the value of CAI for physically handicapped children. Because of their handicaps, many of these children cannot write easily. The computer enabled them to do legible work with ease and increased the likelihood that they could be mainstreamed. With regard to writing, they then become equal to the nonphysically handicapped. Children with muscular dystrophy have trouble writing because of easy fatigue. The word processor can circumvent this problem. Some cerebral-palsied children cannot type in the traditional fashion. With the word processor, they can use single push-button switches that select items from displays on the screen. In addition, the word processor allows for easy correction of errors, an especially valuable asset for disabled people who would have difficulty utilizing correcting devices, such as fluids, tape, cartridges, and erasers.

Severely handicapped individuals can use voice activation of the keys. The computer can even be programmed to recognize the atypical pronunciations and accents of dysarthric children.

DEAF CHILDREN

Parkhurst and MacEachron[19] have used computers to analyze the written language of deaf children. The child types sentences into the computer and observes the product on the display screen. The computer proceeds to analyze the sentence and identifies any errors. The child is then visually instructed to correct the erroneous part of the sentence. The machine thus teaches as well as analyzes. CAI is particularly useful for deaf children because it allows for greater input via the visual mode. Prinz, Nelson, and Stedt[21] were able to use a microcomputer system to help teach two- to six-year-old deaf children to read. They combined vocabulary words with animation and color graphics that interested the children and increased the likelihood of their learning. Foulds[9] also used computers in the education of children who were hearing impaired but not completely deaf. The child would type in the word, and the computer would speak it with the correct pronunciation.

CAI LEARNING FOR OTHER DISABLED CHILDREN

Roe[23] found CAI learning useful for children from disadvantaged neighborhoods who had lost many years of education. The enhanced motivational attraction of the computer increased their learning efficiency and capacity. Haberman[12] provided CAI instruction to a group of socially/emotionally disturbed children and compared their performance with a control group that had received only standard classroom instruction. The CAI group did significantly better. Weir[31] found CAI learning useful in the education of autistic children. Saracho[24] found CAI useful in teaching English to Spanish-speaking migrant children. The experimental group learned English much better than did the control group who received traditional instruction. However, the control group expressed attitudes toward CAI that were more favorable than those of the students who were actually receiving the computerized instruction.

The Future

Many of the computers that are currently used by schools are quite expensive, but it is reasonable to assume that they will drop in cost to the point where practically every student can afford one. Furthermore, the machines are likely to diminish in size (possibly until they are as small as hand calculators) to the point where every student can carry one. Dusewicz[8] states: "Tiny and inexpensive computers and related microelectronic devices may well replace the paper and pencil as the principal tools in the classroom."

There is every reason to believe that, with the aid of computers, people will be working increasingly within their own homes. Considering the waste of time and energy involved in commuting, this certainly makes sense. We are beginning to see a parallel phenomenon take place with regard to children being educated in their homes with the aid of computers. Parents who are dissatisfied with local school facilities now have an option with the home computer. Wollman[34] quotes studies that estimated that 10,000 to 20,000 nondisabled youngsters and 250,000 disabled youngsters were being taught at home. Local school boards have to approve of the home program and agree that it is equivalent to that which is provided in the public school. Generally they are becoming increasingly receptive to such education. The success of such programs, of course, depends on the reliability of parental monitoring. However, since the adults will be working at home more frequently, they will certainly be more available for such supervision. The question is whether they can be uniformly relied on to provide the necessary monitoring. Probably some parents will be capable while others will not be. The problem then will be one of deciding which parents can be relied on and which not and who is to make such decisions. With children spending more time at home, it is possible that parent-child relationships will improve. However, it is also possible that each will spend increasingly more time at his or her own computer. And there is also the possibility that neither will spend much time on educational programs but will devote time instead to computer games. Finally there is always the possibility that all family members will lose interest in the computer and revert back to the old television set.

At present, it is the affluent children who have these games at home; the poor do not. Accordingly, computers may be increasing the gap between the poor and the wealthy. There is no question, however, that if these instruments become widely utilized in poorer schools, poor children are more likely to learn more efficiently.

One of the next steps in education may well be the video disc. Such discs, each costing only about $10, can be programmed to have as much information as one hundred books. Not only would the discs provide information, but they enable the viewer to observe projections from various angles and different vantage points. They could provide visual branching—for example, a child could decide which room of a museum to enter and which pictures to view, and then be given appropriate, descriptive information. The only limitations would be the data programmed onto the disc. The computer has the capability and flexibility to create new types of music and art that were not previously possible; conceivably, this could contribute to even greater artistic creativity.

However, computers have also been used for purposes that cannot but be detrimental. An absurd use of computers is the well-known ELIZA program developed by Joseph Weizenbaum,[32] which purports to provide Rogerian psychotherapy. This is a *reductio ad absurdum* of therapy. Unfortunately, both Weizenbaum and others have taken the program seriously. Intelligent teenagers with an antisocial bent can use computers to penetrate the private networks of government and industry. One group of teenagers penetrated the computer of the Sloan-Kettering Institute in New York City and altered medication dosages being given to seriously ill patients. In 1983 this computer "hacking" was dramatized in the movie *War Games,* which depicted a teenager accessing the computer at his school in order to alter grades and then almost starting a thermonuclear war when he gained entry into a high-level military computer system.

One of the main advantages of the computer is that it is a time saver. It enables us to do things much more efficiently and rapidly. If the children of today are like their parents, they are not likely to use the time that they save for leisurely and more meaningful human involvement. They will probably use the same time to take on increased tasks and do each one more efficiently. Woolley[35] makes the point quite well:

Most of the mechanical and electronic inventions during the past century have been intended to help us get our work done faster and with less strain on our muscles. . . . Much human ingenuity has gone into freeing us from as much labor as possible, so that we might have time for more enjoyable and more rewarding pursuits . . . but it hasn't worked out that way for most of us as the machines have telescoped work time, they have also increased the number of tasks that the people who use them must do. (p. 7)

The computer is just the latest in a series of inventions. There is no question that it has the capability of removing people even further from one another, but it is also true that it has many mind-expanding capabilities and a potential for adding significantly to human pleasure. The children of today have been born into a computer world they cannot avoid. Whether or not they will be better off for this experience remains to be seen.

REFERENCES

1. ASBELL, B. "Writers' Workshop at Age V," *New York Times Magazine,* 26 February 1984, pp. 55ff.

2. BROOKS, D. "Video Games and Social Behavior," in S. S. Baughman and P. D. Clagett, eds., *Video Games and Human Development.* Cambridge, Mass.: Harvard Graduate School of Education, 1983, pp. 14–16.

3. BUDOFF, M., and HUTTEN, L. R. "Microcomputers in Special Education: Promises and Pitfalls," *Exceptional Children,* 49 (1982):123–128.

4. CACHA, F. "Glamorizing and Legitimizing Violence in Software: A Misuse of the Computer," *Educational Technology,* 23 (1983):25–30.

5. CARTWRIGHT, C. A., CARTWRIGHT, G. P., and ROBINE, G. G. "CAI Course in the Early Identification of Handicapped Children," *Journal of Exceptional Children,* 38 (1972):453–459.

6. "Computer-Based Testing," *National Board Examiner,* 31(1984):1–2.

7. DONCHIN, E. "Video Games in Medical Rehabilitation and Learning," in S. S. Baughman and P. D. Clagett, eds., *Video Games and Human Development.* Cambridge, Mass.: Harvard Graduate School of Education, 1983, pp. 30–32.

8. DUSEWICZ, R. A. "Technology in the Education of Young Children," in M. Frank, ed., *Young Children in a Computerized Environment.* New York: Haworth Press, 1982, pp. 3–14.

9. FOULDS, R. A. "Applications of Microcomputers in the Education of the Physically Disabled Child," *Exceptional Children,* 49 (1982):155–162.

10. GARDNER, R. A. *Understanding Children—A Parents' Guide to Child Rearing.* Cresskill, N.J.: Creative Therapeutics, 1973.

11. GREENFIELD, P. "Video Games and Cognitive Skills," in S. S. Baughman and P. D. Clagett, eds., *Video Games and Human Development.* Cambridge, Mass.: Harvard Graduate School of Education, 1983, pp. 19–24.

12. HABERMAN, E. L. "Effectiveness of Computer Assisted Instruction with Socially/Emotionally Disturbed Children," *Dissertation Abstracts International,* 38 (1977):1998–1999.

13. KEGAN, R. G. "Donkey Kong, Pac Man and the Meaning of Life: Reflections in River City," in S. S. Baughman and P. D. Clagett, eds., *Video Games and Human Development.* Cambridge, Mass.: Harvard Graduate School of Education, 1983, pp. 4–7.

14. KOHL, H. "Video Games and Formal Education," in S. S. Baughman and P. D. Clagett, eds., *Video Games and Human Development.* Cambridge, Mass.: Harvard Graduate School of Education, 1983, pp. 47–52.

15. LALLY, M. "Computer-Assisted Teaching of Sight-Word Recognition for Mentally Retarded School Children," *American Journal of Mental Deficiency,* 85 (1981):383–388.

16. LYNCH, W. J. "Video Games in Medical Rehabilitation and Learning," in S. S. Baughman and P. D. Clagett, *Video Games and Human Development.* Cambridge, Mass.: Harvard Graduate School of Education, 1983, pp. 25–28.

17. MALONE, T. W. "What Makes Things Fun to Learn?" in S. S. Baughman and P. D. Clagett, eds., *Video Games and Human Development.* Cambridge, Mass.: Harvard Graduate School of Education, 1983, pp. 49–52.

18. MITCHELL, E. "Video Games and Social Behavior," in S. S. Baughman and P. D. Clagett, eds., *Video Games and Human Development.* Cambridge, Mass.: Harvard Graduate School of Education, 1983, pp. 11–14.

19. PARKHURST, B. G., and MacEachron, M. P. "Computer-Assisted Analysis of Written Language: Assessing the Written Language of Deaf Children: II," *Journal of Communication Disorders,* 13 (1980):493–504.

20. PERKINS, D. N. "Video Games and Informal Settings," in S. S. Baughman and P. D. Clagett, eds., *Video Games and Human Development.* Cambridge, Mass.: Harvard Graduate School of Education, 1983, pp. 33–40.

21. PRINZ, P. M., NELSON, K. E., and STEDT, J. D. "Reading in Young Deaf Children Using Microcomputer Technology," *American Annals of the Deaf,* 127 (1982):529–535.

22. RIZZA, P. J. "Computer Based Education (CBE): Tomorrow's Traditional System," in M. Frank, ed., *Young Children in a Computerized Environment.* New York: Haworth Press, 1982, pp. 29–42.

23. ROE, M. "Living with the Computer," *New York* magazine, 9 January 1984, pp. 23–31.

24. SARACHO, O. N. "The Effects of a Computer-Assisted Instruction Program on Basic Skills Achievement and Attitudes Toward Instruction of Spanish-Speaking Migrant Children," *American Educational Research Journal,* 19 (1982): 201–219.

25. SEARLES, J. E. "Computer Based Education in the Age of Narcissism," in M. Frank, ed., *Young Children in a Computerized Environment.* New York: Haworth Press, 1982, pp. 89–96.

26. SEIDMAN, R. H. "The Effects of Learning the LOGO Computer Programming Language on Conditional Reasoning in School Children," *Dissertation Abstracts International,* 41 (1980):2249.

27. SLABY, E. G. "Video Games and Social Behavior," in S. S. Baughman and P. D. Clagett, eds., *Video Games and Human Development.* Cambridge, Mass.: Harvard Graduate School of Education, 1983, pp. 8–9.

28. SMITH, P. "The Impact of Computerization on Children's Toys and Games," in M. Frank, ed., *Young Children in a Computerized Environment.* New York: Haworth Press, 1982, pp. 73–82.

29. STONE, A. "Video Games and Social Behavior," in S. S. Baughman and P. D. Clagett, eds., *Video Games and Human Development.* Cambridge, Mass.: Harvard Graduate School of Education, 1983, pp. 16–18.

30. TORGESEN, J. K., and YOUNG, K. A. "Priorities for the Use of Microcomputers with Learning Disabled Children," *Journal of Learning Disabilities,* 16 (1983):234–237.

31. WEIR, S. "Video Games in Medical Rehabilitation and Learning," in S. S. Baughman and P. D. Clagett, eds., *Video Games and Human Development.* Cambridge, Mass.: Harvard Graduate School of Education, 1983, pp. 28–32.

32. WEIZENBAUM, J. "ELIZA—A Computer Program for the Study of Natural Language Communication Between Man and Machine," *Communications of the Association for Computing Machinery,* 9 (1966):36–45.

33. ———. "Contextual Understanding by Computers," *Communications of the Association for Computing Machinery,* 10 (1967):474–480.

34. WOLLMAN, J. "Teaching at Home with Help of Computers," *New York Times,* 9 February 1984, pp. C1ff.

35. WOOLLEY, B. "Modern Man Joins Mad Hatter in Race with Clock," *Sunday Express-News* (San Antonio, Texas), 27 February 1983, p. F7.

71 / Child Custody

Richard A. Gardner

Introduction

In recent years the joint custodial concept has enjoyed increasing popularity. For the author, the term joint custody implies a custodial arrangement that attempts to approximate as closely as possible the flexibility in the original two-parent home. In such an arrangement, both parents have equal rights and responsibilities for their children's upbringing, and neither party's rights are superior. Neither parent is designated as the sole or primary parent. There is no structured visitation schedule; the children live in both homes. They do not live in one home and visit the other. Some do use the term joint custody to refer to an arrangement in which there is a structured visitation schedule. Often the arrangement turns out to be one of the traditional custodial arrangements but is given the name joint custody to provide a specious sense of egalitarianism between the parents when there is in fact none or very little.

The joint custodial idea is literally "sweeping the nation." At this point almost every state has either passed legislation in which the joint custody concept, in one form or another, is incorporated or has seriously considered the passage of such statutes. Unfortunately, this practice is often recommended indiscriminately. There are even states in which the judge is required to order a joint custodial arrangement for all divorcing parents unless there are compelling reasons for ordering some other arrangement. It is important for professionals involved in such decisions to be able to distinguish the types of parents for whom the arrangement can be beneficial from those for whom it would be detrimental.[6]

Advantages of Joint Custody

Of all the existing custodial arrangements, joint custody most closely approximates the original marital household. It is free from artificial schedules that are totally unrelated to the vicissitudes of life. There is a free flow of involvement with both parents—obviously a more natural life-style. This offers children (especially older ones) more input into what happens to them, and they are less likely to suffer from the sense of impotence that can be created by the strict schedules of a primary custodial arrangement.

In the primary custodial arrangement, one parent is placed in a position of authority over the other. This inevitably produces resentment. A visiting father whose former wife has primary custody is likely to resent the fact that while he is the primary (if not total) child-support contributor, his access to the children is significantly restricted. In joint custody, however, such a father may feel more motivated to contribute to his children's support. Joint custody also reduces the possibility of the father being viewed as the bearer of gifts and "director of the recreational program" while the mother is viewed as the disciplinarian and child rearer. In joint custody, both parents generally play both roles. Each parent is protected against the terrible sense of loss that the noncustodial parent may feel in the primary custodial arrangement. If, after litigation, one parent has been awarded primary custody, the other parent cannot but feel that he or she has been judged the worse or at least the less adequate parent. This ego-debasing experience is less likely to occur with joint custody.

The Disadvantages of Joint Custody

Joint custody decisions enable judges to avoid a complex and difficult fact-finding task by offering a seemingly benevolent resolution. It certainly is easier for a

judge to award joint custody than to deliberate over all the ambiguous and contradictory "facts" involved in a custody conflict. And judges who circumvent such challenges often justify their actions by considering themselves advanced and modern thinkers. There are some who hold that joint custody has become a judicial "copout"—an arrangement that allows judges to appear egalitarian and benevolent without having to think through the implications of what they are doing. The main drawback to granting joint custody so routinely and indiscriminately is that it may do many children more harm than good. For example, it increases the chances that they will be used as weapons or spies in parental conflicts. Certainly primary custody arrangements cannot protect children from this behavior, but its structure does reduce the opportunities for parents to involve their children in such manipulations. Furthermore, automatic awarding of joint custody seldom takes into consideration the logistics of school attendance. Accordingly, it can cause problems in the educational realm as well.

Another frequent criticism of joint custody is that it may be confusing for a child to be shuttled between two homes—especially when each offers different life-styles, disciplinary measures, rules, and even socioeconomic conditions. Its critics claim that having two homes can give a child a sense of unpredictability and a lack of environmental continuity. This is probably not detrimental to children older than three or four. They generally can adjust well to such transfers, and even younger children are not necessarily harmed by them. What is more important is the nature of the parenting, not the rooms in which the parenting occurs. Even if a young child experiences some mild degree of psychological harm from environmental discontinuity, the disadvantages would be more than outweighed by the advantage of the child's having access to both parents in a less structured and less artificial arrangement. Elsewhere I have discussed various aspects of the joint custodial arrangement.[5,6]

Criteria for Recommending
Joint Custody

Joint custody is viable only when these provisions are satisfied:

1. Both parents are reasonably and equally capable of assuming the responsibilities of child rearing. When

there is a significant disparity between the parents in this area, another custodial arrangement should be considered.

2. The parents must have demonstrated their capacity to cooperate reasonably and meaningfully in matters pertaining to raising their children. They must show the ability to communicate well and be willing to compromise when necessary to ensure the viability of the arrangement.

3. The children's moving from home to home should not disrupt their school situation.

Recommending joint custody requires a certain amount of foresight. Although the first and third provisions may be satisfied by many parents involved in custody disputes, the second is not likely to be. The greater the friction and animosity, the less likely it is that the second requirement will be met.

The animosity between parents is often greatest at the time of their divorce; hence that may not be a good time to recommend a joint custodial arrangement. In general, if the two parents are fighting for primary custody, they are probably poor candidates for joint custody—although such a compromise may appear attractive. Unless one can reasonably predict that the hostilities will die down and cooperation will increase, joint custody should not be recommended. This problem can be prevented to some degree by making joint custodial arrangements temporary and finalizing them only after the parents have had an opportunity to demonstrate that they truly can handle them.

The adversary system may actually reduce parents' capacity to qualify for the joint custodial arrangement. It may worsen parental communication because messages are often relayed through intermediaries—the attorneys. Responses are delayed and the chances of inaccuracy increase. Furthermore, the adversary system tends to polarize parents even further and thereby reduces the likelihood of their cooperating with one another. Attorneys would do well, therefore, to schedule conferences at which both parents and attorneys attempt to reduce animosities and try to work out marital difficulties in a nonadversarial setting. Mediation (which is discussed later) may increase the likelihood that a joint custodial arrangement will be viable.

Basically, one cannot justifiably litigate for joint custody. The very act of litigating renders the claimant(s) an unlikely candidate for it. Sometimes one parent wants joint custody and the other wants sole custody. Occasionally the parent asking for joint custody really wants sole custody but recognizes that he or she is unlikely to obtain it; joint custody may then be proposed as a compromise. Joint custody is in fact a terrible compromise for warring parents. When recommended in such situations, what may actually result is a no-custody arrangement that is merely called joint custody. Neither parent has power or control, and the

children find themselves in a no-man's land exposed to their parents' crossfire and available to both as weapons. In such a situation the likelihood of children developing psychological problems is practically 100 percent.

When children are embroiled in such a no-custody battle, one of the most common ensuing problems arises from their desire to ingratiate themselves with each of the parents. Commonly children will start to lie and tell each parent what they believe will win them favor. Children appear to "know where their bread is buttered" and hope that by supporting each parent's position, they will gain love and affection. In this way they seek to protect themselves from the alienation they fear would follow should they express support for the rival spouse. Such children appear to think about only the immediate benefits of their fabrications and do not consider the long-range untoward effects. Vulnerable and gullible parents will even litigate over what they have been told.

Before the advent of the sex-blind statutes and the joint custody vogue, children and mothers knew that the likelihood of fathers obtaining custody was very small. Accordingly, such problems were far less common. Whatever the disadvantages of the "tender years presumption," it did provide a certain security about the permanence of custodial placement, which in turn lessened the likelihood of custody disputes and of embroiling children in them. Actually, many of the children who are brought into these adversarial confrontations handle it by lying. This happens so frequently that the youngsters lose sight of what their own desires are. They are so used to saying that which would curry favor with the particular parent with whom they are at the moment, and so fearful of saying that which might alienate, that they suppress and repress their own genuine desires. In such situations, the examiner may not be able to ascertain what the child's real preferences are, because the child him- or herself may no longer know what they are.

Not all parents who want custody of their children are motivated by deep love and affection. Specious reasons are often present. A mother, for example, may welcome a joint custodial arrangement because it gives her the opportunity to dump the children on the father more frequently, thereby allowing her to assume less responsibility for raising them. Vengeance can also be a motive. What better way to retaliate against a hated spouse than to deprive him or her of the children? A parent also may request joint custody in order to reduce shame or guilt over the fact that he or she does not want custody at all. Essentially, the parent would much prefer that the other parent have sole custody. Instead, he or she asks for joint custody, hoping that the other parent will assume the major responsibility.

Arguments for Not Providing Any Name at All to the Custodial Arrangement

The term joint custody is variously defined, not only by state statutes but by attorneys, mental health professionals, and clients. As a result, an element of confusion has been introduced—confusion that has resulted in unnecessary litigation and time wasted on irrelevancies. The result has been further expense and psychological trauma to clients, all of which could have been readily avoided.

Often the conflicts are semantic ones. The parties involved in discussing a potential joint custody arrangement may each have a different concept of the meaning of the term—a situation that will predictably cause confusion and waste time. Or attorneys will haggle over the definition of the term and/or whether a particular client's custodial arrangement warrants the designation. In such conflicts the parties become sidetracked into issues that may be basically irrelevant to the decision. Furthermore, what has traditionally been called sole custody may be given the name of joint custody because of the belief that such designation will protect the unfavored party from feelings of lowered self-worth. This may introduce an element of further confusion, especially among those who are reviewing the court rulings and possibly even using such rulings as established precedents.

I believe that the aforementioned problems concerning the joint custodial arrangement could be obviated in a relatively simple way. The semantic problem could be eliminated by strictly avoiding the utilization of *any* of the commonly used terms to refer to the various custodial arrangements previously described. I would recommend that all arrangements be subsumed under a general rubric such as residential and decision-making arrangement. This is essentially what we are concerning ourselves with. We want to decide where the children should be and what powers the parent with whom they are residing should have. All of the traditional terms are attempts to define a particular pattern for the children's residence and visitation and for parental decision-making powers. The use of this general term (or one like it) would enable us to avoid wasting time and energy in arguing over which type of custodial arrangement would be most applicable to a particular family. Rather, we should focus on the particular *substantive* considerations relevant to a given family.

One has to ascertain whether the parents are equally capable of parenting and whether they are equally available to assume parental obligations. One must determine whether they have demonstrated the capacity to cooperate well with one another and to communicate successfully. One has to ask about the feasibility of the child's moving freely back and forth between the two residences while attending the same school. When these issues have been explored, attention should be directed to the question of whether or not the individuals need a court-imposed schedule or whether they can be relied upon to utilize successfully a nonscheduled arrangement. Generally, people who are equally capable as parents and who can communicate and cooperate can be trusted to utilize a nonscheduled arrangement successfully for visitation and place of residence. Those who cannot may need a court-ordered schedule.

The next issue relates to decision-making powers. Are both individuals relatively equal with regard to decision-making capacity? If not generally equal, are there some areas in which one parent should be given priority? Simply to designate one parent as the only one to make primary decisions may not fit in well with the reality of the situation. Of course, considerations of cooperation and communication must also be attended to when deciding about decision-making powers.

The "Parental Alienation Syndrome"

Many children who have been exposed to or embroiled in custody conflicts exhibit manifestations of a psychiatric disturbance that I refer to as the parental alienation syndrome.[7] I have introduced this term to describe a disorder in which the child is obsessed with criticism and denigration of a parent—deprecation that is unwarranted and/or exaggerated. The view that such children are "brainwashed" is a narrow one. It implies that one parent is actively programming the child against the other in a systematic and consciously planned endeavor. While it includes the brainwashing component, the concept of the parental alienation syndrome is more inclusive. In my experience, the prevalence of this disorder has increased markedly. Indeed I see blatant manifestations of it in over 90 percent of the custody conflicts with which I have worked in recent years. I believe that at present it is more common than many of the childhood disorders listed in DSM-III.[1]

CLINICAL MANIFESTATIONS OF THE PARENTAL ALIENATION SYNDROME

Typically the child suffering with the parental alienation syndrome is obsessed with "hatred" of a parent.

(I placed the word hatred in quotes because, as will be discussed, there are still many loving feelings that are suppressed, repressed, or dealt with by reaction formation.) The child may speak of the hated parent with every vilification known and often without guilt or embarrassment over the utilization of the crudest profanities. The denigration of the parent often has the quality of a litany, a prepared speech. At the slightest prompting by a lawyer, judge, mental health professional, or other person involved in the litigation, the child will perform. Not only is there the rehearsed quality, but one can often detect specific phraseology that is not generally utilized by a child of that age. Rather, many terms are those used by the "loved" parent. (Again, "loved" is in quotations because hostility toward that parent may similarly be dealt with by suppression, repression, and reaction formation.)

For months and even years after they have occurred, the child may be preoccupied with minor altercations and indignities experienced in the relationship with the hated parent. These are obviously trivial; generally they are experiences that most children would forget within minutes or hours of their occurrence: "Sometimes he used to tell me to get his things"; "She used to say to me 'Don't interrupt' "; "He makes a lot of noise when he chews at the table." Often, when the examiner asks such children to provide other reasons for the hatred, reasons more compelling than the frivolous ones provided, the child appears to be searching for justifications. And often the loved parent will agree with the child that these professed reasons justify the ongoing animosity.

The professions of hatred are often directly proportional to the proximity of the loved parent. These reach their most extreme form when the loved parent is in the same room as the alienated one. When, however, the child is alone with the allegedly hated parent, he or she may exhibit anything from repeated expressions of hatred, to neutrality, to expressions of affection. Examiners who interview such children should appreciate the fact that the loved parent's proximity will act as an important determinant of what will be said. When seen alone, the child is likely to modify the litany in accordance with which parent is in the waiting room. And judges who see children in chambers do well to appreciate this important phenomenon.

The hatred of a parent often extends to that parent's complete extended family. Uncles, aunts, cousins, and grandparents with whom the child may have had close and meaningful relationships somehow, by extension from the hated parent, are viewed as similarly noxious. Greeting cards remain unanswered. Presents sent to the home remain unopened and even destroyed (usually in the presence of the loved parent). When these relatives call, the child will refuse to take the phone or

will hang up on the caller—sometimes with angry vilifications. (These are more likely to take place if the loved parent is within hearing distance of the conversation.) Here the child is even less capable of providing justifications for the animosity. But rationalizations may still be provided, usually even more absurd than those advanced to justify the hostility toward the hated parent. So great is the anger of such children that they become completely oblivious to the loss of pleasure that could have been derived from these extended family members and to the psychological deprivation they are bringing upon themselves. Again, the loved parent is typically unconcerned with the psychological effects on the child of such separation from relatives who previously provided important psychological input.

Another manifestation is the complete lack of ambivalence. All human relationships are ambivalent, and parent-child relationships are no exception. For these children "mixed feelings" have no place. The hated parent is "all bad" and the loved parent is "all good." When such children are asked to name both good and bad things about each parent, they typically will be able to provide a long list of criticisms of the hated parent but will generally not be able to think of one redeeming quality. The hated parent may have been actively involved in the earlier years of the child's life, and there may have been a deep bond created over many years. The hated parent may provide pictures that clearly demonstrate a joyful and deep relationship —a relationship characterized by significant affection, tenderness, and mutual pleasure. All this seems to have been forgotten. When the child is asked about such enjoyable events, he or she will usually rationalize them as having been forgotten, nonexistent, or feigned: "I really hated being with him then; I just smiled in the picture because he made me. He said he'd hit me if I didn't smile"; "She used to hit me to make me go to the zoo with her." This complete lack of ambivalence is a manifestation of the splitting and reaction formation processes and should make the examiner dubious about the depth of the professed animosity.

FACTORS THAT CONTRIBUTE TO THE
DEVELOPMENT OF THE PARENTAL
ALIENATION SYNDROME

There are two important reasons for the dramatic increase in the prevalence of the parental alienation syndrome. The first relates to the fact that since the mid- to late 1970s, courts have generally appreciated that the "tender years presumption" is basically sexist and that custodial determinations should be made on criteria relating to parenting capacity, regardless of a parent's sex. The second arose from the fact that in the late 1970s and early 1980s the concept of joint custody became ever more popular. Both of these developments have made children's custodial designations far more precarious and unpredictable. Accordingly, custodial parents are more frequently brainwashing their children, and the children themselves have joined forces with the custodial parent in order to produce what they consider to be the most stable arrangement. As mentioned, this syndrome should not be viewed as due simply to brainwashing—that is, the act of deliberately programming a child by one parent against the other in a systematic and consciously planned endeavor. Although this element is often present, it is important to appreciate that there are many other factors that are present as well. In fact, in some cases the brainwashing element may be minimal or even absent, and the disorder arises as the result of one or more of the other contributing factors.

"Brainwashing." At times brainwashing is overt and obvious. The loved parent enters upon a campaign of denigration of the other parent, which may be unrelenting. Under special circumstances the criticisms may even be delusional. However, the child comes to believe completely in the validity of these accusations. Sometimes the lack of contact with the hated parent facilitates the child's total acceptance of the loved parent's criticisms. Fear of rejection by the loved parent —who may be the only remaining parent to whom the child has access—facilitates the child's believing every word.

Subtle and Often Unconscious Programming. There are many ways in which parents may subtly and often unconsciously contribute to their child's alienation from the other parent. A parent may have read a book in which the common advice has been given: "Never criticize the absent parent to the child." A mother may use this advice by saying such things as: "There are things I could say about your father that would make your hair stand on end, but I'm not the kind of a person who criticizes a parent to her children." Or a mother, for example, who requires a father to park at a distance from the home and honk the horn rather than ring the doorbell is implicitly telling the child "The person in that car is a dangerous or undesirable individual, someone whom I would not want to ring the doorbell of my house, let alone enter—even to say hello." The parent who expresses neutrality regarding visitation is basically communicating criticism of the noncustodial parent. The healthy parent recognizes the importance of the children's contact with the noncustodial parent and encourages visitation, even when the child is "not in the mood." The healthy parent does not accept frivolous and inconsequential reasons for not visiting. Under the guise of neutrality, a parent can often foster and support alienation. Under this guise the parent is essentially communicating to the child

that the noncustodial parent is not in a position to provide enough affection, attention, and other positive input to make a missed visitation a loss of any consequence. Such a parent fails to appreciate this author's principle: "Neutrality is as much a position as being on either side."

Here are a few more examples of subtle programming. The father calls, the mother answers, they exchange a few amenities, and then mother calls the child to the phone. In another instance, the father calls, the mother says nothing but immediately becomes angry and says to the child with phone outstretched, "It's your father!" The implication here is that the individual on the phone is not even worthy of a little common courtesy. Even despised individuals who call generally will receive a few more amenities.

One father, the owner of a trucking company, often dealt brutally with truckers, union chiefs, and even underworld Mafia figures. He routinely carried a gun, a practice he considered to be vital to the survival of his company. He described numerous encounters with gangland figures with varying reputations for violence. His fearlessness in these situations was extraordinary. However, this same man claimed complete impotence when it came to forcing his somewhat underweight and scrawny ten-year-old daughter to visit his former wife. His professions of helplessness were often quite convincing to others, and when I pointed out to him the disparity between his ability to impose his opinion on others in the workplace as compared to his home, he still asserted that he had no power over his child.

One could argue that such hostility is common in the divorce situation and that such contributions to the child's alienation are inevitable. I cannot deny this. However, the disorder we are talking about here involves the child being obsessed with resentment above and beyond what might be warranted by the situation. It is this element that differentiates the child who might be justifiably alienated from the one who exhibits a syndrome that warrants a special designation.

Situational Factors. Often situational factors are conducive to the development of the disorder. Most parents know that in a custody conflict time is on the side of the custodial parent. They recognize that the longer the child remains with a particular parent, the greater the likelihood that the child will resist moving to the home of the other. Often adults find change of domicile to be anxiety provoking, and children are even more likely to be tense over such transfer. One way of dealing with such fear is to denigrate the noncustodial parent with a barrage of criticisms that justify the child's remaining in the present custodial home. Consider the case when a mother dies. Her parents— the maternal grandparents—may take over care of the children. Although at first the father may welcome their involvement, there are many cases on record of maternal grandparents litigating for child custody. The children may then develop significant resentment toward the father in order to ensure that they remain with the grandparents, whom the children have come to view as the preferable parents.

In one case with which I was involved, two girls developed this disorder. Their mother, with whom they were living, met a man who lived in Colorado. The father brought her to court in an attempt to restrain her from moving out of the state of New Jersey with the children. Previously there had been a good relationship with the father during visitation; now, however, as their mother became progressively more embroiled in the litigation, the girls gradually developed an increasing hatred toward him. It was clear that this disorder would not have arisen had the mother not met a man whom she wished to marry who lived far away.

Recently we are observing another phenomenon that is contributing to the development of the parental alienation syndrome—the widespread attention being given to the sexual abuse of children by parents. Heretofore, the general consensus among those who work with sexually abused children was that it was extremely rare for a child to accuse a parent falsely of sexually abusing him or her. One reason for this was that children do not routinely have experiences that enable them to describe sexual acts in detail. Children who are able to do so were likely to have had such encounters. However, although child sexual abuse is certainly common, we are now seeing an increase in children's fabricating such experiences. A child's accusation of a parent's sexual abuse has become a powerful weapon in the alienation campaign. A vengeful parent may exaggerate a nonexistent or inconsequential sexual contact and build up a case for sexual abuse—even to the point of reporting the alleged child abuser to investigatory authorities and taking legal action. And the child, in order to ingratiate him- or herself with the litigious parent, may go along with the scheme.

In some cases there has been no particular sexual abuse indoctrination or prompting by the parent; the child originates the complaint. We are living at a time when sexual abuse is being widely discussed on television, in the newspapers, magazines, and even in school prevention programs. Children who are looking for excuses for vilification and/or ammunition for alienation now have a wealth of information provided to them for the creation of their sexual scenarios. When a child is being used as a weapon in a parental conflict, especially when the parents are litigating for custody, examiners must consider the possibility of such fabrication. In making the differentiation the examiner does well to appreciate that children who have genuinely been sexually abused are often quite fearful about re-

vealing the abuse, often because they have been threatened with dire consequences if they were to reveal their experiences. The child who is fabricating such abuse generally does not exhibit such fears and will often freely present in detail the alleged abuses to lawyers, mental health examiners, judges, and so on. Whereas the child who has suffered bona fide sexual abuse has been threatened with the loss of parental affection for such revelation, the fabricating child recognizes that he or she will earn the love and affection of a parent for such descriptions.

Factors Arising Within the Child. Here I refer to factors that initially involve no active contribution on the part of the loved parent, either overt or covert, either conscious or unconscious, either blatant or subtle. Of course, a parent may promulgate the alienation and "get mileage out of it," but initially it is a contribution that results from psychopathological factors within the child. For example, a boy may have repeatedly observed his father beating his mother—sometimes mercilessly. In order to protect himself from similar treatment, the child may profess great affection for his father and alienation from his mother. The professions of love here stem from fear rather than from genuine feelings of affection. This phenomenon is generally referred to as "identification with the aggressor" and is based on the principle: "If you can't fight 'em, join 'em." Those who are knowledgeable about the family situation may express amazement that the child is obsessed with hatred of the mother and love of the father. Another factor that may be operative in this situation is the child's model for what a loving relationship should be like. Love is viewed by the child just described as an exchange of violence, hostility, and pain. In order to be sure of obtaining this "love," the child opts to live with the hostile parent. This is the central mechanism of masochism.[2,3,8,9]

During the course of her parents' divorce litigation, the mother of a thirteen-year-old girl died in an automobile accident. Even prior to her mother's death, the girl had identified with and supported her mother's position; she viewed her father as a rejector and an abandoner. In this regard her mother was supported as well by the maternal grandmother. At the time of the mother's death, however, the girl exhibited what I have described elsewhere[4] as an "instantaneous identification" with her dead mother. This is one of the ways in which children (and even adults) will deal with the death of a parent. It is as if they were saying: "My parent isn't dead; he or she now resides within my own self." With such immediate identification the child takes on many of the dead parent's personality traits, often almost overnight. Such a sequence of events occurred in this case. There was a very rapid transformational process in which the girl abruptly acquired many of her mother's mannerisms. With this she intensified her hatred of her father, even accusing him of having caused the death of her mother. "If you hadn't treated my mother so badly, there wouldn't have been a breakup of the marriage, she wouldn't have had to go visit with her lawyer, and she wouldn't have been killed on the way home from his office." Although there were many other factors involved in her obsessive hatred and complete rejection of her father—a rejection that began on the day of her mother's death—this identification was an important element. Previously she had grudgingly and intermittently seen her father; after her mother's death there was a total cessation of visitation. The maternal grandmother supported this identification and now began to view the girl as the reincarnation of her dead daughter. And in the service of this process she supported the girl in her rejection of her father.

A common mechanism for this kind of alienation is seen when a child feels confident of one parent's love and is not sure of the other's. Generally, the parent who leaves is initially viewed as an abandoner, and the child tends to lose confidence that that parent will continue to show love and affection (the departing parent's professions of continuity notwithstanding). After an initial period of hostility, however, the child may gradually develop an obsessive affection for the departed one and significant animosity toward the parent with whom he or she is living. When this happens, the child then joins with the departed parent in vilifying the custodial parent. Such a reaction is generally related to the child's concern that he or she might lose what little love may still remain in the departed parent's heart. By siding with the noncustodial parent, the child hopes to maintain some kind of affection and continuity. Indeed, there may be a fear that if such a position is not taken, there will be a total abandonment and rejection. And, in fact, this is unfortunately sometimes the case.

Another factor also contributes to the alienation in such situations. The child knows that the custodial parent will tolerate much more hostility than the noncustodial one and can be relied upon to remain loyal, whereas the noncustodial parent provides no such reassurance. Hostilities arising from many sources, both related and unrelated to the divorce, then become vented on the custodial parent. In particular, anger toward the departed parent can become displaced onto the custodial parent. That one is, after all, a much safer target—a target from which significant retaliation is less to be feared.

Examiners who are evaluating alienated children do well to appreciate this complex of factors. Lawyers and courts often ask examiners whether a particular child has been "brainwashed"; not infrequently they will press for a yes-or-no answer. To view such children simply as programmed by one parent against the other is often a gross oversimplification of the situation. Examiners must investigate the more complex factors just outlined.

One of the causes of the parental alienation syndrome has been the failure of legislators and courts to appreciate the importance of early bonding in the parent-child relationship. The desire for sexual egalitarianism in custody decisions has resulted in a situation in which not enough weight is being given to the strong psychological bond that develops between the infant and the primary caretaker (usually the mother) during the formative years. Rather, emphasis has been given to later years of childhood when often both parents have been equally available to take care of the children. I believe that the tenacity with which many mothers fight for their children (even to the point where they brainwash them) and the ferocity with which children fight for their mothers (even to the point of developing scenarios of fabrication) is related to the threat of disruption of this bond. I would therefore recommend that when evaluating custody disputes, preference (not automatic assignment) be given to that parent (regardless of sex) who has provided the greatest degree of child-rearing input during the child's formative years. Because mothers today are still more often the primary child-rearing parents, more mothers would be given parental preference under this guideline. However, if the father was the primary caretaker during the early years of the child's life, he would be considered the preferable custodial parent, unless other factors outweighed this important advantage for him. The implementation of this criterion for resolving custody disputes would, I believe, reduce significantly the incidence of the parental alienation syndrome.

However, mothers who have contributed to the development of this syndrome in their children often have additional, generally pathological, reasons for brainwashing their children—reasons beyond those related to the fear of disruption of their strong psychological ties with their children. These include using the children for vengeful retaliation, inability to tolerate a more egalitarian division of their children's time with the father, and jealousy over a father's new female friend. In such cases therapy is generally warranted. In extreme cases, where the mother is totally unreceptive to treatment, the only recourse may be to remove the children from their mother and place them in the primary custody of the father—with a rigid visitation schedule imposed upon the mother. Elsewhere[7] I have described these therapeutic approaches in greater detail.

I wish to impress upon the reader the fact that my using the mother here as the example of a primary contributor to the parental alienation syndrome stems from my observation that mothers, much more than fathers, have been threatened by the aforementioned legal changes in custody determinations. There are, however, many fathers who also contribute actively to the development of this syndrome in their children; but they represent a smaller segment of the population of brainwashing parents, a fact that is not surprising considering the changes that have placed women at a definite disadvantage in custody disputes.

Concluding Comments

Unfortunately, for most divorced parents the usual practice is to engage the services of an attorney and to initiate an adversarial process as a first step toward resolving divorce conflicts. This, I believe, is an unfortunate tradition. More people are coming to appreciate that there is a preferable option, namely *mediation*. Up until the last few years the legal profession was generally unsympathetic to mediation. It was even considered unethical on the grounds that an attorney serving as a mediator might be biased. More recently, however, this resistance has been reduced significantly by mediation procedures that involve independent attorneys as reviewers of a mediation memorandum and encourage active communication between the mediator and each parent's independent counsel.

Just as adversary litigation may be giving way to mediation, the use of mental health professionals as adversary testifiers in custody litigation is being replaced by their serving as impartial examiners. It is a sad commentary on mental health professionals to note how readily they have agreed to testify as advocates in custody litigation. Many will assert that one parent is better qualified to have custody of the children without having evaluated the other parent! Obviously one cannot say who is the *better* parent unless one has had the opportunity to evaluate *both*. Yet these colleagues una-

shamedly provide such testimony. Fortunately, judges are becoming increasingly wary of such unilateral judgments and are recognizing it as a disservice to the clients, the mental health profession, and the legal profession as well.

I have been a strong proponent of mental health professionals serving only as impartial examiners in custody litigation.[5,7] In my own practice I will appear in such a capacity only after receiving an order from the presiding judge to serve the court in this manner. Generally this requires the agreement of both parents and their attorneys, although a reluctant parent can be ordered to participate if the judge feels strongly enough about the involvement of an impartial examiner. It is only when all reasonable attempts to serve in an impartial role have been unsuccessful that I will consider serving as an advocate; however, before seeing the client, I make no promises as to whether or not I will agree to participate in this way. People with experience in serving courts as impartial examiners may also serve as consultants to mediators. This is an optimal time in which to involve oneself, before the situation has deteriorated to the point where the parents turn to adversarial litigation.

In sum, many changes are rapidly taking place in the area of child custody. The new egalitarianism between parents is certainly an advance. However, like all advances, unanticipated problems have arisen. Most prominent are the psychological problems resulting from elimination of the tender years presumption and the indiscriminate granting of joint custody. We are witnessing a dramatic increase in what I have referred to as the parental alienation syndrome. Our next step must be the improvement of our techniques for preventing and dealing with these now ubiquitous problems. The rapid growth of mediation and the increasing reluctance on the part of mental health professionals to serve as unilateral advocates are also important advances that should lessen the psychological trauma associated with divorce and custody litigation.

REFERENCES

1. AMERICAN PSYCHIATRIC ASSOCIATION. *Diagnostic and Statistical Manual of Mental Disorders,* 3rd ed. (DSM-III). Washington, D.C.: American Psychiatric Association, 1980.

2. GARDNER, R. A. "The Use of Guilt as a Defense Against Anxiety," *Psychoanalytic Review,* 57 (1970):124–136.

3. ———. *Understanding Children—A Parents' Guide to Child Rearing.* Cresskill, N.J.: Creative Therapeutics, 1973.

4. ———. "Death of a Parent," in J. D. Noshpitz, ed., *Basic Handbook of Child Psychiatry,* vol. 4. New York: Basic Books, 1979, pp. 270–283.

5. ———. *Family Evaluation in Child Custody Litigation.* Cresskill, N.J.: Creative Therapeutics, 1982.

6. ———. "Joint Custody Is Not for Everyone," *Family Advocate,* 5 (1982):7–10.

7. ———. *Child Custody Litigation: A Guide for Parents and Mental Health Professionals.* Cresskill, N.J.: Creative Therapeutics, 1986.

8. RADO, S. "An Adaptational View of Sexual Behavior," in *Psychoanalysis of Behavior,* vol. 1. New York: Grune & Stratton, 1956, pp. 186–213.

9. THOMPSON, C. "The Interpersonal Approach to the Clinical Problems of Masochism," in M. R. Green, ed., *Interpersonal Psychoanalysis: The Selected Papers of Clare M. Thompson.* New York: Basic Books, 1964, pp. 183–187.

72 / Kidnapping of Children by Parents

Lee H. Haller

Introduction

Child snatching, child kidnapping, and parental kidnapping are all terms for the abduction or nonconsensual withholding of a child by one parent from the other. It is relatively recently that this has been recognized as a problem, having come to light only in the past decade. Although new in its description, it is an issue of major proportions, with an unofficial estimated frequency of between 25,000 and 100,000 cases per year.[14] One official study indicates that between 250 and 1,000 cases occurred in the Denver, Colorado, area in a single year.[3] Lewis[17] has estimated that many kidnappings have gone unreported since perhaps 60 to 70 percent of them occur before any custody decree has been rendered.

The subject has received much attention in newspapers* and the lay literature.[4,12] However, in spite of the frequency of occurrence and the severity of the trauma to the affected children, little has been published in the professional literature. This chapter discusses what is known about the setting in which abductions take place, the motives of parents who abduct, and how the abductions take place. I also attempt to throw some light on the effect that such behavior has upon children and to review the response of the legal system to this problem.

Setting of Child Kidnapping

Child snatching occurs in the context of an acrimonious dissolution of a marital or quasi-marital relationship. Since there are over one million children affected

*See references 7, 8, 10, 11, 17, 18, and 26.

by parental divorce each year, and perhaps 10 to 15 percent of such divorces are contested, the potential population at risk is enormous.

Within the framework of a contested divorce, children can and do become pawns. Snatching may occur at any point in the process of the breakup of a marital relationship. As described by Katz,[15] child snatching may occur: (1) before finalization of a divorce by a parent who fears losing custody; (2) postdivorce when a parent is unhappy with a custody decree and flees to another state in the hopes of seeking child custody modification; (3) following divorce when the custodial parent may disappear with the child in an effort to deny the noncustodial parent visitation; and (4) when separate states grant conflicting custody awards.

In an effort to define the population of children involved, Agopian[2] studied 91 cases involving 130 abducted children. He found that some 87 percent of the children were eleven years of age or younger. The average age of the abducted child was seven, with 34 percent of the victims being between three and five years of age. He found that 47 percent of the abducted victims were returned to the guardian parent. In contrast, Duckworth[9] estimated that only 10 percent of the children will eventually be recovered. Another troubling statistic reported by one group (Child Find) is that 60 percent of the child victims are either abused or abandoned.[5]

Parental Motive and Behavior

Many different theories and opinions have been put forth to explain why a parent kidnaps his or her child. From Agopian,[2] we know that the kidnapping parent is usually the father. This is not surprising since mothers are granted custody in perhaps 90 percent of the cases. The conscious motives for such behavior have been reported differently, depending on the author's view. For example, in one article parental kidnapping is described as "an angry, vengeful, and impulsive act. The abducting parent is grimly determined to keep the child from the other parent. . . ."[5] In the same speech Dr. Albert Solnit was quoted as stating "clearly, this shows contempt for the child's needs. Abduction shows that the parent doesn't have the child's best interest at heart—it is more his or her own interests." On the other hand, the parents who engaged in this behavior state that they do so out of a wish to be with the children and a fear of losing them through the process of divorce. Parental perceptions of their behavior possess the same validity as do the "facts" in a contested custody case—that is, there is his side, there is her side, and there is the truth.

As far as the professional literature is concerned, Agopian reports on some of the "typical motivations of offenders." These include: "(1) the belief that the child is, or is apt to be, neglected by the custodial parient, (2) the desire to continue a full time parenting role, (3) to punish the other parent who may be blamed for the marital failure, or (4) to induce the withdrawal of the divorce action or initiate a reconciliation." Schetky and Haller,[20] in reporting three cases of parental kidnapping, noted that "ego impairment" was present in all three parents, with two being borderline and one psychotic. They noted, "Such parents may have difficulty differentiating their own needs from the child's needs, have trouble relinquishing bonds to former spouses, and may use primitive defenses of splitting and projection" (p. 284).

Levy[14] describes a case involving yet another parental motivation—fear for the child's well-being. In that instance, mother and father were living together, but with an element of strong marital discord present throughout. On one occasion, the mother abruptly fled the marital home with the child to go live with her parents in another state. She alleged that her son had been repeatedly beaten by the father and was afraid of him.

When looking at the behavior of the abducting parent, it is not difficult to see why children have adverse reactions to the kidnapping experience. Often the abduction takes place unannounced and suddenly. At the time of departure, the child may be told only that he or she and the parent are going on a trip. They thereupon depart without any good-byes to the other parent. Even more traumatic can be the situations where the child is indeed "snatched." For example, many children are taken from their homes or school under some sort of ruse. They are physically grabbed by the parent or an agent of the parent and whisked away.

The abduction is frequently followed by concealment on the part of the parent, as efforts are made to avoid detection. The child may be taken from house to house, from state to state, or even from country to country, with multiple moves in the course of several months. During the abduction and subsequently, the child may be told any number of lies about the parent who was left behind. It is not uncommon for children to report, when they are recovered, that they had been told their original parent had died, or did not love them, or did not want them any more. In some instances young children have even been told that the absent parent was not in fact their parent; a new lover or spouse of the abducting parent may be proffered to the child as the true parent.

In addition, children may be kept out of school for weeks or even months after a kidnapping. Again, this is done to avoid detection. The children are sometimes guarded closely by the abducting parent or by an agent so as to avoid a "snatch-back" by the other parent if their location is discovered. Children may also be told to lie about their background and even about their names. Anecdotal reports in the lay literature describe children who could not even remember their own last name, having been told to lie about it so many different times.[12]

Although these are the dramatic cases, there are multitudinous examples of minor incidents of kidnapping, instances that are all too familiar to the clinician who treats the children of divorced parents. This type of kidnapping involves noncompliance with a visitation schedule. In this instance, for example, a parent who is entitled to a Sunday afternoon visitation and is to return the child by dinnertime will not return the child until much later in the evening, without any notification to the custodial parent. Another example is the custodial parent who takes the child out on an errand or on a vacation when the noncustodial parent is to have visitation, without notifying the visiting parent of these arrangements.

Effects of Kidnapping on Children

In spite of the widespread nature of this problem, little has been written in the professional literature about the effects of kidnapping on the children. Most of the early information came in the lay literature, where experts were quoted who had evaluated or treated children after their return from an abduction. For example, Gill reported[12] the statements of Dr. Jeannette Minkoff, a psychologist in New York. She stated: "Children have described their fears, sadness, loneliness, and hysteria upon realizing they were not being returned to their homes" and "Children have told me they begged, pleaded, and cried in an unsuccessful effort to persuade the kidnapping parent to return them . . ." (p. 147). Gill also reports statements from Peg Edwards, a social worker who has had wide experience with kidnapped children. She is reported as stating that the children's "biggest problem is the fear that when they grow up they won't form healthy relationships." The children lack trust and security, which could cause them to behave poorly in school. She saw the abduction of young children as being a break in the trust that children have in their parents, leading to confusion, guilt, and anger. Edwards stated that the children felt they were to blame, believing they had done something wrong that caused the kidnapping. She reported further difficulties on reunion with the previous custodial parent, including rejection of that parent by the "brainwashed" child (p. 155).

Until very recently the professional literature has yielded only anecdotal reports, and these in the context of a statement about another subject. For example, Miller[19] described a kidnapping that occurred while a child was in therapy. The natural father and mother had been divorced when the patient was age three. At age seven, the child was brought for evaluation. Shortly after treatment was begun, the natural father reappeared after a long absence and wanted to take the child for visitation. It was supposed to be a weekend visit, but he moved her to another state, kept her for seven weeks, and petitioned for custody. During that time he refused to allow the daughter to communicate with her mother, or mother with daughter. Fortunately, the court in the second state referred the entire case back to the original state for evaluation. Thus the child was returned to the mother and a custody evaluation ensued. In the course of this, the therapist was able to see the girl. The experience had reactivated the child's earlier conflicts about the divorce and stirred up fantasies that she was to blame for her father's having left. The kidnapping reinforced previously existing unconscious fears that men were dangerous. Difficulties with aggression and a "bitter oedipal disappointment that [the father] had remarried . . ." (p. 446) were noted. As the therapist interpreted the girl's rage at her father, "she began having nightmares. She dreamed of being a passenger on a hijacked plane" (p. 446). In addition, there were fears of another kidnapping.

In a paper on child custody, Levy[16] reported another case that involved an abduction. His contact with the child postabduction was limited. He reported that the child had exaggerated negative feelings toward the nonpreferred parent. He also noted that the child was unduly anxious and had formed "an exaggerated and unevenly strong alliance with his mother [the kidnap-

ping and custodial parent] against his father [the parent who had been left behind when the mother had abruptly left the house with the child] (p. 229)." Levy did not make any attempt to differentiate which symptoms were a result of parental conflicts from those that might have resulted from the abduction.

In a study of psychically traumatized children, Terr[24] reported the case of a five-year-old girl who had been kidnapped initially by her mother at age three and had been rekidnapped by her father at age five. The girl was interviewed one day after she was rekidnapped. In her mind, there was only one kidnapping, the more recent event. She was "lethargic and confused" about the appearance of a private detective who had kidnapped her. She was not sure she remembered her father, who accompanied her to the interview. A short time later she became a teacher for two imaginary friends "Little Wanda" and "Big Wanda." She "gave them excited and repeated lectures to run away if approached by a stranger" (p. 749). These warnings lasted for approximately eight months. When seen one year after the kidnapping, Wanda related that she believed her "warning games" had started before the second kidnapping. Terr related this as evidence of "post traumatic time skew," which, as she has described elsewhere, is one of the symptoms children manifest after a psychic trauma.[23]

More recently, articles have appeared that have focused specifically on children who are victims of parental kidnapping. Senior, Gladstone, and Nurcombe[21] reported a single case of a two-year-old boy who had been abducted by his natural mother (the noncustodial parent) from his natural father and stepmother. He was taken out of the state for five weeks but was returned because of the difficult behavior he developed. He was seen three months after the abduction. Postabduction symptoms were difficulties falling asleep, frequently awakening terrified and screaming, food refusal, urinating and defecating on the floor with a marked aversion to the toilet, a labile mood, uncontrolled crying, and aggressive behavior directed toward his nine-month-old half brother. The authors reported that "during the day he led his stepmother around the house, searching fearfully for his natural mother. Whenever the doorbell rang, he became very frightened and tearfully cried out his natural mother's name." Prior to the snatching, he had been described as developing normally, being "adventurous, confident, and outgoing. He was toilet trained. He had no sleep or eating difficulties." The authors further reported that subsequently the child "began to confuse his natural mother and stepmother." Also, the child "would repeatedly tell his brother that when *he* was two, [the boy's] natural mother would take *him,* the stepbrother, away" (p. 580). The stepmother also reported believing that when the child was awake at night, he was having fearful hallucinations about the natural mother. The authors describe a brief and focal psychotherapeutic intervention that alleviated the initial symptomatology. However, they reported that the child demonstrated two anniversary reactions and also three "reenactments."

Schetky and Haller[20] reported three cases, two of whom were seen postabduction. Of these two, the first involved a three-year-old girl whose mother took her abruptly from the marital home and went into hiding for two weeks until she was located by detectives. Upon return, the child's behavior was noted to be very regressed, with both daytime and nighttime wetting, acting frightened, clinging to her father during the day, excessive anxiety, rejection of toys in the playroom when interviewed, and personalizing her blanket. Nighttime awakening was also noted as were several spontaneous references to the kidnapping. Over the course of several weeks, her symptoms remitted. In the second case, an eight-year-old girl had been kidnapped by her mother who had gone into hiding for a month. The girl was not evaluated until a year later. At that time she was still terrified of her mother. This fear seemed to be based at least in part on the girl's recollections of physical abuse by the mother and the mother's emotional tirades.

Agopian[12] studied five children and reported at some length on two of them. He concluded that the victims' reaction to the snatching varied considerably, although each child, upon return, was reported as showing some symptomatology. He indicated that the severity of the harm was likely to be affected by "(1) the victim's age at the time of the abduction, (2) type of treatment accorded the victim by the offender, (3) the length of time that the victim is in the offender's control, (4) the victim's life-style and experiences while suppressed, and (5) the type of support and therapy provided the victim upon recovery." One of the cases described was what Terr has termed a "vacation snatch," wherein the child was kept for six weeks beginning with an approved weekend visitation. The little girl was well taken care of and lived in two different residences. Upon return, she was fearful and confused, stating that she knew she was not supposed to go. Subsequent to her recovery, she had "frequent nightmares with visions of monsters." In addition, she was fearful of another abduction and suspicious of strangers. Her symptoms apparently abated relatively quickly. The second case Agopian described involved a child who was abducted at the age of three and one-half, also during a court-approved visitation. Over the subsequent three and one-half years, she lived a nomadic life with multiple moves and at least one name change. Upon recovery, she did not recognize her

mother. She lied frequently, was secretive, had difficulty interacting with peers, and appeared mature beyond her years. It is noteworthy that she remained loyal to the abducting parent. Agopian observed that some victims exhibited resentment toward both parents, feeling "contempt for the offender" and also "resentment toward the custodial parent for not rescuing them quickly."

Finally, Terr[25] reported on eighteen children, eight of whom were "successfully" snatched, three who were involved in abortive snatches, two who had been the object of threatened snatches, and five who were victims of "vacation" snatches. She found that sixteen of the eighteen children experienced some type of emotional effect as a result of the successful or abortive kidnappings. The only two children who did not manifest direct psychiatric symptoms were a pair of siblings. They had been taken by their father but had been told the truth from the beginning and, during their stay with their father, were able to remain in contact with their mother. The author categorized the symptoms into five areas. Eleven of the children showed evidence of psychic trauma (such as repetitive and monotonous play, time skew, reenactment, or dreams).[23] Seven of the children showed evidence of "mental indoctrination (brainwashing)." Seven showed longstanding grief for or rage against an absent parent. Nine children rejected the offending parent and, in two cases, there was an exaggerated identification with or an oedipal wish fulfillment regarding the kidnapping parent. Of particular note is that six out of thirteen of the victims of the "successful" and "vacation" snatches showed psychic trauma or fright, whereas all five of the children involved in abortive or threatened snatches showed this type of symptom. Also, the same five children all rejected the offending parent. In her discussion, Terr noted that the successfully stolen children were frequently indoctrinated (in five of the eight cases) by the kidnapping parent, who convinced the child that the absent parent no longer wanted him or her. Terr commented that "these successfully stolen children grieved or experienced rage for their lost parents, but did not experience fright or post traumatic effects until what looked like the 'real' kidnapping [the second kidnapping] occurred" (p. 154).

The Legal System

From a legal standpoint, the problem of child snatching has arisen largely because, until recently, such commandeering of a child by a parent was completely legal. Furthermore, custody decrees were made by state courts, and the courts of one state were under no obligation to honor the findings of another. Hence a noncustodial parent could kidnap a child, flee to another jurisdiction, file for a custody hearing, and be granted custody in that state. As a result, it was not uncommon for one parent to have custody in one state, while the other parent had custody in another. This failure of the state courts to grant full faith and credit to decrees from sister states encouraged parents to go "forum shopping" in an effort to obtain a favorable judgment.

Over the past four to five years, however, this situation has changed dramatically because of two major pieces of legislation. The first is the Uniform Child Custody Jurisdiction Act (UCCJA).* This model act was drafted in 1968 and has gradually been adopted by every state and the District of Columbia. The UCCJA sets forth specific standards and criteria that must be met for a state to assume jurisdiction in a child custody hearing. The specifics of the act make it highly unlikely that a parent can go "forum shopping" and successfully obtain a new custody determination. Instead, the likely outcome is that the court in the second state will refuse jurisdiction and refer the case back to the state where the initial custody determination was made. Even in cases where no custody decree exists, a parent cannot flee the child's "home state" and get a hearing. With limited exceptions, the UCCJA mandates that in order for a state to obtain jurisdiction a child must be domiciled in that state for six months prior to the commencement of a custody proceeding.

The other major piece of legislation that has been helpful in deterring kidnapping has been the 1980 passage of PL 96-611, the Parental Kidnapping Prevention Act (PKPA). This federal statute was enacted before all the states had adopted the UCCJA. The act has three major sections. The first part mandates that states should give full faith and credit to the child custody determination made by another state and shall not modify that determination, except in limited circumstances. In the second section, the Federal Parent Locater Service (the agency usually used to locate non-custodial parents who are in arrears in paying child support) is made available to states to be used in searching for parents who had kidnapped their children and fled that state. The third section applies when the act of kidnapping is a felony in the state from which the child was taken. It mandates that the Federal Bureau of Investigation (FBI) be brought in to assist in locating any parent who crosses state boundaries after having kidnapped his or her child.

This act was helpful, especially as it limited "havens" for abducting parents when all the states had

*Family Law Reporter, reference file 201: 0009.

not yet enacted the UCCJA. At the outset, however, the latter two sections of the act were not as helpful as had been hoped. This was because states had to enter into agreements with the Federal Parent Locater Service in order to use the service, and the states were somewhat slow in so doing. Also, the FBI was quite reluctant to cooperate, apparently because it viewed the problem as a domestic matter rather than a true crime. However, since the majority of states have now enacted laws making the kidnapping of children by their parents a felony and because subsequent legislation (the Missing Children Act, PL 97-292), has been enacted that requires the FBI to assist in locating missing children, it is now more responsive to requests for assistance.

In spite of this legislation by both the states and the federal government, child kidnapping has not ceased. Parents continue to abduct their children and to flee from state to state, seeking a favorable decision. Furthermore, even though the kidnapping is now a felony, if parents do not seek a new custody order, do not hold a steady job, and keep their children out of school, they are extremely difficult to locate. Once the kidnapping parent and child are located, however, the legislation does help the original custodial parent regain custody of the children. Additionally, the original custodial parent has several avenues open to him or her to litigate successfully against the other parent in a civil action. [22]

Discussion

The emerging professional literature about the problem of child kidnapping tends to confirm the statements made in the lay literature. Both indicate that this behavior causes problems for the children involved. Not surprisingly, the effects that children show are highly variable and seem dependent on several factors. One particularly significant and somewhat surprising findings from Terr's material is that children who were "successfully" snatched in a smooth manner and then indoctrinated did not experience posttraumatic effects until they were kidnapped back by the left-behind parent or an agent of that parent. Given Terr's previous observations that children who were exposed to the psychic trauma of the Chowchilla incident (where children on a school bus were kidnapped by strangers and buried in a truck underground while being ransomed) showed neither amnesia nor denial for the incident, this finding seems especially notable. [23] Certainly one might wonder how the children kidnapped by a parent do experience the initial kidnapping and how they handle indoctrinating statements such as the absent parent did not want or love the child any longer. However, given that the children see the recovery as a kidnapping, Terr has suggested that a uniformed police officer be present when the child is recovered. For young children especially, a police officer can act as a symbol of reassurance and protection.

Also notable is her finding that threatened or abortive snatches were at least as traumatic as successful abductions. This is an extremely significant finding, because threatened kidnappings are quite frequent in the course of, or after, a bitter divorce. For example, the custodial parent may threaten to forbid further visitation, even if court ordered, if the other parent does not pay overdue child support. Or a noncustodial parent may threaten not to return the child from a visitation on time, or at all, unless the custodial parent ceases some behavior that the noncustodial parent finds objectionable. Since these threats are frequently made in the presence of the children, it does not seem surprising that the children exhibit behavior problems both before and after visitation changeover. Similarly, children who have not been kidnapped but who are pawns in a hostile divorce may show effects similar to those seen in children who have been kidnapped, such as mental indoctrination, rage or grief about rejection by one of the parents, or an exaggerated identification with a parent.

Chess and associates[6] looked at how adults were affected by the separation or divorce of their parents that had occurred when the subjects were children. They also studied what effect parental conflict that occurred during the subjects' childhood had on the subjects once they were adults. They found that poor adult adaptation was predicted by early parental conflict, especially when this conflict surrounded child management. Separation and divorce without this conflict were not found to predict adult outcome. It is evident that the act of kidnapping is strong evidence of parental conflict around child management. Hence, from this data, it might be predicted that children who are the victims of child kidnapping may well have difficulties as adults.

Another question raised by Chess and associates surrounds the issue of joint custody, a solution to custody disputes that is being recommended with increasing frequency (see chapters 71 and 73). In some states there is even a presumption in favor of this strategy as the preferred means of resolution. One must wonder how joint custody would work with parents who wind up kidnapping their children. On the one hand, it might be assumed that if parents believed that joint custody would be the recommendation, they would not resort to kidnapping. On the other, we know that joint custody does not necessarily end disputes between the

parents. Indeed, kidnappings have occurred even where joint custody has been awarded.

From a legal standpoint, when the divorce decree gives joint custody to the parents and a kidnapping occurs, it becomes much more difficult, although not impossible, to institute legal action to gain the return of the child. It is best to have some limitations spelled out in the separation and divorce decrees. In particular, it should be clear that neither parent can take the child out of state without at least notifying the other parent as to destination. It might even be wise to mandate that neither parent be allowed to go out of state with the child without the other parent's approval.

In any case, experience teaches that under certain circumstances, even with a joint custody divorce decree, there are parents who will still kidnap their children. In their now-classic book, *Beyond the Best Interests of the Child,*[13] Goldstein, Freud, and Solnit recommended that one parent be awarded sole custody of the children and be given total power to decide whether or not the noncustodial parent would visit and, if visitations were to occur, only under what circumstances. If courts were to follow this recommendation, then visitation would occur only under conditions in which the custodial parent believed the children would be safe. Thus, if the custodial parent were concerned that the other parent might kidnap the children (or harm them in any way), visitation could be denied or limited to supervised visits in the custodial parent's home. Even though this would not eliminate the possibility of the children being kidnapped, it would cut down on opportunities for this to occur. A court-ordered custodial arrangement like this might also encourage the noncustodial parent to be conciliatory, in order to visit the children. Although other recommendations in their book have been widely adopted, this one has not. Perhaps there are cases where such a resolution should be considered.

Finally, the impact on children of having the abducting parent apprehended must be considered. On the positive side, the child will be more easily reunited with the other parent. On the negative side, parents who abduct their children are by that token criminals. As such, they are subject to prosecution and, if convicted, will at least be fined, if not jailed. In addition, the abducting parent may be sued by the other parent in a civil action.[22] What effect might such litigation or jailing of a parent have on the child? Might this not turn out to be another type of psychic trauma?

As child psychiatrists, we can play an important role not only in treating these children postabduction but also in prevention. Frequently we see children who are symptomatic because of disharmony between the parents. As part of our conclusory statements to the parents, we can point out the destructive effects this has on the child and, where appropriate, go on to discuss what might happen to the child if the parents separate, argue over visitation schedules, or kidnap the child for any period of time. Additionally, we can point out that the child may be affected even if kidnapping is brought up only to threaten the other parent. Finally, we can alert our adult psychiatrist colleagues and other mental health professionals who do marital therapy or divorce counseling to be aware of these issues so that they will be equipped to work with parents who seem headed toward an acrimonious divorce. In these ways it is hoped we can help prevent some of these kidnappings, which can be so destructive to the well-being of the children involved.

REFERENCES

1. AGOPIAN, N. W. *Parental Child Stealing.* Lexington, Mass.: Lexington Books, 1981.

2. AGOPIAN, M. "The Impact on Victims of Parental Abduction," Paper presented at the 9th International Congress on Law and Psychiatry, Santa Margherita, Italy, June 20–23, 1983.

3. BACK, S., and BUXTON, J. "The Denver Kidnapping Project: Resources for Prevention and Intervention in the Denver Metropolitan Area," Paper presented at the annual meeting of the Colorado Interdisciplinary Committee on Child Custody, Keystone, Colorado, 11 September 1983.

4. BLACK, B. L. *Somewhere Child.* New York: Viking Press, 1981.

5. ———. "The Frightening Epidemic of Child Snatching", *M.D.,* 26 (1982):162–170.

6. CHESS, S., et al. "Early Parental Attitudes, Divorce and Separation, and Adult Outcome: Finding in a Longitudinal Study," *Journal of the American Academcy of Child Psychiatry,* 22 (1983):47–51.

7. CLIFFORD, G. "Arnold Miller Grieves for his Stolen Son and Fights for Laws that Might Bring Him Back," *People,* 19 March, 1980.

8. DAVIDSON, K. "When Parents Kidnap Their Own Children," *U.S. News and World Report,* 90 (1981):66–67.

9. DUCKWORTH, M. "Child Snatchers Break Hearts, Not Laws," *Sunday Chronicle Herald* (Augusta, Georgia), 20 February 1980.

10. DULLEA, G. "Kid Snatching Goes Worldwide," *Chicago Tribune,* 3 February 1980.

11. FERETTI, T. "Reducing Child Custody Fights," *New York Times,* 20 January 1981.

12. GILL, J. E. *Stolen Children.* New York: Seaview Books, 1981.

13. GOLDSTEIN, J., FREUD, A., and SOLNIT, A. *Beyond the Best Interests of the Child.* New York: Free Press, 1973.

14. GOODMAN, E. "Child Snatching," *Washington Post,* 26 March 1976.

15. KATZ, S. *Child Snatching.* Washington, D.C.: American Bar Association Press, 1981.

16. LEVY, A. "The Meaning of the Child's Preference in Child Custody Determination," *Journal of Psychiatry and Law,* 8(1981):221–234.

17. ———. "On Reducing the Child Snatching Syndrome," *Children Today,* 7(1981):19–21.

18. LEWIS, K. "Parental Kidnapping," *Chicago Tribune,* 3 February 1979.

19. MILLER, E. "Psychotherapy of a Child in a Custody Dispute," *Journal of the American Academy of Child Psychiatry,* 15(1976):441–452.

20. SCHETKY, D., and HALLER, L. "Parental Kidnapping," *Journal of the American Academy of Child Psychiatry,* 22(1983):279–285.

21. SENIOR, N., GLADSTONE, T., and NURCOMBE, B. "Child Snatching: A Case Report," *Journal of the American Academy of Child Psychiatry,* 21(1982):579–583.

22. SOKOLOFF, G. "The Wide World of Torts," in *The First National Conference on Interstate Child Custody in Parental Kidnapping Cases Conference Materials.* Washington, D.C.: American Bar Association Press, 1982.

23. ———. "Psychic Trauma in Children: Observations Following the Chowchilla School-Bus Kidnapping," *American Journal of Psychiatry,* 138(1981):14–19.

24. TERR, L. " 'Forbidden Games': Post-traumatic Child's Play," *Journal of the American Academy of Child Psychiatry,* 20 (1981):741–760.

25. ———. "Child Snatching: A New Epidemic of an Ancient Malady," *Journal of Pediatrics,* 103(1983):151–156.

26. YUENGER, J. "Child Snatching: Tragic Outgrowths of Soaring Divorce," *Chicago Tribune,* 26 March 1978.

73 / Children and the Law: The Psychiatrist as Court Consultant

Elizabeth S. Scott and Andre P. Derdeyn

Introduction

Children are accorded a unique status in the law. While adults are presumed to be legally responsible for their behavior, competent to make decisions, and able to care for themselves and to protect their own interests, children are not. [14] Minors are given more protection and less freedom than adults. [17] They are generally not deemed competent to make medical decisions or binding contracts; their aggressive behavior is treated more leniently than that of adults; and they may be required to attend school and to submit to curfews. Parents are legally entrusted with the care of children; along with this responsibility parents have broad authority to raise their children as they see fit. Under its *parens patriae* authority, however, the state also has broad power to promote the welfare of children, and it may step in to protect them if their parents fail to do so.

Most decisions made by a juvenile court judge involve a determination of the child's best interest. While other interests such as parents' rights, family and individual privacy, and public safety may also be important, promoting the child's welfare is typically a central concern. Thus it is not surprising that child psychiatrists are frequently invited by courts to participate in decisions about children and families.

This chapter focuses on four types of legal decisions for which psychiatrists frequently provide consultation. In delinquency cases, clinicians may assist the court to understand the youth's antisocial behavior and to plan rehabilitative interventions. In divorce custody decisions, consultation may contribute to an understanding of the child's relationship with each parent; observations about the child's needs and the parents ability to meet those needs may also be helpful. Where the state intervenes in the family because of the parents' abusive or neglectful behavior, consultation may focus on such issues as the detriment to the child caused by the parent's behavior and, alternatively, the impact on the child of removal from the home. Clinical opinion on remediation may also be sought. Finally, psychiatrists are invariably involved in the decision that a child requires psychiatric hospitalization—a clinical decision that today often occurs in the context of complex legal regulation.

The Juvenile Justice System and the Child Psychiatrist

HISTORICAL BACKGROUND

As it developed in the early twentieth century, the juvenile justice system was grounded in a benevolent concern for delinquent youth who were perceived as needing treatment rather than punishment. [15] Delinquent behavior was regarded as evidence of psychological, social, or family problems; through the benign ministrations of the juvenile court, youthful offenders could be helped to change their deviant behavior and to move toward a constructive life. The rehabilitative ideal that was central to juvenile court philosophy was based, in part, on optimistic faith in the emerging fields of psychology and psychiatry. Clinicians could assist judges to understand the causes of antisocial behavior; more than that, the clinicians could help devise and implement an individualized treatment plan that would promote behavior change. Court clinics, such as the Judge Baker Guidance Center in Boston, were integral parts of many juvenile courts.

In recent years the traditional juvenile court philosophy has fallen into some disfavor. There is general acknowledgment that rehabilitation has not been very successful in turning youth away from criminal activity. There is much less optimism that intervention focused on the individual offender can effectively combat a problem that is increasingly understood to have complex cultural and social determinants. Further, many commentators have observed that society has not been willing to commit the resources to develop rehabilitative programs that might be effective; in fact, what many delinquent offenders receive is punishment. A shift in juvenile court philosophy is reflected in the recently promulgated Juvenile Justice Standards. This twenty-two-volume code is the product of a comprehensive and far-ranging law reform project of the 1970s. These standards recommend that retribution replace rehabilitation as the primary purpose of juvenile delinquency dispositions—but that the juvenile offender also has a right to rehabilitative services.[10]

Another important development in juvenile justice is that today the juvenile offender is given many of the legal protections accorded adult criminal defendants. In 1967 the landmark Supreme Court case of *In re Gault* (387 U.S. 1) established that juvenile offenders have the right to an attorney and other due-process protections. The *Gault* opinion recognized that juveniles often received little benefit from the informal rehabilitative approach of the juvenile court and were disadvantaged by the lack of basic legal protections.

THE ROLE OF THE PSYCHIATRIST AT DISPOSITION

Despite the movement toward a quasi-criminal system of juvenile justice, important aspects of the rehabilitative model remain. At the dispositional phase of the proceeding, after the youth is adjudicated delinquent, the focus generally remains on rehabilitation. In attempting to understand and address the problems of the youth in question, the judge will generally consider a variety of data about the youth and his or her family, including reports of mental health consultation. Often a dispositional plan is developed that is responsive to the needs of the individual offender.

Psychiatric consultation at disposition may provide valuable assistance to the judge. The central concern of the court may be to elicit clinical opinions and recommendations regarding the causes of the antisocial behavior; the psychiatrist, however, may be reluctant to draw causal inferences. Clearly, any significant areas of dysfunction in the juvenile's life offer an appropriate focus for the evaluation. A diagnosis of psychopathology may be indicated but of equal or greater importance is a broader examination of the youngster's intellectual, emotional, social and familial functioning. In some cases a medical evaluation with an emphasis on neurological functioning may be useful. With some children, evidence of learning disabilities may be important to rehabilitative efforts. Since family dysfunction may

be reflected in the child's acting-out behavior, parents and siblings are therefore essential participants in the evaluative process. Indeed, in a more general way, family relationships are a central focus of any thorough dispositional evaluation. Peer relations may also exert an important influence. It may be relevant to determine whether the behavior is sociosyntonic and the individual offender is part of a delinquent subculture. In addition, issues of poor social skill development may be relevant.

At disposition, the juvenile court has the authority to order a wide range of interventions. One modality is individual psychotherapy, but the concept of treatment for juvenile offenders is much broader than psychotherapy. Group therapy and family therapy may be mandated as well as residential treatment. Drug and alcohol programs may be indicated. Educational interventions may be available under the federal Education for the Handicapped Law, PL 94–142. Vocational school may be a viable option for some adolescents. Where the family situation seems detrimental, the offender may be removed from the home and placed in foster care, a group home, or a residential treatment center. A last resort is placement in a juvenile correctional facility.

While in theory the dispositional plan is individualized to the offender's needs, in practice such factors as the seriousness of the offense and past record are very relevant. A serious offense is much more likely to result in placement in a correctional facility and a minor offense in unsupervised probation.

TRANSFER TO ADULT COURT

Some juvenile offenders are deemed to be not "amenable to treatment" in the juvenile justice system and are transferred to the adult criminal system for trial. Generally, transfer is reserved for serious crimes committed by older offenders (generally age fifteen and older). Adolescents facing transfer are entitled to a hearing at which the judge must find that they are not amenable to treatment as a juvenile.

A finding of amenability to treatment is based on an examination of the nature of the offense, the offender's prior delinquency record, and the presence of prior treatment efforts and the youth's response. The juvenile who is deemed not amenable to treatment is one for whom all appropriate rehabilitative efforts have failed, or whose offense is so serious that the demands of public relations or public safety guide the court to transfer the child to adult criminal court.

At transfer, the psychiatric consultant's role is generally similar to that at disposition. However, the inquiry may here be directed more toward the issue of the potential for behavior change through the rehabilitative interventions available to the juvenile court. If the psychiatrist believes that a particular interventional program is indicated, in the course of a transfer evaluation it may be important to explain its potential effects on the youth's delinquent behavior. Where an offender had previously been offered treatment, the court will be interested in the clinician's view as to why that particular form of treatment had failed to promote behavior change. If the consultant is sufficiently persuasive in describing its potential benefits, the court may respond positively to a recommendation for some form of intervention that has not been previously attempted. However, if psychotherapy has been attempted three times and the youth continues to engage in increasingly serious criminal acts, the court may well decide that he or she is not amenable to psychotherapy.

Consultation in transfer cases raises difficult ethical issues for many child psychiatrists; in particular, they may be reluctant to participate in a proceeding that could result in criminal prosecution of the youthful offender. These evaluations may also raise issues of confidentiality. In some states, damaging evidence introduced at transfer may be used in a later criminal trial; in most, it is available to the juvenile judge if transfer is not ordered. It is important that the juvenile and his or her family undergoing evaluation understand the absence of confidentiality and the uses to which the information may be put.

This area of psychiatric consultation deserves extended deliberation by the various professional associations—the American Academy of Child Psychiatry, the American Psychiatric Association, and the American Academy of Psychiatry and the Law.

TREATMENT IN THE JUVENILE JUSTICE SYSTEM

Mental Health professionals treating juvenile offenders may have concerns unique to this framework and this kind of treatment. The child or parents ordered into treatment may not be ideal patients because of their resistance to a course of therapy that has been imposed upon them. This problem may be compounded by fears that the clinician will report statements made in therapy to the court. Some judges require progress reports of court-ordered psychotherapy; in such cases, clinicians are truly "double agents." However, many judges can be made to understand the importance of confidentiality in treatment and only require reports of missed appointments. The terms of the treatment and any reporting requirements should first be negotiated with the court; once clarified, they should then be clearly explained at the outset to the child and family.

Child Custody Consultation: Neglect, Abuse, and Termination of Parental Rights

In delinquency cases, the child's needs may be balanced against those of public safety. In contrast, when the state intervenes in families because parents abuse or neglect their children, the state's purpose is solely to protect the child. In this situation, however, the *parens patriae* policy of protecting children is balanced against a tradition of respecting family privacy and allowing parents to raise their children as they see fit. The tensions created by these two conflicting policies have often been resolved by actions that are ultimately detrimental to the involved children.[3] Thus the *parens patriae* authority is relatively easily invoked to remove children from parental homes and to place them in foster care. Removal from one's home is, of course, in itself stressful because of separation from parents and the general disruption of the child's life. However, even where the family situation is genuinely harmful, the strong policy favoring parents' rights makes termination of those rights very difficult. Thus a tug-of-war may ensue, with the child becoming subject to a cycle of removals and returns without the stability of a permanent placement either with the natural family or with an adoptive one.[3]

The shortcomings of social policy in this area have been increasingly recognized. The most radical proposal for reform is that offered by Goldstein, Freud, and Solnit in their 1979 book, *Before the Best Interests of the Child.*[7] Consonant with their emphasis on the importance to children of parental autonomy and family privacy, these authors recommend very narrow standards for intervention. Only in cases of severe physical abuse, adjudicated sexual abuse, or neglect leading to repeated serious bodily injury is state interference with the family justified. These authors oppose intervention for neglect and for emotional abuse, and they recommend termination of parental rights only for physical abuse. While no state has adopted the standards proposed by Goldstein, Freud, and Solnit, some recent legislation emphasizes that intervention is appropriate only when the family situation involves demonstrable harm to children.

There is a consensus among critics that if a child is removed, the focus should be on remediating the family situation as quickly as possible so that return is expedited; if this is not considered feasible, parental rights should be terminated in order to free the child for adoption and to break the perpetual cycle of foster care.[18] In many states, laws dealing with foster care and with termination of parental rights have been amended to reflect these concerns. Under some laws, the social services department must develop a foster care plan. This is designed to assist the parents to remediate the conditions that resulted in the child's removal so that the child's return home may occur as quickly as possible. Some states attempt to place time limitations on foster care plans. The goal is that where remediation fails and the child cannot be returned home in a reasonable period of time, parental rights can be terminated and the child freed for adoption. These laws reflect an effort to facilitate permanent placement either with the natural parents or with adoptive parents.

Although substantial changes have occurred in recent years, the law continues to evidence a strong concern for parent's rights and a reluctance to terminate those rights. Even where termination may be in the child's best interest (e.g., when a long-term foster family wishes to adopt), most states require a finding of parental unfitness or of irremediably harmful conditions. In *Santosky v. Kramer* (455 U.S. 745 [1982]), the Supreme Court held that a finding of unfitness on which termination is based must be made by clear and convincing evidence. Most states require that parents be represented by an attorney at termination proceedings.

THE ROLE OF CHILD PSYCHIATRISTS

To the psychiatrist, the law's response to children in cases involving abuse, neglect, and termination of parental rights often seems inadequate and frustrating. However, the psychiatrist may usefully contribute by influencing the court to focus upon the child's needs.

In cases where removal of the child from home is contemplated, the clinician may be called upon to weigh the harm to the child caused by the parents' behavior or by the home environment against the harm caused by removal and placement in another home. The consultant may suggest interventions that address the family's problems while allowing the child to remain in the home.

Whether or not the child is removed from the home, there are a range of remedial interventions that may be utilized to assist the family. Parental psychopathology, marital problems, and environmental stresses may all detract from parenting abilities. The consultant's recommendations for parents may include individual, family, or group therapy; abusive parents' groups; and parenting classes. Recommendations for children may include psychotherapy or other rehabilitative activities.

The clinician may also be consulted concerning a child's return home. Where serious parental problems have not been corrected, consultation may be sought regarding termination of parents' rights. Here the legal issue is whether the conditions that rendered the parents unfit are likely to respond to remedial efforts in a reasonable period of time. Questions posed to the psychiatrist involve the nature, extent, and amenability to change of the parents' personality limitations that are relevant to the capacity to care for the child. When the child's foster parent seeks to establish a more permanent legal relationship, an assessment of this "parent-child" relationship may be sought.

Psychiatrists are often frustrated by the inadequate attention given to preservation of the relationship between the child and his or her psychological parent—that is, the individual to whom the child is bonded psychologically in a parent-child relationship. This may or may not be the biological parent. Removal of a child may be effected without sufficient consideration of the importance to the child of the relationship with the parent. Just as disturbing are situations in which a long-term bond between a child and foster parents is ignored in the service of protecting the rights of natural parents who are virtual strangers to the child. Despite some movement to focus on the welfare of the child rather than the rights of parents, change comes slowly.

Child Custody Consultation: Disputes Between Private Parties

There have been important developments in divorce custody law in recent years, some of which may signify an expanded role for psychiatrists in the custody decision.[2] Over the past two decades the law in most states has moved from a rule that strongly favored mothers for custody—the "tender years" presumption—to an ostensibly sex-neutral "best interest of the child" standard.[13] This recent position encourages the judge to make a careful determination of which custody arrangement will better serve the child's needs. In addition, joint custody, which was unusual ten years ago, is now enthusiastically promoted in many laws as the best arrangement for children after divorce.[16]

THE BEST-INTEREST STANDARD AND THE CHILD PSYCHIATRIST

Under the best-interest standard, the judge may consider any information about the parents, the child, and their relationship that is relevant to the choice of custodian. Under many statutes, the judge has virtually unguided discretion in making the decision. A few states, such as Michigan, attempt to guide the judge by providing criteria to be considered. However, even where the law specifies the factors that must be weighed, the judge decides the weight to be given to each. Moreover, he or she may always consider other criteria deemed relevant to the custody decision.

While the sex-neutral best-interest standard may undo some of the distortions caused by the tender years presumption, in practice it has significant problems. Whether the choice lies between two adequate or two marginal parents, the basis for a decision may be very unclear, and the judge's values and biases may be important determinants.[3] In reaching for a basis for decision, a judge may be influenced by factors of limited relevance to custody, such as life-styles, political views, and sexual practices.

PSYCHIATRIC CONSULTATION

It is not surprising that judges making custody decisions often turn to psychiatrists and other mental health professionals for assistance.[2] A parent seeking custody may also attempt to bolster his or her case by engaging a psychiatrist. However, psychiatric opinion has a more solid clinical foundation and is more persuasive in court if the clinician performs the evaluation for the court or for the guardian *ad litem* (the child's attorney) rather than for one parent. A custody evaluation performed for one parent tends to be of limited clinical value, because usually the only parent seen by the psychiatrist is the one who is paying for the work. In contrast, the psychiatrist who participates as a court consultant tends to approach the task with a higher degree of neutrality and objectivity. All parties then have an incentive to cooperate with the consultant and a more comprehensive assessment may thus be possible.

There are generally three dimensions to psychiatric evaluation in custody disputes: those issues relating to the child, those relating to the parents, and those arising from the relationship between the child and each parent. Within each of these areas, particular elements have received attention in the courts and legislatures in recent years.

In this era when traditional rules (such as automatically giving custody to the mother unless she is unfit) can no longer be relied upon, the child's preference is increasingly emphasized. In many states, if factors are equal, a child of normal intellectual and emotional capabilities is essentially given the right to make the custody decision by about age fourteen. In many instances the older children are probably properly consulted regarding the matter of preference. Some of them, however, and many younger children may need protection from the developing expectation that they

should decide this monumental issue. Psychiatrists can assist by protecting children from pressure from their parents and the court, while facilitating the expression of preference where appropriate.

In weighing parenting capacities, courts often consider issues such as the parents' life-styles and their sexual preference and behavior. To vest custody in a homosexual parent or in a parent living with a paramour may be viewed as contrary to the child's best interest. The parent with unusual political views, religious practices, or living arrangements may also be disfavored. Indeed, one of the few factors that may not be considered is race; the Supreme Court has held that a court may not withdraw custody from a white custodial mother solely because she married a black man (*Palmore v. Sidot;* 466 U.S. 429 [1984]). The psychiatrist may serve an important role in defusing inflammatory issues that might otherwise distort the decision-making process. The consultant can then encourage the judge to focus on the extent to which moral or life-style issues are (or are not) relevant to the determination of a particular child's well-being.

There is a growing recognition of the central importance to the child of maintaining the relationship with his or her "psychological parent," who may or may not be a biological parent.[8] In most families, both parents fill this role. If one parent is in a nurturing and limit-setting role and the other is not, the choice of custodian may be readily resolved. In custody contests between biological parents and third parties (such as grandparents), some states now tend to protect the psychological parent-child relationship, despite the strong traditional legal presumption favoring biological parents.

In a divorce custody dispute where both parents are psychological parents and neither is seriously deficient, the consultant may have a limited role.[13] He or she may describe the character of the child's relationship with each parent, parenting strengths and weaknesses of the mother and father, and special needs of the child. Restraint is desirable lest the consultant, feeling pressure to resolve the issue, go beyond the limits of psychiatric expertise and rely upon his or her values and biases in making any recommendations.

JOINT CUSTODY

The major development in custody law in the past few years has been the emerging prominence of joint custody.[4] In 1975 only one state considered joint custody as a possible disposition; today more than thirty states do so. Joint legal custody involves the sharing by parents of responsibility and authority for their children regarding such issues as medical care, education, and religious instruction. The arrangement may or may not include joint physical custody, where the child is required to spend a substantial amount of time residing with each parent.

We have described a number of factors that have contributed to the current enthusiasm for joint custody.[16] A dramatic increase in the incidence of divorce has occurred in the last twenty years, and there is a growing awareness of the detrimental effects of family breakdown on children. Recent social science research by Hetherington[9] and Wallerstein and Kelly[19] indicates that the destructive impact of divorce may be ameliorated if the child maintains a close relationship with both parents. The important role of the fathers to their children's development is receiving greater recognition. In families in which both parents work, an increasingly common pattern, fathers may have a substantial involvement in child care. Thus some divorcing families have turned to joint custody as a means of minimizing family disruption.

The positive response of the legal system to this custody arrangement is more complex. In some states laws have been passed in response to organized political pressure from fathers' groups. These organizations view joint custody as the only means by which men are likely to obtain custody. Legislatures have responded to their appeal that joint custody preserves family relationships and promotes the child's positive adjustment to divorce. A rule preferring joint custody may also be attractive to the legal system in another way; it offers a means of resolving custody disputes without resorting to the difficult choice between parents.[4]

Some state laws simply make joint custody available if the parents voluntarily choose the arrangement, but a growing number of states are giving joint custody a preferred legal status. Many laws direct courts to consider joint custody if one parent seeks the arrangement and the other parent is opposed. The parent who opposes joint custody may have to overcome the presumption that it is the best arrangement for children. Laws encouraging joint custody are often accompanied by an alternative provision; if one parent is to be given sole custody, the law favors the parent who is more likely to support the child's relationship with the other parent. The combined effect of these provisions may be to coerce unwilling parents to agree to joint custody, an arrangement for which they may be quite unsuited.

As the law has become more favorable toward joint custody, psychiatric opinion is sought increasingly to assess the feasibility of the arrangement for a particular couple and to estimate its probable effects on children. At present, there is no strong research support for joint custody as public policy. However, there is certainly no evidence that children in voluntary joint custody arrangements experience more adjustment problems after divorce than do children in sole custody. Given the observed harmful effects of father absence, this arrangement may well be beneficial for children. But neither the available research nor clinical experience suggests that joint custody is desirable when one of the parents is opposed to the arrangement. Every psychiatrist has seen children from both divorced and intact families who suffer from the effects of conflict between their parents. Research findings suggest that the adjustment problems observed in children from divorced families may be more directly attributable to interparental conflict than to father absence.[9] Several studies indicate that the adjustment of children in single-parent harmonious homes is better than that of children in nuclear families characterized by conflict between the parents.[6] These findings raise serious questions about the desirability of coercive laws that may impose joint custody on a reluctant parent or parents.

The psychiatric consultant may assist the court in assessing the parents' capacity to share custody of their child. Where one parent is adamantly opposed to joint custody, or intense hostility exists between the parents for whatever reason, a sole custody arrangement may be desirable. The consulting psychiatrist may also assist the court in weighing the parents' resistance to joint custody. Many laws that favor joint custody threaten loss of custody to the parent who resists the arrangement and/or is not supportive of the child's relationship with the other parent. While a vindictive parent may indeed not be the optimal parent, a parent's hostility to his or her former spouse may not be the most important consideration in choosing a custodian, as some laws suggest. The psychiatrist can seek to present a balanced picture of each parents' relationship with the child and place the parents' relationship with each other in perspective.

Many psychiatrists who consult in custody disputes believe that their most valuable service may be to assist parents in separating their anger at each other from their concern for their child. While the role of consultant is not a therapeutic one, parents may be helped to focus on their child's needs, to recognize the harm that their conflict may cause, and to alter their behavior accordingly. Indeed, the most successful custody consultations may be those in which the parents resolve the dispute themselves and negate the need for consultation to the court.

Psychiatric Hospitalization of Minors

Traditionally, parents have had authority to make medical decisions for their children, including the authority to consent to the youngsters' admission to a psychiatric facility. The child who resisted had been deemed not competent to make the decision. Recently there has been growing concern that parents may have a conflict of interest with their children on this issue and may inappropriately seek admission for a child whose presence in the home is disruptive.[5]

The United States Supreme Court in 1979 in *Parham v. J.R.* (442 U.S. 584) made clear that such a hearing is not constitutionally required. In upholding a Georgia statute, the Court found that a review of the parents' decision by a neutral factfinder, the director of the hospital, was an adequate protection against inappropriate hospitalization. The Court expressed its faith in parents' good intentions toward their children and assumed that physicians could discern questionable cases and either refuse admission or quickly release the child.

Despite the Supreme Court ruling in *Parham,* some states require judicial hearings. They have decided this is necessary because of the potential stigma and deprivation of liberty inherent in psychiatric hospitalization. Where minors, particularly adolescents, resist their parents' efforts to admit them to a psychiatric hospital, the minors are provided with legal representation. In several jurisdictions minors are treated like adults; the same civil commitment standards apply. In most states, however, the minor is not free to refuse needed treatment as an adult would be simply because he or she is not a danger to self or others. Many statutes direct that any treatment decided on should be the least restrictive alternative. A few state laws include provisions that allow minors to seek admission without their parents' consent. In general, younger children may be admitted on the parents' request, often with formal medical review.

The legal and the psychiatric perspectives concerning psychiatric hospitalization of children may differ.[12] Lawyers tend to see the issue in terms of loss of liberty and stigma, which must be justified by assuring through a hearing that the correct decision has been made. Psychiatrists may place greater emphasis on the child's level of disturbance and need for treatment, and may discount the relevance of his or her resistance to hospitalization. In addition, such a hearing can be disruptive to treatment and to the doctor-patient relationship.[1]

Conclusion

The child psychiatrist may view the prospect of participating in a legal proceeding with considerable ambivalence; the role of court consultant is quite different from that of therapist. Nonetheless, when judges make legal decisions regarding children, psychiatric consultation is often eagerly sought. The psychiatrist who carefully defines the boundaries of his or her expertise and limits observations and opinion accordingly may play a useful role in the process. In most cases, the objective of the court is consonant with the goals of the clinician—to promote the child's welfare.

REFERENCES

1. AMAYA, M., and BURLINGAME, W. V. "Judicial Review of Psychiatric Admissions: The Clinical Impact on Child and Adolescent Inpatients," *Journal of the American Academy of Child Psychiatry,* 20 (1981):761–776.

2. DERDEYN, A. P. "Child Custody Consultation," *American Journal of Orthopsychiatry,* 45 (1975):791–801.

3. ———. "Child Abuse and Neglect: The Rights of Parents and the Needs of Their Children," *American Journal of Orthopsychiatry,* 47 (1977):377–387.

4. DERDEYN, A. P., and SCOTT, E. S. "Joint Custody: A Critical Analysis and Appraisal," *American Journal of Orthopsychiatry,* 54 (1984):199–209.

5. ELLIS, J. W. "Volunteering Children: Parental Commitment of Minors to Mental Institutions," *California Law Review,* 62 (1974): 840.

6. EMERY, R. E., HETHERINGTON, E. M., and DILALLA, L. F. "Divorce, Children, and Social Policy," in H. Stevenson and A. Slegel, eds., *Child Development and Social Policy.* Chicago: University of Chicago Press: 1984, pp. 189–266.

7. GOLDSTEIN, J., FREUD, A., and SOLNIT, A. J. *Before the Best Interests of the Child.* New York: Free Press, 1979.

8. ———. *Beyond the Best Interests of the Child.* New York: Free Press, 1979.

9. HETHERINGTON, E. M., COX, M., and COX, R. "The Aftermath of Divorce," J. Stevens, and M. Mathews, eds., *Mother/Child/Father/Child Relationships.* Washington, D.C.: National Association for the Education of Young Children, 1978.

10. Institute of Judicial Administration/American Bar Association, Juvenile Justice Standards. *Standard Relating to Dispositions.* Cambridge, Mass.: Ballinger, 1980.

11. LEWIS, D. O., et al. "Violent Juvenile Delinquents: Psychiatric, Neurological, Psychological and Abuse Factors," *Journal of the American Academy of Child Psychiatry,* 18 (1979) 307–319.

12. MILLER, D., and BURT, R. A. "Children's Rights on Entering Therapeutic Institutions," *American Journal of Psychiatry,* 134 (1977):153–156.

13. MNOOKIN, R. "Child Custody Adjudication: Judicial

Functions in the Face of Indeterminacy," *Law and Contemporary Problems,* 39 (1975):226.

14. ———. *Child, Family and State.* Boston: Little, Brown, 1978.

15. PAULSEN, M., and WHITEBREAD, C. *Juvenile Law and Procedure.* Reno, Nev.: National Council of Juvenile Court Judges, 1974.

16. SCOTT, E., and DERDEYN, A. P. "Rethinking Joint Custody," *Ohio State Law Journal* 45 (1984):455–498.

17. WADLINGTON, W., WHITEBREAD, C., and DAVIS, S. M. *Children in the Legal System.* Mineola, N.Y.: Foundation Press, 1982.

18. WALD, M. "State Intervention on Behalf of 'Neglected' Children: A Search for Realistic Standards," *Stanford Law Review,* 27 (1975):985.

19. WALLERSTEIN, J. S., and KELLY, J. B. *Surviving the Breakup: How Parents and Children Cope with Divorce.* New York: Basic Books, 1980.

74 / The Rural Child and Child Psychiatry

Theodore A. Petti, Ellen G. Benswanger, and M. Jerome Fialkov

Introduction and Overview

This chapter presents both a historical and a cross-sectional perspective of children, adolescents, and their families residing in rural areas. It describes the context within which mental health–related services are delivered and the complex factors impacting on the social and emotional well-being of these young people. Few child psychiatrists and other mental health professionals have an adequate understanding of the environment within which rural children grow and develop. An extra effort has therefore been made to depict the essence of the rural/urban difference, particularly as it may affect the development of children and the human services delivered to them.

The variety of attempts to define the term rural provide a sense of the inherent richness, complexity, and diversity of the field.* The United States Census Bureau has defined rural as those areas or towns with fewer than 2,500 people and open country outside closely settled suburbs of metropolitan areas. Rural is considered to be synonymous with "nonmetropolitan" areas, or those areas outside of a standard metropolitan statistical area (SMSA) whose central city has a population of at least 50,000. Rural residents make up 30 percent or more of our population and live on up to 89 percent of the land area of the United States.

Rural cultural and belief systems play a major role in the utilization of services and the development of youth in such areas.[7] Rural communities have been described as *gemeinshaft* societies in that they are distinguished by the predominance of small social units,

*See references 4, 6, 7, 18, 25, 35, 41, 45, 49, and 51.

relationships based on kinships and community ties, and homogeneity of interests and beliefs. Remnants of these patterns continue to dominate the quality of life in many contemporary rural communities. Within these settings, the families practice living arrangements that are typical of a "folk" society—great emphasis is placed on conformity to traditional values and adherence to family expectations.[102] Communication tends to be personal, informal, and direct. In many rural communities, orientation to time and space is different from that in urban settings.[7] This outlook is reflected in a personalized perception of distance and duration and a slower pace of daily life.

Rural Children

The nature of rural life and the needs of rural communities vary considerably throughout the United States. Obvious differences exist among the life-styles of children in a New England village, a ranch community in Wyoming, and a rural county in Pennsylvania.[17] Like their urban counterparts, rural children are the product of the diverse factors in their environment. Social, geographic, cultural, economic, and educational elements all play a role.[89] However, certain common themes distinguish rural children from their urban and suburban peers. The high rates of infant mortality, poverty, unemployment, and the lower levels of educational achievement of their parents suggest that rural youth are at greater risk for emotional disorders than are their urban counterparts. Among adults, the incidence of many disorders, particularly depression, has been reported as much higher in rural than in urban areas.[16,27,62,102] The offspring of rural parents with chronically disabling disorders have a heightened vulnerability to a variety of psychopathological conditions.[103] It has been suggested that from an early age rural children are forced to learn nonverbal cues in order to know how their nonverbal parents[60] and other adults are thinking and feeling. They must also become more self-reliant while they are still dependent on others.[40]

Poignant descriptions of rural children and adolescents richly illustrate the differences associated with race, sex, and geography.[40,59,60] The stereotypic image of rural youth growing up in farming communities is misleading; farm youngsters are in fact in the minority. Moreover, increasing numbers of rural youth are being reared in settings outside of the traditional nuclear or extended family.[93] We will not elaborate on the special situation of poverty, poor health, and restricted access to human services of the thousands of children whose parents are rural migrant workers.

The experiences of rural children also distinguish them from their urban counterparts. The dominant urban culture depicted in the mass media and the traditional rural values espoused by their families and acquaintances result in a culture gap between themselves and the older generation, far greater than that experienced by urban youth. Their attempts at change and experimentation conflict with the traditional conservatism and produce intergenerational tension.

In summarizing the findings from several studies of urban-rural differences,[12] beliefs relating to morality, religious convictions, and political philosophy are significantly different in rural communities, with rural folk more likely to hold conservative views on divorce, birth control, and premarital sex and to translate these views into concrete action and community policy. There is less divorce and fewer mothers employed outside of the home in rural as compared to urban locales. Other characteristic values are an emphasis on hard work and mastery of the physical environment; resistance to change; a religiously oriented, fatalistic world view; and reliance on natural helping networks rather than professional caretakers.

In many rural areas enclaves of distinct but idiosyncratic cultural groups, linked by kinship, religious, or social values, coexist with the main stream rural population. This extended kinship pattern is commonly found in Appalachia and the rural southeastern United States. There is greater dependence on authority figures and less dependence on peers,[99] which is also relevant for an understanding of regional rural differences. However, the rural/urban discrepancy in parenting approaches is less than was formerly believed.[92,99] In any case, when children and parents from these groups need mental health services, their life-styles and treatment goals may require urban-trained professionals to consider a different approach to such potent issues as child abuse, incest, alcoholism, and recurrent patterns of psychopathology in families.

In the past, a higher birth rate was characteristic of rural families. More recently, however, the fertility rate has been decreasing so that rural youth have fewer sibs with whom to interact. This change may affect the manner in which country families spend their time and their money and may eventually narrow the gap between urban/rural populations.[19,93]

Studies also indicate that rural children lag behind their urban peers on a majority of cognitive measures including Piagetian conservation tasks, classification and sorting tests, and memory.[43] Given their realistic dependence on external forces,[41] many rural youngsters may have a less internalized concept of locus of control or attributional style. In terms of cognitive style, rural children tend to be more concrete, more passive, less manipulative, and less advanced in the use of strategies to organize and structure information. In some cases these findings may point to actual cognitive deficits. In others they may reflect a misperception of the rural environment and the types of cognitive skills it fosters as well as the inadequacy of standardized tests to measure idiosyncratic abilities and strengths.[43]

Given the physical distances involved, rural youth may miss the opportunity for the "chumship" that Sullivan[96] described as an antidote to internal conflict. Their isolation also limits access to the kinds of cultural, social, and educational opportunities available in the city. The situation may be exacerbated by circumstances limiting their ability to find a satisfying job or to contribute meaningfully to the family or community. Rural youth face the same downward cycle as the areas in which they reside.[17] Many live in homes without electricity or adequate sanitary facilities and are cared for by parents who are unable to provide minimal levels of clothing and health care.[53] Given the bleak environment of their rearing, these youngsters often lack the incentive to improve themselves or to see a hopeful future.[59] The consequence is a climate of boredom and frustration, which provides fertile ground for delinquent behavior, vandalism, alcoholism, and other substance abuse.

Like urban juveniles, rural youth who are substance abusers are more likely to have a delinquent history.[36] Patterns of drug use differ in urban and rural areas, with alcohol as the drug of choice among rural teenagers.[50] Rural youth tend to limit their drug use to alcohol and marijuana and much less frequently abuse other drugs.[36,55]

Human Services in Rural Areas

The identifying characteristics of a given community may be reflected in the structure of its human service system. Distinctive patterns may be observed in the configuration of individual agencies and the links between elements inside and outside of the system. A clear description of these patterns is presented by Williams.[104] Services in a rural community can be classified in terms of "horizontal" or "vertical" linkages. Horizontal patterns of interaction link locally based community programs or organizations with one another. The patterns tend to be personal, direct, and informal.[104] In a rural system, the same person may serve on the board of several agencies simultaneously. Interactions may occur on a regular, informal basis between a number of human service agency workers. These contacts may include resource and information sharing, referrals, or requests for supplementary services. Horizontal linkages are characteristic of small, personalized settings and reflect the positive as well as the negative aspects of intimate, primary relationships.

Local organizations are also related to agencies and units outside of the community by means of "vertical linkages"—for example, the structural ties between a community mental health center and its administrative units at the regional, state, and federal levels. In many rural systems the *gemeinshaft* orientation with its horizontal patterns has been gradually replaced by urban values and goals—reflected in the growth of bureaucratic structures and a corresponding increase in vertical linkage patterns. Connections between local agencies and state and federal units tend to be impersonal and mechanistic. High priorities are given to goal setting, accountability, and professionalism in contrast to the traditional emphasis on mutual needs and individualized care.

The increasing predominance of vertical linkages affects rural communities in significant ways. Rural services receive a large proportion of their funds from external, distant sources. As a result, local folk are only peripherally involved in the policy-setting and decision-making processes. Furthermore, the proliferation of extracommunity influences has affected the nature of the horizontal links within the rural communities. There is increased likelihood that competition for funds, clients, and "turf" will color the horizontal interactions between rural agencies in the same community. The challenge is to develop service delivery models that will incorporate the positive aspects of both the horizontal and vertical patterns.*

The entire constellation of human services is availa-

*See references 9, 20, 33, 75, 76, and 77.

ble in some form to children and families in most rural communities. However, the quality of and accessibility to these services often leaves much to be desired.

Factors affecting delivery of human services to rural settings include a lack of empirical data on the needs of the rural population, geographical limitations and inadequate transportation, shifts in population, the nature of rural culture and belief systems, and the use of inappropriate models in the conceptualization of rural service delivery.

Lack of empirical data about local conditions and needs is a major impediment in planning effective human service programs.[6,19,20,93] It is related to the ineffective interest in rural concerns, the use of urban-based models to carry out the limited research that has been done, and the general absence of rural-based personnel trained to conduct research.

The geography of rural areas is also a critical factor in the delivery of services and in understanding rural people. The distance between families, towns, centers, and human service agencies contributes to social isolation and inaccessability of resources.[6,7,17] Under the Federal Mental Health Centers Act, for example, most rural catchment areas contain over 5,000 square miles (the size of Connecticut). The average size is 17,000 square miles. Administrative units of such dimensions limit the efficacy of centralized service delivery. In catchment areas the size of the entire upper peninsula of Michigan, the use of itinerant professionals is neither feasible nor efficacious in the delivery of special education, court functions, or special services for the physically or multiply handicapped juvenile or adult.[6,26,102] In addition, in many rural areas adverse weather conditions, physical barriers, lack of roads, and uneconomical forms of transportation make travel difficult and expensive for both the providers and recipients of human services.[26]

Low population density leads to increased cost in the delivery of services; this makes the cost benefit ratio of direct service delivery prohibitive.[17] Sparse population also restricts the economic base ordinarily required to support human services.[26] Lack of services may eventuate in the deterioration of rural communities and, with the high rate of rural poverty and unemployment, further exacerbate the problem by contributing to a downward spiral of decreased job opportunities, demoralization, and eventual migration to metropolitan areas.[6,17,41,102] The inability of rural communities to gain adequate access to available funding sources results in a tragic loss of human and economic resources and leads to a sense of futility and hopelessness.

In addition to limited financial resources, rural communities are unable to recruit and retain professional personnel. Those who decide to practice in a rural setting are often treated with distrust and resentment.[94] The existence of a new agency in a nonmetropolitan area may be tenuous as the equilibrium within the community system shifts.[46] Attempts may be made, covert or overt, to hinder its functioning and to exclude the newcomers, who are perceived as invading the turf of both formal and informal service providers. Because of the scarcity of sophisticated urban amenities, both cultural and professional, professional manpower is difficult to recruit to rural areas. The newcomer may expect a higher salary for making the sacrifice, something that community coffers may be unable to provide. Once the "honeymoon" is over, a frequent outcome is the development of resentment on the part of the community and disillusionment for the professional, leading to a state of frustration, dissatisfaction, and "burnout."

Much of the "cultural shock" is due to inadequate professional preparation for rural practice. Once the professional is in the community, problems may arise because of inappropriate assignment within the program, relations within or between programs, isolation from other professionals, and ambiguities about role definition. When the rural agencies are dependent on government subsidies for their existence, the control local governments exert over helping agencies can be extremely frustrating for many professionals.

In communities where the potentially productive and future-oriented segment of the population has migrated to metropolitan areas,[66] those who remain are likely to be dependent and deprived. These are usually the unskilled, the elderly, and children.[102] This results in further depletion of an effective tax base, disproportionate increases in per-capita needs for human services, and an even greater decrease in resources.[41]

Over the past fifteen years a shift toward nonmetropolitan growth has occurred.[6,41,44] This "migration turnaround" has resulted in an increased demand for human services. The new rural immigrants are a mixed group. They do expect the level of services provided in metropolitan areas.[79] This is a large problem in energy-related boom towns of the West.[6] Many of these new settlers are appearing with, or developing, young families. Their racial and cultural backgrounds often differ from the predominant Anglo-Saxon, Protestant rural ethic; with this influx of families come pressures and demands for change.[44,102] The migrant children must adapt to a new culture and different ways of doing things. The native rural children are faced with more sophisticated, often more competitive newcomers who tend to dominate. The impact of one group on the other has not been adequately researched.[80]

Local communities are dominated by personal dynamics that frequently color professional transactions.[26] Conflict with rural power brokers generally spells disaster for rural agencies. The "grassroots" ideology, common to most rural areas throughout the country,[40] clashes directly with the tenets of professionalism.[95] Difficulties then develop around such basic issues such as professional autonomy and confidentiality.[94,95]

Competitive services are rarely present in rural areas. Federal funding agencies and the legislation allocating funds to these areas rarely take urban/rural differences into account. Too often, rural programs are displaced versions of urban models. Consequently, funding for needed services is contingent on providing other services or linkages that may be unnecessary, unavailable, or too costly to deliver. Funds are generally specified as categorical and leave little room for the creative ingenuity of rural professionals to maximize their resources.[6,58,82]

In many rural systems, service mandates and program regulations are simply inappropriate to sparse population density, lack of transportation, or scarcity of personnel.[7] Even the costs of delivering service in nonmetropolitan areas may be higher.[3,27,102] It is ironic that metropolitan areas with less need are often provided more money; relatively poor rural areas may currently be subsidizing the richer urban areas while receiving fewer services.[17]

During the 1980s much progress has been made in recognizing the uniqueness of rural human services. This progress is reflected in the emergence of new professional journals such as the *Journal of Rural Community Psychology, Human Services in the Rural Environment,* and the *American Journal of Rural Health* along with professional organizations such as the American Rural Health Association and the National Association for Rural Mental Health. Collections of essays dealing specifically with rural practice have also been published.[19,51,101]

Health and Mental Health Systems

The most traditional definition equates health with the absence of disease. Knowledgeable analysts examining the relation between health and place of residence have concluded that country living "can be hazardous to your health."[97] This negative assessment is based on the relative and absolute shortage of health and mental health professionals for direct service, supervision, and preventive and education efforts. Rates of chronic diseases, infant mortality, and fatal accidents are highest in rural areas. Facilities for the delivery of traditional medical care are sorely lacking. Rural families are less likely than urban residents to have health insurance coverage, while federal programs, such as Medicare, employ eligibility criteria that discriminate against country dwellers.[4] This makes it more difficult for rural practitioners to attain an adequate income.

While 30 percent of the population lived in rural areas in 1979, only 17 percent of the primary care physicians practiced there; 30 percent fewer nurses and dentists worked in rural than in urban areas.[97] Physicians generally choose neither to reside nor to work in the country. Thus about 80 percent of the 16 million Americans, who live in rural areas are faced with a "critical shortage" of primary physicians. In 1979 over 50 percent of towns with 5,000 to 10,000 population had an internist while only 25 percent had a pediatrician and 17 percent a psychiatrist.[70] Rural children and the mentally ill are deprived of access to specialized medical care.

As rural families often seek mental health care from the general medical sector rather than the specialty sector,[26] The number of generalists or primary care providers is critical. Part of the reason for doctor choice relates to the reluctance to seek help for "mental" reasons. The visibility in rural areas and fears of being labeled as crazy keep many adults from seeking or utilizing mental health facilities. High rates of suicide and alcoholism may be the result of this reluctance to seek help.[98]

The inadequate number of available mental health professionals, especially psychiatrists and psychologists, may be another reason rural residents turn to the medical center for mental health problems. They may seek care away from the rural mental health centers because the center concept itself, based on catchment area and centralized, pluralistic resources, cannot be feasibly implemented in rural locales. For example, it is difficult to integrate family involvement into care programs for rural citizens, and even when the distance is not prohibitive, rural residents are reluctant to go to another town for services or to use a central location as their mental health resource. The relative shortage of community resources renders the centralized concept inadequate. In addition, the lack of knowledge concerning psychiatric disorders inhibits many rural citizens from seeking care at mental health facilities.[11]

Rural mental health centers tend to have fewer staff than are found in urban locales and offer less opportunity to specialize. Typical urban centers have had a full-time equivalent staff of 104.7, whereas the typical rural center employs 44 full-time equivalents. Rural centers use a smaller proportion of psychiatric time than do partially rural or urban centers and depend more heavily on part-time staff.[27] It is noteworthy that the rural staff more closely embody the conceptual philosophy of community mental health centers than do urban staff. They seem to feel a greater sense of

mission and to be more committed to the mental health center ideology. Rural workers endorse higher levels of both organizational and personal activism; they view their centers as being more like social agencies than medical centers.[49] This may be related to the general scarcity of professional skills in rural areas, but may also arise because most rural professionals function as generalists sharing in clinical and administrative roles, as initiators and facilitators, and as educators as well as full participants in rural life.[52,74]

It is unlikely that rural areas will ever receive the professional or financial resources necessary to provide mental health services comparable to those in urban areas. Predominantly rural states contain 33 percent of the children in the United States but have only 4 percent of the mental health clinics providing services to children.[1] Few professionals are trained to work with rural children and their families. Critical reviews emphasize the failure of most training programs to prepare mental health and related professionals for working in nonmetropolitan areas.[6,20,52,58] This is a particular issue for child psychiatrists and other mental health professionals working with children and youth where knowledge of the system is essential to understand the disorder and to plan appropriate treatment strategies.

In most rural mental health settings the traditional therapist-patient relationship in one-to-one psychotherapy is not appropriate.[27] Given the visibility of rural professionals and their patients, the informal patterns of their communication and nature of interagency contacts, rural mental health professionals must learn to balance the prevailing standards of confidentiality and professional responsibility against the demands of the rural system.[46,95] Rural professionals are also expected to interact with their patients and the overall community in a number of roles. These expectations are particularly difficult for highly trained specialists who are unable to feel comfortable with role diffusion.

Fiscal considerations and the inability to recruit or retain professionals in nonmetropolitan locales has resulted in the employment of paraprofessionals, mostly bachelors-level college graduates and masters-level generalists, to provide the bulk of mental health care.[47] Most interventions correspond to the classical one-to-one therapeutic relationship. Supervision is often conducted by professionals who have very little experience or training in the psychiatric assessment and treatment of disturbed children and adolescents.

Qualified child psychiatrists are rarely found in rural counties. Many general psychiatrists in these areas devote a portion of their practice to working with adolescents; they provide supervision to the clinicians who assess and treat children, adolescents, and their families. An emerging pattern in rural western Pennsylvania may be typical of other rural areas of the country. While child psychiatrists provide part-time consultation or direct service to some nonurban counties, most counties lack sufficient input from child psychiatry. A 1979 survey[2] suggests that there has been a decided trend away from the predominant practice of child psychiatry in major metropolitan areas or academic centers. Communities with populations under 10,000 have attracted about 5 percent of the child psychiatrists practicing in such settings as community mental health centers or health maintenance organizations.[85] Significantly more child psychiatrists practicing in nonmetropolitan areas or in midsize cities were board certified than were general psychiatrists from those areas.[61] Frequently, however, child psychiatrists working in rural areas are forced by financial pressures to devote considerable portions of their time to adult work—generally with hospitalized patients.

Most accredited child psychiatry training programs are located in large metropolitan centers or affiliated with urban universities. Few programs offer experiences in rural mental health or include didactic sessions on rural issues.[62] Those programs that do so provide the trainees in psychiatry and child psychiatry with a firsthand opportunity to observe the integration (or in many cases the converse, the failure of coordination) of services. Trainees who become immersed in the training, service, politics, and intra- and intersystems issues become ever more aware of the unique characteristics of practice in rural settings. Such experiences make the trainees more appreciative of the various levels of government that are involved in the delivery of mental health care and the variety of impediments that hamper development of comprehensive human services related to mental health.[62,63]

Some of the stresses that impact on the rural child psychiatrist have been described.[17] These include the inability to practice "ideal medicine" and the need to settle for "pragmatic solutions" to complex problems; the time-consuming nature of providing a range of clinical and nonclinical services to the community with no one else for backup; the need to be a generalist and to practice beyond self-perceived levels of competence "because there is no one else"; the inability to be selective about which patients will be seen for evaluation or treatment; and the real constraints on professional mobility or growth. In addition, the lack of adequate support such as professionally trained clinical child psychologists, child psychiatric social workers, and special education teachers makes the job especially difficult and leads to decreased job satisfaction and the potential for burnout.[17,74]

Rural child psychiatrists are at a great disadvantage in terms of access to continuing medical education.

This has been cited as an important factor leading to migration of physicians from rural areas. The failure of professionals to keep current means that rural patients obtain less than up-to-date care and are unable to benefit from recent advances.

A number of urban teaching programs have extended outreach efforts to rural areas. Some emphasize development of a working knowledge of child and human development, consultation with schools and other child-related agencies oriented toward prevention, and crisis intervention. Other programs have focused on the strengthening of natural helping networks and the development of paraprofessionals and "natural helpers."*

Mental health professionals who are unable to adjust to the slower pace, the lack of anonymity, and the role diffusion characteristic of rural life generally do not remain in such settings. Those remaining quickly learn that the success or failure of a program is dependent less on the training and book learning they bring to their position and more on the immediate response and reaction of the community to their actions and lifestyles as well as the degree to which they can become integrated into the community rather than remaining outsiders.[11]

Welfare and Judicial Systems

Typically most rural children who are dependent or delinquent and who are served by social service agencies are not different from their peers in urban or suburban areas. Since the establishment of the first juvenile court in Chicago, delinquency has been considered an urban phenomenon; as a result most criminological theories have developed from an urban perspective.[23] Statistics have shown that delinquency rates are substantially higher in the cities than in small towns, and higher in both of these than in rural areas.[15] For persons under eighteen, the rate of arrests in cities is slightly higher than in the suburbs, but almost three times greater than the rural arrest rate.[28,29,30]

Crime is less frequent in rural areas for a number of reasons: more stable populations and closely knit families; greater influence of church and school; and people who are less alienated from their communities than are their city counterparts. The judges are more personally related to the population, the culture, and the politics of the area. However, the lower incidence of crime may also reflect less accurate record keeping by rural law enforcement agencies, increased use of informal proc-

*See references 9, 10, 22, 24, 58, 62, 65, and 74.

essing by police, less opportunity for certain kinds of crime, or fewer persons apprehended for crimes committed.

Juvenile crime in rural areas is of a different character than in urban areas; crimes against persons are infrequent, and most rural juvenile offenses are minor property offenses.[73] The only offenses with comparable rates in cities, suburbs, and rural areas are "driving under the influence" and "drunkenness."[31] In a victimization survey of rural Ohio residents, vandalism was the leading crime (38 percent of all crimes), with mailboxes the property most affected. Larceny was the second leading crime.[78]

When one moves from urban to rural communities, the criteria for a "serious" offense change, with minor offenses receiving comparatively greater attention from rural law enforcement agencies. This results in rural juveniles being arrested for offenses that in urban areas would receive little police attention or, at the most, a reprimand and notification of the parents. A study conducted of juveniles detained in adult jails and juvenile detention centers in 187 predominantly rural counties in ten states determined that, according to criteria of the Advisory Committee to the National Institute for Juvenile Justice and Delinquency Prevention,[54] approximately 55 percent would have been ineligible for detention elsewhere. An analysis of the detention rates in New Jersey revealed that of the five counties with the highest detention rates, four were among the most rural in the state.[21]

Often because of limited resources, the only facility available for detention for both serious and minor delinquent offenders, status offenders, and even for children abused by their parents is the county jail, which is used for adult criminals. In order to comply with the federal government's "sight and sound" separation requirement, some juveniles have been secluded in solitary confinement or similar inappropriate settings. As a result of the isolation, detained juveniles are at higher risk for being harmed by others in the same circumstances or of committing self-injurious, even lethal acts.[48]

Psychiatric surveys show markedly lower rates of conduct disorder among rural children and adolescents.[57,59] This urban-rural difference is not confined to disturbances of conduct in young people; it applies as well to emotional disturbances in both young people and their parents.[57,91] Exceptions may be conversion reactions in children[42,83] and depression in adults.[16,27,102]

In all countries statistics consistently show that more boys than girls appear before the courts for delinquent activities. Currently, girls in cities are increasingly more likely to commit, and be apprehended for, the same types of offenses as are boys, albeit less frequently.[14,38] By contrast, in rural areas girls con-

tinue to be viewed in terms of a more traditional, sex-role stereotype and, as a result, are managed by the juvenile court differently from their male counterparts. In a national survey of more than 57,000 institutionalized youth, two-thirds of the girls were status offenders as compared with one-third of the boys. In rural states, this discrepancy may be even greater.[105] Not only are girls sent to institutions more often than boys, but they also remain there longer with indeterminate sentences.

A major issue in rural juvenile justice is the relationship between institutionalization and the availability of resources and services. Predominantly rural states—such as Wyoming and Nevada—have the highest per-capita rates of average daily institutional populations in state-run institutions and camps.[100] As a result, relatively naive rural juveniles may be exposed to more aggressive, streetwise urban delinquents. Such facilities may contain residents who are seriously delinquent and display associated problems including depression, aggression, impulsivity, and overactivity. Staff available at these facilities are generally undertrained and unfamiliar with the necessary tactics for dealing with such youth since most were themselves raised in rural communities. Providing more sophisticated treatment at correctional facilities in rural areas should be a priority for state government.*

Another major population requiring services are those rural children who are abused and neglected. No geographic setting is free of child abuse and neglect, and comparable incidence rates are found in urban, suburban, and rural areas.[69] In a review of substantiated abuse reports in Wisconsin, the rates for nonmetropolitan areas were slightly higher than for metropolitan areas, as was the rate of recurrence of the abuse.[71] The overall incidence rates of abuse and neglect vary little by county type, but the distribution of the major types of maltreatment does differ by geographical area. Of special significance is the higher incidence of sexual abuse in rural areas.[34,69] Similar factors contribute to child maltreatment in both urban and rural communities and will not be detailed.[72,86]

Supportive resources in the form of extended family and social networks provide a measure of protection from child abuse and neglect. For rural families, isolation from informal and formal supports can seriously undermine parent-child relationships. Two types of socially isolated families have been depicted[37]: One type forms part of a "deviant subculture" and remains isolated from traditional supports for generations; and the other type does not establish relationships within a community because of mobility or some other factor that prevents it from putting down roots.[13] These families shy away from social interactions, drawing upon their own resources to deal with crises and life

*See references 33, 39, 64, 76, and 77.

changes.[84] In their Appalachian and Philadelphia studies, Polansky and coworkers[81] found that, when compared to controls, neglectful families were severely isolated socially. Such isolation results in the children lacking the necessary social skills to maintain intimate friendships, thereby perpetuating the isolated life-style across generations. Social isolation may also contribute to sexual victimization, particularly to incest.[8,34]

When borderline cases of abuse and neglect occur, mental health professionals may become involved in rural child welfare. As a rule, clearcut cases of physical abuse with obvious injury or physical neglect with evidence of failure to thrive are diagnosed by physicians. Cases that constitute emotional abuse, more subtle physical neglect, and sexual molestation without physical injury often are referred to mental health clinicians for diagnosis and treatment. The clinician may be asked to confirm that the child has been abused and neglected, to comment on whether the parents and child have diagnosable psychiatric disorders, to determine whether the child should be placed in foster care, and to recommend whether the child and parents can be reunited.[32]

Educational System

Twelve thousand school districts, or 75 percent of the total number of operating school systems in the United States, are located in nonurban areas. They provide education for approximately one-third of all students attending public schools.[68]

Studies of rural education document many of the same general issues and problems characteristic of other rural human services. From the perspective of rural inhabitants, the school that was once "theirs" is seen more and more as being under "outside" control, increasingly dominated by state and federal regulations.[68,79]

The unique aspects of "rural" education can be only partially explained by such factors as size, geographic isolation, values and life-style, and economic and occupational status. The families have been described as resistant to book learning and formal education. Rural schools report deficiencies in both the rate of enrollment of students outside the compulsory age range and the overall level of educational achievement.[56]

In many rural areas there are small pockets of cultural or social groups each with its own cognitive style, linguistic patterns, and educational needs. Before the period of school consolidation, it was not unusual for the children from one large extended family to constitute the majority of students in a small rural school. With the advent of busing and the establishment of consolidated schools, children with differing cognitive styles must be educated under one enormous roof, with uniform curricula, materials, and educational philosophy.[56] The unique abilities and cultural preferences of rural youth may be ignored or disparaged.

Legislation enacted during the past three decades has effected massive changes in rural education. The Supreme Court decision of 1954 and subsequent implementation of the desegregation laws have brought about the abolition of segregated schools, the consolidation of scattered rural districts, widespread busing of students, and substantial improvement in the academic achievement of minorities. The impact of the Education for all Handicapped Children Act, PL 94-142, has been felt in virtually every rural community. The training of circuit-riding specialists, who can bring varied services and specialized instruction to isolated schools, is a major effect.

To implement the various legislative mandates, federal and state governments have offered incentives in the form of funding for specific types of programs. However, rural school districts seldom have the proposal-writing capabilities or grantsmanship skills to compete for these funds or, when funds are obtained, to monitor and evaluate the ensuing programs. Some rural communities have overcome these obstacles and mobilized support for special projects.[68,87] These innovative programs are characterized by similar patterns and processes: a slow, laborious start, colored by intense conflict and upheavals; a high point of achievement and change followed by a leveling-off period; and, eventually, an integration of the new ideas into more traditional practices.

Because the school occupies such a central role in the life of the community, it is likely that the details of these controversial efforts will be displayed prominently by the local news media. Inevitably, children become aware of the intense conflicts over educational policies that rage around them and over which they have no control. However, in the majority of studies of school reform, no consideration is given to the emotional impact of change on the children. It becomes the task of rural mental health specialists to evaluate the consequences of such upheavals in the educational system and to seek to minimize their negative impact on the children.

Future Directions

This chapter has highlighted the factors that have affected the delivery of rural mental health services during the past decade. Programs are gradually evolving that systematically assess needs, upgrade the effectiveness of rural mental health personnel and programs, and improve service delivery.* With changes in demography and the renewed interest of politicians in rural matters, public and private efforts to strengthen rural mental health should be supported.

To remain a relevant and vital force in the care of children and adolescents, child psychiatry must address itself to the rural families that comprise a third of our population and to the training needs of professionals who provide services to those families.[74] Child psychiatry training programs situated in rural areas are frequently the major source of practitioners for rural states. Such programs face loss of their accreditation due to insufficient full-time staff, lack of the comprehensive prerequisites deemed necessary to provide services in urban contexts, or inadequate populations to provide the necessary "teaching cases."[88] To counteract this trend, the discipline of child psychiatry must develop programs to ensure increasing numbers of rural mental

*See references 9, 10, 24, 32, 33, 47, 62, 65, 74, 75, 76, and 77.

health practitioners, adequate professional preparation for work in rural settings, and an upgrading of the skills of those already delivering service.

Rural children will continue to bear an unnecessary and unjustified burden until the necessary research and hard data detailing the incidence, prevalence, and types of psychiatric disorders and the efficacy of intervention strategies and programs are available for policy development and implementation and until training programs address the manpower and other issues specific to rural populations. Academia must accept responsibility for developing such initiatives and for bringing to public awareness the special nature of mental health issues as they impact on the rural family.

ACKNOWLEDGMENT

We would like to acknowledge our gratitude for the inspiration, support, and assistance provided by Meyer Sonis, M.D.

REFERENCES

1. ALBEE, G. "Does Including Psychotherapy in National Health Insurance Represent a Subsidy to the Rich from the Poor?" *American Psychologist,* 32 (1977):719–721.

2. AMERICAN ACADEMY OF CHILD PSYCHIATRY. *A Plan for the Coming Decades.* Washington, D.C.: American Academy of Child Psychiatry, 1983.

3. American Medical Association. "Suit Contends Payment Classification Unfair," *American Medical News,* 23 March 1984, p. 11.

4. American Public Health Association Position Paper. "Improving Health Services for Rural America," *American Journal of Public Health,* 73 (1983): 341–348.

5. ARRINGTON, K. M. "With All Deliberate Speed, 1954–1980," *U.S. Commission of Civil Rights Clearing House Publications 69,* November 1981.

6. BACHRACH, L. L. "Human Services in Rural Areas: An Analytical Review," *Human Services,* 22 July 1981.

7. ———. "Psychiatric Services in Rural Areas: A Sociological Overview," *Hospital and Community Psychiatry,* 34 (1983): 215–226.

8. BAGLEY, C. "Incest Behavior and Incest Taboo," *Social Problems,* 16 (1969):505–519.

9. BENSWANGER, E. G., and FAUST, M. J. "Rural Human Services for Adolescents: Strategies for Systems Change," Paper presented at the 62nd annual meeting of the American Orthopsychiatric Association, New York, April 1985.

10. BENSWANGER, E. G., et al. "Continuing Education as a Link Between Urban and Rural Mental Health Professionals," *Hospital and Community Psychiatry,* 35 (1984):617–619.

11. BERRY, B., and DAVIS, A. E. "Community Mental Health Ideology. A Problematic Model for Rural Areas," *American Journal of Orthopsychiatry,* 48 (1978):673–679.

12. BROWN, D. L. "A Quarter Century of Trends and Changes in the Demographic Structure of American Families," in T. Coward and W. M. Smith, eds., *The Family in Rural Society.* Boulder, Colo.: 1981, Westview Press, pp. 9–26.

13. BROWN, J. S., and SCHWARZWELLER, H. K. "The Appalachian Family," in J. D. Photiadis, and H. K. Schwarzweller, eds., *Change in Rural Appalachia: Implications for Action Programs.* Philadelphia: University of Pennsylvania Press, 1970, pp. 81–97.

14. CLARK, J., and HAUREK, E. "Age and Sex Roles of Adolescents and Their Involvement in Misconduct: A Reappraisal," *Sociology and Social Research,* 50 (1966):495–508.

15. CLINARD, M. B. *Sociology of Deviant Behavior,* 3rd ed., New York: Holt, Rinehart, and Winston, 1968.

16. COCKERHAM, W. C. *Sociology of Mental Disorders.* Englewood Cliffs, N.J.: Prentice-Hall, 1981.

17. COPANS, S., and RACUSIN, R. "Rural Child Psychiatry," *Journal of the American Academy of Child Psychiatry,* 22 (1983):184–190.

18. COWARD, R. T. "Serving Families in Contemporary Rural America: Definitions, Importance, and Future," in R. T. Coward and W. M. Smith, Jr., eds., *Family Services.* Lincoln: University of Nebraska Press, 1983, pp. 3–25.

19. COWARD, R. T., and SMITH, W. M. *The Family in Rural Society.* Boulder, Colo.: Westview Press, 1981.

20. CROSS, H. J., and DENGERINK, H. A. "Introduction," in H. A. Dengerink and H. J. Cross, eds., *Training Professionals for Rural Mental Health.* Lincoln: University of Nebraska Press, 1982, pp. 1–13.

21. DANNEFER, D., and DEJAMES, J. *Juvenile Justice in New Jersey. An Assessment of the New Juvenile Code.* Trenton, N.J.: Department of Human Science, 1979.

22. D'AUGELLI, A. R., and VALLANCE, T. R. "The Help-

ing Community: Promoting Mental Health in Rural Areas Through Informal Helping," *Journal of Rural Community Psychology,* 2 (1981):3–15.

23. DeJAMES, J. "Issues in Rural Juvenile Justice," in J. Jankovic, R. K. Green, and S. D. Cronk, eds., *Juvenile Justice in Rural America.* Washington, D.C.: Law Enforcement Assistance Administration; Office of Juvenile Justice and Delinquency Prevention, 1980, pp. 4–15.

24. DENGERINK, H. A., and CROSS, J. J., eds. *Training Professionals for Rural Mental Health.* Lincoln: University of Nebraska Press, 1982.

25. DUNBAR, E. "Educating Social Workers for Rural Mental Health Settings," in H. A. Dengerink and H. J. Cross, eds., *Training Professionals for Rural Mental Health.* Lincoln: University of Nebraska Press, 1982, pp. 54–69.

26. EDGERTON, J. W. "Models of Service Delivery," in A. W. Childs and G. B. Melton, eds., *Rural Psychology.* New York: Plenum Press, 1983, pp. 275–303.

27. FALCONE, A. M., and ROSENTHAL, T. L. *Delivery of Rural Mental Health Services.* Cleveland: Synapse, Inc., 1982.

28. Federal Bureau of Investigation. *Uniform Crime Reports for the United States, 1971.* Washington, D.C.: U.S. Government Printing Office, 1972, pp. 135, 144, 152.

29. ———. *Uniform Crime Reports for the United States, 1977.* Washington, D.C.: U.S. Government Printing Office, 202, 211, 220, 1978.

30. ———. *Uniform Crime Reports for the United States, 1979.* Washington, D.C.: U.S. Government Printing Office, 1980, pp. 209–211, 218–220, 227–229.

31. ———. *Crime in the United States, 1980.* Washington, D.C.: U.S. Government Printing Office, 1981, pp. 216–218, 240–242, 252–254.

32. FIALKOV, M. J. "The Role of the Mental Health Professional in Permanency Planning for Children in Foster Care," in Panel Discussion entitled Out of Home Placement and the Law: Alliance, Accommodation or Adversaries. Presented at the annual meeting of the American Orthopsychiatric Association, Toronto, April 1984.

33. FIALKOV, M. J., JOSEPH, O., and KNIGHT, M. A. "Delivery of Services to a Coeducational Institution for Juvenile Offenders," Paper presented at the annual meeting of the American Orthopsychiatric Association, Toronto, April 1984.

34. FINKELHOR, D. *Sexually Victimized Children.* New York: Free Press, 1979.

35. FLAX, J. W., et al. "Mental Health and Rural America: An Overview," *Community Mental Health Review,* 3 (1978): 3–15.

36. FORSLUND, M. A. "Drug and Delinquent Behavior of Small Town and Rural Youth," in J. Jankovic, R. K. Green, and S. D. Crank, eds., *Juvenile Justice in Rural America.* Washington, D.C.: U. S. Department of Justice, 1980, pp. 92–97.

37. GARBARINO, J. "The Human Ecology of Child Maltreatment: A Conceptual Model of Research," *Journal of Marriage and the Family,* (November 1977):721–735.

38. GOLD, M. *Delinquent Behavior in an American City.* Belmont, Calif.: Brooks/Cole, 1970.

39. HALPERN, W. I., et al. "Continuity of Mental Health Care to Youth in the Juvenile Justice Network," *Hospital and Community Psychiatry,* 32 (1981):114–117.

40. HARGROVE, D. S. "Mental Health in Rural America," in T. M. Cassidy, M. S. Gordon, and A. Heller, eds., *The Mountains and Valleys Are Mine: A Symposium on Rural Mental Health.* Ridgewood, N. Y.: Bren-Tru Press, 1981, pp. 37–46.

41. HARGROVE, D. S. "The Mental Health Needs of Rural

America," in H. A. Dengerink and H. J. Cross, eds., *Training Professionals for Rural Mental Health.* Lincoln: University of Nebraska Press, 1982, pp. 14–26.

42. HENSLEY, V. R. "Hysteria in Childhood: A Note on Proctor's Incidence Figures 27 Years Later," *American Journal of Orthopsychiatry,* 55 (1985):140–142.

43. HOLLOS, M. "Cross-Cultural Research in Psychological Development in Rural Communities," in A. W. Childs, and G. B. Melton, eds., *Rural Psychology.* New York: Plenum Press, 1983, pp. 45–74.

44. "How America Will Change in the Next Decade," a *U.S. News and World Report,* 92 (1982):51–53.

45. JANKOVIC, J., GREEN, R. K., and CRONK, S. D., eds., *Juvenile Justice in Rural America.* Washington, D.C.: Law Enforcement Assistance Administration, Office of Juvenile Justice and Delinquency Prevention, 1980.

46. JEFFREY, M. J., and REEVES, R. E. "Community Mental Health Services in Rural Areas: Some Practical Issues," *Community Mental Health Journal,* 14 (1978):54–62.

47. JERRELL, J. M. *Mental Health Human Resources Planning and Development Manual.* Pittsburgh: Office of Education and Regional Programming, Western Psychiatric Institute and Clinic, 1983.

48. JOHNSON, R. J. "Youth in Crisis: Dimensions of Self Destructive Conduct Among Adolescent Prisoners," *Adolescence,* 13 (1978):461–482.

49. JONES, J. D., WAGENFELD, M. O., and ROBIN, S. S. "A Profile of the Rural Community Mental Health Center," *Community Mental Health Journal,* 12 (1976): 176–181.

50. KANDEL, D., SINGLE, E., and KOSSLE, R. "The Epidemiology of Drug Use Among New York State High School Students: Distribution, Trends, and Change in Rates of Use," *American Journal of Public Health,* 66 (1976):43–53.

51. KELLER, P. A., and MURRAY, J. D. "Rural Mental Health: An Overview of the Issues," in P. A. Keller and J. D. Murray, eds., *Handbook of Rural Community Mental Health.* New York: Human Sciences Press, 1982, pp. 3–19.

52, KELLER, P. A., and PRUSTMAN, T. D. "Training for Professional Psychology in the Rural Community," in P. A. Keller, and J. D. Murray, eds., *Handbook of Rural Community Mental Health.* New York: Human Sciences Press, 1982, pp. 190–199.

53. KENDALL, R. A., CORNELY, P. J., and SONIS, M. *Children and Youth in Western Pennsylvania.* Pittsburgh: Office of Education and Regional Programming, Western Psychiatric Institute and Clinic, 1980.

54. KIHM, R. C. *Prohibiting Secure Juvenile Detention: Assessing the Effectiveness of National Standards Detention Criteria.* Champaign, Ill.: Community Research Forum, University of Illinois, 1980.

55. KIRK, R. S. "Drug Use Among Rural Youth," in G. M. Beschner, and A. S. Friedman, eds., *Youth Drug Abuse: Problems, Issues and Treatment.* Lexington, Ky.: Lexington Books, 1979, pp. 379–407.

56. KORTE, D. C. "The Quality of Life in Rural and Urban America," in A. W. Childs, and G. B. Melton, *Rural Psychology.* New York:Plenum Press, 1983, pp. 199–216.

57. LAVIK, N. "Urban-Rural Differences in Rates of Disorder: A Comparative Psychiatric Population Study of Norwegian Adolescents," in P. Graham, ed., *Epidemiological Approaches in Child Psychiatry.* London: Academic Press, 1977, pp. 223–251.

58. LIBERTOFF, K. "Natural Helping Networks in the Rural Youth and Family Services," *Journal of Rural Community Psychology,* 1 (1980):4–17.

59. ———. "Reflections on Rural Adolescent Services," in

R. T. Coward, and W. T. Smith, eds., *Family Services.* Lincoln: University of Nebraska, 1983, pp. 171–185.

60. LOOFF, D. H. "Assisting Appalachian Families," in T. M. Cassidy, M. S. Gordon, and A. Heller, eds., *The Mountains and Valleys Are Mine: A Symposium on Rural Mental Health.* Ridgewood, N.Y.: Bren-Tru Press, 1981, pp. 179–189.

61. LOSCHEN, E. L. "Providing Psychiatric Services in a Rural Setting," *International Journal of Mental Health,* 12 (1983): 118–129.

62. MAIURO, R. D., and TRUPIN, E. W. "Rural Internships: A Fixed Role Therapy for the Community Mental Health Professional," *Hospital and Community,* 11 (1980): 497–499.

63. MALCOLM, A. H. "Emotional Erosion Imperils the Farm Family," *New York Times,* 20 November 1984.

64. McMILLEN, M. D. "Report and Recommendations of the Governor's Task Force on the Mental Health of Juvenile Offenders," Harrisburg, Pennsylvania, 1979.

65. MILES, J. E. "A Psychiatric Outreach Project to a Rural Community," *Hospital and Community Psychiatry,* 31 (1980):822–825.

66. MURRAY, J. D., and KUPINSKY, S. "The Influence of Powerlessness and Natural Support Systems on Mental Health in the Rural Community," in P. A. Keller and J. D. Murray, eds., *Handbook of Rural Community Mental Health.* New York: Human Sciences Press, 1982, pp. 62–73.

67. MYERS-WALL, J. A., and COWARD, R. T. "Natural Helping Networks: Their Role in Community Services for Rural Families," in R. T. Coward, and W. M. Smith, Jr., eds., *Family Services.* Lincoln: University of Nebraska Press, 1983, pp. 111–132.

68. NACHTIGAL, P. M. *Rural Education: In Search of a Better Way.* Boulder, Colo.: Westview Press, 1982.

69. National Center on Child Abuse and Neglect. *National Study of the Incidence and Severity of Child Abuse and Neglect.* Washington, D.C.: U.S. Department of Health and Human Services, 1982.

70. NEWHOUSE, J. P., et al. "Where Have All the Doctors Gone?" *Journal of American Medical Association,* 247 (1982): 2392–2396.

71. PADEGITTI, S., GIBBS, L., and OLSON, E. "Forecasting the Reoccurrence of Child Abuse," *Human Services in the Rural Environment,* 6 (1981):32–39.

72. PARKE, R. D., and COLLMER, W. C. "Child Abuse: An Interdisciplinary Analysis," in E. M. Hetherington, ed., *Child Development Research,* vol. 5. Chicago: University of Chicago Press, 1975, pp. 509–590.

73. PAWLAK, E. J. "Juvenile Justice: A Rural-Urban Compassion," in J. Jankovic, R. K. Green, and S. D. Cronk, eds., *Juvenile Justice in Rural America.* Washington, D.C.: Law Enforcement Assistance Administration Office of Juvenile Justice and Delinquency Prevention, 1980, pp. 37–49.

74. PETTI, T. A. "Rethinking Rural Mental Health Policies for Children and Adolescents," manuscript, Pittsburgh, 1984.

75. PETTI, T. A. HOWELL, P., and McINTYRE, A. "The Effective Use of a Consultative Study of Mental Health Related Services for Children and Youth: A Systems Perspective," paper presented at the 62nd annual meeting of the American Orthopsychiatric Association, New York, April 1985.

76. PETTI, T. A., SONIS, M., and APPERSON, L. J. "Linking Community Mental Health Centers with Training Centers for Delinquent Youth: A Pilot Project," Paper presented at the 60th annual meeting of the American Orthopsychiatric Association, Boston, April 4–8, 1983.

77. PETTI, T. A., UDER, E., and NEBEL, D. "Mental Health Services for Incarcerated, Disturbed Delinquents: A Collaborative Effort," manuscript, Pittsburgh, 1984.

78. PHILLIPS, G. H. *Crime in Rural Ohio.* Columbus: Ohio State University, Department of Agricultural Economics and Rural Sociology, 1975.

79. PHOTIADIS, G. D., and SIMONI, J. J. "Characteristics of Rural America," in A. W. Childs, and G. B. Melton, eds., *Rural Psychology.* New York: Plenum Press, 1983, pp. 15–32.

80. PLOCH, L. A. "Family Aspects of the New Wave of Immigrants," in R. T. Coward and W. M. Smith, Jr., *The Family in Rural Society.* Boulder, Colo.: Westview Press, 1981, pp. 40–52.

81. POLANSKY, N. A., et al. *Damaged Parents: An Anatomy of Child Neglect.* Chicago: University of Chicago Press, 1981.

82. The President's Commission on Mental Health. *Task Panel Reports,* vol. 3, Rural Mental Health. Washington, D.C.: U. S. Government Printing Office, *Rural Mental Health.* Washington, D.C.; *1978.*

83. PROCTER, J. "Hysteria in Childhood," *American Journal of Orthopsychiatry,* 28 (1958):394–407.

84. RIEMER, S. A. "Research Note on Incest," *American Journal of Sociology,* 45 (1940):566.

85. ROESKE, N.C.A. "A National Survey of Child Psychiatrists: Their Location, Patient Population, and Sources of Income," *American Academy of Child Psychiatry Newsletter,* Spring (1984):3–6.

86. ROSENBERG, M. S., and REPUCCI, E. D. "Child Abuse: A Review with Special Focus on an Ecological Approach in Rural Communities," in A. W. Childs and G. B. Melton, eds., *Rural Psychology.* New York: Plenum Press, 1983, pp. 305–336.

87. ROSENBLUM, A., and LOUIS, K. S. *Stability and Change: Innovation in an Educational Center.* New York: Plenum Press, 1981.

88. RUSSELL, A. "Implications of Project Future," Paper presented at the annual meeting of the American Academy of Child Psychiatry, San Francisco, October 1983.

89. RUTTER, M. "The City and the Child," *American Journal of Orthopsychiatry,* 51 (1981):610–625.

90. RUTTER, M., et al. "Attainment and Adjustment in Two Geographical Areas I—The Prevalence of Psychiatric Disorder," *British Journal of Psychiatry,* 126 (1975):493–509.

91. RUTTER, M., and QUINLON, D. "Psychiatric Disorders —Ecological Factors and Concepts of Causations," in H. McGirk, ed., *Ecological Factors in Human Development.* Amsterdam: North-Holland, 1977, pp. 173–187.

92. SCHUMM, W. R., and BOLLMAN, S. R. "Interpersonal Processes in Rural Families," in R. T. Coward, and W. M. Smith, Jr., eds., *The Family in Rural Society.* Boulder, Colo.: Westview Press, 1981, pp. 129–145.

93. SMITH, W. M., and COWARD, R. T. "Images of the Future," in R. T. Coward and W. M. Smith, eds., *The Family in Rural Society.* Boulder, Colo.: Westview Press, 1981, pp. 225–229.

94. SOLOMON, G. "The Rural Human Service Delivery System: Entry Issues," *Journal of Rural Community Psychology,* 1 (1980):1–18.

95. SOLOMON, G., HIESBERGER, J., and WINER, J. "Confidentiality Issues in Rural Mental Health," *Journal of Rural Community Psychology,* 2 (1981):17–31.

96. SULLIVAN, H. S. *The Interpersonal Theory of Psychiatry.* New York: W. W. Norton, 1953.

97. THOMPSON, M. C., ed. Rural Health Care," in *Health Policy: The Legislative Agenda.* Washington, D.C.: Congressional Quarterly, 1980, pp. 51–58.

98. TUCKER, G. J., TURNES, J., and CHAPMAN, R. "Prob-

lems in Attracting and Retaining Psychiatrists in Rural Areas," *Hospital and Community Psychiatry,* 32 (1981): 118–120.

99. UREY, J. R., and HENGGELER, S. W. "Interaction in Rural Families," in A. W. Childs and G. B. Melton, eds., *Rural Psychology.* New York: Plenum Press, 1983, pp. 33–44.

100. VINTER, R. D., DOWNS, G., and HALLI, J., *Juvenile Corrections on the States: Residential Programs and Deinstitutionalization, National Assessment of Juvenile Corrections.* Ann Arbor: University of Michigan Press, 1976.

101. WAGENFELD, M. O. *New Directions for Mental Health Services: Perspectives on Rural Mental Health.* San Francisco: Jossey-Bass, 1981.

102. WAGENFELD, M. O., and OZARIN, L. D. "Serving the Underserved Through Rural Mental Health Programs, in H.

C. Schulberg and M. Killilea, eds., *The Modern Practice of Community Mental Health.* San Francisco: Jossey-Bass, 1982, pp. 467–485.

103. WEISSMAN, M. M., et al. "Psychopathology in Children (ages 6–18) of Depressed and Normal Parents," *Journal of the American Academy of Child Psychiatry,* 23 (1984): 78–84.

104. WILLIAMS, A. S. "Changing Patterns of Horizontal and Vertical Linkage," in R. T. Coward, and W. M. Smith, eds., *Family Services: Issues and Opportunities in Contemporary Rural America.* Lincoln: University of Nebraska Press, 1983, pp. 87–101.

105. WOODEN, K. *Weeping in the Playtime of Others: America's Incarcerated Children.* New York: McGraw-Hill, 1976.

75 / Federal Programs and Child Psychiatry

Michael E. Fishman and Larry B. Silver

Introduction

Federal government activity encompasses a broad array of programs that relate to the mental health of American children and adolescents and that are, therefore, relevant to the interests of child psychiatry. These programs operate within a wide spectrum of organizational settings under the auspices of several different federal departments and independent agencies. Some have direct impact on the interests of child psychiatry, whereas others are of more peripheral significance. Some are widely known; others, however, are relatively less generally recognized or understood as aspects of federal activity concerned with child and adolescent mental health. Although the number of programs precludes a description of the entire range of their activities, an effort will be made to consider some of the most relevant. We first describe recent work of the National Institute of Mental Health (NIMH) and its sister Institutes in the Alcohol, Drug Abuse, and Mental Health Administration (ADAMHA). After considering these programs, we review some of the activities in other parts of the federal government directly related to the interests of child psychiatry. Then the focus moves from programs in the Public Health Service to other areas of the Department of Health and Human Services and then to other departments and agencies. After completing this selective review, we examine the relationships between federal activities and more gen-eral developments of interest to child psychiatry. These issues are considered under four headings: financing, service systems, training, and research.

Some Key Federal Programs

NIMH supports activities concerned with research, training, technical assistance, and dissemination of information. The preeminent focus now is on research. The range of efforts related to research is highly diversified and includes a variety of basic, clinical, and applied areas such as the following: studies of etiology, prevalence, course, treatment, and prevention of disorders; research concerned with the organization, staffing, delivery, and financing of services; training of psychiatrists, others with clinical backgrounds, and those from nonclinical fields in research competencies related to mental health. In essentially every area of emphasis within NIMH's range of activities, certain efforts are specifically concerned with children and adolescents. This work is reflected in direct research activity carried out by the institute, in research and training supported in many settings throughout the nation, in collaborative activity with numerous federal and state agencies, and in liaison functions with organizations interested in child mental health. NIMH exerts an influence that goes beyond the magnitude of its dollar outlays; its impact owes much of its authority to a research base, and influences the provision of mental health care to children and adolescents.

In recent years NIMH has been active in a wide variety of areas that have significance for child psychiatry. For instance, it has encouraged child psychiatrists to move into research careers, to prepare for work with relatively underserved populations of children and adolescents, and to work with other service systems. These thrusts parallel closely the objectives identified for child psychiatry in the American Academy of Child Psychiatry's published plan for the future of the profession, "Child Psychiatry: A Plan for the Coming Decades."[1] The same publication cites "existing growth" in child psychiatry research outlined in "The Annual Report on the Child and Youth Activities of the National Institute of Mental Health" for the fiscal years 1980,[8] 1981,[9] and 1982.[10] The report for 1983[5] further describes developments in the referenced research areas. The areas include: primary and secondary prevention with special attention to children at risk, epidemiology, psychopathology, treatment, and basic mechanisms. In prevention, NIMH has recently established a Prevention Center that has devoted over half its resources to the under-eighteen population. In epidemiology, increasing attention is being directed to children and adolescents. Clinical studies are being fostered by a new Center for Studies of Child and Adolescent Psychopathology, and research on psychosocial and pharmacological treatments for youngsters is being encouraged.

Both of NIMH's sister institutes in the Alcohol, Drug Abuse, and Mental Health Administration combine their prime attention to substance abuse with other issues directly relevant to child psychiatry. The National Institute on Alcohol Abuse and Alcoholism (NIAAA) and the National Institute on Drug Abuse (NIDA) have recently joined with NIMH to support research that is focused on combined alcohol, drug abuse, and mental health problems in adolescents. Within the context of its ongoing programs, NIDA devotes attention to children and youth in a wide variety of ways. For instance, considerable attention is being directed toward adolescents in drug use surveys; this includes the well-known high-school senior survey done for NIDA by the University of Michigan Institute for Social Research. Other research in basic, clinical, and applied areas has relevance to children and youth, and some of these studies, such as those focused on treatment of youth, are specifically related to youngsters. In the prevention area, a preponderance of efforts are designed to head off or cut off involvement with drugs among the young. These prevention activities involve multiple strategies including some directed to children and adolescents, some to parents, and some to other important people in children's lives.

NIAAA is also devoting much attention to prevention activity among youth. One major thrust is focusing particular attention on the problem of drinking and driving among youth. Research, conferences, technical assistance, publications, and public education campaigns are being used to focus on prevention of alcohol problems among youngsters. Basic and applied studies supported by the institute include approaches focused specifically on children and families. In the area of treatment, there has been a major effort to mobilize local, state, and community resources to direct additional attention to the treatment needs of youngsters with alcohol problems.

In addition to the three institutes grouped within ADAMHA, there are institutes among those in the National Institutes of Health that support activities germane to child psychiatry. The National Institute of Child Health and Human Development (NICHD) is concerned with the physical health and development of the child and also directs its attention to normative behavioral issues in development during the formative years. In addition, it maintains a specific research focus on mental retardation. The National Institute of Neurological and Communicative Disorders and Stroke (NINCDS) shares an interest with NIMH in supporting research on autism. It also joins NICHD and NIMH in supporting investigations that relate to mental retardation and learning disabilities.

The United States Public Health Service is the chief focus for health issues at the federal level; all the national institutes just cited belong to it. Beyond the institutes mentioned, other programs in the U.S. health establishment are relevant to child psychiatry. Most are of interest because of their attention to physical health matters, but physical health is being addressed increasingly with an eye to related behavioral/emotional issues. The Federal Maternal and Child Health activity exemplifies this positive trend. Recent publications[4,5,6,7] reflect efforts to encourage expanded attention to a variety of psychosocial issues that can present in primary health care settings. These include: social and psychological aspects of genetics, the implications of physically handicapping conditions, the grief of children, and mental and emotional difficulties per se. The role of behavioral/emotional aspects is being addressed in other areas as well, such as in the training of primary health caregivers and in planning for programs that focus on chronic physical illness.

One major federal health-related activity that exists outside the Public Health Service is the realm of health financing. The Health Care Financing Administration (HCFA) is the government agency that superintends both Medicare and Medicaid. These programs support tens of billions of dollars worth of health services. As far as children are concerned, Medicaid is by far the more significant. A review of the mental health benefits under Medicaid indicates that mandatory inpatient hospital services must include psychiatric units of general hospitals.[13] There are also mandatory outpatient and physician services that relate to psychiatric care and that can include children. In addition to mandatory services, there is an extensive list of optional mental health services, which vary from state to state. Most of these provisions have to do with generic problems that may include children. However, there is also a Medicaid program specifically for children and adolescents—the Early and Periodic Screening, Diagnosis and Treatment (EPSDT) program. In 1982 EPSDT expenditures totaled $3.5 billion; this represented 55 percent of all local, state, and federal government spending for child health. The focus of EPSDT includes growth and development; and developmental assessments are intended to address psychosocial as well as physical issues. Hence within this largest of government health programs for the children and adolescents in the United States, the emotional status of the Medicaid-eligible child is one of the significant areas for screening.

The Department of Health and Human Services is not the only federal department involved in major health financing that extends coverage to child psychiatric services. Through the Civilian Health and Medical Programs of the Uniformed Services[2] (CHAMPUS), the Defense Department contributes to the cost of the health care provided to military families by civilian hospitals and doctors. With certain limitations, the services covered include both outpatient and inpatient psychiatric care for the children and adolescents of military families. Among the various resources that can obtain reimbursement for the costs of mental health care are a number of residential treatment centers.

It is clear that the activities of the federal government intersect with the interests of child psychiatry in respect to many health programs. What is perhaps less clear is that there are many federal activities that proceed through systems other than the health system but that also have major implications for the delivery of mental health care to children and youth. Among these systems are those relating to human development or social services, rehabilitative services, education and special education, law enforcement, and juvenile justice. In order to exemplify the breadth and the depth of their potential impact on the work of child psychiatry, two key areas will be briefly considered. One relates to human development services and the other to special education.

In the federal Office of Human Development Services (OHDS) there are four agencies; to a very large degree, two of these focus specifically on child populations. These are, respectively, the Administration for Children, Youth, and Families (ACYF) and the Ad-

ministration on Development Disabilities (ADD); each of these is in turn subdivided into several subsections. ACFY encompasses a varied array of programs including Head Start, the Children's Bureau, and Family and Youth Services. One of the programs within the Children's Bureau is the National Center on Child Abuse and Neglect (NCCAN); Family and Youth Services is associated with federal activities that address the problems of runaways and their families. The Head Start program serves 400,000 three- to five-year-olds; this includes a significant proportion who suffer from handicaps, plus some younger children who are served through parent-child centers. The Children's Bureau distributes funds to states for in-home foster care and adoption services. Under these programs, those who provide parenting for handicapped youngsters, including children who are retarded or mentally ill, can receive federal assistance via the states. ADD, the Administration on Developmental Disabilities, as its name denotes, is particularly concerned with the developmentally disabled including dual-diagnosis mentally retarded (those with concomitant mental illness), autistic children, and the learning disabled. It funds diagnostic and treatment centers directly and provides for services through the states. OHDS has a major program of research, demonstration, evaluation, and training support. In an October 1983 announcement,[3] projects were invited that related to numerous topics of interest to child psychiatry. These included innovative approaches to effective health promotion and avoidance of accidents and substance abuse, furthering family cohesion, preventing and treating child abuse, improving foster care, and facilitating more success with adoptions. The specifics of announcements can vary from year to year, but the 1983 example gives a sense of the range of topics that can be covered.

In the area of special education, the major federal program with implications for child psychiatry is the Education for All Handicapped Children Act (PL 94–142). By now the main thrust of this legislation is familiar to many who work with emotionally disturbed children and youth. The act aims at providing an education for all handicapped children in environments that are as normative as feasible. It requires individualized planning for each handicapped child and addresses not only the children's educational needs but also those related services necessary for that handicapping condition. Among the handicaps covered by the act are learning disability, mental retardation, and emotional disturbance. According to data[14] for the 1982–83 school year, among the children served under PL 94–142 (and under a prior piece of federal legislation providing support to institutionalized handicapped children, PL 89–313), learning disability is the single most-often identified condition; speech impairment was second; mental retardation was third; and emotional disturbances fourth. During that year approximately 4.3 million children, ages three to twenty-one, were served; of these, over 350,000 were identified as emotionally disturbed. The largest category, learning disabled, totaled about 1.75 million; this constituted over 40 percent of all the handicapped listed and 4.4 percent of the total school enrollment. It is also noteworthy that in addition to services for those at the primary and secondary levels, the majority of states are now mandating services for the preschool handicapped population. All this has increased the role of school systems in relating to the needs of handicapped children and youth. By effecting this, PL 94–142 brings such systems more closely in contact with areas of direct interest to child psychiatry and underscores the importance of close cooperation between the mental health and educational systems.

Federal Activity and Recent General Developments

FINANCING

In the area of financing for children's mental health services, federal programs have been given a targeted role—that is, they have been concentrating primarily on low-income, Medicaid-eligible youngsters and on those who qualify for CHAMPUS. For the most part, Medicare has been utilized for the sixty-five and older population and for disabled persons between twenty-one and sixty-five. To a certain degree, federal activities in other areas contribute resources relevant to the mental health of children and youth. These include programs concerned with special education, programs for the developmentally disabled, and provision of social services. A National Medical Care Expenditure Survey was conducted by the National Center for Health Services Research; it yielded data on health insurance for children. Although a 1977 study, it is likely that there have not been major shifts since the original figures, which are summarized in table 75–1. They relate to patterns of coverage for general health care. The situations become significantly more complex when it comes to mental health care for children because private insurance plans vary greatly in their mental health benefits. Even the largest public plan, Medicaid, can vary significantly from state to state. The overall picture has many elements: private carriers, the states, and the federal government; children who are covered by family status, children who are directly eligible, and children who are covered part-time or uncovered; differences between physical and mental health coverages,

between inpatient and outpatient care, and in ways of relating to providers.

Despite the fact that federal financing activity is only a part of this complex picture, it is a particularly significant part because much of it concerns disadvantaged children. This is the case for Medicaid. As previously noted, Medicaid benefits vary according to the individual Medicaid State Plan. Generally, however, inpatient mental health care for the mentally ill is covered in a general hospital setting. In a psychiatric hospital, public or private, mental health inpatient care is covered only for those aged sixty-five or over or under twenty-one, *if* the state chooses to cover one or the other or both of these Medicaid population groups. This is by way of a statutory exception to the Medicaid law, which excludes coverage of inpatient care in an institution for mental diseases. Medicaid also covers care of the mentally ill in skilled nursing facilities and intermediate care facilities (unless they are institutions for mental disease), home health services for the mentally ill, mental health services of physicians and other professional providers licensed by the state and certified as approved Medicaid providers within the state, clinic services for the mentally ill, and a range of care for children and adolescents under Medicaid's Early and Periodic Screening, Diagnosis and Treatment Program (EPSDT).

The EPSDT Program is a mandated set of services in all Medicaid programs for the screening, diagnosis, and treatment of physical and mental defects for individuals under twenty-one. In 1982 eligible recipients of these benefits numbered 9.6 million children and young people under age twenty-one, or 43 percent of the total Medicaid population. It seems fair to say that currently EPSDT is one of the most important mental health benefits available for children and youth. Until 1979 there was debate about the nature of "mental defects" and about the scope of activities to include in diagnosing and treating such defects. As a result, the program focused attention primarily on "physical defects." In lieu of "mental assessment" the term developmental assessment was chosen to focus attention on the behavioral and related psychosocial aspects of the child. In 1981 the American Association of Psychiatric Services for Children contracted with HCFA to develop a model approach to developmental assessment. This was structured in accordance with HCFA's guidelines to states on such assessment.

CHAMPUS benefits apply to mental illness and cover institutional care, partial hospitalization, professional provider services, and certain supplies and services related to covered medical care provided by civilian sources. Inevitably, these benefits are subject to conditions of provider participation. Inpatient hospital care for mental illness is limited to sixty days per year.

TABLE 75-1

Health Insurance Status Public[a] and Private of Children 0–18[b] During 1977

Insurance Category	Number of Children	% of all children 0–18
Children covered by private insurance during whole year	47,517,000	69.0
Children covered by private insurance during part of year and by public insurance for remainder of year only	4,425,000	6.4
Children covered by private insurance for part of year and no coverage for remainder of year	2,631,000	3.8
Children covered by private insurance for part of year, by public insurance only for part of year, and no coverage for part of year	489,000	0.7
Children covered by public insurance only for whole year	5,109,000	7.4
Children covered by public insurance for part of year and no coverage for part of year	2,774,000	4.0
Children with no coverage during whole year	5,919,000	8.6

[a]"Public" includes the Medicare, Medicaid, and CHAMPUS programs.
[b]The total number of children ages 0 to 18 during some part of 1977 was 68,864,000.

Additional days may be covered for the mentally ill, as is a full range of mental health care in CHAMPUS approved residential treatment care (RTC) facilities for children and adolescents (the sixty-day limit does not affect RTCs). Partial hospitalization services are covered as are mental health services of physicians, psychologists, clinical social workers, and nurse practitioners on both an inpatient and outpatient basis. During the treatment period all professional mental health outpatient services are subject to mandatory review at preset intervals. External peer review is additionally required for mental health services exceeding (except for crisis intervention) one hour per day and two hours per week for both inpatients and outpatients. In order to assure the medical necessity or appropriateness of the services being rendered, peer review may be required for mental health care at any time.

The RTC benefit is especially important for child and adolescent mental health care. It covers a wide range of services and supplies, including room and board, patient assessment and diagnostic and treatment services, drugs, medicines, emergency medical care, and social and educational services. CHAMPUS has established special standards for RTCs that govern organization and administration, treatment and residential services, and the physical plant.

Although Medicare has very limited direct relevance to children, a number of developments within this program can have major long-term implications for financing children's mental health services. A case in point is the prospective Medicare payment plan. As a cost-containment effort, the federal government established a plan for prepayment of hospital Medicare costs based on diagnosis-related groups (DRGs). This plan began in October 1983 with a three-year phase-in. Thus far several types of institutions, including psychiatric hospitals and psychiatric units of general hospitals, are excluded from this system; they continue to be paid under the preexisting system.

This approach pays a fixed amount per case based on predetermined rates for specific hospitals and geographic areas. The objective is to reduce hospital costs.

One of the reasons that psychiatric facilities were excluded is the lack of reliable data upon which to base prepayment. HCFA requested that NIMH assist in the assessment of existing data as a first step in developing the necessary information. This assessment of existing data and clarification of what additional data may be needed is now in progress. Special attention will be given to the kind of information that might be needed to develop a suitable approach for children who require hospitalization for mental disorders.

SERVICE SYSTEMS

Since the end of World War II, federal contributions to the development of mental health service systems have been evolving through a series of stages. The experiences of the war helped to catalyze interest in mental health services; indeed, these were a major contributing factor to the founding of NIMH in 1948. In 1955 Congress established a Joint Commission on Mental Illness and Health to study the status of mental health care. The commission report led to the passage of the Community Mental Health Centers (CMHC) Act in 1963. Conceptually, the community-based orientation of this program owed much to the child guidance clinics that had appeared on the scene earlier in the century. These had comprised the first mental health service system specifically for children and youth in the United States. These clinics had been funded largely through private charities and the Commonwealth Fund. However, fifty years later it was the federal government that funded the construction, staffing, and initial operations of these CMHCs. This was worked out through participation in local, regional, and state efforts, both public and private. Each community-based center developed outpatient, inpatient, emergency, partial hospitalization, and consultation-education services; these, in turn, were made available to all individuals within an assigned "catchment" area. By 1976, 548 centers were in existence, servicing about 25 percent of all mental health patients seen. However, in most of these settings, services for children were not highly developed.

In 1965 Congress funded the Joint Commission on the Mental Health of Children. Its mission was to review needs and to recommend plans for action. Following this study, the MHC Act was amended in 1970 to include special funding for child programs. This is noteworthy because, for the first time, U.S. federal money was earmarked specifically for the provision of mental health services to children. During the years 1972 to 1974, 166 programs received such funding.

In 1975 there was a shift in the CMHC's approach to children's services. Initially it had involved earmarked funding; later the children's services were designated as essential, and all funded centers were expected to provide them. This approach continued for the duration of the federally-administered CMHC program. During the latter years of that program, a President's Commission on Mental Health and the Mental Health Systems Act emphasized expanding the focus away from facilities to encompass systems of care. The new emphasis was on networking throughout the states; this was reflected in recommendations that enlarged the role of the states in the federal-state partnership.

Subsequently, the role of the states was further augmented to proportions beyond those envisaged in the Systems Act. This was accomplished by the Block Grant approach, which was adopted in 1981 to supercede the Systems Act. With the introduction of the Block Grant concept, all federal funds for alcohol, drug abuse, and mental health services are provided to states based on a formula. Within broad guidelines afforded by the federal government, each state makes its own decisions as to how to use these funds. At the time of this writing, the Block Grant program was too new to assess adequately with respect to children. There is some preliminary experience to suggest that there will be many issues around apportioning available resources at state levels, and that, within the states, there will need to be continuing attention to striking the kind of balance that recognizes the importance of the under-eighteen population.

In addition to the child guidance clinics and the CMHCs, a large and growing variety of mental health resources serves children and youth. These range from long-established state hospitals through residential treatment centers to new types of private psychiatric facilities. Beyond the mental health system per se, there exist programs that serve mentally ill children under other auspices, such as those within the education system. With so many different kinds of programs operating within a number of different systems, there is a prime need to increase coordination in the delivery of mental health services to mentally ill and emotionally disturbed children and adolescents.

TRAINING

In recent years NIMH has played a significant role in influencing the direction of clinical and research training for child psychiatry. The impact of this institute has in fact transcended the mere provision of financial support; by both reflecting and reinforcing the many professional emphases that flow throughout the field, it has gained in both stature and authority.

In the area of clinical training, NIMH has sought to encourage the targeting of particular groups of children and youth most likely to be affected by shortages. These include: those with serious emotional disturbance; those with combined physical and mental health disorders; those with both mental retardation and emotional disturbance; those especially likely to be underserved because of being abused or neglected, living in inner city or rural areas, or belonging to minority groups. The emphasis on targeting has had to do not only with particular groups of children but also with particular lines of activity engaged in by child psychiatrists. More specifically, recent institute efforts have sought to promote the development of state mental health personnel resources that relate to child and adolescent mental health needs. Concomitantly, NIMH has been encouraging the movement of young psychiatrists into public psychiatry. The latter effort was formulated not only for departments of psychiatry generally but also for divisions of child psychiatry. Thus there has been specific recognition of the importance of preparing a greater proportion of child psychiatrists for service in public settings.

In the area of research training, NIMH has identified [12] many different topics in child mental health that call for continuing development of researchers. These topics fall into the following major research categories: epidemiology, clinical sciences, services, prevention, behavioral sciences, and biological sciences. A number of training mechanisms are being employed by the institute to help build the cadre of investigators who will address pending research needs in child mental health. The mechanisms include the Research Scientist Development Program, the New Investigator Research Award in Prevention, the Clinical Investigator Award, and the Physician Scientist Award. The latter two programs, in particular, are designed to encourage the wedding of clinical and research skills. Child psychiatrists are in an advantageous position to bring their clinical background to a research career. As a result, this has been one of the groups toward which specific efforts have been directed with an eye to encouraging development of investigative skills and pursuit of work in research. The effort to increase the number of child psychiatrist researchers is but one part of a strategy that recognizes the need to produce more researchers who are equipped to operate at the important boundaries, those between the biological and the behavioral, the basic and the clinical, and the developmental and the pathological.

RESEARCH

In recent years there has been growing research activity in child psychiatry. This is reflected at once in the expanding format of the *Journal of the American Academy of Child Psychiatry* and again in the increasing share of NIMH research dollars being directed to children and youth. There are advances in the epidemiological, clinical, developmental, behavioral, and neuroscience fields, and each of these presents new opportunities for research. Simultaneously, methodological gains and new conceptual models are providing more tools with which to address the multiplying research questions. In this context of opportunity and challenge, the federal roles of catalyst and supporter of research continue to contribute significantly to the developing picture. In a 1984 announcement concerned with research and research training in child and adolescent mental health,[12] NIMH outlined a broad range of issues that are both pending business for the child mental health research community and matters of major interest to child psychiatry in general. In each of the categories of inquiry, the announcement described research opportunities that fall within the institute's scope of activity. To exemplify evolving emphases in child-related mental health research, some of the topics will be briefly mentioned.

Epidemiology is one area where there is rapidly growing interest in child psychiatric disorders. Activity in this field should lead to better data on the prevalence and distribution of disorders and dysfunctions among children and adolescents. Through a combination of in-house and in-the-field effort, this is an area where NIMH is pursuing the development of new tools and the generation of new data.

The interest in prevalence and incidence studies extends naturally to a focus on risk factors. In light of the growing concern with prevention, risk factor research is being encouraged by several NIMH research support programs; it is also being addressed within the intramural programs of the institute.

Childhood depression is a disorder whose very existence was once questioned. Now that its existence is generally accepted, its prevalence, characteristics, and course are subjects of keen investigative interest. NIMH is encouraging such attention, as well as concern with the phenomenon of child/adolescent suicide. Research that seeks to clarify the nature of attention deficit disorder, hyperactivity, and conduct disorders is also being encouraged in the field and pursued in-house. Another of the many disorders for whose study NIMH is providing support is autism. Research support is directed not only to learning about the nature of the disorder but also to studying its treatment. Indeed, it is not an exaggeration to say that attention is being directed to research on different treatment approaches that, among them, cover the whole range of childhood disorders.

Beyond the limited sample just cited, there are many other child-related research questions that NIMH is helping to address. Collectively they cover a wide spectrum of basic, clinical, and applied investigative realms. As noted earlier, a number of other federal programs support research efforts, and some of these relate to questions of concern to child psychiatry. In sum, the federal role in research appears to be contributing to both the growing knowledge base and the challenging opportunities for further study regarding the mental health of children and adolescents.

REFERENCES

1. AMERICAN ACADEMY OF CHILD PSYCHIATRY. *Child Psychiatry: A Plan for the Coming Decades.* Washington, D.C.: American Academy of Child Psychiatry, 1983–84.
2. *CHAMPUS Handbook,* No. 6010.46–H, January 1983.
3. *Federal Register,* Part V, 18 October 1983.

4. Health Resources and Services Administration Current Publications, HRS-A-OC 83–1, Division of Maternal and Child Health. *Social and Psychological Aspects of Genetics: A Selected Bibliography,* Code no. G14.
5. Health Resources and Services Administration Current

Publications, HRS-A-OC 83–1, Division of Maternal and Child Health. *Report of the Surgeon General's Workshop on Children with Handicaps and Their Families,* PHS 83–50194.

6. Health Resources and Services Administration Current Publications, HRS-A-OC 83–1, Division of Maternal and Child Health. "Fact Sheet: The Grief of Children" (unnumbered).

7. Health Resources and Services Administration Current Publications, HRS-A-OC 83–1, Division of Maternal and Child Health. *A Reader's Guide for Parents of Children with Mental, Physical, or Emotional Difficulties,* HSA-79–5290

8. National Institute of Mental Health. *Seventh Annual Report on the Child and Youth Activities of the National Institute of Mental Health.* Rockville, Md.: National Institute of Mental Health, 1980.

9. ———. *Eighth Annual Report on the Child and Youth*

Activities of the National Institute of Mental Health, Rockville, Md.: National Institute of Mental Health, 1981.

10. ———. *Ninth Annual Report on The Child and Youth Activities of the National Institute of Mental Health.* Rockville, Md.: National Institute of Mental Health, 1982.

11. ———. *Tenth Annual Report on the Child and Youth Activities of the National Institute of Mental Health.* Rockville, Md.: National Institute of Mental Health, 1983.

12. ———. NIMH Announcement, Support for Child and Adolescent Mental Health Research and Research Training, May 1984.

13. Toff, Gail E. *"Mental Health Benefits Under Medicaid: A Survey of the States."* Intergovernmental Health Policy Project, George Washington University, January 1984.

14. U.S. Department of Education. *Sixth Annual Report to Congress on the Implementation of Public Law 94–142: The Education for All Handicapped Children Act,* 1984.

76 / The Private Practice of Child Psychiatry

William B. Clotworthy, Jr.

Introduction

This chapter provides a broad look at the nature of the private practice of child psychiatry as a source of satisfaction and as a means of livelihood. This type of practice is compared to the private practice of general psychiatry and to the practice of child psychiatry in other settings. The material is also concerned with setting up a practice, with the business side of practice, and with the problems arising from the complications and insecurities of the present economic climate.

mation. It is a privilege to see the world through the eyes of the child, and this adds a fresh dimension to the doctor's day. In line with this is the challenge to keep pace with the ever-changing culture of the child. Most child psychiatrists see patients of all ages, and the ensuing variety is one of the great pleasures of the work. As the ages of the patients vary, so do the appropriate techniques. One moves from the passive mode of psychotherapy with adults to the active interaction with the child in the playroom. Because of their youth and greater flexibility, one might hope to find child cases an easier task, but all too often this advantage is offset in the many cases where it is hard to establish a therapeutic alliance with the child or young person.

The Satisfactions of Child Psychiatry

Thus far, no one has adequately expressed the quality of satisfaction that arises from working as a psychiatrist with children, adolescents, and families. Psychiatric residents are exposed to some work with children to see whether they take to it or not. No one has explored why some say yes. No attempt will be made here to illuminate in any adequate way the rewards of this professional activity. Probably the base for much satisfaction lies in the opportunity in the field for the *child* in the child psychiatrist to find a means of subli-

The Pros and Cons of a Private Office

One of the biggest differences between a private office in the community and salaried work at an agency is the relative isolation in working in private practice. Most psychiatrists feel the need for some professional contacts of the type that are available with an agency or at a university. On the other hand, there are some practical advantages to private practice. Hourly earnings are usually higher, but there is not the security that is present with some, but not all, salaried positions. The private practitioner has the option of setting specific working hours, but frequently work starts early and ends late in order to accommodate young patients' schedules.

Child Versus General Psychiatry

A major issue for child psychiatry is the reluctance of parents to take their children out of school for appointments. There is some reasonable basis for their position; certainly it is not good to miss a considerable amount of schoolwork. Moreover, children who leave school regularly are sometimes targeted for teasing by other children as being different. At times, however, there is no way to avoid taking children out of school for their appointments. Still, child psychiatrists sometimes find it difficult to fill morning time slots.

There are some other economic disadvantages to child versus general psychiatry. The child psychiatrist must have additional office space for a playroom. Children are more frequently sick or the parent may be ill, and either way there are cancellations. Children are usually away more than adult patients, because the child goes to camp or vacations, either with both parents together or with the parents separately, or with friends. Another economic disadvantage faced by child psychiatrists is that fees must be paid by adults at a time in their lives when their budgets are probably the tightest. They are not at the peak of their earning capacity, and they have heavy expenses in raising the children. It is not an uncommon experience in child psychiatry to establish a relationship with a child only to find the parents unable to handle the bill. Another problem for the field is that children's and adolescents' problems often cannot wait until the next appointment, and the child psychiatrist spends a good deal of time on the phone dealing with crises. Another time-consuming practice stems from the need child psychiatrists have for parents to notify them by phone of pertinent events between treatment sessions so that the doctor will be prepared prior to seeing the child. Depending on how this is set up, charges may or may not be made for such telephone time.

Setting Up an Office

Establishing an office requires that important decisions be made—decisions that may effect one's life for years. The neophyte physician must carefully consider a list of factors. Location is among the most important, especially in regard to where child psychiatrists are needed. Maldistribution of general and child psychiatrists has long been a public health problem. Most psychiatrists prefer to congregate in large urban centers to the neglect of smaller cities, towns, and rural areas. The physician will fulfill more unmet needs if he or she establishes an office in the less populous areas. A member of the Rural Child Psychiatry Committee of the American Academy of Child Psychiatry could answer questions about rural and small-town practice.

Should one locate in a metropolitan center, there is usually less competition in the outlying expanding suburbs. Most children will be driven to the psychiatrist's office by parents, but proximity to good public transportation can be very useful. Appropriately aged children and adolescents who visit regularly will often come on their own using public transportation, if the office is accessible. Some child psychiatrists have their offices in their homes, because of physical and financial advantages. However, there are usually significant problems to be overcome in separating the sights and sounds of the patients and the psychiatrist's family. An office in a medical complex, although relatively expensive, has the advantages of providing a clearer medical identity (which can be reassuring to some patients) and closer contacts with medical colleagues in other fields. Whether or not this proximity provides significant contacts can actually depend on the presence or absence of a restaurant attached and patronized by the physicians.

Careful consideration must be given to the amount of office space needed. Most child psychiatrists provide a separate playroom, where the child feels at home and the psychiatrist need not worry about fragile furnishings. If one does family therapy or group therapy, the consultation room must accommodate groups of this size. The playroom's contents vary from one therapist to another, but most include dolls; doll house; puppets; blocks; balls; toy weapons and vehicles; equipment for drawing, cutting, and pasting; and a variety of games that are not too intellectual. Toys that are so intrinsically appealing that they distract the child from expressing his or her inner feelings and drives should be avoided. There should be glue for instant repairing of broken toys.

After opening an office, psychiatrists make their presence known to colleagues and potential referral sources. Staying within the bounds of professional etiquette, this is commonly done through a number of mechanisms: formal mailed announcements of the office opening; listing in the telephone book yellow pages and in local professional directories; listing with local medical society referral services; participation in organizations that bring one in contact with general psychiatrists, other physicians, teachers, and clergymen; talking before parent and teacher groups, psychiatric, and other medical groups and the general public as on television or radio; teaching medical students, psychiatric residents, psychologists, social workers, and teachers; and publishing professional articles. With some ingenuity individual variations can be added to this list. When child psychiatrists appear before the public, they make not only themselves visible but also their field. With its small number of practitioners, child psychiatry has a big problem in making itself better known to the public.

It is important to maintain good relations with one's major referral sources. Examples of good practice with a referring physician are:

1. After the evaluation, send a report of one's findings to the physician, being concise rather than elaborate. Take care about confidentiality, and get a medical release from the parents. Avoid psychiatric jargon, but instead use language used in common with other physicians. Be very specific about one's recommendations.
2. Thank the referring physician.
3. Discuss with the referring doctor what part he or she wishes to play in the ongoing treatment, such as prescription of medication, and what part he or she wishes the child psychiatrist to play. If there is no collaboration during the treatment, send a note at the time of termination to describe the outcome.
4. Some physicians complain that psychiatrists have a condescending attitude; needless to say, avoid this.

In choosing what psychiatric services to offer, a child psychiatrist needs to take into account what type of services are in short supply. For example, the psychotherapy field may be saturated, but many people are looking for a child psychiatrist to do forensic work. The greatest unmet need might be to admit young people to hospitals. In the world of business, this type of analysis and activity is known as marketing. Almost universally psychiatrists do not like this word and find this practice inherently unpleasant, if not beneath their dignity. Some characterize those who put such practices into words and print "hucksters." Whether or not the physician is comfortable with these activities, they are part of surviving in the present economic climate. Even child psychiatrists long established in practice may now find that this kind of market analysis needs to be an ongoing part of their activities.

Hire Help?

The amount of office help one child psychiatrist may employ may range from none to more than one full-time staffer. These differences result from variations in (1) size of practice, (2) whether the type of practice requires few written reports or many, (3) whether it is practical to hire someone to do the bookkeeping or do it yourself, (4) whether an answering service or an answering machine can adequately deal with incoming calls. Most child psychiatrists use answering machines and seem satisfied, while others insist on the costlier but more flexible and personal method of an answering service. Others use a receptionist, especially if in a group. While on vacation, it is vital to arrange coverage by another psychiatric colleague and to tell him or her about those patients who are more likely to call for help.

Solo versus Group Practice

Most child psychiatrists operate as solo practitioners. Where they are part of a group practice, the group usually contains both general and child psychiatrists. There are some advantages to group practice. Partners share such common facilities as waiting rooms, lavatories, a kitchen, and so on. They can share a receptionist, secretary, and bookkeeper. In a group it is easier to be available for emergency services, as a larger number of doctors increases the likelihood that someone can respond promptly to urgent need. This can be an important factor in maintaining good relations with referral sources. Some referring medical doctors for example, dislike taking the time and trouble to hunt for someone to take a case; they prefer to settle their referral problems with one call. This is one reason it is important for the solo practitioner to provide coverage when out of town. Independence of action without the necessity of considering partners is one of the major advantages of a solo practice. In partnerships the majority rules, and this may have unfavorable consequences. Sometimes a partner may be outvoted and pulled unwillingly into projects that he or she does not like or cannot afford.

Fees

Fees for services vary considerably in different parts of the country, usually depending on the local cost of living. The psychiatrist must inquire about the standard fees in the chosen location. Child psychiatrists generally charge the same fees as general psychiatrists. Traditionally some reductions in charges are made for those who cannot afford full fees. Government insurance programs pay close to standard fees for military dependants (Civilian Health and Medical Program of the Uniformed Services, or CHAMPUS), but under Medicaid only a fraction of the standard fee is paid. To be eligible for reimbursement under these programs, the doctor must apply for a provider number from his or her local Medicaid office and from OCHAMPUS, Denver, Colorado 80240. Many child psychiatrists charge more for the initial visit to cover the time spent on the phone at the time of the first inquiry. Charges are usually not made for reports unless they are lengthy. Insurance has, as a rule, not covered the cost of reports. Some child psychiatrists charge more for time spent doing family therapy, while others do not unless there is a cotherapist. The combined fees for an hour of group therapy almost always substantially exceed those for the same time in individual treatment. The length of a session for individual psychotherapy is traditionally forty-five to sixty minutes, and it may be this or 50 percent longer for the initial consultation, for family or for group therapy. Usually charges are made for cancellations without twenty-four hours' notice unless there is a reasonable explanation. Likewise the psychiatrist needs to give reasonable notice for his or her own cancellations.

The hourly rate for forensic child psychiatry tends to run substantially higher. Usually one charges not only for time spent seeing the client and family and time in the courtroom but also for time (1) consulting with lawyers and other involved persons, (2) waiting at court, (3) reading and writing reports, and (4) traveling away from the office.

Insurance and Legal Advice

All psychiatrists in private practice need the protection of malpractice insurance. They are less vulnerable to suit than are many other medical specialties, and their premium rates are proportionally lower. Still there is the possibility of suits from adverse drug response, in connection with a patient's suicide and so on. Also the child psychiatrist should consider having liability insurance for injuries patients might suffer on the office premises. Similarly, it is advisable to have office overhead disability insurance to cover the cost of continuing professional expenses during a prolonged illness. These premiums are tax deductible as business expenses.

Legal advice in connection with the practice may be needed occasionally, and this is apt to be in a rather specialized area of the law. The American Psychiatric Association's Legal Consultation Program has been established to enable clinicians, for a set annual fee, to consult with APA lawyers about such matters as they arise.

Remedying the Problem of Isolation

Many child psychiatrists solve the problem of isolation by working some part of their week in a setting outside the office. They may work as consultants to agencies where they supervise the diagnosis and treatment of children. They may teach in a child psychiatry training program or in programs for other mental health professionals. Some consult to government programs. Again, there may be part-time research opportunities. Frequently physicians will find substantial satisfaction in spreading their influence far beyond the relatively few persons they can see in their offices. This not only helps solve the problem of isolation but offers variety in different settings and different types of cases. In addition, the doctor can find the satisfaction of helping to assure quality services to patients who otherwise might go without.

Responsibility to the Community

Some child psychiatrists limit their practices to middle- and upper-class families. Others feel a responsibility beyond this and seek to offer some form of service to the wider community with its great and varied needs. They may wish to serve the poorer families by being a consultant to a clinic or by taking Medicaid cases. One of the most frequent outside activities is teaching in a child psychiatry training program, thereby following the medical tradition of training young people. Carrying on research is, of course, in some measure its own reward and in addition offers another form of service to the community. Some child psychiatrists provide primary preventive care. They help seek out those children who are in need of treatment but who have not yet been identified as such by consulting with schools and working with teachers. Public education activities such as presentations to parent groups and the public media offer another example.

Responsibility to Professional Organizations

Most child psychiatrists support and participate in their professional organizations. These societies perform several essential functions. One of the most important is to serve as advocate for children and youth. Child psychiatrists need to offer the weight of their expertise in pressing for the needs of children. This includes work for better psychiatric facilities, better programs to prevent mental illness, the implementation of strategies for early identification of children's problems, and so on. In these pursuits child psychiatrists can often provide seasoned experience to legislators seeking advice on mental health matters. Local issues are addressed by local societies and national issues by the American Academy of Child Psychiatry.

Another important function of professional organizations is to address child psychiatry professional matters. There are several mechanisms for the sharing of scientific knowledge and experience in the diagnosis and treatment of psychiatric problems of children and adolescents. These include journals, didactic reviews, grand rounds, and scientific meetings. The American Academy of Child Psychiatry has many committees that deal with scientific topics. Membership in such committees allows colleagues with particular specialized interests to come together regularly to discuss their areas and work toward concrete goals. Another function is to represent the field's economic interests before community bodies in matters such as insurance programs and hospital practices.

Child psychiatrists are commonly active in a wide variety of professional organizations. These include general psychiatry associations, medical societies, psychoanalytic societies, and so on. It is the experience of child psychiatrists that advocacy for children and adolescents can often be achieved most successfully by working through the general psychiatric organizations, the medical societies, or other direct political channels. The activities of these various organizations are broad and varied, and a great deal of effort and commitment is necessary to make it all work. This takes the participation of many psychiatrists. Sometimes the work will be a labor of love, but it will frequently represent a commitment to duty. There are relatively few child psychiatrists, far too few to do the work that needs to be done. The efforts of younger colleagues are therefore particularly welcome and valuable.

assessment techniques such as neuropsychological tests. In the area of treatment, psychopharmacological methods, behavioral techniques, group and family approaches, and a number of novel and beguiling psychotherapies have currently become available. There is much to be assimilated.

In 1980 the Graduate Medical Education National Advisory Committee (GMENAC) reported that of all the medical specialties, child psychiatry was the one most in need of expanding, and they recommended a threefold increase in numbers by 1990.[1] This recommendation was based on need, but the report did not address the question of whether there was an economic base for supporting a large increase in numbers. In light of reductions in insurance benefits and in government funds for children's services, some doubt that there is such a base.

Economically some decidedly negative changes have occurred over the last ten years. Competition has greatly increased, and government policy is encouraging greater competition among physicians. There are many more child psychiatrists, and they are not all busy. There are more psychiatrists and an ever-increasing number of mental health professionals of other types working with children and their families. Many people seek out child psychiatrists because of their medical backgrounds and their extensive training; other parents choose psychologists or social workers, saying, in effect, that the psychiatrist deals with the sickest, and their child is not sick enough to go to a psychiatrist. Whether or not this is so, these parents self-diagnose their child as having minor problems. Thus the public has a distorted image of child psychiatry, an image the field needs to address. One might think that physicians in other fields would be among the most loyal sources of referral to child psychiatrists, but this is not always so. When a mental health referral is necessary, some physicians say that they find it easier to "sell" parents on a psychologist, because it seems to imply that the problem is not too severe. Probably the most dependable sources of referral for many child psychiatrists are the general psychiatrists.

Third-Party Payers

Changes in the Practice of Child Psychiatry

Over the past twenty-five years there have been many changes in the private practice of child psychiatry. A host of new diagnoses have appeared, requiring new

Prior to the 1960s private practice was supported totally by out-of-pocket payment. A family's alternatives were to pay directly, to attend a clinic, or to do without. During the 1960s health insurance was first extended to cover psychiatric hospitalizations and then outpatient psychiatry. Since that time other third-party payers reflecting direct government support—

such as CHAMPUS, Medicare, and Medicaid—have been introduced to help pay the costs.

Third-party coverage has sometimes defrayed 100 percent of the costs of inpatient care. The occasional generous insurance program will cover 365 hospital days a year, while the more frequently encountered arrangement stipulates limitations of various degrees, with some offering as few as thirty days a year. Coverage for outpatient services has ranged from a small percentage of the therapist's fees to as high as 80 percent. As a rule these patients must pay for the first $100 or $200 of medical expenses out of pocket. This so-called deductible expense is for any medical service, not just psychiatric.

The child psychiatrist usually provides some services that are not covered by insurance. Although most insurance companies have been persuaded to pay for time spent with the parents ("collateral services"), they will not pay for consultations with teachers, probation officers, and other key persons in the child's life. Frequently they will not cover the expenses of family therapy in spite of arguments presented to them about the economic benefits of this type of treatment. The entire insurance system is organized around services for a designated patient (including limits for services to a particular family member), and the various carriers have not accepted family treatment as a covered service. They will often agree to family therapy as a form of group therapy with each family member being given a diagnosis and being billed separately. Insurance companies will pay for *medically necessary* services, specifically for the diagnosis and treatment of disorders listed in DSM-III. They do not pay for primary preventive care or for what has been called "personal enhancement." They do pay for psychiatric evaluations to determine whether a disorder exists, provided there are presenting symptoms.

For many people the availability of insurance coverage for psychiatric services has made the difference between having good-quality care or going without. For the psychiatrist, it has had the negative feature of requiring many forms and, occasionally, written reports to the insurance company explaining the need for services. Such reports pose a conflict between the need of the insurance companies to know what they are paying for and the need of the psychiatrist to maintain the patient's confidentiality. During the 1970s this was the subject of considerable controversy. Insurance companies have tried to reassure psychiatrists that clinical reports are handled under the supervision of medical directors and are kept in confidential files. In any case, psychiatrists have now acquiesced to this intrusion on privacy as a price to be paid for the benefits of insurance coverage.

Peer Review

Through the years, insurance companies have found it difficult to deal with the relative lack of specificity in psychiatric diagnosis and treatment in comparison with other medical specialties. They have been especially concerned with the psychiatrist's difficulties in predicting the duration of treatment. They saw great variations in the type, duration, and cost of treatment set by various practitioners for the same diagnosis; all this made them skeptical of the scientific basis of psychiatry.

One of the most important responses to this problem has been the development of psychiatric peer review. Committees have been set up in the American Psychiatric Association and in most district branches of the APA to review questions about the suitability of treatment for specific cases. Most of the subjects for review are referred by insurance companies. In an effort to make administration less complicated, child psychiatry cases have been handled by these same general psychiatry organizations according to their usual routine. Under favorable circumstances, when called upon to review child cases, the peer review committees generally have subcommittees made up of child psychiatrists to perform this function. Confidentiality is maintained as to the name of the patient and the name of the psychiatrist, although this has been known to break down. All in all, over time insurance companies have been increasingly positive in their appraisal of this system, even finding that it has helped contain costs. Incidentally, it has certainly been a meaningful experience for some practitioners to know that at any point they may be called upon to give an accounting of their work with their patient.

Era of Attempts at Cost Containment

Recent years have seen a growing pressure from government and from private industry to contain health care costs, which have commonly risen at a higher rate than has inflation. Psychiatry, along with other branches of medicine, has felt the impact of this concern in the form of reduced benefits and has, in fact, been affected more than other specialties. The reason for this is greater vulnerability rather than some disproportionate responsibility for the increases. To begin with, there is the lack of demand for psychiatric benefits. Most persons do not anticipate psychiatric illness in their own or their family's lives and thus do not demand good psychiatric benefits in their programs. A second factor is that those who do come for treatment and who are hurt by cuts in their benefits are hesitant to raise their voices in protest out of a reluctance to be identified as psychiatric patients. If their psychiatrists should try to speak up for them, the doctors are seen as self-serving. A third factor is the previously mentioned skepticism of insurance companies about the scientific basis on which psychiatry rests. A considerable debate has ensued, and for many years organized psychiatry has been trying to get psychiatric benefits placed on a fair and equitable basis.

Additional mechanisms to contain costs are emerging, which will further impinge on the private practitioner. While by no means new, health maintenance organizations (HMOs) have grown to command a greater proportion of the market. Traditionally these agencies offer only twenty psychiatric outpatient visits a year or less.

Preferred provider organizations (PPOs), which started in California and are spreading rapidly, offer a new cost-cutting mechanism. In PPOs a group from a particular specialty unite for the purpose of offering services to employees of a company, usually at less than the going rate. Many child psychiatrists will soon face the question of whether to join a PPO.

Diagnostically related groups are a mechanism used in hospitals, at this time for Medicare and Medicaid patients, in which a set number of hospital days is allowed for a given diagnostic category. If the patient is out of the hospital earlier, the hospital makes money; if the patient is out later, the hospital loses money. The resultant pressure for hospitals to speed up their procedures is enormous. The potential dangers to the patient's care are of equal proportion. So far psychiatry has been exempt from this system, but attempts are being made to apply it there as well.

Employee assistance programs (EAPs) are probably born as much out of the wish by industry to meet a need as to save money. In these, the company supplies in-house staff to assist and to educate employees regarding health and, in particular, mental health problems. Some preventive work is done by educating employees in health maintenance. There is case finding among the employees, and brief interventions are made. If more extensive therapy is indicated, referral is made to outside practitioners for treatment. This widespread and growing mechanism impinges on the child psychiatrists in that (1) family problems are dealt with within the system and (2) EAPs are staffed almost totally by nonphysicians.

All of these systems move from the traditional ways of providing health care, and many of them threaten the quality of care.

Child Psychiatry's Relative Economic Status

Neither psychiatry nor child psychiatry has ever been one of the more lucrative branches of medicine. Each has consistently competed with pediatrics and family practice for the bottom of the economic ladder. According to a 1983 survey reported in an American Medical Association publication, psychiatry has risen into a position of third from the bottom.[2] This presents a problem in attracting adequate numbers of graduates into the field, especially in these days with increasing proportions of new physicians finding themselves needing to repay loans in the neighborhood of $50,000 to $70,000. It is a responsibility of organized psychiatry and child psychiatry to try to make the field economically attractive, commensurate with the amount of training necessary. The American Academy of Child Psychiatry has formed its Work Group on Consumer Issues to study the economic problems of the child psychiatrist and to make recommendations to its membership. The group has recognized that the day has passed when a child psychiatrist could hang out a shingle and just wait for patients to line up at the door. Some child psychiatrists have hoped that organized psychiatry, through its influence over insurance companies, governmental agencies, and corporations, might reverse the unfavorable trends. After reviewing the outcome of the considerable efforts of psychiatry in this way, the group has concluded that the child psychiatrist's economic state rests more on the individual's shoulders than on organized psychiatry. Thus they recommend the sort of market analyses and practice enhancers described earlier.

In spite of the fact that economic conditions are not as prosperous for the child psychiatrist as was once the case, there are real opportunities to thrive, if one makes the major practical decisions regarding the practice thoughtfully. There are great satisfactions in setting up a practice, working to gain one's share of the market, being one's own boss, and working to understand children and their families and to alleviate their suffering. There are therapeutic advantages to the patient for the therapist to operate in a relatively calm state without pressing worries about survival. This chapter has attempted to point out how these satisfactions will come more smoothly and with more security and equanimity, if the psychiatrist is attentive to the business side of the practice.

REFERENCES

1. GRADUATE MEDICAL EDUCATION NATIONAL ADVISORY COMMITTEE. *The Report to the Secretary, Department of Health and Human Services,* vol. 2. Washington, D.C.: U.S. Department of Health and Human Services, 1980.

2. REYNOLDS, R. A., and OHSFELDT, R. L. *Socio-economic Characteristics of Medical Practice.* Chicago: Center for Health Policy Research, American Medical Association, 1984, p. 108.

NAME INDEX

SUBJECT INDEX

ABAB research design, 204, 206, 207

Abandonment, fear of, 98; in incest victims, 108

Aberfan mining tragedy, 265

ABO blood incompatibility, 245

Abortion, 590, 591

Abreactive therapy, 418

Abuse, 252, 426–431, 567; attention deficit disorder and, 484; of children kidnapped by parents, 646, 649; delinquency and, 586–587; detection of, 426; federal programs on, 673; growth failure and, 277; of impaired infants, 126; of Indian children, 602; prevention of, 429–430; reporting, 426–427; of rural children, 666–667; sexual, see Sexual abuse; symbiotic attachment disorder and, 251; termination of parental rights in cases of, 655–656; trauma of, 268–269; treatment of perpetrators of, 427–428; treatment of victims of, 428–429; tripartite theory of, 281

Accident proneness, 252

Acetazolamide, 473

Acetylcholine, 19, 21; cognitive functions and, 23; in Tourette syndrome, 324

Acting out, 54; as defense against depression, 113, 287; by incest victims, 106, 108

Actions, continuity of, 34–35

Addictive personality, 390

Adjustment disorders, 138, 239

Administration for Children, Youth and Families (ACYF), 673

Administration on Developmental Disabilities (ADD), 673

Adolescents: alternative mental health services for, 526–530; American Indian, 600–612; attention deficit disorder in, 341, 344; autism in, 506, 508; biological tests for affective disorders in, 177–184; bipolar disorder in, 233; borderline conditions in, 453; brief reactive psychosis in, 239; cancer in, 578; change in

body composition of, 67; chronic disease in, 565–568, 570–572; cognitive changes in, 76–77; contraception use by, 592; depression in, 73–74; diagnosis of, 140; disabled, 123–128; encopresis in, 479; epidemiology of mental illness in, 6, 82–88; federal programs for, 672, 673, 677; hospitalization of, 659; identity disorder in, 236, 237; incest with, 105, 108; insomnia in, 472–473; learning disabilities in, 495–496, 498, 501; mood disorders in, 22; narcissistic disorders in, 444, 446, 447, 449; and nuclear threat, 616–627; pregnant, see Teenage pregnancy; psychopharmacology and, 6, 71, 398–405; psychosexual disorders in, 239; psychosis in, 502; rural, 661, 664; schizophrenia in, 23, 234, 371; as siblings of handicapped children, 93; sickle cell anemia in, 97–99, 101–102; sleep apnea in, 473; sleep disorders in, 188–190, 331, 332; sleepwalking in, 476; substance abuse by, 388–393, 520–526; Tourette syndrome in, 468; violence of, 112–116

Adoption: federal programs on, 673; of Indian children, 603; narcissism and, 303; and termination of parental rights, 655–656

Adoption studies: of aggression, 111–112; of anorexia nervosa, 381; of attention deficit disorder, 345

Adrenal cortex, fetal, 28–29

Adrenal function in anorexia nervosa, 378

Adrenal medulla, fetal, 29

Adrenarche, 70

Adrenocorticotropic hormone (ACTH), 21; fetal, 26, 29, 30

Adrenogenital syndrome, 357, 584

Adrenoleukodystrophy, 346

Adult court, transfer of juvenile offenders to, 654–655

Adverse drug reactions, 70

Advocacy, mental health, 528

Affective disorders, 362; attention deficits in, 344; biological tests in, 177–184; computerized axial tomography in, 170; drug-hormone interactions in, 71; eating disorders and, 377–378, 381, 382; epidemiology of, 535; incest and, 105; narcissistic disorders and, 303; positron emission tomography in, 174; psychopharmacology in, 66; regional cerebral blood flow in, 174; see also Depression; Manic-depressive disorder

Affective self, pathway to, 54

Aggression: in anal phase, 62; autism and, 508; behavior therapy for, 407; biochemical changes and, 583; of incest victims, 108; in narcissistic disorders, 296; neurobiology of, 111–112; psychopharmacology and, 399–401; in rapprochement subphase, 43; stability of, 113; testosterone and, 584; see also Violence

Aggressor, identification with, 643

Agoraphobia, 236, 314, 460

AIDS, 245

Al-Anon, 524

Alcohol: dose effect of, 70; excessive somnolence and, 331; violence and, 116

Alcohol, Drug Abuse, and Mental Health Administration (ADAMHA), 671, 672

Alcoholics Anonymous (AA), 389, 391, 520, 521, 524

Alcoholism: adolescent, 521; biological factors in, 389–390; bulimia and, 377, 378, 381, 382; epidemiology of, 535; genetic factors in, 389; among Indians, 601, 602, 608; parental, 586; psychodynamics of, 390, 391; rural, 661, 664

Alprazolam, 418, 476; for panic attacks, 458

Alternative mental health services, 526–530; characteristics of, 527–528; contribution of, 529–530; effectiveness of, 529; legitimization of, 528–529

language acquisition and, 54; object relations and, 42; in practicing subphase, 41; preoedipal castration reactions and, 64; promotion of, in borderline children, 451–453
Ego prostheses, 390
Eighth-month anxiety, 247, 249
Elective mutism, 236, 252
Electroconvulsive therapy, 459
Electroencephalography (EEG): in anorexia nervosa, 377; in attention deficit disorder, 342, 343, 485; in autism, 366; in bulimia nervosa, 384; computerized, 194–200; computerized tomography and, 171, 172; in incest victims, 106; regional cerebral blood flow and, 174; sleep, 178–180, 328, 331–334; in substance abuse, 390; topographic mapping with, 174–176; in Tourette syndrome, 325, 464
Elimination, disorders of, *see* Encopresis; Enuresis
ELIZA program, 636
Empathic failure, 296
Employee assistance programs (EAPs), 684
Encopresis, 237–238, 479–483; differential diagnosis of, 479–480; treatment of, 480–482
Endocrine disorders: in eating disorders, 378–379; encopresis in, 480
Endocrine system, fetal, 26–32
English Common Law, 104
Enkephalins, 21–22
Enriched environment, 6–7
Enuresis, 185, 186, 189–191, 237–238, 328, 332, 333; imipramine for, 489; treatment of, 474–475
Environmental factors: in aggression, 112; in anxiety disorders, 316; in attention deficit disorder, 346–347; in learning disabilities, 359; in narcissistic disorders, 302–303; rural, 660; in Tourette syndrome, 323–324
Environmental failure to thrive, 272
Environmental influences on brain development, 3, 6–13
Environmental retardation, 248
Epidemiology, 534–541; of adolescent mental illness, 6, 82–88; of anxiety disorders, 316; of attention deficit disorder, 339; basics concepts of, 534; of delinquency, 582–583; of depression, 288; of eating disorders, 376; federally-

sponsored research in, 677; of Tourette syndrome, 322
Epidemiology Catchment Area (ECA), 535, 539
Epilepsy: psychomotor, 585; surgical treatment of, 56; *see also* Seizure disorders
Epinephrine, fetal, 29
Episodic dyscontrol syndrome, 116
Epithelial growth factor (EGF), 26
Esophageal atresia, 422
Estradiol, 69; in anorexia nervosa, 378
Estrogens: drug interactions with, 68; fetal, 28, 30; growth hormone and, 71, 181
Event-related potentials (ERPs), 194–195; in attention deficit disorder, 197; in autism, 198; in schizophrenia, 198–199
Evoked potentials, 175; in attention deficit disorder, 343; in Tourette syndrome, 325
Evolution, biological, 243–244
Excessive daytime somnolence (EDS), 331
Explosive disorders, 239
Expressive arts therapy, 516
Extrapyramidal side effects, 509; of haloperidol, 466

Face validity, definition of, 534
Factitious disorders, 239
Failure to thrive, 249, 272–276; developmental classification of, 274–276; treatment of, 421–425
False self, 298–299
Familial sleep paralysis, 332, 333
Family and Youth Services, 673
Family diagnosis, 234
Family pathology, eating disorders and, 380–382
Family Research Project, 529
Family size, failure to limit, 594
Family structures, changes in, 615
Family studies: of anxiety disorders, 316; of autism, 365–366
Family systems theory, 448
Family therapy: for anorexia nervosa, 513–516; in alternative mental health services, 528; for attention deficit disorder, 487, 488; chronic disease and, 570, 571; for depression, 439; for encopresis, 479, 481; for juvenile offenders, 654; for learning disabilities, 497–498; for narcissistic disorder, 447–448; structural, 515; for substance abuse,

524, 525; for Tourette syndrome, 468; for trauma, 417; for violent youth, 116
Fantasies: of annihilation, 621; of borderline children, 450; in computer-assisted instruction, 630; sexual, 263; of siblings of handicapped children, 95
Father-daughter incest, 281–283
Fathers: joint custody and, 685; teenage, 595, 597, 605
Fears: of abandonment, 98–99; nighttime, 186, 187; posttraumatic, 266, 418
Federal Bureau of Investigation (FBI), 415, 650
Federal Maternal and Child Health program, 672
Federal Mental Health Centers Act, 662
Federal Parent Locater Service, 650
Federal programs, 671–678; financing of, 674–675; service systems of, 675–676; training in, 676–677
Fees for services, 680–681
Feingold diet, 490, 500–501
Fels Research Institute, 36
Fenfluramine, 400, 500; for autism, 22
Fetal alcohol syndrome, 245, 346, 358
Fetal development: endocrine factors in, 26–32; risk factors in, 245–247
Fibroblast growth factor (FGF), 26
Filial therapy, 417
Finland, response to nuclear threat in, 624
Fixated sexual offenders, 283
Fluphenazine, 508
Flurazepam, 472; for parasomnias, 476
Follicle-stimulating hormone: in anorexia nervosa, 378, 379; fetal, 26
Food additives, 400, 490, 500–501
Food and Drug Administration, 400, 466
Food refusal: attachment disorders with, 251; dwarfism secondary to, 277
Formal operations period, 225
FORTRAN, 633
Foster Care: federal programs for, 673; for juvenile offenders, 654; for narcissistic children, 444; and termination of parental rights, 655–656
Fragile X syndrome, 232–233; autism and, 366

Subject Index

Household violence, 586–587
Human services, rural, 662–663
Human Services in the Rural Environment (journal), 663
Huntington's chorea, 322, 346
Hyperactivity, 22; behavior therapy for, 405; computer-assisted instruction and, 634; delinquency and, 113; diagnosis of, 161; encopresis and, 482; epidemiology of, 537; fragile X syndrome and, 233; imipramine for, 489–490; in infancy, 252; learning disabilities and, 354, 494–495; psychopharmacology in, 399–402; single-case research on, 206; sleep disorders and, 476; Tourette syndrome and, 320; *see also* Attention deficit disorder
Hyperactivity Rating Scale, 156
Hyperinsulinemia, fetal, 26
Hyperkinesis Index, 156
Hypersomnolence, 190
Hypertelorism, 485
Hypertension, 237
Hypertrophic pyloric stenosis, 245–246, 248
Hyperventilation syndrome, 315
Hypervigilance, 275
Hypnagogic hallucinations, 190, 332
Hypnosis, 418; for sleepwalking, 476; for Tourette syndrome, 468
Hypnotics, 471, 472
Hypochondriasis, 239
Hypoglycemia, 490; learning disabilities and, 500
Hypothalamo-hypophyseal system, fetal development of, 26
Hypothalamus in anorexia nervosa, 378–379, 383–384
Hypothyroidism, 331
Hysterical neurosis, 239; drug responses and, 71

Idealized parental imago, 295
Idealized self-object, 295, 296
Idealizing transference, 445
Identification, 44; with aggressor, 643; with dead parent, 643–644; of mother with infant, 243; with mother's prohibitions, 48; with parents, 92; symbolic play and, 41
Identity disorder, 236, 237
Identity formation, 298–299
Illinois State Psychiatric Institute, 115–116

Illinois Test of Psycholinguistic Abilities, 536
Imipramine, 290, 398–399, 442; for attention deficit disorder, 489–490; for autism, 509; for borderline children, 456; for bulimia nervosa, 517–518; for cataplexy, 473; for conduct disorders, 113; for encopresis, 481–482; for enuresis, 475; for panic attacks, 458; for parasomnias, 476; for separation anxiety disorders, 460–461
Immune system: in autism, 367; handedness and, 357
Impulse control, disorders of, 239; in borderline child, 308–310; in bulimia nervosa, 377, 378; learning disabilities and, 354
Impulse ridden disorder, 235
Incest, 103–111, 280; frequency of, 103–104; interpersonal factors in, 281–283; multiple personality and, 285; posttraumatic symptoms of, 107–109; in rural areas, 667; secret-keeping and, 284–285; sexual victimization factors in, 283; stranger abuse versus, 280–281; as trauma, 106–107, 268; variables affecting impact of, 104–106; *see also* Sexual abuse
Incidence, definition of, 534
Indian Health Service, Indian Children's Program of, 605, 607
Indians, *see* American Indians
Individual differences: in communicative competence, 54; and developmental discontinuity, 34–35; in language acquisition, 57–58
Infants, 242–262; attachment disorders of, 248–252; behavioral disturbances of, 252; communication disorders in, 252; developmental deviations in, 248; healthy responses of, 247–248; impact of parental bipolar disorder on, 291; posttraumatic stress disorder of, 252; psychological development of, 243; psychoneurosis in, 252–253; psychophysiological disorders in, 248; sleep patterns of, 328
Inhibition to unfamiliar, 35–36
Injury, traumatic, 268
Inpatient treatment: of anorexia nervosa, 513; of bulimia nervosa, 517; of psychosis, 504; of substance abuse, 524–526; *see also*

Hospitalization; Residential treatment
In re Gault (1967), 654
Insomnia, 185, 190, 238, 329, 331; treatment of, 471–473
Insulin: for anorexia nervosa, 516; fetal, 26, 29–30
Insulin tolerance test (ITT), 181, 290
Insurance, 682–683
Intelligence tests, 164–168
International Classification of Diseases, 136–139, 230
Interpretation, 440; with borderline children, 450; mutative, 441
Intersubjectivity, 54
Interviewing, structured, *see* Structured interviewing
Interview Schedule for Children (ISC), 150, 152, 288
IQ: autism and, 507–508; as outcome measure, 554, 555, 564; in psychoses, pretreatment evaluation of, 503
Isle of Wight Study, 123, 288, 533, 534, 536–538
Israeli *kibbutzim,* 416

Jactatio capitis nocturna, 333
Jakob-Creutzfeldt disease, 245
Jerusalem Infant Development Study, 234
Johns Hopkins University, 535
Joint custody, 637–640; child snatching and, 651; and parental alienation syndrome, 641–642; psychiatric consultation in decision on, 656–658
Journal of Rural Community Psychology, 663
Journal of the American Academy of Child Psychiatry, 457, 677
Judge Baker Guidance Center, 653
Juvenile Justice and Delinquency Act, 528
Juvenile Justice Standards, 654
Juvenile justice system, 114–115, 581; psychiatric consultation in, 653–655; in rural areas, 665–666

Kaui Longitudinal Study, 125, 128, 339, 533, 534, 536, 538–539
Kiddie-SADS, *see* Schedule for Affective Disorders and Schizophrenia for School Age Children
Kidnapping, parental, 268, 269,

701